# Conversion Information

## Weights and Measures
### Prefixes for Fractions

deci = $10^{-1}$
centi = $10^{-2}$
milli = $10^{-3}$
micro = $10^{-6}$
nano = $10^{-9}$
pico = $10^{-12}$

### Temperature Measures

$8°C = 5/9 × (8°F − 32)$
$8°F = 9/5 × (8°C) + 32$

### Percentage Equivalents

0.1% solution contains 1 mg per mL
1% solution contains 10 mg per mL
10% solution contains 100 mg per mL

### Milliequivalent Conversions

1 mEq Na = 23 mg Na = 58.5 mg NaCl
1 g Na = 2.54 g NaCl = 43 mEq Na
1 g NaCl = 0.39 g Na = 17 mEq Na
1 mEq K = 39 mg K = 74.5 mg KCl
1 g K = 1.91 g KCl = 26 mEq K
1 g KCl = 0.52 g K = 13 mEq K
1 mEq Ca = 20 mg Ca
1 g Ca = 50 mEq Ca
1 mEq Mg = 0.12 g $MgSO_4 \cdot 7H_2O$
1 g Mg = 10.2 g $MgSO_4 \cdot 7H_2O$ = 82 mEq Mg

## Metric Conversions
### Volume Measurements

Teaspoonful = 5 mL
Tablespoonful = 15 mL
Fluid ounce = 30 mL
Pint = 473 mL
Quart = 946 mL

### Linear Measurements

1 mm = 0.04 in
1 in = 25.4 mm = 2.54 cm
1 m = 39.4 in
1 in = 0.025 m

T0210145

1 k̶g = 2.2 lb
1 lb = 0.45 kg

## Weights and Equivalents: Metric System
### Weight

kilogram = kg = 1000 grams
gram = g = 1 gram
milligram = mg = 0.001 gram
microgram = μg = 0.001 milligram
picogram = pg = 0.001 microgram

### Volume

liter = L = 1 L
milliliter = mL = 0.001 L

### Avoirdupois Weight

1 ounce (oz) = 437.5 grains
1 pound (lb) = 16 ounces = 7000 grains

## Metric and Apothecary Equivalents
### Exact Weight Equivalents

| Metric | Apothecary |
| --- | --- |
| 1 mg | 1/64.8 grain |
| 64.8 mg | 1 grain |
| 324 mg | 5 grains |
| 1 gram | 15.432 grains |
| 31.103 gram | 1 ounce (480 grains) |

### Exact Volume Equivalents

| Metric | Apothecary |
| --- | --- |
| 1.00 mL | 16.23 minims |
| 3.69 mL | 1 fluidram (60 minims) |
| 29.57 mL | 1 fluid ounce (480 minims) |
| 473.16 mL | 1 pint (7680 minims) |
| 946.33 mL | 1 quart (15,360 minims) |

# Conversion of Body Weight to Body Surface Area in Dogs

## Kilograms to Pounds and to Body Surface Area in Square Meters

| Body Weight in Kilograms | Body Weight in Pounds | Body Surface Area in Square Meters | Body Weight in Kilograms | Body Weight in Pounds | Body Surface Area in Square Meters |
|---|---|---|---|---|---|
| 1 | 2.2 | 0.1 | 36 | 79.37 | 1.11 |
| 2 | 4.41 | 0.16 | 37 | 81.57 | 1.13 |
| 3 | 6.61 | 0.21 | 38 | 83.77 | 1.15 |
| 4 | 8.82 | 0.26 | 39 | 85.98 | 1.17 |
| 5 | 11.02 | 0.3 | 40 | 88.18 | 1.19 |
| 6 | 13.23 | 0.33 | 41 | 90.39 | 1.21 |
| 7 | 15.43 | 0.37 | 42 | 92.59 | 1.22 |
| 8 | 17.64 | 0.41 | 43 | 94.8 | 1.24 |
| 9 | 19.84 | 0.44 | 44 | 97 | 1.26 |
| 10 | 22.05 | 0.47 | 45 | 99.21 | 1.28 |
| 11 | 24.25 | 0.5 | 46 | 101.41 | 1.3 |
| 12 | 26.46 | 0.53 | 47 | 103.62 | 1.32 |
| 13 | 28.66 | 0.56 | 48 | 105.82 | 1.34 |
| 14 | 30.86 | 0.59 | 49 | 108.03 | 1.36 |
| 15 | 33.07 | 0.62 | 50 | 110.23 | 1.38 |
| 16 | 35.27 | 0.64 | 51 | 112.43 | 1.39 |
| 17 | 37.48 | 0.67 | 52 | 114.64 | 1.41 |
| 18 | 39.68 | 0.7 | 53 | 116.84 | 1.43 |
| 19 | 41.89 | 0.72 | 54 | 119.05 | 1.45 |
| 20 | 44.09 | 0.75 | 55 | 121.25 | 1.47 |
| 21 | 46.3 | 0.77 | 56 | 123.46 | 1.48 |
| 22 | 48.5 | 0.8 | 57 | 125.66 | 1.5 |
| 23 | 50.71 | 0.82 | 58 | 127.87 | 1.52 |
| 24 | 52.91 | 0.84 | 59 | 130.07 | 1.54 |
| 25 | 55.12 | 0.87 | 60 | 132.28 | 1.55 |
| 26 | 57.32 | 0.89 | 61 | 134.48 | 1.57 |
| 27 | 59.52 | 0.91 | 62 | 136.69 | 1.59 |
| 28 | 61.73 | 0.93 | 63 | 138.89 | 1.61 |
| 29 | 63.93 | 0.96 | 64 | 141.09 | 1.62 |
| 30 | 66.14 | 0.98 | 65 | 143.3 | 1.64 |
| 31 | 68.34 | 1 | 66 | 145.5 | 1.66 |
| 32 | 70.55 | 1.02 | 67 | 147.71 | 1.67 |
| 33 | 72.75 | 1.04 | 68 | 149.91 | 1.69 |
| 34 | 74.96 | 1.06 | 69 | 152.12 | 1.71 |
| 35 | 77.16 | 1.08 | 70 | 154.32 | 1.72 |

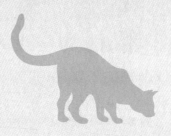

Papich Handbook of

# VETERINARY
# DRUGS

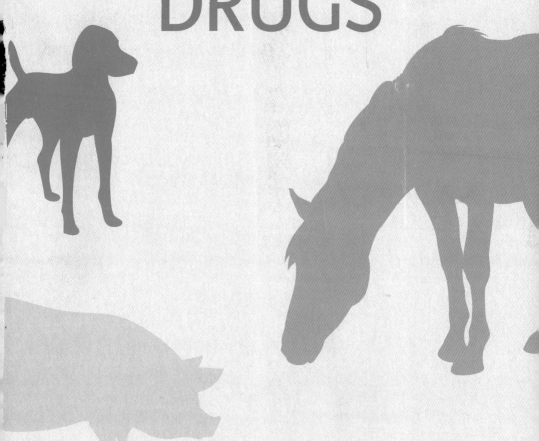

**FIFTH**
EDITION

# Papich Handbook of
# VETERINARY DRUGS

**MARK G. PAPICH**, DVM, MS, DACVCP

Professor of Clinical Pharmacology
Burroughs Wellcome Fund Professorship in Veterinary Pharmacology
College of Veterinary Medicine
North Carolina State University
Raleigh, North Carolina

**ELSEVIER**

Elsevier
3251 Riverport Lane
St. Louis, Missouri 63043

PAPICH HANDBOOK OF VETERINARY MEDICINE, FIFTH EDITION          ISBN: 978-0-323-70957-6
Copyright © 2021 by Elsevier, Inc. All rights reserved.

No part of this publication may be reproduced or transmitted in any form or by any means, electronic or mechanical, including photocopying, recording, or any information storage and retrieval system, without permission in writing from the publisher. Details on how to seek permission, further information about the Publisher's permissions policies and our arrangements with organizations such as the Copyright Clearance Center and the Copyright Licensing Agency, can be found at our website: www.elsevier.com/permissions.

This book and the individual contributions contained in it are protected under copyright by the Publisher (other than as may be noted herein).

---

**Notice**

Practitioners and researchers must always rely on their own experience and knowledge in evaluating and using any information, methods, compounds or experiments described herein. Because of rapid advances in the medical sciences, in particular, independent verification of diagnoses and drug dosages should be made. To the fullest extent of the law, no responsibility is assumed by Elsevier, authors, editors or contributors for any injury and/or damage to persons or property as a matter of products liability, negligence or otherwise, or from any use or operation of any methods, products, instructions, or ideas contained in the material herein.

---

Previous editions copyrighted 2016, 2011, 2007, and 2002.

**Library of Congress Control Number: 2020942037**

*Senior Content Strategist:* Jennifer Catando (Flynn-Briggs)
*Senior Content Development Specialist:* Laura Klein
*Publishing Services Manager:* Catherine Jackson
*Senior Project Manager:* Claire Kramer
*Design Direction:* Patrick Ferguson

Printed in India

Last digit is the print number:  9  8  7  6  5  4  3

Working together
to grow libraries in
developing countries

www.elsevier.com • www.bookaid.org

*This is dedicated to my mother and father, Kathleen and Michael Papich.*
*My goal was to produce a book that helps veterinarians and students,*
*while improving the lives of animals and their owners.*
*My parents taught me to use my knowledge to help others. These*
*values provided the inspiration and motivation to complete this and*
*the previous editions of this book.*

**Mark G. Papich**

# DISCLAIMER

Doses listed are species specific, unless otherwise indicated. There is no assurance for safety and efficacy in other animal species not listed. Many of the doses listed are extralabel or are human drugs used in an extralabel manner. Federal regulations allow use of extralabel veterinary drugs and human drugs in non–food-producing animals when there is a valid veterinarian–client–patient relationship. However, there are restrictions for using these drugs in food-producing animals under the Animal Medicinal Drug Use Clarification Act (AMDUCA) of 1994. Requirements under this act can be found at the website of the American Veterinary Medical Association (AVMA): https://www.avma.org/KB/Resources/Reference/Pages/AMDUCA.aspx. Extralabel use of drugs is prohibited in food-producing animals unless certain requirements are met, which include extended withdrawal times for meat and milk.

Dosages, routes of administration, and indications listed are based on best available evidence at the time of the drug handbook preparation. The author cannot guarantee efficacy or safety of the drugs used according to recommendations in this book. Other patient factors or actions of the drug not known at the time of the book preparation may affect efficacy and safety. Adverse effects of which the author was not aware at the time of the handbook's preparation may be possible from drugs listed in this handbook.

Veterinarians using this handbook are encouraged to check current literature, product label, federal Freedom of Information (FOI) summaries, and the manufacturer's disclosure for information regarding efficacy and any known adverse effects or contraindications not identified at the time of preparation of this handbook.

**Mark G. Papich**

# Preface

The fifth edition of this handbook was developed using a similar style, layout, and format as the previous edition to ease the transition for users of earlier versions. Additions, changes in individual drug monographs, and expanded sections were provided with input and helpful suggestions from veterinarians, drug sponsors, and students or because new information became available in the published literature since the last edition. New drugs that have been approved by the US Food and Drug Administration (FDA) or for which there is new information about their use in the literature have been added. The drugs listed represent the most important medications used in companion animals and livestock. Practically every drug monograph has been updated, and more than 20 new drugs have been added. Some discontinued or outdated medications have been deleted, and readers can refer to previous editions of this book for information on those drugs. As in previous editions, this book includes approved drugs for animals in addition to human medications for which veterinary uses have been identified. Information has been updated on clinical uses and regulatory requirements. The information on drug stability, storage, and compounding has been expanded because medications for animals are often modified from the original source. An increased effort has been made to include evidence-based information on the drug's efficacy and clinical use in the "Indications and Clinical Uses" and "Instructions for Use" sections. To facilitate the location of important information for each medication, the sections are divided into categories for drug interactions, precautions, pharmacology, and clinical use. Tables for quick reference can be found in the appendixes. The appendix tables include antibiotics of choice, drug interactions, regulatory information, information for pharmacists, and a section on drug dose calculations.

The book is designed for busy practitioners and students who want to make the most efficient use of their time and locate accurate and reliable drug information quickly. The format is consistent from drug to drug, and veterinarians and their staff will quickly become familiar with the layout of each drug monograph to rapidly locate concise and accurate information about each medication.

In preparing this handbook, my priorities were ease-of-use, accuracy, and reliability. As in previous editions, the indications for use and drug dosing information were prepared from a review of the literature or input from clinical specialists. In some cases, dosages originated from clinical studies; in other cases, they represent a standard of good clinical practice, even if it is considered extralabel. Manufacturers' recommendations are considered in the dosing recommendations, but other suggestions (extralabel indications and uses) also may be listed where the use and dosage have gone beyond those listed on the product's label. Where dosage recommendations have varied among sources, I have applied my clinical judgment and over 30 years of experience in veterinary clinical pharmacology to derive a scientifically valid dose. In some cases, it may have been necessary to derive a dose based on extrapolations from human medicine, but this was limited to drugs for which the therapeutic index of the drug is high. To derive withdrawal times for food animals, the highest priority has been given to the withdrawal time approved by the FDA. When there was not an FDA-approved withdrawal time, suggestions made by the Food Animal Residue Avoidance Databank (FARAD; www.farad.org) were considered. If neither of these was available, I listed a conservative estimate for a suggested withdrawal time based on the drug's pharmacokinetics and likelihood that it may cause harmful residues.

Each drug is listed alphabetically by its official name (United States Adopted Names [USAN]) that is recognized by the United States Pharmacopeia (USP; www.usp.org). Following each drug name is the brand or trade name and synonyms by which the drug also may be known. Innovator brand names are provided, but not all of the brand names and generic versions available are necessarily listed. The cross-reference table in the front section of the book lists drugs according to their functional classification and condition of use. It may not include all of the known uses for a drug but represents the most common clinical use.

As clinical experience increases and our knowledge of the pharmacology of these drugs expands, new information may become available for the medications listed in this book. I welcome feedback relating to adverse effects observed, clinical experience, and omissions or errors identified. For these and other input and suggestions, I can be reached at mark_papich@ncsu.edu. Adverse drug events also should be reported to the drug sponsor directly or the FDA using this website: www.fda.gov/AnimalVeterinary/SafetyHealth/ReportaProblem/.

# Contents

## Listing of Drugs According to Functional and Therapeutic Classification

| Drug Classification | Drug Name | Brand Name |
| --- | --- | --- |
| Acidifier | Racemethionine (Methionine) | Uroeze, Methio-Form, and generic. Human forms include Pedameth, Uracid, and generic. |
| | Ammonium chloride | Generic |
| Adrenal suppressant | Trilostane | Modrenal, Vetoryl |
| Adrenergic agonist | Ephedrine hydrochloride | Many |
| | Epinephrine | Adrenaline and generic forms |
| | Fenoldopam mesylate | Corlopam |
| | Phenylpropanolamine hydrochloride | Proin, Proin-ER, UriCon, and Propalin tablets and syrup. |
| | Pseudoephedrine hydrochloride | Sudafed |
| Adrenolytic agent | Mitotane | Lysodren, op-DDD |
| Alkalinizing agent | Potassium citrate | Generic, Urocit-K |
| | Sodium bicarbonate | Baking soda, soda mint, citrocarbonate, Arm and Hammer Pure Baking Soda |
| Alpha2-antagonist | Atipamezole hydrochloride | Antisedan |
| | Yohimbine | Yobine |
| Analgesic | Acetaminophen | Tylenol and generic brands |
| | Amantadine | Symmetrel |
| | Gabapentin | Neurontin |
| | Pregabalin | Lyrica |
| | Tramadol | Ultram and generic |
| Analgesic, opioid | Hydrocodone bitartrate | Hycodan |
| | Hydromorphone | Dilaudid, Hydrostat, and generic |
| | Acetaminophen + codeine | Tylenol with codeine and many generic brands |
| | Buprenorphine hydrochloride | Simbadol, Buprenex (Vetergesic in the UK) |
| | Butorphanol tartrate | Torbutrol, Torbugesic |
| | Fentanyl citrate | Sublimaze |
| | Fentanyl transdermal | Duragesic |
| | Meperidine | Demerol |
| | Methadone hydrochloride | Dolophine, Methadose |
| | Morphine sulfate | Extended-release tablets: MS Contin or Oramorph SR, or generic |
| | Oxymorphone hydrochloride | Numorphan |
| | Pentazocine | Talwin-V |
| | Remifentanil | Ultiva |
| | Sufentanil citrate | Sufenta |
| Analgesic, opioid, antitussive | Butorphanol tartrate | Torbutrol, Torbugesic |
| | Codeine | Codeine phosphate, codeine sulfate |
| | Hydrocodone bitartrate | Hycodan |

## Listing of Drugs According to Functional and Therapeutic Classification

| Drug Classification | Drug Name | Brand Name |
| --- | --- | --- |
| Analgesic, nonsteroidal anti-inflammatory drug (NSAID) | Aspirin | ASA, acetylsalicylic acid, Bufferin, Ascriptin, and many generic brands |
| | Carprofen | Rimadyl (Zinecarp is a European brand name) |
| | Deracoxib | Deramaxx |
| | Etodolac | EtoGesic (veterinary); Lodine (human) |
| | Dipyrone | Methampyrone, Metamizole; Zimeta |
| | Firocoxib | Previcox |
| | Flunixin meglumine | Banamine, and generic |
| | Grapiprant | Galliprant |
| | Ibuprofen | Motrin, Advil, Nuprin |
| | Indomethacin | Indocin |
| | Ketoprofen | Orudis-KT (human OTC tablet); Ketofen (veterinary injection); Anafen (outside the US) |
| | Ketorolac tromethamine | Toradol |
| | Meclofenamate sodium; Meclofenamic acid | Arquel, Meclofen |
| | Meloxicam | Metacam (veterinary drug), Mobic (human drug) |
| | Naproxen | Naprosyn, Naxen, Aleve (naproxen sodium) |
| | Phenylbutazone | Butazolidin, PBZ, and generic |
| | Piroxicam | Feldene and generic |
| | Robenacoxib | Onsior |
| | Tepoxalin | Zubrin |
| Anesthetic | Alfaxalone | Alfaxan |
| | Ketamine hydrochloride | Ketalar, Ketavet, Vetalar |
| | Propofol | Rapinovet, Propoflo (veterinary); Diprivan (human) |
| | Tiletamine and Zolazepam | Telazol, Zoletil |
| Anesthetic, sedative alpha$_2$-agonist | Detomidine hydrochloride | Dormosedan |
| | Dexmedetomidine | Dexdomitor, Sileo |
| | Medetomidine hydrochloride | Domitor |
| | Romifidine hydrochloride | Sedivet |
| | Xylazine hydrochloride | Rompun and generic |
| Anesthetic, barbiturate | Methohexital sodium | Brevital |
| | Pentobarbital sodium | Nembutal and generic |
| | Thiopental sodium | Pentothal |
| Anesthetic, inhalant | Enflurane | Ethrane |
| | Halothane | Fluothane |
| | Isoflurane | Aerrane |
| | Methoxyflurane | Metofane |
| | Sevoflurane | Aerrane |
| Antacid | Aluminum hydroxide, and Aluminum carbonate | Aluminum hydroxide gel (Amphogel), aluminum carbonate gel (Basalgel) |

*Continued*

## Listing of Drugs According to Functional and Therapeutic Classification

| Drug Classification | Drug Name | Brand Name |
| --- | --- | --- |
| Antiarrhythmic | Amiodarone | Cordarone |
| | Carvedilol | Coreg |
| | Disopyramide | Norpace (Rythmodan in Canada) |
| | Lidocaine hydrochloride | Xylocaine |
| | Mexiletine | Mexitil |
| | Procainamide hydrochloride | Pronestyl |
| | Quinidine | Quinidine gluconate: Duraquin |
| | Quinidine sulfate | Quinidine polygalacturonate: |
| | Quinidine gluconate | Cardioquin |
| | Quinidine polygalacturonate | Quinidine sulfate: Cin-Quin, Quinora |
| | Tocainide hydrochloride | Tonocard |
| Antiarrhythmic, calcium channel blocker | Diltiazem hydrochloride | Cardizem, Dilacor |
| | Verapamil hydrochloride | Calan, Isoptin |
| Antiarthritic agent | Polysulfated glycosaminoglycan | Adequan Canine Adequan IA, Adequan IM |
| | Chondroitin sulfate | Cosequin, Glycoflex, and other brands |
| | Glucosamine and chondroitin sulfate | Cosequin, Glycoflex, and other brands |
| Antibacterial | Chloramphenicol | Chloramphenicol palmitate, Chloromycetin |
| | Clofazimine | Lamprene |
| | Dapsone | Generic |
| | Florfenicol | Nuflor |
| | Fosfomycin | Monurol |
| | Isoniazid | Isonicotinic acid hydrazide |
| | Linezolid | Zyvox |
| | Methenamine | Methenamine hippurate: Hiprex, Urex, Mesulfin Methenamine mandelate: Mandelamine and generic |
| | Nitrofurantoin | Macrodantin, Furalan, Furatoin, Furadantin, or generic |
| | Polymyxin B | Generic |
| | Pyrimethamine | Daraprim |
| | Rifampin | Rifadin, Rifampicin |
| Antibacterial, aminoglycoside | Amikacin | Amiglyde-V (veterinary), Amikin (human), and generic |
| | Gentamicin sulfate | Gentocin |
| | Neomycin | Biosol |
| | Kanamycin sulfate | Kantrim |
| | Tobramycin sulfate | Nebcin |
| Antibacterial, lincosamide | Lincomycin hydrochloride | Lincocin, Lincomix |
| | Lincomycin hydrochloride monohydrate | |
| | Clindamycin hydrochloride Clindamycin phosphate Clindamycin palmitate | Antirobe, Clindrops, Clintabs, Clinsol, and generic (veterinary); Cleocin (human) |
| Antibacterial, macrolide | Azithromycin | Zithromax |
| | Clarithromycin | Biaxin and generic |
| | Erythromycin | Many brands and generic; Gallimycin-100, Gallimycin-200, Erythro-100 |
| | Gamithromycin | Zactran |

## Listing of Drugs According to Functional and Therapeutic Classification

| Drug Classification | Drug Name | Brand Name |
| --- | --- | --- |
| | Tildipirosin | Zuprevo |
| | Tilmicosin phosphate | Micotil, Pulmotil tilmicosin premix |
| | Tulathromycin | Draxxin, Draxxin 25+C28 |
| | Tylosin | Tylocine, Tylan, Tylosin tartrate |
| Antibacterial, potentiated sulfonamide | Ormetoprim and sulfadimethoxine | Primor |
| | Trimethoprim and sulfadiazine | Tribrissen, Uniprim, Tucoprim, Di-Trim, Equisul-SDT |
| | Trimethoprim and sulfamethoxazole | Bactrim, Septra, and generic forms |
| Antibacterial, antidiarrheal | Sulfasalazine | Azulfidine (Salazopyrin in Canada) |
| Antibacterial, antiparasitic | Metronidazole<br>Metronidazole benzoate<br>Metronidazole hydrochloride | Flagyl and generic |
| Antibacterial, beta-lactam | Amoxicillin | Amoxicillin: Amoxi-Tabs, Amoxi-Drops, Amoxi-Inject, Robamox-V, Biomox, and other brands; Amoxil, Trimox, Wymox, Polymox, (human forms); Amoxicillin trihydrate |
| | Amoxicillin and clavulanate potassium | Veterinary: Clavamox Human: Augmentin |
| | Ampicillin | Human forms include Omnipen, Principen, Totacillin, Polycillin. Injectable forms include Omnipen-N, Polycillin-N, Totacillin-N. Veterinary forms include Amp-Equine, and Ampicillin trihydrate (Polyflex). |
| | Cefaclor | Ceclor |
| | Cefadroxil | Veterinary: Cefa-Tabs, Cefa-Drops, Human dosage form: Duricef |
| | Cefazolin sodium | Ancef, Kefzol, and generic |
| | Cefdinir | Omnicef |
| | Cefepime | Maxipime |
| | Cefixime | Suprax |
| | Cefotetan disodium | Cefotan |
| | Cefovecin | Convenia |
| | Cefoxitin sodium | Mefoxin |
| | Cefpodoxime proxetil | Simplicef (veterinary drug) Vantin (human drug) |
| | Cefquinome | Cobactan, Cephaguard |
| | Ceftazidime | Fortaz, Ceptaz, Tazicef, Tazidime |
| | Ceftiofur crystalline-free acid | Excede |
| | Ceftiofur hydrochloride | Excenel |
| | Ceftiofur sodium | Naxcel |
| | Cephalexin | Keflex, Rilexine, Vetalexin |
| | Cloxacillin sodium | Cloxapen, Orbenin, Tegopen |
| | Doripenem | Doribax |
| | Ertapenem | Invanz |
| | Imipenem and Cilastatin | Primaxin |
| | Oxacillin sodium | Pro-staphli and generic |

*Continued*

## Listing of Drugs According to Functional and Therapeutic Classification

| Drug Classification | Drug Name | Brand Name |
| --- | --- | --- |
| | Penicillin G | Penicillin G potassium or sodium: Many brands<br>Penicillin G benzathine: Benza-Pen, and other names<br>Penicillin G, Procaine: Generic<br>Penicillin V: Pen-Vee |
| | Piperacillin sodium and Tazobactam | Zosyn |
| | Ampicillin and sulbactam | Unasyn |
| | Cefotaxime sodium | Claforan |
| | Dicloxacillin sodium | Dynapen |
| Antibacterial, fluoroquinolone | Ciprofloxacin hydrochloride | Cipro and generic forms |
| | Danofloxacin mesylate | Advocin |
| | Difloxacin hydrochloride | Dicural |
| | Enrofloxacin | Baytril |
| | Levofloxacin | Levaquin |
| | Marbofloxacin | Zeniquin, Marbocyl |
| | Moxifloxacin | Avelox |
| | Norflozacin | Noroxin |
| | Orbifloxacin | Orbax |
| | Pradofloxacin | Veraflox |
| Antibacterial, glycopeptide | Vancomycin | Vancocin, Vancoled |
| Antibacterial, sulfonamide | Sulfachlorpyridazine | Vetisulid |
| | Sulfadiazine | Combined with trimethoprim in Tribrissen |
| | Sulfadimethoxine | Albon, Bactrovet, and generic |
| | Sulfamethazine | Many brands (e.g., Sulmet) |
| | Sulfamethoxazole | Gantanol |
| | Sulfaquinoxaline | Sulfa-Nox |
| Antibacterial, tetracycline | Chlortetracycline | Aureomycin soluble powder, Aureomycin tablets, Aureomycin soluble calf oblets and Calf Scour Bolus, Fermycin |
| | Doxycycline | Vibramycin, Monodox, Doxy Caps, Ronaxan |
| | Minocycline hydrochloride | Minocin |
| | Oxytetracycline | Terramycin, Terramycin soluble powder, Terramycin scours tablets; Biomycin, Oxy-Tet, Oxybiotic Oxy 500, Oxy 1000; long-acting formulations include Liquamycin-LA 200, and Biomycin 200 |
| | Tetracycline | Panmycin, Duramycin powder |
| | Tetracycline hydrochloride | Achromycin V |
| Antibiotic, aminocyclitol | Spectinomycin dihydrochloride pentahydrate | Spectam, Spectogard, Prospec, Adspec |
| | Spectinomycin sulfate tetrahydrate | |

## Listing of Drugs According to Functional and Therapeutic Classification

| Drug Classification | Drug Name | Brand Name |
|---|---|---|
| Anticancer agent | Asparaginase (L-Asparaginase) | Elspar, Asparaginase |
| | Bleomycin sulfate | Blenoxane |
| | Busulfan | Myleran |
| | Carboplatin | Paraplatin |
| | Chlorambucil | Leukeran |
| | Cisplatin | Platinol |
| | Cyclophosphamide | Cytoxan, Neosar, CTX |
| | Cytarabine | Cytosar, Ara-C, Cytosine arabinoside |
| | Dacarbazine | DTIC |
| | Doxorubicin hydrochloride | Adriamycin |
| | Fluorouracil | 5-Fluorouracil, Adrucil |
| | Hydroxyurea | Droxia; Hydrea (Canada) |
| | Lomustine | CeeNu, CCNU |
| | Melphalan | Alkeran |
| | Mercaptopurine | Purinethol |
| | Methotrexate | MTX, Mexate, Folex |
| | Mitoxantrone hydrochloride | Novantrone |
| | Paclitaxel | Paccal |
| | Plicamycin | Mithracin, Mithramycin |
| | Streptozocin | Streptozotocin, Zanosar |
| | Thioguanine | Generic |
| | Thiotepa | Thioplex and generic |
| | Toceranib | Palladia |
| | Vinblastine sulfate | Velban |
| | Vincristine sulfate | Oncovin, Vincasar |
| Anticholinergic | Atropine sulfate | Many generic brands |
| | Glycopyrrolate | Robinul-V |
| | Hyoscyamine | Levsin |
| | Oxybutynin chloride | Ditropan |
| | Aminopentamide | Centrine |
| | N-butylscopolammonium bromide (Butylscopolamine bromide) | Buscopan |
| Anticholinesterase | Pyridostigmine bromide | Mestinon, Regonol |
| | Physostigmine | Antilirium |
| | Neostigmine | Prostigmin, Stiglyn, Neostigmine bromide, Neostigmine methylsulfate |
| Anticoagulant | Dalteparin | Fragmin, LMWH |
| | Dipyridamole | Persantine, Aggrenox |
| | Enoxaparin | Lovenox, LMWH |
| | Heparin sodium | Liquaemin, Hepalean (Canada) |
| | Rivaroxaban | Xarelto |
| | Tissue plasminogen activator (tPA) | tPA, Retavase |
| | Warfarin sodium | Coumadin and generic |

*Continued*

## Listing of Drugs According to Functional and Therapeutic Classification

| Drug Classification | Drug Name | Brand Name |
| --- | --- | --- |
| Anticonvulsant | Bromide | Potassium bromide, sodium bromide |
| | Clonazepam | Klonopin and generic |
| | Clorazepate dipotassium | Tranxene |
| | Felbamate | Felbatol |
| | Imepitoin | Pexion |
| | Levetiracetam | Keppra |
| | Lorazepam | Ativan |
| | Midazolam hydrochloride | Versed |
| | Oxazepam | Serax |
| | Phenobarbital | Luminal, Phenobarbitone, and |
| | Phenobarbital sodium | generic |
| | Phenytoin | Dilantin |
| | Phenytoin sodium | |
| | Primidone | Mylepsin, Neurosyn (Mysoline in Canada) |
| | Valproic acid | Depakene (valproic acid); Depakote |
| | Valproate sodium | (divalproex) (Epival is Canadian brand) |
| | Zonisamide | Zonegran |
| Anticonvulsant, analgesic | Gabapentin | Neurontin and generic |
| | Pregabalin | Lyrica |
| Anticonvulsant, sedative | Diazepam | Valium and generic |
| | Midazolam hydrochloride | Versed |
| Antidiarrheal | Bismuth subsalicylate | Pepto Bismol |
| | Diphenoxylate | Lomotil |
| | Kaolin and pectin | KaoPectate |
| | Loperamide | Imodium, and generic |
| | Mesalamine | Asacol, Mesasal, Pentasa, Mesalazine |
| | Olsalazine sodium | Dipentum |
| | Paregoric | Corrective Mixture |
| | Propantheline bromide | Pro-Banthine |
| | Sulfasalazine | Azulfidine |
| Antidote | Charcoal, activated | ActaChar, Charcodote, Liqui-Char, Toxiban |
| | Deferoxamine mesylate | Desferal |
| | Dimercaprol | BAL in oil; British anti-lewisite |
| | Edetate calcium disodium | Calcium disodium versenate, calcium disodium ethylenediaminetetra-acetate (EDTA) |
| | Flumazenil | Romazicon |
| | Fomepizole | 4-Methylpyrazole, Antizol-Vet, Antizol (human form) |
| | Leucovorin calcium | Wellcovorin and generic |
| | Methylene blue 0.1% | Also called New Methylene Blue |
| | Penicillamine | Cuprimine, Depen |
| | Pralidoxime chloride | 2-PAM, Protopam chloride |
| | Succimer | Chemet |
| | Trientine hydrochloride | Syprine |

## Listing of Drugs According to Functional and Therapeutic Classification

| Drug Classification | Drug Name | Brand Name |
|---|---|---|
| Antiemetic | Aprepitant | Emend |
| | Dolasetron mesylate | Anzemet |
| | Dronabinol | Marinol |
| | Granisetron hydrochloride | Kytril |
| | Maropitant | Cerenia |
| | Meclizine | Antivert, Bonine, Meclozine (British name) |
| | Mirtazapine | Remeron |
| | Ondansetron hydrochloride | Zofran |
| | Trimethobenzamide | Tigan and others |
| Antiemetic, antidiarrheal | Prochlorperazine edisylate Prochlorperazine maleate (each with isopropamide iodide) | Darbazine |
| Antiemetic, phenothiazine | Chlorpromazine | Thorazine, Largactil |
| | Prochlorperazine edisylate Prochlorperazine maleate | Compazine |
| | Trifluoperazine hydrochloride | Stelazine |
| | Triflupromazine hydrochloride | Vesprin, Fluopromazine |
| | Trimeprazine tartrate | Temaril, (Panectyl in Canada), Temaril-P (with prednisolone) |
| | Promethazine hydrochloride | Phenergan |
| Antihistamine | Propiomazine hydrochloride | Tranvet, Largon |
| Antiemetic, prokinetic agent | Metoclopramide hydrochloride | Reglan, Maxolon |
| Antiestrogen | Tamoxifen citrate | Nolvadex |
| Antifungal | Amphotericin B | Fungizone (traditional formulation) and liposomal forms of Amphotec, ABCD, ABELCET, AmBisome |
| | Enilconazole | Imaverol, ClinaFarm-EC |
| | Fluconazole | Diflucan, and generic |
| | Flucytosine | Ancobon |
| | Griseofulvin | Microsize: Fulvicin U/F, Grisactin, Grifulvin Ultramicrosize: Fulvicin P/G, GrisPEG |
| | Itraconazole | Sporanox (Itrafungol for cats is available in Europe) |
| | Ketoconazole | Nizoral |
| | Posaconazole | Noxafil |
| | Terbinafine hydrochloride | Lamisil |
| | Voriconazole | Vfend |
| Antifungal, expectorant | Potassium iodide | Quadrinal |
| Antihistamine | Cetirizine hydrochloride | Zyrtec |
| | Chlorpheniramine maleate | Chlortrimeton, Phenetron, and others |
| | Clemastine fumarate | Tavist, Contac 12-h allergy, and generic |
| | Cyproheptadine hydrochloride | Periactin |
| | Dimenhydrinate | Dramamine (Gravol in Canada) |
| | Diphenhydramine hydrochloride | Benadryl |
| | Hydroxyzine | Atarax |
| | Tripelennamine citrate | Pelamine, PBZ |

*Continued*

## Listing of Drugs According to Functional and Therapeutic Classification

| Drug Classification | Drug Name | Brand Name |
| --- | --- | --- |
| Antihypercalcemic agent | Alendronate | Fosamax |
| | Clodronate disodium | Osphos |
| | Etidronate disodium | Didronel |
| | Pamidronate disodium | Aredia |
| | Tiludronate | Tildren, Skelid |
| | Zoledronate | Zometa |
| Antihyperglycemic agent | Metformin | Glucophage |
| | Glipizide | Glucotrol |
| | Glyburide | Diabeta, Micronase, Glynase, Glibenclamide (British name) |
| Antihyperlipidemic agent | Gemfibrozil | Lopid |
| Anti-inflammatory agent, antipruritic | Oclacitinib | Apoquel |
| Anti-inflammatory agent | Allopurinol | Lopurin, Zyloprim, Allopur (Europe) |
| | Colchicine | Generic |
| | Dimethyl Sulfoxide (DMSO) | DMSO, Domoso |
| | Pentoxifylline | Trental, oxpentifylline |
| | Niacinamide | Nicotinamide, vitamin B3 |
| Anti-inflammatory, corticosteroid | Budesonide | Entocort |
| | Betamethasone | Celestone, betamethasone acetate, betamethasone benzoate |
| | Desoxycorticosterone pivalate | Percorten-V, DOCP, or DOCA pivalate |
| | Dexamethasone | Azium, Dexaject; Dex-A-Vet, Decadron, Dexasone, and generic |
| | Dexamethasone sodium phosphate | Dexaject SP, Dexavet, and Dexasone Tablets include Decadron and generic |
| | Flumethasone | Flucort |
| | Hydrocortisone | Hydrocortisone: Cortef and generic Hydrocortisone sodium succinate: Solu-Cortef |
| | Isoflupredone acetate | Predef 2X |
| | Methylprednisolone | Methylprednisolone: Medrol Methylprednisolone acetate: Depo-Medrol Methylprednisolone sodium succinate: Solu-Medrol |
| | Prednisolone sodium succinate | Solu-Delta-Cortef |
| | Prednisolone | Delta-cortef, PrednisTab |
| | Prednisolone acetate | |
| | Prednisone | Deltasone and generic; Meticorten for injection |
| | Triamcinolone acetonide | Vetalog, Triamtabs, Aristocort |
| | Triamcinolone hexacetonide | Triamcinolone acetonide: Vetalog |
| | Triamcinolone diacetate | |
| Antimyasthenic | Edrophonium chloride | Tensilon and others |
| | Pyridostigmine bromide | Mestinon, Regonol |
| | Physostigmine | Antilirium |
| | Neostigmine | Prostigmin, Stiglyn |

## Listing of Drugs According to Functional and Therapeutic Classification

| Drug Classification | Drug Name | Brand Name |
|---|---|---|
| Antiparasitic | Albendazole | Valbazen |
| | Afoxolaner | NexGuard |
| | Amitraz | Mitaban |
| | Amprolium | Amprol, Corid |
| | Bunamidine hydrochloride | Scolaban |
| | Dichlorvos | Task, Dichlorovos, Atgard, DDVP, Verdisol, Equigard |
| | Diethylcarbamazine citrate | Caricide, Filaribits, Nemacide |
| | Doramectin | Dectomax |
| | Eprinomectin | Eprinex, LongRange, Eprizero, Centragard |
| | Epsiprantel | Cestex |
| | Febantel | Rintal, Vercom |
| | Fenbendazole | Panacur, SafeGuard |
| | Fluralaner | Bravecto |
| | Furazolidone | Furoxone |
| | Ivermectin | Heartguard, Ivomec, Eqvalan liquid, Equimectrin, IverEase, Zimecterin, Privermectin, Ultramectin, Ivercide, Ivercare, Ivermax |
| | Ivermectin and Praziquantel | Equimax |
| | Levamisole hydrochloride | Levasole, Ripercol, Tramisol, Ergamisol |
| | Lotilaner | Credelio |
| | Lufenuron | Program |
| | Lufenuron and milbemycin oxime | Sentinel tablets and Flavor Tabs |
| | Mebendazole | Telmintic, Telmin, Vermox (human drug) |
| | Melarsomine | Immiticide |
| | Metaflumizone | ProMeris |
| | Milbemycin oxime | Interceptor, Interceptor Flavor Tabs, and SafeHeart; milbemycin also is an ingredient in Sentinel |
| | Moxidectin | ProHeart (canine) Quest (equine) Cydectin (bovine) |
| | Nitenpyram | Capstar |
| | Oxfendazole | Benzelmin, Synanthic |
| | Oxibendazole | Anthelcide EQ |
| | Paromomycin sulfate | Humatin |
| | Piperazine | Pipa-Tabs and many generic forms |
| | Praziquantel | Droncit, Drontal (combination with febantel) |
| | Pyrantel pamoate | Nemex, Strongid, Priex, Pyran, Pyr-A-Pam |
| | Pyrantel tartrate | |
| | Sarolaner | Simparica |
| | Selamectin | Revolution |
| | Spinosad | Comfortis |
| | Thenium closylate | Canopar |
| | Thiabendazole | Omnizole, Equizole, TBZ, Thibenzole |
| | Thiacetarsamide sodium | Caparsolate |
| Antiplatelet agent | Clopidogrel | Plavix |

*Continued*

## Listing of Drugs According to Functional and Therapeutic Classification

| Drug Classification | Drug Name | Brand Name |
|---|---|---|
| Antiprotozoal | Atovaquone | Mepron |
| | Diclazuril | Clincox |
| | Diminazene aceturate, Diminazene diaceturate | Berenil, Ganaseg, Veriben |
| | Imidocarb hydrochloride | Imizol |
| | Metronidazole | Flagyl |
| | Nitazoxanide | Navigator (horses) Alinia (human) |
| | Ponazuril | Marquis |
| | Pyrimethamine and Sulfadiazine | ReBalance |
| | Ronidazole | |
| | Tinidazole | Tindamax |
| Antiprotozoal | Toltrazuril | Baycox |
| Antispasmodic | N-butylscopolammonium bromide (butylscopolamine bromide) | Buscopan |
| Antithyroid agent | Carbimazole | Neomercazole |
| | Iopanoic acid | Generic |
| | Ipodate | Calcium ipodate |
| | Methimazole | Tapazole |
| | Propylthiouracil | Generic, Propyl-Thyracil, PTU |
| Antitussive | Hydrocodone bitartrate and homatropine | Hycodan |
| | Dextromethorphan | Benylin and others |
| Antiulcer agent | Misoprostol | Cytotec |
| | Sucralfate | Carafate (Sulcrate in Canada) |
| Antiulcer agent, H2-blocker | Cimetidine hydrochloride | Tagamet (OTC and prescription) |
| | Famotidine | Pepcid |
| | Nizatidine | Axid |
| | Ranitidine hydrochloride | Zantac |
| Antiulcer agent, proton pump inhibitor | Esomeprazole | Nexium |
| | Omeprazole | Prilosec (formerly Losec), human formulation GastroGard and UlcerGard are equine formulations |
| | Pantoprazole | Protonix |
| Antiviral | Acyclovir | Zovirax |
| | Famciclovir | Famvir |
| | Lysine (L-Lysine) | Enisyl-F |
| | Valacyclovir | Valtrex |
| | Zidovudine | Retrovir |
| Antiviral, analgesic | Amantadine | Symmetrel |
| Appetite stimulant | Capromorelin | Entyce |
| | Mirtazapine | Miritaz |
| Behavior-modifying drug | Buspirone hydrochloride | BuSpar |
| | Trazodone | Desyrel |
| | Doxepin | Sinequan |
| Behavior-modifying drug | Imepitoin | Pexion |

## Listing of Drugs According to Functional and Therapeutic Classification

| Drug Classification | Drug Name | Brand Name |
| --- | --- | --- |
| Behavior-modifying drug, tricyclic antidepressant | Amitriptyline hydrochloride | Elavil and generic brands |
| | Clomipramine hydrochloride | Clomicalm (veterinary); Anafranil (human) |
| | Imipramine hydrochloride | Tofranil |
| Behavior-modifying drug, selective serotonin reuptake inhibitor | Fluoxetine hydrochloride | Prozac |
| | Paroxetine | Paxil |
| Beta-agonist | Isoproterenol hydrochloride | Isuprel, isoprenaline hydrochloride |
| Beta-blocker | Atenolol | Tenormin |
| | Bisoprolol | Zebeta |
| | Esmolol hydrochloride | Brevibloc |
| | Metoprolol tartrate | Lopressor |
| | Propranolol hydrochloride | Inderal and generic |
| | Sotalol hydrochloride | Betapace |
| Bronchodilator | Aminophylline | Generic forms |
| | Oxtriphylline | Choledyl-SA |
| | Theophylline | Many brands and generic Theophylline sustained-release is by Inwood Laboratories: Theo-Dur, Slo-bid, Gyrocaps |
| Bronchodilator, beta-agonist | Albuterol sulfate | Proventil, Ventolin Also known as Salbutamol in other countries Torpex Equine Inhaler |
| | Clenbuterol | Ventipulmin |
| | Fluticasone | Flovent, Advair |
| | Metaproterenol sulfate | Alupent, Metaprel, Orciprenaline Sulphate |
| | Terbutaline sulfate | Brethine, Bricanyl |
| | Zilpaterol | Zilmax |
| Calcium supplement | Calcitriol | Rocaltrol, Calcijex |
| | Calcium carbonate | Many brands available: Titralac, Calci-mix, Liqui-cal, Maalox, Tums |
| | Calcium chloride | Generic |
| | Calcium citrate | Citracal (OTC) |
| | Calcium gluconate and Calcium borogluconate | Kalcinate, Calcium borogluconate, AmVet, Cal-Nate, and generic |
| | Calcium lactate | Generic; many brands available |
| Cardiac inotropic agent | Digitoxin | Crystodigin |
| | Digoxin | Lanoxin, Cardoxin |
| | Dobutamine hydrochloride | Dobutrex |
| Cardiac inotropic agent, vasodilator | Pimobendan | Vetmedin |
| Cardiac inotropic agent, beta-agonist | Dopamine hydrochloride | Intropin |
| Cholinergic | Bethanechol chloride | Urecholine |
| Corticosteroid, replacement hormone | Fludrocortisone acetate | Florinef |
| Dermatologic agent | Isotretinoin | Accutane |

*Continued*

## Listing of Drugs According to Functional and Therapeutic Classification

| Drug Classification | Drug Name | Brand Name |
|---|---|---|
| Diuretic | Acetazolamide | Diamox |
| | Chlorothiazide | Diuril |
| | Dichlorphenamide | Daranide |
| | Furosemide | Lasix |
| | Hydrochlorothiazide | HydroDiuril and generic |
| | Mannitol | Osmitrol |
| | Methazolamide | Nepta-zane |
| | Spironolactone | Aldactone |
| | Torsemide | Demadex |
| | Triamterene | Dyrenium |
| Diuretic, laxative | Glycerin | Generic |
| Dopamine agonist | Bromocriptine mesylate | Parlodel |
| | Levodopa | Larodopa, L-dopa |
| | Pergolide | Permax |
| | Pergolide mesylate | |
| | Selegiline hydrochloride | Anipryl (also known as deprenyl and l-deprenyl); human dose form is Eldepryl |
| Emetic | Apomorphine hydrochloride | Generic |
| | Ipecac | Ipecac, Syrup of Ipecac |
| Expectorant, muscle relaxant | Guaifenesin | Glyceryl guaiacolate, Guaiphenesin, Gecolate, Guailaxin, Glycotuss, Hytuss, Glytuss, Fenesin, Humabid LA |
| Fluid replacement | Dextran | Dextran 70 Gentran-70 |
| | Dextrose solution | D5W |
| | Hydroxyethyl starch | HES, Tetrastarch, Hespan |
| | Lactated Ringer's solution | LRS and other names |
| | Pentastarch | Pentaspan |
| | Ringer's solution | Generic |
| | Sodium chloride 0.9% | Generic, normal saline |
| | Sodium chloride 7.2% | Hypertonic saline, HSS |
| Hepatic protectant | S-adenosylmethionine (SAMe) | Denosyl, SAMe |
| | Silymarin | Silybin, Marin, milk thistle |
| Hormone | Cabergoline | Galastop, Dostinex |
| | Colony-stimulating factors | Leukine, Neupogen |
| | Corticotropin | Acthar |
| | Cosyntropin | Cortrosyn, Synthetic ACTH, Tetracosactrin, Tetracosactide |
| | Danazol | Danocrine |
| | Desmopressin acetate | DDAVP |
| | Diethylstilbestrol | DES |
| | Epoetin alpha (erythropoietin) | Epogen, epoetin alfa, "EPO," (r-HuEPO), erythropoietin |
| | Darbepoetin alfa | Aranesp |
| | Estradiol cypionate | ECP, Depo-Estradiol |
| | Estriol | Incurin |
| | Gonadorelin hydrochloride, Gonadorelin diacetate tetrahydrate | Factrel, Fertagyl, Cystolelin, Fertelin, OvaCyst, GnRh, LHRH |
| | Gonadotropin, chorionic | Profasi, Pregnyl, A.P.L. |

## Listing of Drugs According to Functional and Therapeutic Classification

| Drug Classification | Drug Name | Brand Name |
| --- | --- | --- |
| | Growth hormone | Somatrem and Somatropin; brand names include Protropin, Humatrope, Nutropin |
| | Insulin | Lente insulin, Ultralente insulin, Regular insulin, NPH insulin, Protamine zinc insulin (PZI) Humulin Vetsulin (veterinary) PZI Vet (veterinary protamine zinc insulin) |
| | Levothyroxine sodium | Thyro-Tabs, Synthroid equine powders include Equisyn-T4, Levo-Powder, Thyroid Powder, Thyro-L |
| | Liothyronine sodium | Cytomel |
| | Medroxyprogesterone acetate | Depo-Provera (injection); Provera (tablets); Cycrin tablets |
| | Megestrol acetate | Ovaban, Megace |
| | Mibolerone | Cheque-drops |
| | Testosterone | Testosterone cypionate ester: Andro-Cyp, Andronate, Depo-Testosterone Testosterone propionate ester: Testex, (Malogen in Canada) |
| | Urofollitropin | Metrodin, FSH, Fertinex |
| | Vasopressin | Pitressin |
| Hormone antagonist | Finasteride | Proscar |
| Hormone, anabolic agent | Boldenone Undecylenate | Equipoise |
| | Methyltestosterone | Android |
| | Nandrolone decanoate | Deca-Durabolin |
| | Oxymetholone | Anadrol |
| | Stanozolol | Winstrol-V |
| Hormone, progestin | Altrenogest | ReguMate, Matrix |
| | Megestrol acetate | Ovaban, Megace |
| Hormone, thyroid | Thyroid-releasing hormone | TRH |
| | Thyrotropin | Thytropar, Thyrogen, TSH |
| Hormone, labor induction | Oxytocin | Pitocin, Syntocinon (nasal solution), and generic |
| Immunostimulant | Interferon | Virbagen Omega |
| | Lithium carbonate | Lithotabs |
| Immunosuppressive agent | Auranofin | Ridaura |
| | Aurothioglucose | Solganal |
| | Azathioprine | Imuran |
| | Cyclosporine | Atopica (veterinary); Neoral (human); Sandimmune; Optimmune (ophthalmic); Gengraf Other name for cyclosporine is cyclosporin A |
| | Gold sodium thiomalate | Myochrysine |
| | Leflunomide | Arava |
| | Mycophenolate | CellCept |
| | Tacrolimus | Protopic, also known as FK506 |
| Iodine supplement | Iodide | Potassium Iodide |
| | Sodium iodide (20%) | Iodopen |

*Continued*

## Listing of Drugs According to Functional and Therapeutic Classification

| Drug Classification | Drug Name | Brand Name |
| --- | --- | --- |
| Laxative | Bisacodyl | Dulcolax |
| | Cascara sagrada | Nature's Remedy and other brands |
| | Castor oil | Generic |
| | Docusate | Docusate calcium: Surfak, Doxidan |
| | | Docusate sodium: DSS, Colace, Doxan |
| | | Many OTC brands are available |
| | Lactulose | Chronulac |
| | Magnesium citrate | Citroma, CitroNesia (Citro-Mag in Canada) |
| | Magnesium hydroxide | Milk of Magnesia, Carmilax, Magnalax |
| | Mineral oil | Generic |
| | Polyethylene glycol electrolyte solution | Golytely, PEG, Colyte, Co-Lav |
| | Psyllium | Metamucil and others |
| | Senna | Senokot |
| | Ursodiol | Actigall, Ursodeoxycholic acid |
| | Ursodeoxycholic acid | |
| Laxative, antiarrhythmic | Magnesium sulfate | Epsom salts |
| Local anesthetic | Bupivacaine hydrochloride | Marcaine, Nocita, and generic |
| | Mepivacaine | Carbocaine-V |
| Local anesthetic, antiarrhythmic | Lidocaine hydrochloride | Xylocaine |
| Mucolytic, antidote | Acetylcysteine | Mucomyst, Acetadote |
| Muscle relaxant | Atracurium besylate | Tracrium |
| | Dantrolene sodium | Dantrium |
| | Methocarbamol | Robaxin-V |
| | Pancuronium bromide | Pavulon |
| Nutritional supplement | Ferrous sulfate | Ferospace and OTC brands |
| | Iron Dextran | AmTech Iron Dextran, Ferrodex, HemaJect |
| | MCT oil | MCT oil (many sources), medium chain triglycerides |
| | Taurine | Generic |
| | Zinc | Zinc (various forms) |
| Opioid antagonist | Naloxone hydrochloride | Narcan, Trexonil |
| | Naltrexone | Trexan |
| Pancreatic enzyme | Pancrelipase | Viokase, Pancrezyme, Cotazym, Creon, Pancoate, Pancrease, Ultrase |
| Phosphate binder | Sevelamer | generic |
| Potassium supplement | Potassium chloride | Generic |
| | Potassium gluconate | Kaon, Tumil-K, generic |
| | Potassium phosphate | K-Phos, Neutra-Phos-K, and generic |
| Prokinetic agent | Cisapride | Propulsid (Prepulsid in Canada) |
| | Domperidone | Motilium, Equidone |
| | Methylnaltrexone | Relistor |
| | Metoclopramide | Reglan |
| | Tagaserod | Zelnorm |

## Listing of Drugs According to Functional and Therapeutic Classification

| Drug Classification | Drug Name | Brand Name |
| --- | --- | --- |
| Prostaglandin | Cloprostenol | Estrumate, estroPlan |
| | Dinoprost tromethamine | Lutalyse, Dinoprost, Prostin F2 alpha, ProstaMate, Prostaglandin F2alpha, PGF2alpha |
| | Prostaglandin F-2 alpha | Lutalyse, Dinoprost, PG-F2 alpha |
| Respiratory stimulant | Doxapram hydrochloride | Dopram |
| Sedative | Zolpidem | Ambien |
| Tranquilizer, benzodiazepine | Alprazolam | Xanax, Niravam |
| Tranquilizer, Phenothiazine | Acepromazine maleate | ACE, Aceproject, Aceprotabs, Atravet, Promace; it sometimes appears as acetylpromazine |
| Urethral smooth muscle relaxant | Tamsulosin | Flomax |
| Vasodilator | Hydralazine hydrochloride | Apresoline |
| | Irbesartan | Avapro |
| | Isosorbide dinitrate | Isosorbide dinitrate: Isordil, Isorbid, Sorbitrate |
| | Isosorbide mononitrate | Isosorbide mononitrate: Monoket |
| | Isoxsuprine | Vasodilan, and generic |
| | Nitroglycerin | Nitrol, Nitro-bid, Nitrostat |
| | Nitroprusside (Sodium nitroprusside) | Nitropress |
| | Phenoxybenzamine hydrochloride | Dibenzyline |
| | Phentolamine mesylate | Regitine (Rogitine in Canada) |
| | Prazosin | Minipress |
| | Sildenafil | Viagra |
| | Tadalafil | Cialis |
| Vasodilator, ACE inhibitor | Benazepril hydrochloride | Lotensin (human preparation), Fortekor (veterinary formulation) |
| | Captopril | Capoten |
| | Enalapril maleate | Enacard (veterinary), Vasotec (human) |
| | Lisinopril | Prinivil, Zestril |
| | Ramipril | Vasotop |
| | Trandolapril | Mavik |
| Vasodilator, angiotensin receptor blocker | Losartan | Cozaar |
| | Telmisartan | Micardis, Semintra |
| Vasodilator, calcium channel blocker | Amlodipine besylate | Norvasc |
| | Nifedipine | Adalat, Procardia |
| Vasopressor | Arginine vasopressin | Vasopressin, Pitressin |
| | Methoxamine | Vasoxyl |
| | Phenylephrine hydrochloride | Neo-synephrine |

*Continued*

## Listing of Drugs According to Functional and Therapeutic Classification

| Drug Classification | Drug Name | Brand Name |
| --- | --- | --- |
| Vitamin | Ascorbic acid | Vitamin C, sodium ascorbate; there are many brand names available |
| | Cyanocobalamin | Vitamin $B_{12}$ |
| | Dihydrotachysterol | Hytakerol, DHT |
| | Ergocalciferol | Calciferol, Drisdol |
| | Phytonadione | Aquamephyton (injection), Mephyton (tablets), Veta-K1 (capsules), vitamin K1, Phylloquinone; Phytomenadione |
| | Riboflavin | Vitamin $B_2$ |
| | Thiamine hydrochloride | Vitamin $B_1$, Bewon, and others |
| | Vitamin A | Retinol, Aquasol-A, Vitamin AD, vitamin A and D |
| | Vitamin E | Tocopherol, alpha-tocopherol, Aquasol E, and generic |
| | Vitamin K | Aquamephyton (injection), Mephyton (tablets); Veta-K1 (capsules), Veda-K1 (oral and injectable), vitamin K1, Phylloquinone, Phytomenadione |

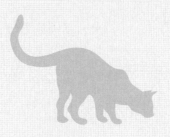

Papich Handbook of

# VETERINARY
# DRUGS

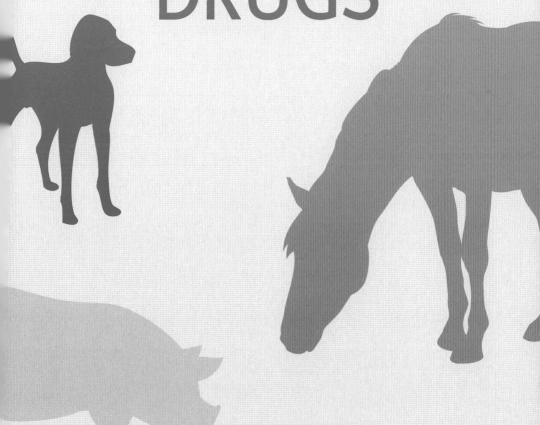

# Acepromazine Maleate
ayss-proe′meh-zeen mal′ee-ate

**Trade and other names:** ACE, AceproJect, AceproTabs, Atravet, and PromAce; it sometimes is called acetylpromazine

**Functional classification:** Tranquilizer, phenothiazine tranquilizer

## Pharmacology and Mechanism of Action
Phenothiazine tranquilizer and sedative. Acepromazine inhibits central dopaminergic receptors to produce sedation and tranquilization. Acepromazine also has antimuscarinic action and blocks norepinephrine at adrenergic receptors (e.g., alpha-receptors). Because of the blockade of alpha-receptors on vascular smooth muscle, it also produces vasodilation. When administered as an anesthetic adjunct, it may produce a decrease in vascular resistance and lower blood pressure but usually does not decrease cardiac output. In horses, IV administration significantly increases the blood flow through digital arteries and laminae. The half-life in horses is approximately 2.5 hours.

## Indications and Clinical Uses
Acepromazine is used as a sedative, a tranquilizer, a pre-anesthetic, and an anesthetic adjunct. When used as an anesthetic pre-anesthetic, it induces muscle relaxation and lowers doses of anesthetic agents used concurrently. In pre-anesthetic protocols, it also may have some anti-arrhythmic effects. In small animals, duration of sedation can occur within 10 minutes and have a 4- to 6-hour duration. In small animals, acepromazine can produce antiemetic effects via dopaminergic blockade. Acepromazine produces arterial smooth muscle relaxation by inhibiting $alpha_1$ receptor–mediated constriction. This effect is used to increase blood flow to tissues, particularly in the metatarsal artery of horses, and produces increased blood flow to the palmar digital artery. This is used for the treatment of horses with laminitis.

Acepromazine has been used as a behavior-modifying agent in animals (e.g., to treat anxiety). However, there are other agents that are preferred for long-term management of behavior disorders in animals that have fewer adverse effects. It should not be used as a first choice to decrease stress in hospitalized animals because there are other preferred agents available. Acepromazine does not provide analgesic activity.

## Precautionary Information
### Adverse Reactions and Side Effects
Sedation and ataxia are common side effects. Extrapyramidal effects (involuntary muscle movements), twitching, dystonia, or Parkinson-like effects are rare but are possible with the administration of phenothiazines to animals. Acepromazine may produce paradoxical excitation, disinhibition, and aggression in some dogs.

Phenothiazines may produce excessive vagal tone in some animals. This may be especially prominent in brachycephalic breeds. Administration of atropine may be used to treat the signs of high vagal tone. Because of alpha-adrenergic antagonism, hypotension is possible in animals. Decreased vascular tone because of $alpha_1$ adrenergic blockade is a prominent effect of acepromazine. This may produce hypotension in susceptible animals.

Dogs with a mutation in the *ABCB1* gene may be deficient for the ABCB1 transporter (p-glycoprotein). These dogs may have increased sensitivity to the effects of acepromazine, resulting in greater sedation scores. Lower doses should be used in these dogs.

In horses, persistent penile prolapse has been reported from use. This effect in horses is unpredictable. Some resources indicate that it is dose dependent with increased likelihood as the dose is increased from 0.01 to 0.1 mg/kg IV. The duration of penile prolapse in horses may be as long as 4 hours with high doses. In rare cases, penile prolapse can lead to permanent paraphimosis. The mechanism is unknown but may be caused by the alpha-adrenergic blockade induced by acepromazine.

**Contraindications and Precautions**

It has been stated in some veterinary textbooks that acepromazine may increase the risk of seizures in animals, and it should be administered cautiously in animals that are prone to seizures. However, a risk of seizures in animals from administration of acepromazine has not been confirmed during clinical use. Seizures were not reported in retrospective studies in which animals prone to seizures were anesthetized and administered acepromazine as an anesthetic adjunct.

Do not use in animals that have problems with dystonia or that have had previous extrapyramidal effects from use of phenothiazines.

Dogs with a mutation in the *ABCB1* gene (previously listed as *MDR1*), which is the gene that codes for the p-glycoprotein membrane transporter, are likely to have prolonged and increased sedation after administration of acepromazine. In these dogs, the dose should be decreased or another sedative selected for use.

Phenothiazines can cause hypotension (via alpha-receptor blockade); therefore, use cautiously with other hypotensive drugs or in conditions that may exacerbate hypotension. When administered as a pre-anesthetic to dogs (0.05 mg/kg), it induces moderate hypotension but does not affect cardiac output significantly.

In pregnancy, it produces only minor reduction in blood flow and oxygen delivery to the fetus when used in late pregnancy in cows.

**Drug Interactions**

Specific drug interactions have not been reported from the use of acepromazine in animals. However, it exacerbates the effects of other sedative drugs and may potentiate other drugs that cause vasodilation. Acepromazine has been used to sedate dogs for glucose tolerance testing (0.1 mg/kg), without adversely affecting the results.

## Instructions for Use

Acepromazine can be administered PO, IV, or IM. The doses used in anesthetic protocols are usually lower than the label dose. When used with general anesthetics, lower doses of general anesthetics can be used, especially when administering barbiturates and inhalant anesthetics. Clinical signs from acepromazine administration are most prominent during the first 3–4 hours after administration but may persist for 7 hours.

## Patient Monitoring and Laboratory Tests

Monitor blood pressure in animals susceptible to hypotension. Acepromazine does not affect adrenal function testing in dogs.

## Formulations
- Acepromazine is available in 5-, 10-, and 25-mg tablets and in a 10-mg/mL injection.
- Acepromazine oral granules and powder are available in Canada.

## Stability and Storage
Store in a tightly sealed container, protected from light, and at room temperature. Stability of compounded formulations has not been investigated.

## Small Animal Dosage
### Dogs
- 0.025–0.1 mg/kg IM, IV, or SQ in a single dose (most common is 0.025 mg/kg). Do not exceed 3 mg total in dogs.
- Sedation: 0.5–2.2 mg/kg q6–8h PO.
- Anesthetic protocols: 0.01–0.05 mg/kg IV, administered with other agents.

### Cats
- 0.025–0.1 mg/kg IM, IV, or SQ in a single dose.
- Sedation: 1.1–2.2 mg/kg q6–8h PO.
- Anesthetic protocols: 0.01–0.05 mg/kg IV, administered with other agents.

## Large Animal Dosage
### Horses
- 0.04–0.1 mg/kg IM. It can be administered q6–12h, but such frequent dosing is not recommended, and an interval of 36–48 hours between doses is preferred. For perioperative use, 0.01–0.05 mg/kg, IM, SQ, or IV.
- Treatment of laminitis: 0.04 mg/kg, IV.

### Cattle
- 0.13–0.26 mg/kg PO, 0.03–0.1 mg/kg IM, or 0.01–0.02 mg/kg IV.

### Pigs
- Adult: 0.03–0.2 mg/kg IV, IM, SQ (single dose).

## Regulatory Information
Withdrawal times: There are no withdrawal times established in the United States. It has been estimated that for extralabel use, establish a withdrawal time of at least 7 days for meat and 48 hours for milk.
Canada: 7 days for meat; 48 hours for milk.
Racing Commissioners International (RCI) Classification: 3

# Acetaminophen
ah-seet-ah-mee′noe-fen

**Trade and other names:** Tylenol and generic brands. Known outside the United States as paracetamol.

**Functional classification:** Analgesic

## Pharmacology and Mechanism of Action
Analgesic drug. Exact mechanism of action is not known. There is evidence that acetaminophen inhibits centrally mediated pain transmission via inhibition of cyclo-oxygenase (COX)-3 a variant of COX-1 found in the central nervous system (CNS). Other evidence indicates that acetaminophen may inhibit prostaglandins in

some cells and tissue in which low concentrations of arachidonic acid are present. The site of acetaminophen action may be the peroxidase enzyme component of prostaglandin $H_2$ synthase. Therefore, COX enzyme inhibition may occur at site-specific tissues, sparing the gastrointestinal (GI) mucosa, platelets, and kidneys but acting centrally.

Acetaminophen may affect inhibitory pain pathways involved in chronic pain and neuropathic pain syndromes. Descending inhibitory pain pathways are mediated by serotonin (5-HT3). Acetaminophen can stimulate the inhibitory pain pathway mediated by serotonin, and these can be blocked by serotonin antagonists. This evidence suggests that acetaminophen may directly activate serotonin receptors. An additional mechanism of action may be by activating transient receptor potential vanilloid 1 (TRPV1) receptors. This action may play a role in some pain syndromes, but the relevance is undetermined for clinical use.

In canine studies, acetaminophen has not produced anti-inflammatory action but has been effective as a mild analgesic agent. The effects of acetaminophen are brief and not as effective as the effects of nonsteroidal anti-inflammatory drugs (NSAIDs).

## Indications and Clinical Uses

Acetaminophen is used as an analgesic and for pain control in dogs. Do not use in cats. It is considered relatively weak as an analgesic. It is often used in combination with an opiate (e.g., codeine), but the contribution of codeine for treatment in animals is undetermined.

## Precautionary Information

### Adverse Reactions and Side Effects

Acetaminophen is well tolerated in dogs at doses listed; however, high doses have caused liver toxicity. It causes severe toxicosis in cats because of their inability to excrete metabolites. Acetaminophen relies on conjugation with glutathione for excretion, and deficiencies in glutathione can lead to toxicity. Treatment of a toxic overdose consists of administration of acetylcysteine (see Acetylcysteine for more details). Clinical signs of toxicity include methemoglobinemia, acute hepatic toxicosis, swelling of paws, and Heinz body anemia.

### Contraindications and Precautions

Do not administer to cats. In people, toxic episodes are more likely when administered with drugs that alter the activity of hepatic drug enzymes. Such a reaction also is possible in animals.

In cats, treatment of intoxication requires prompt treatment with acetylcysteine (see Acetylcysteine), supportive care, and monitoring.

### Drug Interactions

In people, other drugs (especially alcohol) will increase the risk of hepatotoxicosis. It is not known if other drugs increase this risk in animals.

## Instructions for Use

Many nonprescription (over-the-counter) formulations are available. Acetaminophen with codeine also is available, but it is undetermined if this formulation has better analgesic efficacy in animals than acetaminophen alone. See other entries for formulations that contain codeine.

## Patient Monitoring and Laboratory Tests

Monitor liver enzyme levels periodically to look for evidence of hepatotoxicity. In cats that have received acetaminophen, there is a high risk of toxicity, and careful monitoring of liver enzymes and blood cell parameters is needed. Many human hospitals and some diagnostic laboratories can measure acetaminophen concentrations in plasma. In people, treatment is initiated if plasma/serum concentrations are above 200 mcg/mL 4 hours after ingestion.

## Formulations

- Acetaminophen is available in 120-, 160-, 325-, and 500-mg tablets.

## Stability and Storage

Acetaminophen is stable in aqueous solutions. Maximum stability is at pH of 5–7.

## Small Animal Dosage

**Dogs**
- 15 mg/kg q8h PO.

**Cats**
- Contraindicated.

## Large Animal Dosage

**Horses**
- 20 mg/kg PO per day.

**Calves**
- 50 mg/kg PO followed by 30 mg/kg PO q6h.
- No other doses have been reported for large animals.

## Regulatory Information

No regulatory information is available. For extralabel use withdrawal interval estimates, contact Food Animal Residue Avoidance Databank (FARAD) at www.FARAD.org.

RCI Classification: 4

# Acetaminophen + Codeine
ah-seet-ah-mee′noe-fen + koe′deen

**Trade and other names:** Tylenol with codeine and many generic brands

**Functional classification:** Analgesic, opioid

## Pharmacology and Mechanism of Action

Analgesic agent. Exact mechanism of action for acetaminophen is not known; however, as discussed previously (see previous Acetaminophen entry), a centrally mediated mechanism is likely, either via inhibition of central prostaglandin synthesis or effects on serotonergic inhibitory pain pathways. In this formulation, the opiate codeine is added to enhance analgesia. Effects of codeine are not established in animals. Systemic absorption of codeine from oral administration is small in dogs, and codeine may play only a minor role in analgesia.

## Indications and Clinical Uses

Acetaminophen codeine combinations are used for analgesia in dogs (e.g., postoperative use), but the effectiveness of this combination has not been established.

Codeine formulations have also been used as an antitussive. Despite the widespread use of codeine in humans, the efficacy in animals for its antitussive use or analgesic use has not been established.

Oral absorption of codeine in dogs is low. Because codeine is converted to morphine (10% of dose) for its activity and the duration of morphine is short in dogs, the clinical effectiveness of codeine in dogs may be questionable.

## Precautionary Information

### Adverse Reactions and Side Effects

Acetaminophen and codeine formulations are well tolerated in dogs at doses listed because these doses are eliminated quickly. However, high doses can produce liver toxicity.

### Contraindications and Precautions

Do not administer to cats because acetaminophen is known to be toxic to cats. Codeine is a Schedule II controlled substance.

### Drug Interactions

In people, other drugs (especially alcohol) increase the risk of hepatotoxicity. It is not known if other drugs increase this risk in animals but consider this possibility when administering other drugs that may affect hepatic metabolism.

## Instructions for Use

Many generic preparations are available. Consider that other ingredients may be present in some combination tablets (e.g., ibuprofen or caffeine).

## Patient Monitoring and Laboratory Tests

Monitor liver enzyme levels periodically to look for evidence of hepatotoxicity caused by acetaminophen.

## Formulations

- Acetaminophen and codeine combinations are available in oral solution and tablets. A variety of formulations are available (e.g., 300-mg acetaminophen plus 15-, 30-, or 60-mg codeine).

## Stability and Storage

Acetaminophen is stable in aqueous solutions. Maximum stability is at pH of 5–7.

## Small Animal Dosage

### Dogs

Follow dosing recommendations for codeine. Administer dosages of codeine equivalent to 0.5–1.0 mg/kg q4–6h PO.

### Cats

- Contraindicated.

## Large Animal Dosage

- No dose has been reported for large animals.

## Regulatory Information

Acetaminophen + codeine is a Schedule III drug controlled by the Drug Enforcement Agency (DEA). Do not administer to animals intended for food.

# Acetazolamide
ah-seet-ah-zole′a-mide

**Trade and other names:** Diamox, Vetamox (veterinary formulation)

**Functional classification:** Diuretic

## Pharmacology and Mechanism of Action

Carbonic anhydrase inhibitor. Acetazolamide, like other carbonic anhydrase inhibitors, produces diuresis through inhibition of the uptake of bicarbonate in proximal renal tubules via enzyme inhibition. This action results in loss of bicarbonate in the urine and diuresis. The action of carbonic anhydrase inhibitors results in urine loss of bicarbonate, alkaline urine, and water loss.

The pharmacokinetics have been studied in horses. The oral absorption in horses is only 25%, with rapid clearance, and a short half-life of approximately 1 hour.

## Indications and Clinical Uses

Acetazolamide is rarely used as a diuretic. More potent and more effective diuretic drugs are available, such as the loop diuretics (furosemide). It was once recommended for treatment of hydrocephalus in dogs, but it has been ineffective for this use.

Acetazolamide, like other carbonic anhydrase inhibitors, is used primarily to lower intraocular pressure in animals with glaucoma. Methazolamide is used more often than acetazolamide for this purpose, and other treatment regimens are now used more often than carbonic anhydrase inhibitors.

Acetazolamide also is sometimes used to produce more alkaline urine for management of some urinary calculi.

In horses, acetazolamide is used to treat hyperkalemic periodic paralysis (HPP). This is a defect of sodium ion channels in muscle cells, and acetazolamide may alter potassium homeostasis by increasing potassium excretion.

## Precautionary Information

### Adverse Reactions and Side Effects

Acetazolamide can potentially produce hypokalemia in some patients. Significant bicarbonate loss can occur with repeated administration. In dogs, a respiratory reaction has been observed, which is attributed to respiratory acidosis.

### Contraindications and Precautions

Do not use in patients with acidemia. Use cautiously in any animal sensitive to sulfonamides.

### Drug Interactions

Acetazolamide produces alkaline urine, which may affect clearance of some drugs. Alkaline urine may potentiate the effects of some antibacterial drugs (e.g., macrolides and quinolones).

## Instructions for Use

Acetazolamide, in combination with other agents, is usually used to decrease intraocular pressure in the treatment of glaucoma. Acetazolamide has been used to produce alkaline urine to prevent formation of some urinary calculi. However, unless there is supplementation with bicarbonate, the urine alkalinization will not be sustained with repeated administration.

## Patient Monitoring and Laboratory Tests

Monitor patient's ocular pressure when used to treat glaucoma.

## Formulations

- Acetazolamide is available in 125- and 250-mg tablets and a soluble powder for dogs.

## Stability and Storage

Stable if stored in tight containers. Compounded solutions are stable at least 60 days.

## Small Animal Dosage

### Dogs

Note: The approved veterinary formulation lists a dose of 10–30 mg/kg for glaucoma and diuretic uses.

- Glaucoma: 5–10 mg/kg q8–12h PO.
- Other diuretic uses: 4–8 mg/kg q8–12h PO.

### Cats

- 7 mg/kg, q8h, PO.

## Large Animal Dosage

### Horses

- Treatment of HPP: 4 mg/kg IV or 8 mg/kg PO q8–12h.

## Regulatory Information

No regulatory information is available. For extralabel use withdrawal interval estimates, contact FARAD at www.FARAD.org.

RCI Classification: 4

# Acetylcysteine
ah-see-til-sis´tay-een

**Trade and other names:** Mucomyst, Cetylev, and Acetadote; also referred to as N-acetylcysteine

**Functional classification:** Mucolytic, antidote

## Pharmacology and Mechanism of Action

Acetylcysteine decreases viscosity of secretions and is used as a mucolytic agent in eyes and in bronchial nebulizing solutions. Acetylcysteine is a sulfhydryl compound and acts to increase synthesis of glutathione in the liver. Glutathione subsequently acts as an antioxidant and facilitates conjugation to toxic metabolites, particularly the toxic metabolites of acetaminophen. The antioxidant effects also have been used to treat conditions associated with oxidative stress. The pharmacokinetics have been studied in cats. It has a half-life of approximately 1.5 hours and oral absorption of 33%. The clearance is faster than in humans.

## Indications and Clinical Uses

As a donator of the sulfhydryl group, it is used as an antidote for intoxications (e.g., acetaminophen toxicosis in cats). It acts to replenish glutathione in animals that have been intoxicated with drugs that have reactive metabolites. When treating poisoning, it is important that acetylcysteine be administered as soon as possible for optimum effectiveness. Acetylcysteine also has been used to prevent contrast medium–induced nephropathy. Acetylcysteine has been used as a treatment of oxidative stress because it is a scavenger of hydroxyl radicals and hypochlorous acid. It also has been used to treat heavy metal toxicosis when administered with chelating agents. Acetylcysteine can reduce cerebral edema, but this has not produced any established clinical uses.

## Precautionary Information

### Adverse Reactions and Side Effects

Allergic reactions have been reported in people, which resemble anaphylactic reactions when it is given IV. These reactions manifest as skin reactions, bronchospasm, tachycardia, and hypotension. Vomiting has been observed in cats, but this also may be caused by the toxicant (acetaminophen). When delivered via aerosol to the airways of cats, it increases airway resistance and could worsen airway disease in cats.

### Contraindications and Precautions

Acetylcysteine may cause sensitization with prolonged topical administration. It may react with certain materials in nebulizing equipment. Avoid delivering via aerosol to the airways of cats because it might worsen clinical airway disease. Because acetylcysteine is hyperosmolar (2600 mOsmol/L), it must be diluted in sterile water prior to injection. Visually inspect for particulate matter and discoloration prior to injection.

### Drug Interactions

Acetylcysteine acts to donate sulfhydryl groups and may facilitate drug conjugation.

## Instructions for Use

Available as an agent for decreasing viscosity of respiratory secretions, but most common use is as a treatment for intoxications, primarily for cats to treat acetaminophen toxicosis. When treating an intoxication, doses are listed here, but also consult a poison control center for specific guidelines. The doses used in cats (and listed in the dosing section) are extrapolated from dosages used in humans for treatment of intoxication. However, pharmacokinetics are different in cats (shorter half-life and faster clearance), and higher doses may be needed in severe cases. For treatment of oxidative stress, constant rate infusions (CRIs) have been used in which 50 mg/kg is diluted 1:4 in saline solutions and administered IV over the course of 1 hour. Alternatively, the injection can be administered IV as a loading dose (150 mg/kg) over 60 minutes followed by 50 mg/kg over the next 4 hours followed by 100 mg/kg over the next 16 hours (21-hour total treatment time).

When administered by injection, the solution is hyperosmolar and must be diluted first. Diluent for dilution can include 0.45% NaCl, 5% dextrose, or sterile water.

An effervescent tablet of acetylcysteine (Cetylev) also is available and used in people to decrease hepatic injury caused by high doses of acetaminophen.

## Patient Monitoring and Laboratory Tests

When used to treat acetaminophen toxicity, monitor complete blood count (CBC) and liver enzyme concentrations.

## Formulations
- Acetylcysteine is available in a 20% oral solution (200 mg/mL).
- Acetylcysteine tablets are lemon-flavored effervescent tablets for oral administration. 500-mg and 2.5-g tablets.
- Injectable solution: 6 g of acetylcysteine in 30-mL vials for IV use (200 mg/mL).

## Stability and Storage
Acetylcysteine is unstable in air and easily oxidizes. It should be protected from light. Discard open vials after 96 hours. The normal color of the solution ranges from colorless to a slight pink or purple after the stopper is punctured. This color change does not affect the quality of the product. After dilution, the solution can be stored for 24 hours at room temperature. Discard unused portion if stored for longer.

## Small Animal Dosage
### Dogs and Cats
- Antidote: 140 mg/kg (loading dose); then 70 mg/kg q4h IV or PO for five doses.
- Eye solution: 2% solution topically q2h.
- To prevent contrast-medium nephropathy: 17 mg/kg IV bolus followed by 17 mg/kg q12h for 48 hours.
- CRIs have been used to treat oxidative stress (50 mg/kg diluted in saline infused over 1 hour).

## Large Animal Dosage
- No dose has been reported for large animals.

## Regulatory Information
No regulatory information is available. However, because it is short acting and is used primarily for the treatment of intoxications, no withdrawal time is suggested. For further information, contact FARAD at www.FARAD.org.

# Acyclovir
ay-sye´kloe-veer

**Trade and other names:** Zovirax and generic brands

**Functional classification:** Antiviral

## Pharmacology and Mechanism of Action
Antiviral drug. Acyclovir is the prototype of other agents used primarily for treatment of herpes virus infections. These drugs all share a similar mechanism of action but vary in their pharmacokinetics and adverse effects. Acyclovir monophosphate accumulates in cells infected with herpes virus and converted by guanylate cyclase to acyclovir diphosphate and subsequently to the triphosphate form, which is an inhibitor of viral DNA polymerase. This terminates viral enzyme activity. Therefore, acyclovir requires three steps for activation: (1) first, it is converted to the monophosphate form by viral thymidine kinase; (2) conversion to the diphosphate occurs in the host cell; and (3) conversion to the triphosphate form also occurs in the host cell. The triphosphate form is the active compound. It incorporates into the viral DNA to stop viral replication.

*Pharmacokinetics:* The half-lives are 9.6 hours for horses, 2.3 hours for dogs, and 2.6 hours for cats. By comparison, the half-life in humans is 2.5 hours. Unfortunately, it is not absorbed orally in horses (less than 3%), and there are few data to confirm oral absorption in other species. In humans, oral absorption is only 10%. Other forms (e.g., prodrugs and related compounds) are better absorbed in people, and some forms have been used in animals. Information on these drugs (valacyclovir and famciclovir) can be found in other monographs.

## Indications and Clinical Uses

Acyclovir is an antiviral drug. There is variability in susceptibility to acyclovir. Feline herpes virus-1 (FHV-1) is much less efficient (by a factor of 1000) for converting acyclovir to the monophosphate form than human herpes simplex virus (HSV-1). Therefore, it has little efficacy for treating cats with FHV-1. In addition, the oral absorption is very low, producing ineffective plasma drug concentrations. More important, if high concentrations are achieved, toxicity is common in cats.

Equine herpes virus (EHV-1) is more responsive to acyclovir than FHV-1. Unfortunately, it is not absorbed orally in horses (less than 3%). The only effective use is from IV slow infusions (slow infusion necessary to prevent phlebitis). A typical dosage is 10 mg/kg q12h IV infused over 1 hour.

### Precautionary Information
#### Adverse Reactions and Side Effects

The most serious adverse effect in humans is acute renal insufficiency. This may be prevented by slow IV infusion and proper hydration. Phlebitis can occur with IV administration. No adverse effects were identified in limited studies performed in horses, except in one study, the IV infusion caused sweating and muscle tremors when administered rapidly (15 minutes). In cats, significant adverse effects have been observed, which included myelosuppression, hepatotoxicity, and nephrotoxicity.

#### Contraindications and Precautions

Do not use in animals with compromised renal function. Do not use in cats.

#### Drug Interactions

Do not mix with biological solutions (e.g., blood products). Do not mix with fluids that contain bacteriostatic preservatives. Do not use with other nephrotoxic drugs.

## Instructions for Use

To prepare injectable formulation, dilute each vial with 10 or 20 mL of water to make 50 mg/mL. Do not use bacteriostatic water that contains benzyl alcohol or parabens. Further dilute solution to at least 100 mL to a concentration of 7 mg/mL or less.

## Patient Monitoring and Laboratory Tests

Monitor blood urea nitrogen (BUN) and creatinine during use. In horses, doses should be administered to maintain plasma concentrations above 0.3 mcg/mL.

## Formulations

- Acyclovir is available in 400- and 800-mg tablets, 200-mg capsules, 1-g and 500-mg vials for injection (50 mg/mL), and 40-mg/mL oral suspension.

## Stability and Storage

After reconstitution of solution at 50 mg/mL, it is stable for 12 hours at room temperature. More dilute solutions are stable for 24 hours. If refrigerated, a precipitate will form, which should be redissolved at room temperature before use. Store tablets and capsules in a tightly sealed container, protected from light, and at room temperature.

## Small Animal Dosage

### Dogs and Cats

- Dogs: Systemic doses have not been determined and indications for which it might be effective are not established. In rare instances when it has been used, the doses were extrapolated from human use: 3 mg/kg PO five times daily for 10 days, up to 10 mg/kg PO five times daily for 10 days. Alternatively, 10–20 mg/kg IV q8h (slow infusion for 1 hour).
- Cats: Acyclovir is not effective against feline herpes virus infection, it is toxic to cats, and other agents are suggested as alternatives (see Famciclovir).

## Large Animal Dosage

### Horses

- 10 mg/kg q12h IV infused over 1 hour. Even after 20 mg/kg, oral acyclovir is not absorbed in horses well enough for systemic treatment, and other agents may be used for oral treatment (see Valacyclovir).

## Regulatory Information

Because of mutagenicity, it should not be administered to animals intended for food.

# Afoxolaner
a-fox'-olan-er

**Trade and other names:** NexGard

**Functional classification:** Antiparasitic agent (flea and tick insecticide)

## Pharmacology and Mechanism of Action

Afoxolaner belongs to the isoxazolines class of ectoparasiticides. It is effective for treating and preventing infections from fleas, mites, and ticks. It produces selective inhibition of the gamma-aminobutyric acid (GABA) receptor and glutamate-gated chloride channels. The inhibition of the receptor produces changes in chloride channels, hyper-excitement of the parasite, and death. As a GABA antagonist, the effects on chloride transmission in nerve and muscle cells in fleas and ticks produces paralysis and death. Mammals are not affected because of a lack of binding to mammalian GABA receptors.

Efficacy has been demonstrated against a wide range of ectoparasites, including fleas, various mites (including *Demodex* and *Sarcoptes*), and ticks. Fleas, ticks, and mites are exposed and killed during their blood meal. Therefore, the parasite must bite the animal for exposure to the agent. Activity of the isooxazolines has been superior to other ectoparasiticides, including fipronil and imidacloprid.

Other drugs in this class with similar activity, but different pharmacokinetics, include fluralaner, lotilaner, and sarolaner.

## Indications and Clinical Uses

Afoxolaner is indicated to kill adult fleas and is indicated for the treatment and prevention of flea infestations (*Ctenocephalides felis*) and the treatment and control of black-legged tick (*Ixodes scapularis*), American dog tick (*Dermacentor variabilis*), Lone Star tick (*Amblyomma americanum*), and brown dog tick (*Rhipicephalus sanguineus*) infestations in dogs and puppies 8 weeks of age and older, weighing 4 lb of body weight or greater, for 1 month. It is also effective for the treatment of demodicosis caused by the *Demodex* mite.

Because of this action, afoxolaner can reduce the risk that these vectors may pose for disease transmission. For example, it may prevent infections caused by *Borrelia burgdorferi* (Lyme disease) and *Babesia canis*.

The approved label indication for afoxolaner is treatment of fleas and ticks, but extralabel uses, using the approved label dose, have included treatment of generalized demodicosis caused by *Demodex canis*. Dogs with *Demodex* treated with afoxolaner had greater mite reductions than treatment with moxidectin/imidacloprid. Afoxolaner can eliminate sarcoptic mange (*Sarcoptes scabiei*) in dogs.

## Precautionary Information
### Adverse Reactions and Side Effects
Afoxolaner has been safe for use in dogs at least 8 weeks of age. Target animal safety studies performed in dogs indicate good tolerance at the therapeutic dose. Beagle dogs treated at up to five times the therapeutic dose showed no signs of intoxication. In clinical field studies with the isooxazoline group of insecticides, adverse effects reported include vomiting, diarrhea, anorexia, and lethargy.

### Contraindications and Precautions
The isoxazoline group of insecticides have been associated with seizures in animals. Use cautiously in animals that may be prone to seizures. Safety has not been established in breeding or lactating animals.

### Drug Interactions
No drug interactions are reported in animals.

## Instructions for Use
Administer orally once per month. Other measures for flea and tick control in the pet's environment also may be used.

## Patient Monitoring and Laboratory Tests
No specific monitoring is needed.

## Formulations
Afoxolaner is available in chewable tablets containing 11.3, 28.3, 68, or 136 mg of afoxolaner.

## Stability and Storage
Store at room temperature protected from light in manufacturer's packaging.

## Small Animal Dosage
### Dogs
- 2.5 mg/kg (1.14 mg/lb), PO, once per month during flea and tick season. For treatment of *Demodex*, it has been administered twice-weekly.

### Cats
- No dose for cats has been established.

## Large Animal Dosage
- No large animal doses are available.

## Regulatory Information
Although risk of harmful residues is low, do not administer to food-producing animals.

# Aglepristone
ag-le´-pri-stone

**Trade and other names:** Alizine or Alzin

**Functional classification:** Hormone, antiprogestin

## Pharmacology and Mechanism of Action
Aglepristone (RU 46534) is a synthetic steroid antiprogestin related to mifepristone (RU 38486). It has an affinity for progesterone receptors that is three times that of progesterone without producing the same effects as progesterone. When administered, it binds to progesterone receptors to produce an antiprogestin effect and to interrupt and terminate pregnancy.

## Indications and Clinical Uses
Aglepristone has also been used to terminate pregnancy in animals. It has been safe for terminating pregnancy in both dogs and cats. It can also be used to treat mammary hyperplasia in cats, induce parturition in dogs and cats, and treat pyometra. In cats, it was effective to terminate pregnancy when administered with misoprostol. It was more effective in this combination than misoprostol or aglepristone alone.

## Precautionary Information
### Adverse Reactions and Side Effects
After termination of pregnancy in dogs, mucoid discharge may be observed. Other side effects include slight depression, transient anorexia, and mammary gland congestion. Otherwise, there have been no significant adverse effects reported in animals.

### Contraindications and Precautions
Aglepristone terminates pregnancy. It should be handled with caution by women. Owners should be cautioned about risks during pregnancy.

### Drug Interactions
No drug interactions are reported in animals.

## Instructions for Use
For treatment of pyometra, it should be administered on days 1, 2, 7, and 14 by SQ injection.

## Patient Monitoring and Laboratory Tests
No specific monitoring is necessary.

## Formulations
- Aglepristone is not available in the United States at this time. In some European countries, it is available as a 30-mg/mL injection.

## Stability and Storage
Store at room temperature protected from light.

## Small Animal Dosage
### Dogs
- Terminate pregnancy: Two doses of 10 mg/kg (0.33 mL/kg) SQ once daily for 2 days.

## Cats
- Treatment of pyometra: 10 mg/kg SQ, on days 1, 2, 7, and 14.
- Terminate pregnancy (should not be used later than the second trimester): 10 mg/kg SQ, q24h, for two doses. Can be administered with misoprostol at 200 mcg per cat oral q12h until the abortion begins.

## Large Animal Dosage
- No large animal doses are available.

## Regulatory Information
Do not administer to food-producing animals.

# Albendazole
al-ben'dah-zole

**Trade and other names:** Valbazen

**Functional classification:** Antiparasitic

## Pharmacology and Mechanism of Action
Benzimidazole antiparasitic drug. Albendazole binds to intracellular beta-tubulin in parasites and prevents the microtubule formation for cell division.

## Indications and Clinical Uses
Albendazole is used to treat a variety of intestinal helminth parasites. It has been used for treating parasitic infections of the respiratory tract, including *Capillaria aerophila, Paragonimus kellicotti, Aelurostrongylus abstrusus, Filaroides* spp., and *Oslerus osleri*. It is also effective for treatment of *Giardia* in small animals. However, because albendazole has been associated with bone marrow suppression in dogs and cats, other drugs are preferred in small animals for *Giardia*.

## Precautionary Information
### Adverse Reactions and Side Effects
Adverse effects include anorexia, lethargy, and bone marrow toxicity. Leukopenia and thrombocytopenia are possible in dogs and cats. Albendazole has an affinity for rapidly dividing cells and may cause toxicity to bone marrow and intestinal epithelium. High doses have been associated with bone marrow toxicity in dogs and cats, and it should be used cautiously in small animals. In other species, at approved doses, there has been a wide margin of safety.

### Contraindications and Precautions
Adverse effects are more likely when administered for longer than 5 days. Avoid high doses. Pregnancy caution: Do not use during first 45 days of pregnancy.

### Drug Interactions
No drug interactions are reported in animals.

## Instructions for Use
Used primarily as antihelmintic but also has demonstrated efficacy for giardiasis. In small animals, other agents are generally preferred for treating infections caused by *Giardia*.

## Patient Monitoring and Laboratory Tests

Monitor CBC in animals experiencing signs suspicious of adverse effects. If high doses are accidentally administered to small animals, CBC should be examined for evidence of suppression.

## Formulations

- Albendazole is available in a 113.6- and 45.5-mg/mL suspension and 300-mg/mL paste.

## Stability and Storage

Store in a tightly sealed container, protected from light, and at room temperature. Stability of compounded formulations has not been investigated.

## Small Animal Dosage

### Dogs and Cats

- Anthelmintic dosage: 25–50 mg/kg q12h PO for 3 days.
- Respiratory parasites: 50 mg/kg q24h PO for 10–14 days.
- Giardia: 25 mg/kg q12h PO for 2 days.

### Birds

- 50–100 mg/kg once per day for 2–9 days.

## Large Animal Dosage

### Cattle

- Antiparasitic: Single dose of 10 mg/kg oral paste or 10 mg/kg (suspension) PO.

### Horses

- *Dictyocaulus arnfieldi:* 25 mg/kg q12h for 5 days.
- *Strongylus vulgaris:* 50 mg/kg q12h for 2 days.

### Sheep and goats

- Single dose of 7.5 mg/kg oral suspension.

## Regulatory Information

Cattle withdrawal time: 27 days for meat. Do not use in lactating dairy cattle. Sheep withdrawal time: 7 days for meat.

# Albuterol Sulfate
al-byoo´ter-ole sul´fate

**Trade and other names:** Proventil, Ventolin, and Torpex equine inhaler. Also known as Salbutamol outside the United States.

**Functional classification:** Bronchodilator, beta-agonist

## Pharmacology and Mechanism of Action

Beta$_2$-adrenergic agonist. Albuterol stimulates beta$_2$-receptors to relax bronchial smooth muscle. It may also inhibit release of inflammatory mediators, especially from mast cells. This mechanism of action has been beneficial to relax bronchial smooth muscle to relieve bronchospasm and bronchoconstriction.

Albuterol exists as two chiral isomers. The R-isomer is the active bronchodilator form; the S-isomer is associated with adverse effects. The formulation levalbuterol is a formulation containing only the R-isomer.

## Indications and Clinical Uses

Albuterol is indicated in a variety of airway diseases for bronchodilation. Except for equine use, doses are primarily derived from extrapolation of human doses. Efficacy studies for small animal use are not reported. Onset of action is 15–30 minutes, and duration of action may be as long as 8 hours.

Albuterol was previously available as a metered-dose inhaler for horses (Torpex) for treatment of airway disease. It provided immediate relief of bronchospasm and bronchoconstriction in horses. However, the equine formulation is no longer commercially available. The human formulations can be used as a substitute.

## Precautionary Information

### Adverse Reactions and Side Effects

Excessive beta-adrenergic stimulation at high doses results in tachycardia and muscle tremors. Arrhythmias are possible with high doses. All beta$_2$-agonists will inhibit uterine contractions at the end of gestation in pregnant animals. High doses of beta$_2$-agonists can lead to hypokalemia because they stimulate Na$^+$-K$^+$-ATPase and increase intracellular K$^+$, while decreasing serum K$^+$ and producing hyperglycemia. Treatment consists of KCl supplement at a rate of 0.5 mEq/kg/h.

### Contraindications and Precautions

Avoid use in pregnant animals. IM or SQ injections can be painful.

### Drug Interactions

All beta-agonists will interact with and potentiate other drugs that act on beta-adrenergic receptors.

## Instructions for Use

Administration to horses requires an adaptor to facilitate a metered-dose inhaler. For injection, dilute solution to 0.01 mg/mL (10 mcg/mL) before injection and further dilute to 50/50 with saline or 5% dextrose before injection. When used for bronchoconstriction, it is helpful for acute exacerbations, used intermittently, with other drugs (e.g., corticosteroids) administered for maintenance.

## Patient Monitoring and Laboratory Tests

Monitor heart rate and rhythm in animals with cardiovascular disease. Monitor potassium concentrations for evidence of hypokalemia if high doses are administered. Monitor glucose for evidence of hyperglycemia.

## Formulations

- Albuterol is available in 2- and 4-mg tablets and 2-mg/5-mL syrup. Solutions for inhalation are 0.83 and 5 mg/mL. The equine formulation contained 6.7 g of formulated albuterol sulfate in a pressurized aluminum canister. This formulation is no longer commercially available for horses. Human metered-dose inhalers are available in various sizes ranging from 6.7 to 18 g, with 90 mcg per actuation.

## Stability and Storage

Store in well-closed containers and protected from light. Aqueous solutions are stable if kept at an acidic pH (2.2–5).

## Small Animal Dosage

### Dogs and Cats

- 20–50 mcg/kg q6–8h PO, up to a maximum of 100 mcg/kg q6h.

## Large Animal Dosage

### Horses

- Deliver sufficient actuations of the metered-dose inhaler to administer 360 mcg per horse—equivalent to 4 actuations of a 90-mcg human metered-dose inhaler. This dose can be administered up to four times daily.
- Foals: 0.01–0.02 mg/kg q8–12h PO.

## Regulatory Information

Do not administer to animals intended for food.

When treating horses, allow 48 hours or longer for urine clearance in performance animals that may be tested.

RCI Classification: 3

# Alendronate

ah-len´droe-nate

**Trade and other names:** Fosamax and generic

**Functional classification:** Antihypercalcemic

## Pharmacology and Mechanism of Action

Bisphosphonate drug. Drugs in this class include pamidronate, risedronate, zoledronate, and etidronate. New drugs approved to treat navicular syndrome in horses are tiludronate (Tildren) and clodronate (OSPHOS). This is a group of drugs characterized by a germinal bisphosphonate bond. They slow the formation and dissolution of hydroxyapatite crystals. Their clinical use is in their ability to inhibit bone resorption. These drugs decrease bone turnover by inhibiting osteoclast activity, retarding bone resorption, and decreasing the rate of osteoporosis. Alendronate is 100–1000 times more potent than older drugs such as etidronate. Unfortunately, alendronate is poorly absorbed orally (3%–7%), and use of oral formulations in animals may not be effective. In dogs, half-life in plasma is short (1–2 hours), but there is prolonged persistence of the drug in bone, in which the half-life is 300 days.

## Indications and Clinical Uses

Alendronate, like other bisphosphonate drugs, is used in people to treat osteoporosis and treatment of hypercalcemia of malignancy. Most doses for animals have been extrapolated from people (10 mg per person per day, or 70 mg once per week) because no animal-specific studies have identified the optimum dose.

In animals, alendronate is used to decrease calcium in conditions that cause hypercalcemia, such as hyperparathyroidism, cancer, and vitamin D toxicosis. It may be helpful for managing neoplastic complications associated with pathologic bone resorption. It also may provide pain relief in patients with pathologic bone disease. Most experimental work in dogs has been performed with pamidronate rather than alendronate.

## Precautionary Information

### Adverse Reactions and Side Effects

No serious adverse effects have been identified; however, use in animals has been uncommon. In people, esophageal injury and erosion are important problems.

When administering to animals, ensure that the entire medication is swallowed and followed with water.

**Contraindications and Precautions**

Do not administer with foods or medications containing calcium. Food decreases absorption.

**Drug Interactions**

Do not mix with a solution containing calcium (e.g., lactated Ringer's solution). Do not give with foods containing calcium.

## Instructions for Use

When administering oral medication, ensure that the drug is not trapped in the esophagus to avoid injury to esophageal tissue. Food significantly reduces oral absorption. Wait at least 30 minutes before feeding.

## Patient Monitoring and Laboratory Tests

Monitor serum calcium and phosphorus.

## Formulations

- Alendronate is available in 5-, 10-, 35-, 40-, and 70-mg tablets and 70 mg/75 mL oral solution.

## Stability and Storage

Store in a tightly sealed container, protected from light, and at room temperature.

## Small Animal Dosage

**Dogs**

- 0.5–1 mg/kg q24h PO.

**Cats**

- Treatment of ionized hypercalcemia: 5–20 mg per cat PO q7d.

## Large Animal Dosage

- No dose has been reported for large animals.

## Regulatory Information

Withdrawal times are not established for animals that produce food. For extralabel use withdrawal interval estimates, contact FARAD at www.FARAD.org.

# Alfaxalone
al-fax'ah-lone

**Trade and other names:** Alfaxan (previous name was alphaxalone)

**Functional classification:** Anesthetic agent

## Pharmacology and Mechanism of Action

Alfaxalone is a synthetic neuroactive steroid that interacts with GABA receptors in the CNS to produce anesthesia and muscle relaxation. Alfaxalone is related to an older formulation (Saffan) first introduced in 1971, which was alfaxalone plus alfadolone in a combination of neurosteroids. This older formulation was in a castor oil formulation that induced mast cell degranulation and histamine release and produced swollen extremities, anaphylactic reactions, and other signs of histamine release. The new formulation (Alfaxan) available in 2012 overcomes the formulation issue by using a cyclodextrin-solubilizing vehicle, referred to chemically as alfaxalone-2-hydroxypropyl-beta-cyclodextrin (HPCD).

The half-life is short in animals (less than 1 hour), but it exhibits nonlinear pharmacokinetics and may be eliminated more slowly with high doses.

## Indications and Clinical Uses

Alfaxalone is used as a general anesthetic agent. It can be injected directly into the cephalic vein or delivered via CRI. If injected directly, administer over 60 seconds to allow enough time to cross the blood–brain barrier. It has been used successfully as an anesthetic induction agent. It has been used safely with other anesthetic agents (e.g., propofol) and in combination with premedications (e.g., opiates, atropine, phenothiazines, benzodiazepines, and NSAIDs). It can also be used as a maintenance anesthesia agent by administering an initial IV bolus and then repeating the boluses.

## Precautionary Information

### Adverse Reactions and Side Effects

As an anesthetic agent, CNS depression, respiratory depression, and some blood pressure decrease are expected after administration. At CRI doses greater than 0.1 mg/kg/min, it produces noticeable hypotension and hypoventilation. If injected IM, it causes pain and discomfort. SQ injection does not produce a good surgical plane of anesthesia. If injected IM, animals may react to sound, and recovery can include excitement, incoordination, and hyper-reactivity.

### Drug Interactions

No drug interactions are reported in animals. It may be used safely with other anesthetic agents and anesthetic adjuncts.

## Instructions for Use

For induction of anesthesia, use with appropriate monitoring equipment and ventilatory support. IV administration is recommended for alfaxalone for anesthetic purposes. However, for some sedative protocols, IM injection has been used and can be combined with other sedative agents. If administered IM, the peak effect does not occur until 10–15 minutes; therefore, the other agents may be administered at different times. For example, it has been administered with butorphanol (0.4 mg/kg IM) followed by alfaxalone (2 mg/kg IM) 15 minutes later and used for short-term procedures. It has been used in cats IM in combination with ketamine, dexmedetomidine, or butorphanol for short-term surgical procedures of less than 1 hour. There may be pain produced from IM injection. The SQ route of injection should be avoided.

If used for anesthesia induction, it is recommended to include a pre-anesthetic sedative in the protocol. Agents that can be considered are acepromazine, benzodiazepines, opioids, and alpha$_2$ agonists (e.g., dexmedetomidine). If sedative drugs are included in the protocol, the dose listed can be decreased. Note that alfaxalone does not provide analgesia, and other agents can be added to the regimen to provide pain relief.

## Patient Monitoring and Laboratory Tests

Monitor character and depth of anesthesia during use. Monitor blood pressure, heart rate, and body temperature during anesthesia. Apnea may occur after initial induction. Monitor character and rate of respiration.

## Formulations

- Alfaxalone without preservatives is available as a 10-mg/mL injectable formulation, 10-mL vial, with a shelf-life of 6 hours after initial puncture of the stopper.
- Alfaxalone with preservatives is available as a clear aqueous solution with 2-hydroxpropyl-beta-cyclodextrin. It has a pH of 6.5–7. The preservatives are ethanol, benzethonium chloride, and chlorocresol. It is available in 10- and 20-mL vials with a shelf-life of 28 days.

## Stability and Storage

Microbial contamination can occur after opening the preservative-free vial. If the vial does not contain preservatives, the label in the United States says that it must be discarded after 6 hours. However, the Australian label for the same product lists a 7-day duration when refrigerated after a single puncture of the stopper. Avoid multiple punctures and microbial contamination if preservative-free vials are used.

If the vial contains preservatives, it can be stored for 28 days after puncturing the vial. Alfaxalone has been drawn up in the same syringe with other anesthetics and sedatives (e.g., opioids, alpha$_2$ agonists, midazolam) and injected immediately without observed interactions.

## Small Animal Dosage

### Dogs

- Induction: 1.5–4.5 mg/kg IV if dogs did not receive a pre-anesthetic sedative. 0.2–3.5 mg/kg for dogs that received a pre-anesthetic. Always titrate the dose according to the patient response. Generally, the dose is 1–1.2 mg/kg (up to 2 mg/kg) for each 10 minutes of anesthesia. Deliver dose IV over 60 seconds.
- CRI: 6–10 mg/kg/h IV (suitable to use with other anesthetic agents).

### Cats

- 2.2–10 mg/kg (average dose is 4 mg/kg) IV if the cat did not receive a pre-anesthetic sedative. If the cat received a pre-anesthetic sedative, the dose is 1–4 mg/kg IV or IM. Always consider the lower dose first and titrate the dose according to the patient's response. Generally, the dosage is 1–1.3 mg/kg IV (up to 5 mg/kg) delivered over 60 seconds followed by sequential doses of 2 mg/kg as needed.
- Sedation protocols for cats: Inject IM or IV at a dose of 2–3 mg/kg for mild sedation. It may be combined with other sedative agents in the same syringe (e.g., butorphanol at 0.2 mg/kg).
- CRI: Loading dose of 1.7 mg/kg IV followed by CRI of 7–10 mg/kg/h IV.

## Large Animal Dosage

- No large animal doses are available.

## Regulatory Information

Do not administer to food-producing animals. Alfaxalone is a Schedule C-IV controlled substance.

# Allopurinol
al-oh-pyoo′rih-nole

**Trade and other names:** Lopurin, Zyloprim, and Allopur (Europe)

**Functional classification:** Anti-inflammatory

## Pharmacology and Mechanism of Action

Purine analogue. Allopurinol decreases the production of uric acid by inhibiting enzymes responsible for uric acid synthesis. The other use of allopurinol is treating leishmaniasis. In parasites, allopurinol is metabolized to products that disrupt RNA synthesis and interfere with protein synthesis. Allopurinol does not eliminate *Leishmania* or cure the disease, but it may improve cutaneous lesions and induce remission.

## Indications and Clinical Uses

Allopurinol is indicated to decrease formation of uric acid uroliths in at-risk animals. Allopurinol also is used to treat clinical signs associated with leishmaniasis. When used for leishmaniasis, it is administered with pentavalent antimonial compounds such as meglumine antimonite (Glutamine) or sodium stibogluconate (Pentosan). With chronic treatment, allopurinol produces progressive remission and improvement in clinical signs associated with leishmaniasis, which include decreasing the damaging effects of *Leishmania* on the animal's kidneys by decreasing proteinuria and preventing deterioration of glomerular filtration rate. For this use, it is used at 10 mg/kg oral q12h for 6 months or more in combination with meglumine antimoniate at a dosage of 100 mg/kg SQ once daily for 4 weeks. (Meglumine antimoniate is not approved in the United States.)

### Precautionary Information

#### Adverse Reactions and Side Effects

Allopurinol may cause skin reactions (hypersensitivity). In dogs that were treated for leishmaniasis for several months, no adverse effects were reported.

#### Contraindications and Precautions

No contraindications reported for animals.

#### Drug Interactions

Allopurinol may inhibit metabolism of certain drugs. Do not use with azathioprine because it interferes with xanthine oxidase, an important enzyme for metabolizing azathioprine, and enhances toxicity.

## Instructions for Use

In people, allopurinol is used primarily for treating gout. In animals, it is used to decrease formation of uric acid uroliths and for treating signs associated with leishmaniasis. No single drug or combination is completely effective for treating leishmaniasis, but allopurinol improves skin lesions. Allopurinol is usually administered with other drugs for leishmaniasis. For example, it has been administered with either amphotericin B or pentavalent antimonial compounds such as meglumine antimonite (Glutamine) or sodium stibogluconate (Pentosan).

## Patient Monitoring and Laboratory Tests

Dose adjustments for treating leishmaniasis are based on monitoring clinical signs.

## Formulations

- Allopurinol is available in 100- and 300-mg tablets.

## Stability and Storage

Store in well-closed containers at room temperature. Allopurinol is stable for at least 60 days in compounded formulations. Maximum stability in solutions at pH of 3–3.4.

## Small Animal Dosage
### Dogs
- Urate urolith prevention: 10 mg/kg q8h PO; then reduce to 10 mg/kg q24h PO.
- Leishmaniasis: 10 mg/kg q12h PO for at least 4 months and as long as 6 months. For leishmaniasis, some clinicians have used 15 mg/kg q12h, and then if there is a response, have administered 7–10 mg/kg q12–24h PO.

## Large Animal Dosage
### Horses
- 5 mg/kg PO.

## Regulatory Information
No regulatory information is available. For extralabel use withdrawal interval estimates, contact FARAD at www.FARAD.org.

# Alprazolam
al-pray´zoe-lam

**Trade and other names:** Xanax, Niravam, and generic

**Functional classification:** Tranquilizer, CNS depressant

## Pharmacology and Mechanism of Action
Benzodiazepine. Central-acting CNS depressant and anxiolytic (reduces anxiety). Like other benzodiazepines, the mechanism of action is through potentiation of GABA-receptor–mediated effects in the CNS. A drug that has similar effects is diazepam. Similar drugs of this class are also used in veterinary medicine, such as diazepam, midazolam, and lorazepam.

## Indications and Clinical Uses
Alprazolam is used to treat behavior problems in dogs and cats, particularly those associated with anxiety. Alprazolam has been used in dogs for the short-term treatment of anxiety states, such as noise phobias and thunderstorm phobia. For thunderstorm phobia, it may be more effective if combined with long-term clomipramine treatment. In horses, it has been administered orally to control some behavior problems. It has been used in horses is to decrease anxiety and facilitate a mare–foal bonding and acceptance of a foal or orphan foal.

## Precautionary Information
### Adverse Reactions and Side Effects
Sedation is the most common side effect, but alprazolam may also cause paradoxical excitement in dogs. It has been administered safely to horses without producing noticeable ataxia or sedation at a dose of 0.04 mg/kg. In cats, idiopathic fatal hepatic necrosis has been reported from diazepam, but this has not been reported from alprazolam, probably because of differences in metabolism. Alprazolam is not as extensively metabolized as diazepam. Chronic administration in any species may lead to dependence and a withdrawal syndrome if discontinued.

**Contraindications and Precautions**

No serious contraindications. In rare individuals, benzodiazepines have caused paradoxical excitement. Use of benzodiazepines in early pregnancy has been associated with an increased risk of spontaneous abortions and fetal malformations in people. This incidence in animals is unknown. If an animal has been receiving alprazolam for an extended period, do not stop the medication abruptly but decrease the dose over a tapering period to minimize withdrawal signs.

**Drug Interactions**

Other drugs may decrease hepatic metabolism (e.g., ketoconazole, chloramphenicol, and itraconazole).

## Instructions for Use

Use in animals has been primarily derived from empirical use and clinical observation. There are no well-controlled clinical studies or efficacy trials to document clinical effectiveness. Duration of effect is only 2–3 hours in many dogs. Therefore, it is usually used for short-term problems, and if needed, more frequent administration may be required.

When treating noise phobia (thunderstorm phobia), it is helpful in some dogs to administer 0.02 mg/kg of clomipramine 1 hour before a storm in addition to alprazolam.

The Niravam tablets (see the Formulations section) are rapidly dissolving and may be easier to administer to animals that are difficult to medicate. Tablets easily dissolve on the tongue without requiring water and can be cut for accurate dosing.

## Patient Monitoring and Laboratory Tests

Monitor hepatic enzymes in animals with chronic use. Although plasma drug concentrations are usually not measured in animals, 20–40 ng/mL has been associated with therapeutic effects in people.

## Formulations

- Alprazolam is available in 0.25-, 0.5-, 1-, and 2-mg tablets and 1- and 2-mg scored tablets.
- Rapidly dissolving tablets (Niravam) are available in 0.25, 0.5, 1, and 2 mg that can be cut for accurate dosing.

## Stability and Storage

Store in a tightly sealed container, protected from light, and at room temperature. Drug is stable in some compounded formulations for 60 days.

## Small Animal Dosage

**Dogs**

- 0.025–0.05 mg/kg q8h PO. Increase to 0.1 mg/kg if needed. Administration more frequently (q4–6h) has been used in some patients.

**Cats**

- 0.125 mg/cat q12h PO (half of 0.25-mg tablet) or 0.0125–0.025 mg/kg q12h PO and up to q8h.

## Large Animal Dosage

**Horses**

- Loading dose of 0.1 mg/kg initially followed by 0.04 mg/kg q12h PO.

## Regulatory Information

No regulatory information is available. For extralabel use withdrawal interval estimates, contact FARAD at www.FARAD.org.

RCI Classification: 2

# Altrenogest
al-tren´-oh-jest

**Trade and other names:** Regu-Mate, Matrix

**Functional classification:** Hormone

## Pharmacology and Mechanism of Action

Altrenogest is an active synthetic progestin hormone. As a progesterone agonist, it is primarily used to suppress estrus in animals. Suppression of estrus allows for a predictable occurrence of estrous activity after the drug is discontinued. Therefore it is used to induce a normal cycle of estrous activity to facilitate scheduled breeding. When treatment is initiated, 95% of the mares will have an estrous cycle suppressed in 3 days.

## Indications and Clinical Uses

Altrenogest is indicated to suppress estrus in animals to facilitate induction of normal estrous cycle activity. It is used in mares to facilitate scheduled breeding activity. It is also used to suppress estrous behavior in performance horses. When treatment is discontinued, mares exhibiting regular estrous cycles return to estrus within 4–5 days after treatment and continue to cycle normally.

In swine, altrenogest is used for synchronization of estrus in sexually mature gilts that have had at least one estrous cycle. Do not use in gilts having a previous or current history of uterine inflammation (i.e., acute, subacute, or chronic endometritis).

### Precautionary Information

**Contraindications and Precautions**

Do not administer to pregnant animals. Humans handling altrenogest, particularly women, should wear gloves and avoid contact because altrenogest can be absorbed in humans through intact skin. Altrenogest should not be used in mares or gilts with a previous history of uterine problems (metritis).

## Instructions for Use

Administer one dose of altrenogest daily for 15 days, orally on grain or directly on the horse's tongue. In pigs, administer as a top dressing or with feed.

## Patient Monitoring and Laboratory Tests

Monitor for signs of estrous activity. Monitor CBC in cases of overdose.

## Formulations

- Altrenogest is available in an oil solution of 0.22% (2.2 mg/mL).

## Stability and Storage

Store in well-closed containers at room temperature.

## Small Animal Dosage
• No dose available.

## Large Animal Dosage
**Horses**
• 0.044 mg/kg (or 1 mL/110 lb) PO once per day for 15 days.

**Swine**
• Administer 6.8 mL (15 mg altrenogest) per gilt once daily for 14 consecutive days by top dressing on a portion of each gilt's daily feed.

## Regulatory Information
Do not use in horses intended for food. In pigs, gilts must not be slaughtered for human consumption for 21 days after the last treatment. Do not administer to other food-producing animals.

---

# Aluminum Hydroxide and Aluminum Carbonate
ah-loo′mih-num hye-droks′ide, ah-loo′mih-num kar′boe-nate

**Trade and other names:** Aluminum hydroxide gel (Amphojel) and aluminum carbonate gel (Basalgel)

**Functional classification:** Antacid

## Pharmacology and Mechanism of Action
Aluminum is an antacid and phosphate binder in intestine. It is used in both the aluminum hydroxide and aluminum carbonate formulations.

## Indications and Clinical Uses
Aluminum hydroxide is used for its antacid properties to treat or manage GI ulcers. A more common use in small animals is as a phosphate binder. It is indicated in animals with hyperphosphatemia associated with chronic renal failure, often in combination with phosphorus-restricted diets. Although this was once widely available, because of the decreased availability of products containing aluminum, other drugs are used more commonly to decrease hyperphosphatemia in patients, such as calcium carbonate and calcium citrate. A new oral phosphate binder is available in some countries for cats. This product (Lenziaren) consists of a complex of iron oxide/hydroxide and is administered orally to cats.

## Precautionary Information
### Adverse Reactions and Side Effects
These aluminum-containing compounds are generally safe. However, there has been some concern expressed that these drugs may increase the systemic levels of aluminum, which may lead to some forms of aluminum toxicoses. The evidence for this as a clinical problem in veterinary medicine is lacking.

**Contraindications and Precautions**

Aluminum decreases oral absorption of some drugs (e.g., fluoroquinolones, tetracyclines). If fluoroquinolone antimicrobials are used concurrently, separation of oral doses should be considered.

**Drug Interactions**

Aluminum binds and chelates some drugs and prevents GI absorption. Drugs bound to aluminum include tetracyclines and quinolone antibiotics.

## Instructions for Use

Antacid doses are designed to neutralize stomach acid, but duration of acid suppression is short. Although aluminum hydroxide is often used to prevent hyperphosphatemia, this drug may not be available in some pharmacies. A substitute for this indication is calcium citrate or calcium carbonate. An oral product is also available for cats to administer as a phosphate binder (Lenziaren), which is a complex of iron oxide/hydroxide.

## Patient Monitoring and Laboratory Tests

Phosphate plasma levels should be monitored to determine success of therapy.

## Formulations

- Aluminum hydroxide gel is available in a 64-mg/mL oral suspension and 600-mg tablet.
- Aluminum carbonate gel is available in capsules (equivalent to 500-mg aluminum hydroxide).
- Note: Products containing aluminum may no longer be available from many sources, and other products may be used, such as Lenziaren, which is a complex of iron oxide/hydroxide for cats.

## Stability and Storage

Store in a tightly sealed container, protected from light, and at room temperature.

## Small Animal Dosage

**Dogs**

- Aluminum hydroxide gel: 10–30 mg/kg q8h PO (with meals).
- Aluminum carbonate gel: 10–30 mg/kg q8h PO (with meals).

**Cats**

- Aluminum hydroxide gel: 10–30 mg/kg q8h PO (with meals).
- Aluminum carbonate gel: 10–30 mg/kg q8h PO (with meals).

## Large Animal Dosage

**Horses**

- Antacid: 60 mg/kg q8h PO.

## Regulatory Information

No regulatory information is available. Residues from administration to food-producing animals ordinarily are not a concern. However, for extralabel use withdrawal interval estimates, contact FARAD at www.FARAD.org.

# Amantadine
ah-man´tah-deen

**Trade and other names:** Symmetrel and generic brands

**Functional classification:** Antiviral

## Pharmacology and Mechanism of Action

Amantadine is an antiviral drug. The action against viruses is not entirely known. For treating other conditions in people (Parkinson disease), its effects are attributed to an increase in dopamine in the CNS. However, it also is an N-methyl-D-aspartate (NMDA) receptor antagonist. As an NMDA antagonist, it decreases tolerance to other analgesic drugs (e.g., opiates), but it probably does not possess effective analgesic properties when used alone. There are only limited pharmacokinetic data available for animals. The oral formulation is completely absorbed from oral administration in people and animals and crosses the blood–brain barrier. In cats, the half-life is approximately 6 hours; in dogs, the half-life is approximately 5 hours.

## Indications and Clinical Uses

Amantadine is an antiviral drug used to treat influenza infections in people but not used much anymore because many viruses are resistant. It also is used in people to treat Parkinson disease and extrapyramidal reactions, especially those that are drug induced. It also has been used to manage muscular weakness in humans with multiple sclerosis. However, its use in veterinary medicine has primarily been for treating pain in dogs and cats. It is used for treating pain when other drugs have been ineffective or when it is desirable to use in combination with multiple drugs in multimodal therapy analgesic protocols.

## Precautionary Information

### Adverse Reactions and Side Effects

Toxicity has not been seen in dogs and cats until doses are exceeded by at least two times. Rarely, the side effects of anxiety states and dry mouth have been observed. Dizziness, confusion, and other CNS disturbances have been reported in people.

### Contraindications and Precautions

Pregnancy caution: Amantadine is embryotoxic and teratogenic at high doses in laboratory animals. Avoid its use in pregnancy.

### Drug Interactions

Do not use with other drugs that increase dopamine concentrations (e.g., selegiline). If used with other CNS stimulants, it may enhance the effects.

## Instructions for Use

Amantadine for treatment of pain may not be effective when used alone. Administer with another analgesic agent (e.g., NSAID) for best results. In post-surgical patients, it has been used for up to 21 days without adverse effects. Antiviral effects have not been adequately explored in animals. In people, the antiviral dosage is 1.5–3 mg/kg once or twice a day.

## Patient Monitoring and Laboratory Tests

No specific monitoring is necessary.

## Formulations

- Amantadine is available in 100-mg capsules, 100-mg tablets, and 10-mg/mL syrup.

## Stability and Storage

Store in a tightly sealed container, protected from light, and at room temperature. Stability of compounded formulations has not been evaluated.

## Small Animal Dosage

**Dogs**

- For pain treatment, 3–5 mg/kg q12h PO.

**Cats**

- 3 mg/kg q24h PO for treatment of pain, up to a dose of 5 mg/kg in some cases.

## Large Animal Dosage

- No dose has been reported for large animals.

## Regulatory Information

This drug should not be administered to food-producing animals, and no regulatory information is available. For extralabel use withdrawal interval estimates, contact FARAD at www.FARAD.org.

# Amikacin
am-ih-kay'sin

**Trade and other names:** Amiglyde-V (veterinary preparation), Amikin (human preparation), and generic brands

**Functional classification:** Antibacterial

## Pharmacology and Mechanism of Action

Aminoglycoside antibiotic. Action is to inhibit bacteria protein synthesis via binding to 30S ribosome and disrupt the outer membrane in gram-negative bacteria. Amikacin is bactericidal with a broad spectrum of activity except against streptococci and anaerobic bacteria. Amikacin has activity against many bacteria, especially gram-negative bacilli, that are resistant to other drugs. Amikacin may be more active than gentamicin against many gram-negative bacteria, especially enteric species, because it is less susceptible to drug-degrading enzymes produced by bacteria. It is one of the most active of all the aminoglycoside group of antibacterial agents.

*Pharmacokinetics:* In most animals, the half-life is short (1–2 hours), and volume of distribution reflects extracellular body water (e.g., 200–250 mL/kg). Amikacin is not absorbed from oral administration. It is eliminated almost exclusively by renal clearance.

## Indications and Clinical Uses

Amikacin is indicated in bacterial infections, especially for treatment of serious infections caused by gram-negative bacteria. When resistance to gentamicin is anticipated, amikacin is often used in its place because bacteria resistant to gentamicin are still susceptible to amikacin. In horses, amikacin also is used for local administration as an intrauterine lavage to treat metritis and other infections of the genital tract caused by gram-negative bacteria. For this purpose, it has been used as an intrauterine flush. In horses, amikacin also is used for regional limb perfusion.

## Precautionary Information

### Adverse Reactions and Side Effects

Nephrotoxicity is the most dose-limiting toxicity. Ensure that patients have adequate fluid and electrolyte balance during therapy. Ototoxicity and vestibulotoxicity also are possible.

### Contraindications and Precautions

Do not use in animals with renal insufficiency or renal failure. Do not use in dehydrated animals.

### Drug Interactions

Do not mix in vial or syringe with other antibiotics. Amikacin is incompatible with other drugs and compounds when mixed in the same vial or syringe. This effect is particularly important when mixing with other antibiotics. When used with anesthetic agents, neuromuscular blockade is possible.

## Instructions for Use

Once-daily doses are designed to maximize peak-to-minimum inhibitory concentration (MIC) ratio. Consider therapeutic drug monitoring to decrease risk of renal toxicosis. Activity against some bacteria (e.g., *Pseudomonas*) may be enhanced when combined with a beta-lactam antibiotic, but this action is controversial. Nephrotoxicity is increased with persistently high trough concentrations.

## Patient Monitoring and Laboratory Tests

Susceptibility testing: Clinical and Laboratory Standards Institute (CLSI) MIC breakpoint is ≤4 mcg/mL for dogs and horses and ≤ 2 mcg/mL for foals. The canine breakpoint also can be applied to bacterial isolates from cats. Monitor BUN, serum creatinine, and urine for evidence of renal toxicity. Plasma or serum drug concentrations can be monitored to measure for problems with systemic clearance. When monitoring trough levels in patients during once-daily administration, the trough levels should fall below the limit of detection. Alternatively, the half-life and clearance can be measured from samples taken at 1 hour and 2–4 hours post-dosing. Clearance in most animals should be above 1.0 mL/kg/min, and half-life should be less than 2 hours.

## Formulations

• Amikacin is available in 50- or 250-mg/mL injection.

## Stability and Storage

Store in a tightly sealed container, protected from light, and at room temperature. Amikacin will be unstable if mixed with other drugs.

## Small Animal Dosage

### Dogs

• 15 mg/kg q24h IV, IM, or SQ.

### Cats

• 10 mg/kg q24h IV, IM, or SQ.

## Large Animal Dosage

**Horses**

- Adult: 10 mg/kg q24h IV or IM.
- Foal: 20 mg/kg q24h IV.
- Intrauterine use: Administer 2 g (8 mL) diluted in 200-mL sterile saline solution in uterus once per day for 3 days.
- Regional limb perfusion: Doses have ranged from 125 to 500 mg per limb, diluted in 60 mL of saline.

**Cattle (not recommended in food-producing animals)**

- Adult: 10 mg/kg q24h IM, IV, or SQ.
- Calf (younger than 2 weeks of age): 20 mg/kg q24h IV or IM.

## Regulatory Information

Withdrawal times have not been established for extralabel use in animals used for food. Long persistence of drug in tissues (renal) is expected after administration. Amikacin, like other aminoglycoside antibiotics, should not be administered to animals that produce food because of a risk of residue problems. If extralabel doses have been administered, the meat withdrawal time may be as long as 18 months. Contact FARAD at www.FARAD.org for specific withdrawal time information.

# Amino Acid Solution

**Trade and other names:** Travasol

**Functional classification:** Amino acid solution

## Pharmacology and Mechanism of Action

Amino acid solutions are intended to provide amino acid supplement to animals with amino acid deficiency or with liver disorders. This particular solution contains leucine, phenylalanine, lysine, methionine, isoleucine, valine, histidine, threonine, tryptophan, alanine, glycine arginine, proline, tyrosine, and serine.

## Indications and Clinical Uses

In animals, amino acid solutions are infused to provide supplement, particularly for treatment of liver disease.

## Precautionary Information

**Adverse Reactions and Side Effects**

A hyperosmolar state can be induced if the infusion is too aggressive. If neurologic signs appear, the infusion should be stopped. In patients with liver disease or renal failure, hepatic encephalopathy or increases in BUN are possible.

## Instructions for Use

A 10% solution may be diluted in 5% dextrose solution for peripheral vein administration. Otherwise, it should be administered via a central vein.

## Patient Monitoring and Laboratory Tests

No specific monitoring is necessary.

## Formulations

Travasol sterile solution available as 10% amino acid solution in 500 mL, 1000 mL, and 2000 mL containers, which have essential and nonessential amino acids.

## Stability and Storage

Store at room temperature protected from light.

## Small Animal Dosage

### Dogs

- 25 mL of a 10% solution (diluted appropriately) infused IV via a central vein. Administer infusion over 6–8 hours and repeat at 7- to 10-day intervals. Solutions without electrolytes are preferred for treating hepatocutaneous syndrome.
- Note that the human dose is much higher (1 g/kg).

## Large Animal Dosage

- No dose reported.

## Regulatory Information

There is no withdrawal time necessary for food animals.

# Aminopentamide
ah-mee-noe-pent'ah-mide

**Trade and other names:** Centrine

**Functional classification:** Anticholinergic

## Pharmacology and Mechanism of Action

Antidiarrheal drug. Anticholinergic (blocks acetylcholine at parasympathetic synapse). Like other anticholinergic drugs in this class, aminopentamide blocks muscarinic receptors. As a result of blockade, effects of acetylcholine are blocked to inhibit GI secretions and smooth muscle motility. Glandular, respiratory, and other physiologic functions also can be affected. Aminopentamide is an older drug that is not often used as a treatment of diarrhea or GI diseases today.

## Indications and Clinical Uses

Aminopentamide has been used to decrease GI motility and decrease GI secretions in animals. It also has been used to treat diarrhea, but long-term use for this purpose is not recommended.

## Instructions for Use

Dosing guidelines based on manufacturer's recommendation. There have not been any well-controlled studies in animals to establish optimum use and doses.

## Patient Monitoring and Laboratory Tests

Monitor for problems caused by intestinal stasis because of anticholinergic effect.

## Formulations

- Aminopentamide is available in 0.2-mg tablets and 0.5-mg/mL injection.

## Stability and Storage

Store in a tightly sealed container, protected from light, and at room temperature. Stability of compounded formulations has not been evaluated.

## Small Animal Dosage

**Dogs**

- 0.01–0.03 mg/kg q8–12h IM, SQ, or PO.

**Cats**

- 0.1 mg/cat q8–12h IM, SQ, or PO.

## Large Animal Dosage

- No dose has been reported for large animals.

## Regulatory Information

No regulatory information is available. For extralabel use withdrawal interval estimates, contact FARAD at www.FARAD.org.

# Aminophylline
am-in-off'ih-lin

**Trade and other names:** Generic brands

**Functional classification:** Bronchodilator

## Pharmacology and Mechanism of Action

Bronchodilator. Aminophylline is a salt of theophylline, formulated to enhance oral absorption without gastric side effects. It is converted to theophylline after ingestion. The mechanism of action and other properties are the same as theophylline. Consult the theophylline monograph for more details. Theophylline's action is to inhibit phosphodiesterase (PDE) and increase cyclic adenosine monophosphate (cAMP). Other anti-inflammatory mechanisms also may play a role in its clinical effects.

## Indications and Clinical Uses

Aminophylline is indicated for control of reversible airway constriction, to prevent bronchoconstriction, and as an adjunct with other respiratory disease treatment. The uses are similar to the indications for theophylline because it is a salt form of theophylline. It is used for inflammatory airway disease in cats (feline asthma), dogs, and horses. In dogs, the uses include collapsing trachea, bronchitis, and other airway diseases. It has not been effective for respiratory diseases in cattle. The oral forms have mostly been discontinued, and only the injection forms remain. For oral administration, theophylline should be used. Consult the Theophylline section for more information on dosing.

## Precautionary Information

### Adverse Reactions and Side Effects

Aminophylline causes excitement and possible cardiac side effects with high concentrations. Cardiac adverse effects include tachycardia and arrhythmias. GI adverse effects include nausea, vomiting, and diarrhea. CNS adverse effects include excitement, tremors, and seizures.

### Contraindications and Precautions

Although adverse effects appear more common in people than small animals, use cautiously in animals with cardiac arrhythmias. Use cautiously in animals prone to seizures. Horses may become excited from IV administration.

**Drug Interactions**
Use cautiously with other PDE inhibitors such as sildenafil (Viagra) and pimobendan. Many drugs inhibit the metabolism of theophylline and potentially increase concentrations (e.g., cimetidine, erythromycin, fluoroquinolones, and propranolol). Some drugs decrease concentrations by increasing metabolism (e.g., phenobarbital and rifampin).

## Instructions for Use
Therapeutic drug monitoring of theophylline is recommended for accurate dosing during chronic therapy. When dosing with salts or other formulations of theophylline, adjust dose for the amount of the parent drug. The oral forms have been discontinued, and the dosing listed applies to injection formulation. For oral administration, use theophylline.

## Patient Monitoring and Laboratory Tests
Plasma concentrations of theophylline should be monitored in patients receiving therapy with aminophylline. Targeted plasma concentrations range from 10 to 20 mcg/mL, but clinical effects may occur as low as 5 mcg/mL.

## Formulations
- Aminophylline is available in 25-mg/mL injection. A dose of 25 mg/mL of anhydrous aminophylline is equivalent to 19.7 mg of anhydrous theophylline per milliliter. Oral forms have been discontinued; for oral administration, use theophylline instead.

## Stability and Storage
Store in a tightly sealed container, protected from light, and at room temperature. Compounded oral formulations have been stable for 60 days.

## Small Animal Dosage
**Dogs**
- 10 mg/kg q8h IM or IV.

**Cats**
- 6.6 mg/kg q12h IM or IV.

## Large Animal Dosage
**Horses**
- Treatment of recurrent airway obstructions: 12 mg/kg initial dose followed by 5 mg/kg q12h. Aminophylline administered IV to horses has caused transient excitement and restlessness. Give IV administration slowly.

**Cattle**
- 10 mg/kg q8h IV or 23 mg/kg PO, administered once as a single dose.

## Regulatory Information
Cattle: No withdrawal times have been established for food animals.
For extralabel use withdrawal interval estimates, contact FARAD at www.FARAD.org.
RCI Classification: 3

# Amiodarone Hydrochloride
ah-mee-oe´dah-rone

**Trade and other names:** Cordarone

**Functional classification:** Antiarrhythmic

## Pharmacology and Mechanism of Action
Antiarrhythmic drug, Class III. Antiarrhythmic effects are primarily caused by blocking the outward potassium channel in cardiac tissues. Amiodarone prolongs the action potential, delays myocardial repolarization, and delays the refractory period in cardiac tissues. It also may have some alpha-adrenergic receptor, beta-adrenergic receptor, and calcium-channel blocking properties. The IV formulation of amiodarone uses Polysorbate 80 to enhance solubility, which may be responsible for some of the adverse reactions. There is a new noniodinated derivative, dronedarone (Multaq), that is less lipophilic, has a shorter half-life, and may be safer, but there has been no use reported in animals.

*Pharmacokinetics:* Half-life is several days in duration, and in some animals, the half-life may be as long as 100 days with chronic therapy. In horses, the terminal half-life is 38–84 hours.

## Indications and Clinical Uses
Amiodarone is used to treat refractory ventricular arrhythmias. It is reserved for treating life-threatening arrhythmias that have been refractory to other treatments. It has been used as a last resort for recurrent hemodynamically unstable ventricular tachycardia.

In horses, IV amiodarone has been used to treat atrial fibrillation and ventricular arrhythmias.

Amiodarone has been used for Chagas disease in combination with itraconazole. For this use, 15 mg/kg, PO, q12h, for 7 days; then 15 mg/kg PO, q24h for 14 days; then 7.5 mg/kg PO, q24h for 12 months.

## Precautionary Information
### Adverse Reactions and Side Effects
The most common effect in dogs is decreased appetite. Prolonged Q-T interval also is a concern. Other adverse effects include bradycardia, congestive heart failure (CHF), hypotension, atrioventricular block, thyroid dysfunction (decreased triiodothyronine [$T_3$] and tetraiodothyronine [$T_4$]), pulmonary fibrosis, neutropenia, and anemia. Hepatopathy is a serious concern and has been reported in dogs. Doberman dogs were particularly affected by amiodarone when treated for arrhythmias; there was a high incidence of adverse effects that included anorexia, lethargy, hepatic toxicity, and vomiting.

Doses up to 12.5 mg/kg IV have produced no acute cardiovascular reactions; however, with acute IV administration, severe cardiac reactions, hypotension, vasodilation, pruritus, and edema (including swollen extremities) are possible. Adverse effects caused by IV treatment may be caused by the drug vehicle included to enhance solubility, Polysorbate 80, which is known to elicit allergic-type adverse events caused by histamine release. Pretreatment with antihistamines may help to decrease adverse events caused by IV treatment.

No adverse clinical signs were observed in horses after single-administration IV, but for treating atrial fibrillation, mild signs of shifting weight and hind limb weakness were reported.

**Contraindications and Precautions**

Severe reactions, including hepatopathy and cardiac arrhythmias, have been seen in dogs. Use only when arrhythmia has been refractory to other treatments or when dogs are at risk for sudden death.

**Drug Interactions**

Use amiodarone with beta blockers, calcium-channel blockers, and digoxin cautiously because it may slow conduction. Do not mix IV solution with mixtures containing bicarbonate.

## Instructions for Use

Typically, loading doses are administered followed by maintenance dose. Oral dosing in dogs has used 10–15 mg/kg q12h for 1 week and then 5–7.5 mg/kg q12h for 2 weeks followed by a maintenance dose of 7.5 mg/kg q24h. If IV therapy is used, doses should be given slowly; initial infusion rate should not exceed 30 mg/min. Prior to IV treatment, administer antihistamines to prevent allergic-type reactions.

## Patient Monitoring and Laboratory Tests

Because of a concern for adverse effects caused by amiodarone in dogs, therapy should be monitored carefully. It is highly recommended to monitor CBC for anemia and neutropenia and monitor hepatic indices with biochemical profile during treatment. Monitor electrocardiogram during IV treatment because prolonged Q-T interval may occur. Monitor thyroid function during treatment because of adverse effects on thyroid function. Drug monitoring may be available from some laboratories. Therapeutic range of amiodarone in plasma is 1–2.5 mcg/mL.

## Formulations

- Oral: Amiodarone is available in 100-, 200-, and 400-mg tablets.
- Injection: 50-mg/mL injection and a 1.5- and a 1.8-mg/mL injectable under the name Nexterone.
- A new formulation (PM101) uses a different vehicle to enhance solubility rather than Polysorbate 80. This vehicle, beta-cyclodextrin (Captisol), forms a hydrophilic central core and is less likely to elicit an allergic-type reaction.

## Stability and Storage

Store in a tightly sealed container, protected from light, and at room temperature.

## Small Animal Dosage

**Dogs**

- Ventricular arrhythmias: 10–15 mg/kg q12H PO for 1 week and then 5–7.5 mg/kg q12h for 2 weeks followed by a maintenance dose of 7.5 mg/kg q24h.
- Refractory arrhythmias: 25 mg/kg q12h PO for 4 days followed by 25 mg/kg q24h PO.
- Atrial fibrillation: 15 mg/kg loading dose for 5 days followed by 10 mg/kg per day PO thereafter.
- Boxer or Doberman: 200 mg per dog q12h for 1 week PO followed by 200 mg once daily thereafter. Doses as high as two times these rates have been administered but with a higher risk of toxicity.

- Treatment of arrhythmias with injection formulation: 5 mg/kg, slowly IV over 10 minutes. Use cautiously because of risk of adverse effects.

**Cats**
- No dose has been reported for cats.

### Large Animal Dosage
**Horses**
- Treatment of atrial fibrillation or ventricular tachycardia: 5 mg/kg/h for 1 hour followed by 0.83 mg/kg/h for 23 hours IV. Oral absorption was low and inconsistent and has not been recommended.

### Regulatory Information
No regulatory information is available. For extralabel use withdrawal interval estimates, contact FARAD at www.FARAD.org.

# Amitraz
am′ih-traz

**Trade and other names:** Mitaban

**Functional classification:** Antiparasitic

### Pharmacology and Mechanism of Action
Antiparasitic drug for ectoparasites. Amitraz inhibits monoamine oxidase (MAO) in mites. Mammals are resistant to this inhibition. However, administration of amitraz can interact with other MAO inhibitors (MAOIs).

### Indications and Clinical Uses
Amitraz is indicated for the topical treatment of mites, including Demodex. It is applied topically as a dip or sponge-on. It should not be administered systemically. The approved dose is effective in many animals; however, in more resistant cases of Demodex, higher doses have been applied. As the dose increases, the risk of adverse effects also increases. Because of the availability of newer oral agents to treat mites in animals (drugs in the isoxazoline class, such as afoxolaner, fluralaner, sarolaner, and lotilaner), the use of amitraz has declined.

### Precautionary Information
**Adverse Reactions and Side Effects**
Amitraz causes sedation in dogs caused by the agonist activity on alpha$_2$-adrenergic receptors, which may be reversed by yohimbine or atipamezole. When high doses are used, other side effects reported include pruritus, polyuria and polydipsia, bradycardia, hypotension, heart block, hypothermia, hyperglycemia, and (rarely) seizures.

**Contraindications and Precautions**
Adverse effects are more common when high doses are administered.

**Drug Interactions**
Do not administer with MAOIs, such as selegiline (Deprenyl, Anipryl). Do not administer with other alpha$_2$-agonists.

## Instructions for Use

Manufacturer's dose should be used initially, but for refractory cases, this dose has been exceeded to produce increased efficacy.

## Patient Monitoring and Laboratory Tests

Monitor by performing periodic skin scrapings and examining for presence of mites.

## Formulations

• Amitraz is available in 10.6-mL concentrated dip (19.9%).

## Stability and Storage

Store in a tightly sealed container, protected from light, and at room temperature. Stability of compounded formulations has not been evaluated.

## Small Animal Dosage

### Dogs

• 10.6 mL/7.5 L water (0.025% solution). Apply three to six topical treatments every 14 days. For refractory cases, this dosage has been exceeded to improve efficacy. Dosages that have been used include 0.025%, 0.05%, and 0.1% concentration applied once or twice per week. For refractory cases, a dose of 0.125% has been used by applying to only half of the dog's body one day, then to the other half of the body the following day. This alternating schedule has been repeated every day for 4 weeks and up to 5 months to achieve cures but should be considered only in extreme cases.

## Large Animal Dosage

• No dose has been reported for large animals.

## Regulatory Information

No regulatory information is available. For extralabel use withdrawal interval estimates, contact FARAD at www.FARAD.org.

RCI Classification: 3

## Amitriptyline Hydrochloride

am-ih-trip´tih-leen hye-droe-klor´ide

**Trade and other names:** Elavil and generic brands

**Functional classification:** Behavior modification, tricyclic antidepressant

## Pharmacology and Mechanism of Action

Tricyclic antidepressant drug (TCA). Amitriptyline, like other TCAs, acts via inhibition of the uptake of serotonin and other transmitters at presynaptic nerve terminals. The action in cats for treating cystitis is unknown but may be through reducing anxiety, behavior modification, or anticholinergic effects. It has no direct effect on the bladder mucosa.

## Indications and Clinical Uses

Like other TCAs, amitriptyline is used in animals to treat a variety of behavioral disorders (e.g., anxiety). However, there are few studies documenting efficacy in animals, and much of the use is based on anecdotal evidence. For treatment of some disorders, such as obsessive-compulsive disorder (1 mg/kg q12h up to 2 mg/kg), it was not as effective in animals as clomipramine. For treatment of aggressive behavior in dogs (2 mg/kg q12h), there was no difference between amitriptyline and placebo.

Amitriptyline has been used in cats for chronic idiopathic cystitis, a condition that is not well understood. However, when used for short-term treatment of idiopathic cystitis (10 mg per cat q24h) it was not effective. In another study, at 5 mg/cat per day for 7 days (0.55–1.2 mg/kg), there was no difference on recovery from hematuria and pollakiuria between amitriptyline and placebo, leading to a conclusion that short-term treatment is not helpful.

Amitriptyline, like other antidepressants, have been considered for treatment of chronic pain in animals, especially pain that may be maladaptive, or neuropathic in origin. Despite some use of this drug for treatment in people, no studies have established efficacy of amitriptyline in animals for this purpose.

## Precautionary Information

### Adverse Reactions and Side Effects

Amitriptyline has a bitter taste and is difficult to administer orally. Multiple side effects are associated with TCAs, such as antimuscarinic effects (dry mouth and rapid heart rate) and antihistamine effects (sedation). High doses can produce life-threatening cardiotoxicity. In cats, reduced grooming, weight gain, and sedation are possible.

### Contraindications and Precautions

Use cautiously in patients with heart disease.

### Drug Interactions

Do not use with other behavior modification drugs, such as serotonin reuptake inhibitors. Do not use with MAOIs.

## Instructions for Use

Doses are primarily based on empiricism. There are no controlled efficacy trials available for animals. There is evidence for success treating idiopathic cystitis in cats, but more recent studies have been less supportive. Amitriptyline was not effective for treatment of aggressive behavior in dogs, compared with behavior modification alone, and other anti-anxiety drugs for dogs should be considered instead (e.g., fluoxetine, clomipramine). Amitriptyline applied transdermally is not systemically absorbed in cats.

## Patient Monitoring and Laboratory Tests

Monitor patient's cardiovascular status during therapy, such as heart rate and rhythm. Like other TCAs, amitriptyline may decrease total $T_4$ and free $T_4$ concentrations in dogs.

## Formulations

- Amitriptyline is available in 10-, 25-, 50-, 75-, 100-, and 150-mg tablets.
- The injectable formulation is no longer marketed in the United States.

## Stability and Storage

Store in a tightly sealed container, protected from light, and at room temperature. Stability of compounded formulations has not been evaluated.

## Small Animal Dosage

### Dogs

- 1–2 mg/kg q12–24h PO.

Cats
- 2–4 mg per cat/day PO (0.5–1.0 mg/kg PO per day). The dose for cats may be divided into 12-hour intervals.
- Idiopathic cystitis: 2 mg/kg/day PO or a range of 2.5–7.5 mg/cat/day. (This indication is controversial.)

## Large Animal Dosage
- No dose has been reported for large animals.

## Regulatory Information
No regulatory information is available. For extralabel use withdrawal interval estimates, contact FARAD at www.FARAD.org.
RCI Classification: 2

# Amlodipine Besylate
am-loe′dih-peen bess′ih-late

**Trade and other names:** Norvasc

**Functional classification:** Calcium-channel blocker

## Pharmacology and Mechanism of Action
Calcium-channel blocking drug. Amlodipine is a second-generation calcium-channel blocker of the dihydropyridine class. It decreases calcium influx in cardiac and vascular smooth muscle. However, its greatest effect is on vascular smooth muscle by blocking the L-type calcium channels. Through this mechanism, it acts as a vasodilator for treating hypertension.

*Pharmacokinetics:* It has a high volume of distribution and slow systemic clearance, resulting in a half-life of approximately 30 hours. It is well-absorbed orally.

## Indications and Clinical Uses
In both dogs and cats, amlodipine is effective for lowering systemic blood pressure. Therefore, it is used to treat systemic hypertension (high blood pressure). Amlodipine has been considered the drug of choice for many years by clinicians for treating hypertension in cats. Hypertension in cats has been defined as systolic blood pressure greater than 190 mm Hg and diastolic pressure greater than 120 mm Hg. By comparison, angiotensin-converting enzyme (ACE) inhibitors are less effective in cats, and they respond better to amlodipine than to ACE inhibitors. Amlodipine reduces blood pressure in hypertensive cats and can reduce proteinuria but may not improve survival in cats with hypertensive kidney disease. Beta blockers may be added to therapy for cats (e.g., atenolol) to control the heart rate in hypertensive and hyperthyroid cats, but beta blockers do not have a direct anti-hypertensive effect in cats.

Although amlodipine has traditionally been considered the anti-hypertensive drug of choice for cats, recently, the angiotensin II blocker telmisartan has become a preferred agent because of proof of efficacy and available veterinary formulations (see Telmisartan for more information).

**A**

## Precautionary Information

### Adverse Reactions and Side Effects

The most common adverse effect is hypotension. In dogs and cats, gingival hyperplasia has been observed, which may be caused by an up-regulation of circulating androgens or inhibition of transglutaminase. Other mechanisms may be involved but are speculative. Gingival hyperplasia usually resolves after discontinuation of the medication and replacement with another drug (e.g., hydralazine or telmisartan).

In both dogs and cats, amlodipine may activate the renin–angiotensin–aldosterone system (RAAS). When this occurs, ACE inhibitors may be somewhat effective in reducing activation of RAAS, but addition of this medication also may increase risk of hypotension and may decrease renal glomerular pressure. Less common adverse reactions include lethargy, decreased appetite, azotemia, mild hypokalemia, and weight loss. Reflex tachycardia can occur with excessive decrease in blood pressure.

Amlodipine is a calcium-channel blocker, and although the action is more specific for vascular smooth muscle, it may depress the heart in some patients. Therefore, use carefully in patients with heart block or compromised cardiac contractility.

For treatment of a toxic overdose, administer calcium (e.g., calcium gluconate) and vasopressors.

### Contraindications and Precautions

Use cautiously in animals with poor cardiac reserve and that are prone to hypotension. Do not use in dehydrated animals.

### Drug Interactions

Use cautiously with other vasodilators. Drug interactions are possible from concurrent use with phenylpropanolamine, theophylline, and beta-agonists. Concurrent use with ACE inhibitors may increase the risk of hypotension and decreased glomerular pressure.

## Instructions for Use

In cats, efficacy has been established at 0.625 mg/cat once daily. If cats are large size (greater than 4.5 kg) or refractory, increase dose to 1.25 mg/cat q24h PO. In some cats, addition of a beta blocker to slow heart rate may be indicated. The goal of treatment is to decrease systolic pressure to less than 150/90 (systolic/diastolic). See the Patient Monitoring and Laboratory Tests section.

## Patient Monitoring and Laboratory Tests

Monitoring the patient's blood pressure is essential to proper treatment. Cats with high blood pressures of systolic 160–190 mm Hg and diastolic 100–120 mm Hg should be considered at risk of clinical effects from hypertension. When using amlodipine, the target blood pressure should be less than 160 mm Hg. If this is not achieved, increase the dose to 1.25 mg per cat, but maximum dose per cat should not exceed 2.5 mg per cat.

## Formulations

- Amlodipine is available in 2.5-, 5-, and 10-mg tablets. (Tablets are difficult to split for small animals.)

## Stability and Storage
Amlodipine is an unstable drug, and potency and stability are not assured if the original formulation is disrupted or compounded. Store in a tightly sealed container and protect from light.

## Small Animal Dosage
### Dogs
- 2.5 mg/dog or 0.1–0.5 mg/kg q24h PO. The higher dose of 0.5 mg/kg may be needed in refractory cases to reduce blood pressure.

### Cats
- 0.625 mg/cat initially q24h PO and increase if needed to 1.25 mg/cat. The dose of 0.625 mg is one eighth of a 5-mg human tablet. The average recommended dose for most cats is 0.18 mg/kg once daily for hypertension.

## Large Animal Dosage
- No dose has been reported for large animals.

## Regulatory Information
No regulatory information is available. For extralabel use withdrawal interval estimates, contact FARAD at www.FARAD.org.
RCI Classification: 4

# Ammonium Chloride
ah-moe′nee-um klor′ide

**Trade and other names:** Generic brands

**Functional classification:** Acidifier

## Pharmacology and Mechanism of Action
Urine acidifier. After oral administration, ammonium chloride induces acidic urine.

## Indications and Clinical Uses
Compounds containing ammonium are administered to patients to acidify the urine, primarily to manage cystic calculi or chronic urinary tract infections (UTIs).

## Precautionary Information
### Adverse Reactions and Side Effects
Ammonium chloride has a bitter taste when added to food. It may cause acidemia in some patients if administered at high doses.

### Contraindications and Precautions
Do not use in patients with systemic acidemia. Use cautiously in patients with kidney disease. It may be unpalatable when added to some animals' food.

### Drug Interactions
No drug interactions are reported in animals.

## Instructions for Use
Doses are designed to maximize urine acidifying effect.

## Patient Monitoring and Laboratory Tests
Monitor patient's acid–base status.

## Formulations
• Ammonium is available as crystals.

## Stability and Storage
Store in a tightly sealed container, protected from light, and at room temperature. Stability of compounded formulations has not been evaluated.

## Small Animal Dosage
**Dogs**
• 100 mg/kg q12h PO.

**Cats**
• 800 mg/cat or 20 mg/kg (approximately one third to one quarter teaspoon) mixed with food daily.

## Large Animal Dosage
**Horses**
• Acidifier: 100–250 mg/kg q24h PO.

## Regulatory Information
No regulatory information is available. It is not expected to pose a residue risk, and no withdrawal is recommended for food animals.

# Amoxicillin
ah-moks-ih-sill'in

**Trade and other names:** Amoxicillin: Amoxi-Tabs, Amoxi-Drops, Amoxi-Inject, Robamox-V, Biomox, and other brands. Amoxil, Trimox, Wymox, Polymox (human preparation), and amoxicillin trihydrate

**Functional classification:** Antibacterial

## Pharmacology and Mechanism of Action
Beta-lactam antibiotic. Amoxicillin inhibits bacterial cell wall synthesis. Amoxicillin generally has a narrow spectrum of activity that includes streptococci, non–beta-lactamase–producing staphylococci, and other gram-positive cocci and bacilli. Many *Staphylococcus* strains are resistant because of beta-lactamase production. Most enteric gram-negative Enterobacteriaceae bacilli are resistant. Susceptible gram-negative bacteria include some species of *Proteus, Pasteurella multocida,* and *Histophilus* spp. Resistance among other gram-negative bacteria is common.

*Pharmacokinetics:* In dogs, the peak concentration, half-life, volume of distribution (VD/F), and clearance (CL/F) are 11 mcg/mL, 1.3 hours, 0.72 L/kg, and 6.5 mL/kg/min, respectively. In cats, these values are 12 mcg/mL, 1.4 hours, 1.05 L/kg, and 7.8 mL/kg/min, respectively. Amoxicillin oral absorption in small animals is higher than ampicillin (two times higher in some animals). Amoxicillin oral absorption in adult horses is less than 10% and is not recommended. In pigs, oral absorption is approximately 40% with a half-life after oral administration of 45 minutes.

## Indications and Clinical Uses

Amoxicillin is used for a variety of infections in all species, including lower UTIs, soft tissue infections, and pneumonia. It is generally more effective for infections caused by gram-positive bacteria. Because of a short half-life, frequent administration is needed for treating gram-negative infections. Oral absorption in horses is less than 10%, and it is not suitable for treatment of adult horses. However, oral absorption in foals is 36%–43%. Oral absorption in small animals is 50%–60%.

### Precautionary Information

**Adverse Reactions and Side Effects**

Amoxicillin is usually well tolerated. Allergic reactions are possible. Diarrhea and vomiting are common with oral doses. Oral administration to horses or cattle can cause diarrhea or enteritis.

**Contraindications and Precautions**

Use cautiously in animals allergic to penicillin-like drugs.

**Drug Interactions**

Do not mix with other drugs in compounded formulations.

## Instructions for Use

Dose requirements are based on the approved label dose, or the dose used to determine susceptibility testing interpretive categories. Amoxicillin is not a preferred choice for gram-negative infections caused by Enterobacteriaceae bacteria because most are clinically resistant.

## Patient Monitoring and Laboratory Tests

Susceptibility testing: For testing for susceptibility, the CLSI recommends using ampicillin to test for amoxicillin susceptibility. The CLSI breakpoint for susceptible organisms is ≤0.25 mcg/mL for staphylococci, streptococci, and gram-negative bacilli. For uncomplicated canine lower urinary tract pathogens, use a breakpoint of ≤8 mcg/mL (this breakpoint also can be applied to cats for uncomplicated infections). For cattle pathogens, use a breakpoint of ≤0.25 mcg/mL. For equine respiratory pathogens (streptococci), use a break point of ≤0.25 mcg/mL. At this breakpoint for susceptibility (0.25 mcg/mL), gram-negative Enterobacteriaceae bacteria test resistant, and testing of these isolates is unnecessary.

## Formulations

- Amoxicillin is available in 50-, 100-, 150-, 200-, 400-, 500-, and 875-mg tablets and 250- and 500-mg capsules (human preparations). Chewable tablets are available in 125-, 200-, 250-, and 400-mg sizes.
- Amoxicillin trihydrate is available in 50-, 100-, 200-, and 400-mg tablets; 50-mg/mL amoxicillin trihydrate oral suspension; and 100- or 250-mg/mL amoxicillin trihydrate for injection.

## Stability and Storage

Store in a tightly sealed container at room temperature. Oral liquid suspensions are stable for 14 days. Other formulations should be protected from moisture. Optimum stability is at pH 5.8–6.5. Above this pH, hydrolysis occurs.

## Small Animal Dosage

**Dogs and Cats**

- 22 mg/kg q12h PO.

**Cats**
- 12.5 mg/kg q12h PO.

## Large Animal Dosage
**Calves**
- Nonruminating: 10–22 mg/kg q8–12h PO.

**Cattle and horses**
- 6.6–22 mg/kg q8–12h PO (suspension). Note: Oral doses in large animals are not well absorbed (except in foals), and amoxicillin is not recommended by this route.

## Regulatory Information
Withdrawal time (cattle only): 25 days for meat, 96 hours for milk. Amoxicillin intramammary infusion: withdrawal time 12 days for meat, 60 hours for milk.

# Amoxicillin and Clavulanate Potassium
ah-mox-ih-sill´in and klav-yoo-lan´ate poe-tah´see-um

**Trade and other names:** Clavamox (veterinary preparation) and Augmentin (human preparation)

**Functional classification:** Antibacterial

## Pharmacology and Mechanism of Action
Beta-lactam antibiotic and beta-lactamase inhibitor (clavulanate potassium) (beta-lactam and beta-lactamase inhibitor [BLBLI] combination). Amoxicillin activity and spectrum are as described earlier. Clavulanate has no antibacterial effects alone, but it is a competitive, and irreversible inhibitor of the beta-lactamase enzyme that causes resistance among gram-positive and gram-negative bacteria. By adding clavulanate to amoxicillin, the spectrum is extended to include beta-lactamase–producing strains of *Staphylococcus* (non-methicillin resistant) and some strains of gram-negative bacilli. However, unless treating uncomplicated lower UTIs, many of the Enterobacteriaceae are resistant to typical doses of amoxicillin–clavulanate.

## Indications and Clinical Uses
Amoxicillin and clavulanate is a broad-spectrum antibacterial drug used for skin and soft tissue infections, UTIs, wound infections, and respiratory infections. It is indicated for treatment of bacterial infections that may otherwise be resistant to amoxicillin because of bacterial beta-lactamase production. Amoxicillin and clavulanate is particularly useful for treating beta-lactamase–producing strains of *Staphylococcus* spp.

## Precautionary Information
### Adverse Reactions and Side Effects
It is usually well tolerated. Allergic reactions are possible. Diarrhea is common with oral doses and has also caused vomiting in some animals. As the dose of clavulanate increases because of a high proportion of clavulanate in some formulations, vomiting is more likely.

**Contraindications and Precautions**
Use cautiously in animals allergic to penicillin-like drugs. Oral administration to horses and ruminants may produce diarrhea.

**Drug Interactions**
No drug interactions are reported in animals.

## Instructions for Use

Dose requirements are based on the approved label dose, or the dose used to determine susceptibility testing interpretive categories. If treating infections that test in the Intermediate category, more frequent or higher doses are needed. It is not recommended for treatment of infections caused by the Enterobacteriaceae (*Escherichia coli*), because most strains are clinically resistant, unless the infection is in the lower UTI.

Some dermatologists recommend using a higher dose than recommended on the label to treat skin infections (i.e., 25 mg/kg q12h). Oral human dose forms are sometimes substituted for veterinary drugs. Note that veterinary dose formulations contain amoxicillin and clavulanate in a 4:1 ratio. Human dose forms (Augmentin) contain these drugs in ratios of 2:1 to as high as 7:1. Despite the different ratios of amoxicillin to clavulanate in the human formulations, they have been used interchangeably with the veterinary formulations.

## Patient Monitoring and Laboratory Tests

Susceptibility testing: CLSI breakpoint for sensitive organisms is ≤0.25/0.12 mcg/mL for staphylococci, streptococci, *E. coli*, and *Pasteurella multocida*. (The "/" distinguishes the amoxicillin from the clavulanate concentrations.) When treating an uncomplicated lower UTI, a susceptibility breakpoint is ≤8/4 mcg/mL. Although this higher breakpoint is listed only for dogs, it may apply to cats if it is an uncomplicated lower UTI.

## Formulations

- Amoxicillin + clavulanate is available in veterinary dose form: 62.5-, 125-, 250-, and 375-mg tablets and 62.5-mg/mL suspension in a ratio of amoxicillin:clavulanate ratio of 4:1.
- Amoxicillin + clavulanate is available in human dose form: 250/125-, 500/125-, and 875/125-mg tablets.
- Amoxicillin + clavulanate is available in 125/31.25-, 200/28.5-, 250/62.5-, and 400/57-mg chewable tablets
- Oral suspension 125/31.25, 200/28.5, 250/62.5, and 400/57 mg per 5 mL.

## Stability and Storage

Store in a tightly sealed container, protected from light, and below 24°C. Avoid exposure to humidity or moisture. Reconstituted oral products are stable for 10 days. Clavulanate is particularly unstable in compounded formulations, and compounded products can exhibit a dramatic loss of potency, particularly in aqueous suspensions with acidic pH.

## Small Animal Dosage

**Dogs**

- 12.5 mg/kg q12h PO. (Dose is based on combined ingredients: amoxicillin and clavulanate.)

**Cats**
- 62.5 mg/cat q12h PO; equivalent to 12.5 mg/kg amoxicillin and 3.12 mg/kg clavulanate q12h.

**Large Animal Dosage**
- Amoxicillin + clavulanate is only available in an oral formulation. Because these components are not absorbed orally in large animal species, this drug is not recommended.

**Regulatory Information**

No regulatory information is available. However, it is anticipated that withdrawal times are similar to those of amoxicillin.

## Amphotericin B
am-foe-tare'ih-sin

**Trade and other names:** Fungizone (traditional formulation) and liposomal forms of Amphotec, ABLC, ABCD, Abelcet, and AmBisome

**Functional classification:** Antifungal

### Pharmacology and Mechanism of Action

Antifungal drug. Amphotericin B is a fungicidal agent for systemic fungi. Amphotericin B binds to ergosterol in the fungal cell membrane, producing a loss of membrane integrity, leakage of membranes, and cell death. Amphotericin is active against most fungi and some protozoa. There is a conventional formulation of amphotericin B deoxycholate that has been used most often in veterinary medicine. It is the least expensive but the most toxic. Lipid formulations of amphotericin B are now available. The advantage of liposomal formulations over the traditional formulations is that they are less toxic. These new formulations are lipid-based complexes or cholesteryl complexes of amphotericin B that allow higher doses to be administered with less nephrotoxicity. Three lipid formulations are available:
- Amphotericin B lipid complex (Abelcet, ABLC) is a suspension of amphotericin B complexed with two phospholipids at a concentration of 100 mg/20 mL. This formulation was shown to be safe and effective for treating blastomycosis in dogs at a cumulative dose of 8–12 mg/kg by administering 1 mg/kg every other day.
- Amphotericin B cholesteryl sulfate complex (Amphotec, ABCD) is a colloidal dispersion of amphotericin B. It has been effective in studies in which it was administered at doses higher than the traditional amphotericin B formulation.
- The liposomal complex of amphotericin B (AmBisome) is a unilaminar liposomal formulation. When reconstituted, it produces small vesicles of encapsulated amphotericin B. This formulation has been used safely and effectively in some dogs for blastomycosis.

### Indications and Clinical Uses

Amphotericin B is indicated in patients with a variety of systemic mycoses. It is used to treat blastomycosis, coccidioidomycosis, and histoplasmosis. It also has been used to treat leishmaniasis in dogs. It may be administered for treatment of aspergillosis, but this is not a common use in veterinary medicine, and some species of *Aspergillus* are resistant.

## Precautionary Information

### Adverse Reactions and Side Effects

Amphotericin B produces a dose-related nephrotoxicity. It also produces fever, phlebitis, and tremors. Renal toxicity is dose dependent and cumulative. Toxicity is more likely when cumulative doses approach or exceed 6 mg/kg. With repeated use, amphotericin B can cause renal potassium wasting because of loss of potassium in the collecting duct.

### Contraindications and Precautions

Do not use in patients who have renal disease or when renal clearance is not known. Do not use in dehydrated animals or animals with electrolyte imbalances.

### Drug Interactions

When preparing IV solution, do not mix amphotericin B with electrolyte solutions; instead, use 5% dextrose in water. Nephrotoxicity is increased when administered with aminoglycosides.

## Instructions for Use

When administering proprietary forms of liposomal amphotericin B, follow the instructions on the label carefully. Administer IV via slow infusion diluted in 5% dextrose in water and monitor renal function closely. Administer sodium chloride fluid loading IV to patients before therapy to decrease risk of renal toxicosis.

Amphotericin B has been mixed as a solution of amphotericin B in which one vial of 50 mg is mixed with 40 mL of sterile water and 10 mL of Intralipid 10% (soybean oil). Doses of this mixture of 1–2 mg/kg have been used for treating systemic leishmaniasis. For other indications, this mixture has been administered at a dosage of 1–2.5 mg/kg two times per week for 8–10 treatments. This liposomal complex of amphotericin B was used in a study for treatment of canine *Leishmania infantum* at a dose of 3–3.3 mg/kg. Although there was rapid clinical improvement, dogs remained positive for leishmaniasis.

For administration of Abelcet (liposomal formulation), the most common dosage is 0.5 mg/kg IV infused over 90–120 minutes for the first dose. If the first dose is tolerated, increase to 2–3 mg/kg on alternate days. A goal for a total accumulative dose of 12–36 mg/kg, but the patient can be switched to oral azole antifungal agents (e.g., itraconazole) before reaching this limit. For IV use, the dose should be diluted in 5% dextrose to 1 mg/mL for infusion. For some patients, greater dilution (more fluid) can be used to facilitate a slow infusion.

Although intrathecal use is rare, only the conventional formulation should be used for this administration. Start with 0.05 (total dose) q48h and increase to 0.1 and 0.2 mg (total dose) if it is tolerated well. Prepare intrathecal solution with a 5-mg/mL solution in sterile water, further diluting to 0.25 mg/mL by adding 1 mL (5 mg) of the solution to another 19 mL of 5% dextrose and inject directly intrathecally.

## Patient Monitoring and Laboratory Tests

Monitor renal function closely during treatment. After treatment, many animals have an elevated creatinine and BUN. Persistent azotemia may be a cause for discontinuation of treatment and replacement with another antifungal agent. Hypokalemia and hypomagnesemia may occur during use because of renal tubular acidosis.

## Formulations

- The conventional form of amphotericin B is available in a 50-mg injectable vial.
- Liposomal forms are available as 50- and 100-mg injectable vial (Amphotec; lipid complex).
- Amphotericin B phospholipid complex (Abelcet) is available in a 100 mg vial at 5 mg/mL.

## Stability and Storage

Stable if stored in original vial. Amphotericin B for IV infusion reacts with light and should be protected from light during infusions. Store reconstituted solutions in refrigeration. However, unrefrigerated solutions may be stable for up to 1 week. Optimum pH is 6–7.

## Small Animal Dosage

### Dogs

- Conventional formulation: 0.5 mg/kg q48 h IV (slow infusion) to a cumulative dose of 4–8 mg/kg.
- Liposomal formulations: Start with 0.5 mg/kg for the first dose; then increase from 1 to 3 mg/kg/day for subsequent treatments if well tolerated. The IV dose should be infused over 60–120 minutes for up to 9–12 treatments if needed. This dose may be administered three times per week or every other day. A goal for the total cumulative dose for liposomal formulations is 12–36 mg/kg if necessary, but many patients are transitioned to oral azole antifungal agents (e.g., itraconazole) before they reach this limit.
- Intrathecal use: See previous instructions. Start with 0.05 (total dose) q48h and increase to 0.1 and 0.2 mg (total dose).
- SQ dose: 0.5–0.8 mg/kg diluted in 500 mL of 0.45% saline and 2.5% dextrose solution for dogs weighing less than 20 kg and in 1000 mL for dogs weighing more than 20 kg. Drug concentration in fluid should not exceed 20 mg/L. Administer this dose two or three times per week SQ. Note: An important complication from this method is sterile abscess at site of injection.
- *Leishmania* infections: 0.5 mg/kg IV by slow infusion on alternate days for 4 weeks. (To avoid resistance, the World Health Organization has discouraged this use.)

### Cats

- Cats have received similar regimens to those used for dogs (e.g., 0.25-mg/kg conventional formulation). However, many clinicians will start with lower doses in cats. For liposomal formulations in cats, use 1 mg/kg IV three times per week for up to 12 treatments.

## Large Animal Dosage

### Horses

- 0.3 mg/kg IV on day 1 followed by 3 consecutive days and repeat after a 24- to 48-hour drug-free interval. High cost of treatment has prevented common usage in horses.

## Regulatory Information

No regulatory information is available. For extralabel use withdrawal interval estimates, contact FARAD at www.FARAD.org.

# Ampicillin and Ampicillin Sodium
am-pih-sill'in

**Trade and other names:** Omnipen, Principen, Totacillin, and Polycillin (human preparations); Omnipen-N, Polycillin-N, and Totacillin N (injectable preparations); and Amp-Equine and Ampicillin trihydrate (Polyflex), and Ampi-Tab (veterinary preparations)

**Functional classification:** Antibacterial

## Pharmacology and Mechanism of Action

Beta-lactam antibiotic. Ampicillin inhibits bacterial cell wall synthesis. Ampicillin has a narrow spectrum of activity that is similar to that of amoxicillin. Ampicillin spectrum of activity includes streptococci, non–beta-lactamase–producing staphylococci, and other gram-positive cocci and bacilli. Many staphylococci are resistant because of beta-lactamase production. Most enteric gram-negative bacilli of the Enterobacteriaceae are clinically resistant. Susceptible gram-negative bacteria include some species of *Proteus* spp., *Pasteurella multocida,* and *Histophilus* spp.

*Pharmacokinetics:* Pharmacokinetics of ampicillin indicated that the half-life is approximately 1–1.5 hours in most animals. Half-life in horses is 0.6–1.5 hours after IV administration but longer after IM injection. When the trihydrate formulation is injected IM, it produces a lower peak concentration but a longer half-life of 6.7 hours in cattle. Volume of distribution in most species is approximately 0.2–0.3 L/kg. Systemic clearance is approximately 3–5 mL/kg/min in most animals. Oral absorption is less than 50% in dogs and cats and less than 4% in horses. Protein binding is 15%–25% in animals.

## Indications and Clinical Uses

Ampicillin is indicated in patients with infections caused by susceptible bacteria, such as skin and soft tissue infections, UTIs, and pneumonia. Gram-positive bacteria (except beta-lactamase–producing strains of *Staphylococcus* spp.) are usually susceptible. However, infections caused by most gram-negative bacteria of the Enterobacteriaceae are clinically resistant. Fastidious gram-negative bacteria (e.g., *Pasteurella*) are usually clinically susceptible.

## Precautionary Information

### Adverse Reactions and Side Effects

Adverse effects of penicillin drugs are most commonly caused by drug allergy. This can range from acute anaphylaxis when administered IV to other signs of allergic reaction when other routes are used. When used for prophylaxis during surgery, ampicillin can be administered IV to anesthetized patients without affecting cardiovascular parameters. Diarrhea is possible when administered orally, especially with high doses.

### Contraindications and Precautions

Use cautiously in animals allergic to penicillin-like drugs. Ampicillin contains 3 mEq of sodium per gram. Rapid IV bolus injection can produce CNS excitement and convulsive seizures.

### Drug Interactions

Do not mix in vials with other drugs.

## Instructions for Use

Dose requirements are based on the approved label dose or the dose used to determine susceptibility testing interpretive categories. Ampicillin is absorbed approximately 50% less compared with amoxicillin when administered orally. Because of better absorption, amoxicillin is preferred when oral treatment is needed.

When preparing injectable solutions, the stability is dependent on the concentration. Concentrated solutions (250 mg/mL) should be injected within 1 hour of reconstitution either IM, SQ, or slowly (over 3 minutes) IV. Less concentrated solutions prepared in IV fluids (e.g., 30 mg/mL) are stable for longer periods. See the Stability and Storage section for more detail.

## Patient Monitoring and Laboratory Tests

Susceptibility testing: For testing for susceptibility, CLSI breakpoint for susceptible organisms is ≤0.25 mcg/mL for staphylococci, streptococci, and gram-negative bacilli. Most Enterobacteriaceae bacteria (e.g., *E. coli*) test clinically resistant to ampicillin. At this breakpoint for susceptibility (0.25 mcg/mL), gram-negative Enterobacteriaceae bacteria test resistant, and testing of these isolates is unnecessary. When treating an uncomplicated lower UTI, a susceptibility breakpoint for dogs is ≤8 mcg/mL. Although this higher breakpoint is listed only for dogs, it may apply to cats if it is an uncomplicated lower UTI. For cattle pathogens, use a susceptible breakpoint of ≤0.25 mcg/mL. For equine respiratory pathogens (streptococci), use a susceptible breakpoint of ≤0.25 mcg/mL.

## Formulations

- Ampicillin is available in 125-, 250-, and 500-mg capsules.
- Solutions: 125-, 250-, and 500-mg vials of ampicillin sodium. Amp-Equine is available in 1-, 2-, and 3-g vials for injection. (However, this formulation has been discontinued by some suppliers.)
- Although 1- and 2-g vials are primarily for IV use (if available), they may be administered IM when the 250- and 500-mg vials are unavailable. In such instances, dissolve these vials in 3.5 or 6.8 of mL sterile water, for the 1- and 2-g vials, respectively (resulting concentration is 250 mg/mL). When using 1- or 2-g vials for IV administration, dissolve 7.4 or 14.8 mL of sterile water and administer over 15 minutes.
- Suspensions: ampicillin trihydrate suspension (Polyflex) is available in 10- and 25-g vials for injection, and when reconstituted, each milliliter contains ampicillin trihydrate equivalent to 50, 100, or 250 mg of ampicillin.

## Stability and Storage

Store in a tightly sealed container at room temperature.

*Solutions:* After reconstitution of ampicillin sodium, stability is concentration dependent. After reconstitution with sterile water at a concentration of 250 mg/mL, it is stable for 1 hour at room temperature. If diluted to a concentration of up to 30 mg/mL using 0.9% saline or lactated Ringer's solution (e.g., in IV fluids), stability is maintained for 8 hours at room temperature. In refrigerated temperatures, when reconstituted to 30 mg/mL, it is stable for 48 hours in sterile water or 24 hours in sodium chloride or Ringer's solution. At 20 mg/mL, it is stable for 72 hours in sterile water or 48 hours in sodium chloride. If this concentration is prepared in 5% dextrose in water, stability is maintained for only 1 hour.

*Suspensions:* Oral suspensions are stable for 14 days if refrigerated. Ampicillin trihydrate for injection is stable for 12 months refrigerated and 3 months at room temperature. Other formulations should be protected from moisture. Optimum stability is at pH 5.8. Above this pH, hydrolysis occurs.

## Small Animal Dosage

**Ampicillin Sodium, Injectable and Oral**
*Dogs and Cats*
• 10 mg/kg q8h IV, IM, or SQ or 20 mg/kg q8h PO.

**Ampicillin Trihydrate Injection**
*Dogs*
• 10–50 mg/kg q12–24h IM or SQ.
*Cats*
• 10–20 mg/kg q12–24h IM or SQ.

## Large Animal Dosage

**Horses and Ruminants**
*Ampicillin Sodium Injectable*
• 22 mg/kg q12h IM or IV.

**Cattle and Calves**
*Ampicillin Trihydrate*
• 11 mg/kg q12h IM.

**Pigs**
*Ampicillin Trihydrate*
• 15 mg/kg q24h IM

## Regulatory Information

Cattle withdrawal time: 6 days for meat; 48 hours for milk (at 6 mg/kg).
Pig withdrawal time: In Canada, 6 days.

# Ampicillin + Sulbactam
am-pih-sill′in + sul-bak′tam

**Trade and other names:** Unasyn

**Functional classification:** Antibacterial

## Pharmacology and Mechanism of Action

The ampicillin component has the same spectrum and mechanism of action as described previously for ampicillin. This formulation contains ampicillin plus a beta-lactamase inhibitor (sulbactam), also called a BLBLI. Sulbactam has similar activity as clavulanate (ingredient in amoxicillin–clavulanate), but it is not as active as clavulanate against some gram-negative beta-lactamase enzymes (e.g., extended-spectrum beta-lactamase [ESBL] enzymes). Because of the addition of sulbactam, it has a broader spectrum of activity than ampicillin alone. The spectrum includes beta-lactamase–producing strains of *Staphylococcus* spp. and streptococci but few gram-negative bacilli. Most gram-negative Enterobacteriaceae bacteria are clinically resistant.

## Indications and Clinical Uses

This combination is indicated for infections caused by susceptible strains of bacteria. It has been used for acute infections such as pneumonia, sepsis, and prophylaxis in patients with neutropenia. Because of the addition of sulbactam, it has a broader spectrum than ampicillin alone. Therefore, it is used for treating infections for which ampicillin resistance may be expected. Many gram-negative bacilli (e.g., Enterobacteriaceae) have MIC values that are in the clinically resistant range for ampicillin–sulbactam, and other agents should be considered when these bacteria are suspected, such as piperacillin–tazobactam.

Ampicillin–sulbactam can only be administered by injection. For oral use, amoxicillin–clavulanate (e.g., Clavamox and Augmentin) may be used as an equivalent alternative.

---

### Precautionary Information

**Adverse Reactions and Side Effects**

Adverse effects of penicillin drugs are most commonly caused by drug allergy. This can range from acute anaphylaxis when administered to other signs of allergic reaction when other routes are used.

**Contraindications and Precautions**

Use cautiously in animals allergic to penicillin-like drugs.

**Drug Interactions**

Do not mix in vials with other drugs.

---

## Instructions for Use

Dose requirements are based on extrapolation of the approved label dose in people or the dose that is used most often for ampicillin sodium. Concentrated solutions (250 mg/mL) should be injected within 1 hour of reconstitution IM, SQ, or slowly (over 3 minutes) IV. Vials for IM use may be reconstituted in lidocaine hydrochloride to decrease pain from injection. Less concentrated solutions prepared in IV fluids (e.g., 45 mg/mL) are stable for longer periods. See the Stability and Storage section for more details.

## Patient Monitoring and Laboratory Tests

Susceptibility testing: CLSI breakpoint for sensitive organisms is ≤8/4 mcg/mL for staphylococci and gram-negative bacilli, based on the human breakpoint. (The "/" distinguishes the ampicillin from the sulbactam concentrations.) However, CLSI has lower breakpoints for ampicillin in dogs, cats, horses, and cattle, and it is highly likely that the human ampicillin/sulbactam breakpoint is too high to predict susceptibility for isolates from animals. Therefore, the lower susceptibility breakpoint of ampicillin (≤0.25 mcg/mL) should be applied to the use of ampicillin–sulbactam in animals.

## Formulations

- Ampicillin + sulbactam is available in a 2:1 combination for injection and 1.5- and 3-g vials.

## Stability and Storage

Store vial in a tightly sealed container at room temperature. Vials may be reconstituted with sterile water for immediate use at an ampicillin concentration of 250 mg/mL. The vial should be used within 1 hour of reconstitution. When the reconstituted vial is diluted with sterile water or 0.9% sodium chloride at a concentration of 45 mg/mL, stability is maintained for 8 hours at room temperature and 48 hours if refrigerated. Stability is maintained for 8 hours at room temperature and 24 hours refrigerated if lactated Ringer's solution is used. Optimum stability is at pH 5.8. Above this pH, hydrolysis occurs.

## Small Animal Dosage
### Cats and Dogs
- Doses are similar to those used for ampicillin (when dosed according to ampicillin component) 10 mg/kg q8h IV or IM.

## Large Animal Dosage
### Horses and Ruminants
- 11 mg/kg, or 22 mg/kg q12h, IM or IV.

## Regulatory Information
Withdrawal time exists for ampicillin but not sulbactam. Because sulbactam has a similar half-life and presents little risk for toxicity, the withdrawal times listed for ampicillin are suggested.
Cattle withdrawal time: 6 days for meat; 48 hours for milk (at 6 mg/kg).
Pig withdrawal time: In Canada, 6 days.

# Amprolium
am-proe'lee-um

**Trade and other names:** Amprol and Corid

**Functional classification:** Antiparasitic

## Pharmacology and Mechanism of Action
Antiprotozoal drug. This drug is a vitamin $B_1$ or thiamine structural analogue. Amprolium antagonizes thiamine in parasites and is used for treatment of coccidiosis.

## Indications and Clinical Uses
Amprolium is used to control and treat coccidiosis in calves, sheep, goats, puppies, and birds. It is administered orally, often mixed with food.

### Precautionary Information
#### Adverse Reactions and Side Effects
Toxicity is observed only at high doses. CNS signs are caused by thiamine deficiency, which may be reversed by adding thiamine to the diet.

#### Contraindications and Precautions
Do not administer to debilitated animals.

#### Drug Interactions
No drug interactions are reported in animals.

## Instructions for Use
Usually administered as feed additive to livestock. For dogs, 30 mL of 9.6% amprolium has been added to 3.8 L of drinking water for control of coccidiosis.

## Patient Monitoring and Laboratory Tests
No specific monitoring is necessary.

**A**

## Formulations
- Amprolium is available in 9.6% (9.6 g/100 mL) oral solution and a soluble powder in a 22.6-g packet.

## Stability and Storage
Store in a tightly sealed container, protected from light, and at room temperature. Stability of compounded formulations has not been evaluated.

## Small Animal Dosage
### Dogs and Cats
- Treatment of coccidiosis: Add 1.25 g of 20% amprolium powder to daily feed or 30 mL of 9.6% amprolium solution to 3.8 L of drinking water for 7 days.

## Large Animal Dosage
### Calves
- Prevention of coccidiosis: 5 mg/kg q24h for 21 days.
- Treatment of coccidiosis: 10 mg/kg q24h for 5 days PO.

## Regulatory Information
Withdrawal time for cattle (meat): 24 hours before slaughter.
A withdrawal period has not been established for this product in preruminating calves. Do not use in calves to be processed for veal.

# Apomorphine Hydrochloride
ah-poe-mor′feen hye-droe-klor′-ide
**Trade and other names:** Apokyn and generic brands
**Functional classification:** Emetic

## Pharmacology and Mechanism of Action
Emetic drug. Apomorphine is opiate derivative that crosses the blood–brain barrier and stimulates dopamine ($D_2$) or chemoreceptor trigger zone receptors in the vomiting center. It promptly causes vomiting in dogs. Although it is easily absorbed from mucosal surfaces (e.g., conjunctiva of the eye), it is not absorbed orally because of first-pass effects.

## Indications and Clinical Uses
Apomorphine is indicated for inducing emesis in animals that have ingested toxic agents. After SQ administration, the onset of effect is 10 minutes or shorter. It is promptly effective for inducing vomiting in dogs but less so in cats. Apomorphine also is absorbed from mucosal administration after applying to the conjunctiva of the eye. Xylazine often is a more reliable emetic in cats. In dogs, 3% hydrogen peroxide (2.2 mL/kg) was equally effective for inducing emesis. (The dose of 3% hydrogen peroxide is typically 2.2 mL/kg or 1 mL/lb.)

## Precautionary Information
### Adverse Reactions and Side Effects
Apomorphine produces emesis before serious adverse effects can occur, but at higher doses (0.1 mg/kg), sedation can occur, which can mask the signs of some toxic agents. The hydrochloride salt of this formulation has a pH of 3–4 and can be irritating to the ocular conjunctival membranes. At high doses (1 mg/kg), excitement can occur, possibly via stimulation of dopamine ($D_1$ and $D_2$) receptors.

### Contraindications and Precautions
Apomorphine also may decrease vomiting stimulus in vomiting center; therefore, if the initial dose is not effective, emetic effects may be blocked during later attempts to induce vomiting. Use cautiously in cats that may be sensitive to opiates. (Xylazine is a more effective emetic agent in cats.)

### Drug Interactions
No drug interactions are reported in animals. However, some drugs diminish the emetic action of apomorphine (e.g., acepromazine, atropine, and other antiemetics).

## Instructions for Use
Apomorphine should be available in most emergency practices for prompt treatment of poisoning. If not, consult local poison center or pharmacist for availability. Apomorphine can be administered IM, SQ, or to the mucosa (e.g., in the conjunctival sac of the eye). It should not be administered IV because the rapid diffusion to the CNS may block the emetic effects. In dogs, vomiting should occur within 3–10 minutes after administration. Limit administration to once. Consider other agent such as xylazine or dexmedetomidine to induce vomiting in cats.

## Patient Monitoring and Laboratory Tests
No specific monitoring is necessary. If used to induce vomiting from a toxicant, monitor for signs of toxicity because vomiting is able to eliminate less than half of the ingested toxicant.

## Formulations
- Apomorphine is available in 6-mg tablets that can be hydrolyzed prior to use or is available in a 10-mg/mL concentration in a 2-mL ampule or 3-mL preloaded syringes.
- If apomorphine is not available from commercial sources, it has been prepared by compounding pharmacists. One approach is to mix 20 mg apomorphine in a sterile vial with 4.4 mL of sterile water to make a solution of 5 mg/mL. From this solution, drops may be added to the eye to induce vomiting.

## Stability and Storage
Store in a tightly sealed container at room temperature, protected from light. Solutions decompose when exposed to air and light. A green color indicates decomposition. One of the compounded formulations prepared in an aqueous solution (3 mg/mL) was stable at room temperature for 6 months after compounding.

## Small Animal Dosage
### Dogs and Cats (Less effective in cats.)
- 0.03–0.05 mg/kg IM.
- 0.1 mg/kg SQ.

- Dissolve 6-mg tablet in 1–2 mL of 0.9% saline solution and instill directly in the conjunctiva of the eye. After animal vomits, the conjunctiva may be rinsed of residual drug with an eye wash solution.

## Large Animal Dosage
- No dose has been reported for large animals because they typically do not vomit.

## Regulatory Information
Do not administer to animals intended for food.
RCI Classification: 1

# Aprepitant
ap-reh′pih-tant

**Trade and other names:** Emend
**Functional classification:** Antiemetic

## Pharmacology and Mechanism of Action
Aprepitant is a centrally acting antiemetic. Aprepitant is a substance P/neurokinin 1 ($NK_1$) receptor antagonist, similar to the veterinary drug maropitant (Cerenia). It is used primarily in people to prevent vomiting from cancer chemotherapy, such as cisplatin. This drug is effective because chemotherapy drugs and other emetic stimuli release $NK_1$, which is highly emetic. It also blocks vomiting from other stimuli. The use in small animals has been somewhat limited because of the high expense and limited formulations for animals. In dogs, aprepitant is extensively metabolized after administration. Instead, the veterinary drug maropitant (Cerenia) is used much more often.

## Indications and Clinical Uses
Aprepitant is an effective antiemetic for people, particularly when used to treat vomiting associated with cancer chemotherapy. It may be used with corticosteroids (dexamethasone) and serotonin antagonists. However, despite its broad effects to decrease vomiting in people, there are no reports of effective use in dogs or cats. Instead, a similar-acting drug, maropitant (Cerenia), is used in dogs and cats and produces similar antiemetic effects.

## Precautionary Information
### Adverse Reactions and Side Effects
There are no reported adverse effects in animals.

### Contraindications and Precautions
No contraindications reported for animals.

### Drug Interactions
Drug interactions are possible because aprepitant is both an inducer and inhibitor of cytochrome P450 enzymes. Potent inhibitors of cytochrome P450 can potentially affect aprepitant clearance.

## Instructions for Use

Use in patients that are refractory to other antiemetic drugs. It may be combined with other antiemetics.

## Patient Monitoring and Laboratory Tests

No specific monitoring is necessary.

## Formulations

- Aprepitant is available in 80- and 125-mg capsules and as fosaprepitant dimeglumine in a 150-mg vial for IV use.

## Stability and Storage

Do not crush or mix capsules. Store in a tightly sealed container, protected from light, and at room temperature.

## Small Animal Dosage

**Dogs and Cats**

- Start with 1 mg/kg q24h PO and increase to 2 mg/kg in refractory patients.

## Large Animal Dosage

- No dose has been reported for large animals.

## Regulatory Information

No regulatory information is available. For extralabel use withdrawal interval estimates, contact FARAD at www.FARAD.org.

# Ascorbic Acid
ah-skor'bik ass'id

**Trade and other names:** Vitamin C and sodium ascorbate. Many brand names are available.

**Functional classification:** Vitamin

## Pharmacology and Mechanism of Action

Ascorbic acid is vitamin C. It is an important cofactor in a variety of metabolic functions. Vitamin C is used as a supplement in vitamin-deficient animals.

## Indications and Clinical Uses

Ascorbic acid is used to treat vitamin C deficiency and occasionally used as a urine acidifier. Dogs are capable of synthesizing vitamin C, but it is used as a supplement to improve health and performance. There are insufficient data to show that ascorbic acid is effective for preventing cancer, treating infectious diseases, or preventing cardiovascular disease.

## Precautionary Information

**Adverse Reactions and Side Effects**

Adverse effects have not been reported in animals. High doses may increase the risk of oxalate urolith formation.

**Contraindications and Precautions**
No contraindications reported for animals.

**Drug Interactions**
No drug interactions are reported in animals.

## Instructions for Use
Not necessary to supplement in animals with well-balanced diets. However, high doses have been used as adjunctive treatment for some diseases. Evidence shows that at doses of 15 and 50 mg/kg in dogs, the increase in absorption is nonlinear. Therefore, higher doses may not produce proportionately higher blood levels to the lower doses. Comparison of crystalline ascorbic acid and the vitamin C product, Ester-C, produced similar levels of vitamin C in the plasma.

## Patient Monitoring and Laboratory Tests
No specific monitoring is necessary.

## Formulations
- Ascorbic acid is available in tablets of various sizes and injections. Typically, the injection form is 250 mg sodium ascorbate/mL. The formulation of Ester-C appears to be absorbed similarly to the crystalline form of vitamin C.

## Stability and Storage
Light sensitive. It oxidizes, darkens, and decomposes when exposed to air and light. The injectable solution in a vial may build up pressure with storage, which may be decreased by storing in a refrigerator. Otherwise, store at room temperature protected from light.

## Small Animal Dosage
### Dogs and Cats
- Dietary supplementation: 100–500 mg/animal/day PO.
- Urinary acidification: 100 mg/animal q8h PO. Injectable dose ranges from 1 to 10 mL (250 mg/mL), depending on size of animal, IM or IV.
- For treatment of oxidative stress: Dogs: 500–1000 mg/dog q24h, PO; cats: 125 mg/cat, PO, q12h.

### Guinea pigs
- 16 mg/kg twice weekly IM to treat vitamin deficiency.

## Large Animal Dosage
- Vitamin C supplementation: 1–10 mL IM or IV. Repeat daily as needed.
- 1–2 g q24h PO.

## Regulatory Information
Withdrawal time: 0 days for all animals intended for food.

# Asparaginase (L-Asparaginase)
ah-spar′a-jin-aze

**Trade and other names:** Elspar and Asparaginase
**Functional classification:** Anticancer agent

## Pharmacology and Mechanism of Action

Anticancer agent. Neoplastic cells are deficient in asparagine synthase and require extracellular asparagine for DNA and RNA synthesis. L-asparaginase destroys asparagine. Normal cells are capable of synthesizing their own asparagine, but certain malignant cells, especially malignant lymphocytes, are not. Therefore, asparagine is an essential amino acid for cancer cell survival, particularly malignant lymphocytes. Because cancer cells in patients treated with L-asparaginase are depleted of asparagine, this treatment interferes with DNA, RNA, and protein synthesis in cancer cells. It is cell-cycle-specific for the G1 phase of the cell cycle. In dogs, it has a long half-life of 1–2 days.

## Indications and Clinical Uses

Asparaginase has been used in some lymphoma protocols and has been effective for melanoma and mast cell tumors. It has been administered IV, IM, or SQ, but IM administration is preferred over SQ administration. In cats, it also has been used in combination cancer protocols.

### Precautionary Information

**Adverse Reactions and Side Effects**

Asparaginase is a foreign bacterial protein and can cause allergic reactions. Therefore, the most common adverse effect is hypersensitivity (allergic) reactions. Animals have tolerated initial doses but developed hypersensitivity after repeated injections. Hepatotoxic reactions, pancreatitis, and hyperglycemia also have been reported. In some dogs, although rare, increases in ammonia are possible that can lead to hyperammonemic encephalopathy.

**Contraindications and Precautions**

Do not use in animals with known sensitivity (allergic reaction).

**Drug Interactions**

No drug interactions are reported in animals. It has been used with other anticancer drugs.

## Instructions for Use

Asparaginase is usually used in combination with other drugs in cancer chemotherapy protocols (e.g., doxorubicin). IM administration has been more effective than SQ dosing in dogs with lymphoma. Asparaginase has minimal effect on the bone marrow; therefore, it can be used in combination with other myelosuppressive drugs in a protocol. Although it has been used in anticancer protocols, it has shown no benefit when added to cyclophosphamide, doxorubicin, vincristine, and prednisone (CHOP) protocols for lymphoma. Tumor cells can develop resistance by developing a capacity to synthesize asparagine. In cats, it has been used in combination protocols at a dosage of 400 units/kg SQ on day 1 of protocols combined with doxorubicin.

## Patient Monitoring and Laboratory Tests

Monitoring CBC during chemotherapy is recommended.

## Formulations

- Asparaginase is available in 10,000 units per vial for injection. The human form (Elspar) was discontinued in 2012. Distribution of this drug to veterinarians by the manufacturer may be limited, and some pharmacies have prepared compounded formulations. In one study, the compounded formulation was effective in 80% of the cases.

## Stability and Storage
Stable if stored in manufacturer's original vial.

**A**

## Small Animal Dosage
**Dogs (Two-dose regimens have been used.)**
- 400 units/kg SQ or IM weekly.
- 10,000 units/m$^2$ weekly SQ or IM for 3 weeks.

**Cats**
- 400 units/kg weekly SQ or IM.

## Large Animal Dosage
- No dose has been reported for large animals.

## Regulatory Information
Withdrawal times are not established for animals that produce food. This drug should not be used in animals that produce food because it is an anticancer agent.

# Aspirin
as′pir-in

**Trade and other names:** ASA, acetylsalicylic acid, Bufferin, Ascriptin, and many generic brands

**Functional classification:** Nonsteroidal anti-inflammatory drug

## Pharmacology and Mechanism of Action
Nonsteroidal anti-inflammatory drug. Anti-inflammatory action is caused by inhibition of prostaglandins. Aspirin binds irreversibly to the COX enzyme in tissues to inhibit synthesis of prostaglandins. At low doses, it is more specific for COX-1 than COX-2. The sensitivity of COX-1 over COX-2 is the explanation for low aspirin doses used as antiplatelet treatment. However, in some animals, even low-dose aspirin does not inhibit platelet aggregation, possibly because COX-2 can be an additional source of thromboxane (TXA2). Anti-inflammatory effects are attributed to inhibition of COX, but other anti-inflammatory mechanisms attributed to salicylates may also contribute to the anti-inflammatory action, such as inhibition of nuclear factor kappa-β.

*Pharmacokinetics:* The pharmacokinetics are variable in animals with a half-life that ranges from 1 hour in horses, 6 hours in pigs, and 8.5 hours in dogs to 38 hours in cats.

## Indications and Clinical Uses
Aspirin is used as an analgesic, anti-inflammatory, and antiplatelet drug. Aspirin has a long history of use for treating pain and inflammation, especially associated with osteoarthritis. Although it may be effective in animals, other agents specifically approved for animals are much more commonly used nowadays for osteoarthritis and other painful conditions.

At low doses, aspirin is a more specific COX-1 selective inhibitor and antiplatelet drug than other NSAIDs. Therefore, low doses have been used in animals to inhibit platelets and prevent thromboemboli formation. Inhibition of platelets is justified for some diseases because as platelets become hyper-reactive, they can release serotonin and other mediators that may exacerbate vascular diseases and produce blood clots. Although these low doses of aspirin are often used for antiplatelet therapy, aspirin does not provide complete inhibition of platelet stimulation. Low doses (e.g., 1–5 mg/kg) produce inconsistent platelet inhibition in dogs and cats. Some animals are refractory (*aspirin resistance*). Addition of other antiplatelet drugs such as clopidogrel (Plavix) provides more effective inhibition.

Aspirin has been used to prevent complications from heartworm disease (thromboemboli). However, there is no convincing evidence that there is a clinical benefit from this treatment. Some evidence indicates that aspirin may be contraindicated in heartworm disease.

In cats, exposure of feline platelets in vitro to aspirin can have an inhibitory effect. Platelets collected from cats ex vivo after treatment with aspirin (5 mg/kg) had decreased TXA2 production, but platelet aggregation was not affected.

Although aspirin has been available for many years, it is not registered by the Food and Drug Administration (FDA) for use in any species. There are no published controlled studies to document efficacy. Use of aspirin in animals is primarily based on empiricism rather than on published data.

## Precautionary Information
### Adverse Reactions and Side Effects
Narrow therapeutic index. High doses frequently cause vomiting. Other GI effects can include ulceration and bleeding. Aspirin may inhibit platelets and increases risk of bleeding.

### Contraindications and Precautions
Cats are susceptible to salicylate intoxication because of slow clearance. Use cautiously in patients with coagulopathies because of platelet inhibition (e.g., von Willebrand disease). Do not administer to animals prone to GI ulcers.

### Drug Interactions
Some animals are more susceptible to the gastric effects of aspirin if corticosteroids are included in the protocol. Do not administer with other drugs that may cause coagulopathy and increase risk of bleeding problems.

## Instructions for Use
Analgesic and anti-inflammatory doses have primarily been derived from empiricism. Antiplatelet doses are lower because of potent and prolonged effect of aspirin on platelets. The dosing section lists "antiplatelet" doses for aspirin in dogs and cats, but the efficacy of these doses has not been verified through clinical studies. Results from research animals have produced varied results. In some studies, 5–10 mg/kg was considered a consistent antiplatelet dose for dogs; in other studies, 1 mg/kg inhibited platelets in only one third of dogs; and in research dogs, doses as low as 0.5 mg/kg q12h impaired platelet aggregation.

Aspirin is only available in oral form. Because it is a weak acid, it is ordinarily absorbed best in the acidic environment of the upper GI tract; however, considerable absorption also takes place farther in the intestine. In dogs, enteric-coated aspirin reduces gastric irritation, but absorption from this form is erratic and often incomplete. Buffering does not affect absorption but may protect the stomach from injury when high doses are administered. Buffering has less of a beneficial effect when low doses are administered and is not expected to protect the stomach from the more serious effects of GI ulceration, bleeding, and perforations.

## Patient Monitoring and Laboratory Tests

Monitor patients for signs of gastric upset, gastroduodenal ulcers, and bleeding. Effective plasma concentrations: 20–50 mcg/mL for pain and fever and 150–200 mcg/mL for inflammation. Aspirin decreased thyroid concentrations ($T_4$, $T_3$, and free $T_4$) in dogs after 2–4 weeks of dosing but returned to normal in 14 days.

## Formulations

- Aspirin is available in 81-mg (children's aspirin) and 325-mg tablets.
- For large animals, aspirin is available in a 240-grain bolus (14,400 mg) and 3.9-, 15.6-, and 31.2-g tablets.
- Extended-release form for antiplatelet treatment (Durlaza): 16.2 mg capsule. (Do not open or break capsule.)

## Stability and Storage

Store in a tightly sealed container at room temperature. After exposure to moisture, it decomposes to acetic acid and salicylic acid. If stored at pH 7 at 25°C, it has a half-life of 52 hours.

## Small Animal Dosage

### Mild Analgesia

*Dogs*
- 10 mg/kg q12h PO.

*Cats*
- 10 mg/kg q48h PO.

### Anti-inflammatory

*Dogs*
- 20–25 mg/kg q12h PO.

*Cats*
- 10–20 mg/kg q48h PO.

### Antiplatelet

*Dogs*
- Typical doses are in the range of 1–5 mg/kg but have been as high as 5–10 mg/kg q24–48h PO to obtain a greater response. (Convincing evidence of a consistent antiplatelet clinical benefit in dogs is lacking.)

*Cats*
- 80 mg/cat q48h PO. Doses have ranged from 5 mg per cat q72h to 80 mg per cat (one tablet) q72h. No clinical studies have documented efficacy from either dose.

## Large Animal Dosage

### Ruminants

- 100 mg/kg q12h PO. Doses as high as 333 mg/kg have been administered to cattle.

### Swine

- 10 mg/kg q6–8h PO.

### Horses

- 25–50 mg/kg q12h PO (up to 100 mg/kg PO per day).

## Regulatory Information

Extralabel use: Although considered extralabel in animals intended for food, consider a withdrawal time of at least 1 day for meat and 24 hours for milk.

RCI Classification: 4

# Atenolol

ah-ten´oe-lole

**Trade and other names:** Tenormin

**Functional classification:** Beta-antagonist

## Pharmacology and Mechanism of Action

Beta-adrenergic blocker. Relatively selective for beta₁-receptor. Atenolol is a water-soluble beta blocker and relies on the kidneys for clearance. (By comparison, drugs such as propranolol and metoprolol are more lipophilic and rely on the liver for clearance.)

*Pharmacokinetics:* In dogs and cats, oral absorption is 90%. In cats, the half-life is approximately 4–5 hours, with a peak concentration of 1.4–1.9 mcg/mL after a dose of 2.5 mg/kg.

## Indications and Clinical Uses

Atenolol is one of the most commonly administered beta blockers for dogs and cats. Atenolol is used primarily as an antiarrhythmic or for other cardiovascular conditions in which it is needed to slow the sinus rate. In cats, this drug is commonly used to treat heart disease from cardiomyopathy or hyperthyroidism, but it should not be used as monotherapy to treat primary hypertension. Although it is commonly administered to cats with hypertrophic cardiomyopathy to improve clinical signs, it did not slow progression of the disease. In dogs, it has been used for congenital cardiac conditions such as subaortic stenosis and pulmonary stenosis (0.5–1 mg/kg q12h).

## Precautionary Information

### Adverse Reactions and Side Effects

Bradycardia and heart block are possible. Atenolol may produce bronchospasm in sensitive patients.

### Contraindications and Precautions

Use cautiously in animals with airway disease, myocardial failure, and cardiac conduction disturbances. Use cautiously in animals with low cardiac reserve.

### Drug Interactions

Use cautiously with other drugs that may decrease cardiac contraction or heart rate.

## Instructions for Use

Atenolol is reported to be less affected by changes in hepatic metabolism than other beta blockers. Although it is not an FDA-approved drug for dogs and cats, dosing guidelines are based on published reports and experience of experts. In cats, amlodipine (calcium-channel blocker) may be used with atenolol to control hypertension. When administered as a transdermal gel to cats, it produced inconsistent and lower plasma concentrations compared to oral administration.

## Patient Monitoring and Laboratory Tests

Monitor patient's heart rate and rhythm. Although plasma and serum concentrations are not typically monitored, a concentration above 0.26 mcg/mL has been proposed as a target threshold for effective adrenergic beta-receptor blockade.

## Formulations
- Atenolol is available in 25-, 50-, and 100-mg tablets. (Tablets can be split for small animals.)

## Stability and Storage
Store in a tightly sealed container at room temperature. Studies using a compounded flavored oral paste and oral suspension formulation for cats produced similar beta-adrenergic blocking effects as a commercial tablet (2.5 mg/kg). Stability studies indicate that extemporaneously prepared oral suspensions are stable for 14 days, and some compounded oral formulations have been stable for 60 days. Consult compounding pharmacist for beyond-use-day of prepared compounded formulations. Atenolol is water soluble and can be mixed with other water-based vehicles.

## Small Animal Dosage
### Dogs
- 6.25–12.5 mg/dog q12–24h (or 0.25–1.0 mg/kg q12–24h) PO. Start with 1 mg/kg PO q12h initially and lower dose as needed to maintain optimum heart rate. However, doses in dogs also have been increased to 3 mg/kg q12–24h PO for some conditions.

### Cats
- 1–2 mg/kg q12h PO. However, because of tablet size, a common dosage is 6.25–12.5 mg/cat q12–24h PO (one quarter or one half tablet).

## Large Animal Dosage
- No dose has been reported for large animals.

## Regulatory Information
No regulatory information is available. For extralabel use withdrawal interval estimates, contact FARAD at www.FARAD.org.

RCI Classification: 3

# Atipamezole Hydrochloride
ah-tih-pam´eh-zole hye-droe-klor´ide

**Trade and other names:** Antisedan

**Functional classification:** Anesthetic

## Pharmacology and Mechanism of Action
Alpha$_2$-antagonist. It binds to alpha$_2$-receptors to antagonize other drugs that act as agonists, such as dexmedetomidine, medetomidine, and xylazine. Other alpha$_2$-antagonists include yohimbine, but atipamezole is more specific for the alpha$_2$-receptor.

## Indications and Clinical Uses
Atipamezole is used to reverse alpha$_2$-agonists such as dexmedetomidine (Dexdomitor), medetomidine (Domitor), detomidine, and xylazine. Arousal from sedation should occur within 5–10 minutes of injection. It also can be used to reverse sedation caused by amitraz intoxication. In horses, it provides a satisfactory but incomplete reversal of detomidine.

## Precautionary Information

### Adverse Reactions and Side Effects

Atipamezole can cause initial excitement in some animals shortly after reversal. There may be a transient decrease in blood pressure after injection. In horses, it can produce a dose-dependent increase in sweating and hyperexcitability that resolved after 10–15 minutes.

### Contraindications and Precautions

No contraindications reported for animals.

### Drug Interactions

Atipamezole is an alpha$_2$-antagonist. As such, it antagonizes other drugs that bind to the alpha-receptor and prevents their action. Such drugs that may be antagonized include xylazine, medetomidine, dexmedetomidine, romifidine, detomidine, and some alpha$_1$-agonists.

## Instructions for Use

When used to reverse dexmedetomidine or medetomidine, inject the same volume of atipamezole as the volume of dexmedetomidine or medetomidine that was administered. In horses, a wide range of doses has been used (see the dosing section). Typically, the higher dose is more effective for detomidine, but tolazoline antagonizes detomidine in horses more completely and hastens recovery better than atipamezole.

## Patient Monitoring and Laboratory Tests

Monitor cardiovascular status when using alpha$_2$-agonists. Providing oxygen during recovery may help recovery from alpha$_2$-agonists.

## Formulations

• Atipamezole is available in a 5-mg/mL injection.

## Stability and Storage

Store in a tightly sealed container, protected from light, and at room temperature. Stability of compounded formulations has not been evaluated.

## Small Animal Dosage

• Inject the same volume as used for dexmedetomidine or medetomidine. The range of doses (IM or IV) is 0.32 mg/kg for small animals (4 kg, or 8.8 lb), 0.23 mg/kg for medium-sized animals (11 kg, or 24 lb), and up to 0.14 mg/kg for large-sized animals (45 kg or 100 lb).

## Large Animal Dosage

• Horses: The dosage used in horses is 60–80 mcg/kg (0.06–0.08 mg/kg) IV but has ranged up to 150 mcg/kg (0.15 mg/kg). Typically, 100 mcg/kg (0.1 mg/kg) IV is used to reverse detomidine.

## Regulatory Information

Do not administer to animals intended for food.

# Atovaquone

a-toe´-va-kwone´

**Trade and other names:** Mepron

**Functional classification:** Antibacterial, antiprotozoal

## Pharmacology and Mechanism of Action

A

Atovaquone is an antimicrobial agent, an analogue of ubiquinone, that inhibits mitochondrial transport in protozoa by targeting the cytochrome $bc_1$ complex. It also inhibits nucleic acid and adenosine triphosphate (ATP) synthesis in susceptible cells. Atovaquone is active against protozoa such as *Pneumocystis,* for which it is used in people. In cats, it is used to treat *Cytauxzoon felis.* It may not eradicate *Cytauxzoon* but it decreases the parasite burden. In dogs, it has been used to treat *Babesia gibsoni* infections. For treating these infections in dogs and cats, it appears to have an additive or synergistic effect when combined with azithromycin. It is highly lipophilic. Oral absorption in animals is almost 50% but is increased with feeding. The half-life in people is very long (67–77 hours) but is not reported for animals.

## Indications and Clinical Uses

In people, atovaquone is an antiprotozoal that is primarily used in individuals who cannot tolerate sulfonamides. In animals, it has been used, often in combination with azithromycin, to treat refractory protozoan diseases and blood-borne pathogens. It is the drug of choice for the treatment of *B. gibsoni* infections in combination with azithromycin.

Administer with high-fat meal to increase oral absorption.

### Precautionary Information

#### Adverse Reactions and Side Effects

One formulation (Malarone) also contains proguanil HCl. It may increase the risk of diarrhea in dogs when combined with proguanil. Otherwise, adverse effects have not been reported in animals. In people, adverse reactions consist of skin rash, cough, and diarrhea.

#### Contraindications and Precautions

Avoid use in pregnancy.

#### Drug Interactions

No drug interactions are reported in animals. In people, coadministration with rifampin decreases effective concentrations.

## Instructions for Use

There has been only limited experience with use of atovaquone for treatment of infections in animals. A few clinical trials have shown efficacy when combined with azithromycin for treatment of protozoa infections.

## Patient Monitoring and Laboratory Tests

No specific monitoring is necessary.

## Formulations

- Atovaquone is available as a 750-mg/5-mL liquid oral suspension (150 mg/mL). The 250-mg tablets have been discontinued, but it has been compounded into 250 capsules by some compounding pharmacies.

## Stability and Storage

Store at room temperature protected from light. Do not freeze.

## Small Animal Dosage

### Cats

- 15 mg/kg q8h PO in combination with azithromycin (10 mg/kg q24h).

**Dogs**
- Antiprotozoal treatment: 13–15 mg/kg q8h PO for 10 days, usually in combination with azithromycin (10 mg/kg q24h PO).

**Large Animal Dosage**
- No dose reported.

**Regulatory Information**
There is no withdrawal time established for food animals.

## Atracurium Besylate
ah-trah-kyoor´ee-um bess´ih-late

**Trade and other names:** Tracrium

**Functional classification:** Muscle relaxant

### Pharmacology and Mechanism of Action
Neuromuscular blocking agent (nondepolarizing). Atracurium competes with acetylcholine at the neuromuscular end plate. It is used primarily during anesthesia or other conditions in which it is necessary to inhibit muscle contractions. It has a shorter duration of action than pancuronium.

### Indications and Clinical Uses
Atracurium is a paralytic agent used to paralyze skeletal muscle during surgery and mechanical ventilation.

### Precautionary Information

**Adverse Reactions and Side Effects**

Atracurium produces respiratory depression and paralysis. Neuromuscular-blocking drugs have no effect on analgesia.

**Contraindications and Precautions**

Do not use in patients unless it is possible to provide ventilation support. The action of neuromuscular-blocking agents may be antagonized by acetylcholinesterase inhibitors.

**Drug Interactions**

Gentamicin (and possibly other aminoglycosides) potentiates neuromuscular blockade (gentamicin acts at the presynaptic site to decrease release of acetylcholine). No other drug interactions are reported in animals.

### Instructions for Use
Administer only in situations in which careful control of respiration is possible. Doses may need to be individualized for optimum effect. Do not mix with alkalinizing solutions or lactated Ringer's solution.

### Patient Monitoring and Laboratory Tests
Monitoring of respiratory and cardiovascular indices is critical during use. If possible, monitor the oxygenation of the patient during use.

### Formulations
- Atracurium is available in 10-mg/mL injection.

## Stability and Storage
Store in a tightly sealed container, protected from light, and at room temperature. Stability of compounded formulations has not been evaluated.

## Small Animal Dosage
**Dogs and Cats**
- 0.2 mg/kg IV initially; then 0.15 mg/kg q30min.
- CRI: 0.3–0.5 mg/kg IV loading dose followed by 4–9 mcg/kg/min.

## Large Animal Dosage
**Horses**
- 0.05–0.07 mg/kg IV.

## Regulatory Information
Do not administer to animals intended for food.

# Atropine Sulfate
ah'troe-peen sul'fate

**Trade and other names:** Generic brands

**Functional classification:** Anticholinergic

## Pharmacology and Mechanism of Action
Anticholinergic agent (blocks acetylcholine effect at muscarinic receptors), parasympatholytic.

As an antimuscarinic agent, it blocks cholinergic stimulation and causes decrease in GI motility and secretions, decrease in respiratory secretions, increased heart rate (antivagal effect), and mydriasis.

## Indications and Clinical Uses
Atropine is used primarily as an adjunct to anesthesia or other procedures to increase heart rate and decrease respiratory and GI secretions. Atropine is the drug of choice to overcome excess vagal stimulation associated with some clinical conditions. Atropine is used during cardiac arrest to overcome vagal influences. Atropine is also used as an antidote for organophosphate intoxication. In horses, atropine (single dose) may be used to relieve bronchoconstriction in horses with recurrent airway obstruction, also known as equine asthma syndrome. For this use, only a single dose is recommended. N-butylscopolammonium bromide (Buscopan) also is used for this indication.

## Precautionary Information
**Adverse Reactions and Side Effects**
Side effects include xerostomia, ileus, constipation, tachycardia, and urine retention.

**Contraindications and Precautions**
Do not use in patients with glaucoma, intestinal ileus, gastroparesis, or tachycardia. Use high doses (e.g., 0.04 mg/kg) cautiously because it increases oxygen demand.

**Drug Interactions**
Do not mix with alkaline solutions. Atropine antagonizes the effects of any cholinergic drugs administered (e.g., metoclopramide).

## Instructions for Use

Atropine is used ordinarily as an adjunct with anesthesia or other procedures. Compared with lower doses, in dogs, 0.06 mg/kg was more effective than 0.02 mg/kg. Atropine may be used during cardiac resuscitation; however, high doses may cause sustained tachycardia and increased myocardial oxygen demand. During cardiac resuscitation, doses of 0.04 mg/kg IV may be used, but for treating sinus bradycardia, consider lower doses of 0.01 mg/kg.

## Patient Monitoring and Laboratory Tests

Monitor patient's heart rate and rhythm.

## Formulations

- Atropine is available in 400-, 500-, and 540-mcg/mL injection and 15-mg/mL injection.

## Stability and Storage

Store in a tightly sealed container at room temperature.

## Small Animal Dosage

### Dogs

- 0.02–0.04 mg/kg q6–8h IV, IM, or SQ (complete dose range has been from 0.01 mg/kg to 0.06 mg/kg, depending on the indication).
- Sinus bradycardia: 0.005–0.01 mg/kg, but for use during cardiopulmonary resuscitation, up to 0.04 mg/kg.
- Cardiac arrest: 0.04 mg/kg IV (with other supportive measures).

### Cats

- 0.02–0.04 mg/kg q6–8h IV, IM, or SQ.

### Dogs

- For organophosphate and carbamate toxicosis: 0.2–0.5 mg/kg as needed, IV, IM, or SQ.

### Cats

- For organophosphate and carbamate toxicosis: 0.2–0.5 mg/kg as needed, IV, IM, or SQ.

## Large Animal Dosage

Note that in large animals, atropine has a potent effect on inhibiting GI motility.

### Horses

- Antidote to organophosphates or cholinesterase inhibitors: 0.02–0.04 mg/kg IM or SQ; repeat as needed.
- Equine asthma syndrome and recurrent airway obstruction: 0.022 mg/kg, once, IV.

### Pigs

- Antidote to organophosphates or cholinesterase inhibitors: 0.1 mg/kg IV followed by 0.4 mg/kg IM.
- Anesthesia adjunct: 0.02 mg/kg IV or 0.04 mg/kg IM.

### Ruminants

- Antidote to organophosphates or cholinesterase inhibitors: 0.1 mg/kg IV followed by 0.4 mg/kg IM; repeat as needed.
- Anesthesia adjunct to prevent salivation: 0.02 mg/kg IV or 0.04 mg/kg IM.

## Regulatory Information

Withdrawal time: None established in the United States. The manufacturer of large animal products lists 0 days for milk and meat; however, it is listed as 3 days for milk and 14 days for meat in the United Kingdom.

RCI Classification: 3

# Auranofin

or-an′oe-fin

**Trade and other names:** Ridaura

**Functional classification:** Immunosuppressive

## Pharmacology and Mechanism of Action

Used for gold therapy (chrysotherapy). Mechanism of action is unknown but may relate to immunosuppressive effect on lymphocytes.

## Indications and Clinical Uses

Auranofin (gold therapy) is used primarily for immune-mediated diseases. It has been used with some success to control immune-mediated skin diseases, such as pemphigus and immune-mediated arthritis, but evidence of efficacy is lacking for small animal therapy. It has been observed by some clinicians that this product (oral) is not as effective as injectable products such as aurothioglucose.

Auranofin has activity against some protozoan parasites, but the efficacy for treating protozoa, or optimum dose, has not been established in animals.

## Precautionary Information

**Adverse Reactions and Side Effects**

Adverse effects include dermatitis, nephrotoxicity, and blood dyscrasias.

**Contraindications and Precautions**

Do not use in animals with suppressed bone marrow or in animals already receiving bone marrow–suppressing agents.

**Drug Interactions**

No drug interactions are reported in animals.

## Instructions for Use

Use of this drug has not been evaluated in veterinary medicine. No controlled clinical trials are available to determine efficacy in animals. The use in animals is based on anecdotal experience and small observational reports.

## Patient Monitoring and Laboratory Tests

Monitor patient's CBC periodically because gold salts have caused blood dyscrasias.

## Formulations

- Auranofin is available in 3-mg capsules but has been discontinued by some manufacturers.

## Stability and Storage

Store in a tightly sealed container, protected from light, and at room temperature. Stability of compounded formulations has not been evaluated.

## Small Animal Dosage
**Dogs and Cats**
- 0.1–0.2 mg/kg q12h PO.

## Large Animal Dosage
- No dose has been reported for large animals.

## Regulatory Information
Do not administer to animals intended for food.

# Aurothioglucose
or-oh-thye-oe-gloo´kose

**Trade and other names:** Solganal

**Functional classification:** Immunosuppressive

## Pharmacology and Mechanism of Action
Used for gold therapy (chrysotherapy). Mechanism of action is unknown but may relate to immunosuppressive effect on lymphocytes.

## Indications and Clinical Uses
Aurothioglucose (gold therapy) is used primarily for immune-mediated diseases. It has been used with some success to control immune-mediated skin diseases, such as pemphigus and immune-mediated arthritis. However, because of a lack of controlled trials to demonstrate efficacy and adverse effects that have been observed, the use in veterinary medicine has been uncommon.

## Precautionary Information
**Adverse Reactions and Side Effects**
Adverse effects include dermatitis, nephrotoxicity, and blood dyscrasias.

**Contraindications and Precautions**
Do not use in animals with suppressed bone marrow or animals already receiving bone marrow–suppressing agents.

**Drug Interactions**
No drug interactions are reported in animals.

## Instructions for Use
Use of this drug has not been evaluated in veterinary medicine. No controlled clinical trials are available to determine efficacy in animals. This drug is often used in combination with other immunosuppressive drugs such as corticosteroids.

## Patient Monitoring and Laboratory Tests
Monitor patient's CBC periodically because gold salts have caused blood dyscrasias.

## Formulations
- Aurothioglucose has been discontinued and is no longer available. However, some forms still persist (e.g., from compounding pharmacies) in a 50-mg/mL injection.

## Stability and Storage
Store in a tightly sealed container, protected from light, and at room temperature. The stability of compounded formulations has not been evaluated.

## Small Animal Dosage
### Dogs
- Dogs weighing less than 10 kg: 1 mg IM first week, 2 mg IM second week, 1 mg/kg/wk maintenance. Dogs weighing more than 10 kg: 5 mg IM first week, 10 mg IM second week, 1 mg/kg/wk maintenance.

### Cats
- 0.5–1 mg/cat every 7 days IM.

## Large Animal Dosage
### Horses
- 1 mg/kg/wk IM.

## Regulatory Information
Do not administer to animals intended for food.

---

# Azathioprine
ay-za-thye'oe-preen

**Trade and other names:** Imuran and generic

**Functional classification:** Immunosuppressive

---

## Pharmacology and Mechanism of Action
Thiopurine immunosuppressive drug. Acts to inhibit T-cell lymphocyte proliferation. It is active against T cells and B cells and can block both T- and B-cell activation, thus producing immunosuppressive activity. The exact mechanism of action is not known. Azathioprine is initially spontaneously metabolized to 6-mercaptopurine (6-MP). The metabolite 6-MP is further metabolized via thiopurine methyltransferase (TPMT) to 6-methylmercaptopurine (6-MMP), which may be associated with adverse effects, such as liver injury. It is also metabolized via TPMT to other metabolites, including the 6-thioguanine nucleotide (6-TG), which may be responsible for the immunosuppressive effects because it can accumulate in cells and acts as a purine antagonist that disrupts DNA in leukocytes. The concentrations of 6-TG are correlated with therapeutic efficacy. Other cells can use salvage pathways for purine synthesis, but stimulated lymphocytes are not capable of this synthesis.

## Indications and Clinical Uses
Azathioprine is used to treat various immune-mediated diseases in animals, including immune-mediated hemolytic anemia, pemphigus, and inflammatory bowel disease. It is often the first drug of choice, in addition to corticosteroids, for treatment of immune-mediated hemolytic anemia and pemphigus in dogs and is often used for inflammatory bowel disease. It is usually combined with prednisone or prednisolone treatment, but benefits of this combination compared with each drug administered alone has not been confirmed. It is primarily used in dogs and is not recommended in cats. There are some case reports for its successful use to treat immune-mediated disease in horses, but experience is limited. Onset of action is delayed for 4–6 weeks in some human patients. The onset of effects in animals has not been determined, but observations indicate that it occurs more quickly than in people.

## Precautionary Information

### Adverse Reactions and Side Effects

Bone marrow suppression is the most serious concern. Additional adverse effects in dogs include diarrhea, increased risk of secondary infections, and vomiting. Hepatotoxicosis after administration of azathioprine also has been reported. Toxicity may be related to the metabolites, particularly 6-MMP. The incidence of hepatotoxicity may occur in dogs after the first 2–4 weeks of treatment; therefore, this is the most critical time to monitor liver enzymes and bilirubin.

Individuals who have higher sensitivity to the suppressing effects of bone marrow should have the dose reduced. There has been some association with development of pancreatitis when administered with corticosteroids, but this has not been confirmed.

Susceptibility to the adverse effects, and prediction of therapeutic effects in people may be correlated with the levels of the metabolizing enzyme, TPMT. Some people are deficient and have a higher incidence of adverse effects. However, the TPMT levels in dogs are variable and have not been associated with either hepatotoxicity or myelotoxicity. Cats are deficient in TPMT and are particularly susceptible to toxicity.

### Contraindications and Precautions

Ordinarily, it should not be administered to cats, but if treatment is attempted, exercise extreme caution and careful monitoring.

### Drug Interactions

Administer with caution with other drugs that may suppress the bone marrow (e.g., cyclophosphamide and anticancer drugs). There is some evidence that concurrent use with corticosteroids may increase the risk of pancreatitis. Do not administer with allopurinol because antagonism of xanthine oxidase may interfere with metabolism.

## Instructions for Use

Azathioprine is usually used in combination with other immunosuppressive drugs (e.g., corticosteroids) to treat immune-mediated disease. Cats are very sensitive to the bone marrow–suppressing effects of azathioprine. Doses of 2.2 mg/kg to cats have produced toxicity, but some veterinarians have used low dosages of 0.3 mg/kg/day. Alternatively, chlorambucil has been used instead of azathioprine in cats when immunosuppressive action is needed.

## Patient Monitoring and Laboratory Tests

Monitor patient's CBC periodically because some animals are sensitive to the effects of azathioprine and its metabolite, 6-MP. After 2 weeks of treatment, a CBC is essential. Because of risk of hepatotoxicity, monitor hepatic enzymes and bilirubin regularly.

## Formulations

Azathioprine is available in 25-, 50-, 75-, and 100-mg tablets and 10-mg/mL for injection.

## Stability and Storage

Store in a tightly sealed container at room temperature. Compounded oral suspensions are stable for 60 days.

## Small Animal Dosage

### Dogs

- 2 mg/kg q24h PO initially; then 0.5–1 mg/kg q48h. In dogs, dosages as high as 1.5 mg/kg q48h PO have been used with prednisolone.

### Cats (use cautiously)

- Cats are sensitive to bone marrow–suppressing effects, and many clinicians avoid azathioprine in cats altogether. However, if administered to cats, one should start with 0.3 mg/kg q24h PO and adjust the dose to q48h after careful monitoring. Tablet size may be as low as 1/30th to 1/50th of a tablet, which requires careful compounding.

## Large Animal Dosage

### Horses

- 3 mg/kg, PO, q24h.

## Regulatory Information

Do not administer to animals intended for food.

# Azithromycin
ay-zith-roe-my´sin

**Trade and other names:** Zithromax

**Functional classification:** Antibacterial

## Pharmacology and Mechanism of Action

Azalide antibiotic. Similar mechanism of action as macrolides (e.g., erythromycin), which is to inhibit bacteria protein synthesis via inhibition of ribosomal activity. Spectrum of activity is primarily gram-positive cocci, including streptococci and staphylococci. It also has good activity against *Mycoplasma* spp., *Chlamydia* spp., and some intracellular pathogens. The activity against *Toxoplasma* spp. has been questionable.

Azithromycin, like other macrolides, exerts therapeutic benefits not solely explainable by antibacterial activity. Azithromycin has multiple immunomodulatory effects that likely contribute to the therapeutic response in respiratory infections and perhaps other diseases. Even with infections caused by organisms not susceptible to azithromycin in vitro, such as infections caused by *Pseudomonas aeruginosa*, azithromycin has produced benefits by decreasing the virulence properties of the organism (e.g., inhibition of quorum sensing and inhibition of biofilm). Other beneficial effects may be caused by enhanced degranulation and apoptosis of neutrophils and inhibition of inflammatory cytokine production. It also may help clear infections by enhancing macrophage functions.

*Pharmacokinetics:* Pharmacokinetic data show extremely long plasma, tissue, and leukocyte half-lives in dogs, cats, and horses. It is minimally metabolized, and very little active drug is excreted in the urine. Plasma half-life is 15–18 hours in horses, 35 hours in cats, and 30 hours in dogs. The volume of distribution also is large, with values exceeding 10 L/kg. Oral absorption in dogs is 90% but less in cats (58%) and horses (40%–45%). Azithromycin, like other long-acting macrolides, is characterized by low plasma drug concentrations, but much higher (100–200×) concentrations in leukocytes, bronchial secretions, and some tissues.

## Indications and Clinical Uses

Azithromycin is indicated for treatment of bacterial infections. It also has been used in people for a variety of respiratory infections in which the benefits are believed to be partially, if not predominantly, caused by the immunomodulatory properties. Antimicrobial spectrum is primarily against gram-positive bacteria. Azithromycin is not recommended for serious gram-negative infections. It may be used to treat infections caused by *Mycoplasma* and other atypical organisms.

Azithromycin has been used to treat intracellular organisms because of its ability to concentrate in leukocytes. One of the uses has been to treat infections caused by *Rhodococcus equi* in foals. However, in one comparative study, clarithromycin plus rifampin had better clinical success in foals than azithromycin plus rifampin. In foals, azithromycin, administered at a dosage of 10 mg/kg q48h oral during the first 2 weeks after birth has been used prophylactically to decrease *Rhodococcus* spp. infection in foals at high risk (farms with high endemic risk). In horses, azithromycin also has been used to treat proliferative enteritis caused by *Lawsonia intracellularis*.

Azithromycin has been used in cats to treat upper respiratory infections. There are no controlled clinical trials to document success for this use; however, this treatment has been common among veterinarians. Azithromycin administered to cats with infections caused by *Chlamydophila felis* (formerly *Chlamydia psittaci*), at 10–15 mg/kg once daily for 3 days and thereafter two times per week, was not effective for eliminating the organism, although clinical signs improved (perhaps via the immunomodulatory effects). However, azithromycin was not effective in cats for treatment of *Mycoplasma haemofelis* (hemobartonellosis).

When azithromycin was administered to dogs with pyoderma at either 10 mg/kg on day 1 followed by 5 mg/kg on days 2 through 5 or 5 mg/kg given 2 days/wk for 3 weeks, the response was equal statistically to cephalexin at 22 mg/kg twice daily. However, azithromycin is not a preferred drug for treating pyoderma in dogs.

In dairy calves, azithromycin administration significantly suppressed shedding of *Cryptosporidium parvum* and improved clinical signs. However, in cattle and pigs, other injectable long-acting macrolides approved for those species are recommended over azithromycin.

### Precautionary Information

#### Adverse Reactions and Side Effects

Azithromycin has a history of a favorable safety profile after many years of use in people. However, because it is not approved for animals, adverse reaction reports are few and inconsistent. Severe adverse effects to azithromycin have not been reported in publications in which it was administered to animals. However, vomiting is likely with high doses. Diarrhea may occur in some patients. Changes in the consistency of the feces and diarrhea have been reported in horses that were administered recommended doses. The long-term safety in adult horses is not known. A warning occurs on the human label warning of potentially serious cardiac arrhythmias from azithromycin use, but these problems have not been observed in animals.

#### Contraindications and Precautions

Use cautiously in animals with a history of vomiting. Administration to adult horses has been associated with diarrhea. Do not administer IV solution as a bolus or IM.

**A**

**Drug Interactions**

Drug interactions have not been reported in animals. This class of drugs has the potential to inhibit some cytochrome P450 enzymes that are involved in drug metabolism, but azithromycin is less likely than erythromycin or clarithromycin to interfere with cytochrome P450 enzymes.

## Instructions for Use

Azithromycin may be better tolerated than erythromycin. A primary difference from other antibiotics is the high intracellular concentrations achieved and long half-life that allows for intermittent administration. Although azithromycin has been commonly used for infections in dogs and cats, there is insufficient clinical trial evidence for most of these uses. Doses listed in the dosage section are based primarily on anecdotal accounts and clinical experience rather than efficacy studies.

To prepare IV solution, add 4.8 mL of sterile water to each 500-mg vial and shake. Further dilute this solution with either a 500- or 250-mL diluent to a solution of 1 or 2 mg/mL. When administered IV, a 1-mg/mL solution should be administered over a 3-hour period, or 2 mg/mL should be administered over 1 hour.

## Patient Monitoring and Laboratory Tests

Susceptibility testing: CLSI breakpoint for sensitive organisms is ≤2 mcg/mL based on a human clinical breakpoint.

## Formulations

- Azithromycin is available in 250-, 500-, and 600-mg tablets; 100- and 200-mg/5 mL oral suspension; and 500-mg vials for injection. Also, 1-g packets are available for mixing with water.

## Stability and Storage

Azithromycin is stable if maintained in manufacturer's original formulation. Stability has not been reported for compounded formulations. IV solution is stable after reconstitution for 48 hours at room temperature.

## Small Animal Dosage

### Dogs

- A range of dosages has been used, starting with 10 mg/kg once daily PO for 5–7 days and then decreasing to every other day. Alternatively, 5 mg/kg/day has been used by some veterinarians, either once per day or once every other day.

### Cats

- 5–10 mg/kg once daily for 7 days PO followed by administration q48h; or 10–15 mg/kg daily for 3 days followed by the same dose twice weekly PO.
- Upper respiratory infection: 15 mg/kg initially for the first 3 days and then q72h PO.

## Large Animal Dosage

### Horses

- For *R. equi*: 10 mg/kg q24h PO initially for 5 days and then q48h after a response is seen.
- Foals: 10 mg/kg q48h, PO. For foals, the 1-g packet can be mixed with water to create suspension for oral administration.
- Adult horses: 10 mg/kg PO, q48h.

### Cattle

- 10 mg/kg IM.

**Calves**
- For cryptosporidiosis: 33 mg/kg once daily for 7 days PO.

## Regulatory Information

Withdrawal times have not been established for animals producing food, but when administered to cattle, it persisted in milk with a half-life of approximately 160 hours and persisted longer in mastitic milk than in normal milk.

## Benazepril Hydrochloride
ben-ay′zeh-pril hye-droe-klor′ide

**Trade and other names:** Lotensin (human preparation) and Fortekor, Benazecare (veterinary preparation)

**Functional classification:** Vasodilator, angiotensin-converting enzyme (ACE) inhibitor

### Pharmacology and Mechanism of Action
Angiotensin-converting enzyme (ACE) inhibitor. Inhibits conversion of angiotensin I to angiotensin II. Angiotensin II is a potent vasoconstrictor and also produces sympathetic stimulation, renal hypertension, and synthesis of aldosterone. The inhibition of aldosterone decreases sodium and water retention. Benazepril, like other ACE inhibitors, produces vasodilation and decreases aldosterone-induced congestion. ACE inhibitors also contribute to vasodilation by increasing concentrations of some vasodilating kinins and prostaglandins. Unlike enalapril, benazepril has a dual mode of elimination through the kidneys and liver (85% eliminated through the bile), and clearance is not affected in animals with kidney disease. Duration of ACE-inhibiting action is 16–24 hours, despite a short plasma half-life, because of high-affinity binding to ACE.

*Pharmacokinetics:* The half-life in cats is 16–23 hours, which results in once-daily dosing.

### Indications and Clinical Uses
Benazepril, like other ACE inhibitors, is used to treat hypertension and congestive heart failure (CHF). Evidence shows that it may decrease the likelihood of developing cardiomyopathy in some dogs, but other studies failed to show this benefit. For treatment of occult mitral valve disease in dogs, there has not been a benefit of therapy.

It reduces blood pressure in some cats with kidney disease but is less effective in cats with spontaneous hypertension. Therefore, ACE inhibitors such as benazepril are not considered a primary treatment for hypertension in cats. Benazepril has been used in cats to treat proteinuria and hypertension in cats with chronic kidney disease. However, a survival benefit in cats with chronic kidney disease is not demonstrated. In studies in which it has been used in cats with renal insufficiency, it was associated with a small reduction in systemic hypertension, reduced glomerular filtration pressure, decreased glomerular hypertension, reduction in urine protein loss, and an increase in glomerular filtration rate (GFR) but no overall benefits on survival. For cats with kidney disease and hypertension, other agents are preferred such as amlodipine or telmisartan.

In dogs, it produces similar benefits to animals with kidney disease (decreased proteinuria, increased GFR, and lower blood pressure), but it does not increase survival. Despite these limitations, some renal experts recommend including an ACE inhibitor (benazepril or enalapril) in the initial treatment for dogs with proteinuria caused by glomerular disease.

## Precautionary Information

### Adverse Reactions and Side Effects

Benazepril has been well tolerated in dogs and cats with chronic renal failure. However, it may cause azotemia in some patients; carefully monitor renal parameters after initiation of treatment, particularly in patients receiving high doses of diuretics.

### Contraindications and Precautions

Discontinue ACE inhibitors in pregnant animals. ACE inhibitors cross the placenta and have caused fetal malformations and death of the fetus.

### Drug Interactions

Use cautiously with other hypotensive drugs and diuretics. Nonsteroidal anti-inflammatory drugs (NSAIDs) may decrease vasodilating effects. Benazepril, like other ACE inhibitors, may be used with other cardiovascular drugs and furosemide. However, it does not prevent increases in aldosterone (caused by activation of the renin–angiotensin–aldosterone system) in patients treated with furosemide. It is possible that if ACE inhibitors are administered with spironolactone, there may be increases in serum potassium, but this is a rare occurrence in dogs and cats.

## Instructions for Use

Dose is based on approved use in dogs in Europe and Canada. Monitor renal function and electrolytes 3–7 days after initiating therapy and periodically thereafter. In studies in cats, there was no benefit to dosages higher than 0.5–1 mg/kg/day.

## Patient Monitoring and Laboratory Tests

Monitor patients carefully to avoid hypotension. With all ACE inhibitors, monitor electrolytes and renal function 3–7 days after initiating therapy and periodically thereafter. Monitor serum creatinine because some patients will show an increase in creatinine concentrations. Slight increases in creatinine in cats with chronic kidney disease may be tolerable and not a reason to discontinue treatment.

## Formulations

- Benazepril is available in 5-, 10-, 20-, and 40-mg tablets.

## Stability and Storage

Store in a tightly sealed container, protected from light, and at room temperature. Stability of compounded formulations has not been evaluated.

## Small Animal Dosage

### Dogs

- 0.25–0.5 mg/kg q12–24h PO (0.5 mg/kg q24h in most patients). Increase by 0.5 mg/kg if needed, to a maximum of 2 mg/kg q24h.

### Cats

- Systemic hypertension: 0.5–1 mg/kg/day q24h PO. Alternative dosage for cats is 2.5 mg per cat per day for cats up to 5 kg of body weight PO.
- Chronic kidney disease: 0.25–0.5 mg/kg q24h PO.

## Large Animal Dosage

- No dose has been reported for large animals.

## Regulatory Information

Do not administer to animals intended for food.

Racing Commissioners International (RCI) Classification: 3

# Betamethasone

bay-tah-meth'ah-sone

**Trade and other names:** Celestone, BetaVet, betamethasone acetate, and betamethasone benzoate

**Functional classification:** Corticosteroid

## Pharmacology and Mechanism of Action

Potent, long-acting corticosteroid. Anti-inflammatory and immunosuppressive effects are approximately 30 times more than those of cortisol. Anti-inflammatory effects are complex but primarily occur via inhibition of inflammatory cells and suppression of expression of inflammatory mediators.

## Indications and Clinical Uses

Betamethasone is used for treatment of inflammatory and immune-mediated disease. It is used for similar indications as prednisolone and dexamethasone. The equine formulation (BetaVet) is a combination of a slow-release component (betamethasone acetate) and a rapid-acting form (betamethasone sodium phosphate) in a combination for injection intra-articularly for control of pain and inflammation associated with osteoarthritis in horses.

## Precautionary Information

### Adverse Reactions and Side Effects

There are many side effects from corticosteroids, which include polyphagia, polydipsia/polyuria, and hypothalamic–pituitary–adrenal axis suppression. Adverse effects include gastrointestinal (GI) ulceration, hepatopathy, increased risk of diabetes, hyperlipidemia, decreased thyroid hormone, decreased protein synthesis, delayed wound healing, and immunosuppression. Secondary infections can occur as a result of immunosuppression and include demodicosis, toxoplasmosis, fungal infections, and urinary tract infections. In horses, some equine clinicians have suggested that the use may increase risk of laminitis, but this has not been supported with clinical research.

### Contraindications and Precautions

Use cautiously in patients prone to ulcers or infection or in animals in which wound healing is necessary. Use cautiously in diabetic animals, animals with renal failure, and pregnant animals. Do not inject equine product intra-articular if there are signs of infection in the joint.

### Drug Interactions

No drug interactions are reported in animals. However, co-administration with other drugs may increase risk of adverse effects. For example, administration with NSAIDs may increase the risk of GI problems.

## Instructions for Use

Betamethasone is used for similar indications as dexamethasone because of similar potency and duration of effect. Topical forms of betamethasone also are available.

## Patient Monitoring and Laboratory Tests

Monitor complete blood count (CBC) and plasma cortisol.

## Formulations

- Betamethasone is available in 600-mcg (0.6-mg) tablets and 3-mg/mL sodium phosphate injection. (Tablets have been discontinued from some manufacturers and are difficult to obtain.)
- Equine formulation (BetaVet) contains betamethasone sodium phosphate (rapid acting) and betamethasone acetate (slow release) in a suspension for intra-articular use at a concentration of 6 mg/mL (3.15 mg in betamethasone sodium phosphate and 2.85 mg in betamethasone acetate).

## Stability and Storage

Store in a tightly sealed container, protected from light, and at room temperature. Stability of compounded formulations has not been evaluated. After opening the equine product (BetaVet), use once and discard vial after use.

## Small Animal Dosage

### Dogs and Cats

(Oral formulations may not be available.)
- Anti-inflammatory effects: 0.1–0.2 mg/kg q12–24h PO.
- Immunosuppressive effects: 0.2–0.5 mg/kg q12–24h PO.

## Large Animal Dosage

- 0.05–0.1 mg/kg q24h IM or PO.
- Intra-articular injection. The equine intra-articular product can be injected at a dose of 1.5 mL per joint (9 mg).

## Regulatory Information

No withdrawal times are established for animals intended for food (extralabel use). RCI Classification: 4

# Bethanechol Chloride

beh-than′eh-kole klor′ide

**Trade and other names:** Urecholine

**Functional classification:** Cholinergic

## Pharmacology and Mechanism of Action

Muscarinic, cholinergic agonist. Parasympathomimetic. Bethanechol stimulates gastric and intestinal motility. It also stimulates contraction of the urinary bladder via muscarinic receptor activation. Bethanechol, like other carbamoyl esters, resists hydrolysis by acetylcholinesterase to produce a more sustained response. The onset of action is usually 10 minutes after injection and 30–60 minutes after oral administration. Duration of effect is 4–6 hours.

## Indications and Clinical Uses

Bethanechol is used in small animals to increase contraction of the urinary bladder, but efficacy has not been established in well-controlled studies. Adverse effects may preclude this use. In large animals, it may increase GI motility, but the efficacy for treating GI stasis problems is questionable and not recommended.

B

### Precautionary Information

**Adverse Reactions and Side Effects**

High doses of cholinergic agonists increase motility of the GI tract and cause abdominal discomfort and diarrhea. Bethanechol can cause circulatory depression in sensitive animals.

**Contraindications and Precautions**

Do not use in patients with suspected GI or urinary obstruction.

**Drug Interactions**

Anticholinergic drugs (e.g., atropine, scopolamine) antagonize the effects of bethanechol.

## Instructions for Use

Administer injection SQ only. Doses are derived from extrapolation of human doses or via empiricism. There are no well-controlled efficacy studies available for veterinary species.

Bethanechol is no longer available from commercial sources, but some veterinary compounding pharmacists may be able to supply veterinarians.

## Patient Monitoring and Laboratory Tests

Monitor GI function.

## Formulations

- Bethanechol has been available in 5-, 10-, 25-, and 50-mg tablets and 5-mg/mL injection. (Commercial preparations are no longer available but are available through some compounding pharmacies.)

## Stability and Storage

Store in a tightly sealed container at room temperature. Compounded oral suspensions prepared from tablets are not stable.

## Small Animal Dosage

**Dogs**

- 5–15 mg per dog. 2.5 mg per dog for small dogs, 5 mg per dog for medium dogs, and 15 mg for large dogs. All doses administered q8h PO. The dose can be injected SQ, but oral administration is preferred.

**Cats**

- 1.25–5 mg/cat q8h PO.

## Large Animal Dosage

**Horses**

- 0.025 mg/kg SQ, once.

**Cattle**

- 0.07 mg/kg SQ, once.

## Regulatory Information

No withdrawal times are established for animals intended for food (extralabel use). However, the Food Animal Residue Avoidance Databank (FARAD) (1-888-873-2723) recommends a 21-day withdrawal time for slaughter.
RCI Classification: 4

# Bisacodyl
biss-ah-koe′dil

**Trade and other names:** Dulcolax

**Functional classification:** Laxative

## Pharmacology and Mechanism of Action

Laxative and cathartic. Bisacodyl acts via local stimulation of GI motility, most likely by irritation of the bowel.

## Indications and Clinical Uses

Bisacodyl is used as a laxative or for procedures in which bowel evacuation is necessary. It may be used with polyethylene glycol electrolyte solution (e.g., GoLYTELY) to cleanse the bowel prior to endoscopy or surgical procedures.

## Precautionary Information

### Adverse Reactions and Side Effects

Abdominal discomfort. Fluid and electrolyte loss. Avoid chronic use.

### Contraindications and Precautions

Avoid use in patients with renal disease. Do not rely on this medication for long-term treatment of constipation.

### Drug Interactions

No drug interactions are reported in animals.

## Instructions for Use

Bisacodyl is available as an over-the-counter (OTC) tablet. Doses are derived from extrapolation of human doses or via empiricism. There are no well-controlled efficacy studies available for veterinary species. Onset of action is approximately 1 hour after administration.

## Patient Monitoring and Laboratory Tests

Monitor electrolytes in animals if used chronically.

## Formulations

• Bisacodyl is available in 5-mg tablets.

## Stability and Storage

Store in a tightly sealed container, protected from light, and at room temperature. Stability of compounded formulations has not been evaluated.

## Small Animal Dosage
**Dogs and Cats**
- 5 mg/animal q8–24h PO.

## Large Animal Dosage
- No dose has been reported for large animals.

## Regulatory Information
Do not administer to animals intended for food.

# Bismuth Subsalicylate
biz'muth sub-sal-iss'ih-late

**Trade and other names:** Pepto-Bismol

**Functional classification:** Antidiarrheal

## Pharmacology and Mechanism of Action
Antidiarrheal agent and GI protectant. Precise mechanism of action is unknown, but antiprostaglandin action of salicylate component may be beneficial for some forms of enteritis. The bismuth component is efficacious for treating infections caused by spirochete bacteria (*Helicobacter pylori* gastritis). Bismuth subsalicylate in Pepto-Bismol contains five sources of salicylate, which are absorbed systemically after oral administration. Bismuth subsalicylate also may be found in other antidiarrhea preparations, such as kaolin-pectin formulations (e.g., Kaopectate).

## Indications and Clinical Uses
Bismuth subsalicylate is used for symptomatic treatment of diarrhea in small and large animals. Efficacy has not been established for animals. However, in people, it has been shown effective for treating or preventing diarrhea caused by enterotoxigenic *Escherichia coli.*

## Precautionary Information
**Adverse Reactions and Side Effects**

Adverse effects are uncommon. Owners should be warned that bismuth will discolor stools black.

**Contraindications and Precautions**

The salicylate component is absorbed systemically, and overuse should be avoided in animals that cannot tolerate salicylates, such as cats and animals allergic to aspirin.

**Drug Interactions**

No drug interactions are reported in animals. However, it may exacerbate effects of other NSAIDs administered to animals. The bismuth component may prevent oral absorption of some drugs.

## Instructions for Use

Bismuth subsalicylate is available as an OTC product. Doses are derived from extrapolation of human doses or via empiricism. There are no well-controlled efficacy studies available for veterinary species.

## Patient Monitoring and Laboratory Tests

No specific monitoring is necessary.

## Formulations

- Bismuth subsalicylate is available in oral suspension in 262 mg/15 mL or 525 mg/ mL in extra-strength formulation and 262-mg tablets. Two tablespoons (30 mL) contain 270-mg salicylate.

## Stability and Storage

Store in a tightly sealed container, protected from light, and at room temperature. Stability of compounded formulations has not been evaluated.

## Small Animal Dosage

### Dogs and Cats

- 1–3 mL/kg/day (in divided doses) PO.

## Large Animal Dosage

### Calves

- 30 mL per calf, q30min for 8 doses PO.

### Horses

- 1–2 mL/kg q6–8h PO.

## Regulatory Information

No withdrawal times are established for animals intended for food (extralabel use). Because the salicylate component may be systemically absorbed, withdrawal times should be considered for the salicylate component (similar to aspirin).

---

# Bisoprolol Fumarate

bis-oh′-proe-lol

**Trade and other names:** Zebeta

**Functional classification:** Antiarrhythmic, beta blocker

## Pharmacology and Mechanism of Action

Bisoprolol is a synthetic $beta_1$-selective beta-adrenergic receptor blocker with a low affinity for $beta_2$-receptors in bronchial smooth muscle, blood vessels, and fat cells and no intrinsic sympathomimetic activity. Typical cardioselective effects include lower heart rate, decreased cardiac output, and inhibition of renin release by kidneys. At higher doses, it loses $beta_1$ selectivity and inhibits some $beta_2$ receptors to affect bronchial and vascular smooth muscle. Clearance in dogs is balanced (60% metabolized by the liver and 40% excreted unchanged), which distinguishes bisoprolol from lipophilic beta blockers such as carvedilol and metoprolol and from hydrophilic beta blockers such as atenolol. In dogs, bisoprolol has high and consistent oral absorption (91%) and a half-life of 4 hours.

Although bisoprolol prolongs survival in human patients with heart failure, similar studies have not been conducted in dogs or cats.

## Indications and Clinical Uses

Bisoprolol is a beta$_1$ blocker that is somewhat cardioselective and therefore is indicated for conditions that require a reduction in heart rate, heart conductivity, or contractility. Such conditions include tachyarrhythmias and atrial fibrillation. In people, it is used to treat hypertension, but this use of bisoprolol has not been explored in animals.

## Precautionary Information

### Adverse Reactions and Side Effects

Beta blockade results in adverse effects that are attributed to decreased adrenergic tone in the heart. Bradycardia and heart block are possible. At high doses or in sensitive doses, bisoprolol may produce bronchospasm. Treat bradycardia from overdose with atropine.

### Contraindications and Precautions

Use cautiously in animals with airway disease, myocardial failure, and cardiac conduction disturbances. Use cautiously in animals with low cardiac reserve.

### Drug Interactions

Use cautiously with other drugs that may decrease cardiac contraction or heart rate. Concurrent use of rifampin may increase the metabolic clearance of bisoprolol.

## Instructions for Use

Dosing precautions are similar to other beta-blocking drugs.

## Patient Monitoring and Laboratory Tests

Monitor heart rate and rhythm. Monitor blood pressure in patients prone to hypotension.

## Formulations

• Bisoprolol is available in 5- and 10-mg tablets.

## Stability and Storage

Store in a tightly sealed container, protected from light, and at room temperature. Stability of compounded formulations has not been evaluated.

## Small Animal Dosage

### Dogs

• 0.1–0.2 mg/kg q8–12h PO.

### Cats

• No dose has been established for cats.

## Large Animal Dosage

• No dose has been reported for large animals.

## Regulatory Information

No regulatory information is available. For extralabel use withdrawal interval estimates, contact FARAD at www.FARAD.org.

# Bleomycin Sulfate
blee-oh-mye′sin sul′fate

**Trade and other names:** Blenoxane

**Functional classification:** Anticancer agent

## Pharmacology and Mechanism of Action
Anticancer antibiotic agent. It is derived from the fungus *Streptomyces verticillus*. It induces effects in cancer cells by causing oxidative cleavage of DNA, producing single-and double-strand breaks, chromosomal deletions, and fragmentation. It inhibits RNA and protein synthesis. Because it affects rapidly dividing cells, it has been used as an effective anticancer treatment.

## Indications and Clinical Uses
Bleomycin is used for treatment of various sarcomas and carcinomas. In people, it is used in multi-drug combinations for treatment of lymphoma and other forms of cancer. In dogs, it is usually used as a rescue agent for patients with lymphoma after they have already received other cancer treatment protocols. There are few clinical studies in animals to evaluate effectiveness. However, at a dose of 0.5 units/kg either IM or SQ, there was a minimal response to treatment. Low response rate may be attributed to the selection of patients with advance stages of cancer.

## Precautionary Information
### Adverse Reactions and Side Effects
Adverse effects include epithelial lesions (skin ulceration, ulceration of foot pads, and conjunctivitis), GI problems (anorexia, vomiting, diarrhea), elevation of liver enzymes, and kidney injury. Bleomycin causes local reaction at site of injection, pulmonary toxicity, fever, and chills in people.

### Contraindications and Precautions
Do not use in animals with suppressed bone marrow.

### Drug Interactions
No drug interactions are reported in animals. It has been used with other anticancer agents, antihistamines, corticosteroids, and antiemetics.

## Instructions for Use
Injectable solution usually used in combination with other anticancer agents. Dilute in 0.9% sodium chloride prior to administration. After dilution, it may be administered either SQ or IM. Consult anticancer protocols for details regarding use.

## Patient Monitoring and Laboratory Tests
Monitor CBC during treatment. If suppression of blood cells is extreme, withhold the next dose or reduce the dose.

## Formulations
- Bleomycin is available in 15- and 30-unit vials for injection.

## Stability and Storage
Store in a tightly sealed container, protected from light, and at room temperature. Refrigerate vials after opening. Stability of compounded formulations has not been evaluated.

## Small Animal Dosage
### Dogs
- 0.5 Units/kg, IM or SQ, either once, or with other cancer protocols.
- Alternatively, it can be administered at a dosage of 10 units/m$^2$ IV or SQ for 3 days and then 10 units/m$^2$ weekly. (Maximum cumulative dose, 200 units/m$^2$.)

### Cats
- No dose is available for cats.

## Large Animal Dosage
- No dose has been reported for large animals.

## Regulatory Information
Withdrawal times are not established for animals that produce food. Because it is an anticancer agent, do not administer to food-producing animals.

# Boldenone Undecylenate
bole'de-none un-de-sil-en'ate

**Trade and other names:** Equipoise

**Functional classification:** Hormone, anabolic agent

## Pharmacology and Mechanism of Action
Anabolic steroid. Boldenone is a steroid ester designed to maximize anabolic effects while minimizing androgenic action (see also Methyltestosterone). Anabolic agents have been used for reversing catabolic conditions, increasing weight gain, increasing muscling in animals, and stimulating erythropoiesis. Stanozolol is a similar drug used in horses. There are no documented differences in efficacy among the anabolic steroids.

## Indications and Clinical Uses
Boldenone is an anabolic agent. It is used primarily in horses to improve nitrogen balance, reduce overexertion associated with exercise, and improve training. It may also improve appetite and improve weight gain when used with a well-balanced diet. Boldenone is a long-lasting agent, and effects may persist for 6 weeks after an IM injection.

## Precautionary Information
### Adverse Reactions and Side Effects
Adverse effects from anabolic steroids can be attributed to the androgenic action of these steroids. Increased masculine effects are common. Increased aggressiveness may be observed. Increased incidence of some tumors has been reported in people, and 17 alpha-methylated oral anabolic steroids (oxymetholone, stanozolol, and oxandrolone) are associated with hepatic toxicity.

### Contraindications and Precautions
This drug is abused by humans to enhance athletic performance and is a controlled substance. Do not administer to animals intended for food. Do not administer to pregnant animals.

### Drug Interactions
There are no significant drug interactions known; however, use cautiously with other drugs that may affect liver function.

## Instructions for Use

For many indications, use in animals is based on experience in people or anecdotal experience in animals.

## Patient Monitoring and Laboratory Tests

Monitor liver enzymes for signs of hepatic injury (cholestatic) during treatment.

## Formulations

- Boldenone is available in 25- and 50-mg/mL injection in sesame oil.

## Stability and Storage

Store in a tightly sealed container, protected from light, and at room temperature. Do not freeze. Do not mix with aqueous solutions.

## Small Animal Dosage

- Doses have not been reported for small animals.

## Large Animal Dosage

**Horses**

- 1.1 mg/kg IM. Injection may be repeated every 3 weeks.

## Regulatory Information

Do not administer to animals intended for food.
Schedule III controlled drug.
RCI Classification: 4

# Bromide
broe′mide

**Trade and other names:** Potassium bromide and sodium bromide

**Functional classification:** Anticonvulsant

## Pharmacology and Mechanism of Action

Anticonvulsant. Exact mechanism of action is uncertain. Anticonvulsant action is to stabilize neuronal cell membranes. Bromide is a halide salt and may affect neuronal chloride ion channels, causing hyperpolarization of neuronal membranes and raising the seizure threshold. By changing the chloride conductance in neuronal membranes, it may stabilize epileptic foci in the brain. In dogs, oral absorption is 46%. It is not metabolized, and most is eliminated by the kidneys. The half-life is long, which is 11 days in cats, and has ranged from 25 to 46 days in dogs. Bromide is available in two forms: sodium bromide (78% bromide) and potassium bromide (67% bromide).

The use of potassium bromide for seizure control dates back to the 1850s in humans. But in the 20th century, the use of bromide for treating seizure disorders in people diminished because of common adverse effects and availability of other medications.

## Indications and Clinical Uses

Bromide ordinarily is used in patients with seizure disorders that have been refractory to phenobarbital. Usually, patients are treated with both phenobarbital and bromide. However, some patients have been treated with bromide as a single therapy for epilepsy. If bromide is added to phenobarbital therapy, it allows for a reduction in phenobarbital dose (reduce by 25% every 6 weeks). Despite clinical evidence of efficacy, the use of bromide for treating seizures in dogs has declined with the availability of other available agents, such as levetiracetam (Keppra).

Bromide has not been as effective for treating cats with seizure disorders as in dogs, and the use in cats is discouraged. Cats have more adverse effects and are less well controlled; therefore, bromide is rarely recommended for a treatment in cats.

## Precautionary Information

### Adverse Reactions and Side Effects

Common side effects include polyuria/polydipsia, polyphagia, ataxia, sedation, and GI upset. More serious adverse effects are related to high levels of bromide (bromism) and are more specific for the central nervous system (CNS). Signs of toxicosis are CNS depression, delirium, hyperexcitability, weakness, and ataxia. Hind limb stiffness and abnormal gait also may be signs of bromide toxicosis. If adverse effects occur, discontinuation of the medication usually results in resolution of the clinical signs in several days. Resolution may be faster (within hours) with aggressive saline diuresis.

Nausea and pancreatitis have been reported in dogs, and there is evidence that a combination of bromide and phenobarbital in dogs may increase the risk of pancreatitis. However, there is no direct evidence that bromide alone produces pancreatic toxicity. There is no evidence available to indicate that bromide treatment affects thyroid function in dogs.

Some dogs show paradoxical excitement with bromide treatment. In many cats, bronchitis resembling allergic airway disease has been observed. In cats, this may be characterized by coughing.

### Contraindications and Precautions

Consider using sodium bromide, rather than potassium bromide, in patients with hypoadrenocorticism or in any patients in which potassium regulation is a problem. Likewise, consider the sodium content of administration in animals with CHF or hypertension. Diets high in chloride cause a shorter half-life and need for a higher dose. Monitor plasma concentrations and adjust dose as necessary whenever changing diets because increasing chloride in the diet shortens the half-life and vice versa.

### Drug Interactions

Diets high in chloride cause a shorter half-life and need for a higher dose. Administration of bromide interferes with some blood chemistry analysis (e.g., false elevation of chloride).

## Instructions for Use

Bromide usually is administered in combination with phenobarbital. Sodium bromide can be substituted for potassium bromide. When considering doses for sodium bromide, slight dose adjustments should be considered. Potassium bromide is 67% bromide, and sodium bromide is 78% bromide; therefore, the dose of sodium bromide should be approximately 15% less (e.g., 30 mg/kg of potassium bromide is equivalent to 25 mg/kg of sodium bromide).

## Patient Monitoring and Laboratory Tests

Monitor serum bromide concentrations to adjust dose. Effective plasma concentrations should be 1–2 mg/mL (100–200 mg/dL), but if used alone (without phenobarbital), higher concentrations of 2–2.5 mg/mL (200–250 mg/dL) and as high as 4 mg/mL may be needed. Most veterinary laboratories can perform a test for bromide in plasma or serum.

## Formulations

- Bromide is usually prepared as an oral solution. Although there are no commercial forms approved by the US Food and Drug Administration, compounding pharmacists can prepare a solution. To prepare the oral solution, mix 25 g of potassium bromide with 60 mL of purified water; then add a sufficient quantity of corn syrup to make 100 mL. This formulation results in a bromide concentration of approximately 151–185 mg/mL. This solution is stable for 180 days. For sodium bromide oral solution, mix 21.6 g sodium bromide with 60 mL purified water; then add a sufficient quantity of corn syrup to make 100 mL. This formulation results in a concentration of approximately 151–185 mg/mL. This solution is stable for 180 days.
- A pharmacist should prepare the IV solution in sterile water and filter it to remove impurities. To prepare injectable solution, add 3 g of sodium bromide with a sufficient quantity of sterile water to make 100 mL. This formulation results in a bromide concentration of approximately 21–25.6 mg/mL. It is stable for 180 days and should be stored in the refrigerator to decrease the risk of microbial growth.

## Stability and Storage

Store in a tightly sealed container. Compounded formulations in aqueous solutions are stable for at least 180 days. Refrigerate injectable solution to prevent bacterial growth. Do not mix with salt-containing flavorants or solutions.

## Small Animal Dosage

### Cats

- 30 mg/kg q24h PO. (Not recommended for cats.)

### Dogs

- 30–40 mg/kg q24h PO. If administered without phenobarbital, higher doses of up to 40–50 mg/kg may be needed. If animals are on diets high in chloride, higher doses may be needed. Adjust doses by monitoring plasma concentrations.
- Oral loading dose: 600 mg/kg divided over 3–5 days (200 mg/kg once a day for 5 days also has been used), PO. Alternatively, 60 mg/kg/day has been administered for 15 days to achieve a plasma concentration of 100 and 200 mg/dL by 60 days.
- IV loading dose for sodium bromide: 800–1200 mg/kg infused over 8 hours (it is critical to use sodium bromide instead of potassium bromide for this use).

## Large Animal Dosage

### Horses

- 100 mg/kg loading dose followed by 25 mg/kg q24h, PO.
- No dose has been reported for other large animals.

## Regulatory Information

Do not administer to animals intended for food.

# Bromocriptine Mesylate
broe-moe-krip'teen mess'ih-late

**Trade and other names:** Parlodel

**Functional classification:** Dopamine agonist

## Pharmacology and Mechanism of Action

Dopaminergic agonist. Antiprolactin agent. Bromocriptine is a lactation inhibitor. It reduces serum prolactin concentration by inhibition of release from the anterior pituitary gland by binding to dopamine ($D_2$) receptors in the CNS. The binding of $D_2$ receptors restores hormonal function in the pituitary. Through the action on the dopamine pituitary receptors, bromocriptine may decrease corticotropin (adrenocorticotropic hormone [ACTH]) release and has been used in animals (especially horses) for treating pituitary-dependent hyperadrenocorticism (PDH). It has not been effective for treating canine PDH (Cushing syndrome). It also stimulates postsynaptic dopamine receptors and has been used to treat dopamine-deficient neurodegenerative diseases.

## Indications and Clinical Uses

In people, bromocriptine is used for its antiparkinson effect and to inhibit lactation associated with excess prolactin. It also has been used to treat acromegaly. Bromocriptine has been used to treat disorders associated with dopamine deficiency in animals. In dogs, bromocriptine has been used to terminate pregnancy when used in combination with a prostaglandin (dinoprost or cloprostenol). In this combination, it was 100% effective for terminating pregnancy in dogs. Through the action to decrease prolactin, bromocriptine can be used in dogs to decrease milk production in bitches (e.g., to treat pseudopregnancy).

In horses, bromocriptine may decrease ACTH release and has been used in treating equine pituitary pars intermedia dysfunction (Cushing syndrome), but pergolide is usually a preferred treatment.

## Precautionary Information

### Adverse Reactions and Side Effects

Pyometra may occur in dogs after it has been used to induce abortion. Bromocriptine may cause mammary gland enlargement. When terminating pregnancy, bromocriptine is used in combination with prostaglandin $F_2$alpha. Adverse effects (vomiting, nausea, and retching) may occur as a result of the prostaglandin. However, vomiting and retching also can occur through dopamine stimulation of the vomiting center. It can also produce vasodilation and lowering of blood pressure in some animals. Bromocriptine inhibits lactation, which is sometimes a desired clinical effect (e.g., to treat pseudopregnancy).

### Contraindications and Precautions

Except when used for termination of pregnancy, do not use in pregnant animals. Do not use in nursing animals. Women handling bromocriptine should use caution to avoid exposure.

### Drug Interactions

No drug interactions have been reported in animals. However, it exacerbates the effects of selegiline. Do not administer with monoamine oxidase inhibitors (MAOIs).

## Instructions for Use

Use of bromocriptine is limited to treatment of some endocrine disorders. Studies of efficacy are limited and based largely on anecdotal accounts. Bromocriptine has been used to terminate pregnancy in dogs in combination with prostaglandin $F_2$alpha. For this use, administer 15 mcg/kg q12h PO on day 1, 20 mcg/kg 12h PO on days 2 and 3, and 30 mcg/kg q12h PO thereafter for an average of 4–5 days. Ten days may be needed in some dogs for a complete effect. A prostaglandin agent (cloprostenol sodium) should be used at a dosage of 1 mcg/kg q48h SQ during this regimen.

## Patient Monitoring and Laboratory Tests

Monitor pregnant animals carefully, especially if bromocriptine has been used to terminate pregnancy.

## Formulations

- Bromocriptine is available in 5-mg capsules and 2.5-mg tablets. For use in small animals, the commercial tablet of 2.5 mg requires fractioning the tablet into small increments for dosing. The tablet can be dissolved in 10 mL of distilled water in an amber vial to provide a 250-mcg/mL solution.

## Stability and Storage

Store in a tightly sealed container, protected from light, and at room temperature. If an oral solution is prepared from the tablet (see under Formulations), the 250-mcg/mL solution should be stored in an amber vial in a refrigerator and used within 1 week of preparation.

## Small Animal Dosage

### Dogs

- Termination of pregnancy: 15 mcg/kg q12h PO on day 1, 20 mcg/kg 12h PO on days 2 and 3, and 30 mcg/kg q12h PO thereafter for an average of 4–5 days. For treatment success, it should be administered in combination with prostaglandin $F_2$alpha.
- Reducing milk production: 10–100 mcg/kg q12h for 10–14 days.
- Treating pseudopregnancy in bitches: 10–30 mcg/kg, q12h, oral. Lower the dose to 7.5 mcg/kg if adverse effects are observed.
- Other conditions: 20–40 mcg/kg (0.02–0.04 mg/kg) q12h PO.

### Cats

- 20–40 mcg/kg (0.02–0.04 mg/kg) q12h PO.

## Large Animal Dosage

- No dose has been reported for large animals.

## Regulatory Information

Do not administer to animals intended for food.

# Budesonide
byoo-dess'oh-nide

**Trade and other names:** Entocort, Uceris, and generic

**Functional classification:** Anti-inflammatory, corticosteroid

B

## Pharmacology and Mechanism of Action

Budesonide is a locally acting corticosteroid, with high potency that is 15 times more active than prednisolone. It is approved for use in people, but there has been only limited use in small animals. Budesonide granules are contained in an ethylcellulose matrix that is coated with methacrylic acid polymer. This coating does not release the drug until the pH is greater than 5.5. Other forms are available that do not release the medication until the pH is above 7. Therefore, the drug is not usually released until it reaches the distal GI tract. Once released, it accumulates in intestinal cells and is stored by esterification with fatty acids. If any is absorbed, 80%–90% is inactivated by metabolism first-pass effects. Therefore, it has primarily a local effect on the intestine, and systemic glucocorticoid effects are minimized. In humans it has been as effective as other drugs for treatment of Crohn disease.

## Indications and Clinical Uses

In animals, it has been used to treat inflammatory bowel disease. The most common use has been for treating colitis in dogs or inflammatory bowel disease in cats. It has been safe and effective for treating inflammatory bowel disease in dogs, but it may produce some side effects that are similar to prednisone. Other reports of successful treatment are mostly anecdotal.

## Precautionary Information

### Adverse Reactions and Side Effects

There is some systemic absorption, as evidenced by decreased response to ACTH and decreased cortisol after 30-day treatment to dogs at 3 $mg/m^2$. The incidence of adverse effects was similar to prednisone in dogs, but other side effects were not observed, and other variables were not affected. Some mild elevation of liver enzymes may occur in dogs.

### Contraindications and Precautions

No known contraindications. However, some of the drug may be absorbed systemically; therefore, use with caution in animals that should not receive corticosteroids.

### Drug Interactions

Do not administer with drugs that increase stomach pH (antacids, antisecretory drugs). Because budesonide is metabolized by cytochrome P450 enzymes, other drugs that inhibit these enzymes (see Appendix I) may inhibit metabolism.

## Instructions for Use

Use in animals has been limited to anecdotal experience and small clinical studies. The capsules should not be crushed or compounded for animals unless action in the proximal portion of the intestine is desired.

## Patient Monitoring and Laboratory Tests

Monitor corticosteroid effects and, preferably, conduct an ACTH-stimulation test to determine degree of adrenal suppression with chronic use. Some elevations in liver enzymes may occur in dogs.

## Formulations

- Budesonide is available in 3-mg capsule in the conventional form. The new extended-release formulation (Uceris) is a 6- and 9-mg tablet and designed to release at a pH greater than 7.

## Stability and Storage
Store in a tightly sealed container, protected from light, and at room temperature. Do not crush capsules.

## Small Animal Dosage
### Dogs and Cats
- 0.12–0.15 mg/kg q8–12h PO. Dose interval may be increased to q24h when condition improves.
- In dogs, intact 3-mg capsules, once per day, have been administered, but in cats, doses of 0.5–0.75 mg per cat per day are administered by reformulating capsules.
- Full range of doses for dogs: 3–7 kg, 1 mg q24h; 7–15 kg, 2 mg q24h; 15–30 kg, 3 mg q24h; greater than 30 kg, 5 mg q24h.

## Large Animal Dosage
- No dose has been reported for large animals.

## Regulatory Information
No regulatory information is available. Because of minimal systemic absorption expected, no withdrawal time is suggested.
RCI Classification: 4

# Bunamidine Hydrochloride
byoo-nam'ih-deen hye-droe-klor'ide

**Trade and other names:** Scolaban

**Functional classification:** Antiparasitic

## Pharmacology and Mechanism of Action
Bunamidine hydrochloride damages the integrity of protective integument on cestode parasites. It is effective against various species of tapeworms in animals.

## Indications and Clinical Uses
Bunamidine is used as an anticestodal agent to treat tapeworm infections in dogs and cats.

### Precautionary Information
**Adverse Reactions and Side Effects**
Vomiting and diarrhea have occurred after use.

**Contraindications and Precautions**
Avoid use in young animals.

**Drug Interactions**
No drug interactions are reported in animals.

## Instructions for Use
Do not break tablets. Administer tablets on empty stomach. Do not feed animal for 3 hours after administration.

## Patient Monitoring and Laboratory Tests

Monitor fecal samples for evidence of parasites.

## Formulations

• Bunamidine is available in 400-mg tablets.

## Stability and Storage

Store in a tightly sealed container, protected from light, and at room temperature. Stability of compounded formulations has not been evaluated.

## Small Animal Dosage

### Dogs and Cats

• 20–50 mg/kg once PO.

## Large Animal Dosage

• No dose has been reported for large animals.

## Regulatory Information

No regulatory information is available. For extralabel use withdrawal interval estimates, contact FARAD at www.FARAD.org.

## Bupivacaine Hydrochloride
byoo-piv′ah-kane hye-droe-klor′ide

**Trade and other names:** Nocita, Marcaine, Exparel, and generic brands

**Functional classification:** Local anesthetic

## Pharmacology and Mechanism of Action

Local anesthetic. Bupivacaine is a local anesthetic that inhibits nerve conduction via sodium channel blockade. Bupivacaine is a weak base with a pKa of 8; therefore, in tissues, it is non-ionized and highly lipophilic, allowing penetration across membranes. After entering the nerve cell, it is available to bind to sodium channels to produce the anesthetic effect. Bupivacaine has a slow onset of action (15–20 minutes) but is longer acting (6–8 hours) and more potent than lidocaine or other local anesthetics. (By contrast, lidocaine has a rapid onset of less than 5 minutes but a duration of 1–2 hours.) Epidural onset of action of bupivacaine is approximately 15–20 minutes with a duration of 2–4 hours.

Bupivacaine has been formulated in a liposomal suspension injection for dogs and cats to provide pain relief after surgery. The liposomes are composed of lipid bilayers of approximately 10–30 μm in diameter that break down and release the local anesthetic slowly. This product (Nocita) has a long-acting effect that inhibits pain transmission from a postsurgical site after one dose for up to 72 hours.

*Pharmacokinetics:* When injected as the hydrochloride (9 mg/kg) to dogs, the half-life is 10 hours. When injected as the liposomal suspension, the half-life is 26–44 hours, depending on the dose. In cats, the liposomal formulation of bupivacaine has a slow time to peak concentration and a duration of action of at least 72 hours.

## Indications and Clinical Uses

Bupivacaine is used for local anesthesia and epidural analgesia/anesthesia. It is administered by local infiltration or by epidural injection. There is also a liposomal injection as a suspension in multivesicular liposomes (Exparel and Nocita). The human preparation is contained in a foam delivery system (DepoFoam drug delivery), and a liposomal suspension for dogs and cats is administered by local infiltration. After injection of the liposomal formulation into soft tissue, bupivacaine is released from the multivesicular liposomes over a long period of time, providing pain relief for at least 72 hours and up to 96 hours. This formulation is used to infiltrate around a surgical site or near a nerve for a local anesthetic effect. The bupivacaine liposomal suspension for dogs and cats (Nocita) is approved to relieve postoperative pain following cranial cruciate ligament surgery in dogs and onychectomy in cats for 72 hours.

## Precautionary Information

### Adverse Reactions and Side Effects

Adverse effects are rare with local infiltration. High doses absorbed systemically can cause nervous system signs (tremors and convulsions). The toxic dose in cats is 5 mg/kg. In cats, signs of toxicity include bradycardia, arrhythmias, tremors, muscle twitching, and seizures. The dose necessary to stimulate seizures and produce cardiac arrhythmias in dogs is greater than 4 mg/kg, IV. After epidural administration, respiratory paralysis is possible with high doses.

The liposomal formulation injected into surgical sites may produce occasional tissue irritation, but systemic absorption of the liposomal suspension is negligible and far below the concentrations necessary to induce CNS effects such as seizures. Therefore, the absorption of bupivacaine from the liposomal formulation is not expected to produce any systemic adverse effects.

### Contraindications and Precautions

When using for epidural anesthesia, respiratory support should be available. Some formulations contain epinephrine (1:200,000) and should not be administered to animals that are prone to reactions from epinephrine. When using the liposomal suspension, do not administer IV or in a joint.

### Drug Interactions

No drug interactions are reported in animals.

## Instructions for Use

Used for local infiltration or infusion into epidural space. For epidural injection, the volume of injection is approximately 0.2 mL/kg, or not to exceed 6 mL for large dogs. Ordinarily, the dose for a nerve block in small animals does not exceed 1 mg/kg. One may mix 0.1 mEq of sodium bicarbonate per 10-mL solution to increase pH, decrease pain from injection and produce a shorter onset of action. Use immediately after mixing with bicarbonate because of risk of precipitation. Increasing the pH accelerates the onset of anesthetic action.

The liposomal formulation for dogs and cats (Nocita) is intended for single-dose use to infiltrate the surgical site and provide local postoperative analgesia for cranial cruciate ligament surgery in dogs and as a peripheral nerve block to provide regional postoperative analgesia following onychectomy in cats. Use a 25-gauge needle for infiltration and inject slowly into the tissue site. It has also been used extralabel for other surgical sites where pain management may be needed. The dose volume for the liposomal formulation is 0.4 mL/kg, but if this is not sufficient for the surgical site, add up to an equal volume of fluid (saline or lactated Ringer's solution) to increase the volume. Do not use water or mix with other solutions because it could disrupt the liposomes.

## Patient Monitoring and Laboratory Tests
No specific monitoring is necessary.

## Formulations
- Bupivacaine is available in 0.25%, 0.5%, and 0.75% (2.5, 5, and 7.5 mg/mL) solution for injection.
- Exparel (human formulation) local multivesicular liposomes are available in a bupivacaine concentration of 13.3 mg/mL in 10- or 20-mL vials.
- Nocita (veterinary formulation) is a bupivacaine liposome injectable suspension available for dogs and cats in a concentration of 13.3 mg/mL.

## Stability and Storage
Store in a tightly sealed container at room temperature. Avoid mixing with strongly acidic or alkalinic solutions. If solutions change to a yellow, pink, or darker color, they should not be used. If pH is adjusted by mixing with alkalinizing solutions (e.g., bicarbonate), the drug is stable but must be used soon after mixing.

When using the liposomal formulations, puncture the vial only once. Unopened vials should be stored in the refrigerator. After drawing the initial dose into the syringe, it may be stored at room temperature for up to 4 hours, but because it has no preservatives, the syringes should be discarded after 4 hours. Do not freeze the liposomal suspension. The liposomal suspension vials, if unopened, may be kept at room temperature for up to 30 days in sealed, intact (unopened) vials. Do not re-refrigerate.

## Small Animal Dosage
### Dogs and Cats
- Epidural dose: 1–1.5 mg/kg; for nerve blocks, usually 0.2 mL/kg of 0.5% solution is used.
- Multivesicular liposomes: Infiltrate surgical site with 100–200 mg per site. Duration of effect is usually 96 hours.
- Liposomal injectable suspension (13.3 mg/mL): 5.3 mg/kg (0.4 mL/kg) injected by infiltration into the surgical tissues at the time of incisional closure. A single dose is designed to provide up to 72 hours of pain control.
- Use in cats for onychectomy: 5.3 mg/kg per forelimb (0.4 mL/kg per forelimb) to a total dose of 10.6 mg/kg per cat in a four-point nerve block. Inject volumes of 0.02–0.16 mL/kg in the region of the nerves supplying the distal limb, as instructed in the product insert.

## Large Animal Dosage
- Limited to local infiltration for minor surgery.

## Regulatory Information
No withdrawal times are established for animals intended for food (extralabel use). When used for local infiltration, clearance from the animal is expected to be rapid. For extralabel use withdrawal interval estimates, contact FARAD at www.FARAD.org.
RCI Classification: 2

# Buprenorphine Hydrochloride
byoo-preh-nor′feen hye-droe-klor′ide

**Trade and other names:** Buprenex (human form), Simbadol (veterinary form), and Vetergesic (UK veterinary form). Butrans is a human transdermal formulation.

**Functional classification:** Analgesic, opioid

## Pharmacology and Mechanism of Action
Opioid analgesic. Buprenorphine is a partial mu-receptor agonist and kappa-receptor antagonist. It is a thebaine derivative and was originally developed in the 1970s as a treatment for opiate addiction in people because of its properties as a mu-receptor partial agonist. It is 25–50 times more potent than morphine. It has higher binding affinity for the opiate receptor, which may prolong the effects. However, it has a delayed onset of activity, and because of its property as a partial mu-opiate agonist, it has moderate analgesia with a ceiling effect. Buprenorphine has fewer adverse effects than other opiates and may cause less respiratory depression than other opiates.

*Pharmacokinetics:* The pharmacokinetics in dogs have been variable, depending on the study and formulation. The half-life in dogs has ranged from 4 to 9 hours, with a clearance from 5.4 to 24 mL/kg/min. The half-life in cats after IV administration is 7–10 hours, but it is 20–30 hours by other routes. Transmucosal (sublingual) absorption in cats has been previously reported to be over 100%; however, more recent studies indicate that this value may be overestimated and that 23%–32% absorption from this route may be more likely. In horses, the half-life is 7 hours, with a clearance of 8 mL/kg/min, and the absorption from IM administration is highly variable (41%–93%).

Buprenorphine is highly lipophilic with octanol:water partition coefficient of greater than 1000. Protein binding is low (less than 10%).

## Indications and Clinical Uses
Buprenorphine is an opiate analgesic that is used for pain control in dogs, cats, horses, and some exotic and zoo species. It has high binding affinity but lower efficacy (lower ceiling) than pure mu-receptor agonists such as morphine. Buprenorphine has been shown to be effective in animal studies for treating postoperative pain. Duration of analgesia based on plasma values in animals is 3–4 hours, but it may be longer clinically because of slow dissociation from binding sites and higher affinity for the mu-receptor or longer half-life in the CNS. Duration of effect has not been established for all indications in well-controlled studies and has been variable. After injection, it may have a longer time to the onset of effect than other opiates.

In cats, the low doses (0.01–0.02 mg/kg, or 10–20 mcg/kg) given by the IM or IV route are more effective than the SQ route. Studies using the SQ route in cats used higher doses. Higher doses in cats may produce a longer duration of action. For example, a dose of 0.02 mg/kg has a duration of 6–12 hours, but higher doses of 0.12 or 0.24 mg/kg have a duration of 24 hours.

In cats, it has been administered for transmucosal absorption (buccal administration) at a dose of 20 mcg/kg (0.02 mg/kg) and reported to be effective in some studies. However, other studies have shown lower absorption of 23%–32% from transmucosal delivery in cats and lower efficacy; therefore, higher doses of 0.04 mg/kg (40 mcg/kg) transmucosal delivery may be needed q8h to control pain in many cats. In dogs, absorption from transmucosal (gingival) administration is low (47%), and high doses must be administered to achieve analgesic effects. In dogs, 120 mcg/kg administered transmucosally (to the gingiva) is equivalent to 20 mcg/kg IV. At these doses for dogs, the high volume increases the risk of drug loss from the mouth or from swallowing.

Buprenorphine patches for transdermal administration (Butrans) have been used in dogs at a dose of 70 mcg/h, which was equivalent to a SQ dose of 20 mcg/kg. The patch has a slow onset (17 hours of lag time) but a duration of 7 days. However, a 35-mcg/h patch in cats did not produce antinociceptive effects, and plasma drug levels were not detected until 36 hours after placement of the patch. Buprenorphine buccal film (Belbuca) is available in various sizes (see the Formulation section) for application to the buccal membrane in people for relief of pain. However, these film strips have not been evaluated in animals. The oral transmucosal tablets have been administered to cats after first dissolving in water or simple syrup. The bioavailability of this preparation in cats was 57%.

A concentrated solution (1.8 mg/mL) is available for administration SQ to cats at a dosage of 0.24 mg/kg (240 mcg/kg) once per day. This concentrated formulation has also been evaluated in dogs for post-surgical pain and was equivalent to the conventional formulation of 0.3 mg/mL for pain relief when administered at a dose of 20 mcg/kg IM. Buprenorphine SR is available as an unapproved sustained-release biodegradable polymer designed to produce effective concentrations for 72 hours. Injection of Buprenorphine SR in dogs produced concentrations over 1 ng/mL for over 72 hours at a dose of 270 mcg/kg SQ.

In horses, the doses that are analgesic are likely to produce adverse effects (excitement and locomotor activity), which limits the use in horses unless it is administered with sedatives and other analgesics. The adverse effects in horses persist longer than the analgesic effects.

In people, buprenorphine analgesia has been enhanced with the addition of small doses of naloxone (0.001–0.1 mcg/kg), but this effect has not been investigated in animals.

## Precautionary Information

### Adverse Reactions and Side Effects

Adverse effects are similar to other opiate agonists, but there may be less respiratory depression. Sedation is common. Dependency from chronic use of buprenorphine may be less than with pure agonists. The lethal dose in dogs (80 mg/kg) is much higher than the therapeutic dose.

In horses, restlessness, excitatory reactions, head shaking, pawing, shifting leg movements, decreased intestinal motility, and increased locomotor activity are likely and may persist for several hours.

### Contraindications and Precautions

Patients receiving buprenorphine may require higher doses of naloxone for reversal. IV dose in horses may cause behavior reactions (excitement, pacing). There are formulations that vary greatly in concentration from 0.3 mg/mL to 1.8 mg/mL (Simbadol); therefore, pay close attention to the concentration of the formulation to avoid overdoses.

### Drug Interactions

As a partial agonist, buprenorphine may reverse or antagonize some of the mu-receptor effects of other opiates, such as morphine or fentanyl. It may be used with other analgesic agents and NSAIDs.

## Instructions for Use

Buprenorphine is used for analgesia, often in combination with other analgesics or in conjunction with general anesthesia. It has been used safely with acepromazine and alpha$_2$ agonists as a pre-anesthetic. It has been safely used for pain relief in animals in conjunction with NSAIDs. It is longer acting than morphine and only partially reversed by naloxone. When administration is intended to be buccal (transmucosal), it is important that the entire dose be applied to the oral mucosa and not swallowed. Ingested drug will not be effective (only 3%–6% oral absorption). Therefore, as the dose increases, the volume also increases, and there is a higher likelihood that some of the drug will be lost from the mouth or swallowed (e.g., at a dose of 0.03 mg/kg to cats, the volume necessary for administration is 0.45 mL per average cat).

The oral mucosal tablets prepared for people have been used in cats. To prepare these tablets for administration, dissolve a 2-mg tablet in water or simple syrup to a concentration of 0.3 mg/mL. This formulation is stable for 21 days at room temperature. This may be administered to the oral mucosa in cats at a dose of 0.03–0.04 mg/kg.

## Patient Monitoring and Laboratory Tests

Monitor patient's heart rate and respiration. Although bradycardia rarely needs to be treated when it is caused by an opioid, if necessary, atropine can be administered. If serious respiratory depression occurs, the opioid can be reversed with naloxone, but animals receiving buprenorphine may require higher doses of naloxone for reversal. Although plasma or serum concentrations are not typically measured, levels of 4–10 ng/mL have been associated with analgesic efficacy.

## Formulations

- Buprenorphine is available in 0.3-mg/mL injection solution in a 1-mL vial. Simbadol is a veterinary formulation concentrated in 1.8 mg/mL for use in cats but has also been used in dogs.
- Tablets: 2- or 8-mg sublingual tablets (Subutex and Suboxone with naloxone), which has been used in people to treat substance abuse. Suboxone (with naloxone) is also available in a transmucosal/sublingual film.
- Butrans is a 7-day transdermal system (Butrans) that delivers 5-, 10-, and 20-mcg/h to human patients.
- Buprenorphine SR is available as an unapproved injectable sustained-release polymer that is designed for 72-hour delivery in a 10-or 3-mg/mL formulation.
- Buprenorphine buccal film (Belbuca): available in sizes of 75-, 150-, 300-, 450-, 600-, 750-, and 900-mcg buccal film. These have not been evaluated in animals. In people, they are applied q12–24h for pain relief at a maximum dose of 13 mcg/kg.
- Buprenorphine 3 mg/mL oral gel (buccal solution): This formulation has been compounded into a transdermal gel for cats. The formulation that has been tested for stability and potency is as follows: buprenorphine hydrochloride 30 mg, dextrose 500 mg, sodium citrate 20 mg, citric acid monohydrate 25 mg, purified water in a sufficient quantity to make a total of 10 mL. These ingredients are all combined together and mixed well. The pH of the formulation is 3.5–4.2. This product is stable for 90 days after preparation when stored in the refrigerator or room temperature in an amber glass dropper bottle.

## Stability and Storage

Store in a tightly sealed container, protected from light, and at room temperature. Mix with sodium chloride for intravenous infusions. Compounded forms, if prepared as described in the Formulation section, are stable for 90 days.

## Small Animal Dosage

### Dogs

- Conventional formulation (0.3 mg/mL): 0.006–0.02 mg/kg q4–8h IV, IM, or SQ. For analgesia, higher doses are used in the range of 0.03–0.04 mg/kg, IV, IM, or SQ (30–40 mcg/kg).
- Concentrated solution (1.8 mg/mL): 20 mcg/kg, IM or SQ, administered for relief of surgical pain.
- Constant rate infusion (CRI): 20 mcg/kg IV followed by 5 mcg/kg/h infusion.
- Epidural: 0.003–0.006 mg/kg (3–6 mcg/kg).
- Buprenorphine SR: 120–270 mcg/kg (0.12–0.27 mg/kg) SQ (duration of 72 hours).

### Cats

- For analgesia, a dose of 0.01–0.02 mg/kg (10–20 mcg/kg) IV or 0.02 mg/kg (20 mcg/kg) IM. Duration is 4–6 hours typically. Additional doses of 0.02 mg/kg may be administered.
- For sedation, often with other sedative agents, the dose of 0.02–0.04 mg/kg IV or IM is used. It is not as effective for sedation as other combinations of agents.
- CRI: 20 mcg/kg IV followed by 12 mcg/kg/h infusion.
- Subcutaneous administration: The concentrated formulation (Simbadol) can be administered SQ once daily for up to 3 days at a dose of 0.24 mg/kg (240 mcg/kg). This formulation may be administered prior to surgery.
- Buccal (transmucosal) administration: 0.02–0.04 mg/kg (20–40 mcg/kg) q8h. 0.02 mg/kg (20 mcg/kg) is equivalent to 0.066 mL/kg. This may be applied to the cat's gingival or oral mucosa (i.e., sublingual).
- Epidural: 12.5 mcg/kg diluted with saline to a volume of 0.3 mL/kg.
- Buprenorphine SR: 120–270 mcg/kg (0.12–0.27 mg/kg) SQ (duration of 72 hours).

## Large Animal Dosage

### Horses

- 0.005–0.01 mg/kg (5–10 mcg/kg IM); short acting in horses.

### Sheep

- 0.01 mg/kg (10 mcg/kg) IM q6h.

## Regulatory Information

The drug is controlled by the Drug Enforcement Administration. Do not administer to animals intended for food.

Schedule III controlled drug.

RCI Classification: 2

## Buspirone Hydrochloride
byoo-speer'own hye-droe-klor'ide

**Trade and other names:** BuSpar

**Functional classification:** Behavior modification

## Pharmacology and Mechanism of Action

Antianxiety agent of the azapirone class. Buspirone acts as a direct-acting serotonin (5-HT$_{1A}$) agonist. By activating 5-HT$_{1A}$ receptors, buspirone and related drugs alter mood and anxiety. Buspirone is used to treat anxiety and other behavior problems. Other related drugs include gepirone and ipsapirone.

## Indications and Clinical Uses

In veterinary medicine, buspirone has been primarily used for the treatment of urine spraying (urine marking) in cats. In cats, there are published studies demonstrating efficacy. However, some cats relapse after treatment is discontinued. Buspirone also has been used as an antiemetic in cats (4 mg/kg SQ). In dogs, it has occasionally been used to treat behavior problems, such as anxiety disorders.

### Precautionary Information

**Adverse Reactions and Side Effects**

Few side effects are seen in cats compared with other drugs. Some cats show increased aggression, and some cats show increased affection and friendliness to owners. It may produce mild sedation.

**Contraindications and Precautions**

Do not use in animals with sensitivity to serotonin agonists.

**Drug Interactions**

Do not use with other serotonin antagonists, selective serotonin reuptake inhibitors, or MAOIs (e.g., selegiline).

## Instructions for Use

Some efficacy trials suggest effectiveness for treating urine spraying in cats. There may be a lower relapse rate compared with other drugs.

## Patient Monitoring and Laboratory Tests

No specific monitoring is necessary.

## Formulations

- Buspirone is available in 5-, 10-, 15-, and 30-mg tablets.

## Stability and Storage

Store in a tightly sealed container, protected from light, and at room temperature. Stability of compounded formulations has not been evaluated.

## Small Animal Dosage

**Cats**

- 2.5–5 mg/cat q12h PO, which may be increased to 5–7.5 mg per cat twice daily for some cats (0.5–1 mg/kg q12h PO).

**Dogs**

- 2.5–10 mg/dog q24h or q12h PO.
- 1 mg/kg q12h PO.

## Large Animal Dosage

**Horses**

- 100–250 mg/horse q24h PO (0.5 mg/kg).

## Regulatory Information
Do not administer to animals intended for food.
RCI Classification: 2

# Busulfan
byoo-sul′fan

**Trade and other names:** Myleran

**Functional classification:** Anticancer agent

## Pharmacology and Mechanism of Action
Anticancer agent. Busulfan is a bifunctional alkylating agent and acts to disrupt DNA of tumor cells.

## Indications and Clinical Uses
Busulfan is used primarily for lymphoreticular neoplasia.

### Precautionary Information
**Adverse Reactions and Side Effects**
Leukopenia is the most severe side effect.

**Contraindications and Precautions**
Do not use in animals with suppressed bone marrow.

**Drug Interactions**
No drug interactions are reported in animals.

## Instructions for Use
Busulfan is usually used in combination with other anticancer agents. Consult specific protocol for details.

## Patient Monitoring and Laboratory Tests
Monitor CBC in animals during treatment.

## Formulations
• Busulfan is available in 2-mg tablets and a 6-mg/mL injection under the name Busulfex.

## Stability and Storage
Store in a tightly sealed container, protected from light, and at room temperature. Stability of compounded formulations has not been evaluated.

## Small Animal Dosage
**Dogs and Cats**
• 3–4 mg/m$^2$ q24h PO.

## Large Animal Dosage
• No dose has been reported for large animals.

## Regulatory Information
Withdrawal times are not established for animals that produce food. This drug should not be used in food animals because it is an anticancer agent.

# Butorphanol Tartrate
byoo-tor´fah-nole tar´trate

**Trade and other names:** Torbutrol, Dolorex, Butorphine, and Torbugesic

**Functional classification:** Analgesic, opioid

## Pharmacology and Mechanism of Action

Opioid analgesic. Butorphanol is an opiate that acts as kappa-receptor agonist and weak mu-receptor antagonist. As a kappa agonist, butorphanol produces sedation and analgesia in animals. It is considered a mild analgesic compared with pure mu-receptor opiates. It is often used in combination with other anesthetics. It has a short half-life in animals (1–2 hours) and a short duration of analgesia (1–2 hours).

## Indications and Clinical Uses

Butorphanol is used for perioperative analgesia, for chronic pain, and as an antitussive agent. It is considered a weak analgesic compared with drugs that are pure mu-receptor agonists, and some of the observed effects may be caused by sedation rather than analgesia. It can be used, often with other agents, for sedation in patients with anxiety or when sedation is needed. In dogs, at doses of 0.4 mg/kg, butorphanol produces analgesia for a duration of 1 hour or less. As an antitussive, it is more potent than morphine (4×) and codeine (100×). Duration of the antitussive effect is approximately 90 minutes, but the effect may persist for as long as 4 hours. In horses, it may be administered IV, IM, and as a CRI. CRI has been shown effective in controlled studies for relief of abdominal pain in horses.

## Precautionary Information

### Adverse Reactions and Side Effects

Adverse effects are similar to other opioid analgesic drugs, but without significant mu-receptor effects. Sedation is common at analgesic doses. Respiratory depression can occur with high doses. Lethal dose in dogs ($LD_{50}$) is 20 mg/kg, which is much higher than clinical doses. Although bradycardia rarely needs to be treated when it is caused by an opioid, if necessary, atropine can be administered. If serious respiratory depression occurs, the opioid can be reversed with naloxone. Dysphoric effects have been observed with agonist/antagonist drugs; this effect has been observed in cats. Decreased intestinal peristalsis and constipation may occur in some animals. A decrease in intestinal motility may be a particular concern in some horses.

### Contraindications and Precautions

Schedule IV controlled substance. Butorphanol use in birds requires much higher doses than in mammals because of shorter half-life and rapid clearance (e.g., 2–4 mg/kg q2–4h).

### Drug Interactions

Butorphanol is compatible with many other analgesics and is used in combination treatment for analgesia. Because butorphanol is an agonist/antagonist, it may antagonize some effects of drugs that are pure agonists (e.g., fentanyl, morphine, hydromorphone, and oxymorphone). However, the clinical significance of this antagonism has been debated among experts. Do not mix with sodium barbiturates.

## Instructions for Use

Butorphanol is often used in combination with anesthetic agents or in conjunction with other analgesic drugs. For most indications, a dose of 0.4 mg/kg is considered optimum, and there is little justification to increase the dose above 0.8 mg/kg because this is considered the ceiling dose. Butorphanol has a short duration of effect of less than 2 hours and usually only 1 hour. In horses, because butorphanol may cause increased locomotor activity and excitement, xylazine may be administered prior to buprenorphine.

## Patient Monitoring and Laboratory Tests

Monitor patient's heart rate and respiration.

## Formulations

- Butorphanol is available in 1-, 5-, and 10-mg tablets and 0.5- and 1-mg/mL injection. Torbugesic is available as a 10 mg/mL injection; Butorphine for cats is available as a 2-mg/mL injection.

## Stability and Storage

Store in a tightly sealed container, protected from light, and at room temperature. Stability of compounded formulations has not been evaluated.

## Small Animal Dosage

### Dogs

- Antitussive: 0.055 mg/kg q6–12h SQ, 0.011 mg/kg IM, or 0.5–1 mg/kg q6–12h PO.
- Pre-anesthetic or sedative use: 0.2–0.4 mg/kg IV, IM, or SQ. May be used with other sedatives such as acepromazine.
- Analgesic: 0.2–0.4 mg/kg q2–4h IV, IM, or SQ or 1–4 mg/kg q6h PO.
- CRI: Loading dose of 0.2–0.4 mg/kg IV followed by 0.1–0.2 mg/kg/h.

### Cats

- Analgesic: 0.2–0.8 mg/kg q2–6h IV or SQ or 1.5 mg/kg q4–8h PO.
- Sedation: 0.2–0.5 mg/kg IV or IM. Often administered with other sedative agents. When combined with other agents for short-term use, use the lower dose of 0.2 mg/kg.
- CRI: Loading dose of 0.2–0.4 mg/kg IV, followed by 0.1–0.2 mg/kg/h.

## Large Animal Dosage

### Horses

- Pain: 0.2–0.4 mg/kg q3–4h IV. In some instances, lower doses of 0.02–0.1 mg/kg IV or 0.04–0.2 mg/kg IM have been used. Low doses of 0.1 mg/kg IV have been used to minimize the decrease in intestinal motility.
- Sedation: 0.01–0.06 mg/kg IV.
- CRI: 13–24 mcg/kg/h (0.013–0.024 mg/kg) IV.

### Ruminants

- 0.05–0.2 mg/kg IV.

### Cattle

- In combination with xylazine, 0.01–0.02 mg/kg IV.

## Regulatory Information

Drug controlled by DEA, Schedule IV.
Do not administer to animals intended for food.
RCI Classification: 2

# N-Butylscopolammonium Bromide (Butylscopolamine Bromide)

en-byoo-til-skoe-pahl'ah-moe-nee-um broe'mide

**Trade and other names:** Buscopan

**Functional classification:** Antispasmodic

## Pharmacology and Mechanism of Action

Antispasmodic, antimuscarinic, anticholinergic drug. This is a quaternary ammonium compound derived from belladonna alkaloid. Butylscopolamine, like other antimuscarinic drugs, blocks cholinergic receptors and produces a parasympatholytic effect. It affects receptors throughout the body, but it is used more commonly for its GI effects. It effectively inhibits secretions and motility of the GI tract by blocking parasympathetic receptors. It can also relax respiratory smooth muscle. It has a short half-life (15–25 minutes) and short duration of action. As a quaternary ammonium compound, it typically does not cross the blood–brain barrier to produce central nervous system reactions.

## Indications and Clinical Uses

Butylscopolamine bromide is indicated for treating pain associated with spasmodic colic, flatulent colic, and intestinal impactions in horses. It is also used to relax the rectum and reduce intestinal strain to facilitate diagnostic rectal palpation.

This agent also relieves bronchoconstriction caused by airway smooth muscle contraction mediated by vagal activation of muscarinic receptors. When used to treat bronchospasm in horses, it produces a rapid and short-lived improvement in lung function in horses with bronchoconstriction associated with equine asthma syndrome.

## Precautionary Information

### Adverse Reactions and Side Effects

Adverse reactions from anticholinergic drugs are related to their blocking of acetylcholine receptors and producing a systemic parasympatholytic response. As expected with this class of drugs, animals will have increased heart rate, decreased secretions, dry mucous membranes, decreased GI tract motility, and dilated pupils. The effects on intestinal motility usually have less than 2 hours' duration. In target animal safety studies in which doses of 1, 3, and 5 times the approved dose and up to 10 times the dose were administered to horses, the clinical signs described previously were observed. However, at high doses, there were no CBC or biochemical abnormalities or lesions identified at necropsy.

### Contraindications and Precautions

N-butylscopolammonium bromide decreases intestinal motility. Use cautiously in conditions in which decreased motility will be a concern.

### Drug Interactions

N-butylscopolammonium bromide is an anticholinergic drug and therefore antagonizes any other medications that are intended to produce a cholinergic response (e.g., metoclopramide).

## Instructions for Use

Most experience in horses is related to treating spasmodic colic, flatulent colic, and intestinal impactions in horses. It has also been used successfully to alleviate respiratory distress in horses with airway disease associated with bronchospasm. There is no experience in other animals.

## Patient Monitoring and Laboratory Tests

Monitor equine intestinal motility (gut sounds and fecal output) during treatment. Monitor heart rate in treated animals.

## Formulations

- N-butylscopolammonium is available in a 20-mg/mL solution.

## Stability and Storage

Store in a tightly sealed container, protected from light, and at room temperature.

## Small Animal Dosage

- No dose is reported for small animals.

## Large Animal Dosage

**Horses**

- 0.3 mg/kg, slowly IV as a single dose (1.5 mL/100 kg). Onset of action is usually within 2 minutes, with a duration of less than 2 hours.
- To relieve bronchoconstriction: 0.3 mg/kg IV, single dose.

## Regulatory Information

Do not administer to animals intended for food.

# Cabergoline
ca-ber'goe-leen

**Trade and other names:** Galastop (veterinary form) and Dostinex (human form)

**Functional classification:** Serotonin antagonist, prolactin inhibitor

## Pharmacology and Mechanism of Action

Synthetic selective dopamine ($D_2$) agonist used to lower prolactin levels. It is an ergot-derived product with very low affinity for dopamine $D_1$-receptors or other adrenergic receptors (alpha$_1$ and alpha$_2$). Thus, it has specific dopamine $D_2$ antagonistic effects. It also has low affinity for serotonin (5-$HT_1$ and 5-$HT_2$) receptors. Through dopamine antagonism, it reduces serum prolactin release from the anterior pituitary gland. Through the prolactin-inhibiting effect, it is used to treat pseudopregnancy in dogs and decrease milk production. It is more potent than other agents (e.g., bromocriptine) and longer acting. The antiprolactin effect of cabergoline persists longer than bromocriptine and pergolide. Prolactin levels were lowered in dogs for over 50 hours after dosing.

*Pharmacokinetics:* In dogs, peak oral absorption occurs at 1 hour. It is widely distributed to tissues. The half-life in dogs is 19 hours on day 1 but 10 hours on day 28. In people it has a long half-life (100 hours) and approximately 40% protein binding. It can be administered with or without food.

## Indications and Clinical Uses

Cabergoline is used in dogs to treat pseudopregnancy. Clinical studies in dogs showed over 90% efficacy in reduction of mammary gland and improvement in behavior within 10 days. This action is through the inhibition of prolactin, which reduces the signs of pseudopregnancy in dogs and inhibits the development of the mammary gland and lactation. It should be administered once daily (see the dosing section) for 4–6 days initially but can be repeated to fully resolve the problem. In dogs, it is also used for treatment of primary and secondary anestrus. The dosage used for anestrus is 5 mcg/kg PO once daily until 2 days after the onset of proestrus. One study also used a lower dosage of 0.6 mcg/kg PO once daily for treatment of anestrus.

In people, cabergoline is used to treat diseases associated with high levels of prolactin, prolactinoma (prolactin-secreting adenomas), or idiopathic hyperprolactinemia. It is as effective and longer acting than bromocriptine. There are also fewer adverse effects in women compared with treatment with bromocriptine. It has been used in people for symptomatic management of parkinsonian syndrome, but other drugs are usually preferred.

## Precautionary Information

### Adverse Reactions and Side Effects

Because of dopamine agonist effects, adverse effects related to this action are possible. It can cause hypotension in some animals. Gastrointestinal (GI) problems are possible in dogs, with vomiting the most common, especially at doses higher than 5 mcg/kg. Anorexia and lethargy are also possible. These signs do not require discontinuation of treatment.

**Contraindications and Precautions**

Do not use in pregnant animals. Abortion may occur. It may cause hypotension. Use cautiously with other agents that can produce hypotension. Because of the possibility of hypotension, it should be discontinued prior to anesthesia.

*Human warning:* Wash hands after use. Avoid contact with skin and eyes; wash off any splashes immediately. Care should be taken to avoid contact between the solution and women of childbearing age. Women of childbearing age should wear gloves when administering the product.

**Drug Interactions**

There are no direct drug interactions observed in animals, but it should be used with great caution with any other drugs that act as dopamine agonists because it may potentiate the action. If used with dopamine antagonists (e.g., phenothiazines, butyrophenones, metoclopramide), there will be antagonism.

## Instructions for Use

The use in animals is derived from the approved indication in Europe. Start with a once-daily dose for treatment of pseudopregnancy and treat for 4–6 days initially. Repeat the protocol if needed in refractory cases. It can be administered directly in the mouth or administered with food.

## Patient Monitoring and Laboratory Tests

Monitor plasma cortisol concentrations if used long term.

## Formulations

- Cabergoline is available in a veterinary formulation as oral drops. The formulation Galastop is available in 50-mcg/mL concentration in 7- and 15-mL amber bottles. It is also available in a human formulation of 0.5-mg scored tablets.

## Stability and Storage

Store in a tightly sealed container, protected from light, and at room temperature. Do not refrigerate the oral solution. Discard the open container 28 days after opening of the oral liquid.

## Small Animal Dosage

**Dogs**

- Pseudopregnancy: 5 mcg/kg once daily (0.1 mL/kg of the oral liquid).
- Decrease lactation: 5 mcg/kg once daily PO for 5 days.

**Cats**

- Queens: 0.5–1 mL of the oral veterinary liquid per cat (liquid is 50 mcg/mL).

## Large Animal Dosage

- No dose has been reported for large animals. Do not administer to food producing animals.

## Regulatory Information

No regulatory information is available. For extralabel use withdrawal interval estimates, contact Food Animal Residue Avoidance Databank (FARAD) at www.FARAD.org.

# Calcitriol

kal-sih-trye'ole

**Trade and other names:** Rocaltrol and Calcijex

**Functional classification:** Calcium supplement

## Pharmacology and Mechanism of Action

Vitamin D analogue, also called *1,25-dihydroxycholecalciferol*. Calcitriol is normally formed in the kidneys from 25-hydroxycholecalciferol. Action of calcitriol is to increase calcium absorption from the intestine and facilitate a parathyroid hormone (PTH) effect on bone. Low calcitriol levels in animals can cause decreased intestinal calcium absorption. Animals with chronic kidney disease (CKD) (especially cats) and hyperparathyroidism often have low calcitriol levels that require supplementation with this medication. Calcitriol can also inhibit synthesis and storage of PTH.

## Indications and Clinical Uses

Calcitriol is used to treat calcium deficiency and diseases such as hypocalcemia associated with hyperparathyroidism. It is also used to increase calcium in cats that have had parathyroid glands surgically removed. In this use, it is often administered with calcium supplements to the diet. It is used in dogs and cats to manage calcium and phosphorous balance with CKD. Although used by veterinarians to reduce renal secondary PTH concentrations in animals with CKD, this benefit is more controversial and not supported by strong evidence. Supplementation to cats with CKD may help slow progression of disease in some cats, but some cats do not show a benefit. Calcitriol should not be used as a vitamin D supplement.

## Precautionary Information

### Adverse Reactions and Side Effects

Overdose can result in hypercalcemia. High doses can cause soft tissue mineralization.

### Contraindications and Precautions

Do not use in patients that are at risk of hypercalcemia. Capsules made for humans may contain high overdoses for dogs and cats and should be reformulated.

### Drug Interactions

Calcitriol may cause hypercalcemia if used with thiazide diuretics.

## Instructions for Use

When comparing doses with vitamin D, 1 unit of vitamin D is equivalent to 0.025 mcg of cholecalciferol or ergocalciferol (400 units of vitamin D = 10 mcg of cholecalciferol). Doses should be adjusted in each patient according to response and monitoring calcium plasma concentration; thus, the maintenance dose in animals may vary depending on the adjustment to calcium levels. For example, when used for treating dogs with CKD, the average dosage was 2.5 ng/kg/day, but it ranged from 0.75–5 ng/kg/day based on adjustments from measuring calcium concentrations. When used in CKD, it is often used with intestinal phosphate binders (e.g., aluminum hydroxide) and dietary phosphorous restriction. Recommended phosphate concentrations should be maintained at less than 6 mg/dL.

In cats, do not administer simultaneously with a meal to avoid increased calcium absorption. It is best administered in the evening before a meal. If ionized calcium increases above the reference range (above 4.5–5.5 mg/dL), stop treatment and then reintroduce it at a lower dose.

## Patient Monitoring and Laboratory Tests

Monitor plasma ionized calcium concentration. Adjust doses as necessary to maintain normal calcium, phosphorous, and PTH concentrations.

Normal total calcium concentrations in dogs and cats are 9–11.5 mg/dL and 8–10.5 mg/dL, respectively, or 1.2–1.5 mmol/L and 1.1–1.4 mmol/L, respectively. Monitor serum PTH concentrations (assays are available in many diagnostic laboratories). Monitor serum creatinine in animals when used to treat CKD.

## Formulations

- Calcitriol is available as injection (Calcijex) in a 1- and 2-mcg/mL and in 0.25- and 0.5-mcg capsules.
- Calcitriol oral solution is available as 1 mcg/mL (Rocaltrol). This may be diluted for administration to small animals. See the Stability and Storage section for instructions on dilutions.

## Stability and Storage

Store in a tightly sealed container, protected from light, and at room temperature.

*Compounded forms:* Small animal veterinarians have compounded calcitriol in oil to facilitate dosing to small animals. One such recipe uses 1 part oral solution (Rocaltrol) mixed with 9 parts medium-chain triglyceride (MCT) oil or olive oil. Rocaltrol has been mixed with corn oil (1:10 ratio) to prepare a 100-ng/mL oral formulation.

A more complex compounded formulation prepared by some pharmacies uses a diluent prepared from 400 mg of butylated hydroxyanisole (BHA) and 400 mg of butylated hydroxytoluene (BHT) in 2 mL of 100% ethyl alcohol. This should be mixed thoroughly to dissolve BHA and BHT. This mixture is added to 400 mL of extra-light olive oil and mixed thoroughly. This mixture is used as a diluent. 145.5 mL of this diluent is added to 4.5 mL of oral calcitriol (Rocaltrol) 1-mcg/mL oral solution. This mixture produces a 30-ng/mL (0.030 mcg/mL) oral solution. Store in an amber bottle. Beyond-use-date is 6 months from the time of preparation.

## Small Animal Dosage

(Note: To convert from micrograms (mcg) to nanograms (ng) refer to the page facing the inside front cover.)

### Dogs

- Renal secondary hyperparathyroidism in chronic renal failure: 2.5 ng/kg PO once daily. Adjust dose with calcium and PTH measurements. If PTH concentrations remain elevated and calcium is not elevated, increase the dosage to 3.5 ng/kg once daily. The dosage may be increased incrementally up to 5 ng/kg once daily. If dogs cannot be medicated once daily, an alternative dosing regimen is a 10 ng/kg twice per week PO.

### Cats

- Hypocalcemia (after removal of parathyroid glands): 0.25 mcg/cat q48h PO or 0.01–0.04 mcg/kg/day PO (10–40 ng/kg/day).
- Renal secondary hyperparathyroidism: 2.5 ng/kg PO once daily. Adjust dose with calcium and PTH measurements. If PTH concentrations remain elevated and calcium is not elevated, increase the dose to 3.5 ng/kg once daily and incrementally up to a dose of 5 ng/kg/day. Do not exceed 5 ng/kg/day. An alternative dosing regimen that has been used for cats that cannot be

administered once daily is 10 ng/kg twice per week PO. Because the volumes for dosing cats is low, refer to the Formulation section for compounding a more dilute solution.

## Large Animal Dosage
• No dose has been reported for large animals.

## Regulatory Information
No regulatory information is available. For extralabel use withdrawal interval estimates, contact FARAD at www.FARAD.org.

---

# Calcium Carbonate

**Trade and other names:** Titralac, Calci-Mix, Tums, and generic brands

**Functional classification:** Calcium supplement

## Pharmacology and Mechanism of Action
Calcium supplement. Calcium is essential for the functional integrity of several body systems. Calcium carbonate is equivalent to 400 mg of calcium ion per gram. Calcium carbonate neutralizes stomach acid for treating and preventing stomach ulcers.

## Indications and Clinical Uses
Calcium carbonate is used as an oral calcium supplement for hypocalcemia, sometimes used with vitamin D supplements or calcitriol. It contains 40% elemental calcium. It is used as antacid to treat gastric hyperacidity and GI ulcers and as an intestinal phosphate binder for hyperphosphatemia associated with CKD. Pronefra (calcium carbonate and magnesium carbonate) is administered as a palatable phosphate binder in dogs and cats. It is administered as an oral liquid suspension with meals.

## Precautionary Information

### Adverse Reactions and Side Effects
Few side effects. High calcium concentrations are possible. With any calcium supplements, constipation and intestinal bloating can occur.

### Contraindications and Precautions
Do not administer to animals predisposed to forming calcium-containing renal or cystic calculi. When calcium carbonate or calcium citrate is used as a phosphate binder to prevent hyperphosphatemia, caution is advised to avoid hypercalcemia in patients with kidney disease.

### Drug Interactions
Oral administration of calcium supplements may interfere with absorption of other drugs such as fluoroquinolones (e.g., enrofloxacin, orbifloxacin, marbofloxacin, pradofloxacin), bisphosphonates, zinc, iron, and tetracyclines. Use cautiously with thiazide diuretics because this could cause a high increase in calcium concentrations.

## Instructions for Use
Calcium carbonate is equivalent to 400 mg of calcium ion per gram. Doses are primarily derived from extrapolation of human doses. When used as a calcium supplement, doses should be adjusted according to serum calcium concentrations. Administer with food to improve oral absorption. Some tablets also contain vitamin

D. Doses are based on calcium carbonate, not the ion concentration (e.g., a 650-mg tablet contains 260 mg of calcium ion).

## Patient Monitoring and Laboratory Tests

Monitor serum calcium levels, particularly if patients have kidney disease. Normal total calcium concentrations in dogs and cats are 9–11.5 mg/dL and 8–10.5 mg/dL, respectively, or 1.2–1.5 mmol/L and 1.1–1.4 mmol/L, respectively.

## Formulations

Calcium carbonate is available in tablets or oral suspension, most of which are available over the counter (OTC). One gram of calcium carbonate is equivalent to 400 mg of calcium ion. Calci-Mix is available in 1.25-g capsules. OTC tablets are available in 500 and 600 mg and 1, 1.25, and 1.5 g. Oral suspension (Titralac) is 1.25 g/5 mL. The formulation Pronefra also is available as calcium carbonate and magnesium carbonate. It is an oral syrup that may be administered as a phosphate binder in cats. Pronefra is preferred by some cats because it is a palatable liquid suspension with poultry liver flavoring.

## Stability and Storage

Store in a tightly sealed container, protected from light, and at room temperature. Stability of compounded formulations has not been evaluated. Do not mix with other compounds that may chelate with calcium.

## Small Animal Dosage

### Dogs and Cats

- Calcium supplementation: 70–185 mg/kg/day given with food PO.
- Treatment of hypoparathyroidism: 30–60 mg/kg per day in divided doses (with meals).
- Phosphate binder: 60–100 mg/kg/day in divided doses, usually given with food PO.
- Pronefra (calcium carbonate and magnesium carbonate) for use as a phosphate binder. Administer with a meal. Cats: 1 mL per 4.4 kg (8.8 lb) twice a day at mealtime. Dogs: 1 mL/5 kg (11 lb) twice a day at mealtime.

## Large Animal Dosage

- No dose has been reported for large animals. Usually, other calcium salts are used for supplementation in cattle.

## Regulatory Information

No withdrawal times are available. Because this is a normal dietary supplement with little risk from residues, no withdrawal time is suggested for animals intended for food.

# Calcium Chloride

**Trade and other names:** Generic brands

**Functional classification:** Calcium supplement

## Pharmacology and Mechanism of Action

Calcium supplement. Calcium is essential for the functional integrity of several body systems. Injection is 27.2 mg of calcium ion (1.36 mEq) per milliliter.

Calcium chloride increases ionized calcium in blood more than do other calcium salts.

## Indications and Clinical Uses

Calcium chloride is used in acute situations to supplement as electrolyte replacement or as a cardiotonic. It is administered to cows for hypocalcemia (milk fever).

### Precautionary Information

**Adverse Reactions and Side Effects**

Overdose with calcium is possible. Do not administer IV solution SQ or IM because it may cause tissue necrosis. If calcium salts are inadvertently injected perivascularly, flush the area (irrigate) with 0.9% NaCl and apply local corticosteroids. IV administration can cause irritation, and calcium gluconate is preferred for IV use because it is not as irritating as calcium chloride.

**Contraindications and Precautions**

Do not administer by IV injection at a rapid rate because it can cause hypotension, cardiac arrhythmias, and cardiac arrest. Rapid IV administration to cows can cause cardiac arrhythmias and even death.

**Drug Interactions**

Calcium chloride precipitates with sodium bicarbonate. Do not mix with compounds known to chelate with calcium. These include some antibiotics such as tetracyclines and fluoroquinolones (e.g., enrofloxacin, ciprofloxacin). Do not mix calcium salts with medications that contain carbonate, phosphate, sulfate, or tartrate because they may cause chelation.

## Instructions for Use

The injection formulation is 27.2 mg of calcium ion (1.36 mEq) per milliliter. It is usually used in emergency situations. Intracardiac administrations have been performed as an emergency but avoid injections into the myocardium.

## Patient Monitoring and Laboratory Tests

Monitor serum calcium concentration. Normal total calcium concentrations in dogs and cats are 9–11.5 mg/dL and 8–10.5 mg/dL, respectively, or 1.2–1.5 mmol/L and 1.1–1.4 mmol/L, respectively. Monitor heart rate, electrocardiogram (ECG), or both during IV administration.

## Formulations

- Calcium chloride is available in a 10% (100-mg/mL) solution. This supplies 1.36 mEq calcium ion per milliliter or 27.2 elemental calcium per milliliter. Preparations for cattle usually contain 8.5–11.5 g calcium per 500 mL. Many formulations also contain magnesium.

## Stability and Storage

Store in a tightly sealed container, protected from light, and at room temperature. Stability of compounded formulations has not been evaluated. Do not mix with other compounds that may chelate with calcium.

### Small Animal Dosage
**Dogs and Cats**
- 0.1–0.3 mL/kg of 10% solution IV (slowly).
- Treatment of severe hypocalcemia (with tetany and seizures): 5–15 mg/kg elemental calcium over 10–30 minutes IV slowly.

### Large Animal Dosage
**Cows**
- 2 g/100 kg body weight, IV at a rate of 1 g/min.

**Horses**
- 1–2 g per adult horse IV slowly.

### Regulatory Information
No withdrawal times are available. Because this is a normal supplement with little risk from residues, no withdrawal time is suggested for animals intended for food.

## Calcium Citrate

**Trade and other names:** Citracal (OTC)

**Functional classification:** Calcium supplement

### Pharmacology and Mechanism of Action
Calcium supplement. Calcium is essential for the functional integrity of several body systems. It is administered orally to supply calcium to the diet.

### Indications and Clinical Uses
Calcium citrate is used in the treatment of hypocalcemia, such as with hypoparathyroidism. It contains 21% elemental calcium. It also is used as an intestinal phosphate binder for hyperphosphatemia associated with kidney disease.

### Precautionary Information
**Adverse Reactions and Side Effects**
Hypercalcemia is possible with oversupplementation. With any calcium supplements, constipation and intestinal bloating can occur. Constipation and bloating are more likely with calcium citrate than calcium carbonate.

**Contraindications and Precautions**
When calcium carbonate or calcium citrate is used as a phosphate binder to prevent hyperphosphatemia, caution is advised to avoid hypercalcemia in patients with renal failure.

**Drug Interactions**
Oral administration of calcium supplements may interfere with absorption of other drugs such as fluoroquinolones (e.g., enrofloxacin, orbifloxacin, marbofloxacin), bisphosphonates, zinc, iron, and tetracyclines. Calcium citrate does not require acid for absorption and may be administered with ulcer drugs that suppress stomach acid (e.g., omeprazole, $H_2$-blockers).

## Instructions for Use

Doses should be adjusted according to serum calcium concentration. Although calcium carbonate should be administered with a meal, this is not required for calcium citrate.

## Patient Monitoring and Laboratory Tests

Monitor serum calcium levels, particularly if patients have renal failure. Normal total calcium concentrations in dogs and cats are 9–11.5 mg/dL and 8–10.5 mg/dL, respectively, or 1.2–1.5 mmol/L and 1.1–1.4 mmol/L, respectively. If used as a phosphate binder, adjust doses based on serum phosphorous concentrations.

## Formulations

- Calcium citrate is available in 950-mg tablets (contains 200 mg of calcium ion), and 1000-mg tablets. Some forms also contain vitamin $D_3$.

## Stability and Storage

Store in a tightly sealed container, protected from light, and at room temperature. Stability of compounded formulations has not been evaluated. Do not mix with other compounds that may chelate with calcium.

## Small Animal Dosage

**Cats**
- 10–30 mg/kg q8h (with meals) PO.

**Dogs**
- 20 mg/kg/day (with meals) PO.

**Dogs and Cats**
- Phosphate binder (to prevent hyperphosphatemia): 10–20 mg/kg per day in divided doses with meals PO.

## Large Animal Dosage

- No dose has been reported for large animals.

## Regulatory Information

No withdrawal times are available. Because this is a normal dietary supplement with little risk from residues, no withdrawal time is suggested for animals intended for food.

# Calcium Gluconate and Calcium Borogluconate

**Trade and other names:** Kalcinate, AmVet, Cal-Nate, and generic brands

**Functional classification:** Calcium supplement

## Pharmacology and Mechanism of Action

Calcium supplement. Calcium is essential for the functional integrity of several body systems. It is administered orally to supply calcium to the diet but injected for acute conditions in which a rapid increase in serum calcium is needed. Calcium gluconate 10% solution contains 9.3 mg of elemental calcium per milliliter.

## Indications and Clinical Uses

Calcium gluconate and calcium borogluconate are used in the treatment of hypocalcemia, such as with hypoparathyroidism, but are used less commonly than other forms. However, if administered IV, calcium gluconate is not as irritating as calcium chloride. Calcium gluconate and calcium borogluconate are used in diseases that produce electrolyte deficiency. Calcium supplements are administered to cattle for treatment of hypocalcemia (milk fever).

---

### Precautionary Information

#### Adverse Reactions and Side Effects

Hypercalcemia is possible with oversupplementation. Calcium supplements may cause constipation. SQ or IM injections of calcium salts may cause tissue injury and necrosis at the site of injection. If calcium salts are inadvertently injected perivascularly, flush the area (irrigate) with 0.9% NaCl and apply local corticosteroids.

#### Contraindications and Precautions

Do not administer by IV injection at a rapid rate because it can cause hypotension, cardiac arrhythmias, and cardiac arrest. Avoid use in patients that are prone to calcium-containing renal or cystic calculi. Avoid administration of the IV solution IM or SQ because it will cause tissue necrosis and can cause pyogranulomatous panniculitis and adipocyte mineralization at the site of injection.

#### Drug Interactions

Do not mix with bicarbonates (e.g., sodium bicarbonate), phosphates, sulfates, and tartrates because it may cause precipitation. Specific drugs that can precipitate with calcium gluconate include oxytetracycline, promethazine, sulfamethazine, tetracycline, cephalothin, and amphotericin B. Calcium supplements may interfere with the oral absorption of iron, tetracyclines, and fluoroquinolones.

---

### Instructions for Use

The 500-mg tablets contain 45 mg of calcium ion. The 10% injection contains 97 mg (9.3 mg of elemental calcium ion [0.47 mEq]) per milliliter.

### Patient Monitoring and Laboratory Tests

Monitor serum calcium concentration. Normal total calcium concentrations in dogs and cats are 9–11.5 mg/dL and 8–10.5 mg/dL, respectively, or 1.2–1.5 mmol/L and 1.1–1.4 mmol/L, respectively. Monitor heart rate, ECG, or both during IV administration.

### Formulations

- Calcium gluconate is available as 10% (100-mg/mL) injection. Calcium gluconate 10% contains 9.3 mg of calcium ion per milliliter, or 0.465 mEq/mL.
- Tablets: Calcium gluconate is available in tablets in sizes of 325, 500, 650, 975 mg, and 1 g. Each gram contains 90 mg of calcium ion. Chewable tablets intended for human use are available in 650-mg and 1-g tablets.
- Calcium borogluconate is available as 230 mg/mL, 23% solution (AmVet Calcium Gluconate 23% and Cal-Nate). This solution contains 19.14 elemental calcium per milliliter.

### Stability and Storage

Store in a tightly sealed container, protected from light, and at room temperature. Solutions should be clear. If crystals are present, warm vial up to 30°C–40°C (86°F–104°F) to dissolve crystals. Stability of compounded formulations has not been evaluated. Do not mix with other compounds that may chelate with calcium.

## Small Animal Dosage

### Dogs and Cats

- 75–500 mg IV (slowly) or 0.5–1.6 mL/kg IV of the 10% solution (slowly).
- Treatment of severe hypocalcemia (with tetany and seizures): 5–15 mg/kg elemental calcium over 10–30 minutes IV slowly. This dose is equivalent to 0.54–1.6 mL/kg of the 10% solution.

## Large Animal Dosage (Use Calcium Borogluconate)

### Cattle and Horses

- 5–12 g diluted in 500 mL and infused IV slowly.

### Pigs and Sheep

- 20 mg/kg IV slowly.

### Dairy Cows

- 2 g/100 kg body weight slowly at a rate of 1 g/min.

### Horses

- 50–70 mg/kg diluted in 5% dextrose and infused slowly IV.

## Regulatory Information

No withdrawal times are available. Because this is a normal dietary supplement with little risk from residues, no withdrawal time is suggested for animals intended for food.

# Calcium Lactate

**Trade and other names:** Generic brands

**Functional classification:** Calcium supplement

## Pharmacology and Mechanism of Action

Calcium supplement. Calcium is essential for the functional integrity of several body systems. This oral supplement is used to provide animals with dietary calcium to prevent or treat a deficiency. Contains 13% elemental calcium.

## Indications and Clinical Uses

Calcium lactate is used in treatment of hypocalcemia, such as with hypoparathyroidism, and in electrolyte deficiency.

## Precautionary Information

### Adverse Reactions and Side Effects

Hypercalcemia possible with oversupplementation.

### Contraindications and Precautions

Avoid use in patients that are prone to calcium-containing renal or cystic calculi.

### Drug Interactions

Calcium supplements may interfere with the oral absorption of iron, tetracyclines, and fluoroquinolones.

## Instructions for Use

Calcium lactate contains 130 mg of calcium ion per gram.

## Patient Monitoring and Laboratory Tests

Monitor serum calcium concentrations.

## Formulations

- Calcium lactate is available in 325-mg (42.25 mg of calcium ion) and 650-mg (84.5 mg of calcium ion) OTC tablets.

## Stability and Storage

Store in a tightly sealed container, protected from light, and at room temperature. Stability of compounded formulations has not been evaluated. Do not mix with other compounds that may chelate with calcium.

## Small Animal Dosage

**Dogs**

- 0.5 g/day (500 mg) (in divided doses) PO.

**Cats**

- 0.2–0.5 g/day (200–500 mg) (in divided doses) PO.

## Large Animal Dosage

- No dose has been reported for large animals.

## Regulatory Information

No withdrawal times are available. Because this is a normal dietary supplement with little risk from residues, no withdrawal time is suggested for animals intended for food.

# Capromorelin

kap′roe-moe-rel′in

**Trade and other names:** Entyce

**Functional classification:** Appetite stimulant

## Pharmacology and Mechanism of Action

Capromorelin mimics the action of ghrelin, which is a natural hormone produced by the stomach. Dogs can have decreased appetite associated with chronic diseases (cancer, kidney disease, heart disease, and intestinal diseases). Capromorelin is approved in dogs for appetite stimulation. It is a ghrelin-receptor agonist (GRA) that acts on the hypothalamus to mimic the action of endogenous ghrelin to increase appetite in dogs and increase growth hormone. Capromorelin is a growth hormone secretagogue (GHS) with a stimulatory effect on appetite through central effects on the hypothalamus and peripheral pathways through the action on the vagus nerve. Ghrelin increases the insulin-like growth factor (IGF-1), which is stimulated by growth hormone and may reduce cachexia and increase lean muscle mass in animals with chronic diseases. A similar agent evaluated in people is anamorelin, but this has not been evaluated clinically in veterinary medicine.

Other uses for capromorelin have been considered but are not established at this time. Such uses include growth hormone deficiency, cancer, and GI problems.

*Pharmacokinetics:* After oral administration to dogs, it peaks at approximately 1 hour and has a half-life of 1.2 hours. The bioavailability in dogs is 44%, with a volume of distribution (VD) of 2 L/kg. The protein binding is approximately 50% in dogs. Shortly after oral administration, there is a rapid increase in growth hormone followed by an increase in IGF-1. The increase in IGF-1 serves as a negative feedback mechanism to attenuate large spikes in growth hormone. The increase in IGF-1 is maintained with once-daily dosing in dogs at a dose of 3 mg/kg.

## Indications and Clinical Uses

Capromorelin is used to increase appetite in dogs. It should be administered once daily at the approved dose, with no limit to the length of treatment. In severely ill dogs or those with multiple other problems, it may take a few days to see a response. Some dogs may not respond at all. Some clinicians have increased the dose by 1.5 times to obtain a more consistent positive response. If no response is seen in a few days, even with a higher dose, consider discontinuing the drug and pursuing other treatments. In the clinical studies performed to obtain Food and Drug Administration (FDA) approval, at the label dose, it significantly improved appetite and body weight compared with placebo treatment. Other agents that have been used to increase appetite are mirtazapine, cyproheptadine, corticosteroids, and anabolic steroids, but capromorelin is the first drug approved specifically for this indication in dogs.

The current approval is for dogs only. There are no clinical studies in sick cats that can be used to recommend treatment. In healthy research cats, it increased IGF-1, increased appetite, and increased body weight. Future studies may reveal optimum doses and determine safety. It is proposed that it may be useful to stimulate appetite in cats with CKD at a dosage of 2 mg/kg PO once daily. As for dogs, an increase by 1.5 times (3 mg/kg) can be considered in cats that do not respond to the initial dose.

### Precautionary Information

#### Adverse Reactions and Side Effects

In the clinical field trials, the most common adverse effect was diarrhea, vomiting, polydipsia, and hypersalivation. In the target animal safety studies, it was tolerated at 17.5 times the label dose for 12 months in healthy dogs.

#### Contraindications and Precautions

The safety in dogs with liver or kidney disease has not been evaluated. It is metabolized by cytochrome P450 (CYP450) enzymes, and it is possible that other drugs that affect the CYP450 enzymes could alter the pharmacokinetics. It is excreted in both the urine and feces; use with caution in dogs with renal insufficiency or liver disease. Safety has not been evaluated in dogs used for breeding or pregnant or lactating bitches.

The safety has not been evaluated in cats, but it was safe in healthy research cats. There are no known contraindications or restrictions for dogs. It can be used regardless of duration, weight of dog, or age. It can be administered as long as necessary as long as no adverse effects are observed.

#### Drug Interactions

There are no known drug interactions.

## Instructions for Use
Capromorelin is available in a 30-mg/mL oral solution. Dispense the correct dose to pets using the syringe available in the packaging. Rinse the syringe with water between uses.

## Patient Monitoring and Laboratory Tests
Monitor the patient's body weight and appetite. Although guidelines are not available for cats, it is advised to monitor parameters for diabetes in treated cats until other information is available. If cortisol concentrations are measured, there is an increase in cortisol release seen approximately 1 hour after administration of capromorelin; it declines to baseline levels 4 hours after oral administration.

## Formulations
- Capromorelin is available as an oral flavored solution at a concentration of 30 mg/mL. It is available in sizes of 10-, 15-, and 30-mL bottles with a dispensing syringe.

## Stability and Storage
Store in a tightly sealed container, protected from light, at temperatures less than 30°C (86°F). Do not mix with other drugs if compatibility is not known.

## Small Animal Dosage
### Dogs
- 3 mg/kg PO once daily.

### Cats
- Safe clinical doses have not been established. Until a specific feline form is available, consider a dosage of 2 mg/kg PO once daily.

## Large Animal Dosage
- No dose has been reported for large animals.

## Regulatory Information
No withdrawal times are available. Because this is not approved for food animals, it should not be administered to animals intended for food.

# Captopril
kap′toe-pril

**Trade and other names:** Capoten

**Functional classification:** Vasodilator, angiotensin-converting enzyme inhibitor

## Pharmacology and Mechanism of Action
Angiotensin-converting enzyme (ACE) inhibitor. Captopril inhibits conversion of angiotensin I to angiotensin II, leading to vasodilation. Angiotensin II is a potent vasoconstrictor and will stimulate sympathetic stimulation, renal hypertension, and synthesis of aldosterone. ACE inhibitors limit the ability of aldosterone to cause sodium and water retention that contribute to congestion. Captopril, like other ACE inhibitors, causes vasodilation, but ACE inhibitors also contribute to vasodilation by increasing concentrations of some vasodilating kinins and prostaglandins (PGs).

## Indications and Clinical Uses

Captopril, like other ACE inhibitors, has been used to treat hypertension and congestive heart failure. It was once used in dogs, but its use has declined substantially. Captopril was the first ACE inhibitor available for clinical use but has been replaced by other ACE inhibitors such as enalapril, benazepril, and lisinopril. Unlike benazepril and enalapril, there are no clinical studies that have been used to support its clinical use in dogs and cats.

### Precautionary Information

**Adverse Reactions and Side Effects**

Hypotension is possible with excessive doses. Captopril may cause azotemia in some patients, especially when administered with potent diuretics (e.g., furosemide). GI side effects, predominantly anorexia, are common in dogs.

**Contraindications and Precautions**

Discontinue ACE inhibitors in pregnant animals; they cross the placenta and have caused fetal malformations and fetal death.

**Drug Interactions**

Use cautiously with diuretics and potassium supplements. Nonsteroidal anti-inflammatory drugs (NSAIDs) may diminish antihypertensive effect.

## Instructions for Use

Use of captopril has been replaced by enalapril and benazepril in small animal practices, and most clinical experts recommend these other drugs instead of captopril.

### Patient Monitoring and Laboratory Tests

Monitor patients carefully to avoid hypotension. With all ACE inhibitors, monitor electrolytes and renal function 3–7 days after initiating therapy and periodically thereafter.

### Formulations

- Captopril is available in 12.5-, 25-, 50-, and 100-mg tablets.

### Stability and Storage

Store in a tightly sealed container at room temperature. More stable at acidic pH. Oral compounded solutions are stable for 30 days refrigerated. However, tap water should not be used; purified water is necessary to ensure stability.

### Small Animal Dosage

**Dogs**

- 0.5–2 mg/kg q8–12h PO.

**Cats**

- 3.12–6.25 mg/cat q8h PO.

### Large Animal Dosage

- No dose has been reported for large animals.

### Regulatory Information

Do not administer to animals intended for food.
Racing Commissioners International (RCI) Classification: 3

# Carbenicillin
kar-ben-ih-sill'in

**Trade and other names:** Formulations previously marketed were Geopen, Pyopen, and carbenicillin indanyl sodium

**Functional classification:** Antibacterial

**Note:** Carbenicillin is no longer commercially available. Information is included here on the pharmacology and clinical use, but other agents should be substituted for clinical use (e.g., piperacillin–tazobactam).

## Pharmacology and Mechanism of Action

Beta-lactam antibiotic. Carbenicillin has an action similar to ampicillin, which inhibits bacterial cell wall synthesis. Carbenicillin has a broad spectrum of activity that includes both gram-positive and gram-negative bacteria. However, resistance is possible, especially among beta-lactamase–positive strains. The difference between carbenicillin and ampicillin is that it is active against *Pseudomonas aeruginosa,* and other gram-negative bacteria that are resistant to ampicillin and amoxicillin. The activity of piperacillin is greater than carbenicillin and it is preferred for treatment. Half-life of carbenicillin is short, and clearance is rapid in animals; therefore it requires frequent administration.

## Indications and Clinical Uses

Carbenicillin has been used to treat gram-negative infections in animals, including infections caused by *P. aeruginosa,* but carbenicillin has been discontinued and is no longer available. It has been replaced by other broad-spectrum agents such as piperacillin–tazobactam.

## Precautionary Information

**Adverse Reactions and Side Effects**

Carbenicillin, like other penicillin drugs, may cause allergy. Carbenicillin may cause bleeding problems in some animals by interfering with platelets.

**Contraindications and Precautions**

Use cautiously in patients sensitive to penicillins (e.g., allergy).

**Drug Interactions**

No drug interactions are reported in animals. Do not mix in vial with other drugs because inactivation may result.

## Instructions for Use

Carbenicillin has a short half-life and should be administered frequently for optimum bactericidal effect. Carbenicillin injection often is administered with an aminoglycoside when treating *Pseudomonas* infections. Do not mix with aminoglycosides prior to administration, or inactivation will result. Carbenicillin indanyl sodium is the oral formulation of carbenicillin but attains concentrations that are only sufficient for treating urinary tract infections (UTIs). Do not use for systemic infections.

## Patient Monitoring and Laboratory Tests

Culture and sensitivity testing recommended to guide therapy. Clinical and Laboratory Standards Institute (CLSI) breakpoints are ≤128 mcg/mL when testing for *Pseudomonas*-susceptible organisms and ≤16 mcg/mL for other gram-negative organisms.

## Formulations

- Carbenicillin has been unavailable because other drugs are used as a replacement. However, older formulations include 1-, 2-, 5-, 10-, and 30-g vials for injection.

## Stability and Storage

Store in a tightly sealed container, protected from light, and at room temperature. Stable at pH of 6.5, but rate of degradation is greater at higher or lower pH. Use quickly after reconstitution of vials for injection.

## Small Animal Dosage

### Dogs and Cats

- Carbenicillin: 40–50 mg/kg and up to 100 mg/kg q6–8h IV, IM, or SQ.
- Carbenicillin indanyl sodium: 10 mg/kg q8h PO.

## Large Animal Dosage

- No dose has been reported for large animals.

## Regulatory Information

No regulatory information is available. For extralabel use withdrawal interval estimates, contact FARAD at www.FARAD.org.

# Carbimazole

kar-bih'mah-zole

**Trade and other names:** Neomercazole, Vidalta

**Functional classification:** Antithyroid drug

## Pharmacology and Mechanism of Action

Carbimazole is an antithyroid prodrug converted to methimazole after administration. Ten milligrams of carbimazole is equivalent to 6 mg of methimazole. Like methimazole, the action is to serve as substrate for thyroid peroxidase (TPO) and decreases incorporation of iodide into tyrosine molecules. It also inhibits coupling of mono-iodinated and di-iodinated residues to form tetraiodothyronine ($T_4$) and triiodothyronine ($T_3$). Carbimazole has been preferred in some patients because, compared with methimazole, it may have fewer side effects, such as less frequent GI problems. Oral absorption (based on methimazole concentrations) is 88% in cats with a half-life of approximately 5 hours.

## Indications and Clinical Uses

Carbimazole has been used for treating hyperthyroidism, primarily in cats. Carbimazole has been more readily available in Europe, where there is more clinical experience, than in the United States. Experience in the United States is limited because of lack of availability. Sustained-release formulation in Europe (Vidalta) is administered to people as 15 mg once per day followed by 10–25 mg once daily. If switching from methimazole to carbimazole, they are not equivalent.

## Precautionary Information
### Adverse Reactions and Side Effects
In cats, lupus-like reactions are possible, such as vasculitis and bone marrow changes. In people, it has caused agranulocytosis and leukopenia. Other systemic effects reported for methimazole are expected to be similar for carbimazole (e.g., bone marrow effects). See Methimazole for additional information.

### Contraindications and Precautions
Do not use in cats with bone marrow suppression or thrombocytopenia.

### Drug Interactions
No drug interactions are reported in animals.

## Instructions for Use
Carbimazole is used in Europe; clinical experience in the United States is limited. Otherwise, the clinical indications and use are similar as for methimazole.

## Patient Monitoring and Laboratory Tests
Monitor thyroid concentrations to adjust dose. Monitor complete blood count (CBC) periodically for evidence of bone marrow suppression.

## Formulations
- This drug has not been approved in the United States. This drug has been obtained in Europe.

## Stability and Storage
Store in a tightly sealed container, protected from light, and at room temperature. It is not stable in transdermal compounded formulations.

## Small Animal Dosage
### Cats
- 5 mg per cat q8h (induction) followed by 5 mg/cat q12h PO. In Europe, Vidalta (a newer sustained-release brand available) induction usually 15 mg once daily, and maintenance dosage ranges between 10 and 25 mg once daily.

### Dogs
- No dose has been established for dogs.

## Large Animal Dosage
- No dose has been reported for large animals.

## Regulatory Information
Do not administer to animals intended for food.

# Carboplatin
kar-boe-plat'in

**Trade and other names:** Paraplatin and generic

**Functional classification:** Anticancer agent

## Pharmacology and Mechanism of Action

Anticancer agent. Carboplatin is a second-generation platinum compound and is related to cisplatin. The action is similar to cisplatin, but adverse effects may be different. Carboplatin acts as a bifunctional alkylating agent, which interrupts replication of DNA in tumor cells. It induces a non–cell cycle–dependent tumor cell lysis. See Cisplatin for additional information. The major route of elimination is via the kidneys. It has replaced cisplatin in some anticancer protocols because of greater safety. Overall, carboplatin is less toxic than cisplatin with less vomiting, nephrotoxicity, ototoxicity, and neurotoxicity, but it is more myelosuppressive than cisplatin.

## Indications and Clinical Uses

Carboplatin has been used for squamous cell carcinoma and other carcinomas, melanoma, osteosarcomas, and other sarcomas. It has produced a disease-free interval and survival in dogs with osteosarcoma that is similar to other protocols. When used in dogs, myelosuppression has been the most dose-limiting factor. Compared with cisplatin, carboplatin is preferred for cats because it is better tolerated. However, bone marrow suppression is the dose-limiting toxicity in cats. Some forms of carboplatin have been administered locally (e.g., incorporated into beads) and used for treatment of local sarcomas and other tumors.

## Precautionary Information

### Adverse Reactions and Side Effects

Compared with cisplatin, carboplatin is less emetogenic and less nephrotoxic. In dogs, the other most common adverse effects relate to GI system toxicity (gastroenteritis, vomiting, anorexia, and diarrhea). The dose-limiting effect is myelosuppression, anemia, leukopenia, or thrombocytopenia. In dogs, the nadir of myelosuppression occurs at 14 days, but recovery occurs by 21–28 days. In cats, the nadir is 21 days, and recovery occurs by 28 days. Vomiting is not as much of a problem as for cisplatin, but GI toxicosis is still a problem, especially in smaller dogs. Because it is excreted by the kidneys, animals with diminished kidney function may have a higher rate of GI toxicosis.

### Contraindications and Precautions

In one study, small dogs were more prone than larger dogs to adverse effects.

### Drug Interactions

Do not use with other nephrotoxic drugs.

## Instructions for Use

Available for reconstitution for injection. It is stable for 1 month when reconstituted with 5% dextrose. It may be frozen at –4°C to prolong the stability of a reconstituted vial. Do not use with administration sets containing aluminum because of incompatibility. It is usually administered in specific anticancer protocols; consult oncology protocols for specific regimens. In dogs, it has been dosed on a milligram per square meter ($mg/m^2$) dose, which has produced a higher incidence of adverse effects in smaller dogs compared with larger dogs; however, smaller dogs also were more likely to respond. Carboplatin is excreted by the kidneys; therefore it should be avoided in patients with kidney disease, or the dose should be decreased in proportion to reduced glomerular filtration rate and creatinine clearance.

## Patient Monitoring and Laboratory Tests

Monitoring of CBC and platelets is recommended during treatment. Because of high risk of myelosuppression, a CBC is recommended before each treatment and again 7–14 days after each treatment.

## Formulations

- Carboplatin is available in 50-, 150-, and 450-mg vials for injection and a 10-mg/mL infusion.

## Stability and Storage

Store in a tightly sealed container, protected from light, and at room temperature. Stable for 1 month if reconstituted with 5% dextrose solution. It is stable if frozen at –4°C.

## Small Animal Dosage

### Dogs

- 300 mg/m² IV every 3 weeks. Treatment may involve four to six cycles of administration every 3 weeks.

### Cats

- 200–227 mg/m² IV every 4 weeks for four treatments; for a 4-kg cat, the dose is equivalent to 14.7 mg/kg.

## Large Animal Dosage

- No dose has been reported for large animals.

## Regulatory Information

Withdrawal times are not established for animals that produce food. This drug should not be used in animals intended for food because it is an anticancer agent.

# Carprofen
car-proe'fen

**Trade and other names:** Rimadyl, Vetprofen, Zinecarp (Europe), and generic brands

**Functional classification:** Nonsteroidal anti-inflammatory drug

## Pharmacology and Mechanism of Action

Carprofen is an NSAID. Like other drugs in this class, carprofen has analgesic and anti-inflammatory effects by inhibiting the synthesis of PGs. The enzyme inhibited by an NSAID is the cyclo-oxygenase (COX) enzyme. The COX enzyme exists in two isoforms, COX-1 and COX-2. COX-1 is primarily responsible for synthesis of PGs important for maintaining a healthy GI tract, renal function, platelet function, and other normal functions. COX-2 is induced and responsible for synthesizing PGs that are important mediators of pain, inflammation, and fever. (There may be crossover of COX-1 and COX-2 effects in some situations.) Carprofen is relatively COX-1 sparing compared with older NSAIDs, but it is not considered a COX-2–selective agent. It is not known if the specificity for COX-1 or COX-2 determines efficacy or safety. In some studies, carprofen was not a strong inhibitor of peripheral PG synthesis, and because of its high lipophilicity, its effects may be mediated by effects in the central nervous system (CNS).

In horses, carprofen is not as COX-2 selective as it is in dogs. As an analgesic agent, the mechanism of action may involve other mechanisms other than inhibition of PG synthesis.

*Pharmacokinetics:* Carprofen exists as two chiral isomers. The R and S isomers have different pharmacokinetics and different activities. The S isomer is the more active (eutomer) but is cleared faster. Carprofen has been studied extensively in dogs. A summary of more than 10 studies shows an overall average plasma half-life of 5.8 hours, but it is variable among breeds of dogs. The tissue concentrations persist much longer than plasma concentrations. The VD is small because of very high protein binding. The VD is approximately 0.16 L/kg, and systemic clearance is 19 mL/h/kg. The oral absorption is nearly complete.

## Indications and Clinical Uses

Carprofen is one of the most common NSAIDs used in dogs for treatment of musculoskeletal pain and acute pain related to surgery or trauma. It is used primarily for treatment of osteoarthritis and has been administered for long-term treatment safely in many dogs. Long-term safe use in cats has not been established. However, it is registered in Europe for one-time administration in cats at 4-mg/kg injection.

Although use in large animals is uncommon, in cattle, carprofen has been shown to reduce inflammation in cows associated with *Escherichia coli* mastitis at a dose of 0.7 mg/kg IV. In cattle, carprofen is registered in Europe for treatment of fever associated with mastitis and used to reduce inflammation associated with bovine respiratory disease (BRD). Although carprofen has been used in horses, it does not show the same COX-2 selectivity of inhibition as in dogs and has not been a useful analgesic or anti-inflammatory agent.

### Precautionary Information

**Adverse Reactions and Side Effects**

The safety of carprofen in dogs was determined by the sponsor during preclinical studies. The most common adverse effect in dogs has been in the GI tract (vomiting, anorexia, and diarrhea). GI ulcers, perforation, and bleeding are uncommon in dogs but possible. In rare cases, carprofen has caused idiosyncratic acute hepatic toxicity in dogs. Signs of toxicity usually appear 2–3 weeks after exposure. There were no adverse effects on the kidneys when carprofen was evaluated in anesthetized dogs. Carprofen may lower total thyroid ($T_4$) concentrations in dogs but not free $T_4$. In experimental dogs, it has inhibited bone healing in some models (4.4 mg/kg/day × 120 days), but this has not been shown to be a clinical problem. Carprofen has produced toxicity in cats if administered at the same dose rates as for dogs.

**Contraindications and Precautions**

Do not use in cats at doses intended for dogs. Do not administer to animals prone to GI ulcers. Do not administer with ulcerogenic drugs such as corticosteroids. If a patient has had previous adverse effects from NSAIDs, carprofen should be used cautiously.

**Drug Interactions**

Use NSAIDs cautiously with other drugs known to cause GI injury (e.g., corticosteroids). The efficacy of ACE inhibitors and diuretics (e.g., furosemide) may be diminished when administered concurrently with NSAIDs.

## Instructions for Use

Doses are based on clinical investigations in dogs with arthritis and for treatment of pain associated with surgery. Dogs may receive carprofen either once daily (4.4 mg/kg) or twice daily (2.2 mg/kg) with similar effectiveness and safety. The only approved dose for cats is 4 mg/kg as a one-time injection for surgical pain. However, for long-term use, pharmacokinetic extrapolations suggest a long-term dosage of 0.5 mg/kg q24h PO. Long-term safety at this dosage has not been established.

## Patient Monitoring and Laboratory Tests

After administration has begun, one should monitor hepatic enzymes for evidence of drug-induced hepatic toxicity approximately 7–14 days after treatment has started. If liver enzymes are elevated, discontinue the medication and contact the drug manufacturer.

## Formulations

- Carprofen is available in 25-, 75-, and 100-mg caplets; 25-, 75-, and 100-mg chewable tablets; and injectable solution: 50 mg/mL.
- Zinecarp injection has also been available in Europe.

## Stability and Storage

Store in a tightly sealed container, protected from light, and at room temperature. Carprofen has been compounded by mixing tablets with methylcellulose gel (1%), simple syrup, and a suspending and flavoring vehicle to make a 1.25-, 2.5-, and 5-mg/mL suspension. This formulation was stable if stored in the refrigerator or at room temperature for 28 days.

## Small Animal Dosage

### Dogs

- 2.2 mg/kg q12h PO or 4.4 mg/kg q24h PO.
- 2.2 mg/kg q12h SQ or 4.4 mg/kg q24h SQ.

### Cats

- 4 mg/kg given once by injection or 0.5 mg/kg q24h PO for long-term use (safety for long-term use has not been established).

## Large Animal Dosage

### Horses

- 0.7 mg/kg q24h IV (in Europe, oral granules: 0.7 mg/kg PO).

### Cattle

- 1.4 mg/kg SQ, IV.

## Regulatory Information

Withdrawal times have not been established for carprofen in the United States. It is suggested, based on European labeling, that the withdrawal time for meat is 21 days but zero days for milk. Caution is advised when considering carprofen for cattle because it has a longer half-life in cows compared with other animals (30–40 hours). RCI Classification: 4

# Carvedilol
kar-ved′ih-lole

**Trade and other names:** Coreg

**Functional classification:** Antiarrhythmic

## Pharmacology and Mechanism of Action

Antiarrhythmic. Nonselective beta-receptor blocker. Carvedilol is a third-generation adrenergic blocker. Carvedilol blocks both $beta_1$-receptors and $beta_2$-receptors in heart and other tissues. Carvedilol is unique because it also has alpha-receptor–blocking properties that produce relaxation of vascular smooth muscle and vasodilation. It also is reported to have antioxidant properties. Carvedilol prolongs survival in human patients with heart failure, but this effect has not been measured in animals.

*Pharmacokinetics:* In dogs the half-life is short (1.2 hours). Oral absorption is low and variable because of high systemic clearance and first-pass effects. Average oral absorption in one study was only 14% and highly variable, but in another study, it was only 1.6% (range, 0.4%–54%), making the oral use of carvedilol in dogs unpredictable.

## Indications and Clinical Uses

Carvedilol has been used to treat arrhythmias in animals. It is also used to treat systemic hypertension and to block beta-adrenergic cardiac receptors in animals with rapid heart rates. Efficacy has been based on anecdotal accounts, extrapolation from humans, and limited studies in healthy dogs. In healthy dogs, 0.2 mg/kg PO decreased heart rate, and 0.4 mg/kg PO decreased heart rate and lowered blood pressure. At 0.4 mg/kg, the effects in healthy dogs persisted for 36 hours. However, in other studies, doses of 0.3 mg/kg were not effective. In clinical patients, the optimum dose is not known, and long-term benefits have not been established. Because oral absorption is inconsistent in dogs (discussed in the Pharmacology section), the response may be variable. Elimination is rapid after oral administration to dogs, but clinical pharmacodynamic effects may persist for up to 12 hours, possibly from the metabolites.

## Precautionary Information

### Adverse Reactions and Side Effects

Bradycardia can occur resulting from beta-adrenergic receptor blockade. Carvedilol increases risk of myocardial depression and decreased cardiac output. Adverse effects from nonselective beta-adrenergic receptor blockade are possible in other tissues. In research dogs administered doses from 0.3 to 1.0 mg/kg, there was a dose-dependent increase in dizziness, bradycardia, and negative inotropic and chronotropic effects. There was a dose-dependent increase in exercise intolerance at higher doses.

### Contraindications and Precautions

Use carefully in patients with limited cardiac reserve. Do not administer to dehydrated or hypotensive animals. Use carefully in patients with respiratory disease because the $beta_2$-adrenergic blocking properties can worsen bronchoconstriction.

### Drug Interactions

Use with other beta blockers will increase its effect. Do not administer with other drugs that may cause hypotension or depress the heart.

## Instructions for Use

Doses in dogs established through clinical experience and limited trials. In a dose titration study in dogs, the effective dosage was 0.2–0.4 mg/kg q24h PO.

## Patient Monitoring and Laboratory Tests

Monitor patient's heart rate and rhythm carefully during treatment. During the initial phase of dosing, monitor patients for worsening of heart failure.

## Formulations

- Carvedilol is available in 3.125-, 6.25-, 12.5-, and 25-mg tablets.

## Stability and Storage

Store in a tightly sealed container, protected from light, and at room temperature. Carvedilol is not soluble in water. Carvedilol compounded suspension has been prepared by adding 25-mg tablets to water to make a paste and then mixed with simple syrup to make a 2- or 10-mg/mL suspension for oral administration. This suspension has been stable for 90 days at room temperature, protected from light.

## Small Animal Dosage

**Dogs**

- Initial dose: 0.2 mg/kg q24h PO followed by increases up to a maximum of 0.4 mg/kg q12h. There is some evidence that a higher dosage of 1.5 mg/kg q12h PO was more effective, but some dogs are refractory.

**Cats**

- Dose not established.

## Large Animal Dosage

- No dose has been reported for large animals.

## Regulatory Information

No regulatory information is available. For extralabel use withdrawal interval estimates, contact FARAD at www.FARAD.org.

RCI Classification: 3

# Cascara Sagrada

kass-kar'ah sah-grah'dah

**Trade and other names:** Nature's Remedy and generic brands

**Functional classification:** Laxative

## Pharmacology and Mechanism of Action

Stimulant cathartic. Action is believed to be by local stimulation of bowel motility.

## Indications and Clinical Uses

Laxative used to treat constipation or evacuate bowel for procedures.

## Precautionary Information

**Adverse Reactions and Side Effects**

Overuse can cause electrolyte losses.

**Contraindications and Precautions**

Do not use in cases in which there may be intestinal obstruction.

**Drug Interactions**

No drug interactions are reported in animals.

## Instructions for Use

Available in various dietary supplements. This agent is not used clinically very often for GI procedures.

## Patient Monitoring and Laboratory Tests

Monitor electrolytes with chronic therapy.

## Formulations

- Cascara sagrada is available in a variety of strengths, including tablets, capsules, and liquids.

## Stability and Storage

Store in a tightly sealed container, protected from light, and at room temperature. Stability of compounded formulations has not been evaluated.

## Small Animal Dosage

**Dogs**

- 1–5 mg/kg/day PO.

**Cats**

- 1–2 mg/cat/day PO.

## Large Animal Dosage

- No dose has been reported for large animals.

## Regulatory Information

Do not administer to animals intended for food.

# Castor Oil
kas′tar oil

**Trade and other names:** Generic brands

**Functional classification:** Laxative

## Pharmacology and Mechanism of Action

Castor oil is a stimulant cathartic. The action is believed to be by local stimulation of bowel motility. Castor oil is an old preparation used historically as a laxative. Because of availability of more modern laxatives and cathartics, castor oil is not used in animals much anymore.

## Indications and Clinical Uses

Castor oil is used as a laxative to treat constipation or to evacuate the bowel for procedures.

## Precautionary Information

### Adverse Reactions and Side Effects

Overuse can cause electrolyte losses. Castor oil has been known to stimulate premature labor in pregnancy.

### Contraindications and Precautions

Do not use in pregnant animals. It may induce labor. Castor oil has been known to induce histamine release. Monitor patients for signs of histamine reaction.

### Drug Interactions

No drug interactions are reported in animals.

## Instructions for Use

Use in animals is strictly empirical. The doses used are empirical or extrapolated from the human use. It is available as an OTC product. Pet owners should be discouraged from repeated administration to pets.

## Patient Monitoring and Laboratory Tests

No specific monitoring is necessary.

## Formulations

- Castor oil is available in an oral liquid (100%) and 700-mg "Castroclean" capsules.

## Stability and Storage

Store in a tightly sealed container, protected from light, and at room temperature. Stability of compounded formulations has not been evaluated.

## Small Animal Dosage

**Dogs**

- 8–30 mL/day PO.

**Cats**

- 4–10 mL/day PO.

## Large Animal Dosage

- No dose has been reported for large animals.

## Regulatory Information

No regulatory information is available.

# Cefaclor

sef′ah-klor

**Trade and other names:** Generic

**Functional classification:** Antibacterial

## Pharmacology and Mechanism of Action

Cefaclor is a cephalosporin antibiotic. The action is similar to other beta-lactam antibiotics, which is to inhibit synthesis of the bacterial cell wall, leading to cell death. Cephalosporins are divided into first-, second-, third-, and fourth-generation drugs depending on spectrum of activity. Cefaclor is a second-generation cephalosporin with moderate activity against gram-negative bacteria. Cefaclor, like other second-generation cephalosporins, is more active against gram-negative bacteria than first-generation cephalosporins and has been used to treat infections caused by bacteria resistant to first-generation drugs.

There is very little pharmacokinetic information available for dogs or cats to guide dosing. It is moderately absorbed from oral administration and has a half-life of 2–4 hours.

## Indications and Clinical Uses

Cefaclor is not used commonly in veterinary medicine because other cephalosporins are in more widespread use. However, it may be indicated for treatment of infections caused by bacteria that are resistant to first-generation cephalosporins. Although it has been used as oral therapy, the extent of oral absorption and efficacy information is not available for dogs or cats. Dosing regimens and indications are primarily derived from extrapolation and anecdotal information.

## Precautionary Information
### Adverse Reactions and Side Effects
All cephalosporins are generally safe; however, sensitivity can occur in individuals (allergy). Cross-reactivity between penicillin allergy and cephalosporin allergy is low. Rare bleeding disorders have been known to occur with some cephalosporins. Oral administration can potentially produce vomiting and diarrhea in small animals.

### Contraindications and Precautions
Do not use in animals with allergic sensitivity to other beta-lactams, especially other cephalosporins. However, the incidence of cross-sensitivity between penicillins and cephalosporins is small (less than 10% in people). Some cephalosporins should not be used in animals with bleeding problems or that are receiving warfarin anticoagulants. These cephalosporins are those that have an N-methylthiotetrazole (NMTT) side chain and include cefotetan, cefamandole, and cefoperazone. Oral absorption has not been measured in large animals, and cefaclor is not recommended unless information derived from pharmacokinetic or efficacy studies is available.

### Drug Interactions
No drug interactions are reported in animals. However, do not mix with other drugs in a compounded formulation because inactivation may result.

## Instructions for Use
It is used primarily when resistance has been demonstrated to first-generation cephalosporins and other alternatives have been considered. Because there is very little information to guide dosing for cefaclor, other oral cephalosporins should be considered before using cefaclor, such as cefpodoxime or cephalexin.

## Patient Monitoring and Laboratory Tests
Susceptibility testing: CLSI breakpoint for susceptible bacteria is ≤8 mcg/mL for humans, but this may not apply to isolates from animals. The breakpoint for cefazolin could potentially be used to predict activity for treating lower UTIs in dogs.

## Formulations
- Cefaclor is available in 250- and 500-mg capsules and 25-, 37.5-, 50-, and 75-mg/mL oral suspension.

## Stability and Storage
Store in a tightly sealed container, protected from light, and at room temperature. Stability of compounded formulations has not been evaluated.

## Small Animal Dosage
### Dogs
- 15–20 mg/kg q8h PO.

### Cats
- 15–20 mg/kg q8h PO.

## Large Animal Dosage
- No dose has been reported for large animals.

## Regulatory Information
The extralabel administration of cephalosporins to food-producing animals in the United States is a violation of FDA regulations. Withdrawal times are not established for animals that produce food.

# Cefadroxil
sef-ah-drox'il

**Trade and other names:** Cefa-Tabs and Cefa-Drops (veterinary preparations) and Duricef and generic (human preparation)

**Functional classification:** Antibacterial

## Pharmacology and Mechanism of Action

Cephalosporin antibiotic. The action is similar to other beta-lactam antibiotics, which is to inhibit synthesis of the bacterial cell wall, leading to cell death. Cephalosporins are divided into first-, second-, third-, and fourth-generation drugs depending on spectrum of activity. Cefadroxil is a first-generation cephalosporin, and activity and clinical use are similar to cephalexin. Like other first-generation cephalosporins, it is active against *Streptococcus* and *Staphylococcus* spp. and some gram-negative bacilli, such as *Pasteurella* spp. However, if the current susceptibility testing breakpoint for cephalexin (≤2 mcg/mL) is applied to cefadroxil, *E. coli*, and *Klebsiella pneumoniae*, they will likely test as clinically resistant unless they are isolated from the lower urinary tract. It is not active against *P. aeruginosa*. Methicillin-resistant *Staphylococcus* spp. (MRS) that are resistant to oxacillin are resistant to first-generation cephalosporins.

## Indications and Clinical Uses

Like other first-generation cephalosporins, it is indicated for treating common infections in animals, including UTIs, skin and soft tissue infections, pyoderma and other dermal infections, and pneumonia caused by susceptible bacteria. Efficacy against infections caused by anaerobic bacteria is unpredictable. The use in horses is rare. Although there is adequate oral absorption in foals, it is poorly absorbed in adult horses.

## Precautionary Information

### Adverse Reactions and Side Effects

All cephalosporins are generally safe; however, sensitivity can occur in individuals (allergy). Cross-reactivity between penicillin allergy and cephalosporin allergy is low. Rare bleeding disorders have been known to occur with some cephalosporins. Cefadroxil has been known to cause vomiting after oral administration in dogs. Some estimates show that this can occur in up to 10% of treated dogs. If administered orally to adult horses, diarrhea is possible. Oral treatment to horses is.

### Contraindications and Precautions

Do not use in animals with allergic sensitivity to other beta-lactams, especially other cephalosporins. However, the incidence of cross-sensitivity between penicillins and cephalosporins is small (less than 10% in people). Some cephalosporins should not be used in animals with bleeding problems or that are receiving warfarin anticoagulants. These cephalosporins are those that have an NMTT side chain and include cefotetan, cefamandole, and cefoperazone.

### Drug Interactions

No drug interactions are reported in animals. However, do not mix with other drugs in a compounded formulation because inactivation may result.

## Instructions for Use

Spectrum of cefadroxil is similar to other first-generation cephalosporins. The FDA-approved label is appropriate for dosing ranges; however, the availability in most countries has diminished, and cephalexin is used more widely instead. For susceptibility test, use cephalothin or cephalexin as test drug to predict susceptibility to cefadroxil.

## Patient Monitoring and Laboratory Tests

Susceptibility testing: CLSI breakpoint for susceptible organisms is ≤2 mcg/mL using cephalexin as the test to predict susceptibility to cefadroxil. Cephalothin or cephalexin can be used as a marker to test for sensitivity to cefadroxil, but cephalexin is preferred. For urine isolates, a higher breakpoint of ≤16 mcg/mL can be used using cefazolin or other first-generation cephalosporins in the test.

## Formulations

- Cefadroxil is available in 50-mg/mL oral suspension and 50-, 100-, 200-, and 1000-mg tablets for veterinary use. However, availability of veterinary-labeled tablets has been inconsistent. It is also available in 500-mg capsules and 25-, 50-, and 100-mg/mL suspension for human use.

## Stability and Storage

Store in a tightly sealed container, protected from light, and at room temperature. Stability of compounded formulations has not been evaluated. Avoid moisture to prevent hydrolysis.

Suspension is stable for 14 days refrigerated and 10 days at room temperature. Stability of compounded formulations has not been evaluated.

## Small Animal Dosage

### Dogs

- 22 mg/kg q12h PO, up to 30 mg/kg q12h PO.

### Cats

- 22 mg/kg q24h PO.

## Large Animal Dosage

### Foals

- 30 mg/kg q12h PO. Note: Oral absorption is adequate only in foals and not in adults or ruminants.

## Regulatory Information

The extralabel administration of cephalosporins to food-producing animals in the United States is a violation of FDA regulations. Withdrawal times are not established for animals that produce food.

# Cefazolin Sodium

sef-ah′zoe-lin so′dee-um

**Trade and other names:** Ancef, Kefzol, and generic brands

**Functional classification:** Antibacterial

## Pharmacology and Mechanism of Action

Cephalosporin antibiotic. The action of cefazolin is similar to other beta-lactam antibiotics, which inhibits synthesis of the bacterial cell wall, leading to cell death. Cephalosporins are divided into first-, second-, third-, and fourth-generation drugs depending on spectrum of activity. Cefazolin is a first-generation cephalosporin. Like other first-generation cephalosporins, it is active against *Streptococcus* and *Staphylococcus* spp. and some gram-negative bacilli, such as *Pasteurella* spp. Other gram-negative bacilli of the Enterobacteriaceae, such as *E. coli* and *K. pneumoniae*, may test clinically resistant. The difference between cefazolin and other first-generation cephalosporins is that it is slightly more active against gram-negative Enterobacteriaceae, and its spectrum resembles some second-generation drugs. Nevertheless, resistance is common among gram-negative bacteria. It is not active against *P. aeruginosa*. Methicillin-resistant *Staphylococcus aureus* (MRSA) and other staphylococci resistant to oxacillin are resistant to first-generation cephalosporins.

*Pharmacokinetics:* In dogs, the half-life, clearance, and VD are 1.04 hours, 2.9 mL/kg/min, and 0.27 L/kg, respectively. These values in horses are 0.62 hours, 5.07 mL/kg/min, and 0.27 L/kg, respectively. In cats, cefazolin has a half-life of 1.2 hours, VD of 0.3 L/kg, and clearance of 3.4 mL/kg/min. Protein binding in dogs is 19%, but 80% in people.

## Indications and Clinical Uses

Cefazolin, because it is injectable, is the most common drug to be administered prophylactically prior to surgery. It is one of the most frequently injected cephalosporin antibiotics used in small animals. Like other first-generation cephalosporins, it is indicated for treating common infections in animals, including UTIs, soft tissue infections, pyoderma and other dermal infections, and pneumonia. Efficacy against infections caused by anaerobic bacteria is unpredictable.

## Precautionary Information

### Adverse Reactions and Side Effects

All cephalosporins are generally safe; however, sensitivity can occur in individuals (allergy). Cross-reactivity between penicillin allergy and cephalosporin allergy is low. Rare bleeding disorders have been known to occur with some cephalosporins; however, bleeding problems have not been observed from cefazolin. Some cephalosporins have caused seizures, but this is a rare problem. When administered during surgery, it did not adversely affect cardiovascular function in dogs.

### Contraindications and Precautions

Do not use in animals with allergic sensitivity to other beta-lactams, especially other cephalosporins. However, the incidence of cross-sensitivity between penicillins and cephalosporins is small (less than 10% in people). Some cephalosporins should not be used in animals with bleeding problems or that are receiving warfarin anticoagulants. These cephalosporins are those that have an NMTT side chain and include cefotetan, cefamandole, and cefoperazone.

### Drug Interactions

No drug interactions are reported in animals. However, do not mix in a vial or syringe with other drugs because inactivation may result.

## Instructions for Use

Cefazolin is a commonly used first-generation cephalosporin as an injectable drug for prophylaxis for surgery and for acute therapy for serious infections. When performing susceptibility testing, cefazolin should be tested separately because it may be more active than some of the other first-generation cephalosporins. Cefazolin is slightly more active against some gram-negative bacilli compared with other first-generation cephalosporins.

## Patient Monitoring and Laboratory Tests

Susceptibility testing: CLSI breakpoint for susceptible organisms is ≤2 mcg/mL for coagulase-positive staphylococci, *Pasteurella multocida*, streptococci beta-hemolytic group, and *E. coli*. It may be used to predict susceptibility to other first-generation cephalosporins when testing isolates from lower UTIs. The breakpoint for testing urinary isolates is ≤16 mcg/mL.

## Formulations

- Cefazolin is available in 50 and 100 mg/50 mL for injection in 1-g or 500-mg vials. Reconstituted to produce 275 or 330 mg/mL.

## Stability and Storage

Store in a tightly sealed container, protected from light, and at room temperature. If slight yellow discoloration occurs, the solution is still stable. After reconstitution, it is stable for 24 hours at room temperature and 14 days refrigerated. It remains stable if frozen for 3 months.

## Small Animal Dosage

### Dogs and Cats

- 25 mg/kg q6h IV or IM.
- Constant-rate infusion (CRI): 1.3 mg/kg loading dose followed by 1.2 mg/kg/h.
- Perisurgical use: 22 mg/kg IV q2h during surgery.

## Large Animal Dosage

### Horses

- 25 mg/kg q6h IM or IV.

## Regulatory Information

The extralabel administration of cephalosporins to food-producing animals in the United States is a violation of FDA regulations. Withdrawal times are not established for animals that produce food.

# Cefdinir

sef′dih-neer

**Trade and other names:** Omnicef

**Functional classification:** Antibacterial

## Pharmacology and Mechanism of Action

Cephalosporin antibiotic. The action is similar to other beta-lactam antibiotics, which is to inhibit synthesis of the bacterial cell wall, leading to cell death. Cephalosporins are divided into first-, second-, third-, and fourth-generation drugs depending on spectrum of activity. It is an oral third-generation cephalosporin and is active against staphylococci and many gram-negative bacilli.

## Indications and Clinical Uses

Cefdinir is an oral third-generation cephalosporin used in people. Although it has been used as oral therapy, the extent of oral absorption and efficacy information is not available for dogs or cats. Dosing regimens and indications are primarily derived from extrapolation and anecdotal information. It has potential efficacy for infections of the skin, soft tissues, and urinary tract; however, in most instances, other cephalosporins such as cefpodoxime proxetil may be substituted instead.

C

### Precautionary Information

#### Adverse Reactions and Side Effects

All cephalosporins are generally safe; however, sensitivity can occur in individuals (allergy). Rare bleeding disorders have been known to occur with some cephalosporins. Oral cephalosporins can produce vomiting and diarrhea in small animals.

#### Contraindications and Precautions

Do not use in animals with allergic sensitivity to other beta-lactams, especially other cephalosporins. However, the incidence of cross-sensitivity between penicillins and cephalosporins is small (less than 10% in people). Some cephalosporins should not be used in animals with bleeding problems or that are receiving warfarin anticoagulants. These cephalosporins are those that have an NMTT side chain and include cefotetan, cefamandole, and cefoperazone. Oral absorption has not been measured in large animals, and cefdinir is not recommended unless information derived from pharmacokinetic or efficacy studies is available.

#### Drug Interactions

No drug interactions are reported in animals. However, do not mix with other drugs in a compounded formulation because inactivation may result.

## Instructions for Use

Use in veterinary medicine has not been reported. Use and doses are extrapolated from human preparations.

## Patient Monitoring and Laboratory Tests

Susceptibility testing: CLSI breakpoint for susceptible organisms is ≤1 mcg/mL using the human breakpoint. Breakpoints for isolates from animals are not available.

## Formulations

- Cefdinir is available in 300-mg capsules and 25-mg/mL oral suspension.

## Stability and Storage

Store in a tightly sealed container, protected from light, and at room temperature. Stability of compounded formulations has not been evaluated.

## Small Animal Dosage

### Dogs and Cats

- Dose not established. Human dosage is 7 mg/kg q12h PO, and similar dosages of 10 mg/kg q12h PO have been used in animals.

## Large Animal Dosage

- No dose has been reported for large animals.

## Regulatory Information

The extralabel administration of cephalosporins to food-producing animals in the United States is a violation of FDA regulations. Withdrawal times are not established for animals that produce food.

## Cefepime
sef'ah-peem

**Trade and other names:** Maxipime

**Functional classification:** Antibacterial

## Pharmacology and Mechanism of Action

Cefepime is an antibacterial drug of the cephalosporin class. The action against bacterial cell walls is similar to other cephalosporins. Cephalosporins are classified into first-, second-, third-, and fourth-generation based on their activity against gram-negative bacteria. Cefepime is one of the fourth-generation cephalosporins. It has an enhanced, extended spectrum that is greater than that of many of the other generation cephalosporins. Its activity includes gram-positive cocci and gram-negative bacilli. It has been active against organisms resistant to other beta-lactams such as *E. coli* and *Klebsiella* spp. It is active against most *P. aeruginosa*. It is not active against methicillin-resistant staphylococci, *Bacteroides fragilis*, or penicillin-resistant enterococci.

## Indications and Clinical Uses

Cefepime is a fourth-generation cephalosporin. Although it has a broader spectrum than other cephalosporins, the use has been limited in veterinary medicine. Some studies in humans have not shown advantages over other antibacterial agents. Experimental studies have been conducted in foals, adult horses, and dogs to establish doses, but reports of efficacy are not available.

## Precautionary Information

### Adverse Reactions and Side Effects

Cefepime is generally safe. However, clinicians should consider the same possible side effects as for other cephalosporins, which include the possibility of bleeding disorders, allergy, vomiting, and diarrhea.

### Contraindications and Precautions

Do not administer to patients with sensitivity or allergy to cephalosporins. Reduce dose to less frequent intervals (e.g., q12h or q24h) in patients with renal failure.

### Drug Interactions

No drug interactions are reported in animals. However, do not mix in a vial or syringe with other drugs because inactivation may result.

## Instructions for Use

Reconstitute with sterile water, sodium chloride, and 5% dextrose. It may be reconstituted with 1% lidocaine if pain from injection is a problem. Reconstituted solutions are stable for 24 hours at room temperature and 7 days in the refrigerator. Do not mix with other injectable antibiotics. Injection vials also contain L-arginine.

## Patient Monitoring and Laboratory Tests
Susceptibility testing: CLSI breakpoints for susceptible organisms are ≤2 mcg/mL using the human breakpoint for Enterobacteriaceae and ≤8 mcg/mL for testing *P. aeruginosa*. Breakpoints for isolates from animals are not available.

## Formulations
- Cefepime is available in 500-mg, 1-g, and 2-g vials for injection.

## Stability and Storage
Store in a tightly sealed container, protected from light, and at room temperature. Observe manufacturer's recommendations for stability after vial is reconstituted.

## Small Animal Dosage
### Dogs
- 40 mg/kg q6h IM or IV.
- CRI: 1.4 mg/kg loading dose followed by 1.1 mg/kg/h.

## Large Animal Dosage
### Foals
- 11 mg/kg q8h IV.

## Regulatory Information
The extralabel administration of cephalosporins to food-producing animals in the United States is a violation of FDA regulations. Withdrawal times are not established for animals that produce food.

# Cefixime
sef-iks'eem

**Trade and other names:** Suprax

**Functional classification:** Antibacterial

**Note:** Cefixime is no longer commercially available. It is included here because some compounding pharmacies and distributors may still supply some forms. If it is not available, use cefpodoxime proxetil as a substitute.

## Pharmacology and Mechanism of Action
Cefixime is a cephalosporin antibiotic. The action is similar to other beta-lactam antibiotics, which is to inhibit synthesis of the bacterial cell wall, leading to cell death. Cephalosporins are divided into first-, second-, third-, and fourth-generation drugs depending on spectrum of activity. Cefixime is an oral third-generation cephalosporin but is not expected to have the same degree of activity against gram-negative bacilli as injectable third-generation cephalosporins such as cefotaxime or ceftazidime. It has less activity against *Staphylococcus* spp. than many other cephalosporins. The low activity is attributed to lower affinity for staphylococcal penicillin binding protein. When isolates from dogs were tested, cefixime was the least active against *Staphylococcus pseudintermedius* than any of the other cephalosporins tested.

*Pharmacokinetics:* The pharmacokinetics have been studied in dogs. It has an average half-life of approximately 7 hours, with a VD of 0.254 L/kg and clearance of 0.03 L/kg/h. The oral absorption in dogs is 50%–60%. The protein binding is high, at 90%.

## Indications and Clinical Uses

Cefixime is not used clinically often in veterinary medicine because availability of oral products has diminished and because other oral agents are available. Cefixime is one of the few oral third-generation cephalosporins. It has been administered orally in dogs and cats to treat infections of the skin, soft tissues, and urinary tract. It is not as active as cefpodoxime against *Staphylococcus* spp. Because of greater availability of cefpodoxime for animals, it is substituted instead for most indications.

## Precautionary Information

### Adverse Reactions and Side Effects

All cephalosporins are generally safe; however, sensitivity can occur in individuals (allergy). Cross-reactivity between penicillin allergy and cephalosporin allergy is low. Rare bleeding disorders have been known to occur with some cephalosporins. Vomiting and diarrhea are possible from oral cephalosporins.

### Contraindications and Precautions

Do not use in animals with allergic sensitivity to other beta-lactams, especially other cephalosporins. However, the incidence of cross-sensitivity between penicillins and cephalosporins is small (less than 10% in people). Some cephalosporins should not be used in animals with bleeding problems or that are receiving warfarin anticoagulants. These cephalosporins are those that have an NMTT side chain and include cefotetan, cefamandole, and cefoperazone. Oral absorption has not been measured in large animals, and cefixime is not recommended unless information derived from pharmacokinetic or efficacy studies is available.

### Drug Interactions

No drug interactions are reported in animals. However, do not mix with other drugs in a compounded formulation because inactivation may result.

## Instructions for Use

Although not approved for veterinary use, pharmacokinetic studies in dogs have provided recommended doses. Note that breakpoint for sensitivity is lower than for other cephalosporins, indicating that organisms tested as susceptible to other cephalosporins may not be susceptible to cefixime.

## Patient Monitoring and Laboratory Tests

Susceptibility testing: CLSI breakpoint for susceptible organisms is ≤1 mcg/mL using the human breakpoint. Breakpoints for isolates from animals are not available.

## Formulations

- Cefixime is available in 20- or 40-mg/mL oral suspension and 400-mg tablets.

## Stability and Storage

Store in a tightly sealed container, protected from light, and at room temperature. Stability of compounded formulations has not been evaluated.

## Small Animal Dosage

### Dogs and Cats

- 10 mg/kg q12h PO.
- UTI: 5 mg/kg q12–24h PO.

## Large Animal Dosage

- No dose has been reported for large animals.

## Regulatory Information

The extralabel administration of cephalosporins to food-producing animals in the United States is a violation of FDA regulations. Withdrawal times are not established for animals that produce food.

# Cefotaxime Sodium

sef-oh-taks'eem so'dee-um

**Trade and other names:** Claforan and generic

**Functional classification:** Antibacterial

## Pharmacology and Mechanism of Action

Cephalosporin antibiotic. The action of cefotaxime is the same as other beta-lactam antibiotics, which inhibits synthesis of the bacterial cell wall, leading to cell death. Cephalosporins are divided into first-, second-, third-, and fourth-generation drugs depending on spectrum of activity. Cefotaxime is a third-generation cephalosporin. Like other third-generation cephalosporins, it has enhanced activity against gram-negative bacilli, especially Enterobacteriaceae, which may be resistant to first- and second-generation cephalosporins, ampicillin derivatives, and other drugs. It is active against *E. coli*, *K. pneumoniae*, other Enterobacteriaceae, *Pasteurella* spp., and *Salmonella* spp., among others. It is generally not active against *P. aeruginosa*. It is active against streptococci, but *Staphylococcus* spp. are less susceptible. All methicillin-resistant strains of staphylococci will be resistant. Activity against anaerobic bacteria is unpredictable.

## Indications and Clinical Uses

Cefotaxime is used when resistance is encountered to other antibiotics, or in severe infections when highly active antibiotics are needed. The availability has diminished in recent years, and ceftazidime can be used as a substitute. It should not be used for routine infections in veterinary medicine when other drugs will be active. Although cefotaxime is not FDA approved for use in animals, it can be legally administered as an extralabel injectable third-generation cephalosporins used in small animals. The use in large animals is uncommon, and extralabel administration of cephalosporins is illegal in the United States. Cefotaxime has a short half-life and must be injected frequently. It is not absorbed from oral administration.

## Precautionary Information

### Adverse Reactions and Side Effects

All cephalosporins are generally safe; however, sensitivity can occur in individuals (allergy). Cross-reactivity between penicillin allergy and cephalosporin allergy is low. Rare bleeding disorders have been known to occur with some cephalosporins.

### Contraindications and Precautions

Do not use in animals with allergic sensitivity to other beta-lactams, especially other cephalosporins. However, the incidence of cross-sensitivity between penicillins and cephalosporins is small (less than 10% in people). Some cephalosporins should not be used in animals with bleeding problems or that are receiving warfarin anticoagulants. These cephalosporins are those that have an NMTT side chain and include cefotetan, cefamandole, and cefoperazone.

### Drug Interactions

No drug interactions are reported in animals. However, do not mix in a vial or syringe with other drugs because inactivation may result.

## Instructions for Use

Third-generation cephalosporin is used when resistance to first- and second-generation cephalosporins is encountered.

## Patient Monitoring and Laboratory Tests

Susceptibility testing: A CLSI breakpoint for susceptible organisms has not been established for animals. The human susceptible breakpoint of $\leq 1$ mcg/mL for gram-negative Enterobacteriaceae bacteria (e.g., *E. coli*) can be used as an approximation until animal-specific data are available.

## Formulations

- Cefotaxime is available in 500-mg and 1-, 2-, and 10-g vials for injection. Availability of commercial formulations has diminished. Use ceftazadime as an alternative.

## Stability and Storage

Store in a tightly sealed container, protected from light, and at room temperature. Maximum stability is at pH of 5–7. Do not mix with alkaline solutions. Yellow or amber color does not indicate instability. After reconstitution, cefotaxime is stable for 12 hours at room temperature; it is stable for 5 days when stored in plastic syringes or a vial if kept in refrigerator. It is stable for 13 weeks if frozen. IV solutions in 1000 mL are stable for 24 hours at room temperature or 5 days in a refrigerator. Do not refreeze.

## Small Animal Dosage

**Dogs**
- 25 mg/kg q8 h IV, IM, or SQ.
- CRI: 3.2 mg/kg loading dose followed by 5 mg/kg/h.

**Cats**
- 25 mg/kg q8h IV, IM, or SQ.

## Large Animal Dosage

**Foals**
- 40 mg/kg q6h IV bolus injection over 1 minute.
- CRI dose for foals: Administer 4 mg/kg IV loading dose followed by 2.5 mg/kg per hour, IV infusion.

**Horses**
- 25 mg/kg q6h, IV.

## Regulatory Information

The extralabel administration of cephalosporins to food-producing animals in the United States is a violation of FDA regulations. Withdrawal times are not established for animals that produce food.

# Cefotetan Disodium
sef'oh-tee-tan dye-soe'dee-um

**Trade and other names:** Generic

**Functional classification:** Antibacterial

**Note:** Cefotetan has been discontinued from the human market in the United States and may not be available to veterinarians. Consider cefoxitin as a substitute.

## Pharmacology and Mechanism of Action

Cephalosporin antibiotic. The action is similar to other beta-lactam antibiotics, which is to inhibit synthesis of the bacterial cell wall, leading to cell death. Cephalosporins are divided into first-, second-, third-, and fourth-generation drugs depending on spectrum of activity. Cefotetan has been listed with second-generation cephalosporins but is more properly considered with the cephamycin group of cephalosporins, which have greater stability against the beta-lactamases of anaerobic bacteria such as those of the *Bacteroides* group. Cephamycins are not susceptible to inactivation from the extended-spectrum beta-lactamases (ESBLs), but susceptibility tests should be performed to confirm susceptibility. Cefotetan is slightly more active (lower minimum inhibitory concentration [MIC] values) compared with cefoxitin against many bacteria.

## Indications and Clinical Uses

Cefotetan, a second-generation cephalosporin of the cephamycin group, has greater activity against anaerobic bacteria and gram-negative bacilli than other cephalosporins. Therefore it has been used to treat infections in dogs and cats in which enteric gram-negative bacilli or anaerobes are suspected, including abdominal infections and soft tissue wounds and prior to surgery.

## Precautionary Information

### Adverse Reactions and Side Effects

All cephalosporins are generally safe; however, sensitivity can occur in individuals (allergy). Rare bleeding disorders have been known to occur with some cephalosporins.

### Contraindications and Precautions

Do not use in animals with allergic sensitivity to other beta-lactams, especially other cephalosporins. However, the incidence of cross-sensitivity between penicillins and cephalosporins is small (less than 10% in people). Some cephalosporins should not be used in animals with bleeding problems or that are receiving warfarin anticoagulants. These cephalosporins are those that have an NMTT side chain and include cefotetan, cefamandole, and cefoperazone.

### Drug Interactions

No drug interactions are reported in animals. However, do not mix in a vial or syringe with other drugs because inactivation may result.

## Instructions for Use

Cefotetan is a second-generation cephamycin cephalosporin, and if there is no availability, consider cefoxitin as a substitute.

## Patient Monitoring and Laboratory Tests

Susceptibility testing: CLSI breakpoint for susceptible organisms is ≤8 mcg/mL for gram-negative and gram-positive organisms.

## Formulations

- Cefotetan was available in 1-, 2-, and 10-g vials for injection. Formulations may no longer be commercially available.

## Stability and Storage

Store in a tightly sealed container, protected from light, and at room temperature. Observe manufacturer's recommendations for stability after vial is reconstituted.

## Small Animal Dosage
**Dogs and Cats**
- 30 mg/kg q8h IV or SQ.

## Large Animal Dosage
- No dose has been reported for large animals.

## Regulatory Information
The extralabel administration of cephalosporins to food-producing animals in the United States is a violation of FDA regulations. Withdrawal times are not established for animals that produce food.

# Cefovecin
sef-oh-ve'sin

**Trade and other names:** Convenia

**Functional classification:** Antibacterial

## Pharmacology and Mechanism of Action
Cephalosporin antibiotic. The action is similar to other beta-lactam antibiotics, which is to inhibit synthesis of the bacterial cell wall, leading to cell death. Cephalosporins are divided into first-, second-, third-, and fourth-generation drugs depending on spectrum of activity. Cefovecin is considered a third-generation cephalosporin based on structural relationships but may not have the same activity as other injectable third-generation cephalosporins, such as ceftazidime or cefotaxime. Cefovecin has good activity against streptococci, *Staphylococcus* spp., and some gram-negative bacilli. Cefovecin is more active against *S. pseudintermedius* than against *S. aureus*. Concentrations are generally not high enough for treating systemic infections caused by Enterobacteriaceae such as *E. coli*. MIC values are lower for cefovecin than with first-generation cephalosporins. Some Enterobacteriaceae can develop resistance. It is not active against *P. aeruginosa*. MRS are considered resistant to cefovecin. Activity against anaerobic bacteria is unpredictable.

*Pharmacokinetics:* Cefovecin is greater than 99% protein bound in cats and greater than 98% in dogs, which is partly responsible for the long duration. The terminal half-lives are approximately 7 days in cats and 5 days in dogs, and effective concentrations can be maintained in the tissue fluid of these species for 14 days.

## Indications and Clinical Uses
Cefovecin is approved for use in dogs and cats. It is approved in the United States for skin and soft tissue infections but also has been used to treat UTIs, for which it is approved in some countries. The efficacy of cefovecin for treating infections in other sites, such as the respiratory tract, bone, and CNS, has not been established. The high protein binding may limit penetration to some of these sites. In cats, it is approved for treating skin and soft tissue infections that are caused by highly susceptible bacteria such as strains of *P. multocida*. Experience is limited to administration of cefovecin in dogs and cats; the use in other species, such as horses, large animals, birds, and reptiles, is not recommended until specific dosing recommendations are published. Protein binding is lower in these species, which causes a much shorter half-life compared with dogs or cats.

## Precautionary Information
### Adverse Reactions and Side Effects
The animal safety studies have produced few serious adverse reactions. In dogs and cats, vomiting and diarrhea have been observed in a dose-related manner. With approved doses, mild GI upset may be observed for 2–3 days. Injection-site irritation and transient edema occurred with increasing frequency in a dose-related manner and with repeat injections. The long half-life indicates that drug concentrations persist in animals for at least 60 days after an injection, but at this time, this has not produced adverse reactions attributed to a long persistence of drug in tissues. Allergic reactions are possible with any cephalosporin, but cross-reactivity between penicillin allergy and cephalosporin allergy is low.

### Contraindications and Precautions
Do not use in animals with allergic sensitivity to other beta-lactams, especially other cephalosporins. However, the incidence of cross-sensitivity between penicillins and cephalosporins is small.

### Drug Interactions
No drug interactions are reported in animals. However, do not mix in a vial or syringe with other drugs because inactivation may result.

## Instructions for Use
The approved label in the United States indicates that therapeutic concentrations are maintained for an interval of 7 days in dogs. However, pharmacokinetic studies indicated that drug concentrations persist long enough for a 14-day interval for some indications. In Canada and Europe, the approved label dose is 8 mg/kg SQ once every 14 days, and efficacy has been demonstrated with a 14-day interval for administration. The injection may be repeated for infections that require longer than 14 days for a cure (e.g., canine pyoderma).

## Patient Monitoring and Laboratory Tests
Susceptibility testing: The approved CLSI-approved breakpoints for susceptibility testing are ≤0.5 mcg/mL for canine *S. pseudintermedius* isolates from skin and soft tissues and ≤0.12 mcg/mL for *Streptococcus* spp. Isolates of the gram-negative Enterobacteriaceae may test clinically resistant using these breakpoints. The breakpoint is ≤0.12 mcg/mL for feline skin and soft tissue isolates. For isolates from the lower urinary tract in dogs and cats, the susceptible breakpoint is ≤2 mcg/mL.

## Formulations
- Cefovecin is available in 10-mL vials containing 800 mg. When reconstituted, it is 80 mg/mL.

## Stability and Storage
Store in original vial in the refrigerator protected from light. Do not freeze. Once reconstituted, vial should be used within 56 days (the original label had a limitation of 28 days). The reconstituted solution may turn slightly yellow, which does not affect potency.

## Small Animal Dosage
**Dogs and Cats**
- 8 mg/kg SQ every 14 days. For some indications, injections may be repeated at 7 days.

## Large Animal Dosage
- No dose has been established. It is not recommended for large animal species because of pharmacokinetic differences.

## Regulatory Information
Withdrawal times are not established for animals that produce food, and cefovecin should not be administered to food-producing animals. The extralabel administration of cephalosporins to food-producing animals in the United States is a violation of FDA regulations.

# Cefoxitin Sodium
se-fox′ i-tin soe′dee-um

**Trade and other names:** Mefoxitin, Mefoxin, Cefoxil, and generic

**Functional classification:** Antibacterial

## Pharmacology and Mechanism of Action
Cephalosporin antibiotic. The action is similar to other beta-lactam antibiotics, which is to inhibit synthesis of the bacterial cell wall, leading to cell death. Cephalosporins are divided into first-, second-, third-, and fourth-generation drugs depending on spectrum of activity. Cefoxitin has been listed with second-generation cephalosporins but is more properly considered with the cephamycin group of cephalosporins, which have greater stability against the beta-lactamases of anaerobic bacteria such as those of the *Bacteroides* group. Cephamycins also may be stable against some ESBLs but not against AmpC-producing bacteria. A similar drug of the cephamycin group, cefotetan, has been withdrawn from the commercial market and is no longer available. Cefoxitin can be used as a substitute.

*Pharmacokinetics:* In cats, the half-life is 1.6 hours, the VD is 0.3 L/kg, and the clearance is 2.3 mL/kg/min. In horses, these values are 0.82 hours, 0.12 L/kg, and 4.3 mL/min/kg, respectively. In dogs, these values are 1.3 hours, 0.16 L/kg, and 3.2 mL/kg/min, respectively.

## Indications and Clinical Uses
Cefoxitin, a cephalosporin of the cephamycin group, has greater activity against anaerobic bacteria and gram-negative bacilli than other cephalosporins. Therefore, it has been used to treat infections in dogs and cats in which enteric gram-negative bacilli or anaerobes are suspected, including abdominal infections and soft tissue wounds, and prior to surgery. Because cefoxitin is of the cephamycin group of cephalosporins, it may be resistant to many ESBLs and may be used to treat some multidrug-resistant bacterial infections as an alternative to carbapenems. Susceptibility should be confirmed with a test before considering treatment.

## Precautionary Information

### Adverse Reactions and Side Effects

All cephalosporins are generally safe; however, sensitivity can occur in individuals (allergy). Cross-reactivity between penicillin allergy and cephalosporin allergy is low. Rare bleeding disorders have been known to occur with some cephalosporins. Cefoxitin has been administered to dogs during surgery without adversely affecting their cardiovascular function.

### Contraindications and Precautions

Do not use in animals with allergic sensitivity to other beta-lactams, especially other cephalosporins. However, the incidence of cross-sensitivity between penicillins and cephalosporins is small (less than 10% in people). Some cephalosporins should not be used in animals with bleeding problems or that are receiving warfarin anticoagulants. These cephalosporins are those that have an NMTT side chain and include cefotetan, cefamandole, and cefoperazone.

### Drug Interactions

No drug interactions are reported in animals. However, do not mix in a vial or syringe with other drugs because inactivation may result.

## Instructions for Use

Second-generation cephalosporin is often used when activity against anaerobic bacteria is desired. Cefoxitin is similar to another cephamycin, cefotetan, but because cefotetan is no longer available, cefoxitin can be used as a substitute.

## Patient Monitoring and Laboratory Tests

Susceptibility testing: CLSI breakpoint for susceptible organisms is ≤8 mcg/mL using the human breakpoint for Enterobacteriaceae. Breakpoints for isolates from animals are not available. Cefoxitin should not be used to test for methicillin-resistant strains of *S. pseudintermedius* from animals.

## Formulations

• Cefoxitin is available in 1- and 2-g vials for injection (20 or 40 mg/mL).

## Stability and Storage

Store in a tightly sealed container, in the freezer at –25°C to –10°C unless otherwise instructed by the manufacturer. Thaw at room temperature or in refrigerator to dissolve crystals before administration. Do not heat or place in microwave oven. After thawing, solution is potent for 24 hours at room temperature or for 21 days in refrigerator. Protect from light. After it has thawed, do not refreeze.

## Small Animal Dosage

### Dogs and Cats

• 30 mg/kg q8h IM, SQ, or IV. 22 mg/kg IV for presurgical use.

## Large Animal Dosage

### Horses

• 20 mg/kg q4–6h IV or IM.

## Regulatory Information

The extralabel administration of cephalosporins to food-producing animals in the United States is a violation of FDA regulations. Withdrawal times are not established for animals that produce food.

## Cefpodoxime Proxetil

sef-poe-doks'eem prahx'ih-til

**Trade and other names:** Simplicef (veterinary preparation), Vantin (human preparation), and generic

**Functional classification:** Antibacterial

## Pharmacology and Mechanism of Action

Cephalosporin antibiotic. Action is similar to other cephalosporins and beta-lactam antibiotics, which inhibit synthesis of the bacterial cell wall, leading to cell death. Cephalosporins are divided into first-, second-, third-, and fourth-generation drugs depending on spectrum of activity. Cefpodoxime is a third-generation cephalosporin, which indicates greater activity against gram-negative bacilli compared with first-generation cephalosporins. However, cefpodoxime is not as active against many gram-negative bacilli as injectable third-generation cephalosporins such as cefotaxime or ceftazidime. Cefpodoxime has better activity against *Staphylococcus* spp. than other oral third-generation cephalosporins (e.g., cefixime). It is not active against *Enterococcus* spp., MRS, or *P. aeruginosa*. Activity against anaerobic bacteria is unpredictable. It is one of three third-generation oral cephalosporins, but the others are either not available or seldom used. Cefpodoxime is combined with proxetil to produce an ester to improve oral absorption. Therefore, as the ester, it is actually a prodrug that needs to be converted to the active cefpodoxime.

*Pharmacokinetics:* Oral absorption in dogs is 35%. Half-lives are 7.2 hours in horses and 5.7 hours in dogs. Protein binding in dogs is 83%.

## Indications and Clinical Uses

Cefpodoxime is indicated for treatment of skin and other soft tissue infections in dogs caused by susceptible organisms. Efficacy has been established in dogs for treatment of skin and soft tissue infections. Cefpodoxime has greater activity against gram-negative bacilli than first-generation cephalosporins; therefore it may be effective for some gram-negative infections that would not respond to first-generation cephalosporins. Although not currently registered for treatment of UTIs, approximately 50% of administered dose is excreted in urine and expected to be active for treating UTIs caused by common pathogens. Although not registered for cats or tested in cats, no adverse effects have been reported from occasional use. However, oral absorption in cats has not been examined.

## Precautionary Information

### Adverse Reactions and Side Effects

All cephalosporins are generally safe; however, sensitivity can occur in individuals (allergy). Cross-reactivity between penicillin allergy and cephalosporin allergy is low. Rare bleeding disorders have been known to occur with some cephalosporins. Vomiting and diarrhea can occur from oral administration of cephalosporins, but because cefpodoxime proxetil is administered as an inactive pro-drug, the GI reactions may be less than other oral cephalosporins.

### Contraindications and Precautions

This drug is best taken with food to improve oral absorption. Do not use in animals with allergic sensitivity to other beta-lactams, especially other cephalosporins. However, the incidence of cross-sensitivity between penicillins and cephalosporins is small (less than 10% in people). Some cephalosporins should not be used in animals with bleeding problems or that are receiving warfarin anticoagulants. These cephalosporins are those that have an NMTT side chain and include cefotetan, cefamandole, and cefoperazone.

### Drug Interactions

There are no important drug interactions reported for animals, but oral absorption of cefpodoxime in people is inhibited by $H_2$-blockers (e.g., cimetidine and ranitidine) and antacids, which can decrease oral absorption by 30%. Cephalosporins may be administered with other antibiotics to increase the spectrum of activity. However, do not mix with other drugs in a compounded formulation because inactivation may result.

## Instructions for Use

US FDA approval in dogs includes skin and soft tissue infections. It also has been used for UTIs, and based on spectrum and tissue distribution, it has been used for other infections. There has also been occasional anecdotal use in cats on an extralabel basis.

## Patient Monitoring and Laboratory Tests

Susceptibility testing: CLSI breakpoint for susceptible organisms isolated from animals is ≤2 mcg/mL. Strains of *E. coli* and *Klebsiella* spp. that are ESBLs may be clinically resistant. MRS are resistant to cefpodoxime.

## Formulations

• Cefpodoxime proxetil is available in 100- and 200-mg tablets and 10- and 20-mg/mL oral suspension (human preparation).

## Stability and Storage

Store in a tightly sealed container, protected from light, and at room temperature. Stability of compounded tablets has not been evaluated. Avoid exposure to moisture.

## Small Animal Dosage

### Dogs

• 5–10 mg/kg q24h PO.

### Cats

• A dose has not been established by the manufacturer for cefpodoxime proxetil. Some veterinarians have extrapolated from the canine dose.

## Large Animal Dosage

### Horses

- 10 mg/kg oral q6–12h. The 12-hour interval is appropriate for *Klebsiella* spp., *Pasteurella* spp., and streptococci. More frequent intervals may be needed for more resistant organisms.

## Regulatory Information

The extralabel administration of cephalosporins to food-producing animals in the United States is a violation of FDA regulations. Withdrawal times are not established for animals that produce food.

# Cefquinome Sulfate

sefs quin-ome sul' fate

**Trade and other names:** Cobactan and Cephaguard

**Functional classification:** Antibacterial

## Pharmacology and Mechanism of Action

Cephalosporin antibiotic. Cefquinome, like other cephalosporins, inhibits synthesis of the bacterial cell wall, leading to cell death. Cephalosporins are divided into first-, second-, third-, and fourth-generation drugs depending on spectrum of activity. Cefquinome is currently the only fourth-generation cephalosporin approved in any country for use in food animals. In contrast to other cephalosporins, cefquinome is not affected by chromosomal-mediated cephalosporinases of the Amp C type or by plasmid-mediated beta-lactamase from some gram-negative bacilli. Bacteria that produce ESBL and MRS species are resistant.

Cefquinome is currently licensed in Europe but not the United States. Cefquinome has good activity against most gram-negative bacilli, especially Enterobacteriaceae. It has been shown to be active against bovine respiratory pathogens that include *Mannheimia haemolytica, P. multocida,* and *Histophilus somni.* It also is active against pathogens that cause mastitis in cows, including *E. coli, S. aureus, Streptococcus dysgalactiae, Streptococcus agalactiae,* and *Streptococcus uberis.* Activity of cefquinome against equine pathogens includes gram-positive and gram-negative bacteria such as *E. coli, Streptococcus equi* subsp. *zooepidemicus, K. pneumoniae, Enterobacter* spp., *S. aureus, S. equi* subsp. *equi, Clostridium perfringens,* and *Actinobacillus equuli.*

*Pharmacokinetics:* In cattle, cefquinome has a half-life of 2.5 hours and is less than 5% protein bound. Cefquinome is not absorbed after oral administration. In pigs or piglets, the half-life is about 9 hours. Because of low protein binding, cefquinome penetrates into the cerebrospinal fluid (CSF) and the synovial fluid in pigs. In horses, cefquinome has a half-life of 2 hours in adult horses and 1.4 hours in foals with protein binding less than 5%. Absorption from IM injection is almost 100% in adults and 87% in foals. In dogs, cefquinome has a half-life of approximately 1–2 hours from IM and IV administration (longer from IM injection) and 0.85 hours from SQ administration, and absorption is nearly complete from SQ and IM injection. VD is 0.3 L/kg, and protein binding is less than 10%.

## Indications and Clinical Uses

Cefquinome is used in cattle, pigs, and horses to treat infections caused by susceptible pathogens. It is registered in Europe for treatment of respiratory disease, *E. coli* sepsis in calves, and interdigital necrobacillosis (foot rot) in lactating cows in many countries. Cefquinome ointment has been administered intramammary for treatment of *E. coli* mastitis in dairy cattle. In Europe, it is also registered for treatment of swine respiratory disease (SRD), arthritis, meningitis, and dermatitis caused by *P. multocida, Haemophilus parasuis, Actinobacillus pleuropneumoniae, Streptococcus suis, Staphylococcus hyicus,* and other cefquinome-sensitive organisms and mastitis-metritis-agalactia (MMA) syndrome with involvement of *E. coli, Staphylococcus* spp., *Streptococcus* spp., and other cefquinome-sensitive organisms. In horses, it is registered for respiratory infection caused by *S. equi* subsp. *zooepidemicus* and systemic bacterial infection (sepsis) caused by *E. coli*.

The use of cefquinome for small animals is very limited, but in some countries where it is available, it has been injected for short-term treatments.

---

### Precautionary Information

#### Adverse Reactions and Side Effects

All cephalosporins are generally safe; however, sensitivity can occur in individuals (allergy). Cefquinome injection SQ may cause some injection-site reactions.

High doses may produce diarrhea in horses, but if doses are maintained within the range listed in the dosing section, it has been safe in most horses.

#### Contraindications and Precautions

Do not administer to animals prone to sensitivity to beta-lactams.

#### Drug Interactions

No drug interactions are reported in animals. However, do not mix in a vial or syringe with other drugs because inactivation may result.

---

### Instructions for Use

Cefquinome is registered in Europe for treatment of infections in cattle, pigs, and horses. In the United States, without FDA approval, the use would be a violation. Cefquinome in cattle can be administered SQ or IM, depending on the formulation. In pigs, it is administered IM. In horses, the solution can be administered IV initially and then switched to IM injections.

### Patient Monitoring and Laboratory Tests

Monitor CBC if high doses are administered for long periods. Susceptibility testing: CLSI guidelines for susceptible bacteria are not available.

### Formulations

- In countries where cefquinome is available, it is a 7.5% (75-mg/mL) injectable suspension, 2.5% (25-mg/mL) injectable suspension, a powder for reconstitution to be used IV in horses and foals (4.5% or 45 mg/mL in a 30- or 100-mL vial), and an intramammary ointment (75 mg in an 8-g syringe).

### Stability and Storage

After the container is opened, the shelf life is 28 days. For the 4.5% IV solution, the shelf life after reconstitution is 10 days when stored in a refrigerator (2°C–8°C).

## Small Animal Dosage
**Dogs and Cats**
- 2 mg/kg IV, IM, or SQ q12h.

## Large Animal Dosage (Based on Registration Label in Europe)
**Cattle**
- BRD: 2.5 mg/kg IM q48h (1 mL of 7.5% suspension per 30 kg).
- Respiratory disease and foot rot: 1 mg/kg (2 mL per 50 kg of 2.5% suspension) IM once daily for 3–5 days.
- Mastitis (*E. coli*) systemic involvement: 1 mg/kg (2 mL per 50 kg of 2.5% suspension) IM once daily for 2 days.
- Septicemia in calves (*E. coli*): 2 mg/kg (4 mL per 50 kg of 2.5% suspension) IM once daily for 3–5 days.

**Pigs**
- Respiratory infections: 2 mg/kg (2 mL of 2.5% suspension) IM in the neck once daily for 2 days.
- Meningitis, arthritis, or dermatitis in piglets: 2 mg/kg (2 mL of 2.5% suspension) once daily IM for 5 days.

**Horses**
- Respiratory infections caused by *S. equi*: 1 mg/kg (1 mL solution per 45 kg) of solution IV or IM q24h for 5–10 days.
- Systemic infection (especially septicemia in foals) caused by *E. coli*: 1 mg/kg (1 mL per 45 kg) IV or IM q12h for 6–14 days.

## Regulatory Information
For cefquinome suspension, do not use in lactating cattle producing milk for human consumption (during lactation or the dry period). Do not use within 2 months prior to first calving in heifers intended for the production of milk for human consumption. In Europe, the meat withdrawal times are 13 days after 2.5 mg/kg SQ, 5 days after 1 mg/kg IM, and 3 days in pigs. Milk withdrawal time after systemic use is 24 hours. After intramammary administration, the meat withdrawal time is 4 days, and the milk discard time is 5 days. Cefquinome is not approved in the United States, and the extralabel administration of it to food-producing animals in the United States is a violation of FDA regulations.

# Ceftazidime
sef-tah′zih-deem

**Trade and other names:** Fortaz, Ceptaz, Tazicef, and Tazidime

**Functional classification:** Antibacterial

## Pharmacology and Mechanism of Action
Cephalosporin antibiotic. The action is similar to other beta-lactam antibiotics, which is to inhibit synthesis of the bacterial cell wall, leading to cell death. Cephalosporins are divided into first-, second-, third-, and fourth-generation drugs depending on spectrum of activity. Ceftazidime is a third-generation cephalosporin. Not all third-generation cephalosporins are equal in activity. Ceftazidime is active against many gram-negative bacilli of the Enterobacteriaceae and more active against *P. aeruginosa,* than other third-generation cephalosporins. Because other third-generation cephalosporins (e.g., cefotaxime) are not available, ceftazidime is a reasonable alternative for an injectable agent.

*Pharmacokinetics:* Ceftazidime pharmacokinetics have been studied in several veterinary species, including dogs, cats, cattle, horses, and exotic animals. In mammals, the half-life is short (generally 1–2 hours), and the VD reflects extracellular fluid (0.3–0.4 L/kg). Specifically, the half-life in dogs is 1 hour, with a VD of 0.2 L/kg. Protein binding in dogs is 10%.

## Indications and Clinical Uses

Ceftazidime is a third-generation cephalosporin with activity against many gram-negative bacteria resistant to other drugs, especially gram-negative Enterobacteriaceae bacilli (e.g., *E. coli, Klebsiella* spp.) and *P. aeruginosa.* Although it is not an FDA-approved drug for animals, it is used often in zoo, exotic, and companion animals because of its activity against many organisms that are resistant to other drugs. Its activity against *P. aeruginosa,* distinguishes it from other cephalosporins; therefore, it has been used to treat infections in dogs and cats in which enteric gram-negative bacilli or *P. aeruginosa,* are suspected, including abdominal infections, skin infections, soft tissue wounds, and prior to surgery.

## Precautionary Information

### Adverse Reactions and Side Effects

All cephalosporins are generally safe; however, sensitivity can occur in individuals (allergy). Cross-reactivity between penicillin allergy and cephalosporin allergy is low. Rare bleeding disorders have been known to occur with some cephalosporins. Slight irritation or a sting may occur from SQ or IM injections.

### Contraindications and Precautions

Do not use in animals with allergic sensitivity to other beta-lactams, especially other cephalosporins. However, the incidence of cross-sensitivity between penicillins and cephalosporins is small (less than 10% in people). Some cephalosporins should not be used in animals with bleeding problems or that are receiving warfarin anticoagulants. These cephalosporins are those that have an NMTT side chain and include cefotetan, cefamandole, and cefoperazone.

### Drug Interactions

Do not mix in a vial or syringe with other drugs because inactivation may result. In particular, there may be mutual inactivation if mixed with aminoglycosides. If mixed with vancomycin, precipitation may occur.

## Instructions for Use

Ceftazidime may be reconstituted with 1% lidocaine for IM injection to reduce pain. Ceftazidime contains L-arginine. To make up vials containing sodium carbonate, carbon dioxide will form on reconstitution. Venting may be necessary to release gas. Doses listed for dogs and cats are sufficient for treating infections caused by susceptible bacteria, including *P. aeruginosa.*

## Patient Monitoring and Laboratory Tests

Susceptibility testing: CLSI breakpoints for susceptible organisms are ≤4 mcg/mL for testing Enterobacteriaceae (e.g., *E. coli, Klebsiella* spp.) and ≤8 mcg/mL for testing *P. aeruginosa.* Some ESBL-producing strains of *E. coli* or *Klebsiella* spp. may be clinically susceptible to ceftazidime.

## Formulations

- Ceftazidime is available in 0.5-, 1-, 2-, and 6-g vials reconstituted to 280 mg/mL.

## Stability and Storage

Store in a tightly sealed container, protected from light, and at room temperature. Slight discoloration to yellow or amber may occur without losing potency. Do not mix in vial with other drugs, but it may be mixed with IV fluid solutions. When reconstituted with sterile water for injection, it maintains potency for 12 hours at room temperature or for 3 days under refrigeration. Other testing has confirmed stability for 5 days in the refrigerator. Solutions in sterile water for injection can be frozen after reconstitution in the original container and are stable for 3 months when stored at –20°C. If individual dose aliquots are stored in plastic syringes in the freezer for long periods (–18°C) it will retain potency for at least 25 days. After it has thawed, it should not be refrozen.

## Small Animal Dosage

**Dogs and Cats**

- 25 mg/kg q8h IV, SQ, or IM. (There may be some slight sting from SQ and IM injection.)
- Constant IV infusion: Give loading dose of 2 mg/kg followed by 2 mg/kg/h delivered in IV fluids.

## Large Animal Dosage

**Horses**

- 20 mg/kg q8h IV or IM.

## Regulatory Information

The extralabel administration of cephalosporins to food-producing animals in the United States is a violation of FDA regulations. Withdrawal times are not established for animals that produce food.

# Ceftiofur Crystalline-Free Acid
sef'tee-oh-fer

**Trade and other names:** Excede and Naxcel XT

**Functional classification:** Antibacterial

## Pharmacology and Mechanism of Action

Cephalosporin antibiotic. Ceftiofur hydrochloride and ceftiofur sodium have similar action and spectrum. The action is similar to other beta-lactam antibiotics, which is to inhibit synthesis of the bacterial cell wall, leading to cell death. Cephalosporins are divided into first-, second-, third-, and fourth-generation drugs depending on spectrum of activity. Ceftiofur most closely resembles the activity of a third-generation cephalosporin. It has good activity against most gram-negative bacilli, especially Enterobacteriaceae. It has potent activity against bovine and swine respiratory pathogens such as *Mannheimia* spp., *A. pleuropneumoniae, P. multocida, Salmonella enterica, Histophilus somni,* and *Streptococcus* spp. Ceftiofur has activity against some gram-positive cocci, such as streptococci, but activity against staphylococci is not as high as other cephalosporins. Ceftiofur is rapidly metabolized after administration to metabolites such as desfuroylceftiofur, which is active against bacteria, except that it is less active against staphylococci than other cephalosporins and the parent drug ceftiofur.

## Indications and Clinical Uses

Ceftiofur crystalline-free acid is indicated for treatment of SRD caused by *A. pleuropneumoniae, P. multocida, S. enterica, H. parasuis,* and *S. suis.* In cattle, it is used for treatment of BRD caused by *M. haemolytica, P. multocida,* and *H. somni.*

It also can be administered to control respiratory disease in cattle at high risk of developing BRD (metaphylaxis) associated with *M. haemolytica, P. multocida,* and *H. somni.* This formulation also is approved for treating foot rot in cattle (interdigital necrobacillosis) caused by *Fusobacterium necrophorum, Porphyromonas levii,* and *Bacteroides melaninogenicus.* It is approved for treatment of acute metritis in dairy cattle via a two-dose regimen. It is approved for treatment and control of SRD associated with *A. pleuropneumoniae, P. multocida, H. parasuis,* and *S. suis.* This formulation also is approved for use in horses for treatment of respiratory tract infections caused by susceptible *S. equi (S. zooepidemicus)* after administration of two injections. Ceftiofur hydrochloride and ceftiofur crystalline-free acid have also been administered extralabel intramammary to dairy cattle. However, there are specific products designed for intramammary use (Spectramast).

Ceftiofur crystalline-free acid has been administered to zoo and exotic animals for treatment of infections, but the dose has not been established and is extrapolated from use in livestock. The use of this product in small animals has not been reported.

## Precautionary Information

### Adverse Reactions and Side Effects

All cephalosporins are generally safe; however, sensitivity can occur in individuals (allergy). Rare bleeding disorders have been known to occur with some cephalosporins. For ceftiofur, doses that have exceeded the approved label recommendations have caused bone marrow suppression in dogs. Thrombocytopenia and anemia occurred at doses of 6.6 and 11 mg/kg when administered to dogs. High doses have caused diarrhea in horses. Injections of the crystalline-free acid formulation to small animals have caused injection-site lesions in some animals, and this is generally not recommended. In some horses, injections of ceftiofur crystalline-free acid has caused injection-site reactions, consisting of swelling and pain, at the injection site.

### Contraindications and Precautions

Do not administer this formulation (suspension) IV. Do not administer to animals prone to sensitivity to beta-lactams. Do not administer to animals at doses higher than label indication. In horses, do not administer more than 20 mL per injection site. Ceftiofur crystalline-free acid should not be used interchangeably with ceftiofur sodium or ceftiofur hydrochloride without consulting label information for differences in dosing and withdrawal times.

### Drug Interactions

No drug interactions are reported in animals. However, do not mix in a vial or syringe with other drugs because inactivation may result.

## Instructions for Use

Dosing information is available for pigs, horses, and cattle; it is not available for other animals. There is no information on the use of ceftiofur crystalline-free acid in dogs or cats. When administering to cattle, the dose is 6.6 mg/kg. For SQ injection, the injection should be in the middle third of the posterior aspect of the ear or in the posterior aspect of the ear where it attaches to the head (base of the ear) in beef and nonlactating dairy cattle. SQ injection is done in the posterior aspect of the ear where it attaches to the head (base of the ear) in lactating dairy cattle. For horses, administer two IM injections, 4 days apart, at a dose of 6.6 mg/kg. For pigs, administer 5 mg/kg IM in the postauricular region of the neck.

## Patient Monitoring and Laboratory Tests
Monitor CBC if high doses are administered for long periods. Sensitivity testing: CLSI guidelines for susceptible bacteria indicate that susceptible bacteria have MIC values ≤2 mcg/mL. (Note that for some cephalosporins used in humans, the MIC values for susceptibility may be ≤8 mcg/mL.)

## Formulations
• Ceftiofur crystalline-free acid is available in an injectable suspension for cattle at 200 mg/mL ceftiofur equivalents (CE).
• Ceftiofur crystalline-free acid is available in an injectable suspension for pigs at 100 mg/mL CE.

## Stability and Storage
Store at room temperature. Shake well before administration. Protect from freezing. Contents should be used within 12 weeks after the first dose is removed.

## Small Animal Dosage
**Dogs and Cats**
• Dose not established for this product. See Ceftiofur Sodium for small animal dosage.

## Large Animal Dosage
**Cattle**
• 6.6 mg/kg with a single SQ injection in the middle third of the posterior aspect of the ear.

**Horses and Foals**
• 6.6 mg/kg IM in the neck muscle (15 mL per 1000 lb). Administer a second dose in 4 days. Do not administer more than 20 mL in one site.

**Pigs**
• 5.0 mg/kg IM injection in the postauricular region of the neck.

## Regulatory Information
Pig withdrawal times: 14 days.
Cattle withdrawal time (slaughter): 13 days. A withdrawal period has not been established in preruminating calves. Do not use in calves to be processed for veal. Milk withdrawal: zero days. The extralabel administration of cephalosporins to food-producing animals in the United States is a violation of FDA regulations.

# Ceftiofur Hydrochloride
sef′tee-oh-fer hye-droe-klor′ide

**Trade and other names:** Excenel, RTU EZ suspension, and Spectramast DC and Spectramast LC suspension for intramammary treatment

**Functional classification:** Antibacterial

## Pharmacology and Mechanism of Action
Ceftiofur is a cephalosporin antibiotic. Ceftiofur hydrochloride and ceftiofur sodium have similar actions and spectrums. The action is similar to other beta-lactam antibiotics, which is to inhibit synthesis of the bacterial cell wall, leading to cell death. Cephalosporins are divided into first-, second-, third-, and fourth-generation drugs depending on spectrum of activity. Ceftiofur most closely resembles the activity of a third-generation cephalosporin. It has good activity against most gram-negative bacilli, especially Enterobacteriaceae. It has potent activity against bovine respiratory pathogens such as *P.*

*multocida, M. haemolytica* and *H. somni.* Ceftiofur has activity against some gram-positive cocci, such as streptococci, but activity against staphylococci is not as high as other cephalosporins. Ceftiofur is rapidly metabolized after administration to metabolites such as desfuroylceftiofur, which is active against bacteria, except that it is less active against staphylococci than other cephalosporins and the parent drug ceftiofur.

*Pharmacokinetics:* In pigs, ceftiofur hydrochloride has a half-life of 19 hours and a time to peak concentration of 2–3 hours after IM injection. The peak concentration is 23–27 mcg/mL. In cattle, the half-life is 9.3 hours and attains a peak concentration of 11–14 mcg/mL after SQ injection at approximately 1.5–2 hours.

## Indications and Clinical Uses

Ceftiofur hydrochloride is used in cattle and pigs for treatment and control of infections caused by susceptible pathogens. It is registered for treatment of respiratory disease in cattle caused by *M. haemolytica, P. multocida,* and *H. somni.* It is used for interdigital necrobacillosis (foot rot) in cattle caused by *F. necrophorum* or *B. melaninogenicus.* Ceftiofur hydrochloride has been shown to be effective for treatment of acute postpartum metritis in dairy cows when administered at 2.2 mg/kg or for treatment of retained fetal membranes by instilling into the uterus (1 g). Ceftiofur hydrochloride is used for treatment of SRD in pigs caused by *A. pleuropneumoniae, P. multocida, S. enterica,* and *S. suis.* Ceftiofur hydrochloride and ceftiofur crystalline-free acid have also been administered via the intramammary route to dairy cattle. For intramammary use, there is a specific formulation is recommended (Spectramast DC) for the treatment of subclinical mastitis in dairy cattle at the time of dry off associated with *S. aureus, S. dysgalactiae,* and *S. uberis,* and another formulation (Spectramast LC) for treatment of mastitis in lactating cows for treatment of clinical mastitis associated with coagulase-negative staphylococci, *S. dysgalactiae,* and *E. coli.*

Although ceftiofur sodium has been used in horses and dogs to treat infections, there is little experience with administration of ceftiofur hydrochloride in these species. There is a concern that injections of ceftiofur hydrochloride may produce injection-site irritation and lesions.

## Precautionary Information

### Adverse Reactions and Side Effects

All cephalosporins are generally safe; however, sensitivity can occur in individuals (allergy). Rare bleeding disorders have been known to occur with some cephalosporins. For ceftiofur, doses that have exceeded the approved label recommendations have caused bone marrow suppression in dogs. Thrombocytopenia and anemia occurred at doses of 6.6 and 11 mg/kg when administered to dogs. High doses have caused diarrhea in horses.

### Contraindications and Precautions

Do not administer to animals prone to sensitivity to beta-lactams. Do not administer to animals at high doses. Ceftiofur hydrochloride is a sterile suspension and should not be used interchangeably with ceftiofur sodium, which is a solution.

### Drug Interactions

No drug interactions are reported in animals. However, do not mix in a vial or syringe with other drugs because inactivation may result.

## Instructions for Use

Dosing information is not available for species other than pigs and cattle. Dosing in cattle may be extended beyond 3 days if necessary. Alternatively, doses have been administered to cattle for BRD at 2.2 mg/kg at 48-hour intervals. Ceftiofur also is approved for dry-cow and lactating-cow treatment (depending on the formulation). Cows with systemic clinical signs caused by mastitis should receive other appropriate therapy under the direction of a licensed veterinarian. Ceftiofur sodium has been used in horses and dogs, but there is no information available on the use of ceftiofur hydrochloride in these species.

## Patient Monitoring and Laboratory Tests
Monitor CBC if high doses are administered for long periods. Susceptibility testing: CLSI guidelines for susceptible bacteria indicate that susceptible bacteria have MIC values ≤2 mcg/mL. (Note that for some human-labeled cephalosporins, the MIC values for susceptibility may be ≤8 mcg/mL.)

## Formulations
- Ceftiofur hydrochloride is available in 50-mg/mL sterile suspension. Ceftiofur hydrochloride has been marketed in two forms: Excenel RTU and a reformulated form Excenel RTU EZ. These formulations are bioequivalent and interchangeable.
- Sterile suspension for intramammary use. Each plastic syringe of Spectramast DC contains 500 mg of ceftiofur hydrochloride (50 mg/mL). Each syringe of Spectramast LC contains 125 mg of ceftiofur in a 10-mL syringe.

## Stability and Storage
Store at room temperature. Shake well before administration. Protect from freezing.

## Small Animal Dosage
**Dogs and Cats**
Dose not established for this product. See Ceftiofur Sodium for small animal dose.

## Large Animal Dosage
**Cattle**
- 1.1–2.2 mg/kg q24h for 3 days IM or SQ (1–2 mL of suspension per 100 lb). Maximum injection-site volume is 15 mL.
- BRD: 2.2 mg/kg, SQ or IM on days 1 and 3 of treatment (48 hours apart).

**Dairy Cows**
- Intrauterine (retained fetal membranes): 1 g of ceftiofur diluted in 20 mL of sterile water infused in uterus once at 14–20 days after calving.
- Intramammary: Spectramast DC (dry cow): 500 mg (one syringe) injected per quarter at the time of drying off. Spectramast LC (lactating cow): Infuse one syringe (125 mg) into each affected quarter q24h. This may be continued for 8 days.
- Treatment of postpartum metritis: 2.2 mg/kg once daily for 5 days SQ or IM.

**Pigs**
- 3–5 mg/kg q24h for 3 days IM. Maximum injection-site volume is 15 mL.

## Regulatory Information
Cattle withdrawal time: 0 days for milk; 3 days for meat. For the intramammary suspension, a 16-day slaughter withdrawal time should be used.

    Pig withdrawal time: 4 days. The extralabel administration of cephalosporins to food-producing animals in the United States is a violation of FDA regulations.

# Ceftiofur Sodium
sef′tee-oh-fer soe′dee-um
**Trade and other names:** Naxcel
**Functional classification:** Antibacterial

## Pharmacology and Mechanism of Action

Cephalosporin antibiotic. Ceftiofur hydrochloride and ceftiofur sodium have similar action and spectrum. The action is similar to other beta-lactam antibiotics, which is to inhibit synthesis of the bacterial cell wall, leading to cell death. Cephalosporins are divided into first-, second-, third-, and fourth-generation drugs depending on spectrum of activity. Ceftiofur most closely resembles the activity of a third-generation cephalosporin. It has good activity against most gram-negative bacilli, especially Enterobacteriaceae. It has potent activity against bovine and swine respiratory pathogens such as *Mannheimia* spp., *A. pleuropneumoniae, P. multocida, S. enterica, H. somni,* and *Streptococcus* spp. Ceftiofur has activity against some gram-positive cocci, such as streptococci, but activity against staphylococci is not as high as other cephalosporins. Ceftiofur is rapidly metabolized after administration to metabolites such as desfuroylceftiofur, which is active against bacteria, except that it is less active against staphylococci than other cephalosporins and the parent drug ceftiofur.

## Indications and Clinical Uses

Ceftiofur sodium is used in cattle and pigs for treatment and control of infections caused by susceptible pathogens. It is registered for treatment of respiratory disease and interdigital necrobacillosis (foot rot) in lactating cows in many countries. Ceftiofur has been used for treatment of salmonella in calves. At 5 mg/kg q24h IM, it decreased diarrhea and temperature but did not eradicate the organism. Ceftiofur sodium has been administered on an intramammary basis for treatment of coliform mastitis, but this is an extralabel use. It is used in horses for treatment of streptococcal respiratory infections (approved label treatment) and extralabel use for treating other infections such as those caused by gram-negative bacilli, including *E. coli, K. pneumoniae,* and *Salmonella* spp. Higher doses should be used for nonstreptococcal bacteria in horses. Ceftiofur sodium is registered for a daily SQ injection for treatment of UTIs in dogs, but it has not been evaluated for treatment of other infections. Ceftiofur sodium has been administered as a CRI to maintain plasma concentrations above a desired range throughout the infusion period. In food-producing animals, extralabel doses or routes of administration are not allowed. However, when ceftiofur sodium was administered either IM or SQ to cattle, there was similar safety and therapeutic efficacy, with almost identical plasma concentration profiles, from both routes of administration.

## Precautionary Information

### Adverse Reactions and Side Effects

All cephalosporins are generally safe; however, sensitivity can occur in individuals (allergy). Rare bleeding disorders have been known to occur with some cephalosporins. For ceftiofur, doses that have exceeded the approved label recommendations have caused bone marrow suppression in dogs. Thrombocytopenia and anemia occurred at doses of 6.6 and 11 mg/kg when administered to dogs. High doses have caused diarrhea in horses, but if doses are maintained within the range listed in the dosing section, it has been safe in most horses.

### Contraindications and Precautions

Do not administer to animals prone to sensitivity to beta-lactams. Do not administer to animals at high doses.

### Drug Interactions

No drug interactions are reported in animals. However, do not mix in a vial or syringe with other drugs because inactivation may result.

## Instructions for Use

Although dosing information is not available for other species, it has been used safely in dogs, sheep, pigs, horses, and cattle and is expected to be safe for other animals. Ceftiofur sodium is bioequivalent whether administered SQ or IM. In dogs and cats, it has not been evaluated to treat infections other than UTIs in dogs. Higher systemic concentrations may be needed in dogs and cats to treat other infections.

## Patient Monitoring and Laboratory Tests

Monitor CBC if high doses are administered for long periods. Susceptibility testing: CLSI guidelines for susceptible bacteria indicate that susceptible bacteria causing respiratory infections in cattle and pigs have MIC values ≤2 mcg/mL. The breakpoint for *Streptococcus* spp. in horses is ≤0.25 mcg/mL. (Note that for many human-labeled cephalosporins, the MIC values for susceptibility may be ≤8 mcg/mL.)

## Formulations

- Ceftiofur sodium is available in 50-mg/mL vials for injection.

## Stability and Storage

Store in a tightly sealed container, protected from light, and at room temperature. If not reconstituted, it may be stored at 20°C–25°C (room temperature). After reconstitution, solutions are potent for 7 days if refrigerated and 12 hours at room temperature. If solutions are prepared in fluids for CRI, the solution should be replaced q24h. If frozen, solutions are stable for 8 weeks. Do not refreeze. Slight discoloration may occur without losing potency.

## Small Animal Dosage

### Dogs
- UTI: 2.2–4.4 mg/kg q24h SQ.

### Cats
- Dose not established but has been extrapolated from canine dose.

## Large Animal Dosage

### Horses
- 4.4 mg/kg q24h IM or 2.2 mg/kg q12h IM for as long as 10 days. Treatment of some gram-negative infections may require doses at the higher range, and up to 11 mg/kg/day IM has been given to horses.
- CRI: Loading dose of 2.4 mg/kg followed by 0.2 mg/kg/h to achieve a target concentration of 4 mcg/mL.

### Foals
- 5 mg/kg q12h IV or CRI of 1 mg/kg/h IV.

### Cattle
- BRD: 1.1–2.2 mg/kg (0.5–1.0 mg/lb) q24h for 3 days IM. Additional doses may be given on days 4 and 5 if necessary. In cattle, these doses also may be administered SQ, which is bioequivalent to other routes of administration.

### Pigs
- Respiratory infections: 3–5 mg/kg (1.36–2.27 mg/lb) q24h for 3 days IM.

### Sheep and Goats
- 1.1–2.2 mg/kg (0.5–1.0 mg/lb) q24h for 3 days IM or SQ. Additional doses may be given on days 4 and 5 if necessary.

## Regulatory Information
Cattle withdrawal time: 0 days for milk and 4 days for meat.
Sheep and goat withdrawal time: 0 days for meat.
Pig withdrawal time: 4 days.
The extralabel administration of cephalosporins to food-producing animals in the
United States is a violation of FDA regulations.

C

# Cephalexin
sef-ah-lex'in

**Trade and other names:** Keflex, Rilexine, Vetolexin (Canada), and generic brands. (In
European countries, it is spelled *cefalexin*.)

**Functional classification:** Antibacterial

## Pharmacology and Mechanism of Action
Cephalosporin antibiotic. The action is similar to other beta-lactam antibiotics,
which is to inhibit synthesis of the bacterial cell wall, leading to cell death.
Cephalosporins are divided into first-, second-, third-, and fourth-generation drugs
depending on spectrum of activity. Cephalexin is a first-generation cephalosporin
and the most common oral cephalosporin used in veterinary medicine. Like other
first-generation cephalosporins, it is active against *Streptococcus* and *Staphylococcus*
spp. and some gram-negative bacilli, such as *Pasteurella* spp. However, most
Enterobacteriaceae bacteria, such as *E. coli*, and *K. pneumoniae*, test clinically
resistant unless they are from the lower urinary tract. It is not active against *P.
aeruginosa*. *Staphylococcus* spp. resistant to methicillin and oxacillin will be resistant
to first-generation cephalosporins.

*Pharmacokinetics:* In horses, the half-life is short at only 1.6 hours, and oral
absorption is only 5%. In dogs, the oral absorption has ranged from 57% to 90%,
depending on the study. In dogs, the average half-life, oral clearance, VD, and peak
concentration are 2.74 hours, 3.14 mL/kg/min, 0.92 L/kg, and 19.5 mcg/mL,
respectively.

## Indications and Clinical Uses
Like other first-generation cephalosporins, cephalexin is indicated for
treating common infections in animals, including UTIs, soft tissue infections,
pyoderma and other dermal infections, and pneumonia. It is approved in the
United States and other countries for treating skin infections in dogs caused
by *S. pseudintermedius*. There are published efficacy studies documenting its
effectiveness for this indication. Efficacy against infections caused by anaerobic
bacteria is unpredictable.

## Precautionary Information
### Adverse Reactions and Side Effects
Gastrointestinal upset, including vomiting, is the most common adverse effect observed in
small animals. Diarrhea also is possible. It is usually self-limiting and not an indication of a
more serious problem. All cephalosporins are generally safe; however, sensitivity can occur

in individuals (allergy). Cross-reactivity between penicillin allergy and cephalosporin allergy is low. Rare bleeding disorders have been known to occur with some cephalosporins.

**Contraindications and Precautions**

Do not use in animals with allergic sensitivity to other beta-lactams, especially other cephalosporins. However, the incidence of cross-sensitivity between penicillins and cephalosporins is small (less than 10% in people). Some cephalosporins should not be used in animals with bleeding problems or that are receiving warfarin anticoagulants. These cephalosporins are those that have an NMTT side chain and include cefotetan, cefamandole, and cefoperazone.

**Drug Interactions**

No drug interactions are reported in animals. However, do not mix with other drugs in a compounded formulation because inactivation may result.

## Instructions for Use

Cephalexin is approved in most countries for use in dogs, but the use has been extrapolated to cats and other species. The most common use is for treatment of skin and soft tissue infections, but UTIs will respond to cephalexin. The oral absorption in horses is low, and clinical use in horses is rare.

## Patient Monitoring and Laboratory Tests

Susceptibility testing: CLSI breakpoints for susceptible organisms are ≤2 mcg/mL for skin and soft tissue infections and ≤16 mcg/mL for isolates from the lower urinary tract. Cephalothin is no longer recommended as a marker to test for susceptibility to cephalexin. MRS species are clinically resistant to cephalexin. Cephalexin may cause a false-positive test for urine glucose. The test may be positive with test strips that use either the copper reduction test or an enzymatic reaction.

## Formulations

- Cephalexin is available in 250- and 500-mg capsules, 75-, 150-, 300-, and 600-mg chewable tablets (for dogs), 100-mg/mL oral suspension, and 125- and 250-mg/5 mL oral suspension. In Canada, a 100- and 250-mg/mL oral paste is available.

## Stability and Storage

Store in a tightly sealed container, protected from light, and at room temperature. Suspensions should be stored in refrigerator and discarded after 14 days. Cephalexin is compatible with enteral products if used immediately after mixing.

## Small Animal Dosage

**Dogs**

- Pyoderma, other skin and soft tissue infections, and UTIs: 22–25 mg/kg q12h PO.

**Cats**

- 22–25 mg/kg q12h PO.

## Large Animal Dosage

**Horses**

- 30 mg/kg q8h PO for susceptible gram-positive bacteria that have a MIC ≤0.5 mcg/mL.

## Regulatory Information

The extralabel administration of cephalosporins to food-producing animals in the United States is a violation of FDA regulations. Withdrawal times are not established for animals that produce food.

# Cetirizine Hydrochloride
seh-teer'ih-zeen hye-droe-klor'ide

**Trade and other names:** Zyrtec

**Functional classification:** Antihistamine

## Pharmacology and Mechanism of Action

Antihistamine (histamine type-1 [$H_1$] blocker). Cetirizine is the active metabolite of hydroxyzine. Almost all hydroxyzine in dogs is converted to cetirizine. Cetirizine is similar to other antihistamines. It acts by blocking the $H_1$ receptor and suppressing inflammatory reactions caused by histamine. The $H_1$ blockers have been used to control pruritus and skin inflammation, rhinorrhea, and airway inflammation, but clinical efficacy has not been demonstrated in animals for these indications. Cetirizine is considered a second-generation antihistamine to distinguish it from other older antihistamines. The most important difference between cetirizine and older drugs is that it does not cross the blood–brain barrier as readily and produces less sedation. A related drug is levocetirizine (Xyzal), which is the active enantiomer of cetirizine and has twofold higher activity than cetirizine.

*Pharmacokinetics:* In cats, cetirizine is well absorbed after oral administration, with a half-life of 10 hours. In dogs, the half-life is approximately 10–11 hours, and in horses, it is 5.8 hours.

## Indications and Clinical Uses

Cetirizine is used to treat and prevent allergic reactions in people. It is preferred over older drugs because it has fewer side effects. In dogs and cats, it has been considered for pruritus therapy, allergic airway disease, rhinitis, and other allergic conditions. In cats, 1 mg/kg (5 mg/cat) has produced plasma concentrations considered effective. However, it was not effective in decreasing the inflammatory response in cats with hyperresponsive airways (experimentally induced asthma). In dogs, doses of 2 mg/kg suppress histamine response for 8 hours. However, there are no published clinical trials to document efficacy for allergic conditions, pruritus in dogs, or airway diseases.

## Precautionary Information

### Adverse Reactions and Side Effects

Sedation is not as likely as with other antihistamines. However, with higher doses, sedation is still possible. Antimuscarinic effects (atropinelike effects) also are possible, but cetirizine may produce fewer antimuscarinic effects than other antihistamines.

### Contraindications and Precautions

Because antimuscarinic effects (atropinelike effects) are possible, do not use in conditions for which anticholinergic drugs may be contraindicated, such as glaucoma, ileus, or cardiac arrhythmias. Discontinue administration a minimum of 7 days prior to allergen-specific allergy testing in dogs.

### Drug Interactions

Do not use with other antimuscarinic drugs.

## Instructions for Use

Use of cetirizine has been mostly empirical. There are no clinical studies to document efficacy.

## Patient Monitoring and Laboratory Tests
No specific monitoring is necessary.

## Formulations
• Cetirizine hydrochloride is available in 1-mg/mL oral syrup and 5- and 10-mg tablets.

## Stability and Storage
Store in a tightly sealed container, protected from light, and at room temperature. Stability of compounded formulations has not been evaluated.

## Small Animal Dosage
**Dogs**
• 2 mg/kg q12h PO.

**Cats**
• 1 mg/kg daily PO. The most common dose is 5 mg per cat (1 tablet).

## Large Animal Dosage
**Horses**
• 0.2–0.4 mg/kg q12h PO.

## Regulatory Information
No regulatory information is available. For extralabel use withdrawal interval estimates, contact FARAD at www.FARAD.org.

RCI Classification: 4

# Charcoal, Activated

**Trade and other names:** Acta-Char, Charcodote, Liqui-Char, ToxiBan, and generic brands

**Functional classification:** Antidote

## Pharmacology and Mechanism of Action
Adsorbent. It binds to other drugs and prevents their absorption from the intestine. It may reduce the absorption of a poison by as much as 75%.

## Indications and Clinical Uses
Used primarily to adsorb drugs and toxins in intestine to prevent their absorption. Ordinarily, a single dose is administered. In some studies, a single dose was as effective as multiple doses in dogs. Consult a poison control center to determine what other supportive measures should be used if a case of intoxication is treated.

## Precautionary Information
### Adverse Reactions and Side Effects
Not absorbed systemically. Safe for oral administration, except that constipation may occur; however, formulations that contain sorbitol may induce diarrhea.

### Contraindications and Precautions
Used primarily as treatment for intoxication. If administered by gastric administration with a stomach tube, serious complications can occur if it is deposited in the airways.

### Drug Interactions
Charcoal adsorbs most other drugs administered orally to prevent their absorption.

C

## Instructions for Use
Dosing of activated charcoal has used a ratio of 10:1 (charcoal:toxin) to administer for treatment of intoxication. However, more recent evidence indicates that a ratio greater than 40:1 is more appropriate, which may require higher doses than previously thought. Activated charcoal is effective to treat intoxication if administered up to 4 hours after exposure, but after 4 hours, benefits decrease. Charcoal is available in a variety of forms and usually is used as treatment for poisoning. Many commercial preparations contain sorbitol, which acts as a flavoring agent and promotes intestinal catharsis.

## Patient Monitoring and Laboratory Tests
When used as treatment for intoxication, careful monitoring of effects of toxin is necessary because charcoal will not adsorb all of the toxicant.

## Formulations
- Charcoal is available in oral suspension and granules. Strengths of formulations vary from 15 g/72 mL to 50 g/240 mL. Many formulations contain sorbitol, which is a sweetener and also can produce an intestinal cathartic effect.

## Stability and Storage
Store in a tightly sealed container at room temperature. Do not mix with other compounds because it will adsorb other chemicals.

## Small Animal Dosage
### Dogs and Cats
- 1–4 g/kg PO (granules) or 6–12 mL/kg (suspension). Administer a single dose shortly after poisoning. A common dose for dogs is a single dose of 2 g/kg as soon as possible after ingestion of a toxin.

## Large Animal Dosage
- Large animal use is not reported, but it may be considered for treatment of a poisoning. Consider a dose of 1 g/kg PO (granules) or 6–10 mL/kg (suspension) PO.

## Regulatory Information
No residue concerns. Withdrawal time: 0 days.

# Chlorambucil
klor-am'byoo-sil

**Trade and other names:** Leukeran

**Functional classification:** Anticancer agent

## Pharmacology and Mechanism of Action

Chlorambucil is an immunosuppressive agent. Chlorambucil is an alkylating agent of the nitrogen mustard category. It is sometimes used as a substitute for cyclophosphamide. It has a similar action as cyclophosphamide but is one of the slowest acting of the class of nitrogen mustards. As an alkylating agent, it interferes with DNA replication and RNA transcription by alkylation and cross-linking the strands of DNA. When used in metronomic dosing protocols for cancer, it may decrease angiogenesis in tumors.

## Indications and Clinical Uses

Chlorambucil is used for treatment of various tumors and immunosuppressive therapy. Although little has been published on the clinical use of chlorambucil, it may be effective in dogs and cats for immune-mediated disease. However, direct comparisons to other immunosuppressive drugs have not been reported. One of the most frequent uses has been for treatment of immune-mediated skin diseases of cats, for which it has been used to treat cats with pemphigus and eosinophilic granuloma complex (EGC). It is often administered concurrently with corticosteroids. It also has been used to treat inflammatory bowel disease (IBD) in cats and dogs and has been effective for chronic enteropathy characterized by protein losing enteropathy in dogs.

Chlorambucil also has been used as an anticancer agent in some protocols. It also has been used in metronomic dosing protocols. At a dosage of 4 mg/m$^2$ PO q24h, it was well tolerated and produced partial remissions for transitional cell carcinoma.

## Precautionary Information

### Adverse Reactions and Side Effects

Myelosuppression is possible, although most cats tolerate chlorambucil well. Cystitis does not occur with chlorambucil as with cyclophosphamide. Diarrhea and anorexia may occur in some patients. At low doses used in metronomic protocols in dogs, it was well tolerated.

### Contraindications and Precautions

Cytotoxic, potentially immunosuppressive agent. Do not use in animals with suppressed bone marrow.

### Drug Interactions

Chlorambucil will potentiate other immunosuppressive drugs.

## Instructions for Use

Chlorambucil may be combined with prednisolone for treatment of immune-mediated disorders, but it is not known if the combination is more effective than prednisolone alone. It also can be used in dogs as a continuous treatment (everyday dose) at low doses of 4 mg/m$^2$ every day. The cost of chlorambucil has increased dramatically, and some veterinarians have relied on compounded formulations. It is not known if compounded forms are equivalent to the FDA-approved forms.

## Patient Monitoring and Laboratory Tests

Monitor CBC in animals during treatment because myelosuppression is the most serious adverse effect.

## Formulations

- Chlorambucil is available in a 2-mg tablet. The tablet may be difficult to divide for small animals.

## Stability and Storage

Store in a tightly sealed container, protected from light, and at room temperature. Chlorambucil undergoes rapid hydrolysis (within 10 minutes) in the presence of water. Hydrolysis occurs most readily at pH greater than 2. Therefore chlorambucil can decompose rapidly in compounded aqueous formulations, such as those that contain simple syrup and other excipients. Hydrolysis is slower if mixed in alcohol-based solutions. If mixed with alcohol and stored in the freezer, it is stable for 31 days. Exposure to light reduces the drug's stability.

## Small Animal Dosage

### Dogs

- 4 mg/m² q24h PO as a starting dose; then increase the interval to q48h PO. (Equivalent dose is 0.1–0.2 mg/kg.)
- Intestinal disease: Start with 4–6 mg/m² PO q24 for the first 7–21 days; then reduce dose. It may be administered with prednisolone in refractory cases.

### Cats

- Immune-mediated disease: 0.1–0.2 mg/kg (approximately one-half tablet) q24h initially; then q48h PO. Often administered concurrently with corticosteroids. Cats with immune-mediated hemolytic anemia have been treated with 2 mg per cat q48h.
- IBD: 2 mg per cat (one tablet) q48–72h PO.
- Cancer treatment: 2 mg per cat PO q48h.

## Large Animal Dosage

- No dose has been reported for large animals.

## Regulatory Information

Withdrawal times are not established for animals that produce food. This drug should not be used in animals intended for food because it is an anticancer agent.

---

# Chloramphenicol
klor-am fen'ih-kole

**Trade and other names:** Chloramphenicol palmitate, Chloromycetin, Viceton, chloramphenicol sodium succinate, and generic brands

**Functional classification:** Antibacterial

## Pharmacology and Mechanism of Action

Antibacterial drug. Mechanism of action is inhibition of protein synthesis via binding to 50-S ribosome subunit. It has a broad spectrum of activity that includes gram-positive cocci, gram-negative bacilli (including Enterobacteriaceae), and *Rickettsia*. Chloramphenicol is usually regarded as a bacteriostatic drug, and it is important to maintain drug concentrations above the MIC for as long as possible during the dosing interval. However, there is some evidence that against some bacteria, it may have bactericidal effects.

*Pharmacokinetics:* Chloramphenicol is absorbed orally in most animals, except ruminants, with a volume of distribution of 1–2 L/kg in animals. The half-life is approximately 2.4 hours in dogs with a peak concentration of approximately 20 mcg/mL. The half-life is 5 hours in cats. Oral absorption in horses is low and variable, ranging from 21% to 40%, depending on the study. The half-life in horses ranges from approximately 2.5 to 3.5 hours, with a peak concentration from oral administration of 3.5–5.25 mcg/mL, depending on the study. from Chloramphenicol sodium succinate is an injectable solution converted to chloramphenicol by hepatic metabolism, but the injectable form is no longer available.

## Indications and Clinical Uses

Chloramphenicol has been used to treat infections caused by a broad spectrum of organisms, including gram-positive cocci, gram-negative bacilli (including Enterobacteriaceae), anaerobic bacteria, and *Rickettsia*. However, effectiveness against all these organisms has not been verified in clinical studies. Chloramphenicol has been used to treat infections caused by bacteria that are resistant to other common drugs (e.g., MRS in dogs).

Chloramphenicol has been used in horses for oral treatment of a variety of infections. However, recent pharmacokinetic analysis have demonstrated that chloramphenicol has a short half-life, highly variable oral absorption, and *not likely* to reach effective levels considered "susceptible" when tested using current susceptibility breakpoints. Therefore, at an oral dose of 50 mg/kg every 6 hours, chloramphenicol is unlikely to be effective in horses unless the bacteria are highly susceptible with an MIC of ≤2 mcg/mL. Florfenicol acts via a similar mechanism and has been substituted in some animals (see Florfenicol).

## Precautionary Information

### Adverse Reactions and Side Effects

Chloramphenicol has a narrow margin of safety. High doses can produce toxicity in dogs and cats. GI disturbances are rather common. A decrease in protein synthesis in the bone marrow may be associated with prolonged treatment. The effect on the bone marrow is most prominent in cats, especially after 14 days of treatment, but is uncommon in dogs. Bone marrow suppression in animals is reversible. Idiosyncratic aplastic anemia has been described in humans. The incidence of aplastic anemia is rare, but the consequences are severe because it is irreversible. The risk of human exposure led to the ban of chloramphenicol use in food animals. Another problem recognized in dogs is peripheral neuropathy. The mechanism is unknown but may be due to de-myelination of nerve fibers. This causes ataxia and weakness, particularly in the hind limbs of dogs. Large-breed dogs may be more susceptible to this problem. The peripheral neuropathy is reversible if the drug is discontinued.

### Contraindications and Precautions

Avoid use in pregnant or neonatal animals. Avoid long-term use in cats. Because exposure to humans can potentially produce severe consequences, veterinarians should caution pet owners about handling the medications and to ensure that accidental exposure to humans does not occur at home (e.g., to young children).

### Drug Interactions

Chloramphenicol is notorious for producing drug-drug interactions. Chloramphenicol is a CYP450 and CYP2B11 inhibitor and possibly other CYP enzymes in dogs. As such, chloramphenicol decreases the clearance of other drugs that are metabolized by the same metabolic enzymes. Chloramphenicol inhibits the metabolism of opiates, barbiturates, propofol, phenytoin, salicylate, and perhaps other drugs. Therefore, caution should be exercised when administering other drugs metabolized by CYP450 enzymes, particularly anesthetics, concurrently with chloramphenicol.

## Instructions for Use

Chloramphenicol use is based primarily on clinical experience and small observational studies. There were no well-controlled studies that have shown efficacy in animals. Although rarely available commercially, chloramphenicol palmitate requires active enzymes and should not be administered to fasted (or anorectic) animals.

## Patient Monitoring and Laboratory Tests

Susceptibility testing: CLSI breakpoints for susceptible organisms are ≤4 mcg/mL for streptococci and ≤8 mcg/mL for other organisms using the human breakpoint. Caution is advised when using the human breakpoint for interpretation because it may not apply to veterinary use. In horses, bacteria should not be considered susceptible unless the MIC is below 2 mcg/mL, which only includes *Streptococcus equi* and *Actinobacillus equuli*.

## Formulations

- Chloramphenicol palmitate is available in a 30-mg/mL oral suspension. Chloramphenicol is available in 250-mg capsules and 100-, 250-, and 500-mg tablets. Chloramphenicol sodium succinate injection has a concentration of 100 mg/mL (1-g but is no longer available commercially in the United States.

## Stability and Storage

Store in a tightly sealed container, protected from light, and at room temperature. Chloramphenicol tablets or powder dissolved in a water solution are stable for 24 hours. Chloramphenicol palmitate is insoluble in water. Chloramphenicol is stable at a pH of 2–7. Chloramphenicol sodium succinate, if available, is stable for 30 days at room temperature and 6 months if frozen.

## Small Animal Dosage

**Chloramphenicol and Chloramphenicol Palmitate**

Dogs
- 40–50 mg/kg q8h PO.

Cats
- 12.5–20 mg/kg q12h PO (or 50 mg/cat).

**Chloramphenicol Sodium Succinate**

(Rarely available commercially.)

Dogs
- 40–50 mg/kg q6–8h IV or IM.

Cats
- 12.5–20 mg/cat q12h IV or IM.

## Large Animal Dosage

**Horses**
- 35–50 mg/kg q6–8h PO.

## Regulatory Information

It is illegal to administer chloramphenicol to animals that produce food; therefore, no withdrawal times are established.

# Chlorothiazide

klor-oh-thye'ah-zide

**Trade and other names:** Diuril

**Functional classification:** Diuretic

## Pharmacology and Mechanism of Action

Thiazide diuretic. The thiazide diuretics are used infrequently in veterinary medicine. They include hydrochlorothiazide and chlorothiazide. These drugs are sulfonamide analogues and share similar chemical properties, but the pharmacokinetics have not been very well described in animals. The action of thiazides is to inhibit the Na/Cl cotransporter in the luminal side of the distal tubule of the kidney. By inhibiting the cotransporter, $Na^+$ and $Cl^-$ reabsorption is blocked, leading to sodium and water diuresis. Because the action occurs in the distal tubule, these drugs have less of a diuretic effect (less efficacy) than the loop diuretics.

## Indications and Clinical Uses

Chlorothiazide use is not common in animals. There is an approved formulation for dogs (Diuril), but it is not often prescribed. In people, it is used primarily to treat hypertension. In animals, it has been used to treat hypercalciuria (increased calcium in the urine that may lead to urinary calculi). In dairy cattle, it is approved as an oral bolus or injection to treat postparturient udder edema.

Because chlorothiazide decreases renal excretion of calcium, it also has been used to prevent uroliths containing calcium. Dosage regimens used are derived either empirically or from extrapolation of the human dose.

### Precautionary Information

**Adverse Reactions and Side Effects**

Chlorothiazide may cause electrolyte imbalance such as hypokalemia.

**Contraindications and Precautions**

These drugs enhance calcium absorption by decreasing intracellular sodium and enhance the $Na^+/Ca^{2+}$ exchange to decrease calcium excretion in urine. They should never be used in patients with hypercalcemia or at risk of hypercalcemia.

**Drug Interactions**

Avoid administering calcium and vitamin D supplements.

## Instructions for Use

Thiazide diuretics are used rarely in animals. Because they are not as effective as high-ceiling diuretics for producing diuresis, agents such as furosemide are used more often.

## Patient Monitoring and Laboratory Tests

Electrolytes should be monitored during chronic therapy.

## Formulations

- Chlorothiazide is available in 250- and 500-mg tablets, 50-mg/mL oral suspension, and injection vials of 500 mg (with mannitol). Cattle formulation: available as 2-g oral bolus or 25 mg/mL as a hydrochlorothiazide injection.

## Stability and Storage

Store in a tightly sealed container, protected from light, and at room temperature. Reconstituted solutions are stable for 24 hours.

## Small Animal Dosage

**Dogs and Cats**

- 20–40 mg/kg q12h PO.

## Large Animal Dosage

**Cattle**

- For treatment of udder edema, 125–250 mg IV or IM injection once or twice per day or a 2-g oral bolus once or twice per day.

## Regulatory Information

Withdrawal times: for milk: 72 hours (6 milkings); withdrawal time for meat is not established. For extralabel use withdrawal interval estimates, contact FARAD at www.FARAD.org.

RCI Classification: 4

# Chlorpheniramine Maleate
klor-fen-eer′ah-meen mal′ee-ate

**Trade and other names:** Chlor-Trimeton and Phenetron

**Functional classification:** Antihistamine

## Pharmacology and Mechanism of Action

Antihistamine ($H_1$-blocker). Similar to other antihistamines, it acts by blocking the $H_1$ receptor and suppresses inflammatory reactions caused by histamine. The $H_1$-blockers have been used to control pruritus and skin inflammation in dogs and cats, but efficacy for these indications has not been established. Other commonly used antihistamines include clemastine, chlorpheniramine, diphenhydramine, cetirizine, and hydroxyzine.

## Indications and Clinical Uses

Chlorpheniramine is used to prevent allergic reactions and for pruritus therapy in dogs and cats. However, success rates for treatment of pruritus have not been high. In addition to the antihistamine effect for treating allergies, these drugs block the effect of histamine in the vomiting center, vestibular center, and other centers that control vomiting in animals. Use in animals has been primarily derived from empirical use. There is a lack of well-controlled clinical studies or efficacy trials to document clinical effectiveness. Other antiemetic agents are more effective and more commonly used in small animals.

## Precautionary Information

### Adverse Reactions and Side Effects

Antihistamines have a high margin of safety. Sedation is the most common side effect, which is the result of inhibition of histamine N-methyltransferase. Sedation may also be attributed to blocking of other CNS receptors such as those for serotonin, acetylcholine, and alpha-receptors. Antimuscarinic effects (atropine-like effects) also are common, such as dry mouth and decreased GI secretions.

### Contraindications and Precautions

Antimuscarinic effects (atropine-like effects) are common. Do not use in conditions for which anticholinergic drugs may be contraindicated, such as glaucoma, ileus, or cardiac arrhythmias.

### Drug Interactions

No drug interactions are reported in animals.

## Instructions for Use

Chlorpheniramine is included as an ingredient in many OTC cough, cold, and allergy medications.

## Patient Monitoring and Laboratory Tests

No specific monitoring is necessary.

## Formulations

- Chlorpheniramine maleate is available in 4- and 8-mg tablets, 2-mg chewable tablets, and 2-mg/5-mL syrup.

## Stability and Storage

Store in a tightly sealed container, protected from light, and at room temperature. Protect from freezing. Stability of compounded formulations has not been evaluated.

## Small Animal Dosage

### Dogs

- 4–8 mg/dog q12h PO up to a maximum dosage of 0.5 mg/kg q12h.

### Cats

- 2 mg/cat q12h PO.

## Large Animal Dosage

- No dose has been reported for large animals.

## Regulatory Information

Withdrawal times are not established for animals that produce food. For extralabel use withdrawal interval estimates, contact FARAD at www.FARAD.org.

RCI Classification: 4

# Chlorpromazine

klor-proe'mah-zeen

**Trade and other names:** Thorazine and Largactil

**Functional classification:** Antiemetic, phenothiazine

## Pharmacology and Mechanism of Action

Phenothiazine tranquilizer and antiemetic. Chlorpromazine is a centrally acting dopamine antagonist. It inhibits action of dopamine as a neurotransmitter, which may produce some central-acting effects similar to acepromazine and some antiemetic action.

## Indications and Clinical Uses

Use in animals has been primarily derived from empirical use. There are no well-controlled clinical studies or efficacy trials to document clinical effectiveness. Chlorpromazine is most often used as a centrally acting antiemetic for disorders that produce vomiting via a central-acting mechanism. These conditions include administration of emetic cancer chemotherapeutic agents and GI diseases. It is also used for sedation and preanesthetic purposes, although acepromazine has been more commonly used.

## Precautionary Information
### Adverse Reactions and Side Effects
The most common adverse effect is sedation. Like acepromazine, it also may cause alpha-adrenergic blockade and vasodilation, but this effect has not been as well documented as for acepromazine. It may produce anticholinergic effects in some animals. Although phenothiazines are reported to decrease the threshold for producing seizures in some animals, this has not been shown in retrospective studies with acepromazine in animals and has not been reported specifically for chlorpromazine. Like other phenothiazines, it may produce extrapyramidal side effects (involuntary muscle movement) in some individuals. In horses, it has produced undesirable side effects, including violent reactions.

### Contraindications and Precautions
Although a specific risk has not been shown, use with caution in animals with seizure disorders and animals prone to hypotension. Avoid use in horses.

### Drug Interactions
It will potentiate effects from other sedatives.

## Instructions for Use
Chlorpromazine is used for vomiting caused by toxins, drugs, or GI disease. Higher doses than listed in the dose section have been used with cancer chemotherapy (2 mg/kg q3h SQ).

## Patient Monitoring and Laboratory Tests
No specific monitoring is necessary.

## Formulations
- Chlorpromazine is available in a 25-mg/mL injection solution, and 10-, 25-, 50-, 100-, and 200-mg tablets.

## Stability and Storage
Store in a tightly sealed container, protected from light, and at room temperature. Slight discoloration does not affect stability. Some sorption (loss) occurs if stored in polyvinyl chloride (soft plastic) containers.

## Small Animal
### Dogs
- 0.5 mg/kg q6–8h IM or SQ.

### Cats
- 0.2–0.4 mg/kg q6–8h, up to 0.5 mg/kg q8h IM or SQ.

## Large Animal Dosage
### Horses
- Avoid use.

### Cattle
- 0.22 mg/kg IV or 1.1 mg/kg IM, single dose.

### Sheep and Goats
- 0.55 mg/kg IV or 2.2 mg/kg IM, single dose.

### Pigs
- 0.5 mg/kg IM, single dose.

## Regulatory Information
Withdrawal times are not established for animals that produce food. For extralabel use withdrawal interval estimates, contact FARAD at www.FARAD.org.
RCI Classification: 2

# Chlortetracycline
klor-tet' rah-sye-kleen

**Trade and other names:** Aureomycin soluble powder, Aureomycin tablets, Aureomycin soluble calf tablets, Anaplasmosis block, Calf Scour Bolus, Fermycin, and generic brands

**Functional classification:** Antibacterial

## Pharmacology and Mechanism of Action
Tetracycline antibacterial drug. Inhibits bacterial protein synthesis by interfering with peptide elongation by ribosomes by interfering with the 30S ribosome unit. Chlortetracycline is a bacteriostatic agent with a broad spectrum of activity, which includes gram-positive bacteria and *Mycoplasma* spp. One of the organisms treated with chlortetracycline in cattle is *Anaplasma phagocytophilum*, which is a gram-negative bacteria of neutrophils and causes disease in cattle. Most other gram-negative bacilli, particularly enteric Enterobacteriaceae bacteria (e.g., *E. coli*), are clinically resistant. Chlortetracycline is the least well absorbed of all oral tetracyclines in ruminants, and oral administration produces plasma concentrations below the MIC of most common bacteria. Therefore it may be inadequate to treat infections caused by organisms susceptible to other tetracyclines.

### Indications and Clinical Uses
It has been used for routine infections and intracellular pathogens, mostly in livestock. Most of the use is in feed and water and often used as a preventive agent for anaplasmosis. Treatment of serious infections is limited because chlortetracycline is poorly absorbed orally, and other tetracyclines are preferred for systemic treatment of infections. A common use for chlortetracycline is as a feed additive to control respiratory and enteric infections in livestock. The clinical use in small animals and horses is rare.

## Precautionary Information
### Adverse Reactions and Side Effects
Chlortetracycline may bind to bone and developing teeth in young animals. High doses have caused renal injury. Oral administration to horses may produce diarrhea.

### Contraindications and Precautions
Avoid use in young animals, except where permitted by label for young pigs or cattle. Adding chlortetracycline to feed and water of livestock will require a veterinary order using the Veterinary Feed Directive.

### Drug Interactions
Chlortetracycline, like other tetracyclines, binds to other orally administered cations, which prevent its absorption. Oral absorption is decreased if it is administered with products with calcium, zinc, aluminum, magnesium, or iron.

## Instructions for Use

Chlortetracycline is not administered for systemic use in small animals. Doxycycline has replaced most other tetracyclines for treatment in small animals. Most chlortetracycline used is in powdered form and added to feed or drinking water of livestock.

## Patient Monitoring and Laboratory Tests

Susceptibility testing: CLSI tetracycline breakpoints for susceptible organisms are ≤2 mcg/mL for streptococci and ≤4 for other organisms. Tetracycline is used as a marker to test susceptibility for other drugs in this class such as doxycycline, minocycline, and oxytetracycline, but these breakpoints should not apply to chlortetracycline because of its low oral absorption.

## Formulations

- Chlortetracycline is available as a powdered feed additive in 25 or 64 g/lb. It is also available as an anaplasmosis block in 2.5 g/lb and in 25- and 500-mg tablets. (A range of concentrations exists for premix.)

## Stability and Storage

Store in a tightly sealed container, protected from light, and at room temperature. Do not mix with ions that may chelate tetracyclines (calcium, magnesium, iron, aluminum, etc.).

## Small Animal Dosage

### Dogs and Cats

- Rarely used, but doses of 25 mg/kg q6–8h PO have been administered even though there is no evidence of efficacy.

## Large Animal Dosage

### Cattle

- Prophylaxis for anaplasmosis: 0.36–0.7 mg/kg/day (approximately one block per 10 animals).
- Tablets: 11 mg/kg q12h for 3–5 days PO.
- Powdered feed additive: 22 mg/kg/day added to water. Actual dose is affected by feed and water consumption for each animal.

### Pigs

- Powdered feed additive: 22 mg/kg/day added to water. Actual dose is affected by feed and water consumption for each animal.

## Regulatory Information

Cattle withdrawal time for meat: Withdrawal times vary from product to product from 1, 2, 5, or 10 days. Most products list a withdrawal time of 1 day for cattle.

Pig withdrawal time for meat: 1–5 days.

Note that for chlortetracycline, withdrawal times may vary considerably from one product to another. One should consult specific product packaging to determine exact withdrawal time.

# Chondroitin Sulfate
kon-droy′ten sul′fate

**Trade and other names:** Cosequin and Glyco-Flex

**Functional classification:** Nutritional supplement

## Pharmacology and Mechanism of Action

Nutritional supplement for patients with osteoarthritis. According to the manufacturer and supported by some experimental evidence, chondroitin sulfate provides precursors to stimulate synthesis of articular cartilage, inhibits degradation, and improves healing of articular cartilage.

Pharmacokinetic studies have produced conflicting results depending on formulation, species studied, and assay technique. Although some studies have demonstrated adequate oral absorption, there may be limited oral absorption of the intact large molecule. In dogs, oral absorption has been as low as 5%, but in horses, absorption of 22% or 32% has been reported.

It is usually administered in combination with glucosamine. See Glucosamine for further details.

## Indications and Clinical Uses

Chondroitin sulfate is used primarily as a dietary supplement to reduce clinical signs associated with degenerative joint disease. It is usually found in formulations in combination with glucosamine. (See Glucosamine for additional details.) Convincing evidence of clinical efficacy through well-controlled clinical trials is limited. Analyses of published clinical studies in dogs have concluded that there is a moderate level of evidence to indicate some benefit in osteoarthritis, but results may be inconsistent among studies. Benefits of treatment in horses with lameness also have been reported from oral administration of chondroitin–glucosamine supplements.

## Precautionary Information

### Adverse Reactions and Side Effects

Adverse effects have not been reported, although hypersensitivity is possible. Chondroitin is most often administered with glucosamine. See Glucosamine for potential adverse effects.

### Contraindications and Precautions

No contraindications have been reported.

### Drug Interactions

No drug interactions are reported in animals.

## Instructions for Use

Doses are based primarily on empiricism and manufacturer's recommendations. There are limited published trials of efficacy or dose titrations available to determine optimal dose. Doses listed are general recommendations, and products available may vary.

## Patient Monitoring and Laboratory Tests

No specific monitoring is necessary.

## Formulations

- Because several chondroitin sulfate formulations are available, veterinarians are encouraged to carefully examine the product label to ensure proper strength. These products are not FDA approved. Veterinary dietary supplements can be highly variable in quality. One product (Cosequin) is available in regular-strength (RS) and double-strength (DS) capsules. The RS capsules contain 250 mg glucosamine, 200 mg chondroitin sulfate and mixed glycosaminoglycans, 5 mg manganese, and 33 mg manganese ascorbate. The DS tablets contain double of each of these amounts.

## Stability and Storage

Store in a tightly sealed container, protected from light, and at room temperature. Stability of compounded formulations has not been evaluated.

## Small Animal Dosage

Use the product Cosequin RS and DS Strength as a general guide.

**C**

### Dogs

- 1–2 RS capsules per day.
- 2–4 DS capsules for large dogs.

### Cats

- 1 RS capsule daily.

## Large Animal Dosage

- Horses: 12 mg/kg glucosamine, 3.8 mg/kg chondroitin sulfate twice daily PO for 4 weeks, and then 4 mg/kg glucosamine; 1.3 mg/kg chondroitin sulfate thereafter.
- It is common to initiate treatment in horses with a higher dose of 22 mg/kg glucosamine and 8.8 mg/kg chondroitin sulfate daily PO.

## Regulatory Information

Withdrawal times are not established for animals that produce food. Chondroitin sulfate and glucosamine are found naturally, and withdrawal times may not be necessary if these supplements are administered to food animals. For extralabel use withdrawal interval estimates, contact FARAD at www.FARAD.org.

# Cimetidine Hydrochloride

sye-met′ih-deen hye-droe-klor′ide

**Trade and other names:** Tagamet (OTC and prescription)

**Functional classification:** Antiulcer agent

## Pharmacology and Mechanism of Action

Histamine$_2$ antagonist (H$_2$-blocker). Stimulation of acid secretion in the stomach requires activation of histamine type 2 receptors, gastrin receptors, and muscarinic receptors. Cimetidine and related H$_2$-blockers inhibit the action of histamine on the histamine H$_2$-receptor of parietal cells and inhibit parietal cell gastric acid secretion. Cimetidine is the oldest of the H$_2$-receptor blockers available. Cimetidine is rarely, if ever, used clinically anymore. Other agents of this class with more favorable pharmacokinetics and greater potency are used instead (famotidine, ranitidine). Cimetidine can potentially increase stomach pH to help heal and prevent gastric and duodenal ulcers, but evidence that it is effective in dogs, cats, or horses is not available. In animals, the half-life is short, necessitating frequent administration.

## Indications and Clinical Uses

Cimetidine has been used to treat gastric ulcers and gastritis, but the use has declined considerably because of availability of more effective agents, such as proton-pump inhibitors (PPIs). Although it has been administered to animals for treatment of vomiting, this is not an accepted indication. There also are no efficacy data to support its use for preventing NSAID-induced bleeding and ulcers. In dogs and cats, other H$_2$-blockers are preferred, such as famotidine and ranitidine. The PPIs (omeprazole) are preferred for ulcer treatment in horses. For example, studies in horses showed that at 18 g/kg q8h PO, it did not cause healing of ulcers. The poor efficacy may be because of short duration of effect (2–6 hours).

## Precautionary Information

**Adverse Reactions and Side Effects**

Adverse effects have not been reported for animals because it is infrequently used. If they occur, it is more likely if there is decreased renal clearance. In people, CNS signs may occur with high doses.

**Contraindications and Precautions**

Use cautiously with drugs that rely on hepatic metabolism for clearance.

**Drug Interactions**

Cimetidine is a well-known CYP450 enzyme inhibitor. It may increase concentrations of other drugs used concurrently because of inhibition of hepatic enzymes. Cimetidine may increase the pH of the stomach, which can inhibit oral absorption of some drugs (e.g., itraconazole and ketoconazole). Cimetidine inhibits the oral absorption of iron supplements.

## Instructions for Use

Efficacy for treating ulcers in animals has not been established. Frequent dosing may be necessary for suppression of stomach acid. Doses are derived from gastric secretory studies in experimental animals but not tested in clinical patients.

## Patient Monitoring and Laboratory Tests

No specific monitoring is necessary.

## Formulations

• Cimetidine is available in 100-, 150-, 200-, 300-, 400-, and 800-mg tablets; a 60-mg/mL oral solution; and a 150-mg/mL injection.

## Stability and Storage

Store in a tightly sealed container, protected from light, and at room temperature. Do not store injection formulation in refrigerator. Solutions are stable for at least 14 days. Stable if mixed with various enteral products.

## Small Animal Dosage

**Dogs and Cats**

• 10 mg/kg q6–8h IV, IM, or PO.

## Large Animal Dosage

**Horses**

• 3 mg/kg diluted in fluid solution and infused IV over 2 minutes q8h.
• 40–60 mg/kg/day PO. However, oral doses in horses produce inconsistent results.

**Calves**

• Abomasal ulcers in milk-fed calves: 100 mg/kg q8h PO.

## Regulatory Information

Withdrawal times are not established for animals that produce food. For extralabel use withdrawal interval estimates, contact FARAD at www.FARAD.org.

RCI Classification: 5

# Ciprofloxacin Hydrochloride
sip-roe-floks'ah-sin hye-droe-klor'ide

**Trade and other names:** Cipro and generic brands

**Functional classification:** Antibacterial

## Pharmacology and Mechanism of Action
Fluoroquinolone antibacterial. Ciprofloxacin acts to inhibit DNA gyrase and cell DNA and RNA synthesis. Bactericidal. Broad antimicrobial activity. Ciprofloxacin is active against gram-negative bacilli, including Enterobacteriaceae and some gram-positive cocci, including *Staphylococcus*. Ciprofloxacin is more active against *P. aeruginosa,* than other fluoroquinolones, but resistance is possible. Multi-drug resistant bacteria, including gram-negative bacilli of the Enterobacteriaceae, and methicillin-resistant strains of *Staphylococcus* spp., are likely to be resistant to ciprofloxacin and other fluoroquinolones.

*Pharmacokinetics:* Oral absorption of ciprofloxacin in dogs has been variable. Oral absorption may approach 74%–97% but has been as low as 42%. In research dogs, the oral absorption was 58% but with high variability. In research dogs at a dose of approximately 25 mg/kg PO, the peak plasma concentration was 4.4 mcg/mL, terminal half-life was 2.6 hours, and area under the curve (AUC) was 22.5 mcg·h/mL. In a population pharmacokinetic study (patient population), the half-life was 4.3 hours, the peak concentration was 1.2 mcg/mL, and the AUC was 13.8 mcg h/mL at an oral dose of 23 mg/kg. Oral absorption in horses is less than 10% and should not be used orally in horses. In cats, oral absorption is low (22%–33%) and is not effective for gram-positive bacteria even at 10 mg/kg, but at 10 mg/kg q12h, it was able to reach therapeutic targets against susceptible gram-negative bacteria. Other fluoroquinolones approved for animals, such as marbofloxacin and enrofloxacin, have better oral bioavailability.

## Indications and Clinical Uses
Ciprofloxacin, although a human drug, has been used in small animals for treatment of a wide variety of infections, including skin infections, pneumonia, and soft tissue infections. Ciprofloxacin is not approved for animals. However, it can be prescribed by veterinarians as long as it is not administered to animals that produce food or are intended for food. The administration of ciprofloxacin to animals is considered extralabel and subject to other extralabel restrictions. The variable and potentially low ciprofloxacin oral availability for dogs and cats suggests that doses should be higher than the doses currently used for drugs such as enrofloxacin, marbofloxacin, or orbifloxacin. If administered at an oral dose of 25 mg/kg once daily to dogs, the breakpoint for human susceptibility testing will not apply, and bacteria should be considered susceptible only if the MIC is less than 0.06 mcg/mL. Because of the inconsistent oral absorption in dogs, if a human generic fluoroquinolone is used in dogs, levofloxacin is preferred. (See Levofloxacin for more details.)

## Precautionary Information
### Adverse Reactions and Side Effects

High concentrations of fluoroquinolones may cause CNS toxicity, especially in animals with renal failure. Ciprofloxacin causes occasional vomiting. Intravenous solution should be given slowly (over 30 minutes). At high doses, it may cause some nausea, vomiting, and diarrhea. Blindness in cats has not been reported for ciprofloxacin. All of the fluoroquinolones may cause arthropathy in young animals. Dogs are most susceptible to quinolone-induced arthropathy in the age group of 4–28 weeks of age. Large, rapidly growing dogs are the most susceptible.

Intravenous infusions have elicited an anaphylactoid reaction in some dogs. Dogs sensitive to these reactions have shown evidence of hypotension and cardiac abnormalities, including arrhythmia. Observe dogs for signs of reactions during IV infusions.

Administration to horses has caused colic, enteritis, and diarrhea.

### Contraindications and Precautions

Avoid use in young animals because of risk of cartilage injury. Use cautiously in animals that may be prone to seizures, such as epileptics. It is not recommended to administer ciprofloxacin to horses.

### Drug Interactions

Fluoroquinolones may increase concentrations of theophylline and possibly other drugs if used concurrently. Coadministration with divalent and trivalent cations, such as products containing aluminum (e.g., sucralfate), iron, and calcium, may decrease absorption. Do not mix in solutions or in vials with aluminum, calcium, iron, or zinc because chelation may occur.

## Instructions for Use

Doses are based on plasma concentrations needed to achieve sufficient plasma concentration above the MIC. Efficacy studies have not been performed in dogs or cats, and clinical use is based primarily on anecdotal experience and pharmacokinetic and pharmacodynamic analysis. Injectable ciprofloxacin is available in a human preparation, usually 10 mg/mL (in sterile water) or 2 mg/mL (premixed with 5% dextrose). Dilute the concentrated form to 1–2 mg/mL prior to IV use with an IV solution and infuse slowly. Do not infuse concurrently with other medications (e.g., in a piggyback) because inactivation may occur.

## Patient Monitoring and Laboratory Tests

Susceptibility testing: CLSI breakpoint for susceptible organisms has not been determined for animals, but for humans, the breakpoints are ≤0.25 mcg/mL for gram-negative Enterobacteriaceae bacteria and ≤0.5 mcg/mL for *P. aeruginosa*. The human breakpoint for susceptibility should not be applied to dogs and cats. In dogs, at a dosage of 25 mg/kg per day PO, the cutoff for susceptible bacteria is ≤0.06 mcg/mL. Most susceptible gram-negative Enterobacteriaceae bacteria have MIC values less than 0.12 mcg/mL, but the MIC for *P. aeruginosa*, is typically higher (less than 0.5 mcg/mL). *Staphylococcus* spp. typically have MIC values less than 1 mcg/mL.

## Formulations Available
Ciprofloxacin is available in 100-, 250-, 500-, and 750-mg tablets; 500- and 1000-mg extended-release tablets; 50- and 100-mg/mL oral suspension; 10-mg/mL injection; and 2-mg/mL infusion (in dextrose).

## Stability and Storage
Store in a tightly sealed container, protected from light, and at room temperature. Aqueous solutions of 0.5–2 mg/mL retain potency up to 14 days when stored. Do not mix with products that contain ions (e.g., iron, aluminum, magnesium, and calcium).

## Small Animal Dosage
**Dogs**
- 25 mg/kg q24h PO.
- 15 mg/kg q24h IV.

**Cats**
- 20 mg/kg q24h, PO.
- 10 mg/kg q24h IV.

## Large Animal Dosage
- No dosing data are available. Ciprofloxacin has poor oral absorption in horses (less than 10%) and is not recommended.

## Regulatory Information
There are no withdrawal times established because this drug should not be administered to animals that produce food. The extralabel administration of fluoroquinolones to food-producing animals in the United States is a violation of FDA regulations. Withdrawal times are not established for animals that produce food.

# Cisapride
siss′ah-pride

**Trade and other names:** Propulsid (Prepulsid in Canada), not currently available commercially

**Functional classification:** Prokinetic agent

## Pharmacology and Mechanism of Action
Prokinetic agent. Its mechanism is believed to be as an agonist for the 5-hydroxytryptamine (5-HT$_4$) receptor on myenteric neurons (5-HT$_4$ ordinarily stimulates cholinergic transmission in the myenteric neurons). It also acts as an antagonist for the 5-HT$_3$ receptor. Through these mechanisims, or independently, cisapride may enhance release of acetylcholine at the myenteric plexus. Cisapride increases the motility of the stomach, small intestine, and colon. It accelerates the transit of contents in the bowel and intestines. There are some antiemetic effects through antagonism if 5-HT$_3$, but this is not a major use.

## Indications and Clinical Uses
Cisapride is used to stimulate motility for treating gastric reflux, gastroparesis, ileus, and constipation. The most common uses in animals have been to prevent stomach regurgitation, reduce gastroesophageal reflux, decrease postoperative ileus, and treat constipation and megacolon in cats. In dogs, it was shown to be more effective than other treatments for preventing gastroesophageal reflux in anesthetized dogs. It is not

effective to stimulate motility in dogs with megaesophagus. Cisapride has improved recovery of horses with postoperative ileus. Cisapride was removed from the human market and is no longer commercially available. Compounding pharmacies have made cisapride available to veterinarians in compounded forms (see the Formulations section). However, these formulations are not licensed and are unregulated.

## Precautionary Information

### Adverse Reactions and Side Effects
Adverse cardiac effects have been reported in people and are the cause for discontinuation in human medicine. These cardiac effects have not been reported in animals. High overdoses in dogs (18 mg/kg) have produced abdominal pain, aggression, ataxia, fever, and vomiting. With higher overdoses, diarrhea, ataxia, and CNS reactions have been observed.

### Contraindications and Precautions
Contraindicated in patients with GI obstruction. Avoid use in dogs with megaesophagus because it will increase pressure of the lower esophageal sphincter.

### Drug Interactions
Anticholinergic drugs, such as atropine, diminish the action. Cisapride should not be used with drugs that inhibit metabolism (CYP450 inhibitors) or drugs that inhibit P-glycoprotein. Toxicity may result (see list of drugs in Appendixes J and I).

## Instructions for Use
Not currently available commercially. Cisapride was discontinued by the manufacturer in July 2000. However, some veterinary pharmacies can fill some orders or prepare compounded formulations for animals. Consult local compounding pharmacist about availability. Doses are based on extrapolation from human doses, experimental studies, and anecdotal evidence. Efficacy studies have not been performed in dogs or cats.

## Patient Monitoring and Laboratory Tests
In humans, cardiac effects have been reported (arrhythmias). Monitor ECG in susceptible patients.

## Formulations
- Cisapride was once available in a 10-mg tablet but has been discontinued by the manufacturer. Formulations used are prepared by compounding from a pure source. To prepare 1 mg/mL injectable solution (follow United States Pharmacopeia [USP] <797> sterile compounding standards), mix 0.104 g of cisapride monohydrate with 20 mL tartaric acid 6% solution. Add sterile water to make up a 100-mL total volume. Keep the solution in the refrigerator, in a sterile vial, protected from light, and labeled with Beyond Use Date of 14 days post-compounding. A 10-mg/mL oral suspension (follow USP <795> compounding standards) has been prepared by mixing 300 mg (0.3 g) of cisapride monohydrate with 15 mL of Ora Plus and enough Ora Sweet added to make a total of volume of 30 mL. (Oral Plus and Ora Sweet are oral formulation suspending agents and vehicles commonly used in commercial pharmacies.)

## Stability and Storage
Store in a tightly sealed container, protected from light, and at room temperature. Injectable solution should be used within 14 days. An oral suspension of 10 mg/mL in aqueous vehicle was stable for 30 days in a refrigerator.

## Small Animal Dosage

**Dogs**

- 0.1–0.5 mg/kg q8–12h PO (up to 0.5–1.0 mg/kg). 1 mg/kg IV if used to prevent gastroesophageal reflux during anesthesia.

**Cats**

- 2.5–5 mg/cat q8–12h PO (up to 1 mg/kg q8h).

## Large Animal Dosage

**Horses**

- 0.1 mg/kg IV. Note: This formulation is not commercially available, but an IV form has been compounded (see the Formulation section earlier).

## Regulatory Information

Withdrawal times are not established for animals that produce food. This drug should not be used in animals intended for food because it poses a risk to humans.

# Cisplatin
sis-plah′tin

**Trade and other names:** Platinol

**Functional classification:** Anticancer agent

## Pharmacology and Mechanism of Action

Anticancer agent. Cisplatin acts like a bifunctional alkylator of DNA but forms a reactive carbonium ion, and the cross-linking occurs around the platinum ion instead of an alkyl group. It preferentially binds to the N-7 of guanine and adenine bases. As a result of this reaction, interstrand and intrastrand cross-linking of DNA occurs. The result is inhibition of DNA synthesis. A related drug is carboplatin, which is a second-generation platinum compound used in patients who may not tolerate cisplatin.

## Indications and Clinical Uses

Cisplatin is used for treating various solid tumors, including bronchiogenic carcinoma, osteosarcoma, transitional cell carcinoma, and mast cell tumors. It has been shown to be effective for increasing the survival of dogs that have undergone amputations for osteosarcoma.

### Precautionary Information

**Adverse Reactions and Side Effects**

Nephrotoxicity is the most limiting factor to cisplatin therapy. Monitor laboratory indices for kidney injury during treatment. In cats, it causes a dose-related, species-specific, primary pulmonary toxicosis. Vomiting is common in dogs with administration. Cisplatin is one of the most emetic of the cancer agents. Transient thrombocytopenia may occur in dogs. Cisplatin has caused potassium wasting and depletion of magnesium.

**Contraindications and Precautions**

Do not use in cats.

**Drug Interactions**

Cisplatin may be used with other cancer chemotherapy agents in some protocols. Do not use with other nephrotoxic drugs.

## Instructions for Use

To avoid toxicity, fluid loading before administration using sodium chloride should be performed. Antiemetic agents are often administered before therapy to decrease vomiting. For transitional cell and squamous cell carcinomas, dosages used are 40–50 mg/m² every 21–28 days. For osteosarcoma, it has been used at a dosage of 70 mg/m² every 21 days for four treatments.

## Patient Monitoring and Laboratory Tests

Monitor renal function in treated animals. Monitor CBC in patients between treatments.

## Formulations

• Cisplatin is available in a 1-mg/mL injection.

## Stability and Storage

Store in a tightly sealed container, protected from light, and at room temperature.

## Small Animal Dosage

**Dogs**

• 60–70 mg/m² every 3–4 weeks IV. (Administer fluid for diuresis with therapy.)

**Cats**

• Do not use in cats.

## Large Animal Dosage

• No dose has been reported for large animals.

## Regulatory Information

Withdrawal times are not established for animals that produce food. This drug should not be used in animals intended for food because it is an anticancer agent.

# Clarithromycin

klah-rith'roe-mye'sin

**Trade and other names:** Biaxin and generic brands

**Functional classification:** Antibiotic

## Pharmacology and Mechanism of Action

Clarithromycin is a macrolide antibiotic with bacteriostatic activity. It is a substituted 14-carbon macrolide. Clarithromycin was introduced in 1990 as a substitute for erythromycin. Compared with erythromycin, it has higher absorption, a longer half-life, and increased intracellular uptake. The site of action is similar to other macrolide antibiotics, which is the 50-S ribosomal subunit in susceptible bacteria. Spectrum includes primarily gram-positive bacteria. Resistance is expected for most gram-negative bacteria, and Enterobacteriaceae bacteria have intrinsic resistance. Clarithromycin may have higher activity (lower MIC values) for many susceptible bacteria compared with erythromycin or azithromycin.

Clarithromycin, like other macrolides, may have anti-inflammatory properties that are independent of the microbiologic effects (e.g., inhibit neutrophil and eosinophil inflammatory reaction).

*Pharmacokinetics:* Clarithromycin metabolites may contribute to the activity, but these metabolites are not well characterized in animals. It is widely distributed to intracellular and tissue sites with concentrations in most tissues (including the respiratory tract) exceeding the plasma concentration. In foals, the half-life is 4.8–5.4 hours with a VD of 10.5 L/kg and clearance of 1.27 L/kg/h. The oral absorption in foals is 57% with a maximum concentration of 0.5–0.9 mcg/mL.

## Indications and Clinical Uses

The most common use in people is for treatment of *Helicobacter* gastritis and respiratory infections, where it has retained activity against most respiratory tract pathogens (e.g., *Streptococcus* spp., mycoplasma, chlamydia). In small animals, clarithromycin has been used for indications such as skin infections and respiratory infections, but the use in small animals is not common. In foals, clarithromycin has been used for treatment of infections caused by *Rhodococcus equi* (in combination with rifampin). It is more active than other macrolides against *R. equi* and produced better clinical success than azithromycin.

---

### Precautionary Information

**Adverse Reactions and Side Effects**

The most common adverse effects from clarithromycin and related drugs are diarrhea and nausea. Many animals may develop soft feces or mild diarrhea. In studies in healthy foals, diarrhea was uncommon from oral doses and was self-limiting. However, if diarrhea becomes severe, treatment should be discontinued.

**Contraindications and Precautions**

Administer with caution to adult horses, ruminants, rodents, and rabbits because diarrhea and enteritis may develop. Clarithromycin is contraindicated for use in pregnant women. Although problems have not been identified in animals, use with caution in pregnant animals.

**Drug Interactions**

Many macrolide antibiotics are CYP450 enzyme inhibitors and can decrease metabolism of other drugs. For example, in people, it increased digoxin concentrations, and it is possible that it can affect other drugs. Clarithromycin administered to animals may decrease the clearance of other co-administered drugs. For example, clarithromycin decreased clearance of cyclosporine and increased oral absorption of cyclosporine in cats.

Clarithromycin is often administered with rifampin for treatment of horses with *R. equi* infections. Because of induction of enzymes and transporters, co-administration with rifampin decreases plasma drug concentrations of clarithromycin by greater than 90%. (See Rifampin for more details.)

---

## Instructions for Use

Clarithromycin should be given twice daily to animals because of a short half-life and need for a long time above the MIC.

## Patient Monitoring and Laboratory Tests

In the absence of a specific value for clarithromycin, use susceptibility for erythromycin to guide use of clarithromycin. Although the CLSI-derived breakpoint for susceptible bacteria is 1 mcg/mL, cures have been observed when treating respiratory pathogens with MIC values as high as 8 mcg/mL, which is attributed to high respiratory concentrations achieved. MIC values for *R. equi* were 0.12 mcg/mL. Organisms resistant to erythromycin and azithromycin will most likely be resistant to clarithromycin.

## Formulations
- Clarithromycin is available in 250- and 500-mg tablets and 25- and 50-mg/mL oral suspension.

## Stability and Storage
Store in a tightly sealed container, protected from light, and at room temperature. 250-mg tablets have been dissolved in water (50 mL) and administered immediately to foals orally. However, the long-term stability of compounded formulations has not been evaluated.

## Small Animal Dosage
**Dogs and Cats**
- 7.5 mg/kg q12h PO.

## Large Animal Dosage
**Foals**
- 7.5 mg/kg q12h PO (often combined with rifampin at 10 mg/kg q12h).

**Pigs**
- 7.5 mg/kg PO q12h.

## Regulatory Information
No regulatory information is available. For extralabel use withdrawal interval estimates, contact FARAD at www.FARAD.org.

# Clemastine Fumarate
klem′ass-teen fyoo′mar-ate

**Trade and other names:** Tavist and generic brands

**Functional classification:** Antihistamine

## Pharmacology and Mechanism of Action
Antihistamine ($H_1$-blocker). Similar to other antihistamines, it acts by blocking the $H_1$-receptor and suppresses inflammatory reactions caused by histamine. The $H_1$-blockers have been used to control pruritus and skin inflammation in dogs and cats; however, success rates in dogs have not been high. Other commonly used antihistamines include cetirizine, chlorpheniramine, diphenhydramine, and hydroxyzine.

## Indications and Clinical Uses
Clemastine is used primarily for treatment of allergy, but efficacy in animals has not been well established. Some reports have suggested that clemastine is effective for pruritus in dogs, but other agents are preferred for standard treatment. The half-life in dogs is short (3.8 hours), and it has rapid clearance. After oral administration, the oral absorption is only 3% (20%–70% in humans). At a high dose of 0.5 mg/kg PO, it did not suppress intradermal skin reactions. This evidence suggests that oral administration may not be as effective in dogs as previously thought. Oral absorption studies in horses indicated that it is not absorbed when given orally (bioavailability was only 3%), and it would not likely be effective for oral treatment.

C

## Precautionary Information

### Adverse Reactions and Side Effects

Sedation is the most common side effect. Sedation is the result of inhibition of histamine N-methyltransferase. Sedation may also be attributed to blocking of other CNS receptors such as those for serotonin, acetylcholine, and alpha-receptors. Antimuscarinic effects (atropine-like effects) also are possible, such as dry mouth and decreased GI secretions.

### Contraindications and Precautions

No contraindications reported for animals.

### Drug Interactions

No drug interactions are reported in animals.

## Instructions for Use

Clemastine fumarate has been used for short-term treatment of pruritus in dogs, but efficacy is low. It may be more efficacious when combined with other anti-inflammatory drugs.

## Patient Monitoring and Laboratory Tests

No specific monitoring is necessary.

## Formulations

- Clemastine fumarate is available in 1.34-mg tablets (OTC), 2.64-mg tablets (prescription), and 0.1-mg/mL syrup. If the syrup is use, consider that Tavist syrup contains 5.5% alcohol.

## Stability and Storage

Store in a tightly sealed container, protected from light, and at room temperature. Stability of compounded formulations has not been evaluated.

## Small Animal Dosage

### Dogs

- 0.05–0.1 mg/kg q12h PO, up to 0.5–1.5 mg/kg q12h PO.
- Dogs weighing less than 10 kg: half of tablet. (Dose based on q12h treatment and 1.34-mg tablet.)
- Dogs weighing 10–25 kg: 1 tablet. (Dose based on q12h treatment and 1.34-mg tablets.)
- Dogs weighing more than 25 kg: 1.5 tablets. (Dose based on q12h treatment and 1.34-mg tablets.)

## Large Animal Dosage

### Horses

- 50 mcg/kg (0.05 mg/kg) q8h IV. It is not absorbed orally in horses.

## Regulatory Information

Do not administer to animals that produce food.
RCI Classification: 3

# Clenbuterol

klen-byoo′ter-ole

**Trade and other names:** Ventipulmin

**Functional classification:** Bronchodilator, beta agonist

## Pharmacology and Mechanism of Action

Clenbuterol is a beta$_2$-adrenergic agonist, with more selective activity on beta$_2$ receptors than beta$_1$ receptors (beta$_2$/beta$_1$ ratio = 4.0). It is used primarily as a bronchodilator because it stimulates beta$_2$ receptors to relax bronchial smooth muscle. It may inhibit release of inflammatory mediators, especially from mast cells, decrease mucus production by goblet cells, and increase rate of mucociliary transport in the airways. However, effects on mast cells may not be important for inflammatory airway diseases that are mediated primarily by neutrophils. Compared with terbutaline, it has lower efficacy because of lower intrinsic activity and is only a partial agonist. Clenbuterol differs from other beta-agonists because it resists O-sulfate ester conjugation, which leads to a longer half-life compared with other agents. It also has better oral absorption (83%) than other beta-agonists in horses. In horses, the plasma half-life is 13 hours, but in urine, it can be detected for 12 days.

In addition to the effects on respiratory smooth muscle, clenbuterol can produce repartitioning effects, which indicates that it will stimulate development of more muscle (anabolic effect) and less fat (lipolytic effect). The repartitioning effect is caused by leptin- and adiponectin-mediated repartitioning properties that produce an increase in muscle mass. In horses, it decreases the percent body fat and increases muscle mass. The increased muscle mass does not enhance athletic performance and may actually have a negative effect on athletic performance. Because of the effects on muscle, it has been abused in humans (e.g., bodybuilders) and used illegally for weight gain in food-producing animals.

## Indications and Clinical Uses

Clenbuterol is indicated for treatment of animals with reversible bronchoconstriction such as horses with equine asthma syndrome and recurrent airway obstruction (RAO), formerly called chronic obstructive pulmonary disease. The response for treating RAO can be variable. Some horses that do not respond to a low dose respond better at four times the starting dose with a better response rate. At high doses, tachyphylaxis may occur with repeated high doses. Evidence for treating airway disease has been demonstrated in horses, but there are no reports of use in other species. The effects on repartitioning (producing more muscle and less fat) should not be used in performance horses. It should not be used in animals intended for food.

## Precautionary Information

### Adverse Reactions and Side Effects

Clenbuterol may produce excessive beta-adrenergic stimulation at high doses (tachycardia and tremors). Arrhythmias occur at high doses. Chronic use may have adverse effects on cardiac function in healthy horses. There have been conflicting studies on the effects of clenbuterol on athletic performance of horses. In one study at approved doses, it did not have any adverse effects on equine cardiac or skeletal muscle. In other studies, it had negative effects on aerobic athletic performance, faster time to fatigue, decreased cardiac function, and decreased oxygen consumption. The negative effects may occur because after repeated doses it down-regulates the adrenergic beta$_2$ receptor and results in decrease in receptor expression in skeletal muscle and lungs.

### Contraindications and Precautions

Do not administer to animals intended for food. Veterinarians should be warned that clenbuterol is often abused in humans for the purpose of muscle building and weight loss. Subsequently, high doses in humans may cause cardiac toxicity, such as arrhythmias.

### Drug Interactions

Because clenbuterol is a beta-agonist, other adrenergic drugs potentiate the action. In addition, beta-blocking drugs decrease action. Use with caution with any other drug that may stimulate the heart.

## Instructions for Use

Oral administration for horses usually follows the approved label dose. Clenbuterol has not been used in small animals. It is prohibited for use in animals intended for food.

## Patient Monitoring and Laboratory Tests

Monitor heart rate in animals during treatment. Clenbuterol can be detected in urine for 12 days. Effective plasma concentrations are 500 pg/mL.

## Formulations

• Clenbuterol is available in 100- and 33-mL bottles of 72.5-mcg/mL syrup.

## Stability and Storage

Store in a tightly sealed container, protected from light, and at room temperature. Stability of compounded formulations has not been evaluated.

## Small Animal Dosage

### Dogs and Cats

• No dose has been reported for small animals.

## Large Animal Dosage

### Horses

• Equine asthma syndrome (recurrent airway obstruction): 0.8 mcg/kg (0.008 mg/kg) twice daily PO. If initial dose is not effective, increase dose to two, three, and four times the initial dose, up to 3.2 mcg/kg. Duration of effect is approximately 6–8 hours.

## Regulatory Information

There are no withdrawal times established because clenbuterol should not be administered to animals that produce food. In horses, clenbuterol can be detected in urine for 12 days. Although not an approved human drug, it is abused in humans for weight loss and muscle building.

RCI Classification: 3

# Clindamycin Hydrochloride

klin-dah-mye'sin hye-droe-klor'ide

**Trade and other names:** Antirobe, ClinDrops, ClindaTobe, Clintabs, Clinsol, and generic and Cleocin (human form)

**Functional classification:** Antibacterial

## Pharmacology and Mechanism of Action

Antibacterial drug of the lincosamide class (similar in action to macrolides). It shares structural, microbiologic activity, and other properties with lincomycin. It inhibits bacterial protein synthesis via inhibition of bacterial ribosome at the 50S ribosome subunit. Clindamycin is bacteriostatic with a spectrum of activity primarily against gram-positive bacteria and anaerobes. Clindamycin, like the macrolide antibiotics, can concentrate in leukocytes and many tissues. Action of clindamycin is primarily against gram-positive organisms such as *Staphylococcus* spp., *Streptococcus* spp., and gram-positive rods such as *Corynebacterium* spp. Clindamycin also is active against mycoplasma and anaerobic organisms, although not all *Bacteroides* spp. are susceptible. Activity against *Toxoplasma* spp. is controversial. Gram-negative Enterobacteriaceae bacteria and *P. aeruginosa,* are inherently resistant.

*Pharmacokinetics:* In dogs, the VD is 2.5 L/kg, the oral absorption is 73%, and the half-life is 4–4.5 hours after a dose of 5.5 mg/kg and 7–10 hours after a dose of 11 mg/kg.

## Indications and Clinical Uses

Clindamycin is primarily used for gram-positive or anaerobic bacterial infections involving the skin, respiratory tract, or oral cavity. Resistance with *Staphylococcus* spp. may occur with frequent use. It is effective for some oral infections and anaerobic infections. It also has been used for *Mycoplasma* infections. Efficacy of clindamycin for treating toxoplasmosis is controversial. Some studies have shown that clindamycin improved clinical signs, but it did not resolve the infection. Another study showed that clindamycin inhibited killing of *Toxoplasma* organisms by leukocytes. In people, it is a second-choice for treating *Toxoplasma* spp. that requires high doses.

## Precautionary Information

### Adverse Reactions and Side Effects

Oral clindamycin hydrochloride has been associated with esophageal lesions in cats. Oral liquid product may be unpalatable to cats, possibly because of the high alcohol content (8.6%). High doses have caused vomiting and diarrhea in cats. Clindamycin may alter the bacterial population in the intestine and cause diarrhea. In people, it is one of the most common drugs to cause antibiotic associated diarrhea (enteritis) and pseudomembranous colitis caused by *Clostridioides difficile*. Fortunately, this has not been a common problem when treating dogs and cats. However, in animals with fermenting intestinal tracts (horses, ruminants, rodents, rabbits), clindamycin administration can cause serious problems, such as enteritis and diarrhea. It should not be administered orally to these species.

### Contraindications and Precautions

Do not administer to rodents or rabbits because it may cause diarrhea. Do not administer orally to horses or ruminants because diarrhea, enteritis, and perhaps death can result. The oral liquid (Antirobe) contains 8.6% ethyl alcohol, which may be unpalatable to cats. Clindamycin hydrochloride has caused esophageal lesions in cats. When administering orally, be sure that all of the medication passes through the esophagus to the stomach.

### Drug Interactions

Clindamycin injection should not be mixed with other drugs in the same vial, syringe, or IV line.

## Instructions for Use

Most doses are based on manufacturer's drug approval data and efficacy trials. Although every-12-hour frequency is recommended most often for dogs, there are studies that demonstrate efficacy when administered at 11 mg/kg q24h for treatment of pyoderma. An injectable formulation is also available (Cleocin), which is clindamycin phosphate. This may be injected either IV or IM. If administering clindamycin IV, it should be diluted and administered by slow infusion (30–60 minutes). Dilution is usually 10:1 in 0.9% saline. It contains benzyl alcohol, and this vehicle has produced toxic reactions in young infants (and perhaps small animals).

## Patient Monitoring and Laboratory Tests

Susceptibility testing: CLSI breakpoints for susceptible organisms are ≤0.25 mcg/mL for streptococci and ≤0.5 mcg/mL for other organisms.

## Formulations

- Clindamycin is available in oral liquid (Aquadrops) 25 mg/mL; 25-, 75-, 150-, and 300-mg capsules; 25-, 75-, and 150-mg tablets; and 150-mg/mL injection (Cleocin).

## Stability and Storage
Store in a tightly sealed container, protected from light, and at room temperature. Protect from freezing. Reconstituted solutions are stable for 2 weeks. Stability of compounded formulations is at least 60 days.

## Small Animal Dosage

### Dogs
- Staphylococcal infections: 11 mg/kg q12h PO or 22 mg/kg q24h PO. (Label dosage for dogs is 5.5–33 mg/kg q12h PO.)
- Refractory infections: Doses up to 33 mg/kg q12h PO.
- Anaerobic infections and periodontal infections: 11–33 mg/kg q12h PO.
- 10 mg/kg q12h IV or IM. (For IV use, it should be diluted and administered by slow infusion.)

### Cats
- 5.5 mg/kg q12h or 11 mg/kg q24h PO. (Label dosage for cats is 11–33 mg/kg q24h PO.)
- Refractory infections: Doses up to 33 mg/kg q24h PO.
- Anaerobic infections and periodontal infections: 11–33 mg/kg q24h PO.
- Toxoplasmosis: 12.5 mg/kg, up to 25 mg/kg q12h for 4 weeks PO (see Indications and Clinical Uses).
- 10 mg/kg q12h IV or IM. (For IV use, it should be diluted and administered by slow infusion.)

## Large Animal Dosage
- Do not administer clindamycin orally to large animals.

## Regulatory Information
No regulatory information is available. For extralabel use withdrawal interval estimates, contact FARAD at www.FARAD.org.

# Clodronate
cloe-dronate

**Trade and other names:** OSPHOS

**Functional classification:** Antihypercalcemic

## Pharmacology and Mechanism of Action
Clodronate is one of the bisphosphonate drugs. Drugs in this class also include pamidronate, etidronate, tiludronate, ziludronate, and pyrophosphate. The clinical use of this class of drugs resides in their ability to inhibit bone resorption. These drugs decrease bone turnover by inhibiting osteoclast activity, inducing osteoclast apoptosis, retarding bone resorption, and decreasing the rate of osteoporosis. Inhibition of bone resorption is via inhibition of the mevalonate pathway. Bisphosphonates are classified as nitrogen-containing and nonnitrogenous based on the structure, with the nitrogen-containing drugs being more potent. Clodronate disodium is a non-nitrogen, chloro-containing bisphosphonate. After IM injection to horses at the label dose, the half-life was $1.65 \pm 0.52$ hours with a peak at 20 minutes.

## Indications and Clinical Uses
Clodronate is approved in the United States for treatment of bone pain associated with navicular syndrome in horses. Other bisphosphonate drugs are used in people

to treat osteoporosis and treatment of hypercalcemia of malignancy. Other drugs in this class are helpful for managing complications associated with pathologic bone resorption.

The bisphosphonates may provide pain relief in patients with pathologic bone disease. However, they do not have a direct analgesic effect. In horses treated with clodronate or tiludronate they showed clinical improvements in their degree of lameness, but it is unclear whether the reduction in lameness was caused by the effect on bone remodeling, analgesia, or other mechanisms.

Another bisphosphonate is tiludronate (Tildren), also approved for treating navicular disease in horses.

## Precautionary Information

### Adverse Reactions and Side Effects

Reaction to clodronate has only been reported for horses. From field trials, the most commonly reported adverse effects were colic, agitation, and mild neurologic signs, such as tongue rolling and head shaking. Signs of colic usually occur shortly after drug administration (2 hours); therefore, monitor horses for at least 2 hours after injection. In most cases, these signs resolved within 5.5 hours following administration. Clinical pathology abnormalities associated with administration of OSPHOS included elevations in serum blood urea nitrogen, creatinine, glucose, and potassium concentrations and decreases in serum chloride concentrations. In safety studies, the most common adverse effects were clinical signs related to abdominal discomfort (colic), which was dose related (more common at doses that exceeded label dose).

### Contraindications and Precautions

Do not use in horses with kidney disease. Use carefully in conditions associated with hypocalcemia. It is not recommended to administer bisphosphonates to young growing animals. Do not use in pregnant mares because the safety in pregnancy has not been evaluated, and bisphosphonates have caused fetal abnormalities of the bone when administered to laboratory animals.

*Use in young horses:* The manufacturer states that the safety of clodronate in horses younger than 4 years of age has not been evaluated. They also state that the effect of bisphosphonates on the skeleton of growing horses has not been studied; however, bisphosphonates inhibit osteoclast activity, which impacts bone turnover and may affect bone growth. It is recommended *not* to administer bisphosphonates such as clodronate in young performance horses because the change in bone metabolism may predispose young horses to fracture, but one study that examined clodronate and tiludronate in young horses concluded that tiludronate and clodronate did not appear to significantly impact bone tissue on a structural or cellular level using standard dose and administration schedules in young horses.

### Drug Interactions

Do not mix with solutions containing calcium (e.g., lactated Ringer's solution).

## Instructions for Use

Make sure horses are well hydrated prior to use to avoid kidney injury. Observe horses for 2 hours after administration for signs of colic.

## Patient Monitoring and Laboratory Tests

Monitor serum calcium and phosphorus. Monitor urea nitrogen, creatinine, urine-specific gravity, and signs of colic in treated animals.

## Formulations
Clodronate is available as 60 mg clodronate disodium per milliliter in 20-mL vial containing.

## Stability and Storage
Store at controlled room temperature 25°C (77°F) with deviations between 15°C and 30°C (59°F and 86°F) permitted.

C

## Small Animal Dosage
• No doses have been confirmed for dogs or cats, but there are anecdotal accounts of a dose of 20–25 mg/kg IV over 4 hours for treatment of hypercalcemia.

## Large Animal Dosage
**Horses**
• 1.8 mg/kg IM. Maximum dose is 900 mg per horse. Divide the total volume equally into three separate injection sites.

## Regulatory Information
Withdrawal times are not established for animals that produce food. For extralabel use withdrawal interval estimates, contact FARAD at www.FARAD.org.

# Clofazimine
kloe-fah′zih-meen

**Trade and other names:** Lamprene

**Functional classification:** Antibacterial

## Pharmacology and Mechanism of Action
Clofazimine is an antimicrobial agent used to treat feline leprosy. It produces a slow bactericidal effect on *Mycobacterium leprae*.

## Indications and Clinical Uses
Clofazimine has had limited use in veterinary medicine because it is not available in the United States. Its use is limited to treating infections caused by *Mycobacterium* spp., such as feline leprosy. The clinical experience with using clofazimine in cats has been limited, and efficacy has not been compared with other agents.

## Precautionary Information
**Adverse Reactions and Side Effects**
Adverse effects have not been reported in cats. In people, the most serious adverse effects are GI related.

**Contraindications and Precautions**
No contraindications reported for animals.

**Drug Interactions**
No drug interactions are reported in animals.

## Instructions for Use
Doses based on empiricism or extrapolation of human studies.

## Patient Monitoring and Laboratory Tests
No specific monitoring is necessary.

## Formulations
- Clofazimine is not available in the United States but is available in other countries as 50-mg capsules. Some compounding pharmacies will prepare this drug for use in the United States.

## Stability and Storage
Store in a tightly sealed container, protected from light, and at room temperature. Stability of compounded formulations has not been evaluated.

## Small Animal Dosage
Cats
- 1 mg/kg up to a maximum of 4 mg/kg/day PO.

## Large Animal Dosage
- Cattle: 600–1000 mg oral to adult cattle per day (2 mg/kg per day).

## Regulatory Information
No regulatory information is available. For extralabel use withdrawal interval estimates, contact FARAD at www.FARAD.org.

# Clomipramine Hydrochloride
kloe-mip'rah-meen hye-droe-klor'ide

**Trade and other names:** Clomicalm (veterinary preparation) and Anafranil (human preparation)

**Functional classification:** Behavior modification

## Pharmacology and Mechanism of Action
Clomipramine is an antidepressant drug of the tricyclic antidepressant (TCA) class. It is used in people to treat anxiety and depression. The mechanism of action is via inhibition of uptake of serotonin at presynaptic nerve terminals. Beneficial effects may be caused primarily by blocking reuptake of serotonin and modulation of serotonin in areas of the brain that affect anxiety and behavior. Clomipramine has more serotonin-reuptake–blocking effects than other TCA drugs. Side effects result from antimuscarinic effects caused by the active metabolite desmethylclomipramine. However, animals produce less of this metabolite than people do.

*Pharmacokinetics:* In dogs, the half-life is 5 hours after oral administration, with a peak at 1.5 hours, but the half-life may be shorter (2–4 hours) with repeated dosing. The oral absorption in dogs is 20%.

## Indications and Clinical Uses
Like other TCAs, clomipramine is used in animals to treat various behavioral disorders, including obsessive-compulsive disorders (also called canine compulsive disorder) and separation anxiety. In dogs, it has been superior to amitriptyline for treating compulsive disorders; however, it does not appear to be beneficial when used for dominance-related aggression. In cats, with long-term treatment, it has been effective for decreasing urine spraying. It was equally effective as fluoxetine for urine spraying in cats, but treated animals returned to urine marking abruptly after the drug was discontinued. It has not been effective for psychogenic alopecia in cats.

## Precautionary Information
### Adverse Reactions and Side Effects
Reported adverse effects include sedation and reduced appetite. Vomiting may occur in dogs, which can be reduced if administered with a small amount of food. Clomipramine has a bitter taste and some animals may refuse the medication. Other side effects associated with TCAs are antimuscarinic effects (dry mouth, rapid heart rate, and urine retention) and antihistamine effects (sedation). In cats, sedation and weight gain have been observed. The antimuscarinic effects from clomipramine may be caused by an active metabolite. Clomipramine can decrease total $T_4$ and free $T_4$ thyroid concentrations in dogs, but it may still be within normal reference ranges. It has been safe in cats, with no significant adverse effects observed during clinical studies.

Overdoses, especially in dogs that accidentally consume large amounts, can produce life-threatening cardiotoxicity. If an overdose occurs, immediately contact a poison control center.

### Contraindications and Precautions
Use cautiously in patients with heart disease.

### Drug Interactions
Do not use with other behavior-modifying drugs such as serotonin reuptake inhibitors. Do not use with monoamine oxidase inhibitors, such as selegiline or amitraz. Although tramadol can produce some serotonin effects, there have been no reported interactions from administration of tramadol and clomipramine concurrently.

## Instructions for Use
When adjusting doses, one may initiate therapy with a low dose and increase gradually. There may be a delayed onset of 2–4 weeks after initiation of therapy before beneficial effects are observed. After achieving a favorable response, the dose can be gradually lowered in some animals. To reduce incidence of vomiting in dogs, it may be administered with food.

## Patient Monitoring and Laboratory Tests
Monitor animal's heart rate and rhythm periodically during treatment. Like other TCAs, clomipramine may decrease total $T_4$ and free $T_4$ concentrations in dogs.

## Formulations
- Clomipramine is available in 5-, 20-, 40-, and 80-mg tablets (veterinary preparation).
- 25-, 50-, and 75-mg capsules (human preparation).

## Stability and Storage
Store at room temperature. Protect from moisture. It has been compounded in a tuna-flavored liquid for cats without a decrease in efficacy.

## Small Animal Dosage
### Dogs
- 2–4 mg/kg/day, PO, which may be administered as a single dose, or divided into twice-daily doses. Start at lower dose and gradually increase to reach the desired effect. Increases in dose should be made approximately every 14 days until desired effect is observed.

### Cats
- 1–5 mg per cat q12–24h PO (0.5 mg/kg per day) and gradually increase.
- Urine spraying in cats: Up to 5 mg per cat once a day.

## Large Animal Dosage
- No dose has been reported for large animals.

## Regulatory Information
No regulatory information is available. For extralabel use withdrawal interval estimates, contact FARAD at www.FARAD.org.
RCI Classification: 2

# Clonazepam
kloe-nah'zih-pam

**Trade and other names:** Klonopin and generic brands

**Functional classification:** Anticonvulsant

## Pharmacology and Mechanism of Action
Clonazepam is a benzodiazepine with action similar to other benzodiazepines, which is to enhance inhibitory effects of gamma-aminobutyric acid (GABA) in the CNS. Through these GABA effects, it has anticonvulsant action, sedative properties, and effects on some behavioral disorders.

## Indications and Clinical Uses
Clonazepam has been used as an anticonvulsant in dogs and cats, but this use is not common because there are other more effective anticonvulsant agents available. Tolerance may develop to the anticonvulsant effects with long-term use. Like other benzodiazepines, it also is used to treat behavior problems in dogs and cats, particularly those associated with anxiety.

## Precautionary Information

**Adverse Reactions and Side Effects**

Side effects include sedation and polyphagia. Some animals may experience paradoxical excitement.

**Contraindications and Precautions**

No contraindications reported for animals. Use of benzodiazepines in early pregnancy has been associated with an increased risk of spontaneous abortions and fetal malformations in people. This incidence in animals is unknown.

**Drug Interactions**

No drug interactions are reported in animals. However, it potentiates effects from other sedatives and CNS depressants.

## Instructions for Use
The doses used clinically in dogs and cats are based primarily on reports from human medicine, empiricism, or experimental studies. No clinical efficacy studies have been performed in dogs or cats. Some dogs are sensitive to the doses listed in the dosing section and lowered to 0.1–0.2 mg/kg in some animals.

## Patient Monitoring and Laboratory Tests
Samples of plasma or serum may be analyzed for concentrations of benzodiazepines. However, many veterinary laboratories may not have this capability, and laboratories that analyze human samples may be nonspecific for benzodiazepines.

## Formulations
- Clonazepam is available in 0.5-, 1-, and 2-mg tablets. Oral disintegrating tablets are available as 0.125-, 0.25-, 0.5-, 1-, and 2-mg tablets.

## Stability and Storage
Store in a tightly sealed container, protected from light, and at room temperature. Clonazepam, like other benzodiazepines, exhibits adsorption to plastic, especially soft plastic (polyvinyl chloride). Compounded oral products are stable for 60 days.

## Small Animal Dosage
**Dogs**
- 0.5 mg/kg q8–12h PO.

**Cats**
- 0.1–0.2 mg/kg q12–24h PO.

## Large Animal Dosage
- No dose has been reported for large animals.

## Regulatory Information
Do not administer to animals intended for food.
Schedule IV controlled drug.
RCI Classification: 2

# Clopidogrel
kloe-pid′oh-grel

**Trade and other names:** Plavix

**Functional classification:** Antiplatelet drug

## Pharmacology and Mechanism of Action
Clopidogrel is a platelet inhibitor. It is a thienopyridine and inhibits adenosine diphosphate (ADP) receptor–mediated platelet activity. Clopidogrel is metabolized to an active metabolite that exerts its antiplatelet effect. This metabolite blocks ADP from binding to the $P2Y_1$ and $P2Y_{12}$ receptor in a competitive manner, which leads to decreased platelet activity. Binding of ADP to $P2Y_1$ and $P2Y_{12}$ activates a G-protein, which inhibits adenyl cyclase and decreases cyclic adenosine monophosphate (cAMP). Because this mechanism is different from the aspirin-inhibiting effect on platelets, clopidogrel is more effective than aspirin alone. In dog, cats, and horses, oral administration has produced significant inhibitory effects on platelets that are superior to aspirin. Clopidogrel administration also decreased serotonin release from platelets, which may be important in cats because they have highly reactive platelets and serotonin release may contribute to clinical signs of thromboemboli in cats. A related drug is ticlopidine.

*Pharmacokinetics:* In horses the half-life of clopidogrel was 6 hours, but the active metabolite (CAMB) was only 0.5 hours. In dogs, the parent drug (clopidogrel) is not detected in the blood, and the antiplatelet effects are caused by the active metabolite.

## Indications and Clinical Uses

Clopidogrel is used to inhibit platelets in patients that are prone to forming blood clots. In patients with a high risk for thrombi and emboli, clopidogrel inhibits mechanisms that are not affected by aspirin alone. It has been used currently with aspirin treatment, but combined treatment is usually not necessary. Although clopidogrel is more consistently reliable as an antiplatelet drug than aspirin, some animals may be nonresponders (e.g., 33% of horses, 15% of cats). Nevertheless, the consensus opinion by experts recommend that clopidogrel is preferred over aspirin for prevent of arterial thromboemboli in dogs and cats.

In cats, clopidogrel has been recommended to prevent cardiogenic arterial thromboembolism associated with heart disease. Treatment can be initiated in cats based on echocardiogram studies that demonstrate the presence of "smoke" in the left atrium. In cats, clopidogrel produces antiplatelet effects that persist for 3 days after discontinuation of the drug. In dogs, it has been used to prevent embolism caused by heartworm disease and other conditions. In dogs, at a dose of either 0.5 or 1.0 mg/kg, decreased ADP-induced platelet aggregation occurs for 3 days after discontinuation of drug administration in some dogs and longer than 7 days in others. At 2 mg/kg PO q24h, clopidogrel significantly suppressed platelet activity in horses, which persisted for 6 days after the last dose. However, not all horses respond, and effects may not be sustained for 24 hours. This may be caused by rapid elimination of the active metabolite in some horses.

A similar drug is ticlopidine (Ticlid), which should not be used in cats because it produces adverse reactions.

## Precautionary Information

Avoid use in animals that have bleeding problems; use cautiously with other drugs that may inhibit platelets or blood clotting.

### Adverse Reactions and Side Effects

Bleeding problems can occur in susceptible patients, but this has not been reported to be a clinical problem in dogs or cats. In people, pruritus and skin rash have been reported, but this has not been observed in dogs and cats. The taste is bitter, and some cats may refuse oral administration.

### Contraindications and Precautions

Do not use in patients that have a high risk of bleeding. Discontinue several days prior to a planned surgical procedure.

### Drug Interactions

Use cautiously with other drugs that may inhibit blood clotting, such as anticoagulants. In people, omeprazole (oral antiulcer agent) inhibits the conversion of clopidogrel to the active metabolite. This does not occur in dogs. It is not known if this interaction occurs in cats or horses with clinical use.

## Instructions for Use

Administer with or without aspirin in patients prone to thrombi and emboli, but concurrent use with aspirin is not necessary. Because platelets are involved in arterial thromboembolism more than venous thromboembolism, the use for prevention of arterial thromboembolism is better established than the use for venous thromboembolism. The dose in cats of 19 mg is approximately one fourth of a human tablet. It is likely that smaller doses are effective, but they have not been evaluated because it is impractical to divide the human 75-mg tablet into fractions smaller than one fourth. The dosage in dogs is usually 1–2 mg/kg q24h PO. At this dosage, the onset is 2 days, and steady-state is achieved in 5–7 days. Higher doses are often used initially in dogs for the first few days.

## Patient Monitoring and Laboratory Tests
Monitor for bleeding.

## Formulations
- Clopidogrel is available in 75-mg tablets.

## Stability and Storage
Store in a tightly sealed container, protected from light, and at room temperature. Stability of compounded formulations has not been evaluated.

## Small Animal Dosage
### Cats
- 18.75 mg per cat (one fourth of tablet) q24h PO. The taste is bitter for cats, and fractions of the tablets may be placed in gelatin capsules.
- Smaller doses may be effective but have not been evaluated in cats.

### Dogs
- 2 mg/kg q24h PO.
- An oral loading dose may be given at 2–4 mg/kg followed by 1–2 mg/kg q24h PO. In some cases, a higher oral loading dose of 10 mg/kg has been used.

## Large Animal Dosage
### Horses
- Loading dose of 4 mg/kg followed by 2 mg/kg q24h PO.

## Regulatory Information
Do not administer to animals that produce food.

# Cloprostenol Sodium
kloe-pros'te-nole

**Trade and other names:** Estrumate, estroPLAN

**Functional classification:** Prostaglandin

## Pharmacology and Mechanism of Action
Cloprostenol is a synthetic PG, structurally related to $PGF_2$-alpha that produces $PGF_2$-alpha effects. Synthetic prostaglandins are much more potent than natural PGs, and one should not use these at the same dose as natural PGs. $PGF_2$ analogues have a direct luteolytic action on the corpus luteum. After injection, cloprostenol causes functional regression of the corpus luteum (luteolysis). In nonpregnant cycling cattle, this effect will result in starting estrus 2–5 days after injection. In pregnant animals, it terminates pregnancy by inducing luteolysis and decreasing progesterone followed by increasing myometrial contraction and increased uterine evacuation. In animals with prolonged luteal activity that have pyometra, mummified fetuses, or luteal cysts, the luteolysis usually results in resolution of the problem and return to normal cycling.

## Indications and Clinical Uses
Cloprostenol has been used in cattle to induce luteolysis (beef and dairy cattle) to manipulate the timing of the estrus cycle to benefit breeding management practices.

Cloprostenol has been used to terminate pregnancy in any animal that forms a corpus luteum. The indications to terminate pregnancy may be the result from undesired mating and to treat conditions associated with prolonged luteal function (e.g., pyometra, luteal cysts). In horses, it has been administered to induce premature labor in the last 2–4 weeks of pregnancy. Most reports on successful termination of pregnancy have been performed on cattle, horses, and dogs. In dogs, cloprostenol has been administered in combination with other drugs (e.g., cabergoline [Dostinex] and bromocriptine [Parlodel]) to terminate pregnancy. When used to terminate pregnancy, it has been almost 100% effective. In cats, it is effective for treatment of pyometra in cats with an open cervix.

## Precautionary Information

### Adverse Reactions and Side Effects

Induces abortion in pregnant animals. High doses in cattle (50× and 100× dose) have caused discomfort, milk letdown, and some frothing. Endometritis can occur in some animals after treatment for pyometra. When used to treat pyometra in dogs, panting, vomiting, nausea, and diarrhea can be seen 15–45 minutes after injection. In dogs, for termination of pregnancy, side effects have been mild but may include vomiting, nausea, and panting, occurring shortly after the injection and lasting for approximately 15–20 minutes. To avoid vomiting, it is recommended to wait 8 hours after feeding before injection. Abortion may be followed by 1 week (approximately) of mucoid vulvar discharge. There are no long-term effects on fertility. Mammary enlargement and mild milk production may occur in some dogs. In cats, adverse effects after injection include vomiting, vocalization for up to 30 minutes, increased vaginal discharge, and diarrhea.

### Contraindications and Precautions

Synthetic PGs are much more potent than natural PGs, so observe doses carefully to avoid overdose of the synthetic forms. Handle with caution. Women of childbearing age, people with asthma, and persons with bronchial and other respiratory problems should exercise extreme caution when handling this product. Cloprostenol is readily absorbed through the skin and may cause abortion or bronchospasms. Accidental spillage on the skin should be washed off immediately with soap and water.

## Instructions for Use

Give injections to cattle IM. When cloprostenol is injected in cattle, return to estrus activity usually occurs in 3–5 days, at which time animals may be inseminated. In some cases, a second injection may be given 11 days after the first injection (double-injection plan), with estrus occurring at 2–5 days after the second injection. In dairy cattle, it is used with gonadorelin (Fertagyl) to synchronize estrous cycles and allow for a fixed time for artificial insemination (see Gonadorelin and the dosing section below for more information).

When used to terminate pregnancy in cattle, it can be used any time from day 7 to 5 months after breeding, and the fetus is expelled usually after 4–5 days. In dogs, it has been used to terminate pregnancy approximately 30–40 days after breeding. In dogs, when used to terminate pregnancy, it has been used in combination with other drugs (bromocriptine or cabergoline) to allow for a lower dose of 1 mcg/kg, which has fewer side effects. Administer cloprostenol at least 8 hours after feeding to avoid vomiting.

## Patient Monitoring and Laboratory Tests

Monitor for continued vulvar discharge after treatment. Measurement of serum progesterone may be used to monitor therapy, especially if termination of abortion is prolonged.

## Formulations

- Cloprostenol is available in an injectable aqueous solution containing 250 mcg of cloprostenol per milliliter. Dilution in saline is recommended for accurate dosing to dogs and cats.

## Stability and Storage

Store in a tightly sealed container, protected from light, and at room temperature. Stability of compounded formulations has not been evaluated, but prior to injection in small animals, it may be diluted with saline solution to produce a more accurate dose.

## Small Animal Dosage

### Dogs

- Terminate pregnancy: 1–2.5 mcg/kg once daily SQ for 4–5 days, starting on day 25 after mating. (Side effects are lower with 1 mcg/kg.)
- Starting 35–45 days after mating, administer 1 mcg/kg SQ (after 10-fold dilution in saline) on days 1 and 3 of treatment. It can be administered with cabergoline (Galastop) 5 mcg/kg oral q24h on days 1–7 of treatment (see Cabergoline for more information).
- 1 mcg/kg q48h SQ, administered with bromocriptine (see Bromocriptine for additional information).

### Cats

- Terminate pregnancy: 5 mcg/kg SQ once daily for 3 days.

## Large Animal Dosage

### Cattle

- 2 mL (500 mcg) IM once or repeated again 11 days after the first injection.
- Dairy cattle: Administer gonadorelin injection IM (86 mcg) IM on day 0; then administer cloprostenol (500 mcg) IM 6–8 days later. Administer a second gonadorelin injection (86 mcg) 30–72 hours after the last cloprostenol injection and perform artificial insemination 8–24 hours later.

### Horses

- Terminate pregnancy: 2 mL (500 mcg) per horse, IM. In some conditions, repeated injections are administered (e.g., q12h).
- To induce premature labor in the last 2–4 weeks of pregnancy, administer two doses 30 minutes apart (oxytocin also is used for this indication).
- For endometritis, 250 mcg (1 mL) IM twice, 12 hours apart, usually combined with oxytocin.

## Regulatory Information

To be used only by licensed veterinarians. No withdrawal times are listed on approved label for food animals.

# Clorazepate Dipotassium
klor-az'eh-pate dye-poe-tah'see-um

**Trade and other names:** Tranxene and generic

**Functional classification:** Anticonvulsant

## Pharmacology and Mechanism of Action

Clorazepate is a benzodiazepine, related to diazepam. Clorazepate is one of the active metabolites of diazepam, producing similar effects as diazepam but longer acting. After oral absorption, it is quickly converted to the active drug, referred to as nordiazepam or desmethyldiazepam. Similar to diazepam and other benzodiazepines, its action is to enhance inhibitory effects of GABA in the CNS.

## Indications and Clinical Uses

Clorazepate is used for anticonvulsant treatment, sedation, and treatment of some behavioral disorders. The use for treating seizures has diminished because there are other more effective agents available for dogs and cats, but it has been used with other drugs in refractory cases when other drugs are not effective. It is not recommended as a sole treatment for seizure disorders in dogs and cats. When used as an anticonvulsant, tolerance may develop to the anticonvulsant effects with long-term use.

## Precautionary Information

### Adverse Reactions and Side Effects

Side effects include sedation and polyphagia. Some animals may experience paradoxical excitement. Chronic administration may lead to dependence and a withdrawal syndrome if discontinued.

### Contraindications and Precautions

No serious contraindications. In rare individuals, benzodiazepines have caused paradoxical excitement. They may cause fetal abnormalities early in pregnancy, but this has not been reported with veterinary use.

### Drug Interactions

No drug interactions are reported in animals. However, it potentiates effects from other sedatives and CNS depressants.

## Instructions for Use

Doses are based primarily on reports from human medicine, empiricism, or experimental studies. Higher doses may be used for short-term treatment of noise phobia. However, for most indications, no clinical efficacy studies have been performed in dogs or cats.

## Patient Monitoring and Laboratory Tests

Samples of plasma or serum may be analyzed for concentrations of benzodiazepines. If response to clorazepate is measured, the active metabolite, nordiazepam (desmethyldiazepam), should be measured. Plasma concentrations in the range of 100–250 ng/mL have been cited as the therapeutic range for people, but some references have cited this range as 150–300 ng/mL. The optimum range for dogs and cats has not been determined. There are no readily available tests for monitoring in many veterinary laboratories. Laboratories that analyze human samples may have nonspecific tests for benzodiazepines. With these assays, there may be cross-reactivity among benzodiazepine metabolites.

## Formulations Available

• Clorazepate is available in 3.75-, 7.5-, and 15-mg tablets.

## Stability and Storage

Keep in original packaging or store in tightly sealed container, protected from light, and at room temperature. Stability of compounded formulations has not been evaluated, but clorazepate tablets degrade quickly in the presence of light, heat, or moisture.

## Small Animal Dosage

**Dogs**

- 0.5–2 mg/kg q8–12h PO and as frequently as 4 hours. (Total dose is usually 3.75 mg or 7.5 mg.)

**Cats**

- 0.2–0.4 mg/kg q12–24h up to 0.5–2.2 mg/kg q12h PO.

## Large Animal Dosage

- No dose has been reported for large animals.

## Regulatory Information

Do not administer to animals intended for food.
RCI Classification: 2

# Cloxacillin Sodium
kloks-ah-sill'in soe'dee-um

**Trade and other names:** Cloxapen, Orbenin, and Tegopen

**Functional classification:** Antibacterial

## Pharmacology and Mechanism of Action

Cloxacillin is beta-lactam antibiotic, related to the penicillin class. It inhibits bacterial cell wall synthesis by binding to penicillin-binding proteins. Cloxacillin is similar in spectrum and activity as amoxicillin, except that it is resistant to the beta-lactamase enzyme produced by *Staphylococcus* spp. The spectrum is limited to gram-positive bacteria, especially staphylococci. MRS are resistant to cloxacillin. Most gram-negative bacteria are clinically resistant.

## Indications and Clinical Uses

The spectrum of cloxacillin includes gram-positive bacilli, including beta-lactamase–producing strains of *Staphylococcus* spp. Therefore, it has been used to treat staphylococcal infections in animals, including pyoderma. Because of better availability of other beta-lactam drugs for treating gram-positive infections such as those caused by *Staphylococcus* spp., cloxacillin is used infrequently in small animals. The intramammary formulations are used in dairy cattle.

## Precautionary Information

### Adverse Reactions and Side Effects

Adverse effects of penicillin drugs are most commonly caused by drug allergy. This can range from acute anaphylaxis when administered to other signs of allergic reaction when other routes are used. When administered orally (especially with high doses), diarrhea is possible.

### Contraindications and Precautions

Use cautiously in animals allergic to penicillin-like drugs.

### Drug Interactions

No drug interactions are reported in animals. However, do not mix with other drugs because inactivation may result.

## Instructions for Use

Doses based on empiricism or extrapolation from human studies. No clinical efficacy studies available for dogs or cats. Oral absorption is poor; if possible, administer on an empty stomach.

## Patient Monitoring and Laboratory Tests

Culture and sensitivity testing: Use oxacillin as a guide for sensitivity testing. If the strain is susceptible to oxacillin (methicillin-susceptible), cloxacillin and other agents active against *Staphylococcus* spp. can be used (e.g., cephalexin).

## Formulations

• Cloxacillin is available in 250- and 500-mg capsules and 25-mg/mL oral solution.

## Stability and Storage

Store in a tightly sealed container, protected from light, and at room temperature. Stability of compounded formulations has not been evaluated.

## Small Animal Dosage

**Dogs and Cats**

• 20–40 mg/kg q8h PO.

## Large Animal Dosage

• No dose has been reported for large animals. The only formulation approved for food animals is Dariclox, a 20-mg/mL intramammary infusion. The dosage is 10 mL (200 mg) per infected quarter q12h for three treatments.

## Regulatory Information

Dairy cows (intramammary use) withdrawal time for milk: 30 days for dry-cow treatment.

Cattle withdrawal time for meat: 10 days for meat and 48 hours for milk for the lactating cow treatment.

# Codeine
koe′deen

**Trade and other names:** Generic, codeine phosphate, and codeine sulfate

**Functional classification:** Analgesic, opioid, antitussive

## Pharmacology and Mechanism of Action

Codeine is an opiate agonist, analgesic, and antitussive. The mechanism is similar to morphine, except with approximately one tenth the potency of morphine. Codeine is extensively metabolized. In dogs, oral absorption is low (less than 5%), but it is rapidly converted to other metabolites that may have analgesic activity, such as glucuronidated forms of codeine. In people, codeine is partially metabolized to a more active opiate, morphine ($\approx$10%). There is conflicting evidence on whether or not dogs metabolize codeine to morphine. Some dogs convert to small amounts of morphine, but this may be dependent on other co-administered drugs, dog breed, and other factors. The activity of codeine and perhaps some active metabolites is to bind to mu- and kappa-opiate receptors on nerves and inhibit release of neurotransmitters involved with transmission of pain stimuli (e.g., substance P). It also may inhibit release of some inflammatory mediators. Central sedative and euphoric effects are related to mu-receptor effects in brain.

## Indications and Clinical Uses

Codeine, or codeine with acetaminophen, has been used for treatment of moderate pain. It also has been used as an antitussive. Despite the widespread use of codeine in humans, the efficacy in animals for its antitussive or analgesic use has not been established. The limited experience shows that for joint pain in dogs, it is not as effective as oral NSAIDs. Codeine, morphine, and other opiates in dogs have rapid clearance and short half-lives. Therefore, even if absorption is adequate, the duration of action is short, and clinical effectiveness in dogs may be questionable. There is little evidence available for the use in cats. Oral codeine ($\approx$2 mg/kg) did not produce antinociceptive effects in research cats. There is some evidence that horses are capable of conversion of codeine to morphine, which may be useful for treating pain in horses. However, the clinical effectiveness in horses has not been examined.

## Precautionary Information

### Adverse Reactions and Side Effects

Like all opiates, side effects from codeine are predictable. Side effects include sedation, constipation, and bradycardia. Respiratory depression occurs with high doses.

### Contraindications and Precautions

Codeine is a Schedule II controlled substance. Tolerance and dependence occur with chronic administration. High doses (60-mg tablet with acetaminophen) can cause sedation in dogs. Cats are more susceptible to excitement than other species. Some codeine formulations may contain other ingredients (e.g., acetaminophen) that should not be administered to cats.

### Drug Interactions

No drug interactions are reported in animals. However, it potentiates effects from other sedatives and CNS depressants.

## Instructions for Use

Available as codeine phosphate and codeine sulfate oral tablets. Doses listed for analgesia are considered initial doses; individual patients may need higher doses depending on degree of tolerance or pain threshold. When administering acetaminophen–codeine combinations, the high-dose tablet (containing 60 mg codeine) tends to cause sedation in dogs (body weight 20–30 kg), and the lower dose (containing 30 mg) is recommended.

## Patient Monitoring and Laboratory Tests

Monitor patient's heart rate and respiration. Although bradycardia rarely needs to be treated when it is caused by an opioid, if necessary, atropine can be administered. If serious respiratory depression occurs, the opioid can be reversed with naloxone.

## Formulations

- Codeine is available in 15-, 30-, and 60-mg tablets; 5-mg/mL syrup; and 3-mg/mL oral solution. It is also available in formulations with acetaminophen. Note that many of the syrups have other ingredients that may not be appropriate for pets.

## Stability and Storage

Store in a tightly sealed container, protected from light, and at room temperature. Stability of compounded formulations has not been evaluated.

## Small Animal Dosage

**Dogs**

- Analgesia: 0.5–1 mg/kg q4–6h PO.
- Antitussive: 0.1–0.3 mg/kg q4–6h PO.

**Cats**

- Analgesia: 0.5 mg/kg q6h PO. Increase dose as needed to control pain.
- Antitussive: 0.1 mg/kg q6h PO.

## Large Animal Dosage

- No dose has been reported for large animals.

## Regulatory Information

Drug controlled by the Drug Enforcement Administration. Schedule II; some antitussive forms are Schedule V.

RCI Classification: 1

# Colchicine
kol'chih-seen

**Trade and other names:** Colcrys and generic brands

**Functional classification:** Anti-inflammatory agent

## Pharmacology and Mechanism of Action

Anti-inflammatory agent. It inhibits fibrosis and formation of collagen.

## Indications and Clinical Uses

In people, colchicine is used to treat gout. In animals, it has been used as an antifibrotic agent to decrease fibrosis and development of hepatic failure (possibly by inhibiting formation of collagen). However, the efficacy for controlling liver fibrosis in chronic liver disease is questionable and unproven. Anti-inflammatory effects may be caused by inhibition of neutrophil and mononuclear migration. Antifibrotic effects result from blockage of microtubular-mediated transcellular movement of proteins and to inhibit secretion of procollagen molecules into the extracellular matrix. It has also been used in animals to control amyloidosis. In Shar-Pei dogs, colchicine has been used to treat a fever syndrome, possibly because of its use in people for treating Mediterranean fever.

## Precautionary Information

### Adverse Reactions and Side Effects

The most common adverse effects are nausea, vomiting, abdominal pain, and diarrhea. Because there is a risk of vomiting, diarrhea, and decreased appetite in dogs and there is little evidence of antifibrotic effect for chronic liver disease in dogs, the use in dogs with liver disease is discouraged. Colchicine may cause dermatitis in people, but this has not been reported in dogs or cats.

### Contraindications and Precautions

Do not administer to pregnant animals.

### Drug Interactions

There are no drug interactions reported for small animals.

## Instructions for Use
Doses are based on empiricism and anecdotal reports. There are no well-controlled efficacy studies in veterinary species.

## Patient Monitoring and Laboratory Tests
No specific monitoring is necessary.

## Formulations
- Colchicine is available in 600-mcg tablets.

## Stability and Storage
Store in a tightly sealed container, protected from light, and at room temperature. Stability of compounded formulations has not been evaluated.

## Small Animal Dosage
**Dogs and Cats**
- 0.01–0.03 mg/kg q24h PO.

## Large Animal Dosage
- No dose has been reported for large animals.

## Regulatory Information
No regulatory information is available. For extralabel use withdrawal interval estimates, contact FARAD at www.FARAD.org.

# Colony-Stimulating Factors: Sargramostim and Filgrastim
**Trade and other names:** Leukine and Neupogen
**Functional classification:** Hormone

## Pharmacology and Mechanism of Action
Stimulates granulocyte development in bone marrow. Two drugs in this class include filgrastim (rG-CSG) and sargramostim (rGM-CSF).

## Indications and Clinical Uses
Colony-stimulating factors are used primarily to regenerate blood cells to recover from cancer chemotherapy or other bone marrow–suppressing therapy. Their use is uncommon in animals.

## Precautionary Information
**Adverse Reactions and Side Effects**
These agents can cause pain at the injection site. Edema has been reported in people.

**Contraindications and Precautions**
There are none identified in small animals.

**Drug Interactions**
There are no drug interactions reported for small animals.

## Instructions for Use

The doses of these agents have not been studied in animals. If used, the doses are based on limited experimental information and extrapolations from human experience. To prepare sargramostim, add 1 mL to make up 250- or 500-mcg/mL vial. Dilute further with 0.9% saline solution to less than 10 mcg/mL for infusion. Do not shake vial to prevent foaming; gently swirl vial to mix contents.

## Patient Monitoring and Laboratory Tests

Monitor CBC to assess treatment. Treatment can be discontinued when neutrophils recover.

## Formulations

- Colony-stimulating factors are available in 300 mcg/mL (Neupogen) and 250 and 500 mcg/mL (Leukine).

## Stability and Storage

Store in a tightly sealed container protected from light.

## Small Animal Dosage

### Dogs and Cats

- Sargramostim: 250 mcg/m$^2$ (0.25 mg/m$^2$) IV infusion over 2 hours or SQ.
- Filgrastim: 5 mcg/kg (0.005 mg/kg) once daily SQ for 2 weeks or 10 mcg/kg/day.

## Large Animal Dosage

- No dose has been reported for large animals.

## Regulatory Information

Do not administer to animals intended for food.

# Corticotropin
kor-tih-koe-troe′pin

**Trade and other names:** Acthar

**Functional classification:** Hormone

## Pharmacology and Mechanism of Action

Corticotropin (adrenocorticotropic hormone [ACTH]). Corticotropin is a natural peptide hormone, composed of 39 amino acids. The formulation is prepared into a gel for injection. It stimulates normal synthesis of cortisol and other hormones from adrenal cortex. This agent is used primarily for testing the activity of the adrenal gland.

## Indications and Clinical Uses

Adrenocorticotropic hormone is used for diagnostic purposes to evaluate adrenal gland function. Another closely related synthetic product, cosyntropin, is used for the same purpose. The availability of Acthar gel has been limited and is extremely expensive. Therefore, cosyntropin is often used as a substitute (see the Cosyntropin section for more details) and used more frequently. Compounded formulations of corticotropin may not be equivalent.

## Precautionary Information
### Adverse Reactions and Side Effects
Adverse effects unlikely when used as a single injection for diagnostic purposes.

### Contraindications and Precautions
Do not administer IV.

### Drug Interactions
There are no drug interactions reported for small animals.

## Instructions for Use
Doses are established by measuring normal adrenal response in animals. See also Cosyntropin, which is sometimes preferred for clinical use. However, availability and cost of cosyntropin and ACTH are the factors that usually determine which is used in small animals.

## Patient Monitoring and Laboratory Tests
Monitor cortisol concentrations. Post-ACTH cortisol response should be as follows:
- Dogs 5.5–20.0 mcg/dL; greater than 20 mcg/dL is consistent with hyperadrenocorticism.
- Cats 4.5–15 mcg/dL; greater than 15 mcg/dL is consistent with hyperadrenocorticism.

 After treatment for hyperadrenocorticism (e.g., treatment with mitotane), response should be 1–5 mcg/dL. See Trilostane for instructions on monitoring response to trilostane treatment.

## Formulations
- ACTH is available in 80-units (international units [IU])/mL gel. (Extremely expensive)

## Stability and Storage
Store in a tightly sealed container protected from light.

## Small Animal Dosage
### Dogs
- ACTH response test: Collect pre-ACTH sample and inject 2.2 samples and inject 2.2 units (IU)/kg IM. Collect post-ACTH sample at 2 hours.

### Cats
- ACTH response test: Collect pre-ACTH sample and inject 2.2 units (IU)/kg IM. Collect post-ACTH sample at 1.5 and 2 hours.

## Large Animal Dosage
- No dose has been reported for large animals.

## Regulatory Information
No withdrawal times are available. Because clearance is rapid and there is little risk from residues, no withdrawal time is suggested for food animals.

# Cosyntropin
koe-sin-troe′pin

**Trade and other names:** Cortrosyn, synthetic corticotropin, tetracosactrin, and tetracosactide

**Functional classification:** Hormone

## Pharmacology and Mechanism of Action

Cosyntropin (beta-corticotropin) is a synthetic form of the peptide hormone corticotropin (ACTH) that is identical to the N-terminal 24 residues of natural corticotropin. It is also known in international formularies as tetracosactrin or tetracosactide. Whereas cosyntropin is an aqueous solution, ACTH is a gel. Therefore cosyntropin can be administered IV, but ACTH gel cannot. Cosyntropin is also more potent than ACTH. Administration of cosyntropin stimulates secretion of cortisol from adrenal glands. Administration of cosyntropin also stimulates secretion of aldosterone and sex hormones of adrenal origin.

## Indications and Clinical Uses

Cosyntropin is used for diagnostic purposes to evaluate adrenal gland function in dogs, cats, and horses. Maximum peak cortisol secretion occurs at 60–90 minutes in dogs, 60–75 minutes in cats, and 30 minutes in horses. It is used for the same purpose as corticotropin, but in humans, it is preferred over corticotropin because it is less allergenic.

## Precautionary Information

### Adverse Reactions and Side Effects

Adverse effects are unlikely when used as a single injection for diagnostic purposes. In people, cosyntropin is preferred over ACTH gel because cosyntropin is less allergenic.

### Contraindications and Precautions

Maximum dose for dogs should be 250 mcg.

### Drug Interactions

There are no drug interactions reported for small animals.

## Instructions for Use

Use for diagnostic purposes only; it is not intended for treatment of hypoadrenocorticism. Cosyntropin is preferred to ACTH gel because it is available in a formulation that is easier to use in dogs and cats. Preference of cosyntropin versus corticotropin gel is often determined by availability and cost.

In dogs, cosyntropin has been administered at 5 mcg/kg IV or IM and 250 mcg/dog IM. All three protocols produce similar results, and IM injection produces similar results as IV injection. An IV dose of 1 mcg/kg has produced similar results as 5 mcg/kg IV in dogs. In cats, similar response is observed with 125 mcg per cat, or 5 mcg/kg. In horses, 0.1 mcg/kg IV produced maximum response in 30–90 minutes. Compounded formulations of ACTH may produce similar results at 60 minutes postinjection but may have lower cortisol concentrations at 90 and 120 minutes compared with a proprietary formulation. One may split reconstituted Cortrosyn into aliquots of 50 mcg each (250-mcg vial split into 5 aliquots) or 25 mcg each (250-mcg vial split into 10 aliquots) and frozen in plastic syringes.

## Patient Monitoring and Laboratory Tests

Monitor cortisol concentrations. Post-ACTH cortisol response should be as follows:
Dogs: 5.5–20.0 mcg/dL; greater than 20 mcg/dL is consistent with hyperadrenocorticism. More specifically, 5.5–17 mcg/dL normal, 17–25 mcg/dL borderline, 25–30 mcg/dL suggestive, and greater than 30 mcg/dL highly likely for hyperadrenocorticism.

If monitoring sex hormones of adrenal origin, a sample for analysis should be taken at 60 minutes after injection.

Cats: 4.5–15 mcg/dL; greater than 15 mcg/dL is consistent with hyperadrenocorticism.

After treatment for hyperadrenocorticism (e.g., treatment with mitotane), response should be 1–5 mcg/dL.

## Formulations

- Cosyntropin is available in 250 mcg per vial. The lyophilized powder is reconstituted with 1 mL of saline in 2-mL vials for a final concentration of 250 mcg/mL.

## Stability and Storage

Once prepared, this formulation can be kept in the refrigerator for 4 months. Frozen cosyntropin can be stored in plastic syringes as individual dose aliquots for extended periods. For example, a 250-mcg 1-mL dose can be stored in small plastic syringes and frozen at –20°C for up to 6 months or kept in the refrigerator for 4 months. When needed, the 250-mcg aliquot can be added to 24 mL of sterile saline for injection for a final concentration of 10 mcg/mL. Some compounded formulations are stable and have produced reliable results at the 60-minute sample but may be lower at the 120-minute sample compared with the proprietary preparation.

## Small Animal Dosage

### Dogs

- Response test: Collect precosyntropin sample and inject 5 mcg/kg IV or IM and collect postsample at 30 and 60 minutes or one sample may be sufficient, collected at 60 minutes. Maximum dose for dogs should be 250 mcg. The following guidelines can be used for dosing: less than 5 kg, 25 mcg; 5–10 kg, 50 mcg; 10–15 kg, 75 mcg; 15–20 kg, 100 mcg; 20–25 kg, 125 mcg; 25–30 kg, 150 mcg; 30–40 kg, 200 mcg; 40–50 kg, 225 mcg; and more than 50 kg, 250 mcg (1 vial).
- Note: 1 mcg/kg IV has been equivalent as 5 mcg/kg IV for a similar response, but 5 mcg/kg is still the most often recommended dose.

### Cats

- Response test: Collect precosyntropin sample and inject cosyntropin IV or IM and collect postsample either at 60 or 75 minutes after IV administration or at 30 and 60 minutes after IM administration. A dose of 5 mcg/kg produces an equally effective dose to stimulate a maximal response as a dose of 125 mcg per cat.

## Large Animal Dosage

### Horses

- 0.1 mcg/kg IV produces maximum adrenal stimulation, with peak cortisol concentration in 30–90 minutes. Not recommended as a reliable test in horses.

### Foals

- ACTH stimulation test: 0.25 mcg/kg IV. Peak cortisol occurs at 20–30 minutes.

## Regulatory Information

No withdrawal times are available. Because clearance is rapid and there is little risk from residues, no withdrawal time is suggested for animals intended for food.

# Cyanocobalamin
sye-ahn-oh-koe-bahl'ah-min

**Trade and other names:** Cobalamin and vitamin B$_{12}$

**Functional classification:** Vitamin

## Pharmacology and Mechanism of Action
Vitamin B$_{12}$ supplement.

## Indications and Clinical Uses
Vitamin B$_{12}$ has been used to treat some conditions of anemia. Vitamin B$_{12}$ is used to manage vitamin B deficiencies associated with cobalt deficiency, inadequate intake, or intestinal malabsorption. In patients with exocrine pancreatic insufficiency or chronic enteropathies such as IBD, particularly cats, deficiency of cobalamin is common, and supplementation is recommended. Cobalamin deficiency may occur with pancreatic disease because it requires an intrinsic factor (IF) for absorption, and IF is produced by the pancreas. Deficiencies produce metabolic consequences, including anorexia, weight loss, lethargy, central and peripheral neuropathy, villous atrophy, and malabsorption of various vitamins and minerals. Oral supplementation has been effective to normalize serum cobalamin in dogs with intestinal disease.

Vitamin B$_{12}$ is a water-soluble vitamin and absorption in the intestine is a receptor-mediated process. It is dependent on the IF produced by the pancreas, and animals with intestinal disease may have difficulty with absorption. Cats are particularly susceptible because they cannot store cobalamin as well as people, and they lack the binding protein transcobalamin-1. Thus, cats have a much more rapid turnover than people. The half-life in people is 1 year, but in healthy cats, it is 11–14 days, or 4.5–5.5 days in cats with intestinal disease.

## Precautionary Information
### Adverse Reactions and Side Effects
Adverse effects are rare, except in high overdoses, because water-soluble vitamins are easily excreted in the urine.

### Contraindications and Precautions
No contraindications reported for animals.

### Drug Interactions
There are no drug interactions reported for small animals.

## Instructions for Use
Not necessary to supplement in animals with well-balanced diets. But in dogs and cats with intestinal disease, supplementation is recommended. Many cats are deficient if supplementation is not provided (explanation provided above). In these cats, weekly supplementation is recommended.

## Patient Monitoring and Laboratory Tests
Cobalamin concentrations can be measured in most laboratories. Recommended plasma/serum concentrations are 252–908 ng/L in dogs and 290–1500 ng/L in cats. Less than 160 ng/mL in cats is clearly deficient. Monitor CBC when used to treat anemia.

## Formulations

- Cyanocobalamin is available in tablets ranging from 25 to 1000 mcg. Injection formulations range from 1000 to 5000 mcg/mL (1–5 mg/mL). Vitamin B complex solutions may contain 10–100 mcg/mL of vitamin $B_{12}$.

## Stability and Storage

Store in a tightly sealed container, protected from light, and at room temperature. Stability of compounded formulations has not been evaluated.

## Small Animal Dosage

### Dogs

- 100–200 mcg/day PO or 250–500 mcg/day IM or SQ.

### Cats

- 50–100 mcg/day PO or 250 mcg IM or SQ weekly. If levels are maintained with once-weekly injections for 6 weeks, increasing the interval to 2 weeks, 4 weeks, and 6 weeks (incrementally) can be attempted.

## Large Animal Dosage

### Calves and Foals

- 500 mcg once per foal or calf twice weekly IM or SQ.

### Lambs and Pigs

- 500 mcg once per lamb or pig twice weekly IM or SQ.

### Cattle and Horses

- 1000–2000 mcg per horse or cattle once or twice weekly IM or SQ.

## Regulatory Information

No withdrawal times are available. Because clearance is rapid and there is little risk from residues, no withdrawal time is suggested for animals intended for food.

# Cyclophosphamide

sye-kloe-foss'fah-mide

**Trade and other names:** Cytoxan, Neosar, and CTX

**Functional classification:** Anticancer agent

## Pharmacology and Mechanism of Action

Cyclophosphamide is a cytotoxic anticancer agent. Cyclophosphamide is one of the oldest anticancer agents and belongs to the group of nitrogen mustards. The nitrogen mustards are alkylating agents (bifunctional alkylating agents) that alkylate various macromolecules but preferentially alkylate the N-7 of the guanine base of DNA. They are cytotoxic to cancer cells and are toxic to the rapidly dividing cells of the bone marrow. Cyclophosphamide must be metabolized to active metabolites for pharmacologic effect, which requires P450 enzyme activation. The metabolites hydroxyphosphamide and aldophosphamide are cytotoxic. Aldophosphamide is converted at the tissue site to phosphoramide mustard and acrolein. Phosphoramide mustard is responsible for the antitumor effect, and acrolein is responsible for the cytotoxic action that causes toxicity (e.g., hemorrhagic cystitis). The half-life of the parent drug in dogs is 4–6.5 hours.

## Indications and Clinical Uses

Cyclophosphamide is used primarily as an adjunct for cancer chemotherapy and as immunosuppressive therapy. Cyclophosphamide is the most potent of the nitrogen mustards. It is used in chemotherapy protocols for a variety of tumors, carcinomas, sarcomas, feline lymphoproliferative diseases, mast cell tumor, mammary carcinoma, and especially lymphoproliferative tumors (lymphoma). Cancer protocols such as cyclophosphamide, Oncovin, and prednisone (COP) and cyclophosphamide, hydroxydaunomycin, Oncovin, and prednisone (CHOP) incorporate cyclophosphamide as one of the agents.

Cyclophosphamide is also used as continuous treatment for some cancers, also known as metronomic dosing. The advantage of metronomic dosing is decreased adverse effects (lower dose), and other benefits such as decreased angiogenesis in tumors (decreased proliferation), decreased vascular endothelial growth factor (VEGF), and decreased circulating T-regulatory cells (T-reg). However, the benefits of metronomic dosing in small animals has not been established, except for some limited experience. See the dosing section for metronomic protocol.

Cyclophosphamide has been used as an immunosuppressive agent for some forms of immune-mediated disease. Although it has been used for various immune-mediated disorders in animals (immune-mediated hemolytic anemia [IMHA], pemphigus, systemic lupus erythematosus), efficacy has not been reported in controlled studies for these diseases. For treatment of IMHA ($50 \text{ mg/m}^2$), there was no benefit over prednisolone alone.

## Precautionary Information

### Adverse Reactions and Side Effects

Cyclophosphamide is toxic to the bone marrow in a dose-dependent manner. After a single large bolus dose, the nadir of toxicity occurs in 7–10 days, but the effect is reversible because stem cells are usually unaffected. Recovery usually occurs in 21–28 days. Vomiting and diarrhea may occur in some patients. Sterile, hemorrhagic cystitis is a serious and limiting complication to therapy in dogs. It is caused by the toxic effects of metabolites on the bladder epithelium (especially acrolein) that are concentrated and excreted in the urine. Various attempts are used to decrease the injury to the bladder epithelium. Corticosteroids are usually administered with cyclophosphamide to induce polyuria and decrease inflammation of the bladder. The drug mesna (Mesnex, mercaptoethane sulfonate) provides free active thiol groups to bind metabolites of cyclophosphamide in the urine. Furosemide (2.2 mg/kg) administered at the same time as the cyclophosphamide dose may decrease risk of sterile hemorrhagic cystitis. Cats are less susceptible to developing cystitis than dogs. Cyclophosphamide may cause hair loss when used in some chemotherapeutic protocols. Dogs most susceptible are those with continuously growing hair (e.g., poodles and Old English sheepdogs). Cats do not tend to lose hair from cyclophosphamide treatment.

### Contraindications and Precautions

Bone marrow suppressive and immunosuppressive. Use cautiously in animals at risk for infection. Teratogenic and embryotoxic. Do not use in pregnancy.

### Drug Interactions

Use cautiously with other drugs that may cause bone marrow suppression. Although this drug is highly metabolized to active metabolites, it is not known what effect other drugs have on enzyme activity.

C

## Instructions for Use

Cyclophosphamide is usually administered with other drugs (other cancer drugs in cancer protocols or corticosteroids when used for immunosuppressive therapy). Consult specific anticancer protocols for specific regimens. For example, the COAP protocol (COAP is a combination of cyclophosphamide, vincristine, prednisolone, and cytosine arabinoside) uses 50 mg/m$^2$ PO q48h, with vincristine, cytosine arabinoside, and prednisone for 8 weeks, but one CHOP protocol uses 100–150 mg/m$^2$ IV on the first day of the protocol followed by other drugs such as doxorubicin, vincristine, and prednisone. In dogs, the maximum tolerated dose is 500 mg/m$^2$ IV (with autologous bone marrow support).

## Patient Monitoring and Laboratory Tests

Monitor CBC in animals during treatment. Monitor urinalysis in dogs during treatment.

## Formulations

- Cyclophosphamide is available in 25-mg/mL injection and 25- and 50-mg tablets.

## Stability and Storage

Store in a tightly sealed container, protected from light, and at room temperature. Tablets are coated and should not be split to retain stability. Do not let temperatures exceed 30°C. Subject to hydrolysis in aqueous solutions. Use reconstituted solutions within 24 hours at room temperature and within 6 days if refrigerated, although some refrigerated solutions have been stable for 60 days.

## Small Animal Dosage

### Dogs

- Anticancer dosage: 50 mg/m$^2$ ($\approx$2.2 mg/kg) q48h or once daily 4 days/wk PO. Alternatively, some protocols use 150–300 mg/m$^2$ IV and repeat in 21 days.
- Metronomic dosage (continuous administration to suppress T cells): 10–15 mg/m$^2$ q24h PO (approximately 0.3 mg/kg).
- Immunosuppressive therapy: Dogs: 50 mg/m$^2$ q48h PO or 2.2 mg/kg once daily for 4 days/wk.
- Pulse therapy: 200–250 mg/m$^2$ (10 mg/kg) once every 3 weeks. Dividing the 250-mg/m$^2$ dose into three treatments over 3 days may reduce risk of sterile hemorrhagic cystitis.

### Cats

- 6.25–12.5 mg/cat once daily 4 days/wk, PO. In some protocols, the dosage has been increased to 25 mg per cat twice per week PO. Alternatively, doses of 200 mg/m$^2$ have been used.

## Large Animal Dosage

- No dose has been reported for large animals.

## Regulatory Information

Withdrawal times are not established for animals that produce food. This drug should not be used in animals intended for food because it is an anticancer agent.

# Cyclosporine, Cyclosporin A

sye′kloe-spor-een

**Trade and other names:** Atopica (veterinary preparation), Neoral (human preparation), Sandimmune, Optimmune (ophthalmic), Gengraf, and generic brands. In the United States, it is called cyclosporine; the international name is ciclosporin.

**Functional classification:** Immunosuppressive drug

## Pharmacology and Mechanism of Action

Cyclosporine is a commonly used immunosuppressive drug. Cyclosporine binds to a specific cellular receptor on calcineurin and inhibits the T-cell receptor–activated signal transduction pathway. Particularly important are its effects to suppress interleukin-2 (IL-2) and other cytokines (e.g., IL-4 and tumor necrosis factor–alpha) and block proliferation of activated T lymphocytes. The action of cyclosporine is more specific for T cells compared with B cells and affects both helper T cells and cytotoxic T cells. Production of autoantibodies by B cells may be suppressed because this process requires the help of activated T cells. Therefore, calcineurin inhibitors such as cyclosporine may decrease humoral immune response by interfering with T-helper cells instead of interfering directly.

Cyclosporine also inhibits the mitochondrial permeability-transition pores that may attenuate myocardial injury during reperfusion.

*Pharmacokinetics:* The half-lives of cyclosporine are 8–9 hours (average) in dogs and 8–10 hours (average) in cats. However, there is high variability on both species. Oral absorption is low (20%–30%) and may be affected by food and drug interactions. Peak concentration after oral administration occurs at 1–2 hours. The average peak concentration (with high variability) in dogs is approximately 900 ng/mL (600–1200 ng/mL) at 5 mg/kg.

## Indications and Clinical Uses

Systemic uses (usually oral) for cyclosporine include IMHA, atopic dermatitis in dogs, and perianal fistulas. Other diseases have been treated with cyclosporine, such as sebaceous adenitis, idiopathic sterile nodular panniculitis, vesicular cutaneous lupus erythematosus, IMHA, immune-mediated thrombocytopenia, IBD, immune-mediated polyarthritis, myasthenia gravis, idiopathic chronic hepatitis, and aplastic anemia. It has also been used for treatment of granulomatous meningoencephalitis (3–6 mg/kg q12h). For many of these indications, efficacy has not been established through well-controlled clinical studies, and the use is based on anecdotal experience and recommendations from clinical experts.

In dogs, there is strong evidence for effective treatment of atopic dermatitis, for which there is similar efficacy as prednisolone. Treatment response may be delayed for 2 weeks and for as long as 4 weeks in some dogs. During this induction time, it is acceptable to administer other medications (e.g., corticosteroids or oclacitinib) to control pruritus in dogs with atopic dermatitis. There is minimal effectiveness for immune-mediated pemphigus foliaceus (PF) in dogs, but it may have benefits for treating PF in cats. In dogs, some dermatologists have reported improved efficacy when combined with azathioprine for immune-mediated diseases (e.g., PF). Cyclosporine use for keratoconjunctivitis sicca is limited to topical administration.

In cats, cyclosporine has shown beneficial effects for treatment of EGC, IBD, atopic dermatitis (60% effective), oral stomatitis, and airway disease (feline asthma). Cyclosporine (Atopica for cats) is approved for control of feline allergic dermatitis. Higher doses are needed in cats compared with dogs because the oral absorption is more variable. In horses, it is effective as a localized treatment of anterior uveitis.

## Precautionary Information

### Adverse Reactions and Side Effects

The most common adverse effects in dogs and cats are GI problems (vomiting, diarrhea, anorexia, and weight loss). Vomiting is often observed only during initial treatment and may be transient. Hypersalivation has been observed in cats. Cyclosporine may induce shedding of hair and stimulate new hair growth in dogs of a different consistency. Neurotoxicity from high doses has been seen in dogs, which can be seen as tremors. However, this is uncommon from recommended doses. Although kidney injury has been reported with older formulations, it has not been reported from use of current formulations of cyclosporine. Less commonly, cyclosporine can produce gingival proliferation (gingival hyperplasia) in animals, which is caused by a growth factor-mediated proliferation of gingival tissues. There are some reports that administration of azithromycin has been successful to resolve gingival hyperplasia. Occasionally, gingivitis and periodontitis may occur, which can be reversed after discontinuing the drug. There is no confirmed evidence that cyclosporine is a risk factor for neoplasia in dogs or cats.

Calcineurin inhibitors can inhibit pancreatic beta cells and increase risk of diabetes in people. It may increase tissue insulin resistance and impair insulin production or secretion to increase glycemia. However, diabetes has not been reported in pets from clinical use of cyclosporine.

Papillomas have been observed in dogs with chronic use. Unlike other immunosuppressive drugs, it does not cause myelosuppression. Cyclosporine may increase thromboxane $TXA_2$ in platelets and increase platelet activation, but increased risk of thromboembolism has not been associated with cyclosporine treatment in dogs or cats. Aspirin can block this response.

*Effect on vaccination:* At three times the clinical dose, it did not affect the immune response to killed rabies vaccine in dogs, but it failed to increase antibody titers from live parvovirus vaccine. Cats treated with cyclosporine, even at high doses, are capable of mounting a memory humoral immune response to booster vaccination (feline calicivirus, parvovirus, feline leukemia virus [FeLV], feline herpesvirus type 1 [FHV-1], and rabies) that is adequate for protection. However, at high doses, a primary humoral response was not observed within 4 weeks of exposure to a novel antigen (feline immunodeficiency virus [FIV]). Therefore, naïve cats vaccinated before cyclosporine treatment should be able to mount an adequate primary immune response, and subsequent cyclosporine treatment should not affect immune response from booster vaccinations.

*Effect on infections in cats:* Administration to cats at 7.5 mg/kg did not increase the severity of infection by *Toxoplasma gondii* in cats that were previously exposed (seropositive). However, administration of cyclosporine to cats that are naïve (seronegative) may increase the severity of *T. gondii* infection. Naïve cats may have a greater risk of developing clinical toxoplasmosis if they become infected while receiving cyclosporine treatment. Do not administer to cats infected with FeLV or FIV. In cats infected with FHV-1, administration of cyclosporine activated the infection, but the disease was mild and self-limited in most cats.

## Contraindications and Precautions

At high doses, cyclosporine has produced embryotoxic and fetotoxic effects in laboratory animals. It is not recommended to administer to pregnant animals, but there are no specific reports on adverse effects on pregnancy in dogs or cats. It is excreted in milk of lactating animals. Warn animal owners to keep out of reach of children. If used with other drugs, consult the Drug Interactions section for possible interference. A withdrawal time prior to allergen-specific allergy testing in dogs is not necessary.

**Drug Interactions**

Cimetidine, erythromycin, diltiazem, itraconazole, fluconazole, clarithromycin, or ketoconazole may increase cyclosporine concentrations when used concurrently. Dosages of ketoconazole of 2.5–10 mg/kg/day in dogs have been shown to substantially decrease the clearance of cyclosporine and reduce the required dose by one half or more. Grapefruit juice also inhibits clearance and reduces the required dose, although high doses are needed. For example, 10 g of powdered whole grapefruit is needed in dogs to substantially affect exposure (such a large dose of 42 capsules is impractical). Food decreases oral absorption by 15%–22%. Metoclopramide and rifampin (and possibly other drugs that induce enzymes) will lower cyclosporine blood concentrations. There is no evidence that cyclosporine enhances or inhibits allergen-specific immunotherapy (ASIT) treatment.

## Instructions for Use

Atopica (veterinary) and Neoral (human) are identical formulations except the sizes of capsules vary. After animals have been treated with initial doses (see the dosing section) and are stable, doses may be adjusted by increasing the interval to once every other day or every third day rather than lowering the daily dose. Individual doses may be adjusted by monitoring blood concentrations, but monitoring is not necessary for routine use. Most of the experience is with the approved dose to treat atopic dermatitis and allergic dermatitis with doses of 5 mg/kg in dogs and 7 mg/kg in cats. When used to treat animals for immune-mediated disease and organ transplantation, the doses are generally higher, often administered twice daily, and the blood concentrations maintained at a higher level.

Atopica and Neoral oral products are absorbed more predictably than Sandimmune, which is no longer recommended. Atopica and Neoral may produce 50% higher blood concentrations in some patients or reduce the variability in absorption that was associated with the Sandimmune formulations. The injectable formulation has been used infrequently in dogs and cats. It may produce some injection-site reactions such as hair loss, crusts, or injection-site swelling.

There are more than 20 human generic formulations, but none has been tested for bioequivalence in dogs or cats. There is one generic formulation approved for dogs, which is bioequivalent to the proprietary brand. Feeding may reduce oral absorption in dogs but does not decrease efficacy. For cats, it is recommended to administer with food if it does not affect their appetite. If necessary, the oral solution can be diluted to make it more palatable.

To reduce the dose or increase blood concentrations, some veterinarians have administered ketoconazole or other enzyme-inhibiting compounds concurrently.

## Patient Monitoring and Laboratory Tests

Although routine blood concentration monitoring is not necessary, it may be helpful to identify drug interactions, poor absorption, adverse reactions, or poor compliance. However, there has been no correlations established between blood concentrations in dogs and cats and clinical response. When monitoring, collect whole blood in ethylenediaminetetraacetic acid (EDTA; purple top) tube for submission to laboratory. Suggested trough blood concentration range (whole blood assay) is 300–400 ng/mL, although in some studies, levels as low as 200 ng/mL have been effective. Peak concentrations (collected at approximately 2 hours after oral administration of 5 mg/kg) should be in the range of 600–1200 ng/mL. Consult the laboratory to determine if the laboratory result is specific or if it also measures inactive metabolites and requires a conversion. Cyclosporine does not interfere with intradermal skin testing.

## Formulations
- Cyclosporine is available in 10-, 25-, 50-, and 100-mg capsules (Atopica) and 25- and 100-mg microemulsion capsules.
- There is one FDA-approved generic formulation of cyclosporine for dogs, which has shown to be bioequivalent with the proprietary form (original brand). It is approved in the same size capsules as the original formulation.
- Atopica for cats is available as a 100-mg/mL oral solution as a microemulsion. This may be mixed with the cat's food if it does not affect their appetite.
- Human forms are also available as a 100-mg/mL oral solution (Neoral, for microemulsion); 100-mg/mL oral solution and 25- and 100-mg capsules (Sandimmune); and 0.2% ophthalmic ointment (Optimmune). Generic human capsules are available (e.g., Gengraf). The human generic formulations are therapeutically equivalent in people but have not been compared in dogs or cats to Atopica.

## Stability and Storage
Store in a tightly sealed container, protected from light, and at room temperature. It does not require refrigeration but store below 30°C. Freezing capsules at –20°C for 28 days did not affect stability or oral absorption. Compounded ophthalmic products are stable at room temperature for 60 days, but do not refrigerate.

## Small Animal Dosage
### Dogs
- 3–7 mg/kg/day PO. The typical starting dosage is 5 mg/kg/day PO. After the induction period, some dogs with atopic dermatitis have been controlled with dosages as low as 5 mg/kg every other day to every third day.
- For perianal fistulas and immune-mediated diseases (e.g., IMHA), higher doses and more frequent administration have been used (5–8 mg/kg q12h). When a response is observed, the dose and frequency can be reduced.
- For immune suppression associated with organ transplantation, doses should be higher (e.g., 7–10 mg/kg q12h PO).
- IBD: 5 mg/kg PO q12h; then reduce the frequency to q24h after a response is observed.
- Idiopathic chronic hepatitis: 5–8 mg/kg/day, PO.

### Cats
- 7.5 mg/kg per day PO. Some cats can be controlled with administration of this dose every other day or twice weekly. Administer on a small amount of food or at the time of feeding, but if mixed with food, some cats may refuse to eat.
- For immune suppression associated with organ transplantation, doses should be higher (e.g., 3–5 mg/kg q12h PO).

## Large Animal Dosage
- Only local administration has been used in horses (ocular). No other dose has been reported for large animals.

## Regulatory Information
Withdrawal times are not established for animals that produce food. This drug should not be used in animals intended for food because it may have mutagenic potential.

---

# Cyproheptadine Hydrochloride
sih′proe-hep′tah-deen hye-droe-klor′ide

**Trade and other names:** Periactin

**Functional classification:** Antihistamine

## Pharmacology and Mechanism of Action

Cyproheptadine is a phenothiazine with antihistamine and antiserotonin properties. It is not used as a serotonin antagonist in animals but has been used as appetite stimulant (probably by altering serotonin activity in appetite center).

## Indications and Clinical Uses

A common use of cyproheptadine is to stimulate the appetite in sick animals, especially cats, although, evidence based on controlled studies to demonstrate efficacy is not available. For dogs and cats, other appetite stimulants are preferred: mirtazapine for cats and capromorelin for dogs.

Cyproheptadine is used in some cats for treatment of feline asthma if serotonin is considered a component of the airway inflammation. However, in cats with hyperresponsive airways, cyproheptadine failed to reduce eosinophilic inflammation (8 mg per cat q12h). It has been used in some instances for treating inappropriate urination (urine spraying) in cats. Cyproheptadine has been used to treat head shaking in horses. Cyproheptadine has been used to treat equine pituitary pars intermedia dysfunction (Cushing syndrome) at 0.6–1.2 mg/kg, but results have been controversial. It is not effective for treatment of canine pituitary-dependent hyperadrenocorticism (Cushing syndrome). It has been considered as a treatment for animals that have "serotonin syndrome" from antidepressant drugs, although efficacy has not been documented for this use.

## Precautionary Information

### Adverse Reactions and Side Effects

Cyproheptadine may stimulate hunger. It can cause polyphagia and weight gain. Cyproheptadine also has antihistamine effects, antiserotonin effects, and antimuscarinic effects. In some cats, it has stimulated hyperactivity. In horses, it has been used at high doses without adverse effects.

### Contraindications and Precautions

None reported for animals.

### Drug Interactions

There are no drug interactions reported for small animals.

## Instructions for Use

Clinical studies have not been performed in veterinary medicine. Use is based primarily on empiricism and extrapolation from human results. Syrup contains 5% alcohol.

## Patient Monitoring and Laboratory Tests

Monitor weight gain in animals.

## Formulations Available

- Cyproheptadine is available in 4-mg tablets and 2-mg/5-mL syrup.

## Stability and Storage

Store in a tightly sealed container, protected from light, and at room temperature. Do not freeze the syrup. Stability of compounded formulations has not been evaluated.

## Small Animal Dosage

### Dogs and Cats

- Antihistamine: 0.5–1.1 mg/kg q8–12h PO or 2–4 mg/cat PO q12–24h.
- Appetite stimulant: 2 mg/cat PO.

- Feline asthma: 1–2 mg/cat PO q12h.
- Use for inappropriate urination: 2 mg/cat q12h PO; then reduce dosage to 1 mg/cat q12h PO.

### Large Animal Dosage

**Horses**

- 0.5 mg/kg q12h PO.
- Head shaking: 0.3 mg/kg q12h, PO.

### Regulatory Information

No regulatory information is available. For extralabel use withdrawal interval estimates, contact FARAD at www.FARAD.org.

RCI Classification: 4

# Cytarabine

sye-tare′ah-been

**Trade and other names:** Cytosar, Ara-C, and cytosine arabinoside

**Functional classification:** Anticancer agent

### Pharmacology and Mechanism of Action

Cytarabine is an anticancer agent that is also used for immunosuppressive treatment. Cytarabine (Cytosar) is a compound isolated from a sea sponge. It has also been referred to as *cytosine arabinoside* and *Ara-C*. Cytarabine is metabolized to an active drug that inhibits DNA synthesis. Cytarabine is an antimetabolite synthetic nucleoside analogue. Cytarabine A inhibits DNA polymerase in mitotically active cells and produces topoisomerase dysfunction and prevents DNA repair. This action produces the anticancer effects and immunosuppressive properties.

*Pharmacokinetics:* The half-life in dogs is approximately 70 minutes. When administered to dogs, the terminal half-lives of cytarabine are 1.35 hours and 1.15 hours after SQ and CRI, respectively. Peak concentrations are 2.9 mcg/mL and 2.8 mcg/mL after SQ and CRI administration, respectively.

### Indications and Clinical Uses

Cytarabine has been used for lymphoma, leukemia, and myelogenous leukemia in various anticancer drug protocols. It is usually administered as an IM or SQ injection because it has a short half-life ($\approx$20 minutes) when administered IV.

It has also been administered to dogs for treatment of granulomatous meningoencephalomyelitis as an alternative to corticosteroids. Cytarabine penetrates the blood–CSF barrier of dogs and has been reported to improve the temporary and long-term remission and prognosis for dogs diagnosed with meningoencephalitis. Two protocols are used for this indication (see the dosing section). When administered via CRI to dogs, it maintains steady-state concentrations better than a SQ injection.

### Precautionary Information

**Adverse Reactions and Side Effects**

Cytarabine is bone marrow suppressive and can cause granulocytopenia, especially when delivered via CRIs. In addition, it may cause nausea and vomiting.

**Contraindications and Precautions**
Use cautiously in animals administered other bone marrow–suppressing drugs.
**Drug Interactions**
There are no drug interactions reported for small animals.

## Instructions for Use

Cytarabine has been administered to dogs using a variety of protocols (see the dosing section), depending on the study published and dependent on clinician preference. There is not strong evidence that one protocol is superior to another. When treating granulomatous meningoencephalomyelitis, dose protocols (either IV or SQ) have used total doses of 200–400 mg/m² total dose, divided over 2 days, either as SQ injections twice daily for 2 days or an IV infusion with the total dose given over 8 hours.

The dose of cytarabine commonly used in the treatment of meningoencephalitis is a total dose of 200 mg/m², which is lower than that used in the treatment of neoplasia (total dose of 400–600 mg/m²). For meningoencephalitis, veterinary neurologists have recommended 200 mg/m² administered either as four SQ injections of 50 mg/m² given over 2 days or CRI IV administration at 25 mg/m² per hour for 8 hours.

## Patient Monitoring and Laboratory Tests

Monitor CBC to assess toxicity.

## Formulations

- Cytarabine is available in a 100-mg vial for injection.

**Stability and Storage**
Store in a tightly sealed container, protected from light, and at room temperature. Stability of compounded formulations has not been evaluated.

**Small Animal Dosage**
*Dogs (Cancer Protocols, Administered Weekly)*
- 100–150 mg/m² once daily or 50 mg/m² twice daily, each given for 4 days IV or SQ.
- 600 mg/m² IV or SQ, single dose.
- 300 mg/m² per day as a continuous IV infusion over 48 hours (600 mg/m² total).

*Dogs (Granulomatous Meningoencephalomyelitis)*
- 50 mg/m² twice daily for 2 days and repeated every 3 weeks SQ.
- 200 mg/m² total dose administered as 50 mg/m² given four times over 2 days SQ or CRI IV administration at 25 mg/m² per hour for 8 hours.

**Cats**
- 100 mg/m² once daily for 2 days.

## Large Animal Dosage

- No dose has been reported for large animals.

## Regulatory Information

Withdrawal times are not established for animals that produce food. This drug should not be used in animals intended for food because it is an anticancer agent.

# Dacarbazine
dah-kar′bah-zeen

**Trade and other names:** DTIC

**Functional classification:** Anticancer agent

## Pharmacology and Mechanism of Action
Dacarbazine is an anticancer agent used to treat certain types of cancer and as a rescue agent when other anticancer drugs have become ineffective. Dacarbazine, also known as DTIC, acts as a monofunctional alkylating agent; thus, it effectively blocks RNA synthesis. Its action is cell-cycle nonspecific. Its pharmacokinetics are poorly understood in animals. It is a prodrug that is activated to the active anticancer agent by cytochrome P450 enzymes. Differences in enzymes among animals may account for large variation in response among animals.

## Indications and Clinical Uses
DTIC has been primarily used for malignant melanoma and lymphoreticular neoplasms. It is rarely used as a primary agent but is used in protocols with other agents and after other drugs have become ineffective.

## Precautionary Information

**Adverse Reactions and Side Effects**

The most common adverse effects are leukopenia, nausea, vomiting, and diarrhea.

**Contraindications and Precautions**

Do not use in cats.

**Drug Interactions**

There are no drug interactions reported for small animals.

## Instructions for Use
Consult specific anticancer protocol for specific regimens. These are available from oncologists, and oncology textbooks.

## Patient Monitoring and Laboratory Tests
Monitor complete blood count (CBC) during treatment.

## Formulations
- DTIC is available in a 200-mg vial for injection. Dilute the solution in 50–100 mL of 0.9% normal saline for injection.

## Stability and Storage
Store in a tightly sealed container, protected from light, and at room temperature. Stability of compounded formulations has not been evaluated.

## Small Animal Dosage
**Dogs**
- 200 mg/m$^2$ for 5 days every 3 weeks IV or 800–1000 mg/m$^2$ every 3 weeks IV.

## Large Animal Dosage
- No dose has been reported for large animals.

## Regulatory Information
Withdrawal times are not established for animals that produce food. This drug should not be used in animals intended for food because it is an anticancer agent.

---

# Dalteparin
dahl'tah-pare-in

**Trade and other names:** Fragmin and low-molecular-weight heparin

**Functional classification:** Anticoagulant

## Pharmacology and Mechanism of Action
Low-molecular-weight heparin (LMWH), also known as fragmented heparin. LMWH is characterized by a molecular weight of approximately 5000 compared with conventional heparin (unfractionated heparin, or UFH), which has a molecular weight of approximately 15,000. This difference in molecular size affects the absorption, clearance, and activity of LMWH compared to UFH. LMWHs produce their effect by binding to antithrombin (AT) and increasing AT III–mediated inhibition of synthesis and activity of coagulation factor Xa. However, LMWH, unlike conventional heparin, produces less inhibition of thrombin (factor IIa). LMWH's activity is described by the antifactor Xa:anti-factor IIa ratio. For dalteparin, the ratio is 2.7:1 (the conventional UFH ratio is 1:1).

*Pharmacokinetics:* In people, LMWHs have several advantages compared with UFH and include greater anti-Xa/IIa activity, more complete and predictable absorption from injection, longer duration, less frequent administration, reduced risk of bleeding, and a more predictable anticoagulant response. However, in dogs and cats, the half-life of LMWH is much shorter than in humans, reducing some of this advantage. In dogs, the half-life of dalteparin is approximately 2 hours; in cats, it is estimated to be 1.5 hours, which requires much more frequent administration in either species to maintain anti-Xa activity compared to humans.

LMWHs used in veterinary medicine include tinzaparin (Innohep), enoxaparin (Lovenox), and dalteparin (Fragmin).

## Indications and Clinical Uses
Dalteparin, like other LMWHs, is used to treat hypercoagulability disorders and prevent coagulation disorders such as thromboembolism, venous thrombosis, disseminated intravascular coagulopathy (DIC), and pulmonary thromboembolism. Clinical indications are derived from uses of conventional heparin and studies of LMWH in experimental animals or extrapolated from human medicine. In people, enoxaparin has largely replaced dalteparin for routine use.

There has been a lack of clinical studies to evaluate efficacy of LMWH in animals, and there is no clear benefit of LMWH in animals compared with conventional heparin. Doses extrapolated from humans may not be accurate for achieving adequate and consistent anti-Xa activity in dogs and cats. Doses listed in the dosing section are primarily derived from experimental healthy animals.

**D**

## Precautionary Information

### Adverse Reactions and Side Effects

Although better tolerated than regular heparin, bleeding is a risk. LMWHs are associated with a lower incidence of heparin-induced thrombocytopenia (HIT) in people, but HIT from any form of heparin has not been a clinical problem in animals. If excessive anticoagulation and bleeding occur as a result of an overdose, protamine sulfate should be administered to reverse heparin therapy. The protamine dose is 1.0 mg of protamine for every 100 units of dalteparin administered by slow IV infusion. Protamine complexes with heparin to form a stable, inactive compound.

### Contraindications and Precautions

Do not administer IM because it increases a risk of a hematoma at the injection site. Administer SQ only. LMWH is excreted by renal clearance in animals; therefore, if renal disease is present, the elimination will be prolonged. Rebound hypercoagulability may occur after discontinuation of heparin treatment; therefore, it may be advised to taper the dose slowly when discontinuing treatment.

### Drug Interactions

Do not mix with other injectable drugs. Use cautiously in animals that are already receiving other drugs that can interfere with coagulation, such as aspirin, clopidogrel, and warfarin. Although a specific interaction has not been identified, use cautiously in animals that may be receiving certain chondroprotective compounds such as glycosaminoglycans for treatment of arthritis. Some antibiotics, such as cephalosporins, may inhibit coagulation.

## Instructions for Use

Dosing recommendations extrapolated from human medicine are not appropriate for animals, and animal-specific dosing recommendations should be used. Animal owners should be warned that LMWHs are expensive compared with conventional heparin. When dosing, do not interchange doses on a unit-for-unit basis with other heparins.

## Patient Monitoring and Laboratory Tests

Monitor patients for clinical signs of bleeding problems. When administering LMWH, activated partial thromboplastin time (aPTT) and prothrombin time (PT) clotting times are not reliable indicators of therapy, although prolonged aPTT is a sign of overdosing. In people, a-Xa activity is considered the preferred laboratory measure of LMWH activity. However, in studies in which anti-Xa activity was monitored in dogs, it resulted in inconsistent attainment of the targeted range. If the anti-Xa activity is measured, the peak anti-Xa activity occurs 2 hours after dosing, and the target ranges for anti-Xa activity should be 0.5–1.0 units/mL for cats and 0.4–0.8 units/mL for dogs.

## Formulations

- Dalteparin is available in 2500 units of antifactor Xa (16 mg dalteparin sodium) per 0.2 mL in a single-dose syringe, 5000 units of antifactor Xa (32 mg dalteparin sodium) per 0.2 mL in a single-dose syringe, and 10,000 units of antifactor Xa (64 mg dalteparin sodium) per milliliter in a 9.5-mL multiple-dose vial.

## Stability and Storage

Use multiple-dose vial within 2 weeks of initial penetration. Store in a tightly sealed container protected from light.

## Small Animal Dosage
### Dogs
- 150–175 units/kg q8h SQ (see Patient Monitoring and Laboratory Tests for dose adjustment).

### Cats
- 75 units/kg SQ q6h. This dosage may be increased to 150–175 units/kg q4h SQ and up to 180 units/kg q6h, SQ (see Patient Monitoring and Laboratory Tests for dose adjustment).

## Large Animal Dosage
### Horses
- 50 units/kg/day SQ. High-risk patients should receive 100 units/kg/day.

## Regulatory Information
Extralabel withdrawal times are not established. However, 24-hour withdrawal times are suggested because this drug has little risk from residues.

# Danazol
dan′ah-zole

**Trade and other names:** Danocrine

**Functional classification:** Hormone

## Pharmacology and Mechanism of Action
Dalteparin is a gonadotropin inhibitor. It suppresses luteinizing hormone and follicle-stimulating hormone and estrogen synthesis.

Danazol has been used as adjunctive treatment for immune-mediated blood disorders, but the efficacy has not been demonstrated through clinical studies. Its mechanism of action for treating immune-mediated diseases is not understood, but it may interfere with antibody production or the binding of complement or antibody to the platelet or red blood cell. It may also reduce receptors on monocytes for antibodies bound to platelets or red blood cells.

## Indications and Clinical Uses
Danazol has hormone effects (antiestrogen) that are used for endometriosis in women. Danazol (Danocrine) also has been used for treating refractory patients with immune-mediated thrombocytopenia and immune-mediated hemolytic anemia. However, available evidence does not show a benefit in dogs when it has been used to treat immune-mediated hemolytic anemia.

## Precautionary Information
### Adverse Reactions and Side Effects
Danazol's androgenic effects should be considered in treated animals. However, adverse effects have not been reported in animals.

### Contraindications and Precautions
It is absolutely contraindicated in pregnancy.

### Drug Interactions
It has been used with other drugs in the treatment of immune-mediated diseases without reported interactions.

## Instructions for Use
When used to treat autoimmune disease, it is usually used in conjunction with other drugs (e.g., corticosteroids).

## Patient Monitoring and Laboratory Tests
Monitor CBC if used for treatment of immune-mediated diseases.

## Formulations
• Danazol is available in 50-, 100-, and 200-mg capsules.

**D**

## Stability and Storage
Store in a tightly sealed container, protected from light, and at room temperature. Stability of compounded formulations has not been evaluated.

## Small Animal Dosage
**Dogs and Cats**
• 5–10 mg/kg q12h PO.

## Large Animal Dosage
• No dose has been reported for large animals.

## Regulatory Information
Danazol is an anabolic agent and should not be administered to animals intended for food.

Racing Commissioners International (RCI) Classification: 4

---

# Danofloxacin Mesylate
dan-oh-floks´ah-sin mess´ih-late

**Trade and other names:** Advocin (A180 is former name)

**Functional classification:** Antibacterial

## Pharmacology and Mechanism of Action
Danofloxacin, like other fluoroquinolones, has activity against a broad spectrum of bacteria, including gram-negative bacilli, especially Enterobacteriaceae (*Escherichia coli, Klebsiella,* and *Salmonella* spp.) and some gram-positive cocci, such as *Staphylococcus* spp. In particular, it has good activity against pathogens in cattle, such as *Pasteurella multocida, Mannheimia haemolytica,* and *Histophilus somni.*

*Pharmacokinetics:* In cattle, SQ absorption is high. Half-life is 3–6 hours. When used to treat bovine respiratory disease (BRD) in cattle at a dose of 6 mg/kg, danofloxacin had a half-life of 4.2 hours and a peak concentration of 1.7 mcg/mL and produced area under the curve (AUC): minimum inhibitory concentration (MIC) ratio greater than 125.

## Indications and Clinical Uses
Danofloxacin is indicated for the treatment of BRD caused by *P. multocida, M. haemolytica,* and *H. somni.* As a fluoroquinolone with a broad spectrum of activity, other organisms are susceptible. However, extralabel use for other diseases in animals intended for food is prohibited. There are no published reports of danofloxacin use in other animals except some exotic and zoo animals.

## Precautionary Information

### Adverse Reactions and Side Effects

All fluoroquinolones at high concentrations may cause central nervous system (CNS) toxicity. In safety studies in cattle, when high doses were administered, they caused lameness, articular cartilage lesions, and CNS problems (tremors, nystagmus). SQ injections may cause tissue irritation. All of the fluoroquinolones have a potential to produce arthropathy in young animals, and during field trials, danofloxacin was associated with lameness in some calves. Fluoroquinolones have caused blindness in cats, but this has not been reported in any species from danofloxacin.

### Contraindications and Precautions

Do not inject more than 15 mL in one site. Do not use extralabel. Do not use in other species for which safety information is not available. Do not use in animals prone to seizures.

### Drug Interactions

Fluoroquinolones may increase concentrations of other drugs used concurrently through inhibition of drug metabolism, but this has not been shown for danofloxacin. Do not mix in solutions or in vials with aluminum, calcium, iron, or zinc because chelation may occur.

## Instructions for Use

Inject SQ in neck of cattle.

## Patient Monitoring and Laboratory Tests

No specific monitoring is necessary. Clinical and Laboratory Standards Institute (CLSI) breakpoints for sensitive organisms are ≤0.25 mcg/mL for cattle respiratory pathogens. Most organisms have MIC values ≤0.06 mcg/mL.

## Formulations

- Danofloxacin is available in an injectable solution of 180 mg/mL (with 2-pyrrolidone and polyvinyl alcohol).

## Stability and Storage

Store below 30°C, protected from light, and protected from freezing. A slight yellow or amber color is acceptable.

## Small Animal Dosage

### Dogs and Cats

- No small animal dose has been reported.

## Large Animal Dosage

### Cattle

- 6 mg/kg (1.5 mL per 100 lb) once per 48 hours SQ. Or 8 mg/kg, single injection.

### Equine and Swine

- No dose has been reported.

## Regulatory Information

Do not use in calves intended for veal.
Cattle withdrawal time (for meat): 4 days. Not established for milk because it cannot be used in lactating cattle. It is prohibited to use extralabel in food-producing animals.

# Dantrolene Sodium
dan´troe-leen soe´dee-um

**Trade and other names:** Dantrium, Revonto, Ryanodex

**Functional classification:** Muscle relaxant

**D**

## Pharmacology and Mechanism of Action
Dantrolene is used as a muscle relaxant, especially in animals undergoing anesthesia. Dantrolene inhibits calcium leakage from sarcoplasmic reticulum. It is specific for the *RyR1* isoform (sarcoplasmic reticulum channel) in skeletal muscle and *RyR3* in smooth muscle, with minimal effect on the *RyR2* in cardiac muscle. By inhibiting calcium initiation of muscle contraction, it relaxes muscle.

*Pharmacokinetics:* In horses, after oral administration, the half-life of dantrolene was 3–4 hours with a variable peak at 1–6 hours. In dogs, the half-life is 1.25 hours, and pharmacokinetics are markedly different than in people.

## Indications and Clinical Uses
Dantrolene is used as a muscle relaxant. However, in addition to muscle relaxation, it has been used to treat muscle excitability associated with malignant hyperthermia, and it also has been used to relax urethral muscle in cats. Although it has been used in dogs, the efficacy has not been shown, and pharmacokinetic studies show that at a dose of 2.8 mg/kg, it does not produce concentration high enough for activity in canine muscle. Although used as an immunosuppressive agent (via nuclear factor of activated thymocytes [NFAT]–regulated cytokine suppression), it is unlikely to be effective for this use.

In horses, it has improved clinical signs associated with exertional rhabdomyolysis ("tying up"). However, this effect on rhabdomyolysis is mostly based on anecdotal accounts because there are no clinical studies that demonstrate efficacy. It has reduced the release of muscle enzymes (creatine kinase). It can potentially prevent muscle damage in healthy horses. It has been used as a preanesthetic in horses to prevent anesthetic myopathy, but the optimum dose for this problem is undetermined.

## Precautionary Information

### Adverse Reactions and Side Effects
Muscle relaxants can cause weakness in some animals. In people, dantrolene is known to cause muscle weakness, dyspnea, dysphagia, and dizziness. Use of dantrolene in people also has caused hepatitis in some cases. In horses, when administered prior to anesthesia at a dose of 6 mg/kg PO (premedication), it increased plasma potassium concentrations and increased risk of bradycardia and arrhythmias in some horses. Hyperkalemia from dantrolene also has been observed in dogs and pigs.

### Contraindications and Precautions
Do not use in animals with hepatic disease. Use with caution in weak or debilitated animals.

### Drug Interactions
Do not mix or reconstitute the IV solution with acidic solutions because they are incompatible.

## Instructions for Use

It is usually recommended that oral doses should be given on an empty stomach. Doses have been primarily extrapolated from experimental studies or extrapolation of human studies. Few studies are available in veterinary medicine to guide optimum dosing. To relax the urethra in cats, the most effective dose is 1 mg/kg IV.

Equine use has been for muscle relaxation prior to surgery or for exertional rhabdomyolysis. For equine use, the human oral form (usually capsules) is dissolved in water and administered by the oral route. Alternatively, an oral paste can be made from the capsules and administered by the oral route. Capsules and paste formulations are absorbed equally. When administering injections of dantrolene for treatment of malignant hyperthermia in large animals, clinicians should be aware that injectable forms can be expensive, and several vials may be needed because of dilute solution in each vial.

## Patient Monitoring and Laboratory Tests

When used for treatment of malignant hyperthermia, monitor body temperature, acid–base balance, and electrolytes. In people, dantrolene may cause hepatitis, and tests of liver injury (e.g., liver enzymes) and function are monitored. Dantrolene can cause a persistent increase in plasma potassium concentration during anesthesia. The increase in potassium may lead to cardia arrhythmias and should be monitored.

## Formulations

- Dantrolene is available in 100-mg capsules; when reconstituted, the 20-mg vial is equal to 0.33 mg/mL injection. Also available as a more concentrated single-dose vial containing 250 mg reconstituted to 50 mg/mL.

## Stability and Storage

When IV solution is prepared, it is stable for a short time (6 hours). It may be mixed with solutions such as 5% dextrose and 0.9% sodium chloride for IV use. Do not use IV solution if cloudiness or precipitation is present in vial. Compounded oral suspensions are stable for 150 days if mixed with acid solutions (e.g., citric acid). Store in a tightly sealed container, protected from light, and at room temperature.

## Small Animal Dosage

### Dogs

Note: Doses cited below for dogs are from anecdotal experience and extrapolation from humans. Pharmacokinetic studies suggest that these doses are unlikely to produce concentrations high enough to be effective in canine muscle.
- Prevention of malignant hyperthermia: 2–3 mg/kg IV (up to 5–10 mg/kg).
- Malignant hyperthermia crisis: doses of 2.5–3 mg/kg IV rapid bolus (up to 5–10 mg/kg).
- Muscle relaxation: 1–5 mg/kg q8h PO (up to 5–10 mg/kg).
- Urethral relaxation: 1–5 mg/kg q8h PO or 0.5–1.0 mg/kg IV (up to 5–10 mg/kg).

### Cats

- Muscle relaxation: 0.5–2 mg/kg q12h PO.
- Relaxation of urethra: 1–2 mg/kg q8h PO.

## Large Animal Dosage

### Horses

- The most common dose is 500 mg PO per horse, but alternatively, a dose of 4 mg/kg PO has been used in some studies.

### Pigs

- Malignant hyperthermia: 1–3 mg/kg IV once.
- Prophylaxis: 5 mg/kg PO.

## Regulatory Information

For horses, there is a recommended 48- and 168-hour withdrawal time prior to racing for detection in plasma and urine, respectively. For food animals, no regulatory information is available. For extralabel use withdrawal interval estimates, contact Food Animal Residue Avoidance Databank (FARAD) at www.FARAD.org.

RCI Classification: 4

# Dapsone
dap´sone

**Trade and other names:** Also known as diaminodiphenylsulfone and diaphenylsulfone

**Functional classification:** Antibacterial

## Pharmacology and Mechanism of Action

Antimicrobial drug used for treatment of mycobacterium. Its action resembles that of the sulfonamide class of antibacterial agents. It is a competitive antagonist of para-aminobenzoic acid (PABA), which inhibits normal bacterial utilization of PABA for the synthesis of folic acid. Folic acid is needed as an essential molecule for synthesis of other macromolecules in the bacteria.

It may also have some immunosuppressive properties or inhibit function of inflammatory cells, but this function is less well established.

## Indications and Clinical Uses

The original use in human medicine was for treatment of leprosy caused by susceptible strains of susceptible strains of *Mycobacterium leprae*. It is also used for dermatitis herpetiformis. However, the use for treating leprosy in animals is uncommon.

It also has been used for various immune-mediated disorders. It may be effective in people for bullous systemic lupus erythematosus, immune-mediated thrombocytopenia, and pemphigus vulgaris. However, the clinical efficacy for these diseases remains uncertain because of a lack of well-controlled studies.

In veterinary medicine, it has been used for dermatologic diseases in dogs, especially subcorneal pustular dermatosis and dermatitis herpetiformis. It also has been used for canine pemphigus.

## Precautionary Information

### Adverse Reactions and Side Effects

Hepatitis and blood dyscrasias may occur. Because it shares similar properties as a sulfonamide, the same reactions seen with sulfonamides can be seen with dapsone and include anemia, neutropenia, thrombocytopenia, hepatotoxicosis, and skin–drug eruptions. It is toxic to cats and causes neurotoxicosis and anemia.

### Contraindications and Precautions

Do not administer to cats. Do not administer to animals that are sensitive to sulfonamides.

### Drug Interactions

Use caution when administering dapsone with trimethoprim–sulfonamide combinations. (Concurrent administration should be avoided.) Trimethoprim may increase blood concentrations of dapsone because it inhibits excretion and potentiates dapsone adverse effects.

## Instructions for Use
Doses are derived from extrapolation of human doses or empiricism. No well-controlled clinical studies have been performed in veterinary medicine.

## Patient Monitoring and Laboratory Tests
Monitor for signs of hepatic reactions. Monitor CBC occasionally because bone marrow toxicity has occurred in some animals.

## Formulations
- Dapsone is available in 25- and 100-mg tablets. Formulations also may be compounded. See Stability and Storage.

## Stability and Storage
Store in a tightly sealed container, protected from light, and at room temperature. Dapsone may discolor without change in potency. Compounded suspension formulations have been stable for 21 days when mixed with citric acid.

For dosing smaller patients, a 2-mg/mL oral suspension may be made from the tablets in a 1:1 mixture of Ora-Sweet and Ora-Plus. To prepare this formulation, crush eight 25-mg tablets in a mortar and reduce to a fine powder. Add small portions of vehicle and mix to a uniform paste; mix while adding the vehicle in incremental proportions to almost 100 mL; transfer to a calibrated bottle, rinse mortar with vehicle, and add quantity of vehicle sufficient to make 100 mL. Label "Shake well." Stable for 90 days at room temperature or refrigerated.

## Small Animal Dosage
**Dogs**
- 1.1 mg/kg q8–12h PO.

**Cats**
- Do not use.

## Large Animal Dosage
- No dose has been reported for large animals.

## Regulatory Information
No regulatory information is available. For extralabel use withdrawal interval estimates, contact FARAD at www.FARAD.org.

# Darbepoetin Alfa
dar′be-poe′e-tin al′fa

**Trade and other names:** Aranesp

**Functional classification:** Hormone

## Pharmacology and Mechanism of Action
Human recombinant erythropoietin. Hematopoietic growth factor that stimulates erythropoiesis. Darbepoetin is a hyperglycosylated recombinant form of human erythropoietin. It differs from epoetin because it has 5 N-carbohydrate chains, thus producing a longer duration. The longer half-life translates to less often administration. In dogs, it has a three times longer half-life than epoetin. Because of the longer duration, epoetin has largely been replaced in veterinary medicine by darbepoetin.

## Indications and Clinical Uses

Darbepoetin alfa is used to treat nonregenerative anemia. It has been used to treat myelosuppression caused by disease or chemotherapy. It has been used in people to treat anemia associated with chronic kidney disease (CKD) and has been used for this purpose in dogs and cats with CKD. It has been an effective treatment for anemia secondary to CKD in dogs with most dogs achieving a goal of greater than 30% improvement in the packed cell volume (PCV). It also has been effective for this use in cats, at a dosage of 1 mcg/kg per week or higher. For comparison, the typical dosage in people is 2.25 mcg/kg once every 3 weeks or a dosage of 0.45–0.75 mcg/kg per week. When switching from the use of erythropoietin (epoetin alpha) to darbepoetin, a conversion for treatment is: 400 units/wk of epoetin = 1 mcg/kg darbepoetin.

### Precautionary Information

**Adverse Reactions and Side Effects**

Injection-site pain and headache have occurred in people. Adverse effects have included iron deficiency, hypertension, joint pain (arthralgia), gastrointestinal (GI) disturbance, and polycythemia. Because this product is a human-recombinant product, it may induce local and systemic allergic reactions in animals. Human erythropoietin products can cause red cell aplasia caused by neutralizing anti-erythropoietin antibodies that cross-react with other forms of erythropoietin. This is less likely with darbepoetin than epoetin. The feline erythropoietin is 83% homologous to human erythropoietin. Increased red cell aplasia may occur in animals when there is less than 100% homology. Pure red cell aplasia (PRCA) in cats was 25%–30% with epoetin compared with only 8% with darbepoetin. Reported adverse reactions in cats and dogs included vomiting, hypertension, seizures, fevers, and PRCA. Adverse effects in dogs included hypertension, seizures, hyperkalemia (which may be caused by other drugs), and PRCA.

**Contraindications and Precautions**

Do not shake vial vigorously. Do not dilute with other fluids or solutions. Do not use if cloudy. Stop therapy if joint pain, fever, anorexia, or cutaneous reactions are observed. Rotate sites of injection to avoid reactions.

**Drug Interactions**

No interactions are reported.

### Instructions for Use

The use of darbepoetin has been primarily in cats and dogs with anemia caused by CKD. It is preferred over epoetin alpha for this use. Iron supplementation is recommended when used in cats and dogs. By improving anemia, it may increase survival in animals with CKD and improve quality of life. An important adverse effect that may limit the use in animals is PRCA, which is described in the Adverse Reaction section. The doses listed in the dosing section are based on initial treatment. This treatment may be initiated with once-weekly injections for 3–4 weeks until the desired PCV has stabilized. Thereafter, the interval between doses may be increased, but this should not be longer than 21 days.

### Patient Monitoring and Laboratory Tests

Monitor hematocrit. The dose should be adjusted to maintain hematocrit in a range of 25%–35%. Because darbepoetin can cause hypertension, monitor blood pressure in treated animals. An increase may indicate a need for an increase in the antihypertensive drug dose.

## Formulations Available

Darbepoetin alfa is available in a variety of injectable solution concentrations, including: 25, 40, 60, 100, 200, 300, and 500 mcg/mL.

## Stability and Storage

Store in a tightly sealed container, protected from light, and at room temperature. Do not freeze. Do not mix with other solutions or fluids.

## Small Animal Dosage

### Dogs

- Start with 0.5 mcg/kg every 7 days injected SQ. After initial evaluation, increase the dosage to 0.8 mcg/kg once per week if needed; then increase or decrease the dosage as needed by monitoring the patient's PCV.

### Cats

- Start with 1 mcg/kg once per week, injected SQ, until the target PCV is achieved. Then the frequency can be decreased to every 2- to 3-week intervals. Typically, the expected response is a PCV of 25%–35%.

## Large Animal Dosage

No large animal doses are reported.

## Regulatory Information

No withdrawal times are established for food animals. Erythropoietin or derivatives in any form are prohibited to be on the premises of racing horses. RCI Classification: 2

# Deferoxamine Mesylate

deh-fer-oks´ah-meen mess´ih-late

**Trade and other names:** Desferal

**Functional classification:** Antidote, Chelating agent

## Pharmacology and Mechanism of Action

Deferoxamine is a siderophore (iron-binding compound) produced by the bacteria *Streptomyces pilosus*. It is not absorbed well enough from oral administration and must be injected. Because it has strong affinity for trivalent cations, it has chelating properties and is used to treat poisoning from these metal cations. In particular, it is valuable to treat acute iron toxicosis. One molecule of deferoxamine binds to a single atom, forming a complex, referred to as ferrioxamine, that is inactive and can be excreted, primarily through the kidneys. Hepatocytes also can take up deferoxamine and chelate hepatic iron, with the complex excreted in the bile.

There is another similar compound, but it is used less frequently in veterinary medicine. This synthetic chelator, deferasirox, is well absorbed from the GI tract and cleared more slowly, with longer-acting effects.

## Indications and Clinical Uses

Deferoxamine is indicated in cases of severe poisoning, especially iron toxicosis. It also has been used to chelate aluminum and facilitate removal.

## Precautionary Information
### Adverse Reactions and Side Effects
Adverse effects have not been reported in animals. Allergic reactions and hearing problems have occurred in people. Pain at the injection site occurs with SQ injections.

### Contraindications and Precautions
Administer IV formulation slowly to avoid precipitation of cardiac arrhythmias. Deferoxamine is teratogenic. Do not use in pregnant animals unless the benefits outweigh the risks.

### Drug Interactions
Deferoxamine will chelate with cations; avoid mixing with cations prior to administration.

**D**

## Instructions for Use
One hundred mg of deferoxamine binds 8.5 mg of ferric iron. Contact the local poison control center for guidance on dosing after an overdose. Deferoxamine must be injected to be effective. There are no oral forms, but a synthetic chelator, deferasirox, can be taken orally and could be obtained for animals.

## Patient Monitoring and Laboratory Tests
Monitor serum iron concentrations to determine severity of intoxication and success of therapy. Successful therapy is indicated by monitoring urine color (orange-rose color change to urine indicates chelated iron is being eliminated).

## Formulations
• Deferoxamine is available in a 500-mg and 2-g vial for injection.

## Stability and Storage
Deferoxamine is soluble in water. Stable when stored in solution for 14 days. Store in a tightly sealed container, protected from light, and at room temperature. Do not refrigerate and do not mix solutions with other medications.

## Small Animal Dosage
### Dogs and Cats
• 15 mg/kg/h IV infusion, 40 mg/kg IM q4–6h, or 40 mg/kg slow IV injection q4–6h for chelation of iron. The treatment is generally continued 24 hours but can be extended longer based on clinical assessment and monitoring of serum iron concentrations.

## Large Animal Dosage
• No dose has been reported for large animals.

## Regulatory Information
No regulatory information is available. There are no anticipated problems from levels of residues in animals. However, for extralabel use withdrawal interval estimates, contact FARAD at www.FARAD.org.

# Deracoxib
dare-ah-koks'ib

**Trade and other names:** Deramaxx and generic

**Functional classification:** Anti-inflammatory

## Pharmacology and Mechanism of Action

Deracoxib is a nonsteroidal anti-inflammatory drug (NSAID). Like other drugs in this class, deracoxib produces analgesic and anti-inflammatory effects by inhibiting the synthesis of prostaglandins. The enzyme inhibited by NSAID is the cyclo-oxygenase (COX) enzyme. The COX enzyme exists in two isoforms called *COX-1* and *COX-2*. COX-1 is primarily responsible for synthesis of prostaglandins important for maintaining a healthy GI tract, renal function, platelet function, and other normal functions. COX-2 is induced and responsible for synthesizing prostaglandins that are important mediators of pain, inflammation, and fever. However, it is known that there is some crossover of COX-1 and COX-2 effects in some situations, and COX-2 activity is important for some biological effects. Deracoxib, using in vitro assays, is more COX-1 sparing compared with older NSAIDs and is a selective inhibitor of COX-2. The COX-1:COX-2 ratio is high compared with some other drugs registered for dogs. It also is a selective COX-2 inhibitor in cats. It has not been established if the specificity for COX-1 or COX-2 is related to efficacy or safety.

*Pharmacokinetics:* Deracoxib has a half-life of 3 hours in dogs at 2–3 mg/kg and 19 hours at 20 mg/kg. It is highly protein bound. Oral absorption is 90% in dogs. Feeding delays absorption but does not diminish overall absorption. In cats, the half-life is approximately 8 hours.

## Indications and Clinical Uses

Deracoxib is used to decrease pain, inflammation, and fever. It has been used for the acute and chronic treatment of pain and inflammation in dogs. One of the most common uses is osteoarthritis, but it also has been used for pain associated with surgery. Except for experimental studies, the clinical use in cats has not been reported. There has been only limited use of deracoxib in horses, and administration to other large animals has not been reported.

Deracoxib, like other COX-2 inhibitors, may have some antitumor properties. It has produced beneficial effects in dogs with transitional cell carcinoma.

### Precautionary Information

#### Adverse Reactions and Side Effects

Gastrointestinal problems are the most common adverse effects associated with NSAIDs and can include vomiting, diarrhea, nausea, ulcers, and erosions of the GI tract. Gastric and duodenal ulcers have been reported from use of deracoxib in dogs. In field trials with deracoxib, vomiting was the most often reported adverse effect. Renal toxicity, especially in dehydrated animals or animals with preexisting renal disease, has been shown for some NSAIDs. In studies performed in dogs, higher doses (five times the dose) caused azotemia in normal dogs.

#### Contraindications and Precautions

Dogs and cats with preexisting GI or renal problems may be at a greater risk of adverse effects from NSAIDs. Safety in pregnancy is not known, but adverse effects have not been reported. Safety studies are not available for dogs younger than 4 months of age, pregnant animals, or lactating animals. In cats, use only as a single dose.

#### Drug Interactions

Do not administer with other NSAIDs or with corticosteroids. Corticosteroids have been shown to exacerbate the GI adverse effects. Some NSAIDs may interfere with the action of diuretic drugs and angiotensin-converting enzyme (ACE) inhibitors.

## Instructions for Use
Chewable tablets can be administered with or without food. Long-term studies have not been completed in cats; only single-dose studies have been reported.

## Patient Monitoring and Laboratory Tests
Monitor GI signs for evidence of diarrhea, GI bleeding, or ulcers. Because of risk of renal injury, monitor renal parameters (water consumption, blood urea nitrogen, creatinine, and urine-specific gravity) periodically during treatment. Deracoxib does not appear to affect thyroid hormone assays in dogs.

## Formulations
- Deracoxib is available in 12-, 25-, 75-, and 100-mg chewable tablets.

## Stability and Storage
Store in a tightly sealed container, protected from light, and at room temperature. Deracoxib has been mixed in a liquid suspension in water. However, stability of compounded formulations has not been evaluated.

## Small Animal Dosage
### Dogs
- Postoperative pain: 3–4 mg/kg once daily as needed for up to 7 days.
- Chronic use: 1–2 mg/kg once daily PO.

### Cats
- 1 mg/kg PO, single dose.

## Large Animal Dosage
- No dose has been reported for large animals.

## Regulatory Information
Do not administer to animals that produce food.
RCI Classification: 4

# Desmopressin Acetate
dess-moe-press'in ass'ih-tate
**Trade and other names:** DDAVP
**Functional classification:** Hormone

## Pharmacology and Mechanism of Action
Synthetic peptide similar to antidiuretic hormone (ADH), also known as DDAVP. It produces similar effects as natural ADH and is used to treat diabetes insipidus (DI) in animals. This action is related to the stimulation of permeability to water to increase water reabsorption in the distal renal tubule. The difference between desmopressin (DDAVP) and natural ADH is that DDAVP is longer acting and produces fewer vasoconstriction effects.

In addition to the hormone effects, in humans, the administration of DDAVP results in a twofold to fivefold increase in the plasma von Willebrand factor. It may induce a 50% increase in von Willebrand factor in some animals but not as consistently as when administered to people.

## Indications and Clinical Uses

Desmopressin is used as replacement therapy for patients with DI and has been used for treatment of patients with mild to moderate von Willebrand's disease prior to surgery or another procedure that may cause bleeding. However, the response in von Willebrand-deficient dogs is not as consistent or as great as in people.

### Precautionary Information

**Adverse Reactions and Side Effects**

No side effects reported. In people, it has rarely caused thrombotic events.

**Contraindications and Precautions**

There are no specific contraindications.

**Drug Interactions**

Administration of urea and fludrocortisone will increase the antidiuretic effects.

## Instructions for Use

Desmopressin is used only for central forms of DI. Duration of effect is variable (8–20 hours) but typically has a duration of 8–12 hours. It is ineffective for treatment of nephrogenic DI or polyuria from other causes. Intranasal product has been administered as eye drops in dogs. Onset of effect is within 1 hour. Oral tablets are available for humans, but the effects of oral tablets in dogs have not been reported, and the use is extrapolated from the human label.

## Patient Monitoring and Laboratory Tests

Monitor water intake and urinalysis to assess therapy. Desmopressin may be used as a test for DI in animals. To perform this test, administer 2 mcg/kg SQ or IV or 20 mcg intranasally or in the eye. This should be followed by the monitoring of urine concentration and the animal's body weight. Increase in urine-concentrating ability may indicate a diagnosis of DI.

## Formulations

- Desmopressin is available in a 4-mcg/mL injection, acetate nasal solution 100-mcg/mL (0.01%) metered spray, and 0.1- and 0.2-mg tablets (scored).

## Stability and Storage

Store in a tightly sealed container, protected from light, and at room temperature. Stability of compounded formulations has not been evaluated.

## Small Animal Dosage

- DI: 2–4 drops (2 mcg) q12–24h intranasally or in eye. Alternatively, 0.5–2 mcg/dog q12–24h IV or SQ.
- Oral dosage: 0.05–0.1 mcg/kg q12h or as needed. The oral dose may be increased to 0.1–0.2 mcg/kg as needed. Alternatively, administer 0.1 mg (total dose) per dog PO three times daily and adjust dose to control clinical signs (polyuria and polydipsia). If this dose is successful, decrease frequency to twice daily.
- von Willebrand's disease treatment: 1 mcg/kg (0.01 mL/kg) administered SQ or diluted in 20 mL of saline and administered over 10 min IV.

## Large Animal Dosage

- No dose has been reported for large animals.

## Regulatory Information

Withdrawal times are not established. However, this drug has rapid clearance, with little risk from residues; therefore, a short withdrawal time is suggested for food animals.

# Desoxycorticosterone Pivalate
dess-oks-ih-kor-tik-oh-steer'one piv'ah-late

**Trade and other names:** Percorten-V, DOCP, Zycortal, and DOCA pivalate

**Functional classification:** Corticosteroid

**D**

## Pharmacology and Mechanism of Action
Mineralocorticoid with no glucocorticoid activity. Desoxycorticosterone mimics the effects of aldosterone by retaining sodium. The pivalate formulation is a suspension that is absorbed slowly after injection and is used in small animals to produce a long-lasting effect from a single administration.

## Indications and Clinical Uses
Desoxycorticosterone is used as replacement therapy for animals with mineralocorticoid deficiency. It is used for adrenocortical insufficiency (hypoadrenocorticism, also referred to as Addison's disease). Some dogs also may require concurrent glucocorticosteroid therapy when it is used to treat insufficiency.

## Precautionary Information

### Adverse Reactions and Side Effects
Excessive mineralocorticoid effects are possible with high doses of desoxycorticosterone, but hypernatremia is rare. Patients receiving a dose that is too high may have hypokalemia, which may manifest as weakness, lethargy, and potential cardiac problems. Signs of iatrogenic hyperadrenocorticism are not expected with this drug.

### Contraindications and Precautions
Do not use in pregnant animals. It must be used cautiously in patients with congestive heart failure or renal disease. Dogs with congestive heart failure may have exacerbation of clinical signs from treatment with DOCP. In these cases, reduce dose (by half, for example). If the dose is too high, the patient can become hypokalemic (clinical signs include weakness and lethargy). Severe hypernatremia is rare.

### Drug Interactions
Aldosterone antagonists (spironolactone) will blunt the effect.

## Instructions for Use
Initial dose of desoxycorticosterone is based on average response in clinical patients, but individual doses may be based on monitoring electrolytes in patients. The actual interval between doses may range from 14 to 40 days, and the optimum dose may range from 1 to 2.2 mg/kg. In each patient, the optimum dose should be one that maintains the electrolyte concentrations in the desired range throughout the dose interval.

In patients with severe hypovolemia and other signs attributed to acute Addisonian crisis, treat with aggressive sodium-containing fluids before administering this product. Some dogs may also need a glucocorticoid (because desoxycorticosterone had no glucocorticoid effects). In these cases, prednisone supplementation at physiologic doses is appropriate (e.g., 0.2 mg/kg prednisone per day).

When administering the suspension formulation, shake before injection. Desoxycorticosterone has only mineralocorticoid activity. If glucocorticoid activity is needed, administer prednisone at a dosage of 0.2 mg/kg per day.

## Patient Monitoring and Laboratory Tests

If initiating a new treatment, begin monitoring after 14 days. At 14 days, measure the sodium and potassium concentration and adjust the dose to maintain these electrolytes in the normal reference range. Thereafter, monitor serum sodium and potassium as frequently as necessary to adjust the dose and dose interval for each patient.

## Formulations

- Desoxycorticosterone pivalate is available in 25-mg/mL suspension for injection. It is available in a clear vial containing 4 mL. There are two formulations, Percorten-V, and Zycortal, that differ slightly in the amounts of excipients and preservatives.

## Stability and Storage

Store in a tightly sealed container, protected from light, and at room temperature. Stability of compounded formulations has not been evaluated. Do not freeze.

## Small Animal Dosage

### Dogs

- 2.2 mg/kg q25 days SQ or IM. Adjust dose by monitoring electrolytes. The most consistent dosage for DOCP has been 2.2 mg/kg SQ once per 25 days, but many dogs can be managed with a starting dose of 1.5 mg/kg with a target interval ranging from 28 to 30 days.

### Cats

- 2.2 mg/kg SQ every 25 days (adjust dose by monitoring).

## Large Animal Dosage

- No dose has been reported for large animals.

## Regulatory Information

Withdrawal times are not established. However, because of low risk of residues, no withdrawal times are suggested.

RCI Classification: 4

# Detomidine Hydrochloride

deh-toe´mih-deen hye-droe-klor´ide

**Trade and other names:** Dormosedan and Dormosedan Gel

**Functional classification:** Alpha$_2$ analgesic

## Pharmacology and Mechanism of Action

Alpha$_2$-adrenergic agonist. Alpha$_2$ agonists decrease release of neurotransmitters from the neuron. The proposed mechanism whereby they decrease transmission is via binding to presynaptic alpha$_2$ receptors (negative feedback receptors). The result is decreased sympathetic outflow, analgesia, sedation, and anesthesia. Detomidine gel is absorbed from the oral mucous membrane with bioavailability in horses of 22%. Other drugs in this class include xylazine, dexmedetomidine, medetomidine, romifidine, and clonidine. The alpha$_2$-specific effects are measured by comparing the alpha$_1$:alpha$_2$ receptor affinity ratio. The ratios are 1:160 for xylazine, 1:260 for detomidine; 1:360 for romifidine, and 1:1620 for dexmedetomidine. Thus, receptor-binding studies indicate that alpha$_2$/alpha$_1$-adrenergic receptor selectivity for detomidine is much higher than that of xylazine.

*Pharmacokinetics:* In dogs, the half-life from IV administration is approximately 30 minutes, with a volume of distribution of 0.6 L/kg. After application of the mucosal gel to dogs, the peak occurred at 1 hour, the half-life was 40 minutes, and absorption was 34%. After administration of the oral mucosal gel to cats, the peak occurs at 37 minutes, and the half-life was 47 minutes. In horses, the half-life from IV, IM, and the oral mucosal gel was 26 minutes, 53 minutes, and 1.5 hours, respectively. After administration of the oral mucosal gel to horses, the concentrations are below the detection limit in plasma by 24 hours. In calves, the detomidine gel was absorbed approximately 34% and had an onset of effect of approximately 40 minutes.

## Indications and Clinical Uses

Detomidine is used primarily as a sedative, anesthetic adjunct, and analgesia. It is used in horses more often than in other species. When used to treat pain from colic in horses, the duration of effect is approximately 3 hours (20 or 40 mcg/kg). Detomidine also has been administered for epidural analgesia. For pain, detomidine appears to be more potent and longer acting than xylazine.

Detomidine in the gel form (Dormosedan Gel) for horses is administered orally to produce mucosal absorption. It is indicated for producing minor standing sedation to facilitate minor procedures (shoeing, clipping, trimming) or calming a fractious horse. Onset of action is 40 minutes, and duration is 90–180 minutes. The detomidine gel has also been administered intravaginally to horses (40 mcg/kg) and produced reliable sedation. The detomidine gel form for oral mucosal use also has been used successfully in dogs, cats, and calves. These uses and doses are provided in the dosing section. When applied to dogs, cats, and calves, the onset for effect is approximately 40–45 minutes with maximal sedation in 60–75 minutes. The dose can be adjusted in dogs (e.g., 0.5, 1, 2, or 4 mg/m$^2$), depending on the degree of sedation desired. After absorption, it produces a duration of approximately 90 minutes.

## Precautionary Information

### Adverse Reactions and Side Effects

At typical doses, sedation, ataxia, swaying, sweating, and bradycardia are common in horses. It produces vasoconstriction and increased peripheral vascular resistance through the alpha-adrenergic type 2B receptors. This effect increases blood pressure and can lead to reflex bradycardia in all animals tested. Ordinarily, the bradycardia *does not* have to be treated with antimuscarinic agents (e.g., atropine). In small animals, vomiting is common. Vomiting has been observed in 100% of research cats that received detomidine.

Cardiac depression, atrioventricular (AV) block, and hypotension are possible with high doses. In some horses, hyperresponsiveness to stimuli occurs. Diuresis occurs as a consequence of the hyperglycemia produced by alpha$_2$ agonists such as detomidine. Yohimbine (0.11 mg/kg) can be used to reverse effects of alpha$_2$ agonists such as detomidine. In small animals, atipamezole also can be used to reverse effects from detomidine.

### Contraindications and Precautions

Concurrent use of detomidine with sulfonamides IV can lead to cardiac arrhythmias. Xylazine causes problems in pregnant animals, and this also should be considered for other alpha$_2$ agonists. Use cautiously in animals that are pregnant because it may induce labor. In addition, it may decrease oxygen delivery to a fetus in late gestation. Detomidine gel can be absorbed across the skin and from eye and mouth contact in humans. If there is accidental exposure, immediately rinse with soap and water. Contact a physician if there are other concerns.

### Drug Interactions

Other drugs that depress the heart may increase risk for arrhythmias.

## Instructions for Use

Detomidine is used primarily in horses, and although not approved for small animals, extralabel dosages are listed in the dosing section that follows. Atropine (0.01–0.02 mg/kg) has been used to prevent bradycardia but is not necessary for routine use. Detomidine may be administered with other anesthetics, analgesics, sedatives (including butorphanol), and benzodiazepines. When using the mucosal gel in dogs and cats, apply the calculated dose to the oral mucosa (the upper gumline has worked in experimental animals).

## Patient Monitoring and Laboratory Tests

Monitor heart rate and, if possible, the electrocardiogram (ECG) during treatment with this class of drugs. If available, blood pressure monitoring may be indicated in some patients.

## Formulations

• Detomidine is available in a 10-mg/mL injection. Oral gel is 7.6 mg/mL in a 3-mL syringe.

## Stability and Storage

Store in a tightly sealed container, protected from light, and at room temperature. Stability of compounded formulations has not been evaluated.

## Small Animal Dosage

### Dogs

• 5 mcg/kg IV or 10–20 mcg/kg IM.
• Oral mucosal application: The dose can be adjusted for the desired clinical effects. For mild sedation, 0.5 mg/m$^2$; for higher sedation and lateral recumbency, administer 1.0 mg/m$_2$. (Average dose is 35 mcg/kg.) A high dose of 2–4 mg/m$^2$ produces more profound sedation. The gel should be applied applied to the upper gingiva of dogs. Reversal with 0.1 mg/kg of atipamezole IM.

### Cats

• Oral (injectable solution applied transmucosal): 0.5 mg/kg. Administer with ketamine (10 mg/kg) by spraying into cat's mouth.
• Oral (transmucosal gel): for sedation, use 2–4 mg/m$^2$ (anticipate vomiting at this dose). A dose of 4 mg/m$_2$ of the oral mucosal gel in cats is approximately 0.24 mg/kg, or 0.14 mL per cat. Reversal with 0.1 mg/kg of atipamezole IM.

## Large Animal Dosage

### Horses

A dose of 10–20 mcg/kg is equivalent to 5–10 mg per horse.
• Sedation: 20–40 mcg/kg (0.02–0.04 mg/kg) IV or IM. Lower doses of 10–20 mcg/kg are sometimes used in practice initially and then repeated as needed. For example, doses of 10 mcg/kg (0.01 mg/kg) produce slightly less ataxia and sedation. Doses as low as 5 mcg/kg have been used in draft horses.
• Analgesia: 20 mcg/kg (0.02 mg/kg) IV or IM. Duration of analgesia may be longer if a dose of 40 mcg/kg is used.
• Constant-rate infusion (CRI): 10 mcg/kg bolus IV, followed by 0.5 mcg/kg/min for 15 min; then progressively decreasing the rate as needed to 0.1 mcg/kg/min.
• Oral mucosal: 40 mcg/kg (≈2.5 mL to a 1000-lb horse) administered sublingually. This dose has also been used intravaginally in horses.

### Cattle

• 2–10 mcg/kg (0.002–0.1 mg/kg) IV or 5–40 mcg/kg (0.005–0.04 mg/kg) IM.

## Calves
- 30 mcg/kg IV or detomidine oral mucosal gel (equine formulation): 80 mcg/kg.

### Regulatory Information
Cattle withdrawal times (extralabel): 3 days meat; 72 hours milk. For extralabel uses and doses, contact FARAD at www.FARAD.org.
RCI Classification: 3

# Dexamethasone
deks-ah-meth´ah-sone

**Trade and other names:** Azium solution in polyethylene glycol, DexaJect, Dexavet, Decadron, Dexasone, Voren suspension, and generic brands

**Functional classification:** Corticosteroid

## Pharmacology and Mechanism of Action
Corticosteroid. Anti-inflammatory and immunosuppressive effects of dexamethasone are approximately 30 times more potent than cortisol and 6–7 times more potent than prednisolone. Anti-inflammatory effects are complex but primarily via inhibition of inflammatory cells and suppression of expression of inflammatory mediators. The most important use is for treatment of inflammatory and immune-mediated disease. This dexamethasone solution differs from dexamethasone sodium phosphate in that the sodium phosphate form is water soluble and appropriate for IV administration. See the next section for more information about dexamethasone sodium phosphate. Dexamethasone solution is in a polyethylene glycol vehicle that should not be administered rapidly IV.

Dexamethasone-21-isonicotinate is a suspension registered for IM use (usually for horses). After an injection of 10 mg (total dose) to horses, the half-life was 2.5–5 hours, and the volume of distribution (VDss) was 1.7 L/kg. Oral administration of the same dose had a half-life of 4.3 hours and bioavailability (F) of 61%, with a peak concentration at 1.3 hours. In horses, oral absorption is higher in unfed horses, and oral absorption from powder is higher than with solution. The suspension (dexamethasone-21-isonicotinate) has a slow release and produces a 39-hour half-life in horses and suppresses cortisol for 140 hours.

## Indications and Clinical Uses
Dexamethasone is used for treatment of inflammatory and immune-mediated disease. The use of dexamethasone at high doses for treatment of shock is controversial. Most recent evidence does not support administration of dexamethasone for this use unless there is adrenal deficiency. Dexamethasone is often used short term in small animals as an injection (sodium-phosphate form) when oral treatment with prednisone is not possible. Dexamethasone is also used as a diagnostic test of adrenal function. Large animal uses include induction of parturition (cattle) and treatment of inflammatory conditions. In cattle, corticosteroids also have been used in the treatment of ketosis. In horses, dexamethasone has been used to treat equine asthma syndrome, with bronchoconstriction caused by recurrent airway obstruction (RAO).

## Precautionary Information

### Adverse Reactions and Side Effects

Side effects from corticosteroids are many and include polyphagia, polydipsia and polyuria, and hypothalamic–pituitary–adrenal (HPA) axis suppression. Adverse effects include GI ulceration, hepatopathy, increased risk of diabetes, hyperlipidemia, decreased thyroid hormone, decreased protein synthesis, delayed wound healing, and immunosuppression. Secondary infections can occur as a result of immunosuppression and include infections from *Demodex* spp., toxoplasmosis, fungal infections, and urinary tract infections (UTIs). High-dose glucocorticoids in animals with neurologic disease can lead to excitotoxic cell death and oxidative injury via increased excitatory amino acids. In horses, dexamethasone adverse effects have included risk of laminitis, although this effect is controversial and not supported by strong evidence.

### Contraindications and Precautions

Use cautiously in patients prone to ulcers or infection or in animals in which wound healing is necessary. Use cautiously in animals with diabetes or renal failure and in pregnant animals. IV injections should be done slowly because formulations contain polyethylene glycol, which can cause reactions from rapid IV injection (hemolysis, hypotension, and collapse). Do not administer dexamethasone-21-isonicotinate IV (IM use only).

### Drug Interactions

Administration of corticosteroids with NSAIDs increases the risk of GI injury. The pH of the solution is 7–8.5. Do not mix with acidifying solutions, or it may not be compatible. Otherwise, it is compatible with most IV fluid solutions.

## Instructions for Use

For IV administration, the dexamethasone sodium phosphate solution is preferred (Dex-S-P) because of better water solubility for IV use. (See Dexamethasone Sodium Phosphate.) Dosing schedules are based on the condition treated. Anti-inflammatory effects occur at doses of 0.1–0.2 mg/kg, and immunosuppressive effects occur at 0.2–0.5 mg/kg.

Dexamethasone is used to test for hyperadrenocorticism. For the low-dose dexamethasone suppression test, administer to dogs, 0.01 mg/kg (or 0.015 mg/kg in some references) IV, and to cats, 0.1 mg/kg IV; collect samples at 0, 4, and 8 hours. For high-dose dexamethasone suppression test: administer to dogs, 0.1 mg/kg (or 1.0 mg/kg in some references), and to cats, 1.0 mg/kg.

## Patient Monitoring and Laboratory Tests

For the low- and high-dose dexamethasone suppression tests, administer either 0.01 or 0.1 mg/kg and collect cortisol samples at 0, 4, and 8 hours after administration. The normal cortisol concentration after suppression test should be less than 30–40 nmol/L (1.1–1.3 mcg/dL). For the dexamethasone suppression test for horses, administer 0.04 mg/kg IM and collect postcortisol sample 24 hours later. Normal suppression in horses is less than 1 mcg/dL.

## Formulations

- Dexamethasone is available in a 2-mg/mL solution, which contains 500 mg of polyethylene glycol; 0.25-, 0.5-, 0.75-, 1-, 1.5-, 2-, 4-, and 6-mg tablets; 0.1- and 1-mg/mL oral solution; and 10 mg per 15 g powder. Dexamethasone-21-isonicotinate slow-release suspension in an aqueous vehicle is 1 mg/mL.

## Stability and Storage

Store in a tightly sealed container, protected from light, and at room temperature. Dexamethasone formulated in various oral mixtures to enhance flavoring was stable for 26 weeks at room temperature or refrigerated. Dexamethasone sodium phosphate is freely soluble in water, but dexamethasone solution (in polyethylene glycol) is practically insoluble in water.

## Small Animal Dosage

### Dogs and Cats

- Anti-inflammatory: 0.07–0.15 mg/kg q12–24h IV, IM, or PO.
- Oral dosage (cats): 0.1–0.2 mg/kg q24h PO, added to food. After the initial dose, lower to a maintenance dosage of 0.05 mg/kg q48–72h PO.
- Immunosuppressive: 0.125–0.25 mg/kg q24h IV, IM, or PO for initial treatment.
- Pulse dose: 0.5 mg/kg PO for 4 consecutive days; then repeated every 28 days.
- Low-dose dexamethasone suppression test: 0.01 mg/kg IV (dog) and 0.1 mg/kg IV (cat).
- High-dose dexamethasone suppression test: 0.1 mg/kg IV (dog) and 1.0 mg/kg IV (cat).
- Dexamethasone-21-isonicotinate: 0.03–0.05 mg/kg IM.

## Large Animal Dosage

### Cattle and Horses

- 0.04–0.15 mg/kg per day IV or IM. Some product labeling lists a total dose of 5–20 mg/animal, which corresponds to 0.01-0.04 mg/kg/day. However, for some conditions, higher doses may be needed.
- Horses, treatment of equine asthma syndrome (airway disease caused by RAO): 0.05–0.1 mg/kg IV or IM q24h or 0.165 mg/kg PO q24h, usually for 2–3 days, but oral treatment has been continued for 7 days; then tapered to half the dose for another 7 days.
- Induction of parturition (cattle): 0.05 mg/kg (25 mg/animal) as a single dose during the last week or 2 weeks of pregnancy. A dose of prostaglandin (PG) $F_2$ alpha may be administered concurrently (0.5 mg/animal).
- Dexamethasone-21-isonicotinate: 0.01–0.04 mg/kg IM.

### Sheep

- Induction of parturition: 0.15 mg/kg/day IM for 1–5 days during the last week of gestation.

## Regulatory Information

Dexamethasone is approved for use in cattle, but withdrawal times are not established. Although withdrawal times are not listed on the label, at least 96 hours should be used for milk and 4–8 days for meat. Allow at least 3 weeks to eliminate residues from the kidneys and liver and 6 weeks to deplete the drug from the IM injection site. For other extralabel uses, contact FARAD at www.FARAD.org.

RCI Classification: 4

# Dexamethasone Sodium Phosphate

**Trade and other names:** Sodium phosphate: DexaJect SP, Dexavet, and Dexasone; Decadron and generic brand tablets

**Functional classification:** Corticosteroid

## Pharmacology and Mechanism of Action

Dexamethasone is a corticosteroid with anti-inflammatory and immunosuppressive effects that are approximately 30 times more potent than cortisol and 6–7 times more potent than prednisolone. Anti-inflammatory effects are complex but primarily occur via inhibition of inflammatory cells and suppression of expression of inflammatory mediators. The difference among formulations is that dexamethasone sodium phosphate is a water-soluble formulation that can be injected intravenously. Dexamethasone solution is in a polyethylene glycol vehicle that should not be administered rapidly intravenously.

*Pharmacokinetics:* Half-life in plasma for dexamethasone ranges from 3–6 hours, but duration of action is 36–48 hours. The duration of action is not related to plasma pharmacokinetics.

## Indications and Clinical Uses

Use of dexamethasone is for treatment of inflammatory and immune-mediated disease. The use of dexamethasone at high doses for treatment of shock is controversial. Most recent evidence does not support administration of dexamethasone for this use. Large animal uses include induction of parturition (cattle) and treatment of inflammatory conditions. In cattle, corticosteroids also have been used in the treatment of ketosis.

## Precautionary Information

### Adverse Reactions and Side Effects

Side effects from corticosteroids are many and include polyphagia, polydipsia and polyuria, and HPA axis suppression. Adverse effects include GI ulceration, hepatopathy, diabetes, hyperlipidemia, decreased thyroid hormone, decreased protein synthesis, delayed wound healing, and immunosuppression. Secondary infections can occur as a result of immunosuppression and include *Demodex* spp., toxoplasmosis, fungal infections, and UTIs. In horses, additional adverse effects include risk of laminitis.

### Contraindications and Precautions

Use cautiously in patients prone to ulcers or infection or in animals in which wound healing is necessary. Use cautiously, or not at all, in animals receiving NSAIDs because these drugs administered concurrently increase the risk of GI ulceration. Use cautiously in animals with diabetes or renal failure and in pregnant animals.

### Drug Interactions

Administration of corticosteroids with NSAIDs increases the risk of GI injury.

## Instructions for Use

Dosing schedules are based on desired effect. Anti-inflammatory effects are seen at doses of 0.1–0.2 mg/kg, and immunosuppressive effects are seen at 0.2–0.5 mg/kg. Dexamethasone is used for testing hyperadrenocorticism. For the low-dose dexamethasone suppression test (for dogs), use 0.01 mg/kg (or 0.015 mg/kg in some references) IV and 0.1 mg/kg IV (for cats). For the high-dose dexamethasone suppression test in dogs, use 0.1 mg/kg (or 1.0 mg/kg in some references), and in cats, use 1.0 mg/kg. For the test in horses, administer 40 mcg/kg.

## Patient Monitoring and Laboratory Tests

Monitor CBC periodically during treatment to assess effects. For monitoring a low-dose dexamethasone suppression test, collect samples at 4 and 8 hours after dexamethasone. A normal suppression test result should be cortisol less than 30–40 nmol/L (1.1–1.4 mcg/dL). For dexamethasone suppression in horses, collect samples at 17 and 19 hours. Normal horses should have cortisol less than 1.0 mcg/dL.

## Formulations

- Sodium phosphate solution is available as 4 mg/mL, equivalent to 3 mg/mL of dexamethasone base.

**D**

## Stability and Storage

Store in a tightly sealed container, protected from light, and at room temperature. Dexamethasone sodium phosphate in other aqueous solutions has been stable for 28 days. Dexamethasone sodium phosphate is freely soluble in water, but dexamethasone solution (in polyethylene glycol) is practically insoluble in water. If dexamethasone sodium phosphate is mixed with 5% dextrose solution or saline, it is stable for 24 hours.

## Small Animal Dosage

### Dogs and Cats

- Anti-inflammatory: 0.07–0.15 mg/kg q12–24h IV or IM.
- Shock, spinal injury (efficacy is questionable and risks may be high): 2.2–4.4 mg/kg IV.
- Low-dose dexamethasone suppression test: 0.01 mg/kg or 0.015 mg/kg IV (for dogs) and 0.1 mg/kg IV (for cats) and collect sample at 0, 4, and 8 hours.
- High-dose dexamethasone suppression test: 0.1 mg/kg or 1.0 mg/kg IV (for dogs) and 1.0 mg/kg IV (for cats).

## Large Animal Dosage

### Cattle And Horses

- Treatment of inflammation: 0.04–0.15 mg/kg/day IV or IM.
- Ketosis (cattle): 0.01–0.04 mg/kg IV or IM.
- Induction of parturition (cattle): 0.05 mg/kg (25 mg per animal) as a single dose during the last week or 2 weeks of pregnancy. A dose of $PGF_2$ alpha may be administered concurrently (0.5 mg/animal).
- Dexamethasone suppression test in horses: 40 mcg/kg and collect samples at 17 and 19 hours.

### Sheep

- Induction of parturition: 0.15 mg/kg/day IM for 1–5 days during the last week of gestation.

## Regulatory Information

Although withdrawal times are not established, at least 96 hours is required for milk and 4–8 days for meat. However, at least 3 weeks are required to eliminate residues from kidneys and liver and 6 weeks for IM injection site.

# Dexmedetomidine Hydrochloride
dex-meh-deh-toe′mih-deen hye-droe-klor′ide

**Trade and other names:** Dexdomitor (injection) and Sileo (transmucosal gel)

**Functional classification:** Analgesic, alpha₂ agonist

## Pharmacology and Mechanism of Action

Alpha₂-adrenergic agonist. Alpha₂ agonists decrease release of neurotransmitters from the neuron. Dexmedetomidine and medetomidine (Domitor) are very similar in activity. Medetomidine is a racemic mixture containing 50% dexmedetomidine and 50% levomedetomidine. Dexmedetomidine is the active enantiomer of the mixture (D-isomer); therefore, on a mg/mg basis, dexmedetomidine is twice the potency of medetomidine but with the same pharmacological activity and equivalent analgesic and sedative effects.

The proposed mechanism for alpha$_2$ agonists is that they decrease transmission in the CNS through binding to presynaptic alpha$_2$ receptors (negative feedback receptors). The result is decreased sympathetic outflow, analgesia, sedation, and anesthesia. Other drugs in this class include medetomidine, xylazine, detomidine, romifidine, and clonidine. The alpha$_2$-specific effects are measured by comparing the alpha$_1$:alpha$_2$ receptor affinity ratio. The ratios are 1:160 for xylazine, 1:260 for detomidine; 1:360 for romifidine, and 1:1620 for dexmedetomidine. Thus, receptor-binding studies indicate that alpha$_2$/alpha$_1$-adrenergic receptor selectivity for dexmedetomidine is more than 10 times that of xylazine.

The pharmacokinetics have been studied in several species. In horses, the half-life is only 8 minutes with a rapid clearance and volume of distribution of over 1 L/kg. In dogs after injection (IM or IV), the half-life is 0.5–0.7 hours with a clearance of 8 mL/kg/min. In cats, the half-life is 0.5–1.25 hours (depending on the dose) with a clearance of 9–14 mL/kg/min.

The oral mucosal form (Sileo) is a unique formulation approved for application to the oral mucosa (gingiva) of dogs, and extrabel use occurs in cats. In dogs, after oral mucosal application, the peak occurs at 0.6 hours, with bioavailability of 28%. If swallowed, the oral bioavailability is negligible. After absorption from the oral mucosa, the half-life is 0.5–3 hours. Dexmedetomidine is highly protein bound at 93%. Metabolites have no known activity and are excreted in the urine.

## Indications and Clinical Uses

Dexmedetomidine, like other alpha$_2$ agonists, is used as a sedative, anesthetic adjunct, and analgesia. It is approved for use in both dogs and cats. It can be administered to facilitate examinations, diagnostic procedures, treatments, ear and teeth cleaning, and minor surgery. It has been used to sedate animals for intradermal skin testing without affecting results. The oral mucosal gel (oromucosal gel) formulation (Sileo) is approved for the treatment of noise aversion (noise phobia) in dogs. The dose of transmucosal dexmedetomidine needed to produce sedation is higher than the noise-aversion dose. The canine oromucosal gel has also been administered to cats to anxiolytic uses at a dose of 5 mcg/kg (0.25 mL/cat of dosing syringe).

Dexmedetomidine injection is commonly used in cats. In cats, the peak effects are observed in 15–60 minutes, and the recovery occurs by 180 minutes. It has similar clinical effects as medetomidine and can be used for similar indications. It can be administered in combination with ketamine, butorphanol, or opiate agonists for sedation and short-term surgical procedures (see Instructions for Use). In the dosing section, note that many doses listed are lower than the manufacturer's approved label dose.

Dexmedetomidine (and xylazine) can be used to induce vomiting in cats that have ingested a poison at a dose of 10 mcg/kg IM.

## Precautionary Information

### Adverse Reactions and Side Effects

In small animals, vomiting is the most common acute effect. Vomiting is more common in cats than dogs. Alpha$_2$ agonists decrease sympathetic output.

Cardiovascular depression may occur. Like medetomidine, dexmedetomidine can produce an initial bradycardia and hypertension. Although bradycardia is common, it rarely requires treatment with antimuscarinic agents (e.g., atropine). An initial increase in blood pressure may be followed by a decrease in blood pressure caused by decreased sympathetic tone. Lower respiratory rate and body temperature occur in animals during dexmedetomidine sedation. Transient arrhythmias may occur in some animals. Paradoxical excitement may occur in some animals, and animals with high anxiety levels may not respond predictably to alpha₂ agonists. If adverse reactions are observed, reverse with atipamezole (Antisedan) with a dose of 25–300 mcg/kg IM. (See Atipamezole dosing section.) It is not recommended to administer atropine to animals to modify cardiovascular effects. Administration of atropine to dogs with dexmedetomidine resulted in increases in blood pressure and heart rate and deleterious cardiac arrhythmias.

In horses, there are prominent sedative effects, especially in the first 20–30 minutes and decreased intestinal motility that lasted 60 minutes.

**Contraindications and Precautions**

Use cautiously in animals with heart disease. Use may be contraindicated in older animals with preexisting cardiac disease, hypotension, hypoxia, or bradycardia. Use cautiously in animals with respiratory, liver, or kidney disease. Do not use in animals with signs of shock. Use cautiously in animals that are pregnant because alpha₂ agonists have been reported to induce labor. In addition, it may decrease oxygen delivery to fetus in late gestation. Dexmedetomidine can be absorbed through intact human skin; therefore avoid human exposure.

**Drug Interactions**

Do not use with other drugs that may cause cardiac depression. Use with opioid analgesic drugs will greatly enhance the CNS depression. Consider lowering doses if administered with opioids. Anticholinergic drugs (e.g., atropine) may be given in moderate doses *prior* to drug administration to prevent bradycardia induced by alpha₂ agonists, but it is not routinely needed and may prolong initial hypertension. However, administration *simultaneously* with alpha₂ agonists is not recommended. Administration of atropine to dogs with dexmedetomidine resulted in adverse cardiovascular effects.

## Instructions for Use

Dexmedetomidine, medetomidine, and detomidine are more specific for the alpha₂ receptor than xylazine. They may be used for sedation, analgesia, and minor surgical procedures. It is recommended to withhold food for several hours prior to administration of alpha₂ agonists to minimize vomiting.

Lower doses are often administered for cases when less sedation is needed or when combined with other drugs. For example, a dose of 10 mcg/kg IM of dexmedetomidine in combination with ketamine and/or butorphanol has been used for short-term procedures in cats. These combinations induce more sedation and achieved with dexmedetomidine alone, without significant cardiovascular effects. Recommended canine doses for injection are shown in the dosing section.

Dexmedetomidine can also be used with other anesthetics such as propofol, ketamine, thiopental, opiates, benzodiazepines, and inhalant gas anesthetics. However, lower doses (as much as 40%–60%) of other drugs are anticipated when used with dexmedetomidine. It has also been safe and effective in cats as a preanesthetic at a dose of 40 mcg/kg combined with 5 mg/kg of ketamine. In dogs and cats, after procedures in which dexmedetomidine has been used, it can be reversed with atipamezole at a dose of 25–300 mcg/kg (equal to volume of dexmedetomidine used) IM.

Dexmedetomidine oromucosal gel for treatment of noise aversion should be applied 30–60 minutes prior to the noise event that triggers anxiety behavior or at the first sign of anxiety related to loud noise. It may be redosed if necessary after 2–3 hours, but no more than 5 doses should be administered.

## Patient Monitoring and Laboratory Tests

Monitor vital signs during anesthesia. Monitor heart rate, blood pressure, and ECG during anesthesia. Alpha$_2$ agonists will increase blood glucose because of effects on insulin secretion.

## Formulations

- Dexmedetomidine is available in vials containing 0.5-mg/mL injection, and a lower concentration of 0.1 mg/mL in sterile vials. Human formulation is Precedex.
- Dexmedetomidine oromucosal gel (Sileo) contains 0.9 mg/mL dexmedetomidine supplied in a 3-mL syringe with a marked plunger to allow for administration of an accurate dose.

## Stability and Storage

Store in a tightly sealed container, protected from light, and at room temperature. Stability of specific compounded formulations has not been evaluated. However, dexmedetomidine has been combined in the same syringe with ketamine, opioids, and other water-soluble agents and injected without signs of incompatibility. Dexmedetomidine oromucosal gel is available in a preloaded syringe. Once opened, it should be used within 4 weeks.

## Small Animal Dosage

### Dogs

- 125 mcg/m$^2$ IM for preanesthetic, minor sedation, short-term procedures, and analgesia (range, 9 mcg/kg for small dogs to 3 mcg/kg for large dogs).
- 375 mcg/m$^2$ IV or 500 mcg/m$^2$ IM for deeper sedation, analgesia, and minor surgical procedures. For comparison, a dose of 375 mcg/m$^2$ is equivalent to 176 mcg/kg for a 10-kg dog and to 36.75 mcg/kg for a 30-kg dog.
- When calculating doses, the lower doses are used for short-term sedation and analgesia or when combined with other analgesic or anesthetic agents.
- Combination anesthetics: Ketamine (3 mg/kg), dexmedetomidine (15 mcg/kg), and buprenorphine (40 mcg/kg) can be combined for one single IM injection in dogs for short-term surgical procedure or intubation for surgery.
- Oromucosal gel: 125 mg/m$^2$ applied to the gingiva between the cheek and gum. If swallowed, it will not be effective.

### Cats

- IM dose: 40 mcg/kg (0.04 mg/kg) IM (0.35 mL for 4-kg cat). Lower doses (e.g., 10–25 mcg/kg) have been used for short-term sedation and analgesia or when combined with other agents.
- Injectable solution applied to the oral mucosa: 20–40 µg/kg sprayed into the cat's mouth for sedation. (It can be mixed with buprenorphine.)
- IV dose: 5–20 mcg/kg, with degree of sedation increasing with the dose. (This may be used with other agents, such as ketamine 5 mg/kg.)

- Oral mucosal gel (Sileo): 5 mcg/kg applied to the gingiva of cats between cheek and gum (0.25 mL, or "one dot" from the dosing syringe per cat).
- Combinations: Dexmedetomidine can be combined with other agents and administered for short-term procedures. In these protocols, the dose of dexmedetomidine generally ranges from 10 to 20 mcg/kg administered IM with other agents. Examples include 3–5 mg/kg ketamine + 20 mcg/kg dexmedetomidine, butorphanol 0.2 mg/kg + 10 mcg/kg dexmedetomidine, or alfaxalone 2 mg/kg + dexmedetomidine 20 mcg/kg) in one syringe and administered IM 10 minutes prior to a minor procedure. Other combinations have included dexmedetomidine (10 mcg/kg), ketamine (5 mg/kg), and butorphanol (0.2–0.4 mg/kg), or buprenorphine (0.03 mg/kg) injected IM to produce lateral recumbency.
- Constant-rate infusion (CRI): Administer initial dose of 3–10 mcg/kg IM followed by 1 mcg/kg/h CRI.
- Reversal: atipamezole 0.2 mg/kg IM.
- Induction of vomiting: 10 mcg/kg, IM. Lower doses IV also are effective.

### Large Animal Dosage

**Horses**

- Surgery: 5 mcg/kg IV bolus. CRI: 8 mcg/kg/h IV.
- Perioperative analgesia: 1.75–2 mcg/kg/h IV.

### Regulatory Information

Withdrawal times are not established for animals that produce food. The withdrawals time for xylazine in food animals are 4 days for meat and 24 hours for milk. A minimum of these withdrawal periods should be used for dexmedetomidine. For additional extralabel use withdrawal interval estimates, contact FARAD at www.FARAD.org.

RCI Classification: 3

---

# Dextran
deks'tran

**Trade and other names:** Dextran 70 and Gentran-70

**Functional classification:** Fluid replacement

---

## Pharmacology and Mechanism of Action

Synthetic colloid used for volume expansion. Dextrans are glucose polymers and are available as low molecular weight (Dextran 40) and high molecular weight (Dextran 70). Dextran 70 is the most often used. The colloids such as dextrans are large-molecular-weight molecules that remain in the vasculature because of their large size. Therefore, they increase colloid osmotic pressure within the vasculature to prevent intravascular fluid loss and inhibit tissue edema. Other colloids used are hetastarch and pentastarch. See Hydroxyethyl starch for more information on these compounds.

## Indications and Clinical Uses

Dextran is a high-molecular-weight compound administered IV to maintain intravascular volume. It is used for acute treatment of hypovolemia and shock. Duration of effect is approximately 24 hours.

## Precautionary Information

**Adverse Reactions and Side Effects**

There is only limited use in veterinary medicine, and adverse effects have not been reported. The hydroxyethyl starch compounds are used more often in veterinary medicine when colloids are needed for IV use. In people, coagulopathies are possible because of decreased platelet function and antithrombotic effects. Acute renal failure has occurred, and anaphylactic shock also has occurred in people.

**Contraindications and Precautions**

Do not use in animals that are prone to bleeding problems. Dextrans can interfere with cross-matching of blood for transfusion. Cats are more susceptible to fluid overload than dogs, and lower doses must be used in cats.

**Drug Interactions**

Compatible with most IV fluid solutions, including 0.9% saline solution and 5% dextrose solution.

## Instructions for Use

Used primarily in critical care situations, such as hypovolemic shock. It should be delivered slowly via CRI (60–90 minutes). In emergency use, bolus doses of 20 mL/kg can be administered more rapidly.

## Patient Monitoring and Laboratory Tests

Monitor patient's cardiopulmonary status carefully during administration. Dextrans can interfere with cross-matching of blood.

## Formulations

- Dextran is available in 250-, 500-, and 1000-mL solution for injection.

## Stability and Storage

Store in a tightly sealed container, protected from light, and at room temperature. Stability of compounded formulations has not been evaluated.

## Small Animal Dosage

**Dogs**

- 10–20 mL/kg/day IV to effect, over 30–60 minutes.

**Cats**

- 5–10 mL/kg/day IV over 30–60 minutes.

## Large Animal Dosage

**Horses and Cattle**

- 10 mL/kg/day IV.

## Regulatory Information

Withdrawal times are not established. However, this drug presents little risk from residues; therefore, a short withdrawal time is suggested for animals intended for food.

# Dextromethorphan

deks-troe-meth-or'fan

**Trade and other names:** Benylin and other over-the-counter antitussive brands

**Functional classification:** Antitussive

## Pharmacology and Mechanism of Action

Dextromethorphan is a centrally acting antitussive drug. Dextromethorphan shares similar chemical structure to opiates but does not affect opiate receptors and appears to suppress coughing by directly affecting the cough receptor. Dextromethorphan is the d-isomer of levorphan (the l-isomer of levorphan is an opiate with addictive properties, but the d-isomer is not). Dextromethorphan produces mild analgesia and modulates pain via its ability to act as an N-methyl D-aspartate (NMDA) antagonist, but this is unrelated to the antitussive action.

**D**

## Indications and Clinical Uses

Dextromethorphan has been used for suppression of nonproductive cough. However, its efficacy for reducing cough has been questioned because of a lack of proof. Dextromethorphan also has been used as an adjunct for treating pain because of NMDA antagonism, but this is not a practical use in veterinary medicine. Pharmacokinetic studies in dogs indicated that dextromethorphan does not attain effective concentrations after oral administration. Even after IV administration, concentrations of the parent drug and active metabolite persisted for only a short time after dosing. Therefore, routine use in dogs is not recommended until more data are available to establish safe and effective doses. Pharmacokinetic data are available for dogs but have not been reported for cats or any other species.

## Precautionary Information

### Adverse Reactions and Side Effects

Adverse effects from oral administration are not reported in veterinary medicine. High overdose may potentially cause sedation. In healthy research dogs, dextromethorphan produced vomiting after oral doses and severe CNS reactions after IV administration. Some preparations contain alcohol, which can be unpalatable in small animals, especially cats.

### Contraindications and Precautions

There are no contraindications identified for animals. However, pet owners should be cautioned that many over-the-counter (OTC) preparations contain other drugs that may produce significant side effects. For example, some combinations also contain acetaminophen, which can be toxic to cats. Some preparations also contain a decongestant, such as pseudoephedrine or phenylpropanolamine, which can cause excitement and other side effects.

### Drug Interactions

There are no direct interactions identified for dogs. However, interactions are possible when used with other drugs that may interfere with cytochrome P450 metabolism.

## Instructions for Use

Many OTC preparations may contain other ingredients (e.g., antihistamines, decongestants, ibuprofen, and acetaminophen). Adverse effects from each of these ingredients, such as toxic reactions caused by acetaminophen, CNS excitement from decongestants, and GI toxicity from ibuprofen, can occur in animals.

## Patient Monitoring and Laboratory Tests

No specific monitoring is necessary.

## Formulations

- Dextromethorphan is available in syrup, capsules, and tablets in many OTC products. Many preparations are available without a prescription in liquid and tablet form. OTC formulations may vary in concentration but typically contain 2, 5, 10, or 15 mg/mL and in 15- to 20-mg tablets.

## Stability and Storage

Store in a tightly sealed container, protected from light, and at room temperature. Stability of compounded formulations has not been evaluated.

## Small Animal Dosage

### Dogs and Cats

- 0.5–2 mg/kg q6–8h PO. (However, use is not recommended because efficacy at these doses has not been shown.)

## Large Animal Dosage

- No dosing information available. It has little value for treating large animals.

## Regulatory Information

No regulatory information is available. For extralabel use withdrawal interval estimates, contact FARAD at www.FARAD.org.

RCI Classification: 4

# Dextrose Solution

deks´trose

**Trade and other names:** D5W (5% dextrose) and 50% dextrose solution

**Functional classification:** Fluid replacement

## Pharmacology and Mechanism of Action

Dextrose is a sugar added to fluid solutions. It is isotonic as delivered. Five percent dextrose contains 50 g of dextrose per liter. The pH of this solution is 3.5–6.5. Alternatively, 50% dextrose solution can be added to IV fluids to supplement dextrose. For example, 100 mL of 50% dextrose added to 1000 mL supplies 5% dextrose.

## Indications and Clinical Uses

Five percent dextrose is an isotonic fluid solution used for IV administration. Dextrose is considered only for short-term use because it is deficient in electrolytes. After the glucose is metabolized, the water is rapidly distributed out of the vascular space. For emergency treatment of hypoglycemia or to supplement fluids, a 50% dextrose solution (500 mg/mL) is used. Dextrose has been administered as an emergency treatment to lower serum potassium in cases of hyperkalemia. It lowers potassium by inducing insulin release shifting of potassium from extracellular to intracellular stores.

Dextrose has been administered in a 50% solution to treat or prevent periparturient cows with ketosis and hepatic lipidosis or to support anorexic or recumbent cows. However, there is no established benefit of 50% dextrose treatment for prevention of ketosis in dairy cattle as a single treatment of 0.5 or 1.0 L IV. There is a risk of hypophosphatemia with this treatment.

D

## Precautionary Information

**Adverse Reactions and Side Effects**

High doses can produce pulmonary edema.

**Contraindications and Precautions**

Use cautiously in animals with low electrolyte concentrations. Five percent dextrose solution is not a suitable maintenance solution because it does not provide electrolytes. It should not be considered as a replacement solution or a source of energy requirements; it supplies only 170 kcal/L of energy. When aggressive treatment is used with 50% dextrose, it may cause rapid decrease in plasma phosphorous and potassium (intracellular shift).

**Drug Interactions**

No interactions. Five percent dextrose solution is compatible with fluids and most IV drugs.

## Instructions for Use

Dextrose is a commonly used fluid solution administered via CRI. It is often used as a vehicle to deliver IV drugs that are not compatible with electrolytes. However, it is not a maintenance solution. Dextrose 50% solution can also be added to fluids to supply dextrose. For example, 50 mL of 50% dextrose is added to 1000 mL of fluids to achieve a final 2.5% solution.

## Patient Monitoring and Laboratory Tests

Monitor patient's hydration status and evidence of pulmonary edema during infusion. Monitor acid–base status.

## Formulations

- Fluid solution for IV administration is 5% dextrose, which contains 5 g of glucose per 100 mL (50 g/L). Fifty percent dextrose contains 500 mg/mL (50 g/100 mL). For treatment in large animals, add a 500-mL bottle of 50% dextrose to a 5-L bag of IV fluids.

## Stability and Storage

Store in a tightly sealed container at room temperature.

## Small Animal Dosage

**Dogs and Cats**

- Five percent dextrose solution: 40–50 mL/kg q24h IV.
- In emergency hypoglycemic crisis: 1-mL 50% dextrose solution IV diluted with saline.

## Large Animal Dosage

Horses: Treatment of hyperkalemia: 8–16 mg/kg per minute infusion as an emergency treatment for life-threatening hyperkalemia. See the Formulation section for mixing solutions. An infusion can be administered IV over 1 hour. For milder cases, administer 1–2 mg/kg per minute IV.

### Calves, Cattle, and Horses
- Five percent dextrose solution: 45 mL/kg q24h IV.
- Cows: 0.1–0.2 gm/kg/h IV of dextrose 50% solution for 5 days to treat hepatic lipidosis and ketosis.

## Regulatory Information

Withdrawal times are not established. However, this drug presents little risk from residues; therefore, no withdrawal time is suggested for animals intended for food.

---

# Diazepam
dye-ay′zeh-pam

**Trade and other names:** Valium and generic brands

**Functional classification:** Anticonvulsant

## Pharmacology and Mechanism of Action

Diazepam is a sedative and anticonvulsant of the benzodiazepine class. It is a depressant of the CNS. The mechanism of action appears to be via potentiation of gamma-aminobutyric acid (GABA)-receptor–mediated effects in CNS. It does not bind directly to the GABA binding site, but through indirect effects, it potentiates the action of GABA. Diazepam is metabolized to desmethyldiazepam (nordiazepam) and oxazepam. These metabolites also have some centrally acting benzodiazepine effects. In dogs, the IV half-life of diazepam is short (less than 1 hour), but the active metabolites have longer half-lives and persist for much longer. Cats may have decreased capacity for glucuronidation of diazepam and metabolites for clearance and excretion. In cats, the IV half-life is approximately 3.5–5 hours. The protein binding in dogs is high at 94%.

## Indications and Clinical Uses

Diazepam is used for sedation, anesthetic adjunct, anticonvulsant, and behavioral disorders. Although it is used as a muscle relaxant, the action as a muscle relaxant is not as profound as other benzodiazepines, and the efficacy for this use is not established in animals. In cats, diazepam has been administered IV for short-term stimulation of appetite, but other agents are preferred because of risks from repeated IV diazepam in cats. In cats, oral administration has been effective for decreasing urine spraying, but relapses are common when the drug is discontinued.

Diazepam is usually administered orally or intravenously. However, it is also absorbed in dogs from rectal administration and intranasal administration (41% absorption from nasal spray in dogs and 80% from rectal administration).

## Precautionary Information

### Adverse Reactions and Side Effects

Sedation is the most common side effect. In dogs, ataxia and increased appetite can be observed. Diazepam may cause paradoxical excitement and agitation in dogs. In cats, idiopathic fatal hepatic necrosis has been reported. Chronic administration may lead to dependence and a withdrawal syndrome if discontinued. Administration IM or SQ can be painful and irritating. IV injection can cause phlebitis.

### Contraindications and Precautions

Diazepam is highly dependent on liver blood flow for metabolism. Do not administer to patients with impaired liver function. Long-term use in cats should be avoided because of risk of liver toxicity. Its use for ivermectin-induced CNS intoxication is controversial. Use of benzodiazepines in early pregnancy has been associated with an increased risk of spontaneous abortions and fetal malformations in people. This incidence in animals is unknown.

### Drug Interactions

Diazepam is highly lipophilic and will bind to (adsorb) soft plastic containers, infusion, sets, and fluid bags. Storage of diazepam in such containers is not recommended. Diazepam is not soluble in aqueous solutions. Admixing with aqueous solutions or fluids can result in precipitation.

## Instructions for Use

Clearance in dogs is many times faster than in people requiring frequent administration. For treatment of status epilepticus, diazepam solution may be administered intravenously, intranasally, or rectally. Avoid IM administration because of pain from injection and unpredictable absorption.

### Patient Monitoring and Laboratory Tests

Plasma concentrations in the range of 100–250 ng/mL have been cited as the therapeutic range for people, but some references have cited this range as 150–300 ng/mL. Although plasma or serum may be analyzed for concentrations of benzodiazepines, there are no readily available tests for monitoring in many veterinary laboratories. Laboratories that analyze human samples may have nonspecific tests for benzodiazepines. With these assays, there may be cross-reactivity among diazepam and the metabolites desmethyldiazepam and oxazepam.

### Formulations

- Diazepam is available in 2-, 5-, and 10-mg tablets; 5-mg/mL oral solution; and 5-mg/mL solution for injection.

### Stability and Storage

Do not store in soft plastic (polyvinyl chloride [PVC]) containers or fluid bags. Significant adsorption occurs to soft plastic. However, it is compatible with hard plastic, such as syringes. Do not expose to light. Compounded formulations, especially those prepared for transdermal application, may not be stable. Diazepam is practically insoluble in water but is soluble in alcohol and propylene glycol. Diazepam undergoes hydrolysis in water. Diazepam prepared as an oral suspension (1 mg/mL) in various vehicles (pH 4.2) was stable for 60 days.

## Small Animal Dosage

### Dogs and Cats

- Preanesthetic: 0.5 mg/kg IV.
- Status epilepticus: 0.5 mg/kg IV, 0.5–1 mg/kg sprayed intranasal, or 1 mg/kg rectal; repeat if necessary.
- CRI: 15 mcg/kg/min (1 mg/kg/h), which can be decreased by 50% in some animals if excessive side effects are observed.
- Appetite stimulant (cats): 0.2 mg/kg IV.
- Behavior treatment (cats): 1–4 mg/cat q12–24h PO.
- Behavior treatment (dogs): 0.5–2 mg/kg q4–6h PO.

## Large Animal Dosage

### Cattle, Sheep, and Goats

- 0.02–0.08 mg/kg IV, up to 0.5 mg/kg slowly IV. Dose according to desired effect. Cows may be recumbent after 0.5 mg/kg. Do not administer IM.

### Horses

- Seizures: 0.1–0.4 mg/kg IV (start with 50–100 mg per horse). CRI for foals: 1–3 mg/h.

## Regulatory Information

No regulatory information is available. For extralabel use withdrawal interval estimates, contact FARAD at www.FARAD.org.

Schedule IV controlled drug

RCI Classification: 2

---

# Dichlorphenamide

dye-klor-fen′ah-mide

**Trade and other names:** Daranide

**Functional classification:** Diuretic

## Pharmacology and Mechanism of Action

Dichlorphenamide is a carbonic anhydrase inhibitor and used as a diuretic. Dichlorphenamide, like other carbonic anhydrase inhibitors, produces diuresis by inhibiting the reabsorption of bicarbonate in proximal renal tubules via enzyme inhibition. This action results in loss of bicarbonate in the urine and diuresis. The action of carbonic anhydrase inhibitors results in significant urine loss of bicarbonate, alkaline urine, and water. Despite the significant diuretic effect produced, these agents are rarely used as diuretics because other effective agents are available (e.g., furosemide).

## Indications and Clinical Uses

Dichlorphenamide is rarely used as a diuretic any longer. More potent and effective diuretic drugs are available, such as the loop diuretics (furosemide). Dichlorphenamide, like other carbonic anhydrase inhibitors, is used primarily to reduce intraocular pressure in animals with glaucoma. Methazolamide is used more often than dichlorphenamide or acetazolamide for this purpose, and other treatment regimens for glaucoma are used more often than carbonic anhydrase inhibitors. Dichlorphenamide, like other carbonic anhydrase inhibitors, is sometimes used to produce a more alkaline urine for management of some urinary calculi.

## Precautionary Information
### Adverse Reactions and Side Effects
With prolonged use, it depletes bicarbonate if not replenished. Dichlorphenamide is a sulfonamide derivative. Some animals sensitive to sulfonamides may be sensitive to dichlorphenamide. Hypokalemia may occur in some patients. Severe metabolic acidosis is rare.

### Contraindications and Precautions
Use cautiously in animals sensitive to sulfonamides.

### Drug Interactions
Dichlorphenamide produces alkaline urine, which may affect clearance of some drugs. Alkaline urine may potentiate the effects of some antibacterial drugs (e.g., macrolides and quinolones).

## Instructions for Use
Dichlorphenamide is not used as a diuretic, but the use for treating glaucoma or to produce alkaline urine is more common. When used for glaucoma, it has been combined with other antiglaucoma agents.

## Patient Monitoring and Laboratory Tests
Monitor ocular pressure for glaucoma treatment. Monitor serum potassium and acid–base status during treatment.

## Formulations
• Dichlorphenamide is no longer commercially available. However, older forms were available in 50-mg tablets.

## Stability and Storage
Store in a tightly sealed container, protected from light, and at room temperature. Stability of compounded formulations has not been evaluated.

## Small Animal Dosage
### Dogs and Cats
• 3–5 mg/kg q8–12h PO.

## Large Animal Dosage
• No large animal doses are reported.

## Regulatory Information
No regulatory information is available. For extralabel use withdrawal interval estimates, contact FARAD at www.FARAD.org.

RCI Classification: 4

# Dichlorvos
dye´klor-vos

**Trade and other names:** Task, Atgard, DDVP, Verdisol, and Equigard. Also known as dichlorovos.

**Functional classification:** Antiparasitic

## Pharmacology and Mechanism of Action

Dichlorvos is an antiparasitic drug that has been used for many years in animals to treat a wide variety of intestinal parasites. It kills parasites by anticholinesterase action.

## Indications and Clinical Uses

Dichlorvos is used primarily to treat intestinal parasites. Parasites that may be treated include *Toxocara canis* and *Toxascaris leonina* (roundworms), *Ancylostoma caninum*, *Uncinaria stenocephala* (hookworms), and *Trichuris vulpis* (whipworms). However, efficacy against *T. vulpis* may be erratic. In horses, it may be used for the removal and control of bots (*Gastrophilus intestinalis, Gastrophilus nasalis*), large strongyles (*Strongylus vulgaris, Strongylus equinus, Strongylus edentatus*), small strongyles (of the genera *Cyathostomum, Cylicocercus, Cylicodontophorus, Triodontophorus,* and *Poteriostomum*), pinworms (*Oxyuris equi*), and large roundworm (*Parascaris equorum*). In pigs, it is used to treat and control mature, immature, and fourth-stage larvae of the whipworm (*Trichuris suis*), nodular worm (*Oesophagostomum* spp.), large roundworm (*Ascaris suum*), and thick stomach worm (*Ascarops strongylina*).

## Precautionary Information

### Adverse Reactions and Side Effects

Overdoses can cause organophosphate intoxication (treat with pralidoxime chloride and atropine). Signs of toxicity include salivation, diarrhea, difficulty breathing, and muscle twitching.

### Contraindications and Precautions

Do not use in patients with heartworms. Do not administer within 2 days of administration of another cholinesterase-inhibiting drug. Use a split-dosage schedule in animals that are old, heavily parasitized, anemic, or otherwise debilitated. Do not use in young foals, kittens, or puppies weighing less than 2 lb. Its use may exacerbate clinical signs in animals with respiratory disease, such as bronchitis and obstructive pulmonary disease. Do not allow birds access to feed containing this preparation or to fecal excrement from treated animals.

### Drug Interactions

Do not use with other anticholinesterase drugs. Do not use with other antifilarial agents, muscle relaxants, CNS depressants, or tranquilizers.

## Instructions for Use

Administer in about one third of the regular canned dog food ration or in ground meat. Dogs may be treated with any combination of capsules and pellets so that the animal receives a single dose. One half of the single recommended dosage may be given, and the other half may be administered 8–24 hours later. For horses, administer in the grain portion of the ration. It may be administered at one half of the single recommended dose and repeated 8–12 hours later for treatment of old, emaciated, or debilitated subjects or those reluctant to consume medicated feed. Split the dose if heavy parasitism may cause concern over mechanical blockage of the intestinal tract.

## Patient Monitoring and Laboratory Tests

Monitor for parasites as part of a regular parasite control program.

## Formulations

- Dichlorvos is available in 10- and 25-mg tablets. Manufacture of equine formulations has been discontinued, and other forms must be used in horses.

## Stability and Storage
Store in a tightly sealed container, protected from light, and at room temperature. Stability of compounded formulations has not been evaluated.

## Small Animal Dosage
**Dogs**
- 26.4–33 mg/kg once PO.

**Cats**
- 11 mg/kg once PO.

## Large Animal Dosage
**Pigs**
- 11.2–21.6 mg/kg once PO. For pregnant sows, mix into a gestation feed to provide 1000 mg/head daily during the last 30 days of gestation, mixed at a rate of 334–500 g/ton of feed. For other pigs, mix at 334 per ton of feed and feed as sole ration for 2 consecutive days (rate of 8.4 lb of feed per head until the medicated feed has been consumed).

**Horses**
- 31–41 mg/kg once PO.

## Regulatory Information
Do not administer to horses intended for food.
For other animals, no regulatory information is available. For extralabel use withdrawal interval estimates, contact FARAD at www.FARAD.org.

# Diclazuril
dih-klaz´yoor-il

**Trade and other names:** Clincox and Protazil pellets for horses

**Functional classification:** Antiprotozoal

## Pharmacology and Mechanism of Action
Diclazuril is an antiprotozoan drug used most often as a coccidiostat. Diclazuril is in the class of triazinone antiprotozoals that is effective for treating infections caused by *Isospora* spp., *Toxoplasma gondii*, and *Eimeria* spp. and has been used for treating coccidiosis. It also has been used in horses to treat equine protozoal myeloencephalitis (EPM) caused by *Sarcocystis neurona*. Although the exact mechanism of action is currently under investigation, diclazuril exerts its effect on *S. neurona* effect by inhibiting merozoite production.

*Pharmacokinetics:* The pharmacokinetics have been studied primarily in horses, the target animal species. The oral absorption is 1.56% with a half-life of 43–65 hours. Other studies in horses have shown that at a dose of 1 and 0.5 mg/kg, the half-lives are 55 and 87 hours, respectively, with peak concentration of 0.185 and 0.1 mcg/mL, respectively. With repeated dosing to steady state, the half-life from 0.5 and 1.0 mg/kg was 71 and 54 hours, respectively, with peak concentration of 0.97 and 0.9 mcg/mL, respectively. Thus, with chronic dosing, the pharmacokinetic profile was similar with 1.0 and 0.5 mg/kg to horses.

## Indications and Clinical Uses
Dosage information for diclazuril has been based on approved indications, experimental studies, pharmacokinetic data, and clinical experience. Ponazuril is another related agent used for treating EPM in horses.

## Precautionary Information

**Adverse Reactions and Side Effects**

No specific adverse effects have been reported.

**Contraindications and Precautions**

No contraindications have been reported.

**Drug Interactions**

No drug interactions have been reported.

## Instructions for Use

Administer orally to horses. It may be added to feed as pellets.

## Patient Monitoring and Laboratory Tests

No specific monitoring is necessary. The targeted concentration of diclazuril to inhibit merozoite production of *S. neurona* and *Sarcocystis falcatula* in bovine turbinate cell cultures is 0.1 ng/mL to achieve greater than 80% inhibition and 1.0 ng/mL to achieve greater than 95% inhibition.

## Formulations

- Diclazuril pellets for horses is available as 1.56% diclazuril to be mixed as a top dress on feed for treatment of EPM. One 2-lb bucket treats one horse for 28 days. It is also available as a medicated feed additive for poultry.

## Stability and Storage

Store in a tightly sealed container, protected from light, and at room temperature. Stability of compounded formulations has not been evaluated.

## Small Animal Dosage

- No dosing information has been reported for small animals.

## Large Animal Dosage

**Horses**

- Treatment of EPM: 1 mg/kg oral as a top dress on feed for 28 days added to daily ration. It has also been shown that with repeated administration to steady state, 0.5 mg/kg body weight achieves a similar pharmacokinetic profile as dosing at the Food and Drug Administration (FDA)–labeled dose of 1 mg/kg.
- For prevention of EPM: Top dress feed with pellets: 0.5 mg/kg once every 3 or 4 days.

## Regulatory Information

Do not administer to horses intended for food. Withdrawal time for poultry is 5 days. For other animals, no regulatory information is available. For extralabel use withdrawal interval estimates, contact FARAD at www.FARAD.org.

# Dicloxacillin Sodium

dye-kloks-ah-sill´in soe´dee-um

**Trade and other names:** Dynapen and generic

**Functional classification:** Antibacterial

## Pharmacology and Mechanism of Action

Dicloxacillin is a beta-lactam antibiotic and a semisynthetic derivative of penicillin. It resembles ampicillin in activity, except it has greater stability against staphylococcal beta-lactamase. Like other antibiotics in this class, it inhibits bacterial cell wall synthesis by binding to penicillin-binding proteins and weakening the cell wall. The spectrum is limited to gram-positive bacteria, especially staphylococci. It has little, if any, activity against gram-negative bacteria.

**D**

## Indications and Clinical Uses

Dicloxacillin has a relatively narrow spectrum of activity. Like cloxacillin and oxacillin, the spectrum of dicloxacillin includes gram-positive bacilli, including beta-lactamase–producing strains of *Staphylococcus* spp. Therefore it has been used to treat staphylococcal infections in animals, including pyoderma. It is not active against methicillin-resistant *Staphylococcus* spp. Gram-negative Enterobacteriaceae bacteria are clinically resistant. Because of availability of other drugs for small animals to treat this spectrum of bacteria, dicloxacillin is not used commonly. Because it is an oral drug with limited absorption in large animals, its use is limited to small animal oral administration.

## Precautionary Information

### Adverse Reactions and Side Effects

Adverse effects of penicillin drugs are most commonly caused by drug allergy. This can range from acute anaphylaxis when administered to other signs of allergic reaction when other routes are used. When administered orally (especially with high doses), diarrhea is possible.

### Contraindications and Precautions

Use cautiously in animals allergic to penicillin-like drugs.

### Drug Interactions

There are no specific drug interactions. Dicloxacillin is absorbed better on an empty stomach in dogs.

## Instructions for Use

No clinical efficacy studies are available for dogs or cats. In dogs, oral absorption is low and may not be suitable for therapy. Administer on an empty stomach, if possible.

## Patient Monitoring and Laboratory Tests

Use oxacillin as a guide for sensitivity testing. Breakpoints for oxacillin apply to dicloxacillin.

## Formulations

Some formulations have been discontinued. Dicloxacillin has been available in 125-, 250-, and 500-mg capsules and 12.5-mg/mL oral suspension.

## Stability and Storage

Store in a tightly sealed container, protected from light, and at room temperature. Do not mix with other drugs. Reconstituted oral suspension is stable for 14 days refrigerated. Compounded formulations, especially aqueous formulations, may not be stable.

## Small Animal Dosage

### Dogs and Cats

- 11–55 mg/kg q8h PO.

## Large Animal Dosage
• No dose has been reported for large animals. Oral absorption is low.

## Regulatory Information
No regulatory information is available. Because oral absorption is expected to be minimal, when using systemically in food animals, apply similar withdrawal times as for ampicillin. Alternatively, contact FARAD at www.FARAD.org.

# Diethylcarbamazine Citrate
dye-eth-il-kar-bam´eh-zeen sih´trate

**Trade and other names:** Caricide, Filaribits, and Nemacide

**Functional classification:** Antiparasitic

## Pharmacology and Mechanism of Action
Diethylcarbamazine is a heartworm preventative and anthelmintic. It produces neuromuscular blockade in parasite through inhibition of neurotransmitter that causes paralysis of worms. The use has declined substantially because of other agents that are available.

## Indications and Clinical Uses
The commercial tablets (e.g., Caricide) and some other brands used for heartworm prevention have been voluntarily withdrawn by the sponsor. Because of the availability of other heartworm preventatives that are effective and easy to administer (e.g., once per month or less), the use of diethylcarbamazine has diminished significantly. Diethylcarbamazine has been used to prevent infection caused by heartworms in dogs. It has been administered regularly during heartworm season in endemic areas. It is not effective to treat heartworms once infection is established. Other uses of diethylcarbamazine have included control of ascarids infections (*T. canis* and *T. leonina*) and as an aid in treatment of ascarid infections at higher doses (55–110 mg/kg). In cats, diethylcarbamazine has been used to treat ascarid worm infections (55–110 mg/kg).

## Precautionary Information

### Adverse Reactions and Side Effects
Overdoses cause vomiting. If administered to an animal with positive microfilaria, reactions, including pulmonary reactions, are possible. This drug is a piperazine derivative, which is a class of antiparasitic drugs considered generally safe in animals.

### Contraindications and Precautions
Dogs with established heartworm infections caused by *Dirofilaria immitis* should not receive diethylcarbamazine until they have been treated with an adulticide to kill the adult heartworms followed by appropriate microfilaricidal treatment. Reactions can occur in animals with positive microfilaria. However, there are no breed sensitivities or other specific contraindications.

### Drug Interactions
No specific drug interactions are reported.

## Instructions for Use

Specific protocols for heartworm administration may be based on the region of country because the time (season) required for heartworm prevention depends on the duration of active mosquitoes during the year. Although diethylcarbamazine is effective to prevent heartworms, it requires almost continual daily treatment for efficacy. Two or three doses should not be missed. Occasionally, some animals vomit immediately after dosing. Administration with food sometimes decreases this reaction. If diethylcarbamazine treatment has been interrupted, the American Heartworm Society recommends switching chemoprophylaxis to macrocyclic lactones (ivermectin and related drugs).

**D**

## Patient Monitoring and Laboratory Tests

Monitor heartworm status of patient. It is important to test for microfilaria in animals before prescribing. Manufacturers recommend that animals that are currently receiving diethylcarbamazine be checked for microfilaria every 6 months. Reactions can occur in animals with positive microfilaria.

## Formulations

- Although some brands have been withdrawn by the sponsor, some availability of other diethylcarbamazine tablets may vary with manufacturer and brand name and country or region. Not every brand name is available in the sizes listed. Both plain and chewable tablets have been available. Tablet sizes include 30, 45, 50, 60, 100, 120, 150, 180, 200, 300, and 400 mg. Syrup has been available as 60 mg/mL.

## Stability and Storage

Store in a tightly sealed container, protected from light, and at room temperature. Stability of compounded formulations has not been evaluated.

## Small Animal Dosage

**Dogs**
- Heartworm prophylaxis: 6.6 mg/kg q24h PO.
- Treatment of ascarids: 55–110 mg/kg PO as a single treatment (the 110-mg/kg dose may be divided into twice per day).

**Cats**
- Ascarid treatment: 55–110 mg/kg PO. When treating ascarid parasites, consider repeating treatment in 10–20 days to remove immature worms.

## Large Animal Dosage

- No dose has been reported for large animals.

## Regulatory Information

No regulatory information is available.
For extralabel use withdrawal interval estimates, contact FARAD at www.FARAD.org.

# Diethylstilbestrol
dye-eth-il-stil-bess´trole

**Trade and other names:** DES and generic brands

**Functional classification:** Hormone

## Pharmacology and Mechanism of Action

Diethylstilbestrol, known as DES, is a synthetic drug with estrogen effects. It differs from steroid compounds because it does not have a steroid ring, although it has estrogen-like effects. It is used for estrogen replacement in animals. The most common use in dogs is treatment of urinary incontinence. When used to treat urinary incontinence, the action of DES is believed to increase sensitivity of alpha receptors in the urinary sphincter to restore continence.

## Indications and Clinical Uses

Diethylstilbestrol is most commonly used to treat estrogen-responsive incontinence in dogs. Phenylpropanolamine (PPA) has been used in dogs when DES therapy is no longer effective. DES also has been used to induce abortion in dogs. Commercial forms of DES are no longer available, but it is available through some compounding pharmacies. Conjugated estrogens (e.g., Premarin at 20 mcg/kg twice weekly) have been used in some dogs when DES or other estrogens have been unavailable. In addition, there is an approved form of estriol for dogs (Incurin) that can be used instead of DES for treatment of incontinence in female dogs (see Estriol for more details).

## Precautionary Information

### Adverse Reactions and Side Effects

Side effects attributed to excess estrogen may occur. Estrogen therapy may increase risk of pyometra and estrogen-sensitive tumors. Although bone marrow depression (particularly anemia) has been reported from administration of other estrogens in dogs and has been cited as a potential risk, it is a rare complication of DES therapy.

### Contraindications and Precautions

Diethylstilbestrol has been associated with the development of cancer, and human exposure should be minimized as much as possible. This drug is no longer used in people for estrogen replacement and is prohibited in food animals. Although not reported as a significant clinical problem with DES, problems with anemia have occurred with administration of high doses of other estrogens to animals.

### Drug Interactions

No significant drug interactions have been reported for animals. However, in people, administration of estrogens increases thyroid-binding globulin and may decrease the active form of thyroid hormone (tetraiodothyronine [$T_4$]) in patients receiving thyroid supplementation.

## Instructions for Use

Doses listed are for treating urinary incontinence and vary depending on response. Titrate dose to individual patient's response. Although used to induce abortion, it was not efficacious in one study that administered 75 mcg/kg.

## Patient Monitoring and Laboratory Tests

Monitor CBC to detect signs of bone marrow toxicity. Monitor $T_4$ levels if patients are hypothyroid and receiving supplementation.

## Formulations

- DES has been available in 1- and 5-mg tablets and 50-mg/mL injection. DES is no longer marketed commercially in the United States, but it is available from compounding pharmacies.

## Stability and Storage
Store in a tightly sealed container, protected from light, and at room temperature. Stability of compounded formulations has not been reported. However, compounded tablets are available from compounding pharmacies, and anecdotal information indicates that they are effective.

## Small Animal Dosage
**Dogs**
- Dose ranges from 0.1–1 mg per dog q24h PO. The size of the dose is proportional to size of the dog. Continue daily dose for 5 days; then reduce frequency of administration to two or three times per week.

**Cats**
- 0.05–0.1 mg/cat q24h PO.

## Large Animal Dosage
- No dose is available for large animals. Use in animals intended for food is prohibited.

## Regulatory Information
Administering DES to animals that produce food is prohibited.

---

# Difloxacin Hydrochloride
dye-floks′ah-sin hye-droe-klor′ide

**Trade and other names:** Dicural

**Functional classification:** Antibacterial

---

**Note:** Difloxacin is no longer marketed and may not be available in many countries.

## Pharmacology and Mechanism of Action
Difloxacin is a fluoroquinolone antibacterial drug. Its mechanism of action is through inhibition of DNA gyrase in bacteria to inhibit DNA and RNA synthesis. It has bactericidal activity with broad spectrum of activity. Antibacterial activity includes *E. coli*, *Klebsiella* spp., *Pasteurella* spp., and other gram-negative bacilli. Activity against *Pseudomonas aeruginosa* is less than for other gram-negative bacilli. Activity against gram-positive cocci includes *Staphylococcus*. *Streptococcus* and *Enterococcus* spp. are more resistant. Most of the use has been in dogs, with a half-life of approximately 7 hours and a peak concentration of 1.1 mcg/mL. It has had limited use in horses, with an oral half-life of 10.8 hours and bioavailability of 68%.

## Indications and Clinical Uses
Difloxacin, like other fluoroquinolones, has been used for a variety of infections, including skin infections, wound infections, and pneumonia. Unlike other fluoroquinolones, difloxacin does not have high renal clearance. Urine concentrations may not be sufficient for some UTIs.

Despite the features that are typical of other fluoroquinolones, difloxacin has not been in common use and is not available in most countries.

## Precautionary Information

### Adverse Reactions and Side Effects

High concentrations may cause CNS toxicity, especially in animals with renal failure. Difloxacin may cause some nausea, vomiting, and diarrhea at high doses. All of the fluoroquinolones may cause arthropathy in young animals. Dogs are most sensitive at 4 weeks to 28 weeks of age. Large, rapidly growing dogs are the most susceptible. Safety in cats has not been reported. It has not been reported if there is a potential to cause retinal ocular injury in cats.

### Contraindications and Precautions

Avoid use in young animals because of risk of cartilage injury. Use cautiously in animals that may be prone to seizures, such as epileptics. Avoid use in cats unless safety has been established.

### Drug Interactions

Fluoroquinolones may increase concentrations of theophylline if used concurrently. Coadministration with divalent and trivalent cations, such as products containing aluminum (e.g., sucralfate), iron, or calcium, may decrease absorption. Do not mix in solutions or in vials with aluminum, calcium, iron, or zinc because chelation may occur.

## Instructions for Use

Dose range can be used to adjust dose depending on severity of infection and susceptibility of bacteria. Bacteria with low MIC values can be treated with a low dose; susceptible bacteria with higher MIC values should be treated with a higher dose. Difloxacin is primarily eliminated in feces rather than urine (urine is less than 5% of clearance). Sarafloxacin is an active desmethyl metabolite but produced in low amounts. Oral absorption in horses is low and should only be used for bacteria with MIC less than 0.12 mcg/mL.

## Patient Monitoring and Laboratory Tests

Susceptibility testing: CLSI breakpoint for sensitive organisms is ≤0.5 mcg/mL for canine pathogens.

## Formulations

- Difloxacin is no longer marketed and may not be available. It was previously available in 11.4-, 45.4-, and 136-mg tablets. (In some countries, 5% injectable is available.)

## Stability and Storage

Store in a tightly sealed container, protected from light, and at room temperature. Stability of compounded formulations has not been evaluated but has been mixed with simple syrup (100 mg/mL) for horses.

## Small Animal Dosage

### Dogs

- 5–10 mg/kg q24h PO.

### Cats

- No dosing information for cats is available. There is no safety information available.

**Large Animal Dosage**
- Horses: 5 mg/kg PO, q24h.

**Regulatory Information**
Do not administer to animals intended for food.

# Digitoxin
dih-jih-toks´in

**Trade and other names:** Digimerck (European)

**Functional classification:** Cardiac inotropic agent

**Note:** Digitoxin is no longer available commercially and not used clinically. It has been removed from this edition, but readers may consult earlier editions of this handbook for more detailed information on clinical use and dosages.

# Digoxin
dih-joks´in

**Trade and other names:** Lanoxin and Cardoxin

**Functional classification:** Cardiac inotropic agent

## Pharmacology and Mechanism of Action
Digoxin is a cardiac inotropic agent and also is used to regulate cardiac rate and rhythm. Digoxin increases cardiac contractility and decreases heart rate. The mechanism is via inactivation of cardiac muscle sodium–potassium ATPase and increased intracellular availability of calcium, triggering calcium release from sarcoplasmic reticulum. In addition, neuroendocrine effects include sensitization of baroreceptors, which decreases heart rate by increasing vagal tone. Beneficial cardiac effects may be caused by decreased heart rate and suppression of the AV node to inhibit reentrant cardiac arrhythmias via these neuroendocrine effects. An older drug, digitoxin, is no longer available. (Consult older editions of this handbook for information on digitoxin.)

## Indications and Clinical Uses
The use of digoxin for animals in heart failure has declined significantly because pimobendan is more frequently used and is available in a veterinary formulation.

Digoxin has been used for treatment of heart failure in dogs, cats, and occasionally other animals. Because the use for an inotropic effect has declined, the most common use is to decrease the heart rate in animals. This property is used for treatment of supraventricular arrhythmias to decrease ventricular response to atrial stimulation via suppression of the AV node. Digoxin may be used with other drugs for heart failure such as ACE inhibitors (e.g., enalapril), diuretics (furosemide), and vasodilators.

## Precautionary Information

### Adverse Reactions and Side Effects

Digitalis glycosides such as digoxin have a narrow therapeutic index. They may cause a variety of arrhythmias in patients (e.g., AV and ventricular tachycardia) and may produce delayed after depolarization-induced arrhythmias. Heart block (AV block) is possible. Digoxin frequently causes vomiting, anorexia, and diarrhea. Digoxin adverse effects are potentiated by hypokalemia and reduced by hyperkalemia.

### Contraindications and Precautions

Some breeds of dogs (Doberman pinscher) and cats are more sensitive to adverse effects.

### Drug Interactions

High potassium will diminish clinical effect; low potassium will enhance effect and toxicity. Because some animals may also be receiving diuretics, monitor the potassium concentrations during treatment. Digoxin is a substrate for cytochrome P450 enzymes and p-glycoprotein. Many drugs are capable of increasing digoxin concentrations, including quinidine, aspirin, clarithromycin (and other macrolides), and chloramphenicol (see Appendixes I and J for list of inhibitors). Administration of phenobarbital chronically may decrease digoxin concentrations by increasing clearance. Calcium-channel blockers and beta blockers potentiate action on AV node conduction, increasing the risk of AV block. Digoxin is absorbed better in an acid stomach, and proton pump inhibitors or $H_2$ blockers may reduce oral absorption.

## Instructions for Use

When dosing, calculate dose on lean body weight. Doses should be 10% less for elixir because of increased absorption. When used to treat atrial fibrillation in dogs, combined with diltiazem, it may produce greater reduction in ventricular rate than either drug alone.

## Patient Monitoring and Laboratory Tests

Monitor patients carefully. Monitor serum digoxin concentrations in patients to determine optimum therapy. Therapeutic range is 0.8–1.5 ng/mL 8–10 hours after a dose. Some cardiologists recommend concentrations of 0.9–1.0 ng/mL and below for treating heart failure and higher concentrations of to reduce heart rate to 140–160 bpm. Adverse effects are common at concentrations above 3.5 ng/mL, but in some sensitive patients, this may be as low as 2.5 ng/mL. Patients may be monitored with ECG to detect digoxin-induced arrhythmias.

## Formulations

- Digoxin is available in 0.0625-, 0.125-, and 0.25-mg tablets and 0.05- and 0.15-mg/mL elixir.

## Stability and Storage

Store in a tightly sealed container, protected from light, and at room temperature. It is not stable if mixed with low-pH solutions (pH less than 3). Do not compound oral tablets with other medications.

## Small Animal Dosage

**Dogs**

- 0.005–0.011 mg/kg q12h PO (dose used by most cardiologists).
- Alternatively, doses have varied based on dog's body weight: dogs weighing less than 20 kg: 0.005–0.01 mg/kg q12h and if weighing greater than 20 kg: 0.22 mg/m$^2$ q12h PO (subtract 10% for elixir).
- Rapid digitalization: 0.0055–0.011 mg/kg q1h IV to effect.
- Atrial fibrillation: 0.005 mg/kg q12h PO (may be combined with diltiazem at 3 mg/kg q12h PO).

**Cats**

- 0.008–0.01 mg/kg q48h PO. (Approximately one fourth of a 0.125-mg tablet/cat.)

## Large Animal Dosage

**Cattle**

- 22 mcg/kg (0.022 mg/kg) IV loading dose followed by 0.86 mcg/kg/h IV or multiple doses of 3.4 mcg/kg q4h. Plasma concentrations to monitor are similar as for other animals.

**Horses**

- 2 mcg/kg (0.002 mg/kg) IV q12h.
- 15 mcg/kg (0.015 mg/kg) q12h PO.

## Regulatory Information

Do not administer to animals intended for food.
RCI Classification: 4

# Dihydrotachysterol

dye-hye-droe-tak-iss´ter-ole

**Trade and other names:** Vitamin D

**Functional classification:** Vitamin

## Pharmacology and Mechanism of Action

Vitamin D analogue. Vitamin D promotes absorption and utilization of calcium.

## Indications and Clinical Uses

Dihydrotachysterol is used as treatment of hypocalcemia, especially hypoparathyroidism associated with thyroidectomy. The most common use is for replacement in cats that have had thyroidectomy for treatment of hyperthyroidism. Calcitriol and calcium supplements are other drugs used to regulate calcium concentrations in animals (see Calcitriol).

## Precautionary Information

**Adverse Reactions and Side Effects**

Overdose may cause hypercalcemia.

**Contraindications and Precautions**

Avoid use in pregnant animals because it may cause fetal abnormalities.

**Drug Interactions**

No specific drug interactions are reported for animals. However, use cautiously with high doses of preparations containing calcium. Use with caution with thiazide diuretics.

## Instructions for Use

Doses for individual patients should be adjusted by monitoring serum calcium concentrations.

## Patient Monitoring and Laboratory Tests

Monitor serum calcium concentration. Normal total calcium concentrations in dogs and cats are 9–11.5 mg/dL and 8–10.5 mg/dL, respectively, or 1.2–1.5 mmol/L and 1.1–1.4 mmol/L, respectively.

## Formulations

- No formulations are currently available in the United States. It can only be obtained from some compounding pharmacies. Older formulations consisted of 0.125-mg capsules; 0.5-mg/mL oral liquid (20% alcohol); and 125-, 200-, and 400-mg tablets.

## Stability and Storage

Store in a tightly sealed container, protected from light, and at room temperature. Stability of compounded formulations has not been evaluated.

## Small Animal Dosage

### Dog And Cats

- 0.01 mg/kg/day PO.
- Acute treatment: 0.02 mg/kg initially; then 0.01–0.02 mg/kg q24–48h PO thereafter. The dose should be adjusted on the basis of measuring calcium concentrations. Effective doses can range as high as 0.1–0.3 mg/kg.

## Large Animal Dosage

- No large animal doses are reported.

## Regulatory Information

No regulatory information is available. For extralabel use withdrawal interval estimates, contact FARAD at www.FARAD.org.

---

# Diltiazem Hydrochloride

dil-tye′ah-zem hye-droe-klor′ide

**Trade and other names:** Cardizem and Dilacor

**Functional classification:** Calcium-channel blocker

## Pharmacology and Mechanism of Action

Diltiazem is a calcium-channel blocking drug. Diltiazem blocks calcium entry into cells via blockade of voltage-dependent slow calcium channel. Via this action, it produces vasodilation, negative chronotropic effects, and negative inotropic effects. However, the action on cardiac tissue (sinoatrial [SA] node and AV node) predominates over other effects. The effects on vascular smooth muscle—to reduce blood pressure—are not as great as other calcium-channel blocking drugs such as amlodipine.

*Pharmacokinetics:* Half-life in dogs is approximately 3 hours (range, 2.5–4 hours), and it is shorter in horses (1.5 hours).

## Indications and Clinical Uses

Diltiazem is used primarily for control of supraventricular arrhythmias, atrial fibrillation, and hypertrophic cardiomyopathy. It also is used for atrial flutter, AV nodal reentry arrhythmias, and other forms of tachycardia. Diltiazem is more effective on heart tissues (AV node and SA node) than on blood vessels. It can be used with digoxin and the action on cardiac rate and rhythm may be greater when used with digoxin. It should not be used as a primary treatment of hypertension and to produce vasodilation; one of the dihydropyridines calcium-channel blocking drugs (e.g., amlodipine) is preferred. In cats, diltiazem is considered one of the drugs of choice for treatment of feline hypertrophic cardiomyopathy. In dogs, diltiazem has been used to treat acute renal failure. It may improve renal perfusion by decreasing renal vasoconstriction and improving renal perfusion. In horses, diltiazem may be effective for atrial fibrillation. However, treated horses had variable results, and some developed hypotension and sinus arrest. Transdermal administration of diltiazem has not been shown to be effective in cats.

## Precautionary Information

### Adverse Reactions and Side Effects

Hypotension, myocardial depression, bradycardia, and AV block are the most important adverse effects. If acute hypotension occurs, treat with aggressive fluid therapy and administration of calcium gluconate or calcium chloride. It may cause anorexia in some patients. High doses in cats have caused vomiting. When cats were administered 60 mg of Dilacor XR, it produced lethargy, GI disturbances, and weight loss in 36% of cats.

### Contraindications and Precautions

Do not inject rapidly when administering IV. Do not administer to patients with hypotension.

### Drug Interactions

Calcium-channel blocking drugs have been associated with drug interactions in people by interfering with drug metabolism. These interactions have not been documented in veterinary patients but are possible because of similar mechanisms. Therefore, use with caution when administering other drugs that may be p-glycoprotein (efflux protein produced by multi-drug resistance [MDR] gene) substrates. (See Appendixes J and K.) Do not mix IV solutions with furosemide.

## Instructions for Use

Diltiazem is preferred over verapamil in patients with heart failure because of less myocardial depression. When used to treat atrial fibrillation in dogs, combined with digoxin, it may produce greater reduction in ventricular rate than either drug alone. See detailed instructions for cats in the Small Animal Dosage section.

## Patient Monitoring and Laboratory Tests

Monitor heart rate and rhythm during treatment. Monitor blood pressure with acute treatment for atrial fibrillation. If blood concentrations are monitored, to produce a reduction in heart rate, 80–290 ng/mL are necessary in people and 60–120 ng/mL in dogs.

## Formulations

- Diltiazem is available in 30-, 60-, 90-, and 120-mg tablets.
- Diltiazem is also available as 120-, 180-, and 240-mg extended-release capsules and in a 5-mg/mL injection solution.
- Extended-release capsules have three or four tablets in one unit. The capsule may be opened to release the individual tablets for oral dosing in dogs and cats.

## Stability and Storage

Store in a tightly sealed container, protected from light, and at room temperature. Extended-release tablets are difficult to manipulate for pet owners. Compounded transdermal formulations may not be stable. Compounded oral formulations, prepared with various sugars and flavorings, were stable for 50–60 days. Injectable solution may be mixed with IV fluids but should be discarded after 24 hours. Do not freeze.

## Small Animal Dosage

### Dogs

- For most uses: 0.5–1.5 mg/kg q8h PO. For atrial fibrillation, dosages as high as 5 mg/kg q12h PO have been used as monotherapy, or a combination of diltiazem (3 mg/kg q12h PO) plus digoxin (0.005 mg/kg q12h, PO) has been used.
- Atrial fibrillation: 0.05–0.25 mg/kg IV administered every 5 minutes to effect.
- Supraventricular tachycardia: 0.25 mg/kg over 2 minutes IV (repeat if necessary). First, inject 0.25 mg/kg; then wait 20 minutes for response before repeating. To administer a CRI, inject 0.15–0.25 mg/kg IV over 2 minutes; then use a CRI of 0.1–0.2 mg/kg/h, up to a maximum of 0.4 mg/kg/h.
- Acute renal failure: 0.2 mg/kg IV (slowly) followed by 3–5 mcg/kg/min CRI.

### Cats

- 1.75–2.4 mg/kg q8h PO. Most common dosage in cats with immediate-release formulations is 7.5–10 mg per cat q8h PO, with frequency reduced to q12h in some cats.
- Dilacor XR or Cardizem CD: 10 mg/kg once daily PO. Extended-release tablets can be more difficult to use in cats compared to other tablets but have been used at 30 or 60 mg per cat (see later).
- Tablets are difficult to break for use in cats. Note that "XR," "SR," and "CD" all refer to slow-release formulations. Dilacor XR-240 mg contains four 60-mg tablets. XR-180 contains three 60-mg tablets. Slow- and extended-release tablets are not recommended for routine use in cats because they produce inconsistent plasma concentrations that may result in ineffective treatment in some and adverse effects in others. The dose of 30 mg per cat of Dilacor XR (extended-release tablets) produced fewer adverse effects than 60 mg per cat.

## Large Animal Dosage

### Horses

- 0.125 mg/kg IV over at least 2 minutes. Repeat every 10 minutes as needed or until a total dose of 1.1 mg/kg. Doses as high as 1–2 mg/kg have been used in research animals.

## Regulatory Information

No regulatory information is available. For extralabel use withdrawal interval estimates, contact FARAD at www.FARAD.org.

RCI Classification: 4

# Dimenhydrinate
dye-men-hye′drih-nate

**Trade and other names:** Dramamine (Gravol in Canada)

**Functional classification:** Antihistamine

## Pharmacology and Mechanism of Action

Antihistamine ($H_1$-blocker). Diphenhydramine is the active moiety of dimenhydrinate. The pharmacologic properties are the same as diphenhydramine. Dimenhydrinate contains diphenhydramine and chlortheophylline. Dimenhydrinate is a salt consisting of 53.0%–55.5% diphenhydramine and 44.0%–46.5% 8-chlorotheophylline. In people, it is used for treatment of nausea, dizziness, and vomiting associated with motion sickness. Diphenhydramine produces the antinausea effects, and chlorotheophylline, a methylxanthine derivative related to caffeine, is added to reduce drowsiness.

Similar to other antihistamines, diphenhydramine acts by blocking the $H_1$ receptor and suppresses inflammatory reactions caused by histamine. The $H_1$ blockers have been used to control pruritus and skin inflammation in dogs and cats; however, success rates in dogs have not been high. Commonly used antihistamines include clemastine, chlorpheniramine, diphenhydramine, and hydroxyzine. Diphenhydramine also has central-acting antiemetic properties, possibly by acting on the vomiting center or via the chemoreceptor-trigger zone (CRTZ).

*Pharmacokinetics:* The oral bioavailability of diphenhydramine is much higher when administered as the dimenhydrinate salt—as much as 50–70 times in some studies. Diphenhydramine oral bioavailability is 22% in dogs when administered as dimenhydrinate but only 8% when administered alone. The terminal half-life of diphenhydramine from this formulation in dogs is 12 hours. The theophylline component in this formulation is also absorbed and attains levels that can be considered to have therapeutic effects.

## Indications and Clinical Uses

Dimenhydrinate has used to prevent allergic reactions and for pruritus therapy in dogs and cats. However, success rates for treatment of pruritus have not been high. In addition to the antihistamine effect for treating allergies, diphenhydramine, like other antihistamines, acts as an antiemetic via the drug effects on the centers that control vomiting in animals. Antihistamines used as antiemetics are administered for motion sickness, vomiting induced by chemotherapy, and GI disease that stimulates vomiting. Antihistamines are not effective antiemetics for cats. They may be effective in some dogs; however, there are other antiemetics available for dogs and cats that are consistently more effective.

### Precautionary Information

#### Adverse Reactions and Side Effects

Sedation is the most common side effect. Sedation is the result of inhibition of histamine N-methyltransferase. Sedation may also be attributed to the block of other CNS receptors such as those for serotonin, acetylcholine, and alpha receptors. Antimuscarinic effects (atropine-like effects) also are common, including dry mouth and decreased GI secretions. This product also contains a methylxanthine (related to caffeine and theophylline); therefore, excess CNS stimulation could occur with high doses.

#### Contraindications and Precautions

Antimuscarinic effects (atropine-like effects) are common. Do not use in conditions for which anticholinergic drugs may be contraindicated, such as glaucoma, ileus, or cardiac arrhythmias. Do not administer to patients in which theophylline products are contraindicated.

#### Drug Interactions

No drug interactions are reported. However, use with other sedatives and tranquilizers may increase sedation. Some drugs decrease metabolism of theophylline and other methylxanthine drugs (see Appendix I). If these agents are used concurrently with this formulation, adverse effects are possible.

## Instructions for Use

Like other antihistamines, there have been no clinical studies on the use of dimenhydrinate. The use is based on clinical experience and anecdotal accounts. It is primarily used empirically for treatment of vomiting and to prevent allergic reactions.

## Patient Monitoring and Laboratory Tests

No specific monitoring is necessary.

## Formulations

Dimenhydrinate is available in 50-mg tablets and 50-mg/mL injection. Dimenhydrinate is a salt consisting of 53.0%–55.5% diphenhydramine and 44.0%–46.5% 8-chlorotheophylline.

## Stability and Storage

Store in a tightly sealed container, protected from light, and at room temperature. Stability of compounded formulations has not been evaluated.

## Small Animal Dosage

**Dogs**

- 4–8 mg/kg q8–12h PO. IM or IV for the injection form.

**Cats**

- 12.5 mg/cat q8–12h PO. IM or IV for the injection form.

## Large Animal Dosage

- No large animal doses have been reported.

## Regulatory Information

No regulatory information is available. For extralabel use withdrawal interval estimates, contact FARAD at www.FARAD.org.

RCI Classification: 3

# Dimercaprol
dye-mer-cap´role

**Trade and other names:** British anti-lewisite (BAL) in oil

**Functional classification:** Antidote

## Pharmacology and Mechanism of Action

Chelating agent. Dimercaprol is also known as BAL. It is a dithiol chelating agent for chelating with heavy metals. It binds to arsenic, lead, and mercury to treat toxicosis.

## Indications and Clinical Uses

Dimercaprol is used to treat lead, gold, mercury, and arsenic toxicity. There are two formulations: dimercaptopropane-1-sulfonic acid (DMPS) and meso-2,3-dimercaptosuccinic acid. Because these are not readily available, they may be compounded from a bulk source.

## Precautionary Information

### Adverse Reactions and Side Effects
Adverse effects are not reported in veterinary medicine. In people, sterile abscesses occur at the injection site. High doses have caused seizures, drowsiness, and vomiting.

### Contraindications and Precautions
Dimercaprol is used only to treat intoxications.

### Drug Interactions
There are no drug interactions reported, but chelation of metals will occur from administration.

**D**

## Instructions for Use
Administer as soon as possible after intoxicant exposure has been identified. Alkalinization of urine will increase toxin removal. For lead intoxication, dimercaprol may be used with edetate calcium. It may be helpful to contact a Poison Control Center for additional instructions on treatment after an intoxication is identified.

### Patient Monitoring and Laboratory Tests
Heavy metal concentrations can be measured to assess treatment.

### Formulations
• Dimercaprol is available in an injection that must be prepared by compounding.

### Stability and Storage
Store in a tightly sealed container, protected from light, and at room temperature.

### Small Animal Dosage
• 4 mg/kg q4h IM.

### Large Animal Dosage
• 4 mg/kg q4h IM.

### Regulatory Information
Withdrawal time: 5 days for milk and meat (extralabel use).

# Dimethyl Sulfoxide (DMSO)
di-meth-il sulf-oks´ide

**Trade and other names:** DMSO and Domoso

**Functional classification:** Anti-inflammatory

## Pharmacology and Mechanism of Action
Dimethyl sulfoxide (DMSO) is a solvent that is a byproduct of the paper-making process. It is highly hygroscopic (water absorbing). It readily displaces water and penetrates cell membranes, skin, and mucosa easily. It produces anti-inflammatory, antifungal, and antibacterial properties, although this may not translate to clinical applications. The clinical anti-inflammatory action of DMSO is uncertain. It may

produce anti-inflammatory or protective effects on cell membranes via its ability to scavenge oxygen-derived free radicals.

*Pharmacokinetics:* In horses, at a dose of 1 g/kg, the half-life is 8.6 hours. Twenty-six percent of the administered dose was excreted in the urine. In dogs, the half-life is 36 hours.

## Indications and Clinical Uses

DMSO has been administered topically and systemically (IV) for treatment of various inflammatory conditions. It is popular in horses for treatment of laminitis, arthritis, pneumonia, intestinal ischemia, synovitis, and nervous system injuries. Despite popular use, there are no published reports of efficacy for clinical use, and evidence to support use as an anti-inflammatory agent in treatment of clinical disease is primarily anecdotal. There is no evidence to support use to protect ischemic reperfusion injury in the equine intestine, to treat laminitis, or to improve neurologic disease. It does not promote drug penetration across the blood–brain barrier.

## Precautionary Information

### Adverse Reactions and Side Effects

Dimethyl sulfoxide is irritating to skin and mucosal membranes. It is hygroscopic and induces release of histamine in skin. Long-term use has produced ocular lens changes in laboratory animals. Concentrated DMSO, when administered IV, will cause significant hemolysis. IV use also has been associated with hemoglobinemia, acute colic, diarrhea, myositis, muscle tremors, and collapse. These reactions are more likely at doses of 2 g/kg or greater. DMSO produces a strong odor when administered.

### Contraindications and Precautions

Although many veterinarians administer it systemically, DMSO is not approved for this use. It may enhance transdermal absorption of toxicants and contaminants on the skin. Do not administer IV at concentrations greater than 10% or at doses greater than 1 g/kg. Do not administer concentrated solution systemically.

### Drug Interactions

Dimethyl sulfoxide is a strong solvent. It dissolves other compounds. It may act as a penetration enhancer and increase transmembrane penetration of other compounds.

## Instructions for Use

Dilute prior to use to 10% for IV infusion. Doses vary widely among veterinarians. Dose listed of 1 g/kg is common, but ranges of 0.2–4 g/kg have been cited in the literature for horses.

## Patient Monitoring and Laboratory Tests

Monitor CBC during use.

## Formulations

• Available in a solution.

## Stability and Storage

Store in a tightly sealed container, protected from light, and at room temperature. Do not mix with other compounds, unless it is done immediately prior to administration.

## Small Animal Dosage

### Dogs and Cats

• 1 g/kg IV slowly. Do not administer solutions stronger than 10%.

## Large Animal Dosage
### Horses and Cattle
- 1 g/kg IV slowly. Dilute prior to use. Do not administer concentrations greater than 10%. For most conditions, administration is q12h.

### Regulatory Information
Not approved for use in animals intended for food. No withdrawal times are available. If administered to a food-producing animal, contact FARAD for withdrawal time information at www.FARAD.org.
For racing horses, it has changed from RCI Class 5 to Class 4.

**D**

# Diminazene Aceturate and Diminazene Diaceturate
dye´min a zeen
**Trade and other names:** Berenil, Ganaseg, and Veriben
**Functional classification:** Antiprotozoal agent

## Pharmacology and Mechanism of Action
Diminazene is one of the aromatic diamines that is used for antiprotozoal treatment. Others in this group include imidocarb dipropionate, diminazene aceturate, pentamidine isethionate, and phenamidine isethionate. These drugs inhibit DNA synthesis in protozoa. Clinical use is limited in the United States because it is not commercially available. However, it has been tried for some rare infections in dogs, cats, and horses.

*Pharmacokinetics:* In cats, the half-life was 1.7 hours with a peak plasma concentration of 0.5 mcg/mL at 1 hour after IM injection. The half-life is much longer in large animals (29 hours in cattle).

## Indications and Clinical Uses
In dogs, imidocarb and diminazene have been used most widely, primarily for treatment of *Babesia* spp. and *Hepatozoon canis* infections. However, for these infections, imidocarb has been preferred over diminazene because of diminazene's narrow therapeutic index. Another use of diminazene has been for treatment of African trypanosomiasis (*Trypanosoma* spp.).

Diminazene has been used to treat leishmaniasis in humans, but this is not a common use in dogs. It was used in experimental cats infected with *Trypanosoma evansi* at a dose of 3.5 mg/kg via IM injection on 5 consecutive days and was 85.7% effective in eliminating the parasite, and no adverse effects were observed. It was used to treat *Cytauxzoon felis* infection in cats and was effective with two injections administered IM 2 mg/kg within a 1-week interval but was not effective to eradicate the organism. There have been mixed results in dogs for treating *Babesia* infections. It was more effective for *Babesia canis* but not as much for *Babesia gibsoni*.

Diminazene has been used in horses for equine piroplasmosis (*Theileria equi* and *Babesia caballi*). It has been effective in eliminating *B. caballi* infections in horses at 5 mg/kg given twice in a 24-hour interval IM. It was effective in cattle at a dose of 3–5 mg/kg IM for *Babesia* infections and has been used (3.5–7 mg/kg IM) for treating trypanosomiasis.

Availability is an issue with use in the United States. It is available in both aceturate (molecular weight, 515.5) and diaceturate (molecular weight, 587.6) salts, but it is not approved for any animal species.

## Precautionary Information
### Adverse Reactions and Side Effects
Because of limited use, there is not an adverse event profile for diminazene. It can cause pain on injection. In horses, it caused severe injection-site reactions and muscle damage. Single injections in cats for a pharmacokinetic study were well tolerated. But in other studies, reactions in cats included severe ptyalism (salivation) after injection despite atropine administration concurrently. It also produced nausea and vomiting in cats for several hours and increased hepatic enzyme elevations. For these reasons, diminazene is not recommended for cats.

### Contraindications and Precautions
Because of adverse events in cats and lack of demonstration of clinical success, it is not recommended for cats.

### Drug Interactions
There have been no interactions identified in animals.

## Instructions for Use
### Patient Monitoring and Laboratory Tests
If used in animals, monitor the injection site for signs of adverse effects. Monitor the patient's CBC during treatment.

## Formulations
- Diminazene is available in two forms, diminazene aceturate and diminazene diaceturate salts. The powdered formulation of diminazene diaceturate (Veriben) was reconstituted with sterile water to a concentration of 7 mg/mL for IM injection in cats. This formulation contained 3 mg/kg diminazene diaceturate (equivalent to 1.68 mg/kg base or 2.6 mg/kg of diminazene aceturate).

## Stability and Storage
Store in a tightly sealed container, protected from light, and at room temperature. Stability of compounded formulations has not been evaluated.

## Small Animal Dosage
### Dogs
- *Babesia* treatment: 3.5–5 mg/kg q12h for two doses IM.

### Cats
- 4 mg/kg IM q24h for five doses.

## Large Animal Dosage
### Cattle
- Treatment of *Trypanosoma cruzi* or *Babesia*, 3.5–7 mg/kg IM.

### Horses
(See Precautionary Information.)
- Equne piroplasmosis: diminazene diaceturate: 3.5–5 mg/kg IM, q48h for two treatments.
- *Babesia* treatment, diminazene diaceturate: 3–5 mg/kg IM q12h for two treatments.

## Regulatory Information

If administered to food animals, consult FARAD at www.FARAD.org for withdrawal time information. Diminazene is excreted into the milk, with residues for up to 6 days in sheep and goats, and up to 21 days in cattle.

# Dinoprost Tromethamine

dye´noe-prahst troe-meth´ah-meen

**Trade and other names:** Lutalyse, Prostin F2 alpha, ProstaMate, Prostaglandin F2 alpha, and PGF2 alpha

**Functional classification:** Prostaglandin

## Pharmacology and Mechanism of Action

Dinoprost is a PG ($PGF_2$ alpha) that induces luteolysis. $PGF_2$ and its analogues have a direct luteolytic action on the corpus luteum. After injection, it produces a functional regression of the corpus luteum (luteolysis). In nonpregnant cycling cattle, this effect results in estrus beginning 2–5 days after injection. In pregnant animals, it terminates pregnancy. In animals with prolonged luteal activity that have pyometra, mummified fetus, or luteal cysts, the luteolysis usually results in resolution of the problem and return to normal cycling.

## Indications and Clinical Uses

Dinoprost is used for estrus synchronization in cattle and horses by causing luteolysis. In horses and cattle, it is used to control timing of estrus in estrus-cycling females and in clinically anestrus females that have a corpus luteum. In pigs, dinoprost is used to induce parturition when given within 3 days of farrowing. In dogs, dinoprost has been used to treat open pyometra. In cattle, dinoprost has been used for treatment of chronic endometritis.

In large animals, dinoprost is used to induce abortion in the first 100 days of gestation, but use for inducing abortion in small animals has been questioned.

## Precautionary Information

### Adverse Reactions and Side Effects

Prostaglandin $F_2$ alpha causes increased smooth muscle tone, resulting in diarrhea, abdominal discomfort, bronchoconstriction, and increase in blood pressure. In small animals, other side effects include vomiting. Induction of abortion may cause retained placenta.

### Contraindications and Precautions

Do not administer intravenously. Dinoprost induces abortion in pregnant animals. Use caution when handling this drug by veterinarians, animal owners, and technical help. It should not be handled by pregnant women. Absorption through intact human skin is possible. People with respiratory problems also should not handle dinoprost.

### Drug Interactions

According to the label, dinoprost should not be used with NSAIDs because these drugs inhibit synthesis of prostaglandins. However, NSAIDs should not affect concentrations of exogenous $PGF_2$ alpha administered by this product. When using oxytocin concurrently, it should be used cautiously because there is a risk of uterine rupture.

## Instructions for Use

Use in treating pyometra should be monitored carefully. If pyometra is not open, severe consequences may result. When used in cattle, after a single injection, cattle should be bred at the usual time relative to estrus. When administering two injections, cattle can be bred after the second injection, either at the usual time relative to detected estrus or at about 80 hours after the second injection. Estrus is expected to occur 1–5 days after injection if a corpus luteum was present. Cattle that do not become pregnant will be expected to return to estrus in about 18–24 days. When used in cattle to induce abortion, it should be used only during the first 100 days of gestation. Cattle that abort will do so within 35 days after injection.

In pigs, administer within 3 days of predicted farrowing for parturition induction. Farrowing should start in approximately 30 hours.

## Patient Monitoring and Laboratory Tests

When used for estrus synchronization, monitor for signs of estrus. Animals should be bred at usual time relative to estrus.

## Formulations

- Dinoprost is available in a 5-mg/mL solution for IM injection.

## Stability and Storage

Store in a tightly sealed container, protected from light, and at room temperature. Stability of compounded formulations has not been evaluated.

## Small Animal Dosage

### Dogs

- Pyometra: 0.1–0.2 mg/kg once daily for 5 days SQ.
- Terminate pregnancy: 0.025–0.05 mg (25–50 mcg)/kg q12h IM.

### Cats

- Pyometra: 0.1–0.25 mg/kg, once daily for 5 days SQ.
- Terminate pregnancy: 0.5–1 mg/kg IM for two injections.

## Large Animal Dosage

### Cattle

- Terminate pregnancy: 25-mg total dose, administered once IM.
- Estrus synchronization: 25 mg (5 mL), total dose, IM once or twice at 10- to 12-day intervals.
- Pyometra: 25 mg, total dose, administered once IM.

### Horses

- Estrus synchronization: 1 mg/100 lb (1 mg/45 kg) or 1–2 mL administered once IM. Mares should return to estrus within 2–4 days and ovulate 8–12 days after treatment.

### Pigs

- Induction of parturition: 10 mg (2 mL) administered once IM. Parturition occurs within 30 hours.

## Regulatory Information

Do not administer to horses intended for food.
To be used in beef cattle and nonlactating dairy cows only.

# Diphenhydramine Hydrochloride
dye-fen-hye′drah-meen hye-droe-klor′ide

**Trade and other names:** Benadryl and generic

**Functional classification:** Antihistamine

**D**

## Pharmacology and Mechanism of Action
Antihistamine ($H_1$ blocker). Similar to other antihistamines, it acts by blocking the $H_1$ receptor (H1) and suppresses inflammatory reactions caused by histamine. Other commonly used antihistamines include clemastine, chlorpheniramine, and hydroxyzine.

Note that diphenhydramine (Benadryl) and dimenhydrinate (Dramamine) are essentially the same drug. Dimenhydrinate contains diphenhydramine and chlortheophylline. (See Dimenhydrinate for more details.)

## Indications and Clinical Uses
Diphenhydramine, like other antihistamines, blocks histamine type 1 ($H_1$) receptors to prevent action of histamine. It is used to prevent acute allergic reactions and for pruritus therapy in dogs and cats. However, success rates for treatment of pruritus have not been high. Diphenhydramine has been used to treat acute allergy episodes caused by mast cell release, allergy, insect bites, and so on. In addition to the antihistamine effect for treating allergies, these drugs block the effect of histamine in the vomiting center, vestibular center, and other centers that control vomiting in animals. This may control some types of vomiting in dogs but not likely in cats. There are other more effective antiemetics available for dogs and cats that are preferred.

## Precautionary Information

### Adverse Reactions and Side Effects
Sedation is the most common side effect. Sedation is the result of inhibition of histamine N-methyltransferase. Sedation may also be attributed to blockade of other CNS receptors such as those for serotonin, acetylcholine, and alpha-receptors. Antimuscarinic effects (atropinelike effects) also are common, including dry mouth and decreased GI secretions. Excitement has been observed in cats and other animals at high doses. Although it may induce some changes in cardiovascular parameters in some animals with IV administration, this has not been shown to be a problem when injected IV in dogs undergoing mast cell removal surgery.

### Contraindications and Precautions
Antimuscarinic effects (atropinelike effects) are common. Do not use in conditions for which anticholinergic drugs may be contraindicated, such as glaucoma, ileus, or cardiac arrhythmias. Discontinue administration a minimum of 7 days prior to allergen-specific allergy testing in dogs.

### Drug Interactions
There are no specific drug interactions. However, because of anticholinergic (atropinelike) effects, it may counteract drugs that are administered for a parasympathomimetic action (e.g., drugs used to stimulate intestinal motility).

## Instructions for Use
Antihistamine used primarily for allergic disease in animals. These drugs also can be used to treat or prevent vomiting in animals, but antihistamines are not effective antiemetics in cats. Clinical studies documenting efficacy have been limited. Most use is empirical with doses extrapolated from human use.

## Patient Monitoring and Laboratory Tests
No specific monitoring is necessary.

## Formulations
- Diphenhydramine is available OTC in a 2.5-mg/mL elixir, 25- and 50-mg capsules and tablets, and 50-mg/mL injection.

## Stability and Storage
Store in a tightly sealed container, protected from light, and at room temperature. Stability of compounded formulations has not been evaluated. Protect from freezing.

## Small Animal Dosage
### Dogs
- 2.2 mg/kg q8–12h PO, IM, or SQ. For large dogs, this is equivalent to an oral dose of 25 or 50 mg per dog.

### Cats
- 2–4 mg/kg q6–8h PO.
- 1 mg/kg q8h IV or IM.

## Large Animal Dosage
- 0.5–1 mg/kg as a single dose, as needed, IM.

## Regulatory Information
No regulatory information is available. For extralabel use withdrawal interval estimates, contact FARAD at www.FARAD.org.

# Diphenoxylate
dye-fen-oks´ih-late

**Trade and other names:** Lomotil, also called Co-phenotrope

**Functional classification:** Antidiarrheal

## Pharmacology and Mechanism of Action
Diphenoxylate is an opiate agonist. It binds to mu-opiate receptors in intestine and stimulates smooth muscle segmentation in intestine, decreases peristalsis, and enhances fluid and electrolyte absorption. It has little centrally acting effect.

## Indications and Clinical Uses
Diphenoxylate is used for the acute treatment of nonspecific diarrhea. It has a primarily local effect. Loperamide (Imodium) has a similar action and has become more popular for this indication. An additional use, not often used in veterinary medicine, is as an antitussive.

## Precautionary Information

### Adverse Reactions and Side Effects
Adverse effects have not been reported in veterinary medicine. Diphenoxylate is poorly absorbed systemically and produces few systemic side effects. Excessive use can cause constipation.

### Contraindications and Precautions
Do not use in patients with diarrhea caused by infectious causes. Opiates should not be used for chronic treatment of diarrhea.

### Drug Interactions
There are no specific drug interactions reported. However, use cautiously with other opiates and other drugs that may cause constipation (e.g., antimuscarinic drugs).

**D**

## Instructions for Use
Doses are based primarily on empiricism or extrapolation of human dose. Clinical studies have not been performed in animals. Diphenoxylate contains atropine, but the dose is not high enough for significant systemic effects.

### Patient Monitoring and Laboratory Tests
No specific monitoring is necessary.

### Formulations
- Diphenoxylate is available in 2.5-mg tablets that also contain 0.025 mg atropine.
- Oral solution: 2.5 mg plus 0.025 mg atropine in 5 mL of solution (cherry flavored, with 15% alcohol).

### Stability and Storage
Store in a tightly sealed container, protected from light, and at room temperature. Stability of compounded formulations has not been evaluated.

### Small Animal Dosage

#### Dogs
- 0.1–0.2 mg/kg q8–12h PO.
- Antitussive use: 0.2–0.5 mg/kg q12h PO.

#### Cats
- 0.05–0.1 mg/kg q12h PO.

### Large Animal Dosage
- No use in large animals is reported.

### Regulatory Information
No regulatory information is available. For extralabel use withdrawal interval estimates, contact FARAD at www.FARAD.org. Schedule V controlled drug. RCI Classification: 4

# Dipyridamole
dye-peer-id´ah-mole

**Trade and other names:** Persantine

**Functional classification:** Anticoagulant

## Pharmacology and Mechanism of Action

Dipyridamole is a platelet inhibitor. The mechanism of action is attributed to increased levels of cyclic adenosine monophosphate (cAMP) in platelet, which decreases platelet activation. Other more consistently active antiplatelet drugs have replaced dipyridamole as routine treatment (e.g., clopidogrel).

## Indications and Clinical Uses

In people, dipyridamole has been used to prevent thromboembolism and hypercoagulable states. However, the use of dipyridamole has been infrequent in animals. It may be indicated in clinical conditions in which platelet inhibition is desired but other antiplatelet drugs are preferred. It is indicated primarily to prevent thromboembolism. It is more common to administer other platelet inhibitors such as clopidogrel, with and without aspirin.

## Precautionary Information

### Adverse Reactions and Side Effects

Adverse effects have not been reported in animals. However, bleeding problems are expected in animals prone to coagulopathies or receiving other anticoagulants.

### Contraindications and Precautions

Do not use in animals with bleeding problems.

### Drug Interactions

Aspirin may potentiate effects.

## Instructions for Use

Dipyridamole is used primarily in people to prevent thromboembolism. Use in animals has not been reported. When used in people, it is combined with other antithrombotic agents (e.g., warfarin).

## Patient Monitoring and Laboratory Tests

It may be necessary to monitor bleeding times in some animals.

## Formulations

- Dipyridamole is available in 25-, 50-, and 75-mg tablets and 5-mg/mL injection. It is also available combined with aspirin as 200 mg dipyridamole plus 25 mg aspirin (Aggrenox).

## Stability and Storage

Store in a tightly sealed container, protected from light, and at room temperature. Compounded oral formulations have been stable for 60 days.

## Small Animal Dosage

### Dogs and Cats

- 4–10 mg/kg q24h PO.

## Large Animal Dosage

- No use in large animals is reported.

## Regulatory Information

No regulatory information is available. For extralabel use withdrawal interval estimates, contact FARAD at www.FARAD.org.
RCI Classification: 3

## Dipyrone

D

dye-pye'-rone

**Trade and other names:** Methampyrone. Known in many countries as metamizole. Zimeta, equine brand.

**Functional classification:** Analgesic, Antipyretic, nonsteroidal anti-inflammatory drug

## Pharmacology and Mechanism of Action

Dipyrone is an older antipyretic and analgesic often grouped in the NSAID class. In many countries, it is known as metamizole.

In many classifications, it is listed as a NSAID with analgesic and anti-inflammatory properties similar to other NSAIDs through traditional COX inhibition. The COX enzymes exist as two isoforms, COX-1 and COX-2. Inhibition of COX-2 accounts for analgesic and anti-inflammatory effects, although there is also some contribution from inhibition of COX-1. Through these mechanisms, the NSAIDs inhibit synthesis of prostaglandins responsible for many functions in the body, including pain and inflammation.

However, dipyrone appears to be neither a COX-1 or COX-2 inhibitor. It has been considered unique from the traditional NSAIDs by acting through other mechanisms, most likely a central mechanism of inhibiting COX-3, much like the mechanism for acetaminophen. Dipyrone is a pro-drug, which is metabolized to other structurally related pyrazolone compounds. These products produce analgesia and antipyretic effects. It also may activate the opioid system or the endogenous cannabinoid system.

Dipyrone is capable of blocking fever (pyrexia) through prostaglandin-dependent and -independent mechanisms. In horses, it has long been considered an anti-spasmodic agent that is capable of relieving discomfort associated with some types of colic in horses. This mechanism may be through inhibited release of intracellular calcium, but the efficacy for this use has not been tested in clinical trials. *Pharmacokinetics:* In horses dipyrone has a half-life of approximately 4 hours, a volume of distribution of approximately 1.5 L/kg, and a clearance of 230–280 mL/kg/h..

## Indications and Clinical Uses

The most common use for dipyrone has been in horses. The use had diminished because the availability is limited, and there are other NSAIDs used for pain and inflammation in horses. Dipyrone was removed from the US market in 1995 but was approved by the FDA for horses in November 2019 (Zimeta). In the United States, it has not been used in small animals, but it has been in other countries. In horses, the approved use is as an antipyretic agent, but it has also been administered as an analgesic and antispasmodic agent for some forms of colic in horses. The antispasmodic effect has not been shown through well-controlled studies in horses; however, controlled studies and the FDA approval have demonstrated the antipyretic effectiveness.

## Precautionary Information

### Adverse Reactions and Side Effects

Intramuscular and SQ injections can be irritating. Dipyrone should be administered IV. In field trials in horses, it was generally safe with 2 horses out of 107 developing gastric ulcers, and 1 horse out of 107 with right dorsal colitis. There is a risk of dipyrone-induced agranulocytosis, but this has not been reported from use in horses.

Other effects from NSAIDs may be possible, through decreased PG synthesis. When administered to dogs, it has inhibited platelet function for as long as 3 hours and also may prolong bleeding in horses.

### Contraindications and Precautions

Do not use concurrently with other NSAIDs, corticosteroids, or drugs that are ulcerogenic. Do not use in animals in which other NSAIDs are contraindicated. Humans should handle this drug carefully. Human contact should be avoided. In 1977, dipyrone-containing drugs were removed from the human market because of concern of agranulocytosis. Dipyrone is prohibited for use in humans in several countries. However, this effect has not been observe in horses.

### Drug Interactions

NSAIDs such as dipyrone can interact with multiple other drugs, but there are no specific instances identified for dipyrone.

## Instructions for Use

Dipyrone is approved for horses in the United States but is used in small companion animals in other countries. Administer to horses according to the label instructions, IV. Avoid human contact.

## Patient Monitoring and Laboratory Tests

As with use of any NSAID, monitor for NSAID-related adverse effects, such as bleeding, GI problems, and protein loss.

## Formulations

- Dipyrone is available in the United States as a 500 mg/mL IV injection (Zimeta). There has been a 50% injection available in Canada (500 mg/mL). Some compounding pharmacies have prepared it for horses, but these are not recommended because of the availability of an FDA-approved form. It may be available in other countries as metamizole.

## Stability and Storage

Store in a tightly sealed container, protected from light, and at room temperature. Compounded oral formulations have not been evaluated and should be avoided.

## Small Animal Dosage

### Dogs and Cats

- Dogs: 50 mg/kg IV, IM, SQ q12h.
- Cats: safe doses are not established

## Large Animal Dosage

- Horses, antipyrexia use: 30 mg/kg IV, twice-daily (every 12 hours), for up to 3 days.

## Regulatory Information

Do not administer to food-producing animals.

# Dirlotapide
dir-loe′ta-pyed

**Trade and other names:** Slentrol

**Functional classification:** Obesity medication

**Note:** Dirlotapide has been removed from the veterinary market. Consult earlier editions of this handbook for more detailed information on dirlotapide.

# Disopyramide
dye-soe-peer′ah-mide

**Trade and other names:** Norpace (Rythmodan in Canada)

**Functional classification:** Antiarrhythmic agent

## Pharmacology and Mechanism of Action
Disopyramide is an antiarrhythmic agent of Class I group of antiarrhythmic agents. It is similar to other Class I agents in action. Disopyramide blocks the inward sodium channel and depresses myocardial electrophysiologic conduction rate.

## Indications and Clinical Uses
Disopyramide has been used for the control of ventricular arrhythmias. Its use in veterinary medicine is not as common as for other drugs because there are other more commonly used oral agents used for managing cardiac arrhythmias in animals. Studies of efficacy in animals have not been reported.

## Precautionary Information
### Adverse Reactions and Side Effects
Adverse effects have not been reported in animals. High doses may cause cardiac arrhythmias.

### Contraindications and Precautions
At high doses, it may induce arrhythmias in some patients.

### Drug Interactions
No drug interactions are reported for animals. Use cautiously with other drugs that may affect the cardiac rhythm.

## Instructions for Use
Disopyramide is not commonly used in veterinary medicine because of its short half-life in dogs. Other antiarrhythmic drugs are preferred.

## Patient Monitoring and Laboratory Tests
Monitor ECG in treated animals. This drug can be proarrhythmogenic.

## Formulations
- Disopyramide is available in 100- and 150-mg capsules and 10-mg/mL injection (Canada only).

## Stability and Storage
Store in a tightly sealed container, protected from light, and at room temperature. Compounded oral formulations have been stable for 30 days.

## Small Animal Dosage
**Dogs**
- 6–15 mg/kg q8h PO.

**Cats**
- No dose established.

## Large Animal Dosage
- No use in large animals is reported.

## Regulatory Information
No regulatory information is available. For extralabel use withdrawal interval estimates, contact FARAD at www.FARAD.org.

RCI Classification: 4

# Dithiazanine Iodide
dye-thye-az'ah-neen eye'oe-dide

**Trade and other names:** Dizan

**Functional classification:** Antiparasitic

**Note:** Dithiazanine iodide has been removed from the veterinary market. Consult earlier editions of this handbook for more detailed information on dithiazanine iodide.

# Dobutamine Hydrochloride
doe-byoo'tah-meen hye-droe-klor'ide

**Trade and other names:** Dobutrex

**Functional classification:** Cardiac inotropic agent

## Pharmacology and Mechanism of Action
Dobutamine is a potent adrenergic agonist. Dobutamine is a racemic mixture (R and S isomers) that has both beta$_1$- and beta$_2$-adrenergic activity. However, its most important clinical effects are caused by the relative cardioselective agonist activity on beta$_1$ receptors. There are both agonist and antagonist effects on alpha-receptors, the clinical effects of which are uncertain. The primary advantage of dobutamine is that it produces positive inotropic effects without excessive tachycardia. The lack of tachycardia distinguishes it from other sympathomimetic agents. Thus, at appropriate infusion rates, dobutamine can improve contractility without increasing heart rates.

*Pharmacokinetics:* Dobutamine has a short half-life in animals (2–3 minutes). Therefore, it must be given via constant IV infusion and has a short onset of activity.

## Indications and Clinical Uses
Dobutamine is used primarily for the acute treatment of heart failure. It produces an inotropic effect without increasing heart rate. It is usually administered for short-term treatment of heart failure when hospitalization is required (e.g., Class C heart failure class). Short treatment regimens (e.g., 48 hours) can have a residual positive effect in

some animals. In horses, dobutamine is used to improve perfusion of the GI tract and to support cardiovascular function in anesthetized horses.

## Precautionary Information

### Adverse Reactions and Side Effects

Dobutamine may cause tachycardia and ventricular arrhythmias at high doses or in sensitive individuals. If tachycardia or arrhythmias are detected, stop the infusion rate and resume at a lower rate. In horses, 2 mcg/kg/min can cause a significant increase in systemic blood pressure in conscious horses.

### Contraindications and Precautions

Do not use in animals with ventricular arrhythmias. Do not use unless precise infusion and monitoring capabilities are available.

### Drug Interactions

Do not mix with alkaline solutions, such as those containing bicarbonate. Do not infuse in IV line with heparin, cephalosporins, or penicillins. Otherwise, it is compatible with most fluid solutions. Do not administer to animals receiving monoamine oxidase inhibitors (MAOIs) (e.g., selegiline), or withdraw the MAOI before this drug is administered.

### Instructions for Use

Dobutamine has a rapid elimination half-life (minutes) and therefore must be administered via carefully monitored CRI. Dose rates (infusion rate) can be adjusted by monitoring patient response. In dogs, doses as low as 2 mcg/kg/min have improved cardiac output.

### Patient Monitoring and Laboratory Tests

Monitor heart rate and ECG during treatment. Cardiac arrhythmias are possible during infusions, especially at high doses.

### Formulations

• Dobutamine is available in a 250-mg/20-mL (12.5-mg/mL) vial for injection.

### Stability and Storage

Usually dilute in 5% dextrose solution (e.g., 250 mg in 1 L 5% dextrose). A slight pink tinge to the solution can occur without loss of potency; however, do not use if color turns brown.

### Small Animal Dosage

**Dogs**

• 5–20 mcg/kg/min IV infusion. Generally start with low dose and titrate upward.

**Cats**

• 2 mcg/kg/min IV infusion.

### Large Animal Dosage

**Horses**

• During anesthesia to support cardiovascular function: 0.5 mcg/kg/min CRI.
• Higher doses of 5–10 mcg/kg/min (0.005–0.01 mg/kg/min CRI are used for heart failure.
• 5–10 mcg/kg/min (0.005–0.01 mg/kg/min) IV infusion. Observe for increases in heart rate and ventricular arrhythmias. Adjust dose as needed based on patient response and heart rate.

## Regulatory Information

No regulatory information is available. Because of a short half-life, no risk of residue is anticipated in food animals.

RCI Classification: 3

# Docusate
dok'yoo-sate

**Trade and other names:** Docusate calcium: Surfak and Doxidan; Docusate sodium: DSS, Colace, and Doxan; and generic brands

**Functional classification:** Laxative

## Pharmacology and Mechanism of Action

Docusate sodium and docusate calcium are stool softeners. They act as surfactants to help increase water penetration into feces. They act to decrease surface tension to allow more water to accumulate in the stool.

## Indications and Clinical Uses

Docusate is indicated for medical conditions in which softened feces are desirable, such as after intestinal or anal surgery, to help pass hardened feces, and when administering drugs that slow intestinal transit (e.g., opiates). Docusate is indicated for the treatment of constipation. The use of docusate in animals is based purely on anecdotal experience or extrapolations from uses in people. There are no clinical studies with docusate available for animals.

## Precautionary Information

### Adverse Reactions and Side Effects

No adverse effects reported in animals. In people, high doses have caused abdominal discomfort.

### Contraindications and Precautions

Some formulations of docusate calcium and docusate sodium products have contained the stimulant cathartic phenolphthalein, which should be used cautiously in cats. Examine label of products to ensure absence of phenolphthalein.

### Drug Interactions

No specific drug interactions are reported for animals.

## Instructions for Use

Doses are based on extrapolations from humans or empiricism. No clinical studies have been reported for animals.

## Patient Monitoring and Laboratory Tests

No specific monitoring is necessary.

## Formulations

- Docusate calcium is available as 60-mg tablets and 240-mg capsules.
- Docusate sodium is available as 50- and 100-mg capsules and 10-mg/mL liquid.

## Stability and Storage
Store in a tightly sealed container, protected from light, and at room temperature. Stability of compounded formulations has not been evaluated.

## Small Animal Dosage
**Dogs**
- Docusate calcium: 50–100 mg/dog q12–24h PO.
- Docusate sodium: 50–200 mg/dog q8–12h PO.

**Cats**
- Docusate calcium: 50 mg/cat q12–24h PO.
- Docusate sodium: 50 mg/cat q12–24h PO.

## Large Animal Dosage
- Docusate sodium: 10 mg/kg/day PO.

## Regulatory Information
No regulatory information is available for animals intended for food. Because docusate has primarily a locally acting effect in the intestine, there is a minimal risk of residues in animals intended for food.

# Dolasetron Mesylate
doe-lah′seh-tron mess′ih-late (also, dahl-ah′set-rahn)
**Trade and other names:** Anzemet
**Functional classification:** Antiemetic

## Pharmacology and Mechanism of Action
Dolasetron is an antiemetic drug from the class of drugs called *serotonin antagonists*. These drugs act by inhibiting serotonin (5-HT, type 3, 5-HT$_3$) receptors. During chemotherapy, there may be 5-HT released from injury to the GI tract, which stimulates vomiting centrally. The emetic response induced by serotonin is inhibited by this class of drugs. In people, dolasetron is completely metabolized to the active metabolite hydrodolasetron through reduction by carbonyl reductase. This is the major pharmacologically active metabolite in humans. This metabolite is also formed in dogs but not confirmed in cats. This metabolite is 50 times more potent for inhibiting the serotonin receptor than the parent drug. Other serotonin antagonists used for antiemetic therapy include granisetron, ondansetron, and tropisetron.

*Pharmacokinetics:* In cats, the SQ absorption is 37% and has a half-life of 4 hours. The oral absorption is low in cats and is not sufficient to produce antiemetic effects.

## Indications and Clinical Uses
Like other serotonin antagonists, dolasetron is used primarily for its antiemetic effects during chemotherapy, for which they generally have been highly effective. These drugs also may be used to control vomiting from surgery (postoperative nausea and vomiting). It is not effective for xylazine-induced vomiting in cats. These drugs are often used in combination, usually with maropitant (Cerenia), to provide a multi-modal treatment for vomiting in dogs and cats.

## Precautionary Information

**Adverse Reactions and Side Effects**

Dolasetron adverse effects have not been reported in animals. These drugs have little affinity for other 5-HT receptors.

**Contraindications and Precautions**

There are no important contraindications identified in animals.

**Drug Interactions**

No drug interactions have been reported. However, dolasetron is subject to effects from cytochrome P450 inducers and inhibitors. (See Appendixes H and I.) Dolasetron and others in this class have been used concurrently with maropitant without signs of adverse interactions.

## Instructions for Use

Dolasetron has not been studied as much as other antiemetics in veterinary medicine. There are other antiemetics in this class (ondansetron) and other agents (maropitant) that are used more commonly. The dosages are derived from anecdotal experience or extrapolation from human studies, and no clinical studies are reported from animal studies. These drugs are more effective if used to prevent vomiting (administered prior to a chemotherapeutic agent) rather than to treat ongoing vomiting. This class of drugs may be combined with corticosteroids (e.g., dexamethasone) or maropitant to enhance the antiemetic action.

## Patient Monitoring and Laboratory Tests

Monitor GI signs in vomiting patient.

## Formulations

- Dolasetron is available in 50- and 100-mg tablets and 20-mg/mL injection.

## Stability and Storage

Store in a tightly sealed container, protected from light, and at room temperature. It may be added to fluid solutions (compatible in most IV fluid solutions) but do not mix with other IV drugs. Do not use injection after 24 hours when added to fluids. Oral formulations have been added to fruit juice up to 2 hours at room temperature without loss of stability.

## Small Animal Dosage

**Dogs and Cats**

- Prevention of nausea and vomiting: 0.6 mg/kg, q12–24h, IV, SQ, or PO, or 1.2 mg/kg once. Oral absorption is low and may not be sufficient to produce clinical effects.
- Treating vomiting and nausea: 1 mg/kg once daily IV or PO. Oral absorption is low and may not be sufficient to produce clinical effects.

## Large Animal Dosage

- No dose has been reported.

## Regulatory Information

Use in animals intended for food is negligible. No regulatory information is available.

# Domperidone

dahm-pare´ih-done

**Trade and other names:** Motilium and Equidone Gel

**Functional classification:** Prokinetic agent

## Pharmacology and Mechanism of Action

Domperidone is a benzimidazole with dopamine-2 (DA-2) receptor antagonist activity. It may also have some alpha$_1$ adrenoreceptor antagonist and serotonin 5-HT$_3$ antagonist activity.

Domperidone is a GI motility modifier once used in people but withdrawn because of cardiac arrhythmias. (It is still available for people in some countries.) It has actions similar to metoclopramide, although it is chemically unrelated. A difference between metoclopramide and domperidone is that the latter does not cross the blood–brain barrier. Therefore, adverse CNS effects are not as much of a problem with domperidone.

Domperidone stimulates the GI motility by inhibiting DA-2 receptors and possibly through increasing acetylcholine effects. The 5-HT$_3$ antagonist activity also may play a role in GI motility.

Domperidone also has endocrine effects by stimulating secretion of prolactin. It is through this action that domperidone is used to stimulate lactation in horses and treat fescue toxicity. The endocrine effects in horses increases follicular growth in seasonally anestrus mares. There is preliminary evidence that domperidone, via alpha-adrenergic and serotonergic blocking properties, may prevent vasoconstriction and reduction in laminar blood flow in horses with laminitis.

*Pharmacokinetics:* The pharmacokinetics in horses show that absorption is low (1.2%–1.5%), which may limit use for some indications.

## Indications and Clinical Uses

In horses, domperidone is used to treat fescue toxicosis and periparturient agalactia in mares. Fescue toxicosis is caused by a fungus that produces a toxin that causes reproductive problems in horses. The action of domperidone to increase lactation is through the stimulation of prolactin. It increases follicular growth in seasonally anestrus mares and has been used (with altrenogest and estradiol) to induce lactation in barren mares. Domperidone is a dopamine antagonist and has been used to test for pituitary pars intermedia dysfunction (PPID) in horses, but there are other approved treatments (e.g., pergolide). Domperidone has been used for short-term treatment to increase prolactin and aid milk production in nursing dogs and cats.

Domperidone has been used to treat gastroparesis in animals. However, at a dose of 1.1 mg/kg PO in horses, it does not produce a significant intestinal motility stimulating effect, but at 0.2 mg/kg IV, it is effective at restoring motility in experimental horses (no IV form is available).

Domperidone increases digital laminar blood flow in horses. Because of this effect, it has been administered orally to horses as part of a regiment for treating laminitis. Most of this evidence is obtained from healthy research horses, and clinical effects to improve laminitis have not been established.

Domperidone has been used to improve clinical signs in dogs infected with *Leishmania* spp. This effect may occur through prolactin production. Dogs treated with 1 mg/kg q12h for 1 month reduced clinical signs and antibody titers. It also has been used in dogs and cats to increase prolactin and increase milk production in lactating bitches.

## Precautionary Information

### Adverse Reactions and Side Effects

Adverse effects that are seen with metoclopramide are not as common with domperidone because it does not cross the blood–brain barrier as readily as metoclopramide. It causes a transient increase in aldosterone and prolactin secretion. It has also caused a transient increase in plasma adrenocorticotropic hormone (ACTH), which could exacerbate equine Cushing syndrome.

### Contraindications and Precautions

Do not use in patients with GI obstruction. There are no reported adverse effects during pregnancy. It has low milk concentrations in treated animals and no reported adverse effects from offspring during nursing of treated animals.

### Drug Interactions

Acidity is needed for oral administration. Do not administer with stomach antacids, such as omeprazole, cimetidine, or antacids; or acid-suppressing drugs such as omeprazole; or $H_2$ receptor blockers (e.g., famotidine).

## Instructions for Use

Domperidone equine gel is available for use in horses for the treatment of agalactia and fescue toxicosis. It is approved by the FDA for this indication in mares but has questionable efficacy as a prokinetic agent for treatment of ileus in animals.

## Patient Monitoring and Laboratory Tests

No specific monitoring is required, but clinical monitoring of GI motility is important.

## Formulations

• Formulation used in horses is oral gel at 11% (110 mg/mL). In Canada, it is available as 10-mg tablets for people.

## Stability and Storage

Store in a tightly sealed container, protected from light, and at room temperature. Stability of compounded formulations has not been evaluated.

## Small Animal Dosage

• Dog and cat: 2 mg per cat or 2–5 mg per dog q8–12h PO.
• *Leishmania* treatment in dogs: 1 mg/kg q12h for 1 month.
• Treatment to increase prolactin in nursing dogs or cats: 1.5–2 mg/kg for cats and 2.2 mg/kg for dogs, administered PO for 1–3 weeks during nursing.

## Large Animal Dosage

### Horses

• For fescue toxicity and agalactia: Equidone oral gel (11%) administered 10 days prior to foaling at 1.1 mg/kg daily PO, starting 10 days before the scheduled foaling date. (This dose is equivalent to 5 mL per 500 kg or 5 mL per adult horse daily PO of the 11% oral gel.) Continue until foaling. If there is not adequate milk production after foaling, continue for 5 additional days.

- Treatment of laminitis: 1.1 mg/kg PO.
- For testing horses with suspect PPID: Administer 5 mg/kg oral domperidone and collect blood samples at 0, 2, 4, hours for endogenous ACTH measurement. The ACTH reference range is 9–35 pg/mL.

### Regulatory Information

No regulatory information is available. For extralabel use withdrawal interval estimates, contact FARAD at www.FARAD.org.

**D**

# Dopamine Hydrochloride
doe′pah-meen hye-droe-klor′ide

**Trade and other names:** Intropin (discontinued), and generic

**Functional classification:** Cardiac inotropic agent

## Pharmacology and Mechanism of Action

Dopamine is both an adrenergic and dopamine agonist. Dopamine is a neurotransmitter and an immediate precursor to norepinephrine. At low doses, dopamine stimulates the dopamine ($DA_1$) receptors; at moderate doses, it stimulates the adrenergic receptors, and at high doses, it acts as an $alpha_1$-receptor agonist (producing vasoconstriction). At doses that stimulate $DA_1$ receptors, it increases cAMP in smooth muscle cells and causes relaxation and vasodilation. It has been administered to stimulate the heart and to increase urine flow (see next for explanation of renal effects).

## Indications and Clinical Uses

Dopamine is used therapeutically to stimulate myocardium via action on cardiac $beta_1$-receptors. Dopamine infusions will increase both blood pressure and cardiac output. These effects are caused by stimulating cardiac contractility and heart rate by acting as an agonist for $beta_1$-adrenergic receptors. In addition, dopamine increases the release of norepinephrine from nerve terminals (dopamine is a precursor for norepinephrine). It produces a greater chronotropic effect than dobutamine.

It has been proposed that dopamine dilates renal arterioles, increases renal blood flow, and increases the glomerular filtration rate. This effect is proposed to occur via activation of renal dopamine-1 ($DA_1$) receptors. Because of this proposed effect, in the past it has been used for acute renal failure. However, recent evaluation has raised doubts about the clinical effectiveness of dopamine for treatment of acute renal failure. Cats do not have as many $DA_1$ receptors as other animals; therefore it has not been effective in cats to produce diuresis. In addition, evaluation in people and other animals has not produced desired effects. Therefore, there is little support for the use of dopamine to treat acute kidney disease in animals.

## Precautionary Information

**Adverse Reactions and Side Effects**

Dopamine may cause tachycardia and ventricular arrhythmias at high doses or in sensitive individuals.

**Contraindications and Precautions**

Dopamine is unstable in alkaline fluids.

**Drug Interactions**

Do not mix with alkaline solutions. Otherwise, it is compatible with most fluid solutions.

## Instructions for Use

Dopamine has a rapid elimination half-life (minutes) and therefore must be administered via carefully monitored CRI. Because the actions of dopamine are dose dependent, the rate administered is adjusted to reach the desired clinical effect. Dopamine has been administered at doses of 2–10 mcg/kg/min for the acute management of heart failure and cardiogenic shock. When preparing IV solutions, one may admix 200–400 mg of dopamine with 250–500 mL of fluid. Dopamine is unstable in alkaline fluid solutions, such as those containing bicarbonate.

## Patient Monitoring and Laboratory Tests

Monitor heart rate and rhythm while administering dopamine.

## Formulations

• Dopamine is available in 40-, 80-, and 160-mg/mL for IV injection.

## Stability and Storage

Store in a tightly sealed container, protected from light, and at room temperature. It may be added to fluids such as 5% dextrose, saline, and lactated Ringer's solution. It is stable for 24 hours after dilution. Do not use if the solution turns a brown or purple color.

## Small Animal Dosage

**Dogs and Cats**

• 2–10 mcg/kg/min IV infusion. Dose rate is dependent on desired effects.

   Low dose (vasodilation, $D_1$ receptor): 0.5–2 mcg/kg/min; medium dose (cardiac stimulating, $beta_1$-receptor): 2–10 mcg/kg/min; and high dose (vasoconstriction, alpha-receptors): greater than 10 mcg/kg/min.

## Large Animal Dosage

**Horses and Cattle**

• 1–5 mcg/kg/min IV infusion.

## Regulatory Information

No regulatory information is available. Because of a short half-life, no risk of residue is anticipated in food animals.

RCI Classification: 2

# Doramectin
dore-ah-mek'tin

**Trade and other names:** Dectomax

**Functional classification:** Antiparasitic

## Pharmacology and Mechanism of Action
Antiparasitic drug. Avermectins (ivermectin-like drugs) and milbemycins (milbemycin, doramectin, and moxidectin) are macrocyclic lactones and share similarities, including mechanism of action. These drugs are neurotoxic to parasites by potentiating glutamate-gated chloride ion channels in parasites. Paralysis and death of the parasite is caused by increased permeability to chloride ions and hyperpolarization of nerve cells. These drugs also potentiate other chloride channels, including ones gated by GABA. Mammals ordinarily are not affected because they lack glutamate-gated chloride channels, and there is a lower affinity for other mammalian chloride channels. Because these drugs do not penetrate the blood–brain barrier in most animals (see Precautionary Information), GABA-gated channels in the CNS of mammals are not affected. It is effective against nematodes and arthropods but has no effect on flukes or tapeworms.

## Indications and Clinical Uses
Doramectin is used for treatment or prevention of GI parasite (nematode) infections in livestock, lice infestation, lungworm infection, and treatment of scabies. There are reports of a single injection (200–300 mcg/kg) used in cats for treatment of notoedric mange (infections from the mite *Notoedres cati*). In dogs, it has been used for treatment of *Demodex* infection, but there are other agents available that are effective and possibly safer. If used for treatment of *Demodex* infection, the typical time to remission with scheduled treatments is 7–8 weeks, but some dogs require 11 weeks.

## Precautionary Information
### Adverse Reactions and Side Effects
Toxicity may occur at high doses and in breeds in which ivermectin-like drugs cross the blood–brain barrier. Sensitive breeds include collies, Australian shepherds, Shetland sheepdogs, Old English sheepdogs, and some related breeds. Toxicity is neurotoxic, and signs include depression, ataxia, impaired vision, coma, and death. Sensitivity to ivermectin-like drugs may be because of mutation in the blood–brain barrier (p-glycoprotein deficiency). Treatment of hypodermal larvae in cattle may elicit reactions in tissues from dead larvae. These drugs are safe for pregnant animals. No adverse effects were seen in cats treated with doses as high as 345 mcg/kg.

### Contraindications and Precautions
Doramectin is only approved in cattle but there is extralabel use in other animals. Certain breeds of dogs (Shetland sheepdogs and collie-type breeds) are more sensitive to adverse effects than other breeds.

### Drug Interactions
Use cautiously with drugs that may inhibit p-glycoprotein at the blood–brain barrier (see Appendix J).

## Instructions for Use

Doses vary depending on use. In cattle, treatment of hypodermal larvae should begin at the end of fly season. Administration to cattle should use a 16- or 18-gauge needle for SQ administration. For IM injection, use a 1.5-inch needle and inject in the neck muscle. When administering the topical form, remove mud and manure from hide. If it rains within 2 hours of administration, decreased efficacy may occur.

## Patient Monitoring and Laboratory Tests

Monitor for microfilaremia prior to administration in small animals.

## Formulations

- Doramectin is available in a 1% (10-mg/mL) injection and a 5-mg/mL (0.5%) topical transdermal solution.

## Stability and Storage

Store in a tightly sealed container, protected from light, and at room temperature. Stability of compounded formulations has not been evaluated.

## Small Animal Dosage

**Dogs**

- Demodex treatment: 600 mcg/kg once per week for 5–23 weeks SQ or PO.

**Cats**

- Mite infection: 200–270 mcg/kg once SQ.
- 0.1 mL of 1% solution given once SQ.

## Large Animal Dosage

**Cattle**

- 200 mcg/kg (0.2 mg/kg) or 1 mL per 50 kg (110 lb), single injection, IM or SQ.
- Transdermal solution: Give 500 mcg (0.5 mg) per kg or 1 mL per 10 kg (4.5 lb) as a single dose along the animal's back, along the midline.

**Pigs**

- 300 mcg/kg (0.3 mg/kg) or 1 mL per 34 kg (75 lb), single injection, IM.

## Regulatory Information

Cattle withdrawal time (meat): 35 days.
Pig withdrawal time (meat): 24 days.
Do not administer to lactating dairy cattle.
Do not administer to female dairy cattle older than 20 months of age.
Cattle transdermal solution withdrawal time (meat): 45 days. Do not administer to lactating dairy cattle; do not administer within 2 months of calving.

# Doripenem
dor-i-pen'em

**Trade and other names:** Doribax

**Functional classification:** Antibacterial

## Pharmacology and Mechanism of Action

Doripenem is a beta-lactam antibiotic of the carbapenems class with broad spectrum of activity. The action of doripenem on the cell wall is similar to other beta-lactams, which is to bind penicillin-binding proteins (PBPs) that weaken or interfere with cell wall formation. In *E. coli* and *P. aeruginosa*, doripenem binds to PBP 2, which is involved in the maintenance of cell shape, and to PBPs 3 and 4. Carbapenems have a broad spectrum of activity and are among the most active of all antibiotics. Doripenem has similar activity as imipenem and meropenem to include gram-negative bacilli, including Enterobacteriaceae and *P. aeruginosa*. It is slightly more active against *P. aeruginosa*. It also is active against most gram-positive bacteria, except methicillin-resistant strains of *Staphylococcus* spp. It is not active against *Enterococcus* spp.

**D**

## Indications and Clinical Uses

Doripenem is indicated primarily for resistant infections caused by bacteria resistant to other drugs. It is especially valuable for treating resistant infections caused by *P. aeruginosa*, *E. coli*, and *Klebsiella pneumoniae*. Doripenem is only FDA approved for people, and use in animals is extralabel. It has not used in veterinary medicine as commonly as meropenem or imipenem.

---

### Precautionary Information

**Adverse Reactions and Side Effects**

Carbapenems pose similar risks as other beta-lactam antibiotics, but adverse effects are rare. Doripenem does not cause seizures as frequently as imipenem.

**Contraindications and Precautions**

Some slight yellowish discoloration may occur after reconstitution. Slight discoloration will not affect potency. However, a darker amber or brown discoloration may indicate oxidation and loss of potency.

**Drug Interactions**

Do not mix in vial or syringe with other antibiotics or with solutions containing other drugs.

---

## Instructions for Use

Doses in animals have been based on pharmacokinetic studies rather than efficacy trials. To prepare IV injection, mix 500-mg vial with 10 mL of sterile water for injection or sodium chloride 0.9% injection, gently shaking vial to form a suspension (concentration, 50 mg/mL). Withdraw suspension and add to infusion bag containing normal saline 100 mL or dextrose 5%, gently shaking until clear (concentration, 4.5 mg/mL). To prepare 250-mg dose, mix with 10 mL of sterile water for injection or sodium chloride 0.9% injection, gently shaking vial to form a suspension (concentration, 50 mg/mL). Withdraw suspension and add to infusion bag containing normal saline 100 mL or dextrose 5%, gently shaking until clear (concentration, 4.5 mg/mL). Remove 55 mL of this solution from the bag and discard. Infuse the remaining solution (concentration, 4.5 mg/mL).

## Patient Monitoring and Laboratory Tests

Susceptibility testing: Use susceptibility to imipenem to guide testing for doripenem. Enteric gram-negative bacteria usually have MIC values less than 0.5 mcg/mL. *P. aeruginosa* usually have MIC values less than 2 mcg/mL.

## Formulations

• Doripenem is available in a 500-mg vial for injection.

## Stability and Storage

Store vial at 59°F– 86°F. Constituted suspension in vial may be stored for 1 hour prior to dilution in infusion bag. Infusion solution prepared in saline may be stored at room temperature for 8 hours (includes infusion time) or under refrigeration for 24 hours (includes infusion time). Infusion solution prepared in dextrose 5% may be stored at room temperature for 4 hours (includes infusion time) or under refrigeration for 24 hours.

## Small Animal Dosage

**Dogs and Cats**

- 8 mg/kg q8h IV. Infuse over 30 minutes to 1 hour.

## Large Animal Dosage

- No large animal doses have been reported. However, doses similar to the range used in small animals are suggested for foals.

## Regulatory Information

Withdrawal times are not established for animals that produce food. For extralabel use withdrawal interval estimates, contact FARAD at www.FARAD.org.

# Doxapram Hydrochloride

doks´ah-pram hye-droe-klor´ide

**Trade and other names:** Dopram, Respiram

**Functional classification:** Respiratory stimulant

## Pharmacology and Mechanism of Action

Doxapram is a respiratory stimulant. It is a potassium-channel blocking drug and is the oldest known agent (available since the 1960s) in this class used for stimulating respiration. The specific action is to inhibit potassium channels (TASK1, TASK3) on carotid body cells (carotid body chemoreceptors). By blocking these potassium channels, respiratory stimulation is produced by increasing sensitivity to $CO_2$. However, there are other consequences of this channel inhibition, including CNS excitement, sweating, convulsions, and cardiovascular stimulation (increased heart rate and hypertension).

Doxapram is used primarily in emergency during anesthesia or to decrease the respiratory depressant effects of certain drugs (e.g., opiates, barbiturates). It has also been used in veterinary medicine as stimulation of respiration in young horses. There are other drugs that can be used to stimulate opioid-induced respiratory depression. These include ampakines, which stimulate the pre-Bötzinger complex, which is involved in respiratory rhythm generation.

The half-life of doxapram is short (2 hours), but the duration of action is only 5–10 minutes after IV administration.

## Indications and Clinical Uses

Doxapram may stimulate respiration in dogs, cats, and horses during and after general anesthesia. It has been used to stimulate respiration in newborn animals following dystocia or cesarean section surgery. Doxapram increases ventilation (tidal volume, respiratory rate) and reduces acidosis. In horses, it causes cardiac stimulation and respiratory stimulation. There have been reports that administration to neonates may increase their suckling activity shortly after birth and subsequently decrease the incidence of failure of passive transfer of immunoglobulins. The primary use of doxapram in horses is for the treatment of respiratory acidosis in foals caused by hypoxic-ischemic encephalopathy (perinatal asphyxia or neonatal maladjustment syndrome) in neonatal foals. Administration to foals has restored normal ventilation and improved blood pH, $PaO_2$, and respiratory rate in neonatal foals in a dose-dependent manner. Doxapram also has been used in dogs to assist in the diagnosis of laryngeal paralysis.

**D**

## Precautionary Information

### Adverse Reactions and Side Effects
Adverse effects have not been reported in animals. In people, it has caused panic, anxiety, sweating, seizures, and cardiovascular stimulation. CNS stimulation and excitement are possible with high doses or rapid infusions.

### Contraindications and Precautions
Do not use in animals with cardiac or respiratory arrest. Do not use with positive pressure ventilation.

### Drug Interactions
Use with theophylline or aminophylline may increase CNS excitement.

## Instructions for Use
Doxapram has a rapid onset of effect (usually occurs in 20–40 seconds with peak effect at 1–2 minutes) and a short duration of action. The duration of effect varies from 5–12 minutes. Treatment guidelines have been developed primarily for foals. Single-dose injections may be administered, followed by CRIs.

## Patient Monitoring and Laboratory Tests
Monitor patient's heart and respiratory rate.

## Formulations
- Doxapram is available in a 20-mg/mL solution.

## Stability and Storage
Store in a tightly sealed container, protected from light, and at room temperature. The pH is 3.5–5 for IV administration, which may affect compatibility with other drugs. Stability of compounded formulations has not been evaluated.

## Small Animal Dosage
- 5–10 mg/kg IV.
- Neonate: 1–5 mg SQ, sublingual, or via umbilical vein.

## Large Animal Dosage
- Foals: initial IV dose of 0.5 mg/kg followed by a CRI of 0.03–0.08 mg/kg/min for 20 minutes or initiate treatment with 0.05–0.08 mg/kg/min CRI and continue for 8–12 hours.

## Regulatory Information
No regulatory information is available. For extralabel use withdrawal interval estimates, contact FARAD at www.FARAD.org.
RCI Classification: 2

# Doxepin

doks'eh-pin

**Trade and other names:** Sinequan

**Functional classification:** Behavior-modifying drug, tricyclic antidepressant (TCA)

## Pharmacology and Mechanism of Action

Doxepin is a tricyclic antidepressant (TCA). For treatment of depression, this class of drugs is thought to act by increasing synaptic concentrations of norepinephrine and serotonin (5-HT) in the CNS. Doxepin is only a moderate to weak inhibitor of the reuptake of these neurotransmitters. It also has antihistamine ($H_1$) properties. Compared with other drugs in the TCA class, doxepin is used infrequently.

## Indications and Clinical Uses

Doxepin has been used to treat anxiety disorders and dermatologic conditions in dogs and cats. Some use for dermatitis is related to the drug's antihistamine properties. Although it has been used for treating pruritus and dermatitis in small animals, it has not been effective for treating atopic dermatitis in dogs. Doxepin has been used to treat lick granuloma in dogs, which may be through its effects on modifying behavior. There are anecdotal reports of the use of doxepin for treating laryngeal paralysis in dogs, but there are no controlled studies to support this use.

## Precautionary Information

### Adverse Reactions and Side Effects

Tricyclic antidepressants have some antimuscarinic effects that may increase heart rate, cause xerostomia, and affect the GI tract. Some sedation is possible with doxepin.

### Contraindications and Precautions

As with other TCAs, do not administer with other antidepressant drugs. Use cautiously in patients with glaucoma or seizure disorders.

### Drug Interactions

Doxepin may increase sedative effects from antihistamines. Do not administer with MAOIs.

## Instructions for Use

Doxepin has primarily been administered to treat pruritus in dogs. The efficacy for this use has been disappointing. The used for other indications is purely anecdotal and not based on well-designed clinical studies. The dosages used are extrapolated from use in humans.

## Patient Monitoring and Laboratory Tests

No specific monitoring is necessary.

## Formulations

- Doxepin is available in 10-, 25-, 50-, 75-, 100-, and 150-mg capsules and 3- and 6-mg tablets (Silenor). Generic and Sinequan are available in a 10-mg/mL oral solution.

## Stability and Storage

Store in a tightly sealed container, protected from light, and at room temperature. Oral formulations can be mixed with various flavorings, juices, and foods without loss of stability.

## Small Animal Dosage

### Dogs

- 1–5 mg/kg q12h PO. Start with low dose (e.g., 0.5–1 mg/kg) and gradually increase.
- Lick granuloma: 0.5–1 mg/kg q12h PO. (For comparison, antipruritic dose for people is 10–25 mg/person one to three times per day and increased as needed.)

### Cats

- 0.5–1 mg/kg q12–24h. Start with low dose initially.

## Large Animal Dosage

- No large animal doses are reported.

## Regulatory Information

No regulatory information is available. For extralabel use withdrawal interval estimates, contact FARAD at www.FARAD.org.

RCI Classification: 2

# Doxorubicin Hydrochloride
doks-oh-roo′bih-sin hye-droe-klor′ide

**Trade and other names:** Adriamycin

**Functional classification:** Anticancer agent

## Pharmacology and Mechanism of Action

Doxorubicin is an anticancer agent derived from the soil fungus *Streptomyces peucetius*. Doxorubicin is also considered one of the anticancer antibiotics, because it is derived from a fungal source. Other antitumor antibiotics include mitoxantrone, actinomycin D, and bleomycin.

Doxorubicin damages DNA by inhibition of the enzyme topoisomerase II. This enzyme is responsible for DNA functions. When topoisomerase is inhibited, the DNA segments cannot perform transcription, leading to breaks in the DNA strands and cell death. Secondarily, this mechanism causes cell death by blocking synthesis of RNA and proteins. Doxorubicin also forms free radicals ($\cdot$OH) that can attack DNA and lead to oxidation of DNA.

*Pharmacokinetics:* In dogs, the half-life has varied from 8.7 to 11 hours, with a VD of 0.6–0.7 L/kg and clearance of 52–83 L/kg/h. In cats, the pharmacokinetics are highly variable, with half-lives ranging from 11 minutes to 9.5 hours.

## Indications and Clinical Uses

Doxorubicin is a widely used anticancer agent. Doxorubicin is a frequently administered anticancer agent in humans for the treatment of breast tumors, various sarcomas, and osteosarcoma. In veterinary medicine, it has been used for lymphoma, osteosarcoma, and other carcinomas and sarcomas. It is considered one of the most effective single agents in the treatment of lymphoma, but in dogs, the response for T-cell lymphoma is significantly less than for B-cell lymphoma. It is used commonly in cancer protocols with other agents. For example, in the CHOP protocol, the "H" in the protocol refers to doxorubicin (by an older name). For canine lymphoma, some oncologists believe that remission of cancer is best achieved when five treatments are administered (target, 150–180 mg/m² cumulative dose).

In limited studies in horses, it was highly effective for the treatment of some tumors (lymphoma, carcinoma, and sarcoma) as a single agent.

## Precautionary Information

### Adverse Reactions and Side Effects

Adverse effects limit the frequency and cumulative doses that can be administered. Bone marrow toxicity is the major adverse effect that limits the frequency of administration, and cardiotoxicity is the major effect that limits the chronic administration. The nadir of bone marrow depression (leukopenia) is at 7–10 days. The stem cells are usually spared, and recovery occurs within 21 days after each dose. Cardiac toxicity is observed in 4%–8% of cases and is caused by an acute effect during administration seen as arrhythmias and decreased systolic function and a chronic effect that manifests as cardiomyopathy and congestive heart failure. Cardiac toxicity is caused by production of reactive oxygen species that injure cardiac myocytes or blockage of topoisomerase type 2-beta, which leads to mitochondrial dysfunction. Cardiac toxicity is dose related. The risk of chronic cardiac effects increases as total cumulative doses exceed 200–240 mg/m². At doses above 300 mg/m², cardiac toxicity is likely, but in some dogs, cardiac changes can be observed as soon as after 120 mg/m₂ cumulative dose. Most oncologists do not exceed 180 mg/m².

Dexrazoxane (Zinecard) is a potent chelator of iron and has been used to decrease the adverse cardiac effects in some patients. The dose of dexrazoxane is 10 times the doxorubicin dose and is infused over 15 minutes IV.

Alopecia is common in people. However, this effect is seen only in dogs that have continuously growing hair (e.g., poodles). Cats may lose their whiskers.

Gastrointestinal acute side effects (anorexia, vomiting, and diarrhea) are the most common acute side effects after administration. Hypersensitivity (allergic) reactions are not life threatening, but they can occur commonly. They are probably not true allergic reactions but are simply the result of mast cell degranulation that occurs independently of immunoglobulin G (IgG) binding. Signs of this reaction are head shaking (ear pruritus) and generalized urticaria and erythema. Antihistamines can be administered prior to treatment if these signs are anticipated.

Cats are more sensitive to adverse effects than dogs; therefore, lower doses are used in cats. Adverse effects in cats include anorexia, vomiting, and renal injury.

In horses, adverse effects included bone marrow suppression, hair loss, dermatitis, and other skin reactions.

Local reactions may occur if the extravasation of injectable dose is observed. If this occurs, flush the area to dilute the drug. Dexrazoxane may be used to decrease local reaction caused by extravasation by administering 500 mg/m² within 6 hours of extravasation. Local treatments also may be needed.

**Contraindications and Precautions**

Do not use in animals with cardiomyopathy. Monitor CBC in patients before and after treatment. If significant leukopenia (particularly neutropenia of fewer than 1000 cells) is present, withhold treatment or use a lower-dose intensity. Use cautiously in dogs with known mutation deficiency in the MDR membrane transporter (p-glycoprotein, ABCB1 transporter) (e.g., collies and related breeds). These dogs are more prone to toxicity. Boxer dogs are more prone to the cardiac toxicity.

**Drug Interactions**

Doxorubicin is commonly administered with other anticancer drugs, antiemetics, and antihistamines without adverse effects. However, doxorubicin is a p-glycoprotein substrate and should not be used with drugs that are p-glycoprotein inhibitors (e.g., cyclosporine or ketoconazole). (See Appendix J for a list of inhibitors.)

## Instructions for Use

The dose regimen listed in the dosing section may differ for various tumors. To prepare solution, the total dose is diluted in a saline fluid solution of 25 or 50 mL and infused slowly over 15–30 minutes. Alternatively, a 60-minute infusion has been used in which it is diluted in 25, 50, or 100 mL of 0.9 % NaCl. Although some experts have suggested that a long duration of infusion may decrease some adverse effects, data show that a rapid infusion of 15–20 minutes is not more likely to produce adverse effects than an infusion of 60 minutes.

For cats, mix 1 mg/mL in saline solution and administer IV over 5–10 minutes with fluids. In cats, SQ fluids (22 mL/kg) may be administered with doxorubicin. This drug is very irritating, and special care must be made to ensure that extravasation from the vein does not occur.

In chemotherapy protocols, it is sometimes administered with cyclophosphamide. Animals may require antiemetic and antihistamine (diphenhydramine) prior to therapy. Most often, it is administered on a body surface area rate (mg/m$^2$); however, dose according to body weight (mg/kg) may be safer for small dogs (see the Small Animal Dosage section). In cats, additional SQ fluids are administered to prevent renal toxicity.

## Patient Monitoring and Laboratory Tests

Monitor ECG during therapy. ECGs should be performed periodically in dogs to look for evidence of myocardial toxicity. CBC should be monitored regularly and prior to each treatment because of risk of myelotoxicity.

## Formulations

- Doxorubicin is available in a 2-mg/mL injection.

## Stability and Storage

Store in a tightly sealed container, protected from light, and at room temperature.

## Small Animal Dosage

### Dogs

- 30 mg/m$^2$ every 21 days IV.
- Alternatively, doxorubicin may be administered according to body weight: dogs weighing more than 15 kg: 30 mg/m$^2$; dogs weighing less than 15 kg: 1 mg/kg.

## Cats

- 20 mg/m$^2$ ($\approx$1.25 mg/kg) every 3 weeks IV. In some cats, higher doses of 25 mg/m$^2$ appear to be equally tolerated.

## Large Animal Dosage

### Horses

- 70 mg/m$^2$ (0.84–0.96 mg/kg) IV every 3 weeks for six cycles.

## Regulatory Information

Withdrawal times are not established for animals that produce food. This drug should not be used in animals intended for food because it is an anticancer agent.

# Doxycycline Hyclate and Doxycycline Monohydrate
doks-ih-sye´kleen

**Trade and other names:** Vibramycin, Monodox, Doxy Caps, and generic brands

**Functional classification:** Antibacterial

## Pharmacology and Mechanism of Action

Doxycycline is a tetracycline antibiotic. The mechanism of action of tetracyclines is to bind to the 30S ribosomal subunit and inhibit protein synthesis. The action of tetracyclines is usually bacteriostatic. It has a broad spectrum of activity, including many bacteria, some protozoa, *Rickettsia* spp., and *Ehrlichia* spp. Although it is a broad-spectrum antibacterial agent, resistance is common. Most of Enterobacteriaceae bacteria (e.g., *E. coli*) test clinically resistant. *P. aeruginosa* are resistant. *Staphylococcus* spp. may be susceptible, but susceptibility testing is needed to identify clinically susceptible strains.

*Pharmacokinetics:* In dogs, after oral administration, the half-life is 12.6 hours, the volume of distribution is 1.7 L/kg, and oral absorption is 66%, producing a peak concentration of 4.5 mcg/mL. Protein binding in dogs and cats is high (greater than 90%). In horses, oral doxycycline has an average half-life of 10 hours, a volume of distribution (V/F) of 2.3 L/kg, and clearance (CL/F) of 2.03 L/kg/h. The average peak concentration (C$_{MAX}$) after oral administration of 10 mg/kg is 0.5 mcg/mL. The oral absorption in horses is low at only 12%. Protein binding in horses is 70%–80%.

## Indications and Clinical Uses

Doxycycline is usually the drug of choice for treating vector-borne diseases in animals, such as those transmitted by ticks and fleas. Efficacy has been demonstrated in research studies and in some clinical studies. It is used for treating infections caused by bacteria, some protozoa, *Rickettsia* spp., and *Ehrlichia* spp. Doxycycline administered to cats with infections caused by *Mycoplasma* spp. or *Chlamydophila felis* (formerly *Chlamydia psittaci*) at 10–15 mg/kg once daily PO or 5 mg/kg q12h PO, has been effective in eliminating the organism and improving clinical signs. In dogs, 5 mg/kg q12h PO for 3–4 weeks has cleared *Ehrlichia canis* from blood and tissues. Doxycycline is recommended by the American Heartworm Society to be added to treatment of canine heartworm disease and initiated 30 days prior to adulticide treatment. It is used for heartworm disease because of the activity against the organism *Wolbachia*. This may improve microfilaricidal effect when combined with ivermectin, improve response to adulticidal treatment with melarsomine, and decrease injury to pulmonary vessels. In horses, it has been used not only to treat ehrlichiosis but also to treat other diseases (e.g., respiratory infections) when oral treatment is indicated. If doxycycline is too expensive or the availability is limited, other alternatives can be considered, such as minocycline hydrochloride, which has been shown to be an acceptable substitute and more active against some organisms (see Minocycline for more details).

**D**

## Precautionary Information

### Adverse Reactions and Side Effects

Tetracyclines may cause renal tubular necrosis at high doses and can affect bone and teeth formation in young animals. Doxycycline is less likely to cause chelation with calcium and teeth discoloration than other tetracyclines. If administered for a short time, it has not caused teeth discoloration in children.

Doxycycline administered orally to cats has caused esophageal irritation, tissue injury, and esophageal stricture. This may be caused by solid-dose formulations (primarily doxycycline hyclate rather than doxycycline monohydrate) becoming entrapped in the esophagus. Passage into the stomach by giving the cat water or food after administration is recommended to prevent this effect.

Doxycycline given IV to horses has been fatal; however, it has been administered safely to horses PO, although diarrhea is possible. In two equine studies, there were no adverse effects reported from oral administration. In another study, one of the horses in a pharmacokinetic trial developed signs of enteritis and colic.

### Contraindications and Precautions

Ordinarily, tetracyclines should not be administered to young animals because it can affect bone and teeth formation. However, it has been better tolerated in children than other tetracyclines and has been used in children up to 8 years old. Doxycycline is less likely to discolor teeth if used for short-term treatment. If solid-dose forms are administered to cats, lubricate the tablet or capsule or follow with food or water to ensure passage into stomach. Do not administer rapidly IV. Do not administer solution directly IM or SQ. Do not administer IV to horses under any circumstances; acute death has been reported from this use.

Pregnancy precaution: avoid use during pregnancy if possible.

### Drug Interactions

Tetracyclines bind to compounds containing calcium, which decreases oral absorption. However, this is less of a problem with doxycycline than with other tetracyclines. Doxycycline has been mixed with milk prior to oral administration to children without decreasing efficacy. Doxycycline can bind to aluminum-containing products (e.g., sucralfate, antacids), which decreases its oral absorption.

## Instructions for Use

To prepare doxycycline IV infusion solution, add 10 mL to a 100-mg vial or 20 mL to a 200-mg vial and then further dilute for IV use in 100–1000 mL of lactated Ringer's solution, sodium chloride, or 5% dextrose. Infuse over 1–2 hours (see the Stability and Storage section).

## Patient Monitoring and Laboratory Tests

Susceptibility testing: CLSI breakpoints for sensitive organisms are ≤0.25 mcg/mL for testing isolates from dogs. Breakpoints for cats are not established, but similar values are recommended. The breakpoint for testing isolates from horses is ≤0.12 mcg/mL using a dosage of 20 mg/kg PO twice daily. Do not test tetracycline as a surrogate for doxycycline in horses. For other animals, tetracycline can be used as a surrogate for testing. Organisms that are susceptible to tetracycline are also considered susceptible to doxycycline. However, some organisms that are intermediate or resistant to tetracycline may be susceptible to doxycycline or minocycline or both.

## Formulations

- Doxycycline is available in a 10-mg/mL oral suspension; 20-, 50-, 75-, 100-, and 150-mg tablets; and 50- and 100-mg capsules (doxycycline hyclate). Doxycycline monohydrate is available as 50- or 100-mg tablets or capsules. A controlled-release formulation (Oracea) contains 10-mg delayed release and 30-mg immediate release in one capsule.
- Doxycycline hyclate injection is available in a 100- and 200-mg injection vial. The vial should be diluted to 10 mg/mL initially and then to 1 mg/mL before slow IV infusion. Administer IV only and not via the SQ or IM routes.

## Stability and Storage

Store in a tightly sealed container, protected from light, and at room temperature. Avoid mixing with cations such as iron, calcium, aluminum, and zinc. However, doxycycline tablets have been mixed with milk and immediately administered to children without loss of potency.

Doxycycline hyclate for IV injection will retain potency for 48 hours when diluted with sodium chloride or 5% dextrose solution to concentrations between 1 and 0.1 mg/mL if stored at 25°C (room temperature). Protect from direct light exposure, but exposure to fluorescent lights is acceptable for 48 hours. Reconstituted solutions may be stored up to 72 hours if refrigerated and protected from light. If frozen after reconstitution with sterile water, solutions of 10 mg/mL are potent for 8 weeks. If thawed, do not refreeze.

Doxycycline calcium or doxycycline monohydrate commercial oral suspension for people is stable for 2 weeks at room temperature if stored in light-resistant container after reconstitution with water. Doxycycline tablets may be crushed and mixed with drinks or food (milk or pudding), and are stable for 24 hours at room temperature. If doxycycline is prepared in a compounded formulation, it may be unstable. Doxycycline hyclate tablets formulated in Ora Plus and Ora Sweet as a suspension (50:50) retained potency for only 7 days; stability beyond 7 days cannot be assured. Other suspensions prepared for animals also may be unstable. Observe for dark color change (dark brown) as evidence of loss of potency. When doxycycline hyclate and doxycycline monohydrate was compounded in an oil-based suspension, it was stable for 180 days. However, the suspension precipitates in the container and vigorous mixing is suggested prior to administration.

## Small Animal Dosage

### Dogs and Cats

- 5 mg/kg q12h PO or IV. 10 mg/kg q24h PO.
- *Rickettsia* (dogs): 5 mg/kg q12h.
- *Ehrlichia* (dogs): 5 mg/kg q12h for at least 14 days.

- Hemoplasmosis (cats): 10 mg/kg, PO, once daily for 7 days.
- Heartworm treatment (dogs): 10 mg/kg q12h PO administered for 28 days prior to adulticide treatment. It may be administered in combination with ivermectin.

**Birds**
- Mix four 100-mg doxycycline hyclate capsules with 1 L of water (400 mg/L). Shake to make solution and offer as only source of water to birds to eliminate bacteria. Alternatively, 25 mg/kg PO q12h for 3 weeks.

**Large Animal Dosage**
- Horses: 20 mg/kg q12h PO. (*Do not* administer IV.)
- For *Lawsonia intracellularis:* 20 mg/kg PO q24h for 3 weeks.

**Regulatory Information**
No regulatory information is available. For extralabel use withdrawal interval estimates, contact FARAD at www.FARAD.org.

# Dronabinol
droe-nab´ih-nole

**Trade and other names:** Marinol

**Functional classification:** Antiemetic

## Pharmacology and Mechanism of Action
Dronabinol is an antiemetic from the cannabinoid class. In cannabis, there are many active chemicals, but one of the most significant is delta-9-tetrahydrocannabinol (delta-9-THC). This compound is believed to be the most pharmacologically active. Dronabinol is a synthetic form of delta-9-THC that can be administered orally. The site of action is unknown, but there is some evidence that the active ingredient (THC) may affect the CB-1 cannabinoid receptor or possibly opiate receptors or other receptors in the vomiting center.

Dronabinol has good oral absorption, but complete bioavailability is low because of high first-pass effects. The volume of distribution is high.

## Indications and Clinical Uses
Cannabinoids have been used in people who have not responded to any other antiemetic drugs (e.g., patients who are receiving anticancer drugs). This agent and another synthetic form of THC is used to increase the appetite in patients with terminal disease, cancer, and AIDS. Their use has not been reported in veterinary patients, but they have been used by some veterinarians to increase the appetite in cats. The oral synthetic THC agents have not been effective for treatment of chronic pain.

## Precautionary Information

### Adverse Reactions and Side Effects

Cannabinoids are relatively well tolerated in people, but side effects include drowsiness, dizziness, ataxia, and disorientation. Withdrawal signs may occur after abrupt discontinuation after repeated doses. Adverse effects have not been reported in animals because of infrequent use.

### Contraindications and Precautions

No known contraindications.

### Drug Interactions

No drug interactions reported for animals, but cannabinoids are known microsomal enzyme inhibitors.

## Instructions for Use

Dronabinol is a form of synthetic marijuana (THC) and is available as an antiemetic prescription drug. Most clinical use in animals has been anecdotal. It has been administered to decrease vomiting and improve appetite associated with chemotherapy.

## Patient Monitoring and Laboratory Tests

No specific monitoring is necessary.

## Formulations

- Dronabinol is available in 2.5-, 5-, and 10-mg capsules.

## Stability and Storage

Store in a tightly sealed container, protected from light, and at room temperature.

## Small Animal Dosage

### Dogs and Cats

- 5 mg/m$^2$ PO, up to 15 mg/m$^2$ for antiemetic administration prior to chemotherapy.
- Appetite stimulation: start at 2.5 mg before meals.

## Large Animal Dosage

- No dose has been reported for large animals.

## Regulatory Information

Dronabinol is a Schedule III controlled drug. Do not administer to animals intended for food.

# Edetate Calcium Disodium
ed'eh-tate kal'see-um dye-soe'-dee-um

**Trade and other names:** Calcium disodium versenate and calcium disodium ethylenediaminetetra-acetate (EDTA)

**Functional classification:** Antidote

## Pharmacology and Mechanism of Action

Edetate calcium disodium (EDTA) calcium is a chelating agent. It readily chelates with lead, zinc, cadmium, copper, iron, and manganese. Because of the chelation properties, it is used to treat various types of intoxication.

## Indications and Clinical Uses

Edetate calcium disodium is indicated for treatment of acute and chronic lead poisoning. It is sometimes used in combination with dimercaprol.

## Precautionary Information

**Adverse Reactions and Side Effects**

No adverse effects reported in animals. In people, allergic reactions (release of histamine) have occurred after IV administration.

**Contraindications and Precautions**

Do not use edetate disodium to substitute for edetate calcium disodium because it will chelate calcium in the patient. The loss of calcium can be fatal.

**Drug Interactions**

No specific drug interactions are reported. However, it has the potential to chelate other drugs if mixed together.

## Instructions for Use

Edetate calcium disodium may be used with dimercaprol. It is equally effective when administered intravenously or intramuscularly, but IM injection may be painful. Ensure adequate urine flow before the first dose is administered.

## Patient Monitoring and Laboratory Tests

Monitor lead concentrations to assess treatment.

## Formulations

• Edetate calcium disodium is available in a 200-mg/mL injection.

## Stability and Storage

Store in a tightly sealed container, protected from light, and at room temperature. Stability of compounded formulations has not been evaluated.

## Small Animal Dosage

• 25 mg/kg q6h for 2–5 days SQ, IM, or IV.

## Large Animal Dosage

• 25 mg/kg q6h for 2–5 days SQ, IM, or IV.

## Regulatory Information

Withdrawal time: 2 days for meat; 2 days for milk (extralabel).

# Edrophonium Chloride
ed-roe-foe′nee-um klor′ide

**Trade and other names:** Tensilon and generic brands

**Functional classification:** Antimyasthenic, anticholinesterase

## Pharmacology and Mechanism of Action
Edrophonium is a cholinesterase inhibitor. Edrophonium causes cholinergic effects by inhibiting metabolism of acetylcholine. Its effects are acting with fast elimination; therefore, it is used for short-term use only.

## Indications and Clinical Uses
Because edrophonium is short acting, it ordinarily is only used for diagnostic purposes (e.g., myasthenia gravis). It also has been used to reverse neuromuscular blockade of nondepolarizing agents (pancuronium).

## Precautionary Information
### Adverse Reactions and Side Effects
Edrophonium is short acting, and side effects are minimal. Overdose in nonmyasthenia animals may cause salivation, retching, vomiting, and diarrhea. If this is observed, administer atropine at 0.02–0.04 mg/kg. Excessive muscarinic and cholinergic effects may occur with high doses; these may also be counteracted with atropine.

### Contraindications and Precautions
Edrophonium will potentiate effects of other cholinergic drugs. Cats are especially sensitive to edrophonium (see dose differences in the Small Animal Dosage section).

### Drug Interactions
Use cautiously with other cholinergic drugs.

## Instructions for Use
Edrophonium is used primarily for determination of diagnosis of myasthenia gravis. An alternative drug for this purpose is neostigmine methylsulfate (Prostigmin) at 40 mcg/kg IM or 20 mcg/kg IV.

## Patient Monitoring and Laboratory Tests
No specific monitoring is necessary.

## Formulations
- Edrophonium is available in a 10-mg/mL injection.

## Stability and Storage
Store in a tightly sealed container, protected from light, and at room temperature. Stability of compounded formulations has not been evaluated.

## Small Animal Dosage
**Dogs**
- 0.11–0.22 mg/kg IV (maximum dose, 5 mg per dog).

**Cats**
- 0.25–0.5 mg/cat IV.

## Large Animal Dose
- No large animal doses have been reported.

## Regulatory Information
No regulatory information is available. Because of a short half-life, no risk of residue is anticipated in food animals.

Racing Commissioners International (RCI) Classification: 3

E

# Enalapril Maleate
eh-nal'ah-prill mal'ee-ate

**Trade and other names:** Enacard (veterinary preparation) and Vasotec (human preparation)

**Functional classification:** Vasodilator, angiotensin-converting enzyme (ACE) inhibitor

## Pharmacology and Mechanism of Action
Enalapril is an angiotensin-converting enzyme (ACE) inhibitor. Like other ACE inhibitors, it inhibits conversion of angiotensin I to angiotensin II. Angiotensin II is a potent vasoconstrictor and also stimulates sympathetic stimulation, renal hypertension, and synthesis of aldosterone. The ability of aldosterone to cause sodium and water retention contributes to congestion.

Enalapril, like other ACE inhibitors, causes vasodilation and decreases aldosterone-induced congestion, but ACE inhibitors also contribute to vasodilation by increasing concentrations of some vasodilating kinins and prostaglandins.

## Indications and Clinical Uses
Enalapril, like other ACE inhibitors, is used to treat hypertension and congestive heart failure (CHF). Efficacy for treating CHF has been established from clinical trials and can be used with other drugs such as pimobendan, furosemide, digoxin, and spironolactone. If aldosterone breakthrough occurs with administration of ACE inhibitors, spironolactone may be indicated. It is primarily used in dogs. In addition to its use for treatment of CHF, enalapril has been used to delay onset of CHF in dogs with mitral regurgitation. The benefit of enalapril and other ACE inhibitors for occult heart disease is controversial; some studies have shown a benefit, and others have not. Enalapril has been used in some cats in heart failure or with systemic hypertension. Unfortunately, approximately 50% of cats with hypertension do not respond to enalapril, and ACE inhibitors are not considered a primary treatment for hypertension in cats. An angiotensin-receptor blocking drug (e.g., telmisartan) or other vasodilators are preferred in cats.

Angiotensin-converting enzyme inhibitors also have been shown to be beneficial in the management of certain types of kidney disorders (nephropathy) and for renal hypertension. Renal benefits result from limiting systemic and glomerular capillary hypertension, the antiproteinuric effect to decrease in urine protein-to-creatinine ratio and retarding the development of glomerular sclerosis and tubulointerstitial lesions. ACE inhibitors have decreased proteinuria in patients, but long-term benefits on survival have not been established. The benefits of ACE inhibitor treatment in cats with chronic renal disease are somewhat modest and have little effect on survival time or long-term prognosis.

Large animal uses have not been established, but in horses, the metabolite enalaprilat at 0.5 mg/kg IV completely inhibited ACE activity but did not change blood pressure or other hemodynamic variables in response to exercise.

## Precautionary Information

### Adverse Reactions and Side Effects

Enalapril may cause azotemia in some patients, but this effect is uncommon. Nevertheless, monitor renal parameters in patients receiving ACE inhibitors, especially if they are receiving diuretics.

### Contraindications and Precautions

Discontinue ACE inhibitors in pregnant animals; they cross the placenta and have caused fetal malformations and death of the fetus.

### Drug Interactions

Use cautiously with other drugs known to cause hypotension. The use may exacerbate effects of diuretics. Nonsteroidal anti-inflammatory drugs (NSAIDs) may potentially decrease vasodilating effects, but this has not been shown in studies in animals.

## Instructions for Use

The doses of enalapril are based on clinical trials conducted in dogs. For dogs, generally start with once-daily administration and increase to q12h if needed (see the dosing section). In some dogs with mild disease, start with 0.25 mg/kg q12h and then increase to 0.5 mg/kg q12h at the first recheck. Other drugs used for treatment of heart failure, such as pimobendan and spironolactone, may be used concurrently.

## Patient Monitoring and Laboratory Tests

Monitor patients carefully to avoid hypotension. With all ACE inhibitors, monitor electrolytes and renal function 3–7 days after initiating therapy and periodically thereafter.

## Formulations

- Enalapril is available as Vasotec (human preparation) in 2.5-, 5-, 10-, and 20-mg tablets and as Enacard (veterinary preparation) in 1-, 2.5-, 5-, 10-, and 20-mg tablets.

## Stability and Storage

Store in a tightly sealed container, protected from light, and at room temperature. Enalapril, compounded in a variety of oral suspensions and flavorings, was stable for 60 days. Above a pH of 5, degradation occurs more quickly.

## Small Animal Dosage

### Dogs

- 0.5 mg/kg q12–24h PO. In some animals, it may be necessary to increase dose to 1 mg/kg/day, administered as 0.5 mg/kg q12h.

### Cats

- 0.25–0.5 mg/kg q12–24h PO.
- 1–1.25 mg/cat/day PO.

## Large Animal Dosage

- Horses: Although enalapril has been examined in research horses, there are no clinical studies available to establish doses.

## Regulatory Information

No regulatory information is available. For extralabel use withdrawal interval estimates, contact Food Animal Residue Avoidance Databank (FARAD) at www.FARAD.org.

RCI Classification: 3

# Enflurane
en-floor´ane

**Trade and other names:** Ethrane

**Functional classification:** Inhalant anesthetic

## Pharmacology and Mechanism of Action

Inhalant anesthetic. Like other inhalant anesthetics, the mechanism of action is uncertain. Enflurane produces a generalized, reversible, depression of the central nervous system (CNS). The inhalant anesthetics vary in their solubility in blood, their potency, and the rate of induction and recovery. Those with low blood/gas partition coefficients are associated with the most rapid rates of induction and recovery. Enflurane has a vapor pressure of 175 mm Hg (at 20°C), a blood/gas partition coefficient of 1.8, and a fat/blood coefficient of 36.

## Indications and Clinical Uses

Enflurane, like other inhalant anesthetics, is used for general anesthesia in animals. It has a minimum alveolar concentration (MAC) value of 2.37%, 2.06%, and 2.12% in cats, dogs, and horses, respectively.

## Precautionary Information

### Adverse Reactions and Side Effects

Like other inhalant anesthetics, enflurane produces vasodilation and increased blood flow to cerebral blood vessels. This may increase intracranial pressure. Like other inhalant anesthetics, it produces a dose-dependent myocardial depression with accompanying decrease in cardiac output. It also depresses respiratory rate and alveolar ventilation. Like other inhalant anesthetics, it increases the risk of ventricular arrhythmias, especially in response to catecholamines.

### Contraindications and Precautions

No specific contraindications are reported for animals.

### Drug Interactions

Other sedatives and anesthetics (e.g., opiates, benzodiazepines, phenothiazines, alpha$_2$ agonists) will lower the requirement for inhalant gas anesthesia.

## Instructions for Use

Titrate dose for each individual with anesthetic monitoring.

## Patient Monitoring and Laboratory Tests

Monitor anesthesia parameters. During anesthesia, monitor heart rate and rhythm and respiratory rate.

## Formulations

• Enflurane is available as a solution for inhalation.

## Stability and Storage

Store in a tightly sealed container, protected from light, and at room temperature.

## Small Animal Dosage

• Induction: 2%–3%.
• Maintenance: 1.5%–3%.

## Large Animal Dosage
• MAC value: 1.66%.

## Regulatory Information
No withdrawal times are established for food animals. Clearance is rapid, and short withdrawal times are suggested. For extralabel use withdrawal interval estimates, contact FARAD at www.FARAD.org.

# Enilconazole
en-il-kah′nah-zole

**Trade and other names:** Imazalil, Imaverol, and Clinafarm-EC

**Functional classification:** Antifungal

## Pharmacology and Mechanism of Action
Enilconazole is an azole antifungal agent for topical use only. It was originally used in agriculture to prevent fungal infections in crops. In some drug references, it is known as imazalil or chloramizole. Like other azoles, enilconazole inhibits membrane synthesis (ergosterol) in fungus and weakens the cell wall. It is highly active against dermatophytes. It is used topically on animals and in the environment to treat and prevent fungal infections.

## Indications and Clinical Uses
Enilconazole is only used topically. It is used as a topical agent for treatment of dermatophytes; as a spray, it is used to treat the environment. It may be applied to animal bedding, stalls, and cages. In addition to dermatologic use, enilconazole has been instilled into the nasal sinuses of dogs for treatment of nasal aspergillosis.

## Precautionary Information
### Adverse Reactions and Side Effects
Adverse effects have not been reported. However, it is reported that if used on cats, they should be prevented from licking fur after application until the drug has dried.

### Contraindications and Precautions
No specific contraindications are reported.

### Drug Interactions
No specific interactions are reported. However, like other azoles, systemic treatment may result in cytochrome P450 enzyme inhibition.

## Instructions for Use
Enilconazole is only used topically. Imaverol is available in Canada as 10% emulsion. In the United States, Clinafarm EC is available for use in poultry units as 13.8% solution. Dilute solution to at least 50:1 and apply topically every 3–4 days for 2–3 weeks. Enilconazole also has been instilled as 1:1 dilution into the nasal sinus for nasal aspergillosis. In addition, enilconazole has been used in a diluted form as a spray to kill fungi on bedding, equine tack, and cages.

## Patient Monitoring and Laboratory Tests
No specific monitoring is necessary.

## Formulations Available
- Enilconazole is available as 10% or 13.8% emulsion.

## Stability and Storage
Store in a tightly sealed container, protected from light, and at room temperature. Stability of compounded formulations has not been evaluated. When the emulsion is mixed, it should be used immediately and not stored.

## Small Animal Dosage
- Nasal aspergillosis: 10 mg/kg q12h instilled into nasal sinus for 14 days (10% solution diluted 50/50 with water).
- Dermatophytes: Dilute 10% solution to 0.2% and wash lesion with solution four times at 3- to 4-day intervals. Solution may be sponged directly on animal. Allow solution to air dry.

## Large Animal Dosage
**Horses**
- Dilute 10% solution to 0.2% and wash lesions with solution four times at 3- to 4-day intervals.
- Treatment of aspergillus rhinitis: Infuse in nasal catheter a 2% solution q12h (25–100 mL).

## Regulatory Information
No regulatory information is available. For extralabel use withdrawal interval estimates, contact FARAD at www.FARAD.org.

# Enoxaparin Sodium
en-oks´ah-pare-in

**Trade and other names:** Lovenox and low-molecular-weight heparin (LMWH)

**Functional classification:** Anticoagulant

## Pharmacology and Mechanism of Action
Enoxaparin is a low-molecular-weight heparin (LMWH) is also known as *fragmented heparin*. LMWH is characterized by a molecular weight composed of approximately 5000 compared with conventional heparin (unfractionated heparin, UFH) with a molecular weight of approximately 15,000. Subsequently, the absorption, clearance, and activity of LMWH differ from UFH. LMWHs produce their effect by binding to antithrombin (AT) and increasing AT III–mediated inhibition of synthesis and activity of coagulation factor Xa. However, LMWH, unlike conventional heparin, produces less inhibition of thrombin (factor IIa). LMWH's activity is described by the anti-factor Xa: antifactor IIa ratio. Enoxaparin has a ratio of 3.8:1 (the conventional UFH ratio is 1:1). In people, LMWHs have several advantages compared with UFH and include greater anti-Xa/IIa activity, more complete and predictable absorption from injection, longer duration, less frequent administration, reduced risk of bleeding, and a more predictable anticoagulant response. However, in dogs and cats, the half-life of LMWH is much shorter than in humans, reducing some of this advantage. In dogs, the half-life of enoxaparin is approximately 5 hours; in cats, it is estimated to

be 1.9 hours, which requires much more frequent administration in either species to maintain anti-Xa activity compared with humans. LMWH used in veterinary medicine include tinzaparin (Innohep), enoxaparin (Lovenox), and dalteparin (Fragmin). In people, enoxaparin has replaced dalteparin as the preferred LMWH for clinical use.

## Indications and Clinical Uses

Enoxaparin, like other LMWHs, is used to treat hypercoagulability disorders and prevent coagulation disorders such as thromboembolism, venous thrombosis, disseminated intravascular coagulopathy, and pulmonary thromboembolism. In dogs and cats, there is insufficient evidence to show that LMWH is superior to UFH for treatment. Clinical indications are derived from uses of conventional heparin or extrapolated from human medicine. There have been few clinical studies to examine efficacy of LMWH in animals. Previously published doses extrapolated from humans have been shown *not* to produce adequate and consistent anti-Xa activity in dogs and cats; therefore, specific doses for dogs and cats, rather than extrapolated from human medicine, should be used.

## Precautionary Information

### Adverse Reactions and Side Effects

Although enoxaparin is better tolerated than regular heparin, bleeding is a risk. However, LMWHs produce fewer bleeding problems than administration of conventional heparin. LMWHs are associated with a lower incidence of heparin-induced thrombocytopenia (HIT) in people, but HIT from any form of heparin has not been a clinical problem in animals. If excessive anticoagulation and bleeding occur as a result of an overdose, protamine sulfate should be administered to reverse heparin treatment. The protamine dose is 1.0 mg protamine for every 1.0 mg enoxaparin administered by slow IV infusion. Protamine complexes with heparin to form a stable, inactive compound.

### Contraindications and Precautions

Do not administer IM to prevent hematoma; administer SQ only. LMWH is excreted by renal clearance in animals; therefore, if renal disease is present, the elimination will be prolonged. Rebound hypercoagulability may occur after discontinuation of heparin treatment; therefore, it may be advised to taper the dose slowly when discontinuing treatment.

### Drug Interactions

Do not mix with other injectable drugs. Use cautiously in animals that are already receiving other drugs that can interfere with coagulation, such as aspirin, warfarin, and factor Xa inhibitors. Although a specific interaction has not been identified, use cautiously in animals that may be receiving certain chondroprotective compounds such as glycosaminoglycans for treatment of arthritis. Some antibiotics, such as cephalosporins, may inhibit coagulation.

## Instructions for Use

Dosing recommendations extrapolated from human medicine are not appropriate for animals. Animal owners should be warned that LMWHs are expensive compared with conventional heparin. When dosing, do not interchange doses on a unit-for-unit basis with heparin or other LMWHs because they differ in manufacturing process, molecular weight distribution, anti-Xa and anti-IIa activities, units, and dosage.

## Patient Monitoring and Laboratory Tests

Monitor patients for clinical signs of bleeding problems. When administering LMWH, activated partial thromboplastin time (aPTT) and prothrombin time clotting times are not reliable indicators of therapy, although prolonged aPTT is a sign of overdosing. Anti-Xa activity is considered the preferred laboratory measure of LMWH activity in people, but the use of this parameter is controversial in animals. Peak anti-Xa activity occurs 3–4 hours after dosing, and the target range for anti-Xa activity should be 0.5–1.0 units/mL for cats and 0.5–2.0 units/mL for dogs.

## Formulations

- Enoxaparin is available as 100 mg/mL in the following sizes: 30 mg in 0.3-mL, 40 mg in 0.4-mL, 60 mg in 0.6-mL, 80 mg in 0.8-mL, 100 mg in 1-mL, and 300 mg/3-mL injection; and 150 mg/mL with 120 mg/0.8 mL and 150-mg/mL injection.

## Stability and Storage

Store in a tightly sealed container protected from light. The pH of the injection is 5.5–7.5.

## Small Animal Dosage

### Dogs

- 0.8 mg/kg SQ q6h (see Patient Monitoring and Laboratory Tests for dose adjustment). The dose may need to be adjusted because this may not achieve adequate anti-Xa levels in all dogs.

### Cats

- 0.75–1 mg/kg SQ q12h, up to 1.25 mg/kg SQ q6h. Every 6 hours is preferred by many experts. (See Patient Monitoring and Laboratory Tests for dose adjustment.)

## Large Animal Dosage

### Horses

- Prophylaxis: 0.5 mg/kg q24h SQ and 1 mg/kg q24h SQ for high-risk patients.

## Regulatory Information

Extralabel withdrawal times are not established. However, 24-hour withdrawal times are suggested because this drug has little risk from residues.

# Enrofloxacin
en-roe-floks′ah-sin

**Trade and other names:** Baytril and generic

**Functional classification:** Antibacterial

## Pharmacology and Mechanism of Action

Enrofloxacin is a fluoroquinolone antibacterial drug. Enrofloxacin acts via inhibition of DNA gyrase in bacteria to inhibit DNA and RNA synthesis. It is a bactericidal with a broad spectrum of activity. In most animal species, enrofloxacin is metabolized, at least partially, to ciprofloxacin. Ciprofloxacin is an active desmethyl metabolite of enrofloxacin and may contribute in an additive fashion to the antibacterial effects. At the peak concentration, ciprofloxacin may account for approximately 10% and 20% of the total concentration in cats and dogs, respectively, and is variable in other animals. Susceptible bacteria include *Staphylococcus* spp., *Escherichia coli, Proteus* spp., *Klebsiella* spp., and *Pasteurella* spp. *Pseudomonas aeruginosa* is moderately susceptible but requires higher concentrations. Cattle and swine respiratory pathogens are susceptible. Enrofloxacin has poor activity against *Streptococcus* spp. and anaerobic bacteria. Other atypical bacteria such as *Mycoplasma* spp. may be variably susceptible.

*Pharmacokinetics:* The pharmacokinetics of enrofloxacin have been studied in every domestic animal and many zoo and exotic animals. In dogs, the half-life (approximate values) ranges from 3 to 5 hours, with a volume of distribution (VD) of 2.5–5 L/kg, and peak concentrations of 1.5–2 mcg/mL after a dose of 5 mg/kg. It has high oral absorption of 75%–80%. In cats, enrofloxacin has a half-life of 4–7 hours, with a VD of 3–6 L/kg, and peak concentration of 1–1.5 mcg/mL after a dose of 5 mg/kg. Oral absorption approaches 100%. In cattle, the half-life has a wide range of 3–9 hours, depending on the study and type of cattle. The VD is 1.5–2.5 L/kg, and peak concentration is 0.7–1 mcg/mL. In pigs, the half-life is 6–12 hours, the VD is 1.5–3.5 L/kg, and peak concentration is 0.6–1.2 mcg/mL. From several studies in horses, the average half-life is 8 hours, and oral clearance (CL/F) is 0.4 L/kg/h, with a peak concentration of 1.4 mcg/mL after an average dose of 6 mg/kg. The average oral absorption is 60%. Plasma protein binding rates in animals are 60% in cattle, 34% in dogs, 22% in horses, and 23% in pigs.

## Indications and Clinical Uses

Enrofloxacin, like other fluoroquinolones, is used to treat susceptible bacteria in a variety of species. Treatment has included infections of skin and soft tissue, urinary tract infections in dogs and cats, *Chlamydophila felis* infections in cats, and ulcerative colitis caused by *E. coli* in dogs. Enrofloxacin has been shown effective for treating *Rickettsia* infections in dogs. However, it is not effective for treating *Ehrlichia* infections (see Doxycycline). In horses, it has been used for a variety of soft tissue infections and respiratory infections, although this use is based primarily on anecdotal experience. Enrofloxacin is approved for the treatment and control of swine respiratory disease (SRD) associated with *Actinobacillus pleuropneumoniae, Pasteurella multocida, Haemophilus parasuis,* and *Streptococcus suis.* It is approved in weaned pigs where colibacillosis associated with E. coli has been diagnosed. It is also approved for treatment of bovine respiratory disease (BRD) associated with *Mannheimia haemolytica, P. multocida,* and *Haemophilus somni.* Enrofloxacin is also used in most exotic animal species because of its safety and activity against a wide variety of pathogens.

## Precautionary Information

### Adverse Reactions and Side Effects

High concentrations may cause CNS toxicity. Animals with kidney disease may be more susceptible. It may cause occasional vomiting and, at high doses, may cause some nausea and diarrhea. All of the fluoroquinolones may cause arthropathy in young animals. Dogs are most sensitive at 4 weeks to 28 weeks of age. Large, rapidly growing dogs are the most susceptible. Cats are relatively resistant to cartilage injury, but foals are susceptible. Blindness in cats that is caused by retinal degeneration has been reported from enrofloxacin. Affected cats have had permanent blindness. This may be a dose-related effect. Cats administered doses of 20 mg/kg developed retinal degeneration but did not at 5 mg/kg. Therefore, dose restrictions in cats have been used. Administration of concentrated solution (100 mg/mL) given orally to horses has caused oral mucosal lesions. When injected, this solution (pH 10.5) may be irritating to some tissues.

Problems reported in people from use of fluoroquinolones include tendon injury and rupture (mostly Achilles tendon) and aortic artery dissection and rupture. These events occur as a result of fluoroquinolone's ability to upregulate cell matrix metalloproteinases, resulting in a reduction of collagen fibrils of types I and III collagen, which comprise the majority of collagen in tendons and the aorta. Fluoroquinolones can affect glucose homeostasis in people with diabetes. However, despite the reports of these effects in people, there are no reported instances of these problems in animals with current use.

**Contraindications and Precautions**
Avoid use in young dogs because of risk of cartilage injury. Do not administer to young foals; injury to articular cartilage has been reported. Use cautiously in animals that may be prone to seizures, such as those with epilepsy. Do not administer to cats at doses greater than 5 mg/kg/day. Avoid use in older cats.

**Drug Interactions**
Fluoroquinolones may increase concentrations of theophylline and possibly other drugs if used concurrently. Coadministration with divalent and trivalent cations, such as products containing aluminum, magnesium (e.g., antacids), iron, and calcium, may decrease absorption. Sucralfate suspension, but not intact tablets, may inhibit oral absorption because aluminum chelates with enrofloxacin.

Do not mix in solutions or in vials with aluminum, calcium, iron, or zinc because chelation may occur. Enrofloxacin may precipitate in an IV line if injected directly into IV fluids.

## Instructions for Use
A low dosage in dogs and cats of 5 mg/kg/day is used for susceptible organisms with minimum inhibitory concentration (MIC) values of 0.5 mcg/mL for all indications. The dose can be increased for bacteria with higher MIC values, but bacteria with MIC values greater than 2 mcg/mL are resistant. Maximum dosage for cats is 5 mg/kg once daily but can be increased up to 20 mg/kg once daily for dogs. The injectable solution is not approved for IV use, but it has been administered via this route safely if given slowly. Enrofloxacin was not absorbed in cats after transdermal application in a pluronic gel vehicle.

Concentrated enrofloxacin solution (cattle formulation at 100 mg/mL) is basic (pH 10.5); therefore, it can be irritating to some animals when injected intramuscularly. Do not inject more than 20 mL at each site. Also, this formulation may precipitate out of solution if pH is decreased by other solutions.

## Patient Monitoring and Laboratory Tests
Susceptibility testing (from the Clinical and Laboratory Standards Institute [CLSI]): For dogs and cats, the breakpoint for susceptible organisms is ≤0.5 mcg/mL, and bacteria above 2 mcg/mL are clinically resistant. For cattle, the breakpoint for susceptible bacteria (BRD pathogens) is ≤0.25 mcg/mL. For pigs, the breakpoint for susceptible bacteria is ≤0.25 mcg/mL for SRD pathogens but ≤0.5 mcg/mL for *Streptococcus suis*. For horses, the breakpoint for susceptible bacteria is ≤0.12 mcg/mL at an oral dose of 7.5 mg/kg once daily. These breakpoints may be applied to other species when specific breakpoints are not available.

## Formulations
Enrofloxacin is available in 22.7- and 68-mg tablets; Taste Tabs are 22.7, 68, and 136 mg. It is also available in a 22.7-mg/mL injection and a 100-mg/mL preparation for large animals (Baytril-100).

## Stability and Storage
Store in a tightly sealed container, protected from light, and at room temperature. Stability of compounded formulations have been evaluated, and it was found to be stable with many mixtures. A 1% solution diluted in other vehicles (chlorhexidine, salicylic acid, EDTA, and water) was stable for 28 days. However, do not mix with solutions that contain ions that may chelate with enrofloxacin (iron, magnesium, aluminum, and calcium). If administered intravenously, it is recommended to first dilute

the solution in fluids (e.g., 1:10 dilution) and infuse slowly. The 100-mg/mL solution is alkaline and contains benzyl alcohol and l-arginine as a base (pH 10). The pH of this solution is alkaline, and if the pH is lowered, the drug may precipitate. The 22.7-mg/mL formulation has a pH of 11.5 and may not be compatible with some solutions.

## Small Animal Dosage
### Dogs
- 5–20 mg/kg/day IM, PO, or IV. Higher doses are used for bacteria with high MIC values in the intermediate range of susceptibility. For uncomplicated lower urinary tract infection, 18–20 mg/kg once daily PO every 3 days.

### Cats
- 5 mg/kg/day PO or IM. Avoid IV use in cats. Do not exceed 5 mg/kg in cats.

### Exotic Animals
- Usually 5 mg/kg/day IM or oral in reptiles every other day or every third day.

### Birds
- 15 mg/kg q12h IM or PO.

## Large Animal Dosage
### Horses
- 5 mg/kg q24h IV.
- 7.5 mg/kg q24h PO.
- 5 mg/kg of 100 mg/mL solution (Baytril-100) IM once per day (rotate injection sites).

### Cattle (BRD)
- Single dose: 7.5–12.5 mg/kg once SQ (3.4–5.7 mL/100 lb).
- Multiple dose: 2.5–5 mg/kg SQ (1.1–2.3 mL/100 lb) once daily for 3–5 days.

### Swine (SRD)
- 7.5 mg/kg IM or SQ behind the ear once. Do not administer more than 5 mL per injection site.

## Regulatory Information
Cattle withdrawal time: 28 days for meat. Not to be used in lactating dairy cattle or calves intended to be used as veal. Do not use in female dairy cattle 20 months of age or older. Pig withdrawal time: 5 days.
Extralabel use of fluoroquinolones in animals that produce food is illegal.

# Ephedrine Hydrochloride
eh-fed′rin hye-droe-klor′ide

**Trade and other names:** Generic brands

**Functional classification:** Adrenergic agonist

## Pharmacology and Mechanism of Action
Ephedrine is an adrenergic agonist. The most common use is as a decongestant. Ephedrine acts as an agonist on alpha-adrenergic receptors and beta$_1$-adrenergic receptors but has less effect on beta$_2$ receptors. The effects as a decongestant are attributed to action on alpha$_1$ adrenergic receptors and constriction of blood vessels on mucous membranes. Therefore, it also is used to constrict blood vessels for other indications.

## Indications and Clinical Uses

Ephedrine is used as a vasopressor (e.g., when it is administered during anesthesia). It also has been used as a CNS stimulant. Oral formulations have been used to treat urinary incontinence because of action on bladder sphincter muscle. However, this is no longer recommended, and most oral dose forms are no longer available.

### Precautionary Information

**Adverse Reactions and Side Effects**

Adverse effects are related to excessive adrenergic activity (e.g., peripheral vasoconstriction and tachycardia, or alternatively, reflex bradycardia).

**Contraindications and Precautions**

Use in animals with cardiovascular disease is not recommended.

**Drug Interactions**

No specific drug interactions are reported. However, ephedrine potentiates any other adrenergic agonist.

**E**

## Instructions for Use

The most current use is from injection primarily in acute situations to increase blood pressure. Oral use for urinary incontinence in dogs has diminished because of lack of available formulations and other agents to treat urinary incontinence (e.g., phenylpropanolamine).

### Patient Monitoring and Laboratory Tests

Monitor heart rate and rhythm in patients.

### Formulations

- Most formulations of ephedrine have been removed from the market. Previously available as a 25- and 50-mg/mL injection.

### Stability and Storage

Store in a tightly sealed container, protected from light, and at room temperature.

### Small Animal Dosage

**Dogs**

- Urinary incontinence: 4 mg/kg or 12.5–50 mg/dog q8–12h PO.
- Vasopressor: 0.75 mg/kg IM or SQ; repeat as needed.

**Cats**

- Urinary incontinence: 2–4 mg/kg q12h PO.
- Vasopressor: 0.75 mg/kg IM or SQ; repeat as needed.

### Large Animal Dosage

- No large animal doses are reported.

### Regulatory Information

Withdrawal time: No withdrawal times are established. Ephedrine is metabolized after administration, and a short withdrawal is recommended.

RCI Classification: 2

# Epinephrine
eh-pih-nef′rin

**Trade and other names:** Adrenaline and generic brands

**Functional classification:** Adrenergic agonist

## Pharmacology and Mechanism of Action

Epinephrine is a prototype for an adrenergic agonist. Also called adrenaline. Epinephrine is a nonselective agonist for alpha-adrenergic and beta-adrenergic receptors. The alpha-adrenergic effects increase vascular resistance and act as a potent vasopressor. The beta$_1$-receptor effects stimulate the heart. The beta$_2$-adrenergic effects increase bronchodilation and decrease inflammatory mediators in the airways. Epinephrine is a potent adrenergic agonist with a prompt onset and a short duration of action. Compared with norepinephrine, epinephrine has more profound beta-receptor activity. As a result, compared with norepinephrine, epinephrine is more likely to cause increases in heart rate and tachyarrhythmias than norepinephrine.

## Indications and Clinical Uses

Epinephrine is used primarily for emergency situations to treat cardiopulmonary arrest and anaphylactic shock. It is administered IV, IM, or endotracheal for acute use. Vasopressin (arginine vasopressin) has replaced epinephrine as a vasopressor in some cardiopulmonary resuscitation (CPR) protocols. Epinephrine has been used in horses to test for diagnosis of anhidrosis, but terbutaline sulfate challenge is used more frequently for this test.

## Precautionary Information

### Adverse Reactions and Side Effects

An overdose of epinephrine causes excessive vasoconstriction and hypertension. High doses can cause ventricular arrhythmias. When high doses are used for cardiopulmonary arrest, an electrical defibrillator should be available.

### Contraindications and Precautions

Avoid repeated administration in patients to prevent excessive adrenergic receptor stimulation.

### Drug Interactions

Epinephrine interacts with other drugs that are used to either potentiate or antagonize alpha-adrenergic or beta-adrenergic receptors. It is incompatible with alkaline solutions (e.g., bicarbonate), chlorine, bromine, and salts of metals or oxidizing solutions. Do not mix with bicarbonates, nitrates, citrates, and other salts.

## Instructions for Use

Doses are based on experimental studies, primarily in dogs. Clinical studies are not available, but the doses and protocols are developed from the experience of clinical use. IV doses are ordinarily used, but endotracheal administration is acceptable when IV access is not available. When the endotracheal route is used, the dose is higher (up to 10 times the IV dose for CPR), and the duration of effect may be longer than with IV administration. When administering an endotracheal dose, one can dilute the dose in a volume of 2–10 mL of saline. The intraosseous route also has been used, and doses are equivalent to IV doses. There appears to be no advantage to intracardiac injection compared with IV administration. Solutions are available in 1:1000 and 1:10,000 (either 1 mg/mL or 0.1 mg/mL). Generally, only the 1:10,000 solution is given IV. 1:1000 solutions are intended for IM use. Avoid the SQ route of administration because the vasoconstriction produced delays absorption from this site.

For CPR, the doses have been controversial (see the dosing section). There is a low dose (10 mcg/kg or 0.01 mg/kg) and a high dose (100 mcg/kg or 0.1 mg/kg). Generally, start with the low dose every 3–5 minutes IV in CPR; then use the high dose after prolonged CPR.

## Patient Monitoring and Laboratory Tests

Monitor heart rate and rhythm during treatment.

## Formulations

- Epinephrine is available in a 1-mg/mL (1:1000) injection solution and 0.1-mg/ mL (1:10,000) injection solution. The 1:10,000 is often used IV, and the 1:1000 solution is used IM or SQ. Ampules for people are designed to deliver 1 mg/ person (approximately 14 mcg/kg).

## Stability and Storage

It is compatible with plastic in syringes. When solution becomes oxidized, it turns brown. Do not use if this color change is observed. It is most stable at pH of 3–4. If the pH of the solution is greater than 5.5, it becomes unstable.

## Small Animal Dosage

- Cardiac arrest: 10–20 mcg/kg IV or 100–200 mcg/kg (0.1–0.2 mg/kg) endotracheal (may be diluted in saline before administration). The low dose of 10–20 mcg/kg IV initially may be used and increased to 100 mcg/kg IV for prolonged CPR.
- Anaphylactic shock: 5–10 mcg/kg IV or IM or 50 mcg/kg endotracheal (may be diluted in saline).
- Vasopressor therapy: 100–200 mcg/kg (0.1–0.2 mg/kg) IV (high dose) or 10–20 mcg/kg (0.01–0.02 mg/kg) IV (low dose). Administer low dose first; if no response, use high dose.
- Constant-rate infusion (CRI): 0.05 mcg/kg/min IV.
- During emergency use, the dose may be repeated every 5–15 minutes, but the maximum doses in dogs are 0.3 mg total for dogs weighing less than 40 kg and 0.5 mg total for dogs weighing more than 40 kg body weight.

## Large Animal Dosage

- 1 mg/mL (1:1000) solution most often used.
- Anaphylactic shock (cattle, pigs, horses, and sheep): 20 mcg/kg (0.02 mg/kg) IM or 1 mL/45 kg (1 mL/100 lb). 5–10 mcg/kg (0.005–0.01 mg/kg) IV or 0.25–0.5 mL/45 kg (100 lb).

## Regulatory Information

No withdrawal times are established. Epinephrine is rapidly metabolized after administration, and zero days is recommended for withdrawal.
RCI Classification: 2

# Epoetin Alfa (Erythropoietin)
ee-poe'eh-tin

**Trade and other names:** Procrit, Eprex, and Erythropoietin

**Functional classification:** Hormone

## Pharmacology and Mechanism of Action

Epoetin alfa is a human recombinant form of erythropoietin. Erythropoietin is a hematopoietic growth factor that stimulates erythropoiesis. It is used in clinical patients where stimulation of red blood cell production is needed.

## Indications and Clinical Uses

Epoetin alfa is used to treat nonregenerative anemia. It has been used to treat myelosuppression caused by disease or chemotherapy. It also has been used to treat chronic anemia associated with chronic renal failure. The value of epoetin alpha to improve anemia in cats with chronic renal failure has been established in several studies.

In some animals, anemia is also caused by iron deficiency and can be combined with ferrous sulfate at a dose of 50–100 mg per cat daily. Darbepoetin alfa (Aranesp), a similar drug, also has been used in small animals (see Darbepoetin Alfa). Because of several advantages, many experts now prefer darbepoetin instead of epoetin alfa.

## Precautionary Information

### Adverse Reactions and Side Effects

Because this product is a human-recombinant product, it may induce local and systemic allergic reactions in animals. Injection-site pain and headache have occurred in people. Seizures also have occurred. Delayed anemia may occur because of cross-reacting antibodies against animal erythropoietin (reversible when drug is withdrawn). Antiepoetin antibodies may increase with long-term use, which may occur in as high as 30% of treated cats, leading to failure of treatment.

### Contraindications and Precautions

Stop therapy with epoetin when joint pain, fever, anorexia, or cutaneous reactions are observed.

### Drug Interactions

No interactions are reported.

## Instructions for Use

The use of epoetin alfa has been limited primarily to dogs and cats. The only form currently available is a human-recombinant product. It is used in animals when hematocrit falls below 25%. In cats, 100 units/kg SQ three times a week is administered until a target hematocrit of 30%–40% is attained. Thereafter, twice-weekly injections are used. Maintenance dose is usually in a range of 75–100 units/kg SQ once or twice a week. Consider switching to darbepoetin if long-term use is needed.

## Patient Monitoring and Laboratory Tests

Monitor hematocrit. Dose should be adjusted to maintain hematocrit in a range of 30%–34%.

## Formulations Available

- Epoetin alfa is available in a range of strengths, including 2000-, 3000-, 4000-, 10,000-, 20,000-, and 40,000-units/mL injection.

## Stability and Storage

Store in a tightly sealed container, protected from light, and at room temperature. Stability of compounded formulations has not been evaluated.

## Small Animal Dosage

### Dogs

- 35 or 50 units/kg three times a week, up to 400 units/kg/wk SQ (adjust dose to maintain hematocrit of 30%–34%).

### Cats

- Start with 100 units/kg SQ three times weekly; reduce to twice weekly and then to once weekly when target hematocrit of 30%–40% is attained. In most cats, maintenance dosage is 75–100 units/kg SQ twice weekly.

## Large Animal Dosage

- No large animal doses are reported.

## Regulatory Information

No withdrawal times are established for food animals. Erythropoietin in any form is prohibited to be on the premises of racing horses. RCI Classification: 2

# Eprinomectin
e-prin-o-mek´tin

**Trade and other names:** Eprinex, LongRange, Eprizero, and Centragard

**Functional classification:** Antiparasitic

## Pharmacology and Mechanism of Action

Eprinomectin is an antiparasitic drug of the avermectin class. Avermectins (ivermectin-like drugs), such as eprinomectin and milbemycins (milbemycin and moxidectin), are macrocyclic lactones and share similarities, including mechanism of action. These drugs are neurotoxic to parasites by potentiating glutamate-gated chloride ion channels in parasites. Paralysis and death of the parasite are caused by increased permeability to chloride ions and hyperpolarization of nerve cells. These drugs also potentiate other chloride channels, including ones gated by gamma-aminobutyric acid (GABA). Mammals ordinarily are not affected because they lack glutamate-gated chloride channels, and there is a lower affinity for other mammalian chloride channels. Because these drugs ordinarily do not penetrate the blood–brain barrier, GABA-gated channels in the CNS of mammals are not affected. Eprinomectin is active against intestinal parasites (roundworms, hookworms, and tapeworms), mites, bots, heartworm microfilaria, and developing larvae. Eprinomectin can prevent disease caused by the heartworm *Dirofilaria immitis*. It has no effect on trematode or cestode parasites.

## Indications and Clinical Uses

Eprinomectin is indicated for treating cattle with gastrointestinal (GI) nematodes, roundworms, lungworms, cattle grubs (all stages), lice, mange mites, and flies. The duration of the sustained-release injection for GI parasites and lungworms is 100–120 days. The injection formulation can also be administered SQ for the treatment, protection, and control of *Bunostomum phlebotomum* for 150 days after treatment.

Eprinomectin is combined with praziquantel in a transdermal solution for cats for prevention of heartworm disease caused by *D. immitis* and treatment and control of roundworms, hookworms, and tapeworms.

## Precautionary Information

**Adverse Reactions and Side Effects**

Toxicity may occur at high doses and in canine breeds in which this class of drugs crosses the blood–brain barrier. Toxicity is neurotoxic, and signs include hypersalivation, depression, ataxia, difficulty with vision, coma, and death. Sensitivity to this class of drugs occurs in certain breeds because of a mutation in the multidrug resistance gene (ABCB1, formerly MDR1 gene) that codes for the membrane pump P-glycoprotein. This mutation affects the efflux pump in the blood–brain barrier. Neurologic signs also may occur when other animals are administered high doses.

**Contraindications and Precautions**

Animals with high numbers of microfilaremia may show adverse reactions to high doses. Do not administer to dogs at high doses if they are sensitive to the ivermectin class of drugs.

**Drug Interactions**

Do not administer with drugs that could potentially increase the penetration of these drugs across the blood–brain barrier. Such drugs include ketoconazole, itraconazole, cyclosporine, and calcium-channel blockers.

## Instructions for Use

Eprinomectin is approved in cattle for treating GI nematodes, roundworms, lungworms, cattle grubs (all stages), lice, mange mites, and flies. It is approved as a transdermal solution in cats for preventing heartworms and GI parasites in combination with praziquantel.

Eprinomectin is used in animals for internal and external parasites. Dosage regimens vary, depending on the species, formulation, and parasite treated.

## Patient Monitoring and Laboratory Tests

Monitor for microfilaremia prior to administration in small animals. For other parasitic infections, confirm successful treatment with fecal examinations or skin scrapings.

## Formulations

- Eprinomectin is available as a pour-on for cattle in a solution containing 5 mg/mL of eprinomectin. Available in 250-mL, 1-L, 2.5-L, and 5-L plastic bottles.
- 5% solution (50 mg/mL) extended-release for injection in 50-, 250-, and 500-mL bottles.
- Eprinomectin is combined with praziquantel in a transdermal solution for cats consisting of 4 mg/mL of eprinomectin and 83 mg/mL of praziquantel.

## Stability and Storage

Store in a tightly sealed container, protected from light, and at room temperature. Stability of compounded formulations has not been evaluated.

## Small Animal Dosage

**Dogs**

- Heartworm preventative: The dose for heartworm prevention in dogs has not been established.

**Cats**

- Heartworm preventative: 0.5 mg/kg of eprinomectin and 10 mg/kg of praziquantel. This solution is applied on the skin.

## Large Animal Dosage

Horses: Doses have not been established for horses.

**Cattle (Beef and Dairy)**

- Pour-on: 1 mL/10 kg of body weight (500 mcg/kg). Pour along the backline of the cattle from the shoulder to the tailhead.
- Injection: 1 mg/kg injected SQ.

## Regulatory Information

Cattle pour-on product: milk withdrawal time, zero days; preslaughter withdrawal time, zero days.
Cattle injectable product: 48 days withdrawal slaughter time.

# Epsiprantel
ep-sih-pran'til

**Trade and other names:** Cestex

**Functional classification:** Antiparasitic

## Pharmacology and Mechanism of Action

Epsiprantel is an anticestodal agent similar to praziquantel. The action of epsiprantel on parasites is related to neuromuscular toxicity and paralysis via altered permeability to calcium. Susceptible parasites include canine cestodes *Dipylidium caninum* and *Taenia pisiformis* and feline cestodes *D. caninum* and *T. taeniaeformis*.

## Indications and Clinical Uses

Like praziquantel, epsiprantel is used primarily to treat infections caused by tapeworms.

## Precautionary Information

### Adverse Reactions and Side Effects

Vomiting occurs at high doses. Anorexia and transient diarrhea have been reported. Epsiprantel is safe in pregnant animals.

### Contraindications and Precautions

Do not use in animals younger than 7 weeks of age. All doses are single dose.

### Drug Interactions

No drug interactions are reported.

## Instructions for Use

Administer as directed to treat tapeworm infections.

## Patient Monitoring and Laboratory Tests

No specific monitoring is necessary.

## Formulations

- Epsiprantel is available in 12.5-, 25-, 50-, and 100-mg coated tablets.

## Stability and Storage

Store in a tightly sealed container, protected from light, and at room temperature. Stability of compounded formulations has not been evaluated.

## Small Animal Dosage

**Dogs**

- 5.5 mg/kg PO.

## Cats
- 2.75 mg/kg PO.

## Large Animal Dosage
- No large animal doses are reported.

## Regulatory Information
No regulatory information is available. For extralabel use withdrawal interval estimates, contact FARAD at www.FARAD.org.

---

# Ergocalciferol
er-go-kal-sif'-role

**Trade and other names:** Calciferol and Drisdol

**Functional classification:** Vitamin

## Pharmacology and Mechanism of Action
Ergocalciferol is a vitamin D analogue. This agent is used as a supplement when vitamin D is needed. Vitamin D promotes absorption and utilization of calcium.

## Indications and Clinical Uses
Ergocalciferol is used for vitamin D deficiency and as treatment of hypocalcemia associated with hypoparathyroidism. Calcitriol often is used in place of ergocalciferol in dogs and cats. See Calcitriol for more information.

### Precautionary Information
**Adverse Reactions and Side Effects**
Overdose may cause hypercalcemia.

**Contraindications and Precautions**
Avoid use in pregnant animals because it may cause fetal abnormalities. Use cautiously with high doses of preparations containing calcium.

**Drug Interactions**
No drug interactions are reported.

## Instructions for Use
Ergocalciferol should not be used for renal secondary hypoparathyroidism because of an inability to convert to active compound. Doses for individual patients should be adjusted by monitoring serum calcium concentrations.

## Patient Monitoring and Laboratory Tests
Monitor serum calcium concentration. Normal total calcium concentrations in dogs and cats are 9–11.5 mg/dL and 8–10.5 mg/dL, respectively, or 1.2–1.5 mmol/L and 1.1–1.4 mmol/L, respectively.

## Formulations
- Ergocalciferol is available in 50,000 units per capsule.

**Conversion of Units**

To convert: 1.0 units ergocalciferol is equivalent to 0.025 mcg ergocalciferol or cholecalciferol.

**Stability and Storage**

Store in a tightly sealed container, protected from light, and at room temperature. Stability of compounded formulations has not been evaluated.

**Small Animal Dosage**

• 500–2000 units/kg/day PO.

**Large Animal Dosage**

• No large animal doses are reported.

**Regulatory Information**

No regulatory information is available. For extralabel use withdrawal interval estimates, contact FARAD at www.FARAD.org.

# Ertapenem
er-tah-pen´em

**Trade and other names:** Invanz

**Functional classification:** Antibacterial

## Pharmacology and Mechanism of Action

Ertapenem is a beta-lactam antibiotic of the carbapenem (penem) class with a broad spectrum of activity. Its action on cell walls is similar to other beta-lactams, which is to bind penicillin-binding proteins (PBPs) that weaken or interfere with cell wall formation. In *Escherichia coli,* it has strong affinity toward PBPs 1a, 1b, 2, 3, 4, and 5, with preference for PBPs 2 and 3. Ertapenem is stable against hydrolysis by a variety of beta-lactamases, including penicillinases, cephalosporinases, and extended spectrum beta-lactamases. The antibacterial spectrum includes gram-negative bacilli, including Enterobacteriaceae. Ertapenem is not as active against *P. aeruginosa* as other carbapenems. It is also active against most gram-positive bacteria, except methicillin-resistant strains of *Staphylococcus* and *Enterococcus* spp.

*Pharmacokinetics:* In people, the half-life is longer than other carbapenems (4 hours) because of high protein binding (95%), which allows for less frequent dosing. However, in dogs, these advantages do not exist. The protein binding in dogs is 46%, the VD is 0.28 L/kg, and the half-life is only 1.3 hours.

## Indications and Clinical Use

Ertapenem is indicated primarily for resistant infections caused by bacteria resistant to other drugs. It may be valuable for treating resistant infections caused by *E. coli* and *Klebsiella pneumoniae* but is not useful for *P. aeruginosa.* The use of ertapenem has not been as common as for meropenem or imipenem. High protein binding and a long half-life in people have allowed less frequent administration compared with other carbapenems. However, dosing protocols have not been tested in dogs and cats.

## Precautionary Information

### Adverse Reactions and Side Effects

Carbapenems pose similar risks as other beta-lactam antibiotics, but adverse effects are rare. There is a risk of CNS toxicity (seizures and tremors) with high doses.

### Contraindications and Precautions

Some slight yellowish discoloration may occur after reconstitution. Slight discoloration will not affect potency. However, a darker amber or brown discoloration may indicate oxidation and loss of potency.

### Drug Interactions

Do not mix in vial or syringe with other antibiotics.

## Instructions for Use

Doses in animals have been based on extrapolation from human studies rather than efficacy trials.

## Patient Monitoring and Laboratory Tests

Susceptibility testing: CLSI breakpoint for susceptible organisms in humans is ≤4 mcg/mL. Veterinary breakpoints are not established. Most bacteria have an MIC less than 2 mcg/mL. Sensitivity to imipenem can be used as a marker for ertapenem.

## Formulations

• Ertapenem is available in a 1-g vial for injection.

## Stability and Storage

Store in a tightly sealed container, protected from light, and at room temperature.

## Small Animal Dosage

### Dogs and Cats

• 30 mg/kg qh8 (q8h) IV or SQ.

## Large Animal Dosage

• No large animal doses have been reported.

## Regulatory Information

Withdrawal times are not established for animals that produce food. For extralabel use withdrawal interval estimates, contact FARAD at www.FARAD.org.

# Erythromycin

eh-rith-roe-mye′

**Trade and other names:** Gallimycin-100, Gallimycin-200, Erythro-100, and generic brands

**Functional classification:** Antibacterial

## Pharmacology and Mechanism of Action

Erythromycin is one of the oldest macrolide antibiotics. It is the prototype of this class and not used much clinically except for some forms used in livestock. Like other macrolides, it inhibits bacteria by binding of the 50S ribosome and inhibits bacteria protein synthesis. The spectrum of activity of erythromycin is limited primarily to gram-positive aerobic bacteria; it has little or no effect on gram-negative bacteria. The spectrum of activity also includes *Mycoplasma* spp. In cattle, it is also active against respiratory pathogens such as *Pasteurella multocida, Mannheimia haemolytica,* and *Histophilus somni* but is not used much clinically for this indication.

Erythromycin's effects on GI motility are via stimulation of motilin receptors to increase smooth muscle activity.

*Pharmacokinetics:* In dogs, the half-lives are 1.3 hours IV and 2.9 hours PO, with only 11% bioavailability. In cats, the half-life is less than 1 hour. In horses, the oral absorption is only 8%–26%, which contributes to diarrhea, and the half-life is short, necessitating frequent dose intervals.

## Indications and Clinical Uses

Erythromycin has been used in a variety of species to treat infections caused by susceptible bacteria. Infections treated include respiratory infections (pneumonia), soft tissue infections caused by gram-positive bacteria, and skin and respiratory infections. In foals, it has been used to treat *Rhodococcus equi* pneumonia, often in combination with rifampin. In some species, including horses, it has been used at low doses to stimulate intestinal motility, but demonstration of this activity has been limited in clinical patients. In horses, the dose of erythromycin to stimulate GI motility is lower than the antibacterial dose (1 mg/kg), but the clinical efficacy for this use has not been shown. In experimental calves, 8.8 mg/kg IM significantly increased rumen motility. At a dose of 10 mg/kg IM in cows undergoing surgery for left displaced abomasum, it increased rumen contractions.

The use of erythromycin has diminished because of decreased availability of some dose forms (erythromycin estolate), adverse effects in small animals (frequent vomiting), a short half-life that requires frequent dosing, and diarrhea in horses. Other macrolides have become used more often in each species. For example, azithromycin and clarithromycin are used in small animals and horses, and tilmicosin, gamithromycin, tildipirosin, and tulathromycin are used more often in cattle instead of erythromycin.

## Instructions for Use

There are several forms of erythromycin, including the ethylsuccinate and estolate esters and stearate salt for oral administration. However, the estolate form is only available as a suspension. There are no convincing data to suggest that one form is absorbed better than another, and the same dosage is applied for all. Only erythromycin gluceptate and lactate are to be administered IV (gluceptate is rarely available). A motilin-like effect to stimulate GI motility occurs at low doses and has been studied primarily in experimental horses. Erythromycin may be administered to cattle in conjunction with surgical procedures to stimulate rumen motility postsurgery.

## Precautionary Information

### Adverse Reactions and Side Effects

Diarrhea in large animals is the most common adverse effect. This is believed to be caused by a disruption of the normal bacterial intestinal flora and more common from oral administration. Nursing mares have developed diarrhea through exposure to treated foals. Hyperthermia (febrile syndrome) in association with erythromycin treatment has been observed in foals.

In small animals, the most common side effect is vomiting (probably caused by cholinergic-like effect or motilin-induced motility). In small animals, it also may cause diarrhea. In rodents and rabbits, the diarrhea caused by erythromycin can be serious and even fatal.

**Contraindications and Precautions**

Do not administer orally to rodents or rabbits. Do not administer erythromycin solutions intended for IM administration by IV injection. Only the gluceptate and lactobionate salts should be used intravenously (gluceptate is rarely available).

**Drug Interactions**

Erythromycin, like other macrolides, is known to inhibit the cytochrome P450 enzymes and may decrease the metabolism of other coadministered drugs. See Appendixes H and I.

## Patient Monitoring and Laboratory Tests

Susceptibility testing: CLSI breakpoints for sensitive organisms are ≤0.25 mcg/mL for streptococci and ≤0.5 for other organisms, using the human breakpoint. A veterinary breakpoint has not been established. Susceptibility to erythromycin tends to predict susceptibility to other macrolide antibiotics.

## Formulations

- Erythromycin is available in several forms that contain either a 250- or 500-mg erythromycin base. Oral formulations include 25- and 50-mg/mL erythromycin estolate suspension, 40-mg/mL erythromycin ethylsuccinate suspension, 400-mg ethylsuccinate tablets, and 250- and 500-mg erythromycin stearate tablets.
- IV formulations include erythromycin lactobionate, but erythromycin gluceptate is rarely available.
- Erythromycin phosphate, a feed additive available as a powder, has been administered in horses and shown to produce adequate absorption. Erythromycin phosphate is 260 mg/g, which is equivalent to 231-mg erythromycin base per gram.

## Stability and Storage

Store in a tightly sealed container, protected from light, and at room temperature. Protect from freezing. Erythromycin base is most stable at a pH of 7–7.5. In acidic solution, it may decompose. Ethylsuccinate formulations are stable for 14 days.

## Small Animal Dosage

**Dogs and Cats**

- 10–20 mg/kg q8–12h PO.
- Prokinetic effects (GI): 0.5–1 mg/kg q8–12h PO or IV.

## Large Animal Dosage

**Horses**

- *R. equi*: Erythromycin phosphate or erythromycin estolate 37.5 mg/kg q12h PO or 25 mg/kg q8h PO. Note that in horses, erythromycin base (plain tablets) are poorly absorbed, and other forms should be used. (See Instructions for Dosing regarding dosage forms.)
- Erythromycin lactobionate injection: 5 mg/kg q4–6h IV. To stimulate GI motility: 1 mg/kg.

**Cattle**
- Abscesses, pododermatitis: 2.2–8.8 mg/kg q24h IM.
- Pneumonia: 2.2–8.8 mg/kg q24h IM or 15 mg/kg q12h IM.
- Stimulate rumen motility: calves, 8.8 mg/kg IM; cows, 10 mg/kg IM.

## Regulatory Information

Cattle withdrawal times: 6 days meat (at 8.8 mg/kg). Do not use in female dairy cattle older than 20 months of age. Do not slaughter treated animals within 6 days of last treatment. To avoid excess trim, do not slaughter within 21 days of last injection. In Canada, withdrawal times are 14 days for meat and 72 hours for milk.

**E**

# Esmolol Hydrochloride
ez´moe-lole hye-droe-klor´ide

**Trade and other names:** Brevibloc

**Functional classification:** Beta blocker, antiarrhythmic

## Pharmacology and Mechanism of Action

Esmolol is a short-acting beta-adrenergic blocker. It is most selective for the beta$_1$ receptor. The difference between esmolol and other beta blockers is the short duration of action, which is attributed to metabolism by red blood cell esterases. It has a half-life of only 9–10 minutes; thus, it is impractical for long-term use.

## Indications and Clinical Uses

Esmolol is indicated for short-term control of systemic hypertension and tachyarrhythmias. It has been used for emergency therapy or short-term treatment. Long-term treatment is not possible because of the short half-life. Ordinarily, if an animal shows a positive response to esmolol, it can be switched to longer-acting beta blockers (e.g., propranolol or atenolol).

## Precautionary Information

### Adverse Reactions and Side Effects

Adverse effects related to beta$_1$-blocking effects on the heart include myocardial depression, reduced cardiac output, and bradycardia.

### Contraindications and Precautions

When administering to patients with dilated cardiomyopathy, consider the risk of negative cardiac effects. Use cautiously in patients with bronchospasm. Esmolol is contraindicated in patients with bradycardia or atrioventricular block.

### Drug Interactions

Use cautiously with digoxin, morphine, or warfarin.

## Instructions for Use

Esmolol is indicated for short-term IV therapy only. Doses are based primarily on empiricism or extrapolation of human dose. No clinical studies have been reported in animals.

## Patient Monitoring and Laboratory Tests

Monitor heart rate and rhythm during treatment.

## Formulations
- Esmolol is available in 10-mg/mL injection.

## Stability and Storage
Store in a tightly sealed container, protected from light, and at room temperature. Stability of compounded formulations has not been evaluated.

## Small Animal Dosage
### Dogs and Cats
- 0.5 mg/kg (500 mcg/kg) IV, which may be given as 0.05–0.1 mg/kg slowly every 5 minutes.
- CRI: 0.5 mg/kg slowly over a 30- to 60-second period followed by 50- to 200-mcg/kg/min infusion.

## Large Animal Dosage
### Horses
- 0.2 mg/kg over 1 minute IV. After 10 minutes, administer 0.5 mg/kg over 1 minute IV.
- CRI: 0.5 mg/kg IV followed by 25 mcg/kg/min IV.

## Regulatory Information
Withdrawal times are not reported. However, because of short duration of action and rapid metabolism, a short withdrawal period is suggested.
RCI Classification: 3

# Esomeprazole
es-oh-mep rah-zole

**Trade and other names:** Nexium

**Functional classification:** Antiulcer agent

## Pharmacology and Mechanism of Action
Esomeprazole is a proton pump inhibitor (PPI). Omeprazole exists in two chiral isomers: the S- and R-isomer. The S-isomer is biologically active; thus, esomeprazole represents the active form (S-isomer). Esomeprazole inhibits gastric acid secretion by inhibiting the $K^+/H^+$ pump (potassium pump) located on the apical membrane of the gastric parietal cell. This action inhibits secretion of $H^+$ into the stomach. Like other PPIs, it produces a longer duration of acid suppression than other antiulcer drugs (e.g., $H_2$ blockers). Other PPIs include pantoprazole (Protonix), lansoprazole (Prevacid), omeprazole, and rabeprazole (Aciphex). They all act via similar mechanism and are equally effective. PPIs also have some effect for inhibiting *Helicobacter* organisms in the stomach when administered with antibiotics.

In people, esomeprazole is metabolized more slowly than omeprazole, producing greater exposure, with less variability. Otherwise, esomeprazole is almost identical to omeprazole in clinical effects.

*Pharmacokinetics:* In dogs, the half-life is approximately 1 hour with a VD of 0.25–0.3 L/kg, and clearance of 0.24–0.4 L/kg/h. Oral absorption is 70%–80% and increases with multiple doses.

## Indications and Clinical Uses

Esomeprazole, like other PPIs, is used for treatment and prevention of GI ulcers and to decrease the esophageal irritation from gastroesophageal reflux. It has not been used in dogs, cats, or horses as often as omeprazole but is expected to be equally effective if equipotent doses are administered. In people, there is evidence that it might produce better results than omeprazole. See Omeprazole for more detailed information.

In most studies, the PPIs have more consistently produced stomach pH that is above the minimum that is associated with ulcer healing compared with other agents such as histamine $H_2$ blockers. Therefore, the PPI group of drugs is preferred over histamine $H_2$ blockers for treating and inhibiting gastric ulcers, but there is no evidence available to show that esomeprazole is more effective than other PPIs in dogs, horses, or cats. There is some evidence in experimental animals, but not confirmed in clinical studies, that it might produce more consistent acid suppression than omeprazole. In studies performed in healthy dogs, 0.5 mg/kg or 1 mg/kg q12h increased the stomach pH above 3 for 75% of the dosing interval and above pH 4 for 67% of the dose interval. These pH thresholds are often cited as the targets for therapeutic effects. In horses it may be more effective than omeprazole for treatment of ulcers in the glandular portion of the stomach (EGGD), but more work is needed before recommendations can be made.

Esomeprazole is available in an injectable formulation and may be substituted for injectable pantoprazole if necessary.

### Precautionary Information

#### Adverse Reactions and Side Effects

The use of esomeprazole has not been as common as with omeprazole. Therefore, adverse effects have not been reported in animals with esomeprazole. However, adverse effects are assumed to be similar during long-term use as for omeprazole, and readers can consult the section on omeprazole for other information.

#### Contraindications and Precautions

No contraindications have been reported for animals. There are concerns that long-term administration of PPIs in people can lead to *Clostridium*-associated diarrhea, risk of fractures, and hypomagnesemia. This has not been reported in animals. Long-term administration of PPIs in people can lead to bacterial overgrowth in the stomach and intestine, but it is not known if this is a risk in animals.

#### Drug Interactions

Although esomeprazole has not been associated with drug interactions in animals, PPIs may inhibit some drug-metabolizing enzymes (cytochrome P450 enzymes). Because of stomach acid suppression, do not administer with drugs that depend on stomach acid for absorption (e.g., ketoconazole and itraconazole).

## Instructions for Use

Omeprazole is the most common drug of this class used in animals, but esomeprazole is expected to be equally effective if equipotent doses are administered. Other PPIs include pantoprazole (Protonix), lansoprazole (Prevacid), and rabeprazole (Aciphex). Little clinical experience with these other products is reported for veterinary medicine.

## Patient Monitoring and Laboratory Tests
Esomeprazole and PPIs are generally considered safe. No routine tests for monitoring adverse effects are recommended. If gastrin concentrations are measured, a 7-day withdrawal from esomeprazole treatment should be used; otherwise, there is a significant increase in serum gastrin concentrations from esomeprazole treatment.

## Formulations
- Oral forms: Esomeprazole is available in 20- and 40-mg delayed-release capsules; 2.5-, 5-, 10-, 20-, and 40-mg powder for delayed-release suspension, and 24.65- and 49.3-mg delayed-release capsules.
- Oral packets containing granules: There are also packets available in sizes of 2.5-, 5-, 10-, 20-, 40-mg. To prepare this oral form, empty the contents of each 2.5- or 5-mg packet into a container with 5 mL of water or empty the 10-, 20-, or 40-mg packet into a container with 15 mL of water. Stir and leave for 2–3 minutes until it thickens. Then it may be administered orally. Store at room temperature.
- Injection forms: 20- and 40-mg esomeprazole sodium vials for injection. Reconstitute with 5 mL of normal saline and inject IV. For IV infusion, this may be further diluted for IV infusion (e.g., 100 mL). Fifty mL of 0.9% saline may be mixed with a 40-mg vial to produce a concentration of 0.8 mg/mL, which may be infused IV. Discard fluid bag after 5 days. Five mL of 0.9% saline may be mixed for a concentration of 8 mg/mL and injected IV. After dilution in normal saline, Ringer's solution, or 5% dextrose, the solutions are stable in fluid bags for 48 hours at room temperature or 120 hours if refrigerated.

### Stability and Storage
Esomeprazole should be maintained in the manufacturer's original formulation (capsules or suspension) for optimum stability and effectiveness. After reconstitution of the injectable solutions retain in refrigerator or room temperature.

## Small Animal Dosage
### Dogs
- 20 mg/dog q24h PO, 1–2 mg/kg q12h PO, or 0.5–1 mg/kg IV q12h.

### Cats
- 1 mg/kg q12h PO or IV.

## Large Animal Dosage
### Horses
- Treat ulcers: 4 mg/kg once daily for 4 weeks PO. (But doses as low as 2 mg/kg might be equally effective.)
- Prevent ulcers: 1–2 mg/kg q24h PO.
- Treatment of ulcers: Loading dose of 1 mg/kg PO followed by 0.5 mg/kg/day for 14–28 days.

## Regulatory Information
Not intended for administration to animals that produce food. Oral absorption in ruminants is not established. Withdrawal times are not established for animals that produce food. For extralabel use withdrawal interval estimates, contact FARAD at www.FARAD.org.
RCI Classification: 5

# Estradiol Cypionate
ess-trah-dye´ole sip´ee-oh-nate
**Trade and other names:** ECP, Depo-Estradiol, and generic brands
**Functional classification:** Hormone

## Pharmacology and Mechanism of Action
Estradiol is a semisynthetic estrogen compound. Its effects mimic those of estrogen in animals. Estradiol is used for estrogen replacement in animals. It also has been used to induce abortion in animals.

## Indications and Clinical Uses
The most common use in small animals has been to terminate pregnancy. The estradiol cypionate formulation was highly effective to terminate pregnancy (95%) but was associated with serious adverse effects and is no longer recommended. Estradiol cypionate is longer acting and more potent than other estrogen formulations. Estradiol valerate injection (20 mg/mL) is also available for human medicine to treat hypoestrogenism.

## Precautionary Information
### Adverse Reactions and Side Effects
Estradiol has a high risk of causing endometrial hyperplasia and pyometra. There is a dose-dependent risk of bone marrow toxicity in animals, particularly in dogs. Estradiol cypionate injections have produced leukopenia, thrombocytopenia, and fatal aplastic anemia. Because stem cells can be affected, the bone marrow toxicity may not be reversible. These adverse effects can be severe, and other agents should be used instead of estradiol cypionate if possible.

### Contraindications and Precautions
Estradiol is contraindicated in pregnancy unless used to terminate pregnancy. Do not administer to ferrets. Do not administer to animals unless careful monitoring of complete blood count (CBC) is possible.

### Drug Interactions
No drug interactions are reported for animals. It should not be used with other drugs that may suppress the bone marrow. In people, it has been recommended that these estrogen compounds should not be used with other drugs that may cause hepatotoxicity. Estradiol may increase cyclosporine concentrations.

## Instructions for Use
To terminate pregnancy, 22 mcg/kg is administered once IM during days 3–5 of estrus or within 3 days of mating. However, in one study, a dose of 44 mcg/kg was more efficacious than a dose of 22 mcg/kg when given during estrus or diestrus.

## Patient Monitoring and Laboratory Tests
Monitor CBC for evidence of bone marrow suppression.

## Formulations
- Estradiol is available in a 2-mg/mL injection. Estradiol valerate is available as a 20-mg/mL injection in 5-mL vials.

## Stability and Storage

Store in a tightly sealed container, protected from light, and at room temperature. Stability of compounded formulations has not been evaluated.

## Small Animal Dosage

**Dogs**
- 22–44 mcg/kg IM (total dose not to exceed 1 mg).

**Cats**
- 250 mcg/cat IM, between 40 hours and 5 days of mating.

## Large Animal Dosage
- No large animal doses have been reported.

## Regulatory Information

Do not use in food-producing animals.

---

# Estriol
ess-tree-ole

**Trade and other names:** Incurin and Theelol (previously called Oestriol)
**Functional classification:** Hormone

## Pharmacology and Mechanism of Action

Estriol is a natural estrogen hormone. It differs from diethylstilbestrol (DES) and other estrogens because it is naturally occurring and occupies the receptor for a shorter duration compared with synthetic compounds such as estradiol and DES. When used to treat urinary incontinence, its effects are believed to be caused by increasing sensitivity of alpha-adrenergic receptors in urinary smooth muscle.

## Indications and Clinical Uses

Estriol is an estrogen replacement. In small animals, it has most often been used to treat urinary incontinence that is associated with estrogen deficiency in female dogs. This problem is most common in dogs that have undergone ovariohysterectomy. An advantage of estriol is that one tablet can be used to treat all sizes of dogs, and if they respond to initial dosing, the frequency of administration can be tapered to the lowest effective level. Another approved drug for treating urinary incontinence in dogs is phenylpropanolamine (PPA) (see Phenylpropanolamine). It may be used instead of or concurrently with estriol.

## Precautionary Information

### Adverse Reactions and Side Effects

In field studies, the most common adverse effects were loss of appetite, vomiting, excessive water drinking, and swollen vulva. Estriol has not been associated with pyometra or bone marrow suppression compared with estradiol.

### Contraindications and Precautions

Estriol is contraindicated in pregnancy. Do not administer to ferrets.

### Drug Interactions

No drug interactions are reported for animals. It should not be used with other drugs that may suppress the bone marrow. In people, it has been recommended that these estrogen compounds not be used with other drugs that may cause hepatotoxicity, but such an interaction has not been shown in dogs for estriol.

## Instructions for Use

To treat urinary incontinence, it has been used in combination with PPA; however, the addition of PPA to the treatment regimen may not improve efficacy compared to estrogen drugs used alone.

## Patient Monitoring and Laboratory Tests

Monitor CBC for evidence of bone marrow suppression.

## Formulations

• Estriol is available as a 1-mg tablet.

## Stability and Storage

Store in a tightly sealed container, protected from light, and at room temperature. Stability of compounded formulations has not been evaluated.

## Small Animal Dosage

### Dogs

• 2 mg per dog PO q24h (may be combined with PPA). After starting with 2 mg per dog per day, after 1 week, reduce dose to 1.5 mg per dog per day for 1 week, then 1 mg per dog per day for 1 week, and a gradually tapered regimen and increased interval (every other day, every third day, and so on) until a goal of 0.5 mg per dog once per week is achieved.

### Cats

• No dose has been established.

## Large Animal Dosage

• No large animal doses have been reported.

## Regulatory Information

Do not use in food-producing animals.

# Etidronate Disodium

eh-tih-droe′nate dye-soe′dee-um

**Trade and other names:** Didronel

**Functional classification:** Antihypercalcemic agent

## Pharmacology and Mechanism of Action

Etidronate disodium is a bisphosphonate drug and used to treat bone disorders. This group of drugs is characterized by a germinal bisphosphonate bond. They slow the formation and dissolution of hydroxyapatite crystals. Their clinical use resides in their ability to inhibit bone resorption. These drugs decrease bone turnover by inhibiting osteoclast activity and retard bone resorption and decrease the rate of osteoporosis. Other drugs in this class used in animals are alendronate, zoledronate (Zometa), pamidronate, clodronate (Osphos), and tiludronate (Tildren).

## Indications and Clinical Uses

The bisphosphonate group of drugs, which includes etidronate, is used primarily in people to treat osteoporosis and hypercalcemia of malignancy. In animals, they are used to decrease calcium in conditions that cause hypercalcemia, such as cancer and vitamin D toxicosis. Studies in people have shown that bisphosphonates may have action in cancer-induced bone disease that is more significant than the effect on osteolysis and bone resorption and may decrease the tumor burden. In dogs, more experimental work has been performed with pamidronate than other drugs in this group. Some bisphosphonates have been used to treat navicular disease and bone spavin in horses. There are two bisphosphonates approved for treating horses, which are used more often than other bisphosphonates. These drugs for horses include clodronate (Osphos) and tiludronate (Tildren) (see Tiludronate and Clodronate).

## Precautionary Information

### Adverse Reactions and Side Effects

Adverse effects are not reported for animals, but use has been uncommon and not sufficient to record a full range of possible adverse effects. In people, GI problems are common. Esophageal lesions have occurred because of reaction from contact with mucosa. If used in animals, ensure that tablets are completely swallowed.

### Contraindications and Precautions

No contraindications have been identified in animals. There are concerns about the use of these agents in young horses. Consult the sections on clodronate (Osphos) and tiludronate (Tildren) for more information.

### Drug Interactions

No drug interactions have been reported in animals. If mixed with other solutions or drugs, avoid mixtures containing calcium.

## Instructions for Use

At high doses, etidronate may inhibit mineralization of bone. In people, alendronate has replaced etidronate because of side effects. There are no clinical studies demonstrating efficacy of etidronate in animals; the use is extrapolated from human medicine and anecdotal experience.

## Patient Monitoring and Laboratory Tests

Monitor serum calcium and phosphorus. Monitor urea nitrogen, creatinine, and urine-specific gravity in treated animals and food intake.

## Formulations

- Etidronate is available in 200- and 400-mg tablets.

## Stability and Storage

Store in a tightly sealed container, protected from light, and at room temperature. Stability of compounded formulations has not been evaluated.

## Small Animal Dosage

### Dogs

- 5 mg/kg/day PO.

### Cats

- 10 mg/kg/day PO.

## Large Animal Dosage

- No large animal doses have been reported.

## Regulatory Information

Withdrawal times are not established; 24-hour withdrawal times are suggested because this drug has little risk from residues.

# Etodolac

ee-toe´doe-lak

**Trade and other names:** EtoGesic (veterinary preparation) and Lodine (human preparation)

**Functional classification:** Nonsteroidal anti-inflammatory drug

**Note:** This drug is no longer on the market for veterinary use. It has been replaced by other NSAIDs. A description is included here because some human forms may still be available.

**E**

## Pharmacology and Mechanism of Action

Etodolac is in the class of NSAIDs. Like other NSAIDs, etodolac has analgesic and anti-inflammatory effects by inhibiting the synthesis of prostaglandins. The enzyme inhibited by NSAIDs is the cyclo-oxygenase (COX) enzyme. The COX enzyme exists in two isoforms: COX-1 and COX-2. COX-1 is primarily responsible for synthesis of prostaglandins important for maintaining a healthy GI tract, renal function, platelet function, and other normal functions. COX-2 is induced and responsible for synthesizing prostaglandins that are important mediators of pain, inflammation, and fever. However, it is understood that there is some crossover of COX-1 and COX-2 effects in some situations, and COX-2 activity is important for some biological effects.

*Pharmacokinetics:* In dogs, etodolac has a half-life of 7.6–14 hours, depending on the study and feeding conditions. In dogs, it shows either little preference for COX-2 or COX-1 (nonselective) or slight COX-2 selectivity in vitro. It is not known if selectivity for COX-2 affects efficacy or risk of adverse effects. In horses, etodolac is relatively COX-2 selective and is more potent than in dogs. The half-life in horses is only 3 hours, and a duration of effect of approximately 24 hours has been observed in horses with lameness.

## Indications and Clinical Uses

Etodolac is indicated for treatment of osteoarthritis in dogs. It also is used as an analgesic and may be used for other painful conditions. Like other NSAIDs, etodolac is expected to reduce fever. Uses in cats have not been established. Etodolac has been used in some horses to relieve pain associated with abdominal surgery and to treat lameness (e.g., caused by navicular disease). Dose regimens are different for horses compared with other animals.

## Precautionary Information

### Adverse Reactions and Side Effects

Nonsteroidal anti-inflammatory drugs may cause GI ulceration. Other adverse effects caused by NSAIDs include decreased platelet function and kidney injury. In clinical trials with etodolac at recommended doses, some dogs showed weight loss, loose stools, or diarrhea. At high doses (above label dose), etodolac caused GI ulceration in dogs. Etodolac has been associated with keratoconjunctivitis sicca (KCS) in dogs, which in some cases has been severe. Resolution of KCS has occurred in only 10%–15% of cases after discontinuing medication. Improvement in KCS was greater if treatment duration was short. In horses, at high doses, GI toxicity has been observed.

### Contraindications and Precautions

Do not administer to animals prone to GI ulcers. Do not administer with other ulcerogenic drugs, such as corticosteroids. Do not administer to dogs that may be prone to developing KCS. Do not administer to animals with compromised renal function.

**Drug Interactions**
Use NSAIDs cautiously with other drugs known to cause GI injury (e.g., corticosteroids). The efficacy of ACE inhibitors and diuretics (furosemide) may be diminished when administered concurrently with NSAIDs. Etodolac may cross-react with sulfonamides in sensitive animals.

## Instructions for Use

Administer as directed and avoid concurrent use of other medications that may increase GI toxicity. Most of the use in dogs has been associated with treatment of osteoarthritis. In horses, it has been shown experimentally to improve lameness associated with navicular disease. When used in horses for this purpose, it was given at 23 mg/kg PO once or twice daily for 3 days. Treated horses improved with either regimen and showed no signs of adverse effects. Experimental horses treated with 20 or 23 mg/kg did not demonstrate adverse effects, but long-term safety has not been reported.

## Patient Monitoring and Laboratory Tests

Monitor for signs of GI ulcers and bleeding. Monitor tear production periodically in dogs treated with etodolac and observe for ocular signs of KCS. Monitor liver enzymes in dogs treated with NSAIDs periodically for signs of liver toxicosis. Monitor urea nitrogen and creatinine in treated animals for signs of kidney injury. Etodolac has had varying effects on tetraiodothyronine ($T_4$), free $T_4$, and thyroid-stimulating hormone concentrations in dogs. One study showed no effect, and another study showed a decrease in $T_4$ and free $T_4$ in treated dogs after 2 weeks.

## Formulations

Etodolac is available in 150- and 300-mg tablets. Injectable 100 mg/mL. Human formulations include a 400-mg tablet and 200- and 300-mg capsules. Some formulations are no longer marketed in veterinary medicine.

## Stability and Storage

Store in a tightly sealed container, protected from light, and at room temperature. Etodolac is insoluble in water but is soluble in alcohol or propylene glycol.

## Small Animal Dosage

**Dogs**
- 10–15 mg/kg once daily PO or 10–15 mg/kg injection SQ as a single dorsoscapular injection.

**Cats**
- Dose not established.

## Large Animal Dosage

**Horses**
- 23 mg/kg q24h PO. Long-term safety with this regimen has not been established (see Instructions for Dosing).

## Regulatory Information

No withdrawal times have been established. For extralabel use withdrawal interval estimates, contact FARAD at www.FARAD.org.
RCI Classification: 4

# Famciclovir
fam-sye′kloe-veer

**Trade and other names:** Famvir

**Functional classification:** Antiviral

## Pharmacology and Mechanism of Action
Famciclovir is an antiviral drug used in people most often for treating infections caused by the herpes virus. Famciclovir is a synthetic purine analogue (acyclic nucleoside analogue). It is the diacetyl 6-deoxy derivative of penciclovir and converted to the antiviral drug penciclovir via di-deacetylation and oxidation. The conversion of famciclovir to penciclovir may be inefficient in cats, and oral absorption to the active drug is approximately 10% in cats and can be variable. After conversion in cats, penciclovir has a half-life of approximately 3.6–4.7 hours.

Penciclovir has antiviral activity against herpes virus types 1 (HSV1) and 2 (HSV2). The action is related to the affinity for the enzyme thymidine kinase, which converts penciclovir into penciclovir triphosphate, which inhibits viral DNA polymerase to prevent DNA chain elongation, thus inhibiting viral DNA chain elongation. It is considered virustatic. It is used for treatment of various forms of herpes virus infection in humans and also has been used for treatment of viral infections in animals, particularly feline herpes virus 1 (FHV1). FHV1 is resistant to acyclovir and valacyclovir; therefore, famciclovir (penciclovir) is the most promising oral drug to treat cats with FHV1 infection.

## Indications and Clinical Uses
The most common use of famciclovir in veterinary medicine is to treat FHV1 associated with conjunctivitis, rhinosinusitis, keratitis, and FHV1-associated dermatitis. Famciclovir has been effective in cats with experimentally induced or spontaneous herpetic disease.

*Optimum doses for cats:* Early studies with oral administration of famciclovir at 62.5 mg per cat failed to produce high enough blood concentrations of penciclovir to be consistently effective. Most experts recommend dosages of 90 mg/kg PO q8–12h. The most consistent positive results have been from 90 mg/kg q8h. Most of these recommendations are derived from small observational studies. There has been conflicting results in shelter cats. In one study, a single dose of 125 or 500 mg to cats (16–52 or 92–227 mg/kg, respectively) at the time of shelter entry did not reduce shedding of FHV1 DNA or clinical disease scores compared with placebo. In another study, a dose of 30 or 90 mg/kg for 1 week did not reduce clinical signs of upper respiratory disease but reduced FHV1 shedding. In other studies, there were improvements in conjunctivitis, decreased conjunctival inflammation, decreased ocular discomfort, and decreased tearing. When treating cats with conjunctivitis or upper respiratory disease, a tetracycline (minocycline or doxycycline) may be administered concurrently.

## Precautionary Information
### Adverse Reactions and Side Effects
Adverse effects observed from famciclovir in cats include mild anemia. Mild increase in white blood cells may be seen. No adverse effects were identified in limited studies performed in cats.

**Contraindications and Precautions**
Reduce dose in animals with compromised renal function. Safety in pregnant cats has not been studied.

**Drug Interactions**
No interactions identified.

## Instructions for Use
The dose listed for cats is based on limited studies in which 62.5 mg per cat was studied initially, but later evidence suggested that a more effective dosage is at least 125 mg per cat (or higher) q8–12h PO. Duration of treatment is undetermined, but generally 2 weeks may be needed.

## Patient Monitoring and Laboratory Tests
Monitor blood urea nitrogen (BUN) and creatinine during use.

## Formulations
- Famciclovir is available in 125-, 250-, and 500-mg tablets. It has been compounded into smaller tablets for kittens. A compounded oral suspension may be made by mixing 20 of the 500 mg famciclovir tablets (10 g), with 100 mL of a 1:1 mixture of Ora-Plus and Ora-Sweet. The final oral suspension is 100 mg/mL and is stable for 90 days if stored in a refrigerator. Label to indicate that it should be well shaken before use. Other compounded formulations for animals have not shown consistent quality or strength.

## Stability and Storage
Store tablets and capsules in tightly sealed container, protected from light, and at room temperature.

## Small Animal Dosage
### Cats
- Treatment of feline herpes virus: The preferred dose is 90 mg/kg q12h, and some experts recommend q8h. Higher doses of 500 mg per cat (92–227 mg/kg) also have been used. Lower dosages should be used in kittens (30–50 mg/kg q12h PO).

## Large Animal Dosage
### Horses
- No doses have been established.

## Regulatory Information
Because of mutagenicity, it should not be administered to animals intended for food.

# Famotidine
fah-moe′tih-deen

**Trade and other names:** Pepcid and generic

**Functional classification:** Antiulcer agent

## Pharmacology and Mechanism of Action
Histamine$_2$ antagonist (H$_2$ blocker). Stimulation of acid secretion in the stomach requires activation of histamine type 2 receptors (H$_2$ receptor), gastrin receptors, and muscarinic

receptors. Famotidine and other $H_2$ blockers inhibit the action of histamine on the histamine $H_2$ receptor of parietal cells and inhibit gastric parietal cell gastric acid secretion. Famotidine increases stomach pH to help heal and prevent gastric and duodenal ulcers.

## Indications and Clinical Uses

Famotidine, like other $H_2$-receptor blockers, is used to treat ulcers and gastritis in a variety of animals. Although it is often used for animals with vomiting, there are no efficacy data to indicate that it is effective as an antiemetic. There are no efficacy data to support its use for preventing nonsteroidal anti-inflammatory drug (NSAID)–induced bleeding and ulcers. Famotidine has been used by veterinarians as a preferred $H_2$ blocker, but there is a lack of evidence to demonstrate superiority over other drugs in this class. Some studies have demonstrated efficacy at 1 mg/kg in dogs, while other studies have not demonstrated differences between famotidine and a placebo in dogs for increasing stomach pH. The target goal for stomach pH is greater than 3 for 75% of the dose interval or a pH greater than 4 for 67% of the dose interval. With oral doses, famotidine often does not meet these targets. Most evidence supports a lack of efficacy in dogs at a dosage of 1 mg/kg administered q12h, but it is more effective if administered as a constant-rate infusion (CRI) (1 mg/kg IV loading dose followed by 8-mg/kg/day infusion). In dogs, it may have short-term effects on acid suppression, but it had a diminished effect if administered for more than 12 days. It had less effect to maintain the stomach pH above 3 on day 1 of dosing compared with day 12. Therefore, if used, famotidine may be better for short-term use than long-term administration.

The use in large animals has received little attention. Omeprazole is preferred in horses for stomach acid suppression. In cattle, the half-life of famotidine is short and requires frequent administration (e.g., q6h) for effectiveness.

Proton pump inhibitors (PPIs) such as omeprazole, esomeprazole, and others are more effective for consistently suppressing stomach acid secretion and are preferred over histamine $H_2$ antagonists for dogs, horses, and cats.

## Precautionary Information

### Adverse Reactions and Side Effects

Adverse effects usually are seen only with decreased renal clearance. In people, central nervous system (CNS) signs may occur with high doses. The IV solution contains benzyl alcohol, aspartic acid, and mannitol. Give IV injections slowly to cats (over 5 minutes) because rapid IV injections may cause hemolysis.

### Contraindications and Precautions

Intravenous solutions contain benzyl alcohol. IV injections to small animals, especially cats, should be done slowly.

### Drug Interactions

Famotidine and other $H_2$-receptor blockers block secretion of stomach acid. Therefore, they interfere with oral absorption of drugs dependent on acidity, such as ketoconazole, itraconazole, and iron supplements. Unlike cimetidine, famotidine is not associated with inhibition of microsomal P450 enzymes.

## Instructions for Use

Administer with food for best absorption. Clinical studies for famotidine have not been performed; therefore, optimal doses for ulcer prevention and healing are not known. Dose recommendations are extrapolated from human use, studies in experimental animals, or from anecdotal experience. Experimental studies in dogs have shown that doses of 0.1–0.2 mg/kg may inhibit stomach acid secretion, but most other studies have shown that higher doses of 1.0 mg/kg are needed to suppress stomach acid. Even at this dose, it has not been effective for reaching therapeutic targets in dogs but is more effective if administered as a CRI. For IV use, dilute with IV solutions (e.g., 0.9% saline) to a total volume of 5–10 mL.

## Patient Monitoring and Laboratory Tests
No specific monitoring is necessary.

## Formulations
- Famotidine is available in 20- and 40-mg tablets, 8-mg/mL oral suspension, and 10-mg/mL injection.

## Stability and Storage
Store in a tightly sealed container, protected from light, and at room temperature. Famotidine is soluble in water. Compounded formulations in cherry syrup have been stable for 14 days. Diluted IV solutions in saline are stable for 48 hours at room temperature.

## Small Animal Dosage
### Dogs
- 0.5 mg/kg q12h PO, IV, SQ, or IM. A dosage of 40 mg/dog q12h has been used empirically. Higher dosages of 1 mg/kg q12h have been recommended for more reliable suppression of stomach acid.
- CRI: 1 mg/kg IV loading dose followed by 8 mg/kg/day CRI.

### Cats
- 0.2 mg/kg q24h, up to 0.25 mg/kg q12h IM, SQ, PO, or IV (slowly over 5 minutes).

## Large Animal Dosage

### Horses
- 1–2 mg/kg q6–8h PO or 0.2–0.4 mg/kg IV q6h.

### Cattle
- 0.4 mg/kg IV q6h.

## Regulatory Information
No restrictions on use in animals not intended for food.
Racing Commissioners International (RCI) Classification: 5

# Febantel
feh-ban'tel

**Trade and other names:** Rintal and Vercom. Drontal Plus also contains two other drugs.

**Functional classification:** Antiparasitic

## Pharmacology and Mechanism of Action
Febantel is an antiparasitic that interferes with carbohydrate metabolism in parasitic worms. It suppresses mitochondrial reactions via inhibition of fumarate reductase and interferes with glucose transport. It is metabolized to a benzimidazole compound that binds to structural protein tubulin and prevents polymerization to

microtubules, which results in incomplete digestion and absorption of nutrients by the parasite.

## Indications and Clinical Uses

Febantel is indicated in the control and treatment of larvae and adult stages of intestinal nematodes. In horses, it is used for removal of large strongyles (*Strongylus vulgaris, Strongylus edentatus, Strongylus equinus*), ascarids *(Parascaris equorum,* sexually mature and immature), pinworms (*Oxyuris equi,* adult and fourth-stage larvae), and the various small strongyles.

In dogs and cats, it is used for treatment of hookworms (*Ancylostoma caninum* and *Uncinaria stenocephala*), ascarids (*Toxocara canis* and *Toxascaris leonina*), and whipworms (*Trichuris vulpis*). In dogs, it is used in combination with praziquantel for treatment of hookworms (*A. caninum* and *U. stenocephala*), whipworms (*T. vulpis*), ascarids (*T. canis* and *T. leonina*), and tapeworms (*Dipylidium caninum* and *Taenia pisiformis*).

A formulation of febantel, pyrantel, and praziquantel (Drontal Plus) has been used in cats for treatment of *Giardia* spp., roundworms, hookworms, and whipworms. In cats, it is also used in combination with praziquantel for removal of hookworms (*A. tubaeforme*), ascarids (*Toxocara cati*), and tapeworms (*D. caninum* and *Taenia taeniaeformis*).

---

### Precautionary Information

**Adverse Reactions and Side Effects**

Ordinarily, adverse effects have been rare. Vomiting and diarrhea may occur after dosing.

**Contraindications and Precautions**

Do not use in pregnant animals. Do not use in animals with liver or kidney dysfunction.

**Drug Interactions**

No drug interactions have been reported.

---

## Instructions for Use

For horses, the paste may be administered on the base of the tongue or added to a portion of the normal grain ration. For most effective results, retreat in 6–8 weeks. Febantel suspension may be used in combination with trichlorfon oral liquid when combining 1 part febantel suspension with 5 parts trichlorfon liquid.

## Patient Monitoring and Laboratory Tests

No specific monitoring is necessary.

## Formulations

- Febantel is available in an equine paste: 45.5% febantel (455 mg/mL), suspension: 9.3% febantel (2.75 g/ounce), and 27.2- and 163.3-mg tablets.
- Febantel is also available in combinations; each gram of paste contains 34 mg of febantel and 3.4 mg of praziquantel.
- Chewable tablets are available for small animals in three sizes containing febantel, pyrantel pamoate, and praziquantel in the following sizes: 22.7 mg praziquantel, 22.7 mg pyrantel, and 113.4 mg febantel; 68.0 mg praziquantel, 68.0 mg pyrantel, and 340.2 mg febantel; and 136.0 mg praziquantel, 136.0 mg pyrantel, and 680.4 mg febantel.

## Stability and Storage
Store in a tightly sealed container, protected from light, and at room temperature.

## Small Animal Dosage
**Dogs**
- 10 mg/kg febantel alone or in combination with 1 mg/kg praziquantel PO with food once daily for 3 days.
- Puppies: 15 mg/kg febantel alone or in combination with 1.5 mg/kg praziquantel PO with food once daily for 3 days.
- For treatment of *Giardia* infection, it has been combined with pyrantel (27–35 mg/kg febantel + 27–35 mg/kg pyrantel) q24h PO for 3 days.

**Cats**
- 10 mg/kg febantel alone or in combination with 1 mg/kg praziquantel PO in the food once daily for 3 days.
- Kittens: 15 mg/kg febantel alone or in combination with 1.5 mg/kg praziquantel.

## Large Animal Dosage
**Cattle**
- 7.5 mL/100 kg body weight PO.

**Sheep and Goats**
- 1 mL/20 kg body weight or 5 mL/25 kg PO.

**Horses**
- 6 mg/kg PO.

## Regulatory Information
Not for use in horses intended for food. No other regulatory restrictions are listed. If administered to food producing animals, consult Food Animal Residue Avoidance Databank (FARAD) for withdrawal time recommendations (www.FARAD.org).

# Felbamate
fel′bah-mate

**Trade and other names:** Felbatol and generic

**Functional classification:** Anticonvulsant

## Pharmacology and Mechanism of Action
Felbamate is an anticonvulsant, used infrequently in animals. The action to treat seizures in animals may be via antagonism at the N-methyl-D-aspartate (NMDA) receptor and block effects of excitatory amino acids.

*Pharmacokinetics:* There has not been much work performed on pharmacokinetics in animals. The half-life in dogs is 5–6 hours, which may require more frequent administration compared with use in people.

## Indications and Clinical Uses
Felbamate is used to treat epilepsy in dogs when they are refractory to other anticonvulsants. Other drugs are typically used first before attempting to add felbamate. It has been used in conjunction with other anticonvulsants. However, the use in animals has declined because of the availability of other drugs to treat refractory seizures, such as levetiracetam, zonisamide, gabapentin, and pregabalin.

## Precautionary Information
### Adverse Reactions and Side Effects
In dogs, it has increased risk of liver injury. It also may cause tremors, salivation, restlessness, and agitation (usually at the high doses). Keratoconjunctivitis sicca also has been reported in dogs. Some blood abnormalities, such as neutropenia lymphopenia and thrombocytopenia, have been reported. In people, the most severe reactions have been hepatotoxicity and aplastic anemia.

### Contraindications and Precautions
It may increase phenobarbital concentrations. It may be more likely to cause liver injury when used with phenobarbital.

### Drug Interactions
Possible interactions exist with drugs that either alter or are substrates for hepatic cytochrome P450 enzymes. (See Appendixes H and I.) It may increase phenobarbital concentrations if used concurrently.

## Instructions for Use
Dosing has been empirically in dogs. The use in dogs is based on small observational studies. There are no controlled studies to document efficacy, but it is usually administered when animals have been refractory to other drugs, such as phenobarbital or bromide.

## Patient Monitoring and Laboratory Tests
Monitoring of plasma concentrations is helpful to assess therapy. Assays may be available in some commercial laboratories. Ideal plasma concentrations have not been established for animals. However, concentrations in humans of 24–137 mcg/mL in plasma have been effective (mean, 78 mcg/mL). Monitor complete blood count (CBC) and chemistry panels periodically (e.g., every 6 months).

## Formulations
- Felbamate is available in 120-mg/mL oral suspension and 400- and 600-mg tablets.

## Stability and Storage
Store in a tightly sealed container, protected from light, and at room temperature. Stability of compounded formulations has not been evaluated.

## Small Animal Dosage
### Dogs
- Start with 15–20 mg/kg q8h PO; increase as needed to control seizures. Maximum dosage is approximately 70 mg/kg q8h PO.
- Small dogs: 200 mg/dog q8h PO; increase to a maximum dosage of 600 mg/dog q8h.
- Large dogs: 400 mg/dog q8h. Increase dose gradually by 200-mg (15-mg/kg) increments until seizure control. Maximum dosage for large dogs is 1200 mg/dog q8h.

## Large Animal Dosage
- No large animal doses have been reported.

## Regulatory Information
No withdrawal times have been established. For extralabel use withdrawal interval estimates, contact FARAD at www.FARAD.org.
RCI Classification: 3

# Fenbendazole
fen-ben′dah-zole

**Trade and other names:** Panacur and Safe-Guard

**Functional classification:** Antiparasitic

## Pharmacology and Mechanism of Action
Fenbendazole is a benzimidazole antiparasitic drug. Like other benzimidazoles, fenbendazole produces a degeneration of the parasite microtubule and irreversibly blocks glucose uptake in parasites. Inhibition of glucose uptake causes depletion of energy stores in the parasite, eventually resulting in death. Mammals are spared from adverse effects because there is no effect on glucose metabolism in mammals.

## Indications and Clinical Uses
Fenbendazole is effective for treatment of numerous helminth intestinal parasites in animals, including *Toxocara, Toxascaris, Ancylostoma,* and *Trichuris* spp. In dogs, it is effective for most intestinal helminth parasites and against nematodes. In dogs, it also has been used for pulmonary helminths (lungworms), but a longer duration of treatment is needed. Fenbendazole has been effective for treatment of *Giardia* infection, but higher doses are needed and there may be failure rates as high as 50%. It is effective in cats for treatment of lungworms, flukes, and a variety of helminth parasites. In horses, it is used for the control of large strongyles, small strongyles, pinworms, and ascarids. In pigs, it is effective for lungworms, large roundworms, nodular worms, small stomach worms, and kidney worms. In beef and dairy cattle, it is effective for control of lungworms, stomach worms, barberpole worms, stomach worms,  and various intestinal worms.

## Precautionary Information
### Adverse Reactions and Side Effects
Fenbendazole has a good safety margin, but vomiting and diarrhea have been reported. When evaluated at doses of three and five times the recommended dose at three times the recommended duration, fenbendazole was well tolerated, and no adverse effects were reported in the target species. It has been safe to use during pregnancy. There have been reports of pancytopenia associated with fenbendazole administration, but these are rare.

### Contraindications and Precautions
No known contraindications. It may be used in all ages of animals.

### Drug Interactions
There are no known drug interactions.

## Instructions for Use
Dose recommendations are based on clinical studies by the manufacturer. Granules may be mixed with food. Paste may be given to horses and cattle. Presence of food does not affect oral absorption. In studies for treatment of *Giardia* infection, it was safer than other treatments but less effective.

## Patient Monitoring and Laboratory Tests
Fecal monitoring may be performed to determine the efficacy of treatment for intestinal parasites.

## Formulations

- Fenbendazole is available in 22.2% (222 mg/g) (Panacur) granules, 10% oral paste (92 g/32 oz), and 100-mg/mL oral suspension. Some formulations (e.g., Panacur Plus) may contain other ingredients such as ivermectin and praziquantel.

## Stability and Storage

Store in a tightly sealed container, protected from light, and at room temperature. Stability of compounded formulations has not been evaluated.

## Small Animal Dosage

**Dogs**

- 50 mg/kg/day for 3 days PO. Duration may be extended to 5 days for severe parasitic infestations. For pulmonary helminths (lungworms) in dogs, increase the duration of this dosage to 10–14 days.
- *Giardia* treatment: 50 mg/kg q24h for 3–5 days.

**Cats**

- 50 mg/kg/day for 3 days PO.
- Duration may be extended to 5 days for severe parasitic infestations.

## Large Animal Dosage

**Horses**

- Intestinal parasites, such as strongyles, pinworms, and ascarids: Panacur granules or paste is administered at a dose of 5.1 mg/kg (2.3 mg/lb) PO. Two packets of 1.15 g each will treat a 450-kg (1000-lb) horse. Panacur paste can be administered to horses at a dose of 5 mg/kg PO. Retreatment at 6–8 weeks may be necessary. For treatment of ascarids (*Parascaris equorum*) in horses, a higher dose of 10 mg/kg is recommended.

**Sheep and Goats**

- 5 mg/kg PO.

**Cattle**

- 5 mg/kg PO or 5 mg/kg/day provided in feed for 3–6 days.

## Regulatory Information

Cattle withdrawal time (meat): 8 days. There is no withdrawal period for milk. Goat withdrawal time: 6 days meat; 0 days milk. For additional withdrawal time information, contact FARAD at www.FARAD.org.

# Fenoldopam Mesylate
fe-nol'doe-pam

**Trade and other names:** Corlopam

**Functional classification:** Vasodilator

## Pharmacology and Mechanism of Action

Fenoldopam is a dopamine agonist. It is specific for the dopamine $D_1$ receptors, without effects on alpha- or beta-adrenergic receptors, and therefore has been used to produce smooth muscle relaxation and vasodilation in vascular beds that have $D_1$ receptors (peripheral arteries and kidneys). It has no activity on $D_2$ receptors and only a small effect on alpha-adrenergic receptors. Because of this activity, fenoldopam has more specificity than dopamine, which has been used for similar indications. The most common use of fenoldopam is for increasing renal perfusion to treat acute renal failure.

*Pharmacokinetics:* The half-life in animals is very short (1–7 minutes in dogs), with very high clearance (60 mL/min/h); therefore, it is usually administered via CRI.

## Indications and Clinical Uses

The use of fenoldopam in veterinary medicine is limited to a few research studies (primarily in cats and dogs), small observational studies, and some anecdotal evidence of efficacy for treating acute kidney injury (AKI). In healthy dogs at a dose of 0.8 mcg/kg/min (CRI), it produced a significant increase in glomerular filtration rate, and renal plasma flow without inducing hypotension. This effect likely is produced through its action as a renal vasodilator and improvement in renal plasma flow. Despite this effect in healthy animals, at this time, there is insufficient evidence to recommend for routine treatment in patients with kidney failure as there has been no demonstrated difference in survival associated with treatment. In people, fenoldopam has replaced dopamine as a treatment of AKI. It is also used in people to treat severe hypertension, to prevent renal ischemia, and to increase gastrointestinal (GI) perfusion, as well as being a treatment for AKI. The use is limited to short-term in-hospital use when rapid treatment of hypertension is needed. These indications in people have not been fully explored for use in animals.

## Precautionary Information

### Adverse Reactions and Side Effects

It has been generally safe and well-tolerated in dogs and cats, but these studies were in healthy animals. The most common side effect is hypotension. The half-life of fenoldopam is short; therefore, if hypotension is observed, decrease the infusion rate. Other adverse effects described for small animals include reflex tachycardia and mild hypokalemia. Rarely, it has caused facial twitching and hypersalivation in cats. In people, adverse effects can include increased intraocular pressure (risk in glaucoma), low potassium, and tachycardia.

### Contraindications and Precautions

No known contraindications.

### Drug Interactions

Use cautiously with other vasodilators; excessive hypotension can occur. Do not use with beta blockers.

## Instructions for Use

Administer by CRI. There is no need to administer bolus doses because the onset of effects should occur within 15 minutes of starting the CRI. Dose recommendations are based on some limited research studies and anecdotal clinical experience from veterinarians. There have been no well-controlled studies of efficacy in animals, and the use is largely extrapolated from human recommendations. It is recommended that the solution be added to fluids (e.g., 5% dextrose) to make a 40-mcg/mL solution for infusion. For example, add 1 mL (10 mg) to 250 mL.

## Patient Monitoring and Laboratory Tests

Monitor patient's heart rate and blood pressure during treatment.

## Formulations

• Fenoldopam is available as a 10-mg/mL injection. The pH range is 2.8–3.8.

## Stability and Storage

Fenoldopam solution can be mixed with sodium chloride solution (0.9%) or 5% dextrose solution for infusion. After being mixed in fluids, it is stable under normal ambient light and temperature conditions for at least 24 hours. After 24 hours, discard the solution.

## Small Animal Dosage
**Dogs**
- 0.8 mcg/kg/min CRI.

**Cats**
- 0.5–0.8 mcg/kg/min CRI.

## Large Animal Dosage
**Foals**
- 0.04 mcg/kg/min.

## Regulatory Information
There are no withdrawal times established for food animals. Because fenoldopam has a very short half-life, residues in food animals are not expected to be a problem.

F

# Fentanyl Citrate (Note: Transdermal Fentanyl Is Listed Separately in the Next Section)
fen′tah-nil sih′trate

**Trade and other names:** Sublimaze and generic brands; Fentora buccal tablets

**Functional classification:** Analgesic, opioid

## Pharmacology and Mechanism of Action
Fentanyl is a synthetic opioid analgesic. Fentanyl is approximately 80–100 times more potent than morphine. Fentanyl is an agonist for the mu-opiate receptors on nerves and inhibits release of neurotransmitters involved with transmission of pain stimuli (e.g., substance P). The central sedative and euphoric effects are related to mu-receptor effects in the brain. Fentanyl has a wide safety profile with doses as high as 300 times the recommended dose not being lethal in spontaneously breathing dogs. It is highly lipophilic (approximately 1000 times more lipophilic than morphine) and has low protein binding in dogs (15.6%), which produces rapid diffusion into the CNS.
*Pharmacokinetics:* In dogs, the half-life is approximately 2–6 hours (depending on the study); in cats, it is approximately 2.5 hours. Clearance is high, approximately equal to hepatic blood flow, and oral absorption is very low. Fentanyl can be absorbed from the skin or oral mucous membrane, but it is not orally bioavailable if swallowed.

## Indications and Clinical Uses
Fentanyl citrate is used as an IV bolus or as a CRI in animals for relief of pain, an adjunct for anesthesia, or as a sedative in combination with other CNS sedatives. After administration by the IV route, fentanyl will produce antinociceptive effects for approximately 2 hours. Most of the doses are based on empirical observations, small retrospective observational studies, and experimental studies in research animals. Oral buccal tablets have been used in people for treatment of breakthrough pain, but there has been only anecdotal experience with this use in animals. See Fentanyl, Transdermal for information about the transdermal form. Clinical use is primarily in dogs and cats. In horses at doses needed to produce analgesia, it is associated with a high degree of restlessness, tachycardia, increased locomotor activity, and excitement if sedative drugs are not administered concurrently (see Adverse Reactions and Side Effects). In horses, there has been poor efficacy at lower doses.

## Precautionary Information

### Adverse Reactions and Side Effects

Fentanyl has adverse effects similar to morphine. Like all opiates, side effects attributed to mu-opiate receptor effects are predictable and unavoidable. Side effects include sedation, constipation, and bradycardia. Respiratory depression occurs with high doses. As with other opiates, a slight decrease in heart rate is expected. In most cases, this decrease does not have to be treated with anticholinergic drugs (e.g., atropine), but it should be monitored. In horses, undesirable and even dangerous behavior can follow rapid IV opioid administration. Horses should receive a sedative if fentanyl is administered IV, such as a preanesthetic of acepromazine or an alpha$_2$-agonist.

### Contraindications and Precautions

Fentanyl citrate is a Schedule II controlled substance. This agent is highly abused in people and responsible for many opioid-related deaths in people. Tolerance and dependence occur with repeated administration. Cats and horses are prone to excitement after administration, especially when fentanyl is administered by the IV route.

### Drug Interactions

There are no specific drug interactions, but fentanyl decreases other anesthetic requirements. Fentanyl potentiates other opiates and CNS depressants.

## Instructions for Use

Fentanyl injection is widely used in dogs and cats and some exotic species for management of pain and as an anesthetic adjunct. It is administered IV, via CRI; IM; and SQ. (Transdermal formulations are included in the next section.) For SQ administration, the pH of the solution (5.2) can elicit pain. The pain can be decreased by adding bicarbonate solution 1:10 and 1:20 dilution to increase pH to 8.0 for injection. Oral transmucosal (buccal) forms are available for human administration but have not been adequately tested in animals.

## Patient Monitoring and Laboratory Tests

Monitor analgesic response. Monitor patient's heart rate and respiration. Although bradycardia rarely needs to be treated when it is caused by an opioid, atropine can be administered if necessary. If serious respiratory depression occurs, the opioid can be reversed with naloxone.

## Formulations

- Fentanyl citrate is available as a 250-mcg/5 mL injection (50 mcg/mL).
- Fentora buccal tablets are 100, 200, 400, 600, and 800 mcg.

## Stability and Storage

Store in a tightly sealed container, protected from light, and at room temperature. Store in an appropriate locked compartment for Schedule II Controlled Substances. It is soluble in water and slightly soluble in alcohol. When compounded into a transmucosal gel, it has not been effective. The pH of fentanyl citrate is 5.2. If bicarbonate solution is added (1:10 or 1:20 dilution), the pH increases to 8.0, which may decrease pain from injection if injected immediately after mixing.

## Small Animal Dosage

### Dogs and Cats

- Anesthetic uses: 0.02–0.04 mg/kg q2h IV, SQ, or IM; if administered with acepromazine or diazepam, use 0.01 mg/kg IV, IM, or SQ.

- Analgesic agent, 0.005–0.01 mg/kg q2h IV, IM, or SQ.
- Cat premedication prior to surgery: 2–5 mcg/kg IV(0.002–0.005 mg/kg IV).
- CRI for pain control in cats: Start with a 3–5 mcg/kg (0.003–0.005 mg/kg) IV loading dose, then 2–5 mcg/kg/h, and increase up to 7 mcg/kg/h if necessary to control pain.
- CRI for pain control in dogs: Start with 0.003–0.005 mg/kg IV (3–5 mcg/kg) loading dose followed by 0.005 mg/kg/h (5 mcg/kg/h) and increase to 10 mcg/kg/h if necessary to control pain.
- CRI for maintenance of surgery in dogs: Administer 10 mcg/kg IV initially, then start CRI at 5 mcg/kg/h, and increase to 50 mcg/kg/h, if needed.

### Large Animal Dosage
**Small Ruminants**
- 5–10 mcg/kg (0.005–0.010 mg/kg) IV.

### Regulatory Information
Schedule II controlled drug by Drug Enforcement Administration (DEA). No withdrawal information is available for food-producing animals. Consult FARAD if withdrawal times are needed for food producing animals (www.FARAD.org).
RCI Classification: 1

# Fentanyl, Transdermal
fen′tah-nil

**Trade and other names:** Duragesic (patches)

**Functional classification:** Analgesic, opioid

### Pharmacology and Mechanism of Action
Fentanyl is a synthetic opiate analgesic, discussed in detail in the previous section. Fentanyl is approximately 80–100 times more potent than morphine. Fentanyl is an agonist for the mu-opiate receptors on nerves and inhibits release of neurotransmitters involved with transmission of pain stimuli (e.g., substance P). The central sedative and euphoric effects are related to mu-receptor effects in the brain. Fentanyl transdermal has the same properties as fentanyl citrate administered by IV, but in this formulation, it is administered transdermally to produce pain relief and as an adjunct to other drugs in peri-operative patients and in patients with chronic pain. The fentanyl transdermal patch system delivers fentanyl through the skin at a constant rate to produce systemic effects. The fentanyl transdermal solution is rapidly absorbed in dogs to produce a peak concentration and maintains effective concentrations for treatment of pain for 4 days.

Fentanyl transdermal solution (50 mg/mL) previously available for use in dogs (Recuvyra) has been withdrawn by the manufacturer. Patches are available that deliver 25, 50, 75, and 100 mcg/h.

*Pharmacokinetics:* Absorption across the skin can be variable in animals (e.g., rate of release of fentanyl has varied from 27%–98% [mean, 71%] of the theoretical value). Cats absorbed the fentanyl at an average rate of approximately one third of the theoretical delivery rate, but one patch maintains consistent concentrations of fentanyl in the plasma for at least 118 hours. Fentanyl transdermal patches (two or three 100-mcg/h patches) have been applied to the skin of horses to relieve pain. In horses, the duration is less than in dogs or cats and may have to be reapplied q48h.

## Indications and Clinical Uses

Transdermal absorption from fentanyl patches has been demonstrated for cats, dogs, horses, and goats. In dogs, fentanyl transdermal patches (50 mcg/h) are appropriate for most average-size dogs. Transdermal fentanyl patches have been shown in clinical studies to be effective to relieve postoperative pain in dogs. The patches have been well tolerated in cats, except for some mild opioid-related effects when the full patch (25 mcg/h) is applied. Fentanyl patches (25 mcg/h) were effective and safe to relieve pain from onychectomy surgery in cats. Cats that have received fentanyl patches have had improvement in temperament, attitude, and appetite. Transdermal fentanyl has been used alone or combined with NSAIDs for treating severe pain in horses and may provide pain relief that is superior to NSAIDs alone.

## Precautionary Information

### Adverse Reactions and Side Effects

Severe adverse effects have not been reported. Typical opiate effects can be anticipated. The patch may cause slight skin irritation at the site of application. If patch delivery of fentanyl is high, some signs of opiate overdose may occur (e.g., excitement in cats or sedation in dogs); however, these reactions are rare. Adverse effects have not been reported from the use in horses. If adverse effects are observed in animals (e.g., respiratory depression, excess sedation, or excitement in cats), remove the patch and, if necessary, administer naloxone hydrochloride (0.4-mg/mL solution at a dose of 0.04 mg/kg).

### Contraindications and Precautions

Transdermal fentanyl is a Schedule II controlled substance. Use cautiously in animals of small body weight (e.g., small toy dogs and young or debilitated cats). Fentanyl has high potency and abuse potential in people. The patches have been abused in people and have caused deaths. Animal owners should be advised of the high risks to humans if transdermal patches is applied to humans. Fentanyl is absorbed through intact human skin.

### Drug Interactions

There are no specific drug interactions, but transdermal fentanyl decreases other anesthetic requirements. Transdermal fentanyl potentiates other opiates and CNS depressants.

## Instructions for Use

Transdermal fentanyl incorporates fentanyl into adhesive patches applied to the skin of dogs and cats. Studies have determined that patches release sustained levels of fentanyl for 72–108 hours in dogs and cats. One 100-mcg/h patch is equivalent to 10 mg/kg of morphine q4h IM. Studies have determined that 25-mcg/h patches are appropriate for most cats, but if the rate of delivery is too high for cats and adverse reactions are suspected, covering half the adhesive surface area reduces the rate of delivery. A single 50-mcg/h patch is appropriate for dogs weighing 10–20 kg. In horses, two or three 100-mcg/h patches achieved rapid plasma concentrations within effective ranges in adults, but it was highly variable. Duration of effect in horses is less than in dogs or cats at only 48 hours. Follow the manufacturer's recommendations carefully when applying patches and disposing of used patches.

## Patient Monitoring and Laboratory Tests

Monitor the patient's heart rate and respiration. Although bradycardia rarely needs to be treated when it is caused by an opioid, atropine can be administered if necessary. If serious respiratory depression occurs, the opioid can be reversed with naloxone (0.04 mg/kg). Monitor for signs of excitement in cats.

## Formulations

- Transdermal fentanyl patches are available in 25-, 50-, 75-, and 100-mcg/h patches. In May 2009, the formulation was switched to a matrix vehicle instead of a reservoir system. These have been bioequivalent to previous formulations in people.
- Fentanyl transdermal solution (Recuvyra) has been withdrawn by the manufacturer and is no longer available.

## Stability and Storage

Store in a tightly sealed container, protected from light, and at room temperature. Do not open the fentanyl patch membrane.

**F**

## Small Animal Dosage

**Dogs**

- Patches: 10–20 kg: 50-mcg/h patch q72h. Higher size patch (75- or 100-mcg patch) may be used in large dogs, but there is no evidence showing a relationship between size of the patch and dog size.

**Cats**

- 25-mcg patch per cat q120h. For small cats, half of the patch surface can be covered to reduce surface area and decrease amount absorbed.

## Large Animal Dosage

**Horses**

- Patches: In adult horses, two or three transdermal patches of 100 mcg/h each (10 mg of fentanyl, equivalent to 35–110 mcg/kg delivered transdermally).
- Patches: In foals, one transdermal patch of 100 mcg/h.

**Sheep and Goats**

- 100-mcg/h patch, or approximately 2.5 mcg/kg/h, depending on goat size. (Absorption has been inconsistent.)

## Regulatory Information

Schedule II controlled drug by the DEA.
Fentanyl should not be administered to animals that produce food. Withdrawal times are not established.

---

# Ferrous Sulfate
fare′us sul′fate

**Trade and other names:** Ferospace and generic brands (over-the-counter)

**Functional classification:** Mineral supplement, iron supplement

## Pharmacology and Mechanism of Action

Ferrous sulfate is a common iron supplement. This supplement replaces iron in animals that are deficient or with iron-deficiency anemia.

## Indications and Clinical Uses

Iron supplements are indicated in patients with diseases caused by iron deficiency, such as iron deficiency anemia. Oral iron supplements are considered one of the primary means of treatment iron deficiency in dogs and cats. The supplements most often used are ferrous sulfate or ferrous gluconate.

## Precautionary Information

### Adverse Reactions and Side Effects
High doses cause stomach ulceration. Feces become dark with oral administration.

### Contraindications and Precautions
Do not use in animals prone to gastric ulcers. High doses or accidental ingestion may cause severe ulcers and perforation and should be treated as an emergency.

### Drug Interactions
Iron supplements interfere with oral absorption of other drugs such as fluoroquinolones, tetracyclines, and other drugs that may chelate with iron. Histamine $H_2$ antagonists, PPIs such as omeprazole, and oral antacids decrease oral absorption because an acid environment favors absorption.

## Instructions for Use
The recommendations for iron supplementation are based on dose needed to increase hematocrit. In some animals, injectable iron dextran is used instead of oral therapy.

Note that doses are often expressed in mg of elemental iron in the formulation. There are two forms of ferrous sulfate: tablets, and a dried form (desiccated). Ferrous sulfate tablets contain approximately 20% elemental iron; ferrous sulfate desiccated (dried) contains approximately 30% elemental iron.

## Patient Monitoring and Laboratory Tests
Monitor hematocrit, serum iron levels, and total iron-binding capacity.

## Formulations
- Over-the-counter oral formulations are available; 250-mg ferrous sulfate contains 50 mg of elemental iron.
- 1 g of the dried form (desiccated form) contains 300 mg of elemental iron. Or each tablet of 200 mg of dried ferrous sulfate contains 65 mg of elemental iron.
- Injectable forms are usually iron dextran. (Iron dextran is listed in a separate section.)

## Stability and Storage
Store in a tightly sealed container, protected from light, and at room temperature. Do not mix with other drugs because chelation may occur. Ferrous sulfate is soluble in water.

## Small Animal Dosage
### Dogs
- 100–300 mg/dog q24h PO. Usually administered with a meal.

### Cats
- 50–100 mg/cat q24h PO.

## Large Animal Dosage
- No large animal doses have been reported.

## Regulatory Information
Extralabel withdrawal times are not established. However, 24-hour withdrawal times are suggested because this drug has little risk from residues.

# Finasteride
fin-ass′ter-ide

**Trade and other names:** Proscar

**Functional classification:** Hormone antagonist

## Pharmacology and Mechanism of Action
Finasteride is a synthetic steroid type-II 5 alpha reductase inhibitor. It inhibits conversion of testosterone to dihydrotestosterone (DHT). A similar drug in this class (but not evaluated in veterinary medicine) is dutasteride (Avodart). In people, finasteride is most often administered to decrease prostate size in patients with benign prostatic hypertrophy. It may reduce risk of prostate cancer, but this effect is controversial.

## Indications and Clinical Uses
Because DHT stimulates prostate growth, finasteride has been used for benign prostatic hypertrophy (BPH). In dogs with BPH, finasteride has been shown to reduce prostatic size without adversely affecting testosterone production or semen quality. It may be used concurrently with tamsulosin, an antagonist of alpha$_{1A}$-adrenoreceptors in the prostate smooth muscle to improve urine flow.

## Precautionary Information
### Adverse Reactions and Side Effects
No adverse effects have been reported in dogs.

### Contraindications and Precautions
Finasteride is contraindicated in pregnant animals.

### Drug Interactions
No drug interactions are reported for animals. Finasteride may be used with smooth muscle relaxants that are intended to relax prostate and urethral smooth muscle to improve urine flow. Such drugs include tamsulosin, which is an antagonist of alpha$_{1A}$-adrenoreceptors in the prostate smooth muscle.

## Instructions for Use
Doses are based on clinical studies in dogs, and information for other animals has not been reported. One study in dogs found significant effects at 0.1 mg/kg q24h. Another study used a dosage range of 0.1–0.5 mg/kg q24h and reported reduction in prostate size.

## Patient Monitoring and Laboratory Tests
No specific monitoring is necessary.

## Formulations
• Finasteride is available in 1- and 5-mg tablets.

## Stability and Storage
Store in a tightly sealed container, protected from light, and at room temperature. Stability of compounded formulations has not been evaluated.

## Small Animal Dosage
- 0.1 mg/kg q24h PO.
- Dogs 10–50 kg: 5-mg tablet per dog q24h PO.

## Large Animal Dosage
- No large animal doses have been reported.

## Regulatory Information
No withdrawal times are established. Do not use in animals intended for food.

# Firocoxib
feer-oh-koks'ib

**Trade and other names:** Previcox and Equioxx

**Functional classification:** Anti-inflammatory

## Pharmacology and Mechanism of Action
Firocoxib is an NSAID used in dogs and horses. Like other drugs in this class, firocoxib produces analgesic and anti-inflammatory effects by inhibiting the synthesis of prostaglandins. The enzyme inhibited by the NSAID is the cyclo-oxygenase (COX) enzyme. The COX enzyme exists in two isoforms: COX-1 and COX-2. COX-1 is primarily responsible for synthesis of prostaglandins important for maintaining a healthy GI tract, renal function, platelet function, and other normal functions. COX-2 is induced and responsible for synthesizing prostaglandins that are important mediators of pain, inflammation, and fever. However, it is understood that there is some crossover of COX-1 and COX-2 effects in some situations, and COX-2 activity is important for some biological effects. Firocoxib, using in vitro assays, is more COX-1 sparing compared with older NSAIDs and is a selective inhibitor of COX-2. The COX-1:COX-2 ratio is greater than for other drugs, indicating that firocoxib is a selective COX-2 inhibitor in dogs, horses, and cats. It has not been established if the specificity for COX-1 or COX-2 produces superior efficacy or safety compared to other less selective NSAIDs.

*Pharmacokinetics:* Firocoxib has half-lives of 7.8 hours in dogs, 9–12 hours in cats, 11 hours in foals, 30–40 hours in adult horses, and 6.7 hours in calves. Because of shorter half-life, the concentrations are lower in foals compared with adult horses. It is highly protein bound (96%–98%). Oral absorption is 38% in dogs, 79%–100% in horses, approximately 100% in calves, and 54%–70% in cats. Feeding delays absorption but does not diminish overall absorption. In horses, oral absorption is 79%–100% with oral paste at a dose of 0.1 mg/kg and 88% when the canine tablets are administered (no significant difference in absorption between oral paste and tablets). Fasted horses have higher absorption than fed horses.

## Indications and Clinical Uses
Firocoxib is used to decrease pain, inflammation, and fever. It has been used for the acute and chronic treatment of pain and inflammation in dogs. One of the most common uses is osteoarthritis, but it also has been used for pain associated with surgery. In horses, it is used for osteoarthritis and for pain associated with surgery. In cats, firocoxib has been demonstrated to be effective for attenuating acute febrile responses, but the use in cats is limited to short-term or long-term use at low doses.

## Precautionary Information

### Adverse Reactions and Side Effects

Gastrointestinal problems are the most common adverse events associated with NSAIDs and can include vomiting, diarrhea, nausea, ulcers, and erosions of the GI tract. Both acute and long-term safety and efficacy have been established for firocoxib in dogs and horses prior to approval. In field trials, vomiting was the most often reported adverse effect in dogs. In studies performed in dogs, higher doses (five times the normal dose) caused GI problems. In studies of young juvenile dogs, administration of firocoxib was associated with periportal fatty hepatic changes in some animals. Renal toxicity, especially in dehydrated animals or animals with preexisting kidney disease, has been observed for some NSAIDs. Behavior changes have occurred in dogs and horses, but they are rare.

In horses, adverse effects have included oral ulcerations, renal papillary necrosis, and GI effects after 42 days of dosing, but mucosal recovery after intestinal ischemia was less than other nonselective NSAIDs. In horses, GI problems (diarrhea, loose stool) have been reported in field trials, but they are rare at approved doses. At doses exceeding the labeled dose or duration in horses, ulcers, azotemia, renal injury, erosions of skin and oral mucosa, and prolonged bleeding times have been observed.

### Contraindications and Precautions

Animals with preexisting GI problems or renal problems may be at a greater risk of adverse effects from NSAIDs. There is no information on the safety of firocoxib in the treatment of breeding, pregnant, or lactating animals, but adverse effects have not been reported in breeding animals.

In horses, do not exceed recommended duration of treatment. During animal safety studies in horses, toxicity occurred at recommended doses if administration exceeded 30 days.

### Drug Interactions

Do not administer with other NSAIDs or with corticosteroids. Corticosteroids have been shown to exacerbate the GI adverse effects. Some NSAIDs may interfere with the action of diuretic drugs and angiotensin-converting enzyme (ACE) inhibitors.

## Instructions for Use

Use according to manufacturer's dosing guidelines. Chewable tablets can be administered with or without food. Long-term studies have not been completed in cats, and only single-dose studies have been reported. The canine tablets have been administered orally to horses, with no significant differences in absorption compared with oral paste. Although this use is not allowed according to US Food and Drug Administration (FDA) regulations, the oral tablets have been bioavailable in horses.

## Patient Monitoring and Laboratory Tests

Monitor GI signs for evidence of diarrhea, GI bleeding, or ulcers. Because of risk of renal injury, monitor renal parameters (water consumption, BUN, creatinine, and urine-specific gravity) periodically during treatment.

## Formulations

- Firocoxib is available in 57- and 227-mg tablets.
- Equine oral paste is available as 8.2 mg/g of paste (0.82% w/w).

- Equine injection is available as 20-mg/mL solution for IV use (with polyethylene glycol and glycerol vehicle).

## Stability and Storage

Store in a tightly sealed container, protected from light, and at room temperature. Stability of compounded formulations has not been evaluated. It is not ionized, and solubility is not affected by pH.

## Small Animal Dosage

### Dogs
- 5 mg/kg once daily PO.

### Cats
- 1.5 mg/kg once PO. Long-term safety in cats has not been determined.

## Large Animal Dosage

### Horses
- 0.1 mg/kg q24h PO for up to 14 days.
- IV: 0.09 mg/kg IV once daily (2 mL per 1000 lb, or 2.6 mL/1250 lb; 1.5 mL/750 lb).

### Calves
- An approved dose is not established, but 0.5 mg/kg PO or IV has been used q24h.

## Regulatory Information

Withdrawal time is not established for food animals, but 26 days for slaughter has been used for calves in other countries. Do not administer to horses that are used for human consumption.

In racing horses, it is not permitted to be used 12 hours prior to competition.

# Florfenicol
flore-fen'ih-kole

**Trade and other names:** Nuflor, Nuflor Gold, and Resflor (flunixin and florfenicol) Aquaflor (fish formulation)

**Functional classification:** Antibacterial

## Pharmacology and Mechanism of Action

Florfenicol is a thiamphenicol derivative with the same mechanism of action as chloramphenicol (inhibition of protein synthesis). However, it is more active than either chloramphenicol or thiamphenicol and may be more bactericidal than previously thought against some pathogens (e.g., bovine respiratory disease [BRD] pathogens). Florfenicol has a broad spectrum of antibacterial activity that includes all organisms sensitive to chloramphenicol, gram-negative bacilli, gram-positive cocci, and other atypical bacteria such as mycoplasma. Florfenicol is highly lipophilic, which provides high enough concentrations to treat intracellular pathogens and cross some anatomic barriers (penetration across the blood–brain barrier in cattle is 46%).

*Pharmacokinetics:* The half-life of florfenicol is 2–3 hours in cattle after IV administration, but it is prolonged (18 hours) after IM injection and 27 or 62 hours (depending on the study) after 40 mg/kg SQ. The peak concentration in cattle after 40 mg/kg SQ is 5.5 mcg/mL. In dogs, the half-life is shorter, with values of 1.1 and 1.2 after IV and oral administration, respectively. The half-lives in cats are approximately 4 hours and 7.8 hours after IV and oral administration, respectively. The protein binding is small.

## Indications and Clinical Uses

Because florfenicol is a derivative of chloramphenicol, it has been used in situations in which chloramphenicol is unavailable or illegal. (Chloramphenicol is illegal to use in food animals in the United States.) Florfenicol has been shown to be effective for treatment of BRD in cattle associated with *Mannheimia haemolytica, Pasteurella multocida,* and *Histophilus somni.* Administration of florfenicol (40 mg/kg once SQ) at time of arrival to the feedlot decreased the incidence of BRD. It also is used for treatment of bovine interdigital phlegmon (foot rot, acute interdigital necrobacillosis, and infectious pododermatitis) associated with *Fusobacterium necrophorum* and *Bacteroides melaninogenicus* and for treatment of infectious bovine keratoconjunctivitis caused by *Moraxella bovis.* Resflor Gold contains both florfenicol and flunixin. It is used for the same BRD pathogens and provides anti-inflammatory activity with the addition of flunixin meglumine, including BRD-associated pyrexia in beef and nonlactating dairy cattle.

In pigs, florfenicol is used for treatment of swine respiratory disease (SRD) caused by *Actinobacillus pleuropneumoniae, Pasteurella multocida, Salmonella choleraesuis,* and *Streptococcus suis.* In cats, effective concentrations can be achieved with twice-daily administration. In dogs, the half-life is short, and frequent administration is necessary to produce effective concentrations. Florfenicol also has been administered to fish. There is a feed-additive formulation that also has been approved for fish (10–15 mg/kg body weigh/day for 10 consecutive days).

---

## Precautionary Information

### Adverse Reactions and Side Effects

Florfenicol use in dogs and cats has been limited; therefore, adverse effects have not been reported. Long-term use should be avoided in dogs and cats. Chloramphenicol has been linked to dose-dependent bone marrow depression, and similar reactions may be possible with florfenicol. However, there is not a risk of aplastic anemia as for chloramphenicol. At high doses, florfenicol may cause testicular degeneration. In horses, doses of 20 mg/kg q48h IM changed the bacterial flora and increased risk of diarrhea.

### Contraindications and Precautions

Long-term use in animals may cause bone marrow suppression. Administration to horses has caused diarrhea, colitis, and elevations in bilirubin. Administration to horses is not recommended. Do not administer more than 10 mL in a single site.

### Drug Interactions

No drug interactions are reported for animals. However, chloramphenicol is well known to inhibit cytochrome P450 enzymes and decrease metabolism of other drugs (see Appendix I). Therefore, it is possible—but not documented—that florfenicol could cause drug interactions.

---

## Instructions for Use

The florfenicol dose form available is only approved for use in cattle and pigs (with an exception for the oral form for fish). The doses, intervals, and indications for livestock have been established through well-controlled studies and FDA evaluation and approval.

However, there is insufficient information available for dogs and cats. The doses listed below in the dosing section have not been thoroughly evaluated in small animals and were derived only from pharmacokinetic studies in healthy animals. Sustained effect in cattle from IM and SQ administration does not appear to be long lasting in dogs. Injectable formulation for cattle has been administered orally to small animals, if necessary, but the taste is bitter.

## Patient Monitoring and Laboratory Tests

Monitor CBC for evidence of bone marrow depression. Clinical and Laboratory Standards Institute (CLSI) breakpoints for florfenicol susceptible organisms are ≤2 mcg/mL for bovine and swine respiratory pathogens and ≤4 meg/mL for *Streptococcus suis.*

## Formulations

- 300-mg/mL injectable solution (cattle). Nuflor Gold contains 300 mg/mL of florfenicol with excipients triacetin and 2-pyrrolidone added. Nuflor contains 300 mg/mL of florfenicol with propylene glycol added as an excipient.
- 23-mg/mL solution to be added to drinking water for pigs (400 mg/gallon).
- Type A medicated feed formulation contains 500 g/kg (227.27 g/lb) to be added to fish feed.
- Flunixin is combined with florfenicol in Resflor Gold, which has 300 mg of florfenicol and 16.5 mg of flunixin per milliliter with vehicles of 2-pyrrolidone, 35-mg malic acid, and triacetin.

## Stability and Storage

Store in a tightly sealed container, protected from light, and at room temperature. Light yellow or straw color does not affect potency. Stability of compounded formulations has not been evaluated.

## Small Animal Dosage

### Dogs

- 20 mg/kg q6h IM or PO.

### Cats

- 22 mg/kg q8h IM or PO.

## Large Animal Dosage

### Cattle, Bovine Respiratory Disease

- 20 mg/kg q48h SQ or IM (in the neck).
- 40 mg/kg SQ as a single injection or q72h SQ in the neck region (also combined with flunixin at 2.2 mg/kg and Nuflor Gold at 40-mg/kg single injection).

### Horses

- Although florfenicol has been administered, some references cite adverse effects after administration. Until more safety data become available, it is suggested to avoid use of florfenicol in horses.

### Sheep

- 20–30 mg/kg IM or 40 mg/kg SQ administered daily for 3 days.

### Pigs

- 15 mg/kg IM in the neck q48h.
- Administer in drinking water at 400 mg/gallon (100 parts per million) for 5 consecutive days.

**Fish**
- 10–15 mg/kg body weight/day for 10 consecutive days

## Regulatory Information

Cattle withdrawal time (meat): 28 days if administered IM; 38 days if administered SQ. Nuflor Gold withdrawal time (40 mg/kg SQ) is 44 days. Sheep: Apply at least 42-day slaughter withdrawal time. Do not use in calves to be processed for veal; not to be used in dairy cattle 20 months of age or older or in veal calves younger than 1 month. A withdrawal period has not been established in preruminating calves, but FARAD (www.FARAD.org) recommends 90 days. Do not use in dairy cattle. If administered intramammary, 5 days is needed for depletion. Pig withdrawal time: 16 days after last treatment when administered in water; 13 days after last treatment when administered with feed.

# Fluconazole
floo-kahn′ah-zole

**Trade and other names:** Diflucan and generic brands

**Functional classification:** Antifungal

## Pharmacology and Mechanism of Action

Fluconazole is an oral azole antifungal drug. It has fungistatic properties. Fluconazole inhibits ergosterol synthesis in fungal cell membrane to inhibit fungal cell growth. It has activity against dermatophytes, systemic fungi, and yeasts, including *Candida, Coccidioides,* and *Cryptococcus* spp. However, it has weak activity against molds such as *Aspergillus* and *Zygomycetes* spp. The two triazole rings on fluconazole make it less lipophilic and more water soluble than other azole antifungal agents. It is less protein bound than other azole antifungal drugs.

*Pharmacokinetics:* Compared with other oral azole antifungals, fluconazole is absorbed more predictably and completely, even on an empty stomach. The half-life in dogs, cats, and horses is approximately 14–15, 13–25, and 38 hours, respectively.

## Indications and Clinical Uses

Fluconazole is effective against dermatophytes, yeasts, and a variety of systemic fungi. In dogs, cats, horses, and exotic animals, it is used to treat systemic fungal infections, yeast infections, and dermatophytes, including *Malassezia* dermatitis. In cats, it has been used to treat *Cryptococcus* infection and histoplasmosis. In dogs, it is not as active against coccidioidomycosis as other azole antifungal drugs, but it has been effective in some patients. Higher dosages may be needed (e.g., 10 mg/kg q12h) for coccidioidomycosis. It has been as effective as for treatment of blastomycosis in dogs with efficacy similar to itraconazole. Because it is water soluble, it is excreted in the urine in an active form and has been used to treat fungal cystitis.

## Precautionary Information

### Adverse Reactions and Side Effects

Adverse effects have not been reported from fluconazole administration, but it is a human-label drug, and a complete adverse event profile is not available. Compared with ketoconazole, it has less effect on endocrine function. However, increased liver enzyme concentrations and hepatopathy are possible.

**Contraindications and Precautions**

Use cautiously in pregnant animals. At high doses in laboratory animals, it has caused fetal abnormalities.

**Drug Interactions**

Fluconazole can be an inhibitor of cytochrome P450 enzymes, which can increase other drug concentrations. It causes an increase in cyclosporine concentrations in dogs. It may decrease the metabolism of other drugs, such as anesthetics, sedatives (e.g., midazolam), and analgesics (tramadol). Horses administered fluconazole had prolonged recovery from anesthesia, presumably caused by decreased anesthetic metabolism.

## Instructions for Use

Doses for fluconazole are primarily based on studies performed in cats for treatment of cryptococcosis. Efficacy for other infections has not been reported. The primary difference between fluconazole and other azoles is that fluconazole attains higher concentrations in the CNS. Oral absorption of fluconazole is more predictable than itraconazole and ketoconazole and less affected by administration without food.

## Patient Monitoring and Laboratory Tests

Monitor hepatic enzymes periodically in treated animals. Susceptibility testing is possible, but ranges are only established for *Candida* spp. Fluconazole may cause mild elevations of liver enzymes in some dogs.

## Formulations

* Fluconazole is available in 50-, 100-, 150-, and 200-mg tablets; 10- and 40-mg/mL oral suspension; and 2-mg/mL IV injection.

## Stability and Storage

Fluconazole is stable for 14 days after reconstituting oral suspension. Because it is water soluble at a concentration of 8–10 mg/mL, it also may be compounded in formulations for administration to small animals. Tablets have been crushed and mixed with liquid vehicles for oral administration. However, long-term stability of compounded formulations beyond 15 days has not been determined. Suspensions made for animals in concentrations of 30 and 100 mg/mL by compounding pharmacies had poor accuracy and precision of the formulation.

## Small Animal Dosage
**Dogs**
* 5 mg/kg q12h PO or IV. In refractory cases, increase dosage to 10 mg/kg q12h PO or IV.
* Blastomycosis: 10 mg/kg/day.
* *Malassezia* treatment: 5 mg/kg q12h PO.

**Cats**
* 50 mg/cat per once daily PO; in refractory cases, increase to 50 mg per cat q12h PO (10 mg/kg q12h). In most cases, it is administered once daily.

## Large Animal Dosage
**Horses**
* 5 mg/kg q24h PO.

## Regulatory Information
No withdrawal times are established for animals intended for food (extralabel use). Consult FARAD if extralabel withdrawal information is needed (www.FARAD.org).

# Flucytosine
floo-sye′toe-seen

**Trade and other names:** Ancobon

**Functional classification:** Antifungal

F

## Pharmacology and Mechanism of Action
Flucytosine is an antifungal drug, usually administered with other agents. The action is to penetrate fungal cells, where it is converted to fluorouracil, which acts as antimetabolite.

## Indications and Clinical Uses
Flucytosine is an antifungal drug that has been limited in veterinary medicine to treat cryptococcal meningitis. It should be used in combination with amphotericin B (but not azole antifungal drugs) for treatment of cryptococcosis to improve efficacy and decrease resistance. The use is primarily confined to treatment of cryptococcosis in cats because it causes toxic reactions in dogs.

## Precautionary Information

**Adverse Reactions and Side Effects**

Anemia and thrombocytopenia are the most common adverse effects. Cutaneous and mucocutaneous eruptions have been observed with use of flucytosine in dogs. Therefore, it is not recommended for use in dogs.

**Contraindications and Precautions**

No specific contraindications have been identified for animals. Use in dogs is not recommended because of eruptions of skin reactions.

**Drug Interactions**

No drug interactions are reported for animals.

## Instructions for Use
Flucytosine is used primarily to treat cryptococcosis in animals. Efficacy is based on its ability to attain high concentrations in cerebrospinal fluid. Flucytosine may be synergistic with amphotericin B.

## Patient Monitoring and Laboratory Tests
Monitor CBC during treatment.

## Formulations Available
• Flucytosine is available in 250- and 500-mg capsules.

## Stability and Storage
Store in a tightly sealed container, protected from light, and at room temperature. Compounded oral suspensions have been stable for 60 days.

## Small Animal Dosage

**Cats (Not Recommended For Dogs)**
- 25–50 mg/kg q6–8h PO, up to a maximum dosage of 100 mg/kg q12h PO.
- Cryptococcal meningitis: 20–40 mg/kg q6h PO.

## Large Animal Dosage
- No large animal doses have been reported.

## Regulatory Information
No withdrawal times are established for animals that are intended for food (extralabel use).

# Fludrocortisone Acetate
floo-droe-kor'tih-sone ass'ih-tate

**Trade and other names:** Florinef

**Functional classification:** Corticosteroid

## Pharmacology and Mechanism of Action
Fludrocortisone is a corticosteroid administered orally to animals with mineralocorticoid deficiency. It is used for mineralocorticoid replacement therapy. Fludrocortisone has high potency of mineralocorticoid activity compared with glucocorticoid activity. Fludrocortisone acts to mimic the action of aldosterone in the body, specifically to increase reabsorption of sodium in renal tubules.

## Indications and Clinical Uses
Fludrocortisone is used as replacement therapy in animals with adrenocortical insufficiency (Addison disease). It has high mineralocorticoid potency compared with the glucocorticoid potency. Desoxycorticosterone pivalate (DOCP) is used as an alternative in dogs when an intermittent injectable is desired rather than daily oral doses of fludrocortisone. One injection of DOCP can last 25 days or longer, which avoids daily administration of fludrocortisone. In cats, fludrocortisone has been used to treat primary hyperaldosteronism.

## Precautionary Information

**Adverse Reactions and Side Effects**

Adverse effects are primarily related to glucocorticoid effects with high doses. Polyuria and polydipsia may occur in some animals. Long-term treatment for hypoadrenocorticism may result in glucocorticoid side effects. Administration of fludrocortisone causes a significant reduction in urine aldosterone.

**Contraindications and Precautions**

Although used as a mineralocorticoid, it may produce glucocorticoid side effects. Use cautiously in animals that may be at risk for corticosteroid side effects.

**Drug Interactions**

No drug interactions are reported for animals.

## Instructions for Use
Dose should be adjusted by monitoring patient response (i.e., monitoring electrolyte concentrations). In some patients, it is administered with a glucocorticoid (e.g., prednisolone/prednisone at a dosage of 0.2–0.3 mg/kg/day), accompanied with

sodium supplementation. However, because it has retained some glucocorticosteroid activity, some animals may not require additional supplementation with glucocorticoids when receiving fludrocortisone.

### Patient Monitoring and Laboratory Tests

Monitor the patient's electrolytes (especially sodium and potassium). Dose adjustment should be based on electrolyte monitoring to maintain these within a desired range. Fludrocortisone is used as a diagnostic test for primary hyperaldosteronism in cats. This suppression test can be performed as a confirmatory test in cats with basal urine aldosterone:creatinine ratio greater than $7.5 \times 10^{-9}$; suppression less than 50% indicates inappropriate aldosterone secretion. See the dosing section for protocol.

### Formulations

- Fludrocortisone is available in 100-mcg (0.1-mg) tablets.

### Stability and Storage

Store in a tightly sealed container, protected from light, and at room temperature. It is insoluble in water. When crushed tablets were prepared in various suspensions, they were stable for 14 days.

### Small Animal Dosage

**Dogs**

- 10 mcg/kg/day PO (0.01 mg/kg). The dosage can be increased to 30 mcg/kg/day (0.03 mg/kg) PO if necessary based on electrolyte monitoring.

**Cats**

- 0.1–0.3 mg/cat q24h PO (100–300 mcg per cat).
- To test for primary aldosteronism, administer 0.05 mg/kg q12h for 4 days and measure effect with urine aldosterone-to-creatinine ratio. (The range is greater than $7.5 \times 10^{-9}$ in cats with hyperaldosteronism.)

### Large Animal Dosage

- No large animal doses have been reported.

### Regulatory Information

Extralabel withdrawal times are not established. However, 24-hour withdrawal times are suggested because this drug has little risk from residues.
RCI Classification: 4

# Flumazenil
floo-may′zeh-nil
**Trade and other names:** Romazicon
**Functional classification:** Antidote

### Pharmacology and Mechanism of Action

Flumazenil is a benzodiazepine receptor antagonist. Flumazenil blocks the action of benzodiazepines, such as diazepam, from the action on the gamma-aminobutyric acid (GABA) receptor. Therefore, this medication has no primary use but is used to treat overdoses of benzodiazepines.

## Indications and Clinical Uses

Flumazenil has no therapeutic benefits of its own, but it is used as a reversal agent after benzodiazepine administration in people (not commonly used in veterinary medicine). Because of high first-pass effects, it cannot be administered orally; it must be injected.

### Precautionary Information

**Adverse Reactions and Side Effects**

No adverse effects reported in animals.

**Contraindications and Precautions**

Flumazenil may precipitate a seizure if used with tricyclic antidepressants (TCAs) or other drugs that can lower seizure threshold.

**Drug Interactions**

Flumazenil may increase risk of seizures when used with other drugs known to inhibit the inhibitory neurotransmitter GABA.

### Instructions for Use

Flumazenil is used primarily to block effects of benzodiazepine drugs. It has been used to reverse overdoses of benzodiazepines (e.g., diazepam). Although it has been used experimentally for treating hepatic encephalopathy, its efficacy for this condition is not established.

### Patient Monitoring and Laboratory Tests

No specific monitoring is necessary.

### Formulations

- Flumazenil is available in a 100-mcg/mL (0.1-mg/mL) injection.

### Stability and Storage

Store in a tightly sealed container, protected from light, and at room temperature. Stability of compounded formulations has not been evaluated.

### Small Animal Dosage

**Dogs and Cats**

- 0.02 mg/kg (20 mcg/kg) IV.
- To reverse benzodiazepines: 0.2 mg (total dose), as needed, IV.

### Large Animal Dosage

**Horses, Cattle, Swine, and Sheep**

- To reverse benzodiazepines: 20 mcg/kg IV (0.02 mg/kg).

### Regulatory Information

Do not use in animals intended for food.

# Flumethasone

floo-meth'ah-sone

**Trade and other names:** Flucort, Fluosmin suspension, and Anaprime suspension

**Functional classification:** Corticosteroid

## Pharmacology and Mechanism of Action

Flumethasone is a potent glucocorticoid anti-inflammatory drug. Potency is listed by one reference as approximately 15 times that of cortisol and in other veterinary references as 30 times that of cortisol and 6–7 times the potency of prednisolone. Anti-inflammatory effects are complex but primarily via inhibition of inflammatory cells and suppression of expression of inflammatory mediators. It is not used as commonly as prednisone or dexamethasone. The major use of flumethasone is for treatment of inflammatory and immune-mediated disease.

## Indications and Clinical Uses

Flumethasone, like other corticosteroids, is used to treat a variety of inflammatory and immune-mediated diseases. The dosing section contains the range of doses for replacement therapy, anti-inflammatory therapy, and immunosuppressive therapy. Flumethasone is used more often in large animals than small animals. Large-animal uses include treatment of inflammatory conditions, especially musculoskeletal disorders, and is used intra-articularly. In horses, flumethasone has been used for treatment of equine asthma syndrome accompanied by recurrent airway obstruction (RAO; formerly called chronic obstructive pulmonary disease). In cattle, corticosteroids have been used in the treatment of ketosis.

## Precautionary Information

### Adverse Reactions and Side Effects

Side effects from corticosteroids are many and include polyphagia, polydipsia and polyuria, and hypothalamic–pituitary–adrenal axis suppression. Adverse effects include GI ulceration, hepatopathy, diabetes, hyperlipidemia, decreased thyroid hormone, decreased protein synthesis, and delayed wound healing and immunosuppression. Secondary infections can occur as a result of immunosuppression and include demodicosis, toxoplasmosis, fungal infections, and urinary tract infections (UTIs). In horses, additional adverse effects include risk of laminitis.

### Contraindications and Precautions

Use cautiously in patients prone to ulcers or infection and in animals in which wound healing is necessary. Use cautiously in animals with kidney disease or diabetes and in pregnant animals. The manufacturer has warned that corticosteroids administered orally or parenterally to animals may induce the first stage of parturition when administered during the last trimester of pregnancy and may precipitate premature parturition followed by dystocia, fetal death, retained placenta, and metritis.

### Drug Interactions

Administration of corticosteroids with NSAIDs will increase the risk of GI injury.

## Instructions for Use

Doses are based on severity of underlying disease. For example, anti-inflammatory conditions require lower doses than immune-mediated conditions. For all conditions, cats often require higher doses than dogs. Note that the approved label dose for cattle and horses is in the range of 1.25–5 mg per animal or approximately 0.003–0.006 mg/kg (3–6 mcg/kg) for an adult animal. Considering that the potency of flumethasone may be similar to dexamethasone, many experts believe that the dose should be higher, in the range of 0.04–0.15 mg/kg to obtain a full therapeutic effect. The manufacturer's label dose for dogs and cats is approximately 0.01–0.02 mg/kg/day, PO, IV, IM, or SQ. But based on comparative potency, the manufacturer's dose may be low for some conditions.

## Patient Monitoring and Laboratory Tests

Monitor liver enzymes, blood glucose, and renal function during therapy. Monitor patients for signs of secondary infections. Perform an adrenocorticotropic hormone (ACTH) stimulation test to monitor adrenal function.

## Formulations

Flumethasone is available in a 0.5-mg/mL solution for injection, 0.0625-mg tablets for small animal use, 2 mg/mL flumethasone acetate suspension for small animals, and 2-mg/mL liquid suspension for intra-articular use in horses.

## Stability and Storage

Store in a tightly sealed container, protected from light, and at room temperature. Stability of compounded formulations has not been evaluated.

## Small Animal Dosage

### Dogs and Cats

• Anti-inflammatory uses: 0.15–0.3 mg/kg q12–24h PO, IV, IM, or SQ. Note that the manufacturer's label dosage is 0.06–0.25 mg per dog per day, and 0.03–0.125 mg per cat per day ($\approx$0.01–0.02 mg/kg), but this may be low based on relative potency.

## Large Animal Dosage

### Horses

• 1.25–2.5 mg per animal as a single dose IM or IV ($\approx$0.003–0.006 mg/kg). This is the dose frequently listed on the product label. However, many experts prefer doses of 0.04–0.15 mg/kg as a single dose IV or IM.
• Intra-articular use in horses: 6–10 mg per joint of the 2-mg/mL suspension.

### Cattle

• 1.25–5 mg/animal as a single dose IV or IM. This is the dose frequently listed on the product label. However, many experts prefer doses of 0.04–0.15 mg/kg as a single dose IV or IM.

## Regulatory Information

There are no US withdrawal times established. Consult FARAD if withdrawal times are needed for food producing animals (www.FARAD.org). In Canada, cattle withdrawal time (meat): 4 days.
RCI Classification: 4

# Flunixin Meglumine

floo-nix'in meg'loo-meen

**Trade and other names:** Banamine, Banamine-S, Resflor (with florfenicol), and Hexasol (with oxytetracycline)

**Functional classification:** Nonsteroidal anti-inflammatory drug

## Pharmacology and Mechanism of Action

Flunixin is a potent NSAID widely used in large animals. Like other NSAIDs, it produces analgesic and anti-inflammatory effects by inhibiting the synthesis of prostaglandins. The enzyme inhibited by NSAID is the COX enzyme. The COX enzyme exists in two isoforms: COX-1 and COX-2. COX-1 is primarily responsible for synthesis of prostaglandins important for maintaining a healthy GI tract, renal function, platelet function, and other normal functions. COX-2 is induced and responsible for synthesizing prostaglandins that are important mediators of pain, inflammation, and fever. However, it is understood that there is some crossover of COX-1 and COX-2 effects in some situations, and COX-2 activity is important for some biological effects. Flunixin is not selective for either COX-1 or COX-2. Other anti-inflammatory effects may occur (e.g., effects on leukocytes) but have not been well characterized.

*Pharmacokinetics:* In horses, the half-life is 2 hours, oral absorption of paste is 77%, and absorption of granules is 85%. However, access to hay delays peak concentrations and oral absorption from granules and paste mixed with feed may be more erratic. In adult cattle, the half-life is 3–4 hours IV but 6 hours in calves. The half-life is longer when administered IM or SQ compared to IV administration. Oral absorption in cattle is 60%. There are age-related differences in pharmacokinetics in cattle, with young calves showing a slower clearance and longer half-life than older calves. In healthy weaned calves, the half-life was 6–7 hours, but in veal calves, the half-life was 13 hours, with a volume of distribution of 0.6 L/kg.

The transdermal formulation of flunixin exhibits different pharmacokinetics in cattle than the injectable form. The half-lives of the transdermal form are 9.3 and 13.2 hours in 2- and 8-month-old calves, respectively, with absorption of 40% and 63%, respectively. After transdermal application of 3.3 mg/kg to Holstein calves, the bioavailability is 48% with a half-life of 6.4 hours.

## Indications and Clinical Uses

Flunixin is used primarily for short-term treatment of moderate pain and inflammation. It has been used to treat abdominal pain in horses and to decrease signs of sepsis in horses. In horses, as an adjunctive treatment for sepsis, it is often used at a low dose of 0.25 mg/kg. The dose of 0.25 mg/kg is not an "antiendotoxin" dose, as is popularly characterized, because it does not directly inhibit endotoxin. But at this low dose, it may inhibit prostaglandins responsible for hemodynamic effects during sepsis in horses.

It is approved in the United States for treatment of pyrexia in cattle associated with BRD and to decrease clinical signs associated with coliform mastitis, as well as control of inflammation associated with endotoxemia. Flunixin has been used as a single dose for treatment of diarrhea in dairy calves. The transdermal formulation is the only NSAID approved in the United States for treatment of pain in cattle.

Flunixin at 2.2 mg/kg IV in cows with endotoxin mastitis did not affect milk production, but it decreased fever and improved rumen motility. Flunixin has been used as an adjunctive treatment, with antibiotics, for treatment of BRD in which it reduces inflammatory lung reactions and reduces BRD-associated pyrexia. Resflor Gold contains both florfenicol and flunixin in the same formulation. Hexasol contains oxytetracycline and flunixin in the same formulation.

In pigs, flunixin is used for pyrexia associated with SRD.

In dogs and cats, flunixin has been used occasionally, but treatment is usually confined to one or two treatments because of risk of GI toxicity (ulcers and perforation). Generally, other NSAIDs that have a better safety profile are used in dogs and cats.

## Precautionary Information

### Adverse Reactions and Side Effects

Most severe adverse effects are related to the GI system. Flunixin causes gastritis and GI ulceration with high doses or prolonged use. Reduced renal perfusion has also been documented. In horses, flunixin administration may affect recovery after ischemic injury to the intestine. In horses, if given IM, it can result in myositis and abscess at the injection site. It can also cause irritation and injection-site lesions if injected SQ or IM in cattle. If used in dogs, treatment should not go beyond 4 consecutive days.

### Contraindications and Precautions

Avoid use in pregnant animals near term. Do not use in calves to be processed for veal. Do not use in bulls intended for breeding because reproductive effects in this class of cattle have not been studied. Flunixin is approved for IV treatment in some food animals, but if the dose is administered IM or SQ, there is an increased risk of meat residues. Administration to cows with mastitis showed that elimination may be prolonged more than healthy cows, thus increasing the risk of violative residues, even when withdrawal times are followed. Do not use for treating heat stroke in animals.

### Drug Interactions

Ulcerogenic effects are potentiated when administered with corticosteroids. Coadministration with phenylbutazone will increase the risk of hypoproteinemia and gastric ulcers in horses. Flunixin, like other NSAIDs, may interfere with the action of diuretics such as furosemide and ACE inhibitors.

Coadministration with enrofloxacin in dogs increased flunixin plasma concentrations because of reduced clearance.

## Instructions for Use

Flunixin use in food producing animals must follow the label instructions for the condition treated. Treatment interval in all animals is limited to once daily to avoid adverse effects on GI tract and kidney. It is not approved for small animals in the United States but has been approved for use in small animals in Europe for short-term use.

## Patient Monitoring and Laboratory Tests

Monitor treated animals for signs of GI bleeding and ulcers during treatment. Monitor serum albumin in horses because repeated administration of NSAIDs has caused hypoproteinemia in some horses.

## Formulations

- 250-mg packet granules in a 10-g packet.
- 10- and 50-mg/mL injection.
- Paste formulation, with each 30-g syringe containing flunixin meglumine equivalent to 1500 mg of flunixin.
- Flunixin is combined with florfenicol in Resflor Gold, which has 300 mg florfenicol and 16.5 mg flunixin per milliliter with vehicles of 2-pyrrolidone, 35-mg malic acid, and triacetin.
- Flunixin is combined with oxytetracycline in Hexasol, with 300-mg/mL oxytetracycline and 20-mg/mL flunixin.
- Transdermal formulation: 50 mg/mL.

## Stability and Storage

Store in a tightly sealed container, protected from light, and at room temperature. Stability of compounded formulations has not been evaluated.

## Small Animal Dosage

**Dogs and Cats**

- 1.1 mg/kg once IV, IM, or SQ.
- 1.1 mg/kg/day 3 day/wk PO.
- Ophthalmic use (associated with ocular surgery): 0.5 mg/kg once IV.

## Large Animal Dosage

**Horses**

- 1.1 mg/kg q24h for up to 5 days IV or IM. Note: In foals, it has been shown that doses as low as 0.25 mg/kg inhibit prostaglandin synthesis during sepsis. Horses with colic are also often treated with low dosages of 0.25 mg/kg IV q8h.
- Paste: 1.1 mg/kg q24h PO.
- Granules: 1.1 mg/kg/day PO (one packet per 500 lb).

**Cattle**

- 1.1–2.2 mg/kg (slowly) once a day for up to 3 days IV. It may administered as a single once-daily dose or divided and administered q12h for up to 3 days.
- Veal calves: 2.2 mg/kg IV.
- In combination with florfenicol (Resflor Gold): 40 mg/kg of florfenicol and 2.2 mg/kg of flunixin administered SQ.
- Transdermal: 3.33 mg/kg applied topically to the skin. Apply only once along the dorsal midline.

**Pigs**

- 2.2 mg/kg once IM.

## Regulatory Information

**Cattle**

- For the FDA-approved IV injection formulation, the withdrawal times are 4 days for meat and 36 hours for milk. Risk of residues is higher if dose is administered IM or SQ, and the withdrawal time should be extended if other routes are used (see more details later).
- For the transdermal form administered to cattle at 3.33 mg/kg, the slaughter withdrawal time is 8 days. It should not be used in female dairy cattle 20 months of age or older, including dry dairy cows. It should not be used in suckling beef calves, dairy calves, and veal calves.
- For the formulation containing oxytetracycline and flunixin, the slaughter withdrawal time is 21 days when administered IM or SQ in beef cattle, non-lactating dairy cattle, calves, and yearlings.
- If the injection formulation is administered by other routes, FARAD recommends that after administration of a single dose to adult cattle by the IV, IM, SQ, or PO route, a milk withdrawal time of 84 hours for the IV route and 96 hours for the other routes, and 7 days for meat should be used. If multiple doses are administered, FARAD recommends a meat withdrawal time of 60 days. Because of differences in pharmacokinetics, FARAD (www.FARAD.org) recommends a meat withdrawal time of at least 14 days when flunixin is administered to dairy heifers, beef steers, and veal calves.

**Pigs**

- After administration of formulations that do not have a swine label, such as 2.2 mg/kg IM once, FARAD recommends a meat withdrawal time of 13–15 days.

- After oral or IV administration to pigs, of 2.2 mg/kg, FARAD recommends a meat withdrawal time of 21 days.
- If a specific swine-labeled dose form is used (Banamine-S), the withdrawal time is 12 days.

RCI Classification: 4

# Fluorouracil
floo-roe-yoo′rah-sil

**Trade and other names:** 5-Fluorouracil and Adrucil

**Functional classification:** Anticancer agent

## Pharmacology and Mechanism of Action

Fluorouracil is an anticancer agent also referred to as 5-fluorouracil (5-FU). 5-FU is an analogue of thymidine and uracil, which are bases of DNA and RNA, respectively. When used as an anticancer agent, it acts as an antimetabolite and disrupts DNA and RNA to inhibit cancer cell growth. Fluorouracil is used in veterinary anticancer protocols such as carcinomas, osteosarcoma, hemangiosarcoma, transmissible venereal tumor, and mast cell tumors.

## Indications and Clinical Uses

Fluorouracil is used in various cancer protocols in dogs but infrequently compared with other agents. It has been used as a component with other combination cancer regimens.

## Precautionary Information

### Adverse Reactions and Side Effects

The toxicity from fluorouracil is most evident in rapidly growing cells (bone marrow, intestinal epithelium, and epithelial cells). Fluorouracil causes mild leukopenia, thrombocytopenia, and CNS toxicity. In dogs, it has caused GI sloughing, vomiting, respiratory distress, myelosuppression, behavioral changes, seizures, other neurologic signs, and cardiac abnormalities.

Dogs have been accidentally exposed by consuming topical formulations intended for people. Doses of 40 mg/kg in dogs result in death, and doses of 20, 10, and 5 mg/kg have caused high, intermediate, and low toxic effects in dogs, respectively.

### Contraindications and Precautions

Do not use in cats.

### Drug Interactions

No drug interactions are reported for animals because of the limited use. However, with any anticancer agent, drug interactions are possible.

## Instructions for Use

Consult anticancer treatment protocol for precise dosage and regimen.

Patient monitoring and laboratory tests: Monitor CBC for evidence of bone marrow toxicity.

## Formulations
- Fluorouracil is available in a 50-mg/mL vial. It is also available in topical forms as 0.5%, 1%, 2%, and 5% solutions and 1% and 5% creams. The topical forms are used in people for skin tumors and keratosis.

## Stability and Storage
Store in a tightly sealed container, protected from light, and at room temperature. Stability of compounded formulations has not been evaluated.

## Small Animal Dosage
**Dogs**
- 150 mg/m$^2$ once per week IV.

**Cats**
- Do not use.

## Large Animal Dosage
- No large animal doses have been reported.

## Regulatory Information
Withdrawal times are not established for animals that produce food. This drug should not be used in food animals because it is an anticancer agent.

**F**

---

# Fluoxetine Hydrochloride
floo-oks′eh-teen hye-droe-klor′ide

**Trade and other names:** Prozac (human formulation) and Reconcile (veterinary formulation)

**Functional classification:** Behavior modification, selective serotonin reuptake inhibitor

## Pharmacology and Mechanism of Action
Fluoxetine is an antidepressant drug and used for behavior problems in animals. Fluoxetine, like other drugs in this class, is a selective serotonin reuptake inhibitor (SSRI). Its mechanism of action is through selective inhibition of serotonin reuptake and downregulation of 5-HT$_1$ receptors. SSRIs are more selective for inhibiting serotonin reuptake than the TCAs; therefore there may be fewer effects on other receptors compared with other behavior-modifying drugs.

*Pharmacokinetics:* Fluoxetine is metabolized to norfluoxetine, which is an active metabolite. Oral absorption in dogs is 72% with a half-life of 6–10 hours. The metabolite norfluoxetine has a longer half-life of 48–57 hours. In cats, oral absorption is 100% with a half-life of 34–47 hours; the metabolite norfluoxetine has a half-life of 51–55 hours. Absorption in cats from transdermal administration is only 10%. Another SSRI used in animals is paroxetine (Paxil).

## Indications and Clinical Uses
Fluoxetine, like other SSRIs, is used to treat behavioral disorders such as separation anxiety, canine compulsive behaviors, and dominance aggression. In cats, it has been effective for decreasing urine spraying (1 mg/kg/day). In trials comparing fluoxetine with clomipramine for treating urine marking in cats, both drugs were equally effective for long-term use. However, the urine marking returned after discontinuation of

the drug. In both dogs and cats, SSRIs have been used for pain syndromes, such as neuropathic pain, but there are no studies of efficacy published to confirm efficacy for this indication. In horses, fluoxetine has been used for "cribbing behavior" and other behavior disorders, but efficacy is based on small observational studies.

## Precautionary Information

### Adverse Reactions and Side Effects

Fluoxetine has fewer adverse effects (especially antihistamine and antimuscarinic effects) compared with other antidepressant drugs. During clinical trials in dogs, adverse reactions included vomiting, decreased appetite, lethargy, depression, trembling, and shaking in some dogs; the most common were lethargy and decreased appetite. In rare cases, it may cause seizures. Adverse effects are more common at doses above 8–10 mg/kg, but occasionally, some of these signs may be seen at lower doses. In dogs, at high doses of 10–20 mg/kg, it caused tremors, anorexia, aggressive behavior, nystagmus, emesis, and ataxia. Seizures can occur at doses above 25 mg/kg.

In cats, nervousness or increased anxiousness has been observed. In cats, 5 mg/kg produced tremors, and 3 mg/kg produced anorexia and vomiting. However, in trials used for treating urine spraying, few adverse effects were reported, and cats have tolerated doses up to 50 mg/kg.

### Contraindications and Precautions

Use cautiously in animals prone to aggression because it may decrease inhibition. In early pregnancy, it appears to be safe but has caused pulmonary hypertension in experimental animals late in pregnancy. Serotonin reuptake inhibitors can increase the risk of bleeding by inhibiting serotonin uptake by platelets, but this has not been reported in animals.

### Drug Interactions

Do not use with other behavior-modifying drugs such as other SSRIs or TCAs. Do not use with monoamine oxidase inhibitors (MAOIs). Administration with selegiline may induce a reaction. Because it is highly metabolized by the liver, it may be subject to interactions caused by cytochrome P450 inhibitors. (See Appendix I.)

## Instructions for Use

Always use in conjunction with a comprehensive behavior modification protocol. Clinical efficacy of fluoxetine for separation anxiety in dogs has been established from clinical studies. Because of a long half-life, accumulation in plasma may take several days to weeks. There may be a delay in the onset of action of 2 weeks. Do not apply transdermally; absorption is low, and it may cause skin irritation.

In some animals, paroxetine (Paxil) is preferred, which is a human formulation available in tablets and has been used for smaller-size animals.

Sudden discontinuation of serotonin reuptake inhibitors can produce other behavior problems, such as anxiety, signs of agitation and nervousness. If treatment is discontinued, gradually withdraw the medication.

## Patient Monitoring and Laboratory Tests

Use in animals has been relatively safe, and one should only monitor behavior changes.

## Formulations

- Fluoxetine is available in human formulations of 10-, 20-, and 40-mg capsules; 10-, 20-, and 60-mg tablets; and 4-mg/mL oral solution. The veterinary formulations have been available in sizes of 8-, 16-, 32-, and 64-mg tablets.

## Stability and Storage

Store in a tightly sealed container, protected from light, and at room temperature. It is soluble in water at 14 mg/mL and in alcohol at 100 mg/mL. Fluoxetine hydrochloride solution has been mixed with various juices and flavorings and found to be stable for 8 weeks. In one trial, it was mixed in tuna-flavored water for cats and retained effectiveness.

## Small Animal Dosage

**Dogs**
- 1–2 mg/kg once daily PO.

**Cats**
- 0.5–4 mg/cat q24h PO (0.5–1 mg/kg/day). Start with 1/4 tablet (2.5 mg) per cat and increase as needed.
- Urine marking: 1 mg/kg q24h PO and increase to 1.5 mg/kg if there has been inadequate response.

## Large Animal Dosage
- Horses: 0.25–0.5 mg/kg PO once daily, mixed with grain.

## Regulatory Information

Do not administer to animals intended for food.
RCI Classification: 2

# Fluralaner

floor ′ah-lan′er

**Trade and other names:** Bravecto

**Functional classification:** Antiparasitic, Ectoparasiticide

## Pharmacology and Mechanism of Action

Fluralaner belongs to the isooxazolines class of ectoparasiticides. It is effective for treating and preventing infections from fleas, mites, and ticks. It produces selective inhibition of the GABA receptor and L-glutamate–gated chloride channels. This inhibition of the receptor produces changes in chloride channels, hyperexcitement of the parasite, and death. Mammals are not affected because of a lack of binding to mammalian GABA receptors.

Efficacy has been demonstrated against a wide range of ectoparasites, including fleas, various mites (including *Demodex* and *Sarcoptes* spp.), and ticks. The parasite must bite the animal for exposure to the agent. Activity of the isooxazolines has been superior to other ectoparasiticides, including dieldrin, fipronil, deltamethrin, and imidacloprid.

*Pharmacokinetics:* Fluralaner has a long half-life in dogs. After topical or oral administration, the peak concentration occurs between 2 hours and 3 days. The half-life ranges between 14 and 29 days with a bioavailability from either route of approximately 25%.

Other drugs in this class with similar activity but different pharmacokinetics include afoxolaner, lotilaner, and sarolaner.

## Indications and Clinical Uses

Fluralaner, like the other isooxazolines is active against fleas, mites, and ticks. After oral administration or topical application, it can start killing fleas within

2–4 hours, with practically 100% of the fleas killed by 8 hours. The chew tablet for dogs has an approved indication for killing adult fleas and to prevent flea infestations (*Ctenocephalides felis*). It is also approved for treatment and control of tick infestations. Because of this action, fluralaner can reduce the risk that these vectors may pose for disease transmission. For example, it may prevent infections caused by *Borrelia burgdorferi* (Lyme disease) and *Babesia canis*.

The approved label indication for fluralaner is treatment of fleas and ticks, but extralabel uses, using the approved label dose, have included treatment of generalized demodicosis caused by *Demodex canis*. In a clinical study, there were greater reductions in mites from treatment with fluralaner compared with treatment with moxidectin and imidacloprid . A single dose was effective for eliminating sarcoptic mange (*Sarcoptes scabiei*) in dogs. It has also been effective for eliminating ear mites (*Otodectes cynotis*) in dogs and cats.

The proper use of fluralaner involves administration of an oral chew tablets, administered with or without food, or application of a topical solution. A topical solution containing both fluralaner and moxidectin is available for cats (Bravecto Plus) for prevention of heartworm, roundworms, hookworms, and fleas and ticks.

Exotic species: There have been successful accounts of treatment in zoo or exotic species, without adverse effects, such as rabbits, bears, and other zoo mammals.

## Precautionary Information

### Adverse Reactions and Side Effects

Adverse effects have been rare from administration of fluralaner. It has been safe in dogs at least 6 months of age. Collie breeds and other herding breeds with genetic mutations of the *MDR* gene or *ABCB1* gene can be treated safely with fluralaner. It can also be used with other ectoparasiticides such as ivermectin and milbemycin.

Adverse effects reported from the manufacturer's safety studies (some at high doses) of the chewable tablet include vomiting, diarrhea, lethargy, and reduced appetite. According to the manufacturer, it should not be used in puppies or kittens younger than 6 months of age, but they performed safety studies in puppies 8–9 weeks of age at five times the clinical dose and there were no adverse effects.

For the topical solution, the most common adverse effects included vomiting, hair loss, diarrhea, lethargy, decreased appetite, and moist dermatitis or rash and scabs or ulcerated lesions on the skin. It was safe in adult cats and kittens older than 6 months of age. In safety studies in kittens at least 11–13 weeks of age, it was safe at five times the dose.

There is a concern about neurologic adverse effects, including seizures, from administration of isooxazolines in dogs. This has been reported primarily with sarolaner, but the manufacturer of fluralaner warns that it should be used cautiously in dogs or cats with a history of seizures. In cats, neurologic problems were observed in 2 of 244 cats involved with a field study.

### Contraindications and Precautions

There are no known contraindications. Fluralaner was studied at three times the dose in laboratory animals, and adverse effects on breeding, pregnancy, or lactation were not observed. However, safety in breeding cats has not been studied. Because of risk of seizures, use cautiously in animals prone to seizures.

### Drug Interactions

There are no known drug interactions with fluralaner. It has been administered safely with vaccines, anthelmintics, antibiotics, and corticosteroids. It should not be used concurrently with other drugs in the isooxazoline class because this may increase the risk of neurologic problems.

## Instructions for Use

Doses for fluralaner are established from the approved label dosing. Interval of dosing is based on efficacy studies. It is effective for treatment of fleas and most ticks for 12 weeks but not beyond 8 weeks for the Lone Star tick (*Amblyomma americanum*). It can eliminate sarcoptic mange with a single dose. In cats, it was effective for fleas and ticks for 12 weeks but not beyond 8 weeks for the American dog tick (*Dermacentor variabilis*).

The oral chew tablets can be administered with, or without food. To administer the topical solution, follow the instructions on the product label. The hair between the shoulder blades on dogs or behind the head on cats should be parted and the contents of the solution should be applied to the skin. Avoid contact with the application site until it has dried.

## Patient Monitoring and Laboratory Tests

There is no routine monitoring required. Monitor response to treatment through clinical examination of skin at regular check-ups.

## Formulations

- Fluralaner is available in a flavored chew tablet for dogs in 112.5-, 250-, 500-, 1000-, and 1400-mg sizes.
- Fluralaner is available as a topical solution with 280 mg of fluralaner per milliliter in each tube. Each tube is packaged separately in sizes of 112.5-, 250-, 500-, 1000-, and 1400-mg per tube.
- Fluralaner topical solution for cats. Each tube is formulated to administer a 40-mg/kg dose. Each milliliter contains 280 mg of fluralaner in sizes of 112.5-, 250-, and 500-mg per tube.
- Fluralaner and moxidectin topical solution for cats is available as 280 mg fluralaner and 14 mg moxidectin per milliliter.

## Stability and Storage

Fluralaner should be stored in a dry place at controlled temperatures less than 25°C.

## Small Animal Dosage

### Dogs

- 25 mg/kg once every 12 weeks for either oral chew tablets or topical solution.
- Treatment of *Demodex* infection: 25 mg/kg at 12-week intervals.

### Cats

- 40 mg/kg topical solution applied every 12 weeks.
- The combination of fluralaner and moxidectin for cats (Bravecto Plus) should be applied at a dose of 40 mg/kg fluralaner and 0.9 mg/kg moxidectin every 2 months.

## Large Animal Dosage

No large animal doses have been established.

## Regulatory Information

No withdrawal times are established for animals intended for food (extralabel use).

# Fluticasone Propionate

floo-tik′ah-sone proe-pee-oe-nayt

**Trade and other names:** Flovent

**Functional classification:** Corticosteroid

## Pharmacology and Mechanism of Action

Fluticasone is a potent glucocorticoid anti-inflammatory drug with potency 18 times that of dexamethasone. It is usually administered as a topical (local) application, most often for inflammatory airway disease. In patients with inflammatory airway diseases, glucocorticoids have potent anti-inflammatory effects on the bronchial mucosa. Glucocorticoids bind to receptors on cells and inhibit the transcription of genes for the production of mediators (cytokines, chemokines, adhesion molecules) involved in airway inflammation. Glucocorticoids decrease the synthesis of inflammatory mediators such as prostaglandins, leukotrienes, and platelet-activating factor, which also may be important in these diseases. Glucocorticoids also play a role in enhancing the action of adrenergic agonists on $beta_2$ receptors in the bronchial smooth muscle, either by modifying the receptor or augmenting muscle relaxation after a receptor has been bound. Corticosteroids also may prevent downregulation of $beta_2$ receptors.

Topical (inhaled) corticosteroids such as fluticasone or budesonide are used to avoid systemic effects. They typically have high first-pass effects and low systemic exposure if swallowed. Because of low systemic effects, fluticasone produces fewer systemic steroid effects than prednisolone, such as effects on water consumption, appetite, and systemic immunity.

## Indications and Clinical Uses

Fluticasone is used as an inhaled (topical) corticosteroid for treatment of airway disease. Most of the use has been established for cats, but it also could be used for dogs, horses, or other animals in which a special adapter can be used to deliver the drug via a metered-dose inhaler (MDI). In dogs and cats, the most common use is for inflammatory airway diseases such as asthma, bronchitis, or bronchospasm. For example, if a cat is given 2 puffs twice a day of a potent inhaled corticosteroid (e.g., budesonide, fluticasone) and allowed 5–7 breaths (10 seconds) from a chamber (spacer), it may reduce the need for oral prednisolone in cats with feline asthma. When doses were compared in experimental cats, the low dosage of 44 mcg twice daily was as effective as 110 or 220 mcg twice daily.

In horses, the most common use is for equine asthma syndrome characterized by RAO.

### Precautionary Information

#### Adverse Reactions and Side Effects

Although fluticasone systemic absorption is low, some systemic exposure will occur in animals. Side effects can occur but are not expected to be as severe as with systemic corticosteroids. Adrenal suppression is expected to occur in treated animals (suppressed ACTH response) but may recover once treatment is discontinued.

#### Contraindications and Precautions

Use cautiously in patients with oral or respiratory tract infections because immunosuppression may occur.

#### Drug Interactions

Some systemic effects are possible but minimal. Administration of corticosteroids with NSAIDs will increase the risk of GI injury.

### Instructions for Use

The use is based on administration of fluticasone for treatment of airway diseases. It is delivered via an MDI. These inhalers can be used in animals if special adaptations, such as a spacer device, which are available for cats, dogs, and horses, are used. When treating dogs and cats, doses listed in the dosing section can be used initially and are then adjusted depending on response.

## Patient Monitoring and Laboratory Tests
Monitor liver enzymes, blood glucose, and renal function during therapy. Monitor patients for signs of secondary infections. Perform ACTH stimulation test if it is necessary to monitor adrenal function. Fluticasone, although minimally absorbed systemically, will suppress the ACTH response.

## Formulations
• MDI at 44, 110, or 220 mcg per puff.

## Stability and Storage
Store in original container (MDI). Do not puncture container or attempt to remove drug from pressurized container. Stability of compounded formulations has not been evaluated.

## Small Animal Dosage
**Dogs**
• Start with 220 mcg per dose q12h delivered with an MDI. As patient is stabilized, decrease dose gradually to 110 mcg per dose, lower if possible.

**Cats**
• Start with 44 mcg per dose (1 puff from a 44-mcg inhaler) twice daily. Increase the dose as needed to 110 mcg and then to 220 mcg.

## Large Animal Dosage
**Horses**
• 1–2 mg per horse (6–12 puffs from 220-mcg inhaler) twice daily for airway disease.
• For long-term management in horses, start with 2 mg per horse q24h; then gradually taper to 1.5 mg per horse every other day.

## Regulatory Information
There are no US withdrawal times established.
RCI classification: not established.

# Fomepizole
foh-meh′pih-zole
**Trade and other names:** 4-Methylpyrazole, Antizol-Vet, and Antizol (human preparation)
**Functional classification:** Antidote

## Pharmacology and Mechanism of Action
Fomepizole, which is also known as 4-methylpyrazole, is an antidote for ethylene glycol (antifreeze) and methanol intoxication. It inhibits the dehydrogenase enzyme that converts ethylene glycol to toxic metabolites.

## Indications and Clinical Uses
Fomepizole is used for treatment of acute ethylene glycol toxicosis in dogs and cats. In people, it is used for this purpose but also is registered for methanol poisoning.

It should be used early for maximum success. Fomepizole was safe and effective in dogs in clinical trials if used within 8 hours of poisoning. In cats, it is effective if administered at high doses within 3 hours of ethylene glycol ingestion. When fomepizole is unavailable, ethanol can be used as an alternative.

## Precautionary Information

**Adverse Reactions and Side Effects**
No adverse effects have been reported.

**Contraindications and Precautions**
Treatment should be initiated early for optimum effect. In cats, treatment should be initiated within 3 hours using a dose that is higher than for dogs.

**Drug Interactions**
Fomepizole will inhibit the metabolism of other drugs and compounds that share a similar pathway as alcohol. Use cautiously with any other coadministered drugs.

## Instructions for Use

The only use documented is for emergency management of ethylene glycol intoxication. Experimental studies have demonstrated effectiveness in dogs and cats (high doses in cats). In cats, administration of ethanol infusion is also effective. Administer 0.9% sodium chloride before administration of fomepizole. If used for treating methanol intoxication, include administration of folinic acid (Leucovorin) at a dose of 1 mg/kg.

## Patient Monitoring and Laboratory Tests

Monitor renal function during treatment. Monitor urine output. Some human hospitals have assays for monitoring ethylene glycol in patients. These assays can be used to monitor treated cats.

## Formulations

- Note: The veterinary-approved product has recently been withdrawn by the manufacturer. The human formulation, or ethanol, can be used as an alternative. Fomepizole is available in a 1-g/mL solution (Antizol), a human preparation. 1.5 g may be added to 30 mL saline solution for injection (50 mg/mL).

## Stability and Storage

Store in a tightly sealed container, protected from light, and at room temperature. Stability of compounded formulations has not been evaluated.

## Small Animal Dosage

**Dogs**
- 20 mg/kg initially IV, then 15 mg/kg at 12- and 24-hour intervals, and then 5 mg at 36 hours.

**Cats**
- 125 mg/kg initially followed by 31.3 mg/kg at 12, 24, and 36 hours after the initial dose. Continue doses q12h until ethylene glycol is no longer detected. If analysis of ethylene glycol is not available, treat with 31 mg/kg q12h through 60 hours.

## Large Animal Dosage

- No large animal doses have been reported.

## Regulatory Information

No withdrawal times are established for animals intended for food. There is little risk of residues in food animals.

# Fosfomycin Tromethamine
fos-foe-mye'sin troe-meth'ah-meen

**Trade and other names:** Monurol

**Functional classification:** Antibacterial (urinary)

## Pharmacology and Mechanism of Action

Fosfomycin is a urinary antimicrobial. It inhibits cell walls of susceptible bacteria and may decrease virulence by inhibiting the adherence of bacteria to bladder mucosa. It produces adequate concentrations in urine to manage UTIs. The concentrations in other tissues may not be high enough for treatment of non-UTIs. In people, it is used as a single dose to treat an acute UTI. For gram-negative urinary pathogens, the mutation frequency for resistance is high. This raises concerns related to the potential for the development of resistance to fosfomycin during therapy.

*Pharmacokinetics:* In dogs, the half-life is short (1.1 hours IV and 2–3 hours PO), with good oral absorption.

## Indications and Clinical Uses

Fosfomycin has been used as treatment or adjunctive treatment for UTIs. In women, it is used as a single dose to treat acute UTIs. Although this may be an accepted treatment for people, the use in animals has been primarily derived from empirical use and small observational studies. There are no well-controlled clinical studies or efficacy trials to document clinical effectiveness.

## Precautionary Information

### Adverse Reactions and Side Effects

No adverse effects have been reported, but use in animals has been very limited. It has been safe and well tolerated in dogs up to 120–200 mg/kg.

### Contraindications and Precautions

Do not administer in dry form; mix with water. There are no other known contraindications. Fosfomycin should not be substituted for antibiotics with established efficacy.

### Drug Interactions

No known drug interactions, but the use in animals has been very rare and not sufficient to assess potential drug interactions.

## Instructions for Use

Fosfomycin has been used to treat UTIs in animals, primarily when other drugs have failed or were inactive as a result of resistance. Alternatively, fosfomycin has been used intermittently (pulse therapy) to prevent recurrences of UTIs. The efficacy of any of these indications is not established in animals and based on only small observational studies or anecdotal use.

## Patient Monitoring and Laboratory Tests

Monitor UTI with culture and urinalysis. The susceptibility testing breakpoints may not apply to bacteria isolated from animals.

## Formulations

- Fosfomycin is available in a 3-g packet. The packet also contains saccharin and sucrose for flavoring. This packet may be mixed with water and administered immediately orally.

## Stability and Storage
Store in original package, protected from light, and at room temperature. Stability of compounded formulations has not been evaluated.

## Small Animal Dosage
**Dogs**
- Precise doses are not established for dogs; 75–150 mg/kg q12h PO has been recommended based on pharmacokinetic studies. Additional cited doses used are empiric and include a recommendation of a 3-g packet divided equally into three daily doses (1 g dissolved in 30 mL) and administered daily to dogs.

**Cats**
- No doses have been established for cats.

## Large Animal Dosage
- No large animal doses have been reported.

## Regulatory Information
No withdrawal times are established for animals intended for food.

# Furazolidone
fyoo-rah-zole′ih-done
**Trade and other names:** Furoxone
**Functional classification:** Antiparasitic

## Pharmacology and Mechanism of Action
Furazolidone is an oral antiprotozoal drug with activity against *Giardia* spp., and it may have some activity against bacteria in the intestine. It is used for only local treatment of intestinal parasites; it is not used for systemic therapy.

## Indications and Clinical Uses
Furazolidone has been used to treat protozoal intestinal parasites. However, because efficacy and safety of other oral antiprotozoal drugs are better established, they are used more often.

## Precautionary Information
**Adverse Reactions and Side Effects**
Adverse effects are not reported in animals. In people, mild anemia, hypersensitivity, and disturbance of intestinal flora have been reported.

**Contraindications and Precautions**
No contraindications reported for animals.

**Drug Interactions**
Do not use with MAOIs.

## Instructions for Use
Clinical studies have not been reported for animals. Doses and recommendations are based on extrapolation from humans. Other drugs, such as fenbendazole, may be preferred for treating *Giardia* infections.

## Patient Monitoring and Laboratory Tests
No specific monitoring is necessary.

## Formulations
- Furazolidone has been discontinued in the United States. It may be available through some compounding pharmacies. The previously available tablet was 100 mg.

## Stability and Storage
Store in a tightly sealed container, protected from light, and at room temperature. Stability of compounded formulations has not been evaluated.

## Small Animal Dosage
- 4 mg/kg q12h for 7–10 days PO.

## Large Animal Dosage
- No large animal doses have been reported.

## Regulatory Information
No regulatory information is available. For extralabel use withdrawal interval estimates, contact FARAD at www.FARAD.org.

# Furosemide
fyoo-roe′seh-mide

**Trade and other names:** Lasix and generic brands
**Functional classification:** Diuretic

## Pharmacology and Mechanism of Action
Furosemide is a loop diuretic that inhibits the $Na^+/K^+/2Cl^-$ cotransporter in the ascending thick loop of Henle. It is often called *a high-ceiling diuretic* because it is more effective than other diuretics. Furosemide decreases the sodium, chloride, and potassium reabsorption from the tubule. Subsequently, these ions are retained in the renal tubule and presented to the distal nephron. Dilute urine is produced because water is retained in the tubule when it reaches the distal tubule. In addition, there is an associated urine loss of $Mg^{2+}$ and $Ca^{2+}$. An additional mechanism of action is via prostaglandin synthesis. Furosemide increases intrarenal prostaglandin production (e.g., $PGI_2$), which increases renal blood flow. Synthesis of prostaglandins also may cause vasodilation in other tissues. Torsemide is another diuretic in the same class as furosemide. It has greater potency than furosemide and can be used in refractory cases.

*Pharmacokinetics:* The plasma half-life in animals is short (1.5–3 hours); therefore, this is a short-acting drug, with a maximum onset of effect of 1–2 hours and a duration of 2–4 hours. Oral absorption can be highly variable but in dogs is as high as 77%. SQ absorption is as high as other injectable routes. In horses, oral absorption is so low that this is not a viable method of administration.

## Indications and Clinical Uses
In small animals, furosemide is the drug of choice to treat conditions that cause edema, including pulmonary edema, liver disease, heart disease, and vascular disease. It is recommended in dogs with clinical signs of stage C heart disease, to be used initially, until the patient's clinical signs have improved. Furosemide increases potassium and calcium excretion and is used to treat hyperkalemia and hypercalcemia.

The use of furosemide for AKI treatment has no benefit or effect on patient outcome based on available evidence. Furosemide promotes urine output by decreasing reabsorption of sodium but does not increase glomerular filtration rate.

In horses, furosemide has been used to treat edema and syndromes associated with congestion. The most common use in horses is pretreatment prior to racing. Although it appears to produce faster racing times, the mechanism is unclear. It may decrease body weight via water loss and may decrease exercise-induced pulmonary hemorrhage (EIPH). The efficacy to reduce EIPH has been controversial in horses, but there is reported evidence to support this effect. In cattle, furosemide also is used for treating conditions of edema (e.g., udder edema) and for treatment of heart failure and pulmonary hypertension.

In all animals, duration of effect is short, approximately 2–4 hours. Because of short duration, CRIs can produce greater efficacy in some animals.

## Precautionary Information

### Adverse Reactions and Side Effects
Adverse effects are primarily related to diuretic effect (loss of fluid and electrolytes). In dogs, hyponatremia is more common than hypokalemia. Tolerance and activation of the renin–angiotensin–aldosterone system (RAAS) occur with repeated administration, in which the diuretic effect is attenuated. When administered to dogs at a dosage of 2 mg/kg q12h, it significantly increased RAAS activity by day 5 of treatment. When the RAAS is activated, increased concentrations of aldosterone can have persistent and deleterious effects on vasculature and cardiac remodeling. SQ injection may cause irritation (stinging) at the injection site.

### Contraindications and Precautions
Administer conservatively in animals receiving ACE inhibitors to decrease the risk of azotemia. Repeated administration may increase aldosterone levels via activation of RAAS.

### Drug Interactions
Concurrent use with aminoglycoside antibiotics or amphotericin B may increase risk of nephrotoxicity and ototoxicity. Administration of NSAIDs with furosemide may diminish the effect. The pH of solution is 8–9.8. Furosemide is stable with alkaline drugs but it should not be mixed with acidifying drug solutions with a pH less than 5.5.

## Instructions for Use
Recommendations for use of furosemide are based on extensive clinical use of furosemide in animals. The onset of effect after an injection is usually 5 minutes, with the peak at 30 minutes to 2 hours and a duration of approximately 2–4 hours. CRIs in dogs and horses can be more effective than intermittent bolus. Long-term repeated administration may attenuate the effects because of tolerance and activation of the RAAS.

## Patient Monitoring and Laboratory Tests
Monitor electrolyte concentrations (particularly potassium) and hydration status in patients during treatment.

## Formulations
- Furosemide is available in 12.5-, 20-, 40-, 50-, and 80-mg tablets; 20-, 40-, and 80-mg tablets (human preparation); 10-mg/mL oral solution (syrup); and 50-mg/

ml injection. Tablets usually can be easily split. A 2-g bolus is available for large animals, but oral absorption is uncertain.

## Stability and Storage

Store in a tightly sealed container, protected from light, and at room temperature. Do not mix with acidic solutions. It is compatible in plastic syringes and infusion sets. Furosemide is poorly soluble in water but may be mixed with 5% dextrose, 0.9% saline, or lactated Ringer's solution at a concentration of 10 mg/mL for IV administration. These solutions are stable for 8 hours. It is more soluble if the pH is greater than 8, but it readily precipitates when pH is less than 5.5. Compounded oral formulations in syrups and other flavorings are stable if kept at alkaline pH or in alcohol. However, lower pH results in instability of formulation. If discoloration occurs, discard formulation.

**F**

## Small Animal Dosage

### Dogs

- 2–6 mg/kg q8–12h (or as needed) IV, IM, SQ, or PO. A common initial dose when treating heart failure patients is 2 mg/kg q12h PO; then lower to 1–2 mg/ kg q12h PO.
- In acute cases in which intensive treatment is needed, administer 2 mg/kg IV followed by 2 mg/kg every 30 minutes until improvement is seen.
- CRI: 0.66 mg/kg bolus dose IV followed by 0.66 mg/kg/h for 8 hours. Alternatively, a dose of 2 mg/kg in 5% glucose can be infused over an 8-hour period IV.

### Cats

- Start with 1 mg/kg; then increase as needed, within a range of 1–4 mg/kg q8–24h IV, IM, SQ, or PO.

## Large Animal Dosage

### Horses

- 1 mg/kg q8h or 250–500 mg/horse at 6- to 8-hour intervals IM or IV.
- CRI: 0.12 mg/kg IV followed by 0.12 mg/kg/h IV.
- Prevention of EIPH: 0.5 or 1 mg/kg IV, administered 4 hours prior to exercise or administered 24 hours preracing. Consult local racetrack jurisdiction for restrictions on administration.

### Cattle

- 500 mg/animal once a day or 250 mg/animal twice a day IM or IV.

## Regulatory Information

Cattle withdrawal times: 2 days meat and 48 hours milk.
Horses: Most racing regulations specify that a 250-mg/horse dose may be given by a single IV injection no later than 4 hours before racing post time. In most horses, this does not produce violations above 100 ng/mL urine threshold at 4 hours. Check local racetrack jurisdiction for restrictions for administration on race day.

# Gabapentin
gab′ah-pen-tin

**Trade and other names:** Neurontin and generic brands

**Functional classification:** Anticonvulsant, analgesic

## Pharmacology and Mechanism of Action

Gabapentin is used as both an anticonvulsant and analgesic. Gabapentin is an analogue of the inhibitory neurotransmitter gamma-aminobutyric acid (GABA); however, it is not an agonist or antagonist for the GABA receptor. The mechanism of anticonvulsant action and analgesic effects is not clear, but there is evidence that the mechanism of action appears to be via blocking calcium-dependent channels. Gabapentin inhibits the alpha-2-delta ($\alpha_2\delta$) subunit of the N-type voltage-dependent calcium channel on neurons. Through inhibition of these channels, it reduces the calcium influx that is needed for release of neurotransmitters—specifically, excitatory amino acids—from presynaptic neurons. Blocking the channels has little effect on normal neurons, but it may suppress stimulated neurons involved in seizure activity and pain.

Another related drug is pregabalin (Lyrica), which is used in people for neuropathic pain and has also been used in dogs.

*Pharmacokinetics:* Half-lives in dogs and cats are only 3–4 hours and 2.8 hours, respectively, which may necessitate frequent administration. In horses, the half-life has ranged considerably, depending on the study. In one study, it was 6.7–12 hours; and in another, it was 3–4 hours. In a study examining doses of 10–160 mg/kg, the half-life ranged from 11–15 hours. Oral absorption in horses was only 16% resulting in lower plasma concentrations in horses compared to other animals. Gabapentin is eliminated entirely by renal clearance in people, but there is 30%–40% hepatic metabolism in dogs. Therefore, drugs that affect liver metabolism or severe liver disease may decrease gabapentin clearance in dogs.

## Indications and Clinical Uses

Gabapentin is used as an anticonvulsant, sedative, anxiolytic, and to treat chronic pain syndromes, including neuropathic pain. It is used to treat neuropathic pain that does not respond to nonsteroidal anti-inflammatory drugs (NSAIDs) or opioids. However, studies demonstrating efficacy for pain treatment in dogs and cats are currently lacking. It was not effective for postoperative pain in dogs and was not effective in a thermal nociceptive study in experimental cats at doses up to 30 mg/kg. However, it has been effective in one study in dogs with syringomyelia.

In cats, it has also been used to reduce anxiety in cats prior to traveling, visits to the veterinarian, or other stressful events with evidence from clinical studies that it may be helpful for this indication. For this use, administer 100 mg per cat ($\approx$20–30 mg/kg) 90 minutes prior to a stressful event (e.g., visit to a veterinary office). The peak effect occurs in 2–3 hours. This use may decrease stress-related behavior and aggression and improve compliance of cats.

In dogs, gabapentin has gained attention, as adjunctive treatment, for treating anxiety, phobias, panic disorders, and compulsive disorders. It is used when other agents (selective serotonin reuptake inhibitors [SSRIs] or tricyclic antidepressants [TCAs]) have not been effective and has been used concurrently with SSRIs or TCAs).

In horses, gabapentin has been used to treat laminitis and other pain syndromes, but efficacy has not been shown in well-controlled studies. The use is based on anecdotal or small observational case studies. It has low and variable oral absorption in horses, and the doses have varied widely (5–20 mg/kg two or three times daily). In calves, it has a long half-life but is not effective for analgesia in dehorning procedures.

When used to treat epilepsy, gabapentin (or pregabalin) is rarely used as a single agent but is considered when the seizures have become refractory to other drugs. Neurologists consider gabapentin an "add-on" for treating seizures in animals, but it is not very effective when used alone. When included in a regimen as an add-on, it is not as effective as zonisamide or levetiracetam.

## Precautionary Information

### Adverse Reactions and Side Effects

Sedation and ataxia are reported adverse effects. As dose increases in dogs (see the dosing section), sedation is more likely. In people, a withdrawal syndrome from abrupt discontinuation has been described, but it is not reported in animals. However, based on this concern in people, gradual withdrawal should be considered. When high doses are administered (see the dosing section), adverse effects include ataxia, decreased appetite, vomiting, and diarrhea. Some of these effects are transient, but if they persist, lower the dose by one-half or consider another alternative.

The oral solution contains xylitol, which is an artificial sweetener that can be toxic to dogs and produces hypoglycemia and liver injury with high doses exceeding 0.1 g/kg. With standard doses of gabapentin oral solution, the toxic level of xylitol is not likely to be exceeded, but one should be cautious about adding other drugs that also contain xylitol.

### Contraindications and Precautions

No known contraindications in animals. However, because this is only licensed as a human drug, the full extent of adverse effects and precautions in animals is not known. Any discontinuation of this medication should be done with a gradual taper, rather than a sudden withdrawal.

### Drug Interactions

Antacids decrease oral absorption. If antacids are administered, there should be 2 hours between dosing of each drug. Other drug interactions are possible based on experience in people, but these have not been documented in animals. If an animal is scheduled for an anesthetic procedure, consider lower doses of the anesthetic or sedative used for anesthesia.

## Instructions for Use

Gabapentin has been used in some animals as an anticonvulsant when they are refractory to other drugs. It can be used with other drugs such as phenobarbital and bromide. It also has been used to treat neuropathic pain syndromes and can be used with NSAIDs and opioids. Efficacy for each of these indications is anecdotal or based on small uncontrolled observational studies; there are no controlled studies published to show efficacy for treating pain syndromes in animals. Gabapentin has been administered to cats to reduce anxiety and fear associated with stressful events. For this use, administer gabapentin orally 2–3 hours prior to the anticipated stressful event.

## Patient Monitoring and Laboratory Tests

No specific monitoring is necessary. If plasma/serum drug concentrations are monitored, the targeted trough concentration is 2 mcg/mL in dogs.

## Formulations

- Gabapentin is available in 100-, 300-, and 400-mg capsules; 100-, 300-, 400-, 600-, and 800-mg scored tablets; and 50-mg/mL oral solution. A gastroretentive tablet is available (Gralise) that releases for 10 hours in people and is used once daily but has not been evaluated in dogs or cats.
- Transdermal formulations have been examined in cats but are not absorbed sufficiently to produce efficacy.

## Stability and Storage

If stored at high temperatures and high humidity, there may be degradation within 9 weeks. Split tablets and intact tablets are stable after storage at room temperature for 9 weeks. Stability of compounded formulations has not been evaluated.

## Small Animal Dosage

### Dogs

- Anticonvulsant dosage: 10–20 mg/kg q8h PO. The higher dose may be needed in some dogs to control seizures.
- Neuropathic pain: Start with 5–15 mg/kg q12h PO and increase dosage gradually to as high as 40 mg/kg q8–12h PO if necessary.
- Treatment of behavior disorders: (often used concurrently with SSRI or TCA drugs) 5–30 mg/kg up to three times daily. Start at the low end and titrate up to achieve the desired event but avoid adverse effects. Dose changes should occur about 7 days apart. For short-term treatment to achieve anxiolysis, doses have been as high as 30–60 mg/kg 1–2 hours before an event that is anticipated to trigger anxiety in a dog.

### Cats

- Anticonvulsant dosage: 5–10 mg/kg q12h PO. The dosage has been increased to 20 mg/kg q8–12h in some cats to control seizures.
- Neuropathic pain: 5–10 mg/kg q12h PO.
- Treatment of anxiety: 100 mg per cat PO (20–30 mg/kg). Administer 90 minutes prior to a stressful event (such as a veterinary visit) with a peak effect at 2–3 hours.

## Large Animal Dosage

### Horses

- Neuropathic pain: 2.5 mg/kg q12h PO, increased to higher doses if needed (see laminitis dose).
- Laminitis: 2.5 mg/kg q8h, q12h, or q24h, increased to higher doses as needed. Doses of 10 mg/kg and higher administered q8–12h reached concentrations that are effective in other animals.

## Regulatory Information

No regulatory information is available. For extralabel use withdrawal interval estimates, contact Food Animal Residue Avoidance Databank (FARAD) at www.FARAD.org.
Racing Commissioners International (RCI) Classification: 3

# Gamithromycin
gam-ith-roe-mye'sin
**Trade and other names:** Zactran
**Functional classification:** Antibacterial

## Pharmacology and Mechanism of Action

Gamithromycin is an antibacterial agent of the macrolide class of drugs. It is a 15-membered ring (like azithromycin and tulathromycin) macrolide. Like other macrolides, it inhibits bacterial protein synthesis by binding to the ribosomal 50S subunit. The spectrum of activity for gamithromycin is limited to gram-positive bacteria and some gram-negative bacteria that cause respiratory diseases in cattle (e.g., *Mannheimia haemolytica*, *Mycoplasma* spp., and *Pasteurella multocida*). It also has activity against *Rhodococcus equi* and *Streptococcus equi* in horses. Like other long-acting macrolides, gamithromycin has high penetration into leukocytes. Other anti-inflammatory effects attributed to macrolide antibiotics may explain the clinical effects for respiratory infections, such as reduced inflammatory effects and cytokine expression in leukocytes.

*Pharmacokinetics:* The half-life is long (e.g., 51-hour plasma half-life and 90-hour [4-day] half-life in lungs), which prolongs the drug concentration at the site of infection. It has high penetration to tissues, including respiratory tissues, and leukocytes. The half-life is shorter in foals than adult horses with a half-life of 39 hours and 64 hours in plasma and respiratory fluids, respectively.

## Indications and Clinical Uses

In cattle, gamithromycin is used for treatment of bovine respiratory disease (BRD) caused by *M. haemolytica, P. multocida,* and *Histophilus somni.* It is also effective for treating infections caused by *Mycoplasma* spp. It also may be used for control of respiratory disease in beef and nonlactating dairy cattle at high risk of developing BRD (metaphylaxis) associated with *M. haemolytica* and *P. multocida.*

In horses, experimental studies indicate that it may have efficacy for treating infections caused by *S. equi* and *R. equi.* For this use, it may be substituted for erythromycin or azithromycin and administered with rifampin.

## Precautionary Information

### Adverse Reactions and Side Effects

Serious adverse reactions have not been observed. Injection-site reactions are possible in some animals, with swelling or irritation at the injection site. When injected in horses, 58% had pain at the injection site, and there were mild signs of colic in some (6%) of the horses.

### Contraindications and Precautions

No specific contraindications have been reported.

### Drug Interactions

No drug interactions have been reported.

## Instructions for Use

In cattle, administer as a single SQ injection in the neck. In horses, an injection IM can be administered every 6–7 days to maintain effective concentrations in respiratory fluids.

## Patient Monitoring and Laboratory Tests

Clinical and Laboratory Standards Institute (CLSI) breakpoint for susceptibility is ≤4.0 mcg/mL.

## Formulations

- Gamithromycin is available in a 150-mg/mL solution for injection.

## Stability and Storage

Store in a tightly sealed container, protected from light, and at room temperature.

## Small Animal Dosage

- No small animal doses have been established.

## Large Animal Dosage

**Cattle**

- 6 mg/kg SQ (neck) as a single injection (2 mL per 110 lb).

**Pigs**

- Not recommended.

## Horses

- For treatment of *Streptococcus zooepidemicus* or *R. equi:* 6 mg/kg IM administered every 7 days if needed.

## Regulatory Information

No milk withdrawal times are established; do not use in lactating dairy cattle and do not use in female dairy cattle 20 months of age or older.
Do not treat cattle within 35 days of slaughter. No withdrawal period has been established for young preruminating calves; do not use in veal calves.

# Gemfibrozil
jem-fih′broe-zil
**Trade and other names:** Lopid
**Functional classification:** Antihyperlipidemic agent

## Pharmacology and Mechanism of Action

Gemfibrozil is a fibric acid derivative that lowers cholesterol, reduces plasma triglyceride and very-low-density-lipoprotein (VLDL), and increases high-density lipoproteins. The cholesterol-lowering effects results from activation of the nuclear transcription factor peroxisome proliferator-activated receptor-alpha (PPAR-alpha). This receptor regulates the genes that control lipid and glucose metabolism, inflammation, and endothelial function. These agents decease triglyceride, VLDL, and cholesterol. This agent can be used to lower severe hypertriglyceridemia and used in people to lower cholesterol, but the use in animals is uncommon.

## Indications and Clinical Uses

It is used for treatment of hyperlipidemia. It has been used in dogs for treatment of some hyperlipidemia syndromes, but the efficacy has not been reported.

## Precautionary Information

### Adverse Reactions and Side Effects

Adverse effects have not been reported in animals. In people, GI effects are common.

### Contraindications and Precautions

No reported contraindications in animals, but in people, it is contraindicated in patients with gallbladder disease. It should be used cautiously in patients with kidney disease. It should be avoided in pregnant animals.

### Drug Interactions

No drug interactions are reported for animals. In people, it may potentiate the effects of other drugs. The use with statins may increase the risk of myopathy.

## Instructions for Use

Used primarily in people to treat hyperlipidemia, but it is used occasionally in dogs. Clinical studies have not been performed in animals.

## Patient Monitoring and Laboratory Tests

Monitor cholesterol concentrations.

## Formulations
- Gemfibrozil is available in 600-mg tablets in the United States and 300-mg capsules in Canada only.

## Stability and Storage
Store in a tightly sealed container, protected from light, and at room temperature. Stability of compounded formulations has not been evaluated.

## Small Animal Dosage
**Dogs and cats**
- 7.5 mg/kg q12h PO.

## Large Animal Dosage
- No large animal doses have been reported.

## Regulatory Information
No regulatory information is available. For extralabel use withdrawal interval estimates, contact FARAD at www.FARAD.org.

G

# Gentamicin Sulfate
jen-tah-mye′sin sul′fate
**Trade and other names:** Gentocin, Garasol, Garacin, and generic
**Functional classification:** Antibacterial

## Pharmacology and Mechanism of Action
Gentamicin is an aminoglycoside antibiotic. Like other aminoglycosides, the action is to inhibit bacteria protein synthesis via binding to 30S ribosome. Through this action, it causes a misreading of the genetic code and inhibits bacterial protein synthesis. Another mechanism important for gram-negative bacteria is to disrupt the cell surface biofilm, particularly on gram-negative bacteria, to produce disruption, loss of cell wall integrity, and a rapid bactericidal effect. Magnesium and calcium are important to cross-bridge adjacent lipopolysaccharide molecules. Positive-charged aminoglycosides competitively displace $Ca^{2+}$ and $Mg^{2+}$ and destabilize the bacteria outer membrane. Therefore, death of the bacteria is caused by a cell surface effect rather than inhibition of the ribosome. This property is not as prominent for gram-positive bacteria unless administered with a cell wall–disrupting agent such as vancomycin or a beta-lactam antibiotic. Gentamicin spectrum of activity includes most gram-negative bacterial isolates in animals, particularly gram-negative Enterobacteriaceae. It is not very active against streptococci and anaerobic bacteria. It has action on *Staphylococcus* spp. but is not a preferred treatment for these bacteria.

*Pharmacokinetics:* The pharmacokinetics have been studied in many domestic and exotic animal species. The half-life is typically 1–2 hours in mammals, and the volume of distribution is approximately 0.2–0.3 L/kg. Clearance is via glomerular filtration and is similar to the glomerular filtration rate (GFR) in animals. Clearance is impaired in patients with kidney disease.

## Indications and Clinical Uses
Gentamicin has a rapid, bactericidal action and is indicated for acute serious infections, such as those caused by gram-negative bacilli. Gentamicin has been

administered IM, SQ, and IV. It is not absorbed after oral administration, and this use is restricted to labeled use in pigs for treatment of diarrhea. Gentamicin, like other aminoglycosides, can be used with beta-lactam antibiotics because it broadens the spectrum when used with drugs such as penicillins, ampicillin, or cephalosporins. Although gentamicin is generally active against most gram-negative bacilli, amikacin is more consistently active against resistant strains. The use should be avoided in food-producing animals because of risk of residues. The only approved use in food animals is oral treatment in pigs for swine dysentery.

## Precautionary Information

### Adverse Reactions and Side Effects

Nephrotoxicity is the most dose-limiting toxicity. Ensure that patients have adequate fluid and electrolyte balance during therapy. Electrolyte depletion increases the risk of nephrotoxicity. Kidney injury is increased with persistently high trough concentrations. High levels of calcium and protein in the diet decrease the risk of nephrotoxicity. Ototoxicity and vestibulotoxicity also are possible but have not been often reported in animals. With high doses, neuromuscular toxicity is possible, although rare.

### Contraindications and Precautions

Do not administer to animals with compromised renal function, renal insufficiency, kidney disease, or renal failure. Kidney disease impairs renal clearance of gentamicin and increases the risk of kidney injury. Use in young animals is acceptable, but higher doses may be necessary.

### Drug Interactions

When gentamicin is used with anesthetic agents, neuromuscular blockade is possible. Do not mix in vial or syringe with other antibiotics; otherwise, inactivation can occur. Ototoxicity and nephrotoxicity are potentiated by loop diuretics such as furosemide.

## Instructions for Use

Dosing regimens in most animals emphasize once-daily administration to maximize efficacy and decrease adverse effects. Once-daily administration is as efficacious and possibly more effective than administration more than once per day. The once daily treatment is also safer because of less kidney exposure, as multiple treatments. Activity against some bacteria (e.g., *Pseudomonas aeruginosa*) may be enhanced when combined with a beta-lactam antibiotic, such as ceftazidime, but there is no strong evidence that it is synergistic with beta-lactam antibiotics when treating other bacteria.

## Patient Monitoring and Laboratory Tests

Susceptibility testing: The CLSI minimum inhibitory concentration breakpoint for susceptibility testing is $\leq 2$ mcg/mL. Monitor blood urea nitrogen, creatinine, and urine for evidence of renal toxicity. Blood levels can be monitored to measure for problems with systemic clearance. When monitoring trough levels in patients that are administered gentamicin once per day, the trough levels should be near or below the limit of detection. Alternatively, measure half-life from samples taken at 1 hour and 2–4 hours postdosing. Clearance should be approximately equal to the GFR (greater than 1.0 mL/kg/min), and the half-life should be less than 2 hours.

## Formulations
- Gentamicin is available in a 50- and 100-mg/mL solution for injection, a 50-mg/mL oral solution for pigs, and a 5-mg/mL injection for turkeys.

## Stability and Storage
Store in a tightly sealed container, protected from light, and at room temperature. Gentamicin is soluble in water. Do not mix with other drugs, especially in a vial, syringe, or fluid administration set. Inactivation may occur. Avoid long-term storage in plastic containers.

## Small Animal Dosage
### Dogs
- 9–14 mg/kg q24h SQ, IM, or IV.

### Cats
- 5–8 mg/kg q24h SQ, IM, or IV.

## Large Animal Dosage
### Horses
- Adult: 4–6.6 mg/kg q24h IM or IV.
- Foals younger than 2 weeks: 12–14 mg/kg q24h IM or IV.

### Pigs
- 15 mg/kg for young pigs and 10 mg/kg for older pigs once daily SQ or IM.
- Colibacillosis, swine dysentery: 1.1–2.2 mg/kg for 3 days in drinking water.

### Calves
- Younger than 2 weeks: 12–15 mg/kg q24h IV or IM.
- Adult cattle: 5–6 mg/kg q24h IM or IV.

## Regulatory information
With the exception of licensed products for pigs, aminoglycosides should not be administered to food animals because of residue concerns.

Withdrawal time for pigs: 3 days for meat at 1.1 mg/kg PO and 40 days for meat at 5 mg/kg IM; 14 days for meat at 5 mg/kg PO.

If gentamicin is administered systemically to cattle, an extended withdrawal time is necessary because of persistence of residues in the kidney. FARAD recommends 18 months. After systemic administration of 5 mg/kg, milk withdrawal time should be 5 days. If gentamicin is administered intramammarily (500 mg per quarter), a milk withdrawal time of at least 10 days and a meat withdrawal time of 180 days should be used.

Contact FARAD for additional information at www.FARAD.org.

# Glipizide
glip-ih′zide

**Trade and other names:** Glucotrol

**Functional classification:** Antidiabetic agent, hypoglycemic agent

## Pharmacology and Mechanism of Action
Glipizide is a sulfonylurea oral hypoglycemic agent. This drug acts to increase secretion of insulin from beta cells of the pancreas, probably by interacting with

sulfonylurea receptors on beta cells or by inhibiting adenosine triphosphate (ATP)–sensitive potassium channels on the pancreatic beta cells, which increases insulin secretion. These drugs also may increase sensitivity of existing insulin receptors. Glipizide is used to manage diabetes in people but is infrequently used in animals, except occasional use in cats.

*Pharmacokinetics:* Studies in cats showed that glipizide had a half-life of 17 hours and effective plasma concentration for 50% efficacy ($EC_{50}$) of 70 mcg/mL.

## Indications and Clinical Uses

Glipizide is used as oral treatment in the management of diabetes mellitus, particularly in cats. The use in other animals is rare. The response rate in cats is approximately 44%–65% (some reports are 30% or lower). The response rate in dogs is poor. It has been more common to administer the sulfonylurea class of drugs in cats than other oral hypoglycemic drugs because the sulfonylureas have had better efficacy. Glipizide is the most common of this class used in animals. Other oral hypoglycemic drugs include acetohexamide, chlorpropamide, glyburide (DiaBeta, Micronase), gliclazide, and tolazamide. Metformin is of the biguanide class of oral drugs for diabetes and has not had efficacy as high as glipizide in cats.

Glipizide transdermal absorption from a pluronic transdermal gel (pluronic organogel [PLO]) vehicle is poor in cats (less than 20%) and inconsistent. This route is not recommended.

## Precautionary Information

### Adverse Reactions and Side Effects

Adverse effects are dose related. These include vomiting, anorexia, increased bilirubin, and elevated liver enzymes in some cats (15%). It may exacerbate deposits of amyloid in the feline pancreas and increase the loss of pancreatic beta cells. Glipizide may cause hypoglycemia but less so than insulin. In people, increased cardiac mortality is possible, but this has not been reported in cats.

### Contraindications and Precautions

Many cats do not respond and will require insulin therapy. Do not rely on glipizide in cats that are not stable or if they are dehydrated or debilitated. Do not rely on glipizide for treatment of diabetes in dogs.

### Drug Interactions

Many drug interactions have been reported in people. It is not known if these occur in animals because of infrequent use. Use cautiously with beta blockers, antifungal drugs, anticoagulants, fluoroquinolones, sulfonamides, and others.

## Instructions for Use

Oral hypoglycemic agents are successful in people only for noninsulin-dependent diabetes. There has been only limited use in animals. Because response to oral hypoglycemic agents in cats is unpredictable, it is recommended to use a trial first of at least 4 weeks. If the cat responds, the drug can be continued; otherwise, insulin may be indicated. Feed cats a high-fiber diet when using oral hypoglycemic agents. Transdermal glipizide (5-mg dose) in a PLO gel was evaluated in cats. Although the transdermal formulation produced a modest change in glucose concentrations, systemic absorption was only 20%.

## Patient Monitoring and Laboratory Tests

Monitor blood glucose levels to determine if the drug is effective. Monitor liver enzymes. It may increase alanine transaminase and alkaline phosphatase.

## Formulations
- Glipizide is available in 5- and 10-mg tablets.

## Stability and Storage
Store glipizide in a tightly sealed container, protected from light, and at room temperature. Stability of compounded formulations has not been evaluated.

## Small Animal Dosage
### Dogs
- No effective dose available.

### Cats
- 2.5–7.5 mg/cat q12h PO. Usual dose is 2.5 mg/cat initially; then increase to 5 mg/cat q12h.

## Large Animal Dosage
- No large animal doses have been reported.

## Regulatory Information
No regulatory information is available. For extralabel use withdrawal interval estimates, contact FARAD at www.FARAD.org.

G

# Glucosamine Chondroitin Sulfate
gloo-koe′seh-meen kahn-droy′ten sul′fate

**Trade and other names:** Cosequin, Glyco-Flex, and generic brands

**Functional classification:** Nutritional supplement

## Pharmacology and Mechanism of Action
Glucosamine is an amino sugar synthesized from glucose and glutamine. It is a source of glucosamine-6-phosphate and N-acetylglucosamine. It is an intermediate compound, converted to an ester that is incorporated into articular cartilage. Therefore, it is a direct precursor in the formation of glycosaminoglycans in cartilage. Glucosamine is usually administered as a combination of glucosamine HCl and chondroitin sulfate. Other forms include glucosamine sodium sulfate and glucosamine potassium sulfate. These compounds are regulated as dietary supplements that modify disease and are not regulated as drugs. Glucosamine has been promoted to stimulate synthesis of synovial fluid, inhibit degradation, and improve healing of articular cartilage. Additional information is available in the section on chondroitin sulfate of this handbook.

*Pharmacokinetics:* Bioavailability studies have produced varying results depending on formulation, assay technique, and species. Oral absorption of glucosamine has varied, ranging from 12% in dogs to only 2.5% (125 mg/kg) or 6% (20 mg/kg) in horses. Although in vitro studies have demonstrated benefits to articular cartilage, some studies have questioned whether oral glucosamine is absorbed systemically intact to a high enough extent to provide beneficial effects. Oral absorption may be affected by the form administered because glucosamine sulfate may be better absorbed than glucosamine hydrochloride.

## Indications and Clinical Uses
Glucosamine is used primarily as a disease-modifying agent in the management of degenerative joint disease in animals. It is regarded as a dietary supplement and

has no claims of efficacy. It is usually found in formulations in combination with chondroitin sulfate. (See Chondroitin Sulfate for additional details.) Analyses of published clinical studies in dogs have concluded that there is a moderate level of evidence to indicate some benefit in osteoarthritis, but results may be inconsistent among studies. In some studies, the response was no better than a placebo treatment. Benefits of treatment in horses with lameness also have been reported from oral administration of chondroitin–glucosamine supplements. In human medicine, the American College of Rheumatology has strongly recommended against the use of glucosamine for osteoarthritis. Although it has been promoted for other uses, there is a lack of supporting evidence that systemic administration is effective for reducing recurrent urinary tract infections in animals (via a beneficial effect on bladder mucosa).

## Precautionary Information

### Adverse Reactions and Side Effects

In some animals, soft stools and intestinal gas have been reported. In experimental rodents, injections of glucosamine can cause hyperglycemia, insulin resistance, and a decrease in the metabolic action of insulin via the hexosamine pathway. However, the clinical relevance of these findings has not been shown when oral dietary supplements are administered. Clinical studies in dogs have shown that short-term (21 days) administration of glucosamine does not affect glycemic control or cause diabetes mellitus in dogs. Otherwise, adverse effects have not been reported, although hypersensitivity is possible.

### Contraindications and Precautions

The safety of glucosamine has not been established in diabetic animals or obese animals that may be prone to developing diabetes. Otherwise, there are no known precautions.

### Drug Interactions

No drug interactions are reported. Glucosamine- and chondroitin-containing products may be used safely with NSAIDs.

## Instructions for Use

The doses recommended are based primarily on empiricism and manufacturer's recommendations. There are few published trials of efficacy or dose titrations available to determine optimal dose. Doses listed are general recommendations and may vary among products. Products may vary in their stability, purity, and potency. Use products from a reputable supplier. When comparing products, glucosamine hydrochloride is more bioavailable than glucosamine sulfate.

## Patient Monitoring and Laboratory Tests

No routine patient monitoring is necessary. There is no evidence that glucosamine administration will increase serum glucose in animals with oral treatment. Glucosamine is produced by glucose in the body, but this is an irreversible reaction.

## Formulations

- Several formulations are available. Veterinarians are encouraged to carefully examine the product label to ensure proper strength. One product (Cosequin) is available as regular-strength (RS) and double-strength (DS) capsules. RS contains 250 mg of glucosamine, 200 mg of chondroitin sulfate, mixed glycosaminoglycans, 5 mg of

manganese, and 33 mg of manganese ascorbate. The DS tablets contain double of each of these amounts.
- Products for horses contain 3.3 g per scoop, equal to 1800 mg of glucosamine and 570 mg of chondroitin.

## Stability and Storage
Store in a tightly sealed container, protected from light, and at room temperature. Products may vary in stability and potency.

## Small Animal Dosage
- General dosing requirements for glucosamine: 22 mg/kg/day PO, increased to 44 mg/kg/day PO in patients that do not initially respond. Alternatively, a better response may be anticipated by starting with the higher dose.
- Many preparations are administered in combination with chondroitin. For general dosing, use the Cosequin RS and DS strength as a general guide.

### Dogs
- 1–2 capsules per day and 2–4 capsules for large dogs.

### Cats
- 1 capsule daily.

## Large Animal Dosage
### Horses
- 12 mg/kg glucosamine + 3.8 mg/kg chondroitin sulfate twice daily PO for 4 weeks; then 4 mg/kg glucosamine + 1.3 mg/kg chondroitin sulfate thereafter. It is common to initiate treatment in horses with a higher dosage of 22 mg/kg glucosamine + 8.8 mg/kg chondroitin sulfate daily PO.

## Regulatory Information
No regulatory information is available. Because of low risk of residues, no withdrawal times are suggested.

# Glyburide
glye′byoor-ide

**Trade and other names:** DiaBeta, Micronase, Glynase, and Glibenclamide (British name)

**Functional classification:** Antidiabetic agent, hypoglycemic agent

## Pharmacology and Mechanism of Action
Glyburide is a sulfonylurea oral hypoglycemic agent; it is also known as glibenclamide. This drug acts to increase secretion of insulin from the pancreas, probably by interacting with sulfonylurea receptors on beta cells or by interfering with ATP-sensitive potassium channels on pancreatic beta cells, which increases secretion of insulin. These drugs also may increase sensitivity of existing insulin receptors. It is used as oral treatment in the management of diabetes mellitus, particularly in cats, but not used in dogs. The response rate is approximately 40%. Sulfonylurea drugs include glipizide (Glucotrol) and glyburide (DiaBeta, Micronase). Metformin is also used but is of the biguanide class of oral drugs for diabetes.

## Indications and Clinical Uses
Oral hypoglycemic agents are successful in people only for non–insulin-dependent diabetes. There has been only limited use in animals. Glyburide is not effective in dogs but has been used in some cats. Some cats may initially respond to oral hypoglycemic agents but eventually need insulin treatment. Similar drugs include acetohexamide, chlorpropamide, glipizide, gliclazide, and tolazamide. There is more experience with glipizide than with other drugs, and it should be used as the first choice (see Glipizide for more details).

---

### Precautionary Information
**Adverse Reactions and Side Effects**
It may cause dose-related vomiting, anorexia, increased bilirubin, and elevated liver enzymes in some cats. Glyburide causes hypoglycemia but less so than insulin. In people, increased cardiac mortality is possible.

**Contraindications and Precautions**
There are no known contraindications in animals.

**Drug Interactions**
Many drug interactions have been reported in people. It is not known if these occur in animals because clinical use has been rare. Use cautiously with beta blockers, antifungal drugs, anticoagulants, fluoroquinolones, and sulfonamides.

---

## Instructions for Use
Because response to oral hypoglycemic agents in cats is unpredictable, it is recommended to use a trial first of at least 4 weeks. If the cat responds, the drug can be continued. Otherwise, insulin may be indicated. Feed cats a high-fiber diet when using oral hypoglycemic agents.

## Patient Monitoring and Laboratory Tests
Monitor blood glucose levels to determine if the drug is effective. Monitor liver enzymes.

## Formulations
- Glyburide is available in 1.25-, 2.5-, and 5-mg tablets (DiaBeta and Micronase). Glynase is available in 1.5-, 3-, and 6-mg micronized tablets.

## Stability and Storage
Store in a tightly sealed container, protected from light, and at room temperature. Stability of compounded formulations has not been evaluated.

## Small Animal Dosage
**Dogs**
- No effective doses have been reported.

**Cats**
- 0.2 mg/kg daily PO. Alternatively, start with 0.625 mg (half of a 1.25-mg tablet) per cat once daily.

## Large Animal Dosage
- No large animal doses have been reported.

## Regulatory Information
No regulatory information is available. No withdrawal information is available.

# Glycerin
glih'ser-in
**Trade and other names:** Generic
**Functional classification:** Diuretic, laxative

## Pharmacology and Mechanism of Action
Glycerin has been administered to lower ocular pressure to treat acute glaucoma. However, IV mannitol is used more frequently for this purpose. Glycerin has been used as a laxative; it lubricates the stools and adds water to intestinal contents.

## Indications and Clinical Uses
Glycerin is an osmotic agent that draws water into the intestine or renal tubule. Administered systemically, it acts as an osmotic diuretic agent, preventing water reabsorption from the renal tubules. Administered orally, it is not absorbed but acts as an osmotic laxative, drawing water into the intestine. The use of glycerin is uncommon in animals.

## Precautionary Information
**Adverse Reactions and Side Effects**
Glycerin may cause dehydration with frequent use or high doses.

**Contraindications and Precautions**
Do not administer to dehydrated animals.

**Drug Interactions**
No drug interactions are reported for animals.

## Instructions for Use
Although glycerin may lower ocular pressure, other drugs are used to treat acute glaucoma.

## Patient Monitoring and Laboratory Tests
Monitor ocular pressures. Monitor electrolytes in treated animals.

## Formulations Available
• Glycerin is available in an oral solution or 40-mg/mL emulsion.

## Stability and Storage
Store in a tightly sealed container, protected from light, and at room temperature. Stability of compounded formulations has not been evaluated.

## Small Animal Dosage (Dogs and Cats)
• 1–2 mL/kg q8h PO.

## Large Animal Dosage
• No large animal doses have been reported.

## Regulatory Information
No regulatory information is available. Because of the low risk of residues, no withdrawal times are suggested.

# Glycopyrrolate

glye-koe-peer′oe-late

**Trade and other names:** Robinul-V

**Functional classification:** Anticholinergic

## Pharmacology and Mechanism of Action

Glycopyrrolate is an anticholinergic agent (blocks acetylcholine effect at muscarinic receptor), parasympatholytic. Glycopyrrolate produces atropine-like effects systemically. However, glycopyrrolate may have less effect on the central nervous system (CNS) compared with atropine because of lower penetration to CNS. It may produce a longer duration of action than atropine. The major use is as an adjunct to anesthetic agents to decrease secretions or increase heart rate.

## Indications and Clinical Uses

Glycopyrrolate is used to inhibit vagal effects and increase heart rate in animals. It also decreases respiratory, salivary, and GI secretions. It may be used as an adjunct to anesthesia when it is necessary to override vagal stimulus. In horses, glycopyrrolate has a half-life of 7–19 hours, but this varies depending on the breed of horse.

## Precautionary Information

### Adverse Reactions and Side Effects

Adverse effects are attributed to antimuscarinic (anticholinergic) effects. Side effects of therapy include xerostomia, ileus, constipation, tachycardia, and urine retention. CNS effects are less than with atropine.

### Contraindications and Precautions

Do not use in patients with glaucoma, intestinal ileus, gastroparesis, or tachycardia.

### Drug Interactions

No specific drug interactions are reported for animals. However, it is expected that glycopyrrolate, like other anticholinergic drugs, antagonizes drugs that stimulate respiratory and GI secretions and GI motility.

## Instructions for Use

Glycopyrrolate is often used in combination with other agents, particularly anesthetic drugs. Although some anesthetic agents such as alpha$_2$ agonists and opioids are associated with bradycardia, it is rarely necessary to administer anticholinergic agents such as glycopyrrolate to reduce the bradycardia.

## Patient Monitoring and Laboratory Tests

Monitor heart rate during treatment.

## Formulations

• Glycopyrrolate is available as a 0.2-mg/mL injection.

## Stability and Storage

Store in a tightly sealed container, protected from light, and at room temperature. Stability of compounded formulations has not been evaluated.

## Small Animal Dosage
**Dogs and cats**
- 0.005–0.01 mg/kg IV, IM, or SQ.

## Large Animal Dosage
**Cattle and Horses**
- Use during anesthesia: 0.005–0.01 mg/kg IM or SQ or 0.0025–0.005 mg/kg IV. A common dose is 1 mg per horse.

## Regulatory Information
No regulatory information is available. For extralabel use withdrawal interval estimates, contact FARAD at www.FARAD.org.

RCI Classification: 3

G

# Gold Sodium Thiomalate
gold soe'dee-um thye-oh-mah'late

**Trade and other names:** Myochrysine

**Functional classification:** Immunosuppressive

## Pharmacology and Mechanism of Action
Gold sodium thiomalate is a gold salt uses for diseases that respond to gold therapy (chrysotherapy). The mechanism of action is unknown, but it may relate to immunosuppressive effect on lymphocytes or suppression of sulfhydryl systems.

## Indications and Clinical Uses
Gold therapy is used primarily for immune-mediated diseases (e.g., dermatologic disease) in animals. In people, it has been used for rheumatoid arthritis. In animals, there is a lack of controlled clinical trials to document efficacy, and the use is based only on anecdotal experiences and extrapolation of the use in people. Its use in animals is uncommon. Other immunosuppressive drugs are used more frequently.

## Precautionary Information
**Adverse Reactions and Side Effects**
Adverse effects include dermatitis, nephrotoxicity, and blood dyscrasias.

**Contraindications and Precautions**
Use cautiously in animals with bone marrow suppression or renal disease.

**Drug Interactions**
Use with penicillamine will increase risk of hematologic adverse effects.

## Instructions for Use
Clinical studies have not been performed in animals. Aurothioglucose generally is used more often than gold sodium thiomalate.

## Patient Monitoring and Laboratory Tests
Complete blood count (CBC) should be monitored periodically during treatment.

### Formulations Available
- Note: Most forms of this drug are no longer approved and may not be available commercially. Gold sodium thiomalate has been available in 10-, 25-, and 50-mg/mL injection.

### Stability and Storage
Store in a tightly sealed container, protected from light, and at room temperature. Stability of compounded formulations has not been evaluated.

### Small Animal Dosage
**Dogs and cats**
- 1–5 mg per animal IM first week, then 2–10 mg IM second week, and then 1 mg/kg once per week IM for maintenance.

### Large Animal Dosage
- No large animal doses have been reported.

### Regulatory Information
No regulatory information is available. For extralabel use withdrawal interval estimates, contact FARAD at www.FARAD.org.

# Gonadorelin Hydrochloride and Gonadorelin Diacetate Tetrahydrate
goe-nad-oh-rell'in hye-droe-klor'ide and goe-nad-oh-rell'in dye-ass'eh-tate tet-ra-hye'drate

**Trade and other names:** Factrel, Fertagyl, Cystorelin, Fertilin, OvaCyst, GnRh, and LHRH

**Functional classification:** Hormone

### Pharmacology and Mechanism of Action
Gonadorelin is a hormone that stimulates synthesis and release of luteinizing hormone (LH) and, to a lesser degree, follicle-stimulating hormone. It is used to manage reproductive conditions in animals.

### Indications and Clinical Uses
Gonadorelin is used to induce luteinization and ovulation in animals. Gonadotropin has been used to manage various reproductive disorders in which stimulation of ovulation is desired. The use is mostly confined to large animals. In dairy cattle, it is used to treat ovarian follicular cysts.

### Precautionary Information
**Adverse Reactions and Side Effects**

Adverse effects have not been reported in animals, but effects are possible because of excessive effects from LH.

**Contraindications and Precautions**

Do not administer to pregnant animals. Extreme care should be used by people, particularly women, handling this medication. Human exposure may pose a risk to pregnant women.

**Drug Interactions**

No drug interactions in animals are reported.

## Instructions for Use

For treatment of dairy cattle, with the diacetate tetrahydrate form, administer 100 mcg per cow as a single IM or IV injection for treatment of ovarian cysts. For the hydrochloride formulation, administer 100 mcg IM for the treatment of cystic ovaries (ovarian follicular cysts) in cattle to reduce the time to first estrus. In dairy cows, it may be used with dinoprost tromethamine or cloprostenol injection to synchronize estrous cycles to allow fixed-time artificial insemination in lactating dairy cows.

## Patient Monitoring and Laboratory Tests

Monitor treated cattle for ovulation.

## Formulations

- Gonadorelin is available in 50-mcg gonadorelin diacetate tetrahydrate per milliliter (equivalent to 43 mcg/mL of gonadorelin) or 50-mcg gonadorelin (as hydrochloride) in aqueous solution.

## Stability and Storage

Store in a tightly sealed container, protected from light, and at room temperature. Stability of compounded formulations has not been evaluated.

## Small Animal Dosage

**Dogs**
- 50–100 mcg/dog/day q24–48h IM.

**Cats**
- 25 mcg/cat once IM.

## Large Animal Dosage

**Cattle**
- 100 mcg/cow IM or IV once (equivalent to approximately 2 mL per cow for gonadorelin diacetate tetrahydrate). In lactating dairy cows, 100–200 mcg/cow (2–4 mL) IM may be used.

## Regulatory Information

No withdrawal times are necessary (zero days).

# Gonadotropin, Chorionic
go-nad-o-tro′pin, kor-ee-ahn′ik

**Trade and other names:** Profasi, Pregnyl, A.P.L., Follutein, Ferti-Cept, Chortropin, Chorulon, and Improvest

**Functional classification:** Hormone

## Pharmacology and Mechanism of Action

Gonadotropin is a hormone also referred to as *human chorionic gonadotropin* (hCG). The action of hCG is identical to that of LH. It is used when diseases or reproductive management requires stimulation of LH.

## Indications and Clinical Uses

Gonadotropin is used to induce luteinization in animals. It has been used to manage various reproductive disorders when stimulation of ovulation is desired. Most of the use has been in large animals, but there are some conditions treated in dogs and cats in which stimulation of luteinization is necessary. In cows, it is used for treatment of nymphomania (frequent or constant heat) caused by cystic ovaries.

In pigs, it is used for induction of fertile estrus (heat) in prepuberal (noncycling) gilts or for induction of estrus in healthy weaned sows experiencing delayed return to estrus. It is also used in pigs for the temporary immunologic castration (suppression of testicular function) and reduction of boar taint in intact male pigs intended for slaughter.

## Precautionary Information

### Adverse Reactions and Side Effects
Adverse effects have not been reported in animals.

### Contraindications and Precautions
Do not administer to pregnant animals. Extreme care should be used by people, particularly women, handling this medication. Human exposure may pose a risk to pregnant women.

### Drug Interactions
No specific drug interactions are reported.

## Instructions for Use
When used in horses, most ovulate 32–40 hours after treatment. In cows, it may be repeated in 14 days if the animal's behavior or rectal examination of the ovaries indicates the necessity for re-treatment. In pigs, use only in gilts older than 5½ months that weigh at least 85 kg (185 lb). Delayed return to estrus is most prevalent after the first litter. The effectiveness has not been established after later litters. Delayed return to estrus often occurs after periods of adverse environmental conditions, and sows mated after such conditions may farrow smaller than normal litters.

## Patient Monitoring and Laboratory Tests
Monitor treated patients for signs of luteinization and estrus.

## Formulations
- hCG and the cattle formulation is available in 5000-, 10,000-, and 20,000-unit vials for injection to be diluted in 10 mL of diluent. The swine formulation consists of 400 units of serum gonadotropin and 200 of chorionic gonadotropin as a freeze-dried powder to be reconstituted with 5 mL of sterile aqueous diluent.

## Stability and Storage
Store in a tightly sealed container, protected from light, and at room temperature. Stability of compounded formulations has not been evaluated.

## Small Animal Dosage
### Dogs
- 22 units/kg q24–48h IM or 44 units once IM.

### Cats
- 250 units/cat once IM.

## Large Animal Dosage
### Horses
- Ovulation induction: 2500–5000 units per mare IM or IV.

### Cattle (Cows)
- 10,000 units as a single, deep IM injection; 500–2500 units for intrafollicular injection; 2500–5000 units IV.

**Pigs (Sows)**
- Conditions of use: 400 units of serum gonadotropin with 200 units of chorionic gonadotropin per 5 mL dose per animal SQ.

## Regulatory Information
No regulatory information is available for food animals. A tolerance for residues of gonadotropin in uncooked edible tissues of cattle or of fish is not required. Because of low risk of residues, no withdrawal times are suggested.

# Granisetron Hydrochloride
grah-nih′seh-tron hye-droe-klor′ide

**Trade and other names:** Kytril

**Functional classification:** Antiemetic

## Pharmacology and Mechanism of Action
Granisetron is an antiemetic drug from the class of drugs called *serotonin antagonists.* These drugs act by inhibiting serotonin (5-HT, type 3) receptors. During chemotherapy, 5-HT may be released from injury to the GI tract that stimulates vomiting centrally, which is blocked by this class of drugs. These drugs also have been used to treat vomiting from other forms of gastroenteritis. They have been effective in people for various forms of vomiting and nausea, particularly vomiting and nausea from cancer chemotherapeutic agents. Although there are no well-controlled clinical studies in animals, the use is based on experiences in people and observations from clinical specialists. Compared with other serotonin antagonists, granisetron is used less frequently than ondansetron. Other serotonin antagonists used for antiemetic therapy include dolasetron, azasetron, and tropisetron.

## Indications and Clinical Uses
Granisetron, like other serotonin antagonists, is used primarily as an antiemetic during chemotherapy, for which it has been effective. It can be used concurrently with maropitant, which acts through a different mechanism. These combinations are used commonly in small animals. Granisetron may be administered prior to chemotherapy to prevent nausea and vomiting or for GI diseases that stimulate vomiting in dogs and cats. Use in animals has been primarily derived from empirical use. There are no well-controlled clinical studies or efficacy trials to document clinical effectiveness.

## Precautionary Information
### Adverse Reactions and Side Effects
None reported in dogs or cats. The use of granisetron is uncommon, and a full listing of adverse effects is not available. These drugs have little affinity for other serotonin receptors.

### Contraindications and Precautions
No contraindications reported in animals.

### Drug Interactions
No interactions are reported. It may be used with cancer chemotherapy agents. There are no known drug interactions in animals, but use has been infrequent for these to be fully documented.

## Instructions for Use

There have been only limited uses of this class of antiemetic drugs in veterinary patients. Most doses have been extrapolated from human uses. Granisetron and other serotonin receptor antagonists may be combined with maropitant.

## Patient Monitoring and Laboratory Tests

No specific monitoring is necessary.

## Formulations

• Granisetron is available in 1-mg tablets, 1-mg/mL injection, and 0.5-mg/mL oral solution.

## Stability and Storage

Store in a tightly sealed container, protected from light, and at room temperature. Discard opened vial after 30 days. Compounded solutions are stable in various fluids for 24 hours. Oral compounded formulations have been prepared in juices, syrups, and flavorings and were stable for 14 days.

## Small Animal Dosage

### Dogs and Cats

• 0.01 mg/kg IV or 0.02 mg/kg PO. (Oral doses have been extrapolated from people: 2 mg/person PO as single dose.)

## Large Animal Dosage

• No large animal doses have been reported.

## Regulatory Information

No regulatory information is available for food animals. Because of low risk of residues, no withdrawal times are suggested.

# Grapiprant

grap′ah-prant

**Trade and other names:** Galliprant

**Functional classification:** Analgesic, anti-inflammatory

## Pharmacology and Mechanism of Action

Grapiprant belongs to a unique class called "piprants" that can technically be considered NSAIDs but act through a different mechanism than other NSAIDs. Grapiprant is used in dogs as an alternative to other traditional NSAIDs.

Grapiprant is a non-cyclo-oxygenase (COX)–inhibiting agent. Instead of inhibiting production of prostaglandins, it blocks the prostaglandin (PG) receptor. After inflammation is triggered and PGs are synthesized, $PGE_2$ exerts its effects via four receptors (EP1–4). The EP4 receptor is responsible for some of the sensitization of sensory neurons and signs of inflammation. Although other receptors are activated during inflammation, the EP4 receptor has been identified as the primary receptor responsible for mediating pain and inflammation associated with osteoarthritis. In dogs, grapiprant has high binding affinity for the EP4 receptor and binds competitively at a single site. The effective dose in dogs was based on pharmacokinetic–pharmacodynamic analysis and extrapolation from laboratory animal models of pain. Reduction in inflammation was demonstrated in studies with rats as a model.

*Pharmacokinetics:* The pharmacokinetics have been studied in dogs, cats, and horses. The half-lives are 3–9 hours, 1.4–6 hours, and 4–11 hours, respectively.

## Indications and Clinical Uses

Grapiprant is approved for dogs to treat pain and inflammation associated with osteoarthritis. It has also been used to treat other painful conditions. Clinical use is based on the approved indication, field studies, and published reports. It was safe and effective compared with placebo treatment when used in dogs to reduce signs associated with osteoarthritis.

Grapiprant is the first from this group approved for any animal or human. There is no approval at this time for cats, but new studies are emerging that may help for treatment of cats in the future.

The use in horses has been examined only through pharmacokinetic studies. These studies showed that at a dose of 2 mg/kg PO, it did not achieve concentrations considered effective in other animals. There are no studies that have demonstrated efficacy in horses.

**G**

## Precautionary Information

### Adverse Reactions and Side Effects

Adverse effects were reported from the field studies used for US Food and Drug Administration approval. Adverse reactions in dogs have been minimal and are typical as for traditional NSAIDs. These may include vomiting, diarrhea, and decreased appetite. These events have been mild and usually transient. In a safety study with research dogs, they tolerated a dose equivalent to 30 mg/kg of the tablet for 9 months with adverse effects attributed to the gastrointestinal (GI) tract as mild and infrequent.

### Contraindications and Precautions

Like other NSAIDs, grapiprant should be used cautiously in dogs with a history of GI disease.

### Drug Interactions

There are no known drug interactions from grapiprant.

## Instructions for Use

Grapiprant can be used in animals with a history of pain and inflammation associated with osteoarthritis.

## Patient Monitoring and Laboratory Tests

No specific monitoring is necessary. As with other NSAIDs, monitor liver enzymes and renal parameters during regular check-ups.

## Formulations

• Grapiprant tablets are available in 20-, 60-, and 100-mg tablets.

## Stability and Storage

Store in the manufacturer's packaging.

## Small Animal Dosage
### Dogs
- Osteoarthritis, pain, and inflammation: 2 mg/kg once daily. There is no limit to the duration of treatment.

### Cats
- Safe and effective doses have not been established for cats.

## Large Animal Dosage
### Horses
- Safe and effective doses have not been established for horses. The canine dose (2 mg/kg) did not achieve effective concentrations in horses.

### Other Large Animals
- There are no reports of use in food animals.

## Regulatory Information
No regulatory information is available. Grapiprant should be avoided in food animals. If administered to a food animal, consult FARAD for withdrawal time information (www.FARAD.org).

# Griseofulvin
grizs-ee-oh-ful'vin

**Trade and other names:** Microsize: Fulvicin U/F, Grisactin, and Grifulvin; ultramicrosize: Fulvicin P/G and Gris-PEG

**Functional classification:** Antifungal

## Pharmacology and Mechanism of Action
Griseofulvin is an antifungal drug unrelated to other common antifungal drugs such as oral azoles. After systemic administration, griseofulvin is deposited in the keratin precursor cells of the skin and hair. It is rapidly taken up into these tissues within 4–8 hours or 48–72 hours (depending on the study) after administration. After it is incorporated into these cells, mitosis of the fungal cells is inhibited by effects on the mitotic spindle, and eventually fungal cells are killed. Griseofulvin persists in skin and hair for prolonged periods and is used to treat dermatophytes. It also has a predilection to accumulate in inflammatory sites of the skin and may be effective for treating some noninfectious, inflammatory dermatoses other than dermatomycosis.

## Indications and Clinical Uses
Griseofulvin is one of the drugs of choice when systemic treatment is needed for dermatophyte infections caused by *Microsporum* spp. and *Trichophyton* spp. in dogs and cats. It is sometimes used in combination with topical therapy. Griseofulvin is not effective for the treatment of yeasts or bacteria. At least 4 weeks, and sometimes 3 months or more, is needed for successful therapy. Its use has been replaced by azole antifungal drugs in most cases (itraconazole, fluconazole, etc.), so the use of griseofulvin has declined.

## Precautionary Information

### Adverse Reactions and Side Effects

Adverse effects in animals include teratogenicity in cats, anemia and leukopenia in cats, anorexia, depression, vomiting, and diarrhea. In cats, feline immunodeficiency virus (FIV) infection may increase the risk of bone marrow toxicosis. Whether the bone marrow problems are caused by high doses or this is an idiosyncratic (non–dose-related) reaction is not understood. These effects resolve in cats when treatment is stopped, but irreversible idiosyncratic pancytopenia has been reported.

### Contraindications and Precautions

Do not administer to pregnant cats. Caution should be used when administering griseofulvin to cats with viral infections (FIV) because this may exacerbate bone marrow effects.

### Drug Interactions

Griseofulvin is an enhancer of cytochrome P450 drug enzymes. Therefore, other concurrent drugs may be metabolized and cleared more quickly if given with griseofulvin.

## Instructions for Use

A wide range of doses has been reported. Doses listed here represent the current consensus. Oral absorption is favored in the presence of fat, and administration of the drug with a high-fat meal can tremendously enhance the extent of absorption. Two formulations are available: microsize and ultramicrosize. Administration of a formulation made up of fine particles (microsize) is preferred because the small particles improve oral absorption. Veterinary formulations are generally composed of microsize preparations, and this is reflected in the dosage regimens. If the ultramicrosized preparations are used, the dose may be decreased by half. Shake oral suspension well before using. Consider 25 mg/kg q12h initially and then increase to 50–60 mg/kg q12h for problem cases.

## Patient Monitoring and Laboratory Tests

Monitor CBC for evidence of bone marrow toxicity.

## Formulations

- Griseofulvin is available in 125-, 250-, and 500-mg microsize tablets; 25-mg/mL oral suspension; 125-mg/mL oral syrup; and 125-, and 250-mg, ultramicrosized tablets. It is also available as microsized griseofulvin powder in 15-g pouches that contain 2.5 g of the active ingredient.

## Stability and Storage

Store in a tightly sealed container, protected from light, and at room temperature. Griseofulvin is insoluble in water but is soluble in alcohol.

## Small Animal Dosage

### Dogs

- Microsize: 25 mg/kg q12h PO up to a maximum dosage of 50–60 mg/kg q12h. Start with 25 mg/kg q12h PO and then increase to 50–60 mg/kg q12h PO for refractory cases.
- Ultramicrosize: 30 mg/kg/day in divided treatments PO.

**Cats**
- Microsize formulation: 25 mg/kg q12h PO.

## Large Animal Dosage
**Horses**
- Dermatophytosis: 5.6 mg/kg q24h of the oral microsize powder, which may be mixed with feed. Treatment should be continued for a minimum of 10 days.

## Regulatory Information
No regulatory information is available for food animals. Because of potential for teratogenic effects, do not administer to food animals.

# Growth Hormone

**Trade and other names:** Somatrem, Somatropin, Protropin, Humatrope, and Nutropin

**Functional classification:** Hormone

## Pharmacology and Mechanism of Action
Growth hormone, also known as hCG. It is administered to correct growth hormone deficiency in animals. Somatrem is a biosynthetic somatropin.

## Indications and Clinical Uses
Growth hormone is used to treat growth hormone deficiencies, but this use is rare in veterinary medicine.

## Precautionary Information
**Adverse Reactions and Side Effects**
Growth hormone is diabetogenic in all animals. Excess growth hormone causes acromegaly.

**Contraindications and Precautions**
Except for diabetes, there are no other contraindications reported in animals.

**Drug Interactions**
No drug interactions are reported in animals.

## Instructions for Use
There is only limited clinical experience in animals. Dose form must be reconstituted with sterile diluent before use.

## Patient Monitoring and Laboratory Tests
Monitor glucose periodically during treatment.

## Formulations
- Growth hormone is available in 5- and 10-mg/vial (1 mg is equal to 3 units).

## Stability and Storage
Prepared solution is stable if refrigerated for 14 days. Otherwise, it is stable for only 24 hours.

## Small Animal Dosage
**Dogs and cats**
- 0.1 units/kg three times a week for 4–6 weeks SQ or IM. (Usual human pediatric dosage is 0.18–0.3 mg/kg/week SQ or IM.)

## Large Animal Dosage
- No large animal doses have been reported.

## Regulatory Information
Do not administer to animals that produce food.

G

# Guaifenesin
gwye-fen′eh-sin

**Trade and other names:** Glyceryl guaiacolate, Guaiphenesin, Gecolate, Guailaxin, Glycotuss, Hytuss, Glytuss, Fenesin, Humibid LA, and Mucinex

**Functional classification:** Expectorant; muscle relaxant

## Pharmacology and Mechanism of Action
Guaifenesin, which is also known as glyceryl guaiacolate, is a compound that has been an older traditional therapy for treating cough in people, although the efficacy has been questioned for this effect. For respiratory disease, it is administered orally to produce an expectorant effect. This effect is presumably via stimulation of vagal transmission to produce less viscous bronchial secretions and enhance ciliary clearance. There are no studies to evaluate efficacy of the expectorant action in animals.

As an anesthetic adjunct, it is used as a preanesthetic with barbiturates and other injectable anesthetic agents. It is a central-acting skeletal muscle relaxant and causes sedation and relaxation via depression of nerve transmission. A distinct advantage of griseofulvin is that it provides profound muscle relaxation without adverse cardiovascular and respiratory depression associated with other anesthetic agents.

*Pharmacokinetics:* Pharmacokinetic information is limited, but half-lives are 60–84 minutes in ponies and 60–108 minutes in horses. Duration of action in horses is approximately 30 minutes. After PO administration to horses, the half-life is 1.3–4.8 hours.

## Indications and Clinical Uses
Guaifenesin is administered IV (particularly in large animals) as an adjunct to anesthesia. Most often, it is used prior to induction of general anesthesia in horses. An example of this use in horses is "GKX," which is 1000–2000 mg of ketamine, 500 mg of xylazine, and 5% of guaifenesin mixed and added to 1 L to infuse at 2 mL/kg/h IV or anesthesia. When administered with propofol to horses, it helped to prevent adverse anesthetic events that occur when propofol is administered as a sole agent.

Guaifenesin is also administered orally in animals as an expectorant. It has been administered orally to horses (3.5 mg/kg) to clear mucus from airways. Supporting data for an expectorant effect are lacking, but it may increase the volume and reduce the viscosity of secretions in the trachea and bronchi. It may also facilitate removal of secretions.

## Precautionary Information

### Adverse Reactions and Side Effects

Minor leakage outside the vein from an IV injection does not cause tissue injury. However, thrombophlebitis from IV injection may occur. Hypotension may occur from high doses. Some hemolysis has been observed from IV infusion, but this is not significant at a concentration less than 15%. In horses, when used alone for anesthetic induction, it may cause excitement, myotonus, and paddling. Therefore, it is often used with other agents in horses. A vagal effect (e.g., stimulation of secretions) may occur when the drug is used as an expectorant.

### Contraindications and Precautions

Do not administer IV if visible precipitate is observed.

Oral formulations for people (cough and cold remedies) may contain other ingredients such as dextromethorphan or decongestants (e.g., phenylephrine or pseudoephedrine). Do not use these combinations in animals sensitive to these drugs, and if possible, use only formulations that contain guaifenesin.

### Drug Interactions

No significant drug interactions are reported. It has been safely used with acepromazine, xylazine, detomidine, ketamine, thiopental, and pentobarbital.

## Instructions for Use

For anesthetic purposes, it is used with other agents. For IV infusion, 5% guaifenesin is prepared from powder (50 g/L) dissolved in sterile water. It dissolves more readily if the water is warm. Infusion of 110 mg/kg can produce transient recumbency. It can be administered with a variety of other anesthetic agents for the benefit of producing a smoother induction in horses. One such combination is Equine "Triple-Drip" listed in the dosing section. It also has been administered with propofol to horses (3 mg/kg of propofol and 90 mg/kg of guaifenesin infused over 3 minutes).

## Patient Monitoring and Laboratory Tests

Monitoring of animals during anesthesia (heart rate, rhythm, and respiratory rate) is suggested. Hypotension is possible; therefore, blood pressure should be monitored.

## Formulations

- Guaifenesin is administered as an IV solution prepared prior to infusion from powder to a 5% solution.
- Expectorant formulations: 100- and 200-mg tablet; 600-mg extended-release tablets; and 20-mg/mL and 40-mg/mL oral solution. Human over-the-counter formulations may contain other ingredients such as dextromethorphan and decongestants.
- Guaifenesin oral: Guaifenesin powder can be mixed with water (60 mL) for oral administration to horses.

## Stability and Storage

Guaifenesin is soluble in water and in alcohol. It is more soluble in warm water. It precipitates if the temperature is 22°C or colder. It should be administered orally shortly after preparation because stability is short. However, 10% solutions have been stable for as long as 7 days. For IV use, it has been mixed with xylazine and ketamine without apparent loss of stability.

## Small Animal Dosage
**Dogs**
- Expectorant: 3–5 mg/kg q8h PO.
- Anesthetic adjunct: 2.2 mL/kg/h of a 5% solution IV. Administered with alpha$_2$ agonists and ketamine.

**Cats**
- Expectorant: 3–5 mg/kg q8h PO.

## Large Animal Dosage
**Horses**
- 2.2 mL/kg of a 5% solution (110 mg/kg) infused IV to horses prior to other anesthetic agents, such as ketamine. Guaifenesin solution may be infused rapidly.
- Constant-rate infusion: 2.2 mL/kg/h of 5% solution (50 mg/mL).
- Induction dose (with propofol): 90 mg/kg IV administered over 3 minutes followed by propofol 3-mg/kg IV bolus.
- Equine "triple-drip": 1 L of 5% guaifenesin in dextrose, mixed with 500 mg of xylazine and 2 g of ketamine. Administer as 1.1 mL/kg for induction and then 2–4 mL/kg/h infusion IV. Use yohimbine if necessary to speed recovery.
- PO (powder mixed with water): 3.5 mg/kg q12h.

## Regulatory Information
Withdrawal time (extralabel): 3 days for meat and 48 hours for milk.
RCI Classification: 4

# Halothane
hal'oe-thane

**Trade and other names:** Fluothane

**Functional classification:** Inhalant anesthetic

## Pharmacology and Mechanism of Action
Halothane is one of the older inhalant anesthetics. Halothane is a multi-halogenated ethane. It is characterized by rapid induction and recovery, high potency, and few adverse effects. Like other inhalant anesthetics, the mechanism of action is uncertain. They produce generalized, reversible depression of the central nervous system (CNS). The inhalant anesthetics vary in their solubility in blood, their potency, and the rate of induction and recovery. Those with low blood/gas partition coefficients are associated with the most rapid rates of induction and recovery. Halothane has a vapor pressure of 243 mm Hg (at 20°C), a blood/gas partition coefficient of 2.3, and a fat/blood coefficient of 51. Because of high solubility in fat, its clearance from the body is slower than other agents.

## Indications and Clinical Uses
Halothane, like other inhalant anesthetics, is used for general anesthesia in animals. It has minimum alveolar concentration (MAC) values of 1.04%, 0.87%, and 0.88% in cats, dogs, and horses, respectively. However, it is rarely used today and has been replaced by newer inhalant anesthetics (e.g., isoflurane) in many veterinary practices.

## Precautionary Information
### Adverse Reactions and Side Effects
Like other inhalant anesthetics, halothane produces vasodilation and increased blood flow to cerebral blood vessels. This may increase intracranial pressure. Also, like other inhalant anesthetics, it produces a dose-dependent myocardial depression, with an accompanying decrease in cardiac output. It also depresses respiratory rate and alveolar ventilation. In addition, like other inhalant anesthetics, it increases the risk of ventricular arrhythmias, especially in response to catecholamines. Hepatotoxicity has been reported in people.

### Contraindications and Precautions
Administer with caution to patients with cardiovascular problems.

### Drug Interactions
No specific drug interactions. Use of other anesthetics in conjunction with halothane lowers the requirement for the halothane dose.

## Instructions for Use
Use of inhalant anesthetics requires careful monitoring. Dose is determined by depth of anesthesia.

## Patient Monitoring and Laboratory Tests
Monitor patient's heart rate and rhythm and respiration during anesthesia.

## Formulations
- Halothane is available in a 250-mL bottle.

## Stability and Storage
Halothane is highly volatile and should be stored in a tightly sealed container.

## Small Animal Dosage
- Induction: 3%
- Maintenance: 0.5%–1.5%.

## Large Animal Dosage
- MAC value: 1%.

## Regulatory Information
No withdrawal times are established for food animals. Clearance is rapid, and short withdrawal times are suggested. For extralabel use withdrawal interval estimates, contact Food Animal Residue Avoidance Databank (FARAD) at www.FARAD.org.

# Hemoglobin Glutamer (Oxyglobin)
hee′moe-gloe-bin gloot′am-er

**H**

**Trade and other names:** Oxyglobin

**Functional classification:** Iron supplement, hemoglobin substitute

## Pharmacology and Mechanism of Action
Hemoglobin glutamer (bovine) is used as oxygen-carrying fluid in dogs with varying causes of anemia. Oxyglobin is an ultrapurified polymerized bovine hemoglobin. The molecular weight is 64,000–500,000 (average, 200,000). Osmolality is 300 mOsm/mL. Colloid osmotic pressure is higher than other colloids, with a colloid osmotic pressure of 43.3.

*Pharmacokinetics:* The half-life in dogs is approximately 24 hours (range, 18–43 hours). It is metabolized by macrophages, and 95% of a dose is eliminated in 5–9 days.

## Indications and Clinical Uses
Hemoglobin glutamer has been used to treat anemia caused by blood loss, hemolysis, and decreased blood cell production. Although approved for dogs, it also has been used in cats. The availability has varied, and in some countries, it is no longer commercially available, or availability can fluctuate. Because of limited availability from the manufacturer, the use has become infrequent.

## Precautionary Information

### Adverse Reactions and Side Effects
Circulatory overload is possible, especially with high doses and rapid administration. Patients at the most risk of circulatory overload are those with cardiac disease, respiratory disease, risk of hypertension, cerebral edema, oliguria or anuria caused by renal failure, and cats. Pulmonary hypertension has been observed because of depletion of nitric oxide (NO) and volume overload. Because cats are more sensitive to the adverse effects than dogs, lower dose rates should be used in cats. Other adverse effects have been skin and mucous membrane discoloration, vomiting, diarrhea, and anorexia. Discoloration of skin and mucous membranes can persist for 3–5 days.

### Contraindications and Precautions
Hemoglobin glutamer should not be used in dogs with advanced heart disease. Administer with caution to cats because of an increased risk of pulmonary hypertension.

### Drug Interactions
Do not administer with other drugs via the same infusion set. Do not mix with other drugs.

## Instructions for Use
Administer using aseptic technique. In 5–7 days, 90% of dose is eliminated.

## Patient Monitoring and Laboratory Tests
Use of Oxyglobin does not require cross-matching, but because these patients are usually critically ill, they should be monitored carefully. Monitoring packed cell volume or hematocrit is not useful for assessing response to Oxyglobin therapy. Oxyglobin will interfere with other monitoring tests, such as blood chemistry analysis (colorimetric assays). Doses of 30 mL/kg are listed by the manufacturer, but many veterinarians use 10–15 mL/kg.

## Formulations
- Hemoglobin glutamer has been available in 13-g/dL polymerized hemoglobin of bovine origin in 60- and 125-mL single-dose bags. Availability may be limited, or it may only be available in certain countries. Check with local distributors to determine availability.

## Stability and Storage
At room temperature, hemoglobin glutamer has a 3-year shelf-life. After it is opened, a 125-mL bag should be used within 24 hours because of oxidation of hemoglobin to methemoglobin. Do not freeze.

## Small Animal Dosage
**Dogs**
- One-time dose of 10–30 mL/kg IV or up to a rate of 5–10 mL/kg/h.

**Cats**
- One-time dose of 3–5 mL/kg IV, slowly. Maximum rate is 5 mL/kg/h and not to exceed 13–20 mL/kg in 24 hours.

## Large Animal Dosage
No doses reported. Do not use in racehorses.

## Regulatory Information
No regulatory information is available. Because of low risk of residues, no withdrawal times are suggested. However, hemoglobin glutamer (Oxyglobin) is prohibited to be on the premises of racing horses.

Racing Commissioners International (RCI) Classification: 2

# Heparin Sodium
hep'ah-rin soe'dee-um

**Trade and other names:** Unfractionated heparin (UFH), Liquaemin and Hepalean (Canada)

**Functional classification:** Anticoagulant

## Pharmacology and Mechanism of Action
Heparin, also referred to as unfractionated heparin (UFH), is one of the oldest and best-known anticoagulants. Heparin produces its action by increasing antithrombin III–mediated inhibition of synthesis and activity of factor Xa. Heparin differs from low-molecular-weight heparin (LMWH) by an equal antifactor Xa/antifactor IIa ratio. (See Enoxaparin and Dalteparin as examples.) Heparin has a ratio of 1:1, but the LMWHs have ratios of 2:1 or higher.

Low-molecular-weight heparins are characterized by a molecular weight composed of approximately 5000 compared with conventional heparin (unfractionated heparin, UFH) with a molecular weight of approximately 15,000. In people, there is an advantage of LMWH over conventional heparin because the LMWHs have longer half-lives, and less frequent administration is needed. However, this may not be an advantage for dogs and cats. Consult the description of LMWH for more information such as the sections on enoxaparin (Lovenox) and dalteparin (Fragmin).

## Indications and Clinical Uses

Heparin is administered to prevent and treat hypercoagulability disorders and prevent coagulation disorders such as thromboembolism, venous thrombosis, disseminated intravascular coagulopathy, and pulmonary thromboembolism. The use in specific situations in animals is primarily anecdotal or derived from the clinical experience and opinions of experts. No outcome-based studies to evaluate efficacy have been published to support specific guidelines for therapy. Although the LMWHs have shown advantages for human medicine, there are no studies in veterinary medicine that have shown an advantage of LMWH over UFH. Use for prevention of thrombosis in canine patients with immune-mediated hemolytic anemia was not initially effective (50–300 units/kg SQ q6h), but when doses were adjusted based on anti-Xa activity, it was more effective and doses in individual dogs were as high as 560 mg/kg q6h. In horses, it is used to prevent thrombosis in patients at risk, but efficacy has not been measured at the recommended doses.

## Precautionary Information

### Adverse Reactions and Side Effects

Adverse effects caused by excessive inhibition of coagulation result in bleeding. Heparin-induced thrombocytopenia, a problem in people, has not been cited as a problem in animals. If excessive anticoagulation and bleeding occur as a result of an overdose, protamine sulfate should be administered to reverse heparin therapy. Protamine should be administered by slow IV infusion. It complexes with heparin to form a stable, inactive compound.

### Contraindications and Precautions

Do not use in animals unless able to monitor bleeding because it may be life threatening. Do not inject intramuscularly because it may create a hematoma.

### Drug Interactions

Use cautiously in animals that are already receiving other drugs that can interfere with coagulation, such as aspirin and warfarin. Although a specific interaction has not been identified, use cautiously in animals that may be receiving certain chondroprotective compounds, such as glycosaminoglycans for treatment of arthritis.

## Instructions for Use

Dose adjustments should be performed by monitoring clotting times. For example, dose is adjusted to maintain activated partial thromboplastin time (aPTT) at 1.5–2 times normal. For information on other forms of heparin, such as LMWHs, see Enoxaparin and Dalteparin. Duration of anticoagulant effect may vary among patients, but in general, a 200-unit/kg dose in dogs has a duration of effect of approximately 6 hours.

Only the SQ route of administration has been investigated in cats and the IV or SQ route in dogs. The IM route of administration is not recommended because of risk of hematoma formation.

**H**

The doses listed in the dosing section are based primarily on anecdotal experience and opinions of experts. Optimum doses are not established and likely vary in each individual. The doses vary depending whether it is intended for prevention in high-risk patients or treatment of ongoing coagulopathy. In high-risk patients, for prevention, it has been administered at doses as high as 500 units/kg SQ followed by reduced doses such as those listed in the dosing section q8–12h (see the dosing section for more information).

Heparin also has been used to prepare heparinized saline solutions for flushing catheters. The advantage of using heparinized saline instead of regular saline for flushing saline has not been shown in clinical studies. However, the dose for providing this solution is listed in the dosing section.

## Patient Monitoring and Laboratory Tests
Monitor effect using aPTT or anti-Xa activity. Dose is adjusted to maintain aPTT at 1.5–2 times normal. Target range for anti-Xa activity is 0.35–0.70 units/mL. If anti-Xa activity is greater than 0.7 units/mL, reduce dose by 25%.

## Formulations
- Heparin sodium is available in 1000- and 10,000-units/mL injection.

### Fluid supplementation
- To prepare heparinized saline solutions for IV use: the recommended mixture ranges from 0.25 to 10 units/mL of fluids. This is equivalent to adding 0.25 mL of heparin (1000 units/mL concentration) per 1000 mL of fluids, or 1 mL heparin (10,000 units/mL concentration) per 1000 mL of fluids, respectively. (Note: The advantage of adding heparin to fluid solutions for flushing IV catheters has not been demonstrated in clinical studies.)

## Stability and Storage
Store in a tightly sealed container, protected from light, and at room temperature.

## Small Animal Dosage
### Dogs
- Low-dose prophylaxis: 70–100 units/kg q8h SQ.
- Treatment of ongoing coagulopathy: 100–200 units/kg IV or SQ loading dose; then 150–300 units/kg q6h SQ. Adjust dose via monitoring of anti-Xa response and increase to 500–600 units/kg if necessary. In more severe cases, start with 500 units/kg SQ as the initial dose and then administer 500 units/kg q12h.
- Constant-rate infusion (CRI): Loading dose of 100 units/kg IV followed by CRI 20–30 units/kg/h. (Total dose of 480–720 units per 24 hours.)

### Cats
- Low-dose prophylaxis: 70–100 units/kg q8h SQ.
- 250 units/kg SQ q6h. The dose can be gradually increased up to 500 units/kg if necessary.

## Large Animal Dosage
- 125 units/kg SQ or IM q8–12h. (Lower dosages of 80 units/kg SQ q12h also have been used in horses.)

## Regulatory Information
No regulatory information is available for food animals. Because of low risk of residues, no withdrawal times are suggested.

# Hydralazine Hydrochloride
hye-drahl'ah-zeen hye-droe-klor'ide

**Trade and other names:** Apresoline

**Functional classification:** Vasodilator

## Pharmacology and Mechanism of Action
Hydralazine is a vasodilator used when patients have become refractory to other vasodilators. Hydralazine relaxes vascular smooth muscle and reduces blood pressure. In arteriolar vascular beds, it relaxes vascular smooth muscle to reduce vascular resistance and improves cardiac output. The mechanism of action is not certain. It may generate NO or act via other smooth muscle–relaxing properties. The peak effect occurs approximately 3–5 hours after administration, and the duration of effect on blood vessels is approximately 12 hours.

## Indications and Clinical Uses
Hydralazine is used to dilate arterioles and decrease cardiac afterload. It is primarily used for treatment of congestive heart failure (CHF), valvular disease of the heart, and other cardiovascular disorders characterized by high peripheral vascular resistance. It may be used with other cardiac drugs such as angiotensin-converting enzyme (ACE) inhibitors and pimobendan. Use in animals has been primarily derived from empirical use and small observational studies. There are no well-controlled clinical studies or efficacy trials to document clinical effectiveness. The most common use is as a vasodilator when canine patients have become refractory to other common cardiovascular agents such as ACE inhibitors and pimobendan. Candidates for hydralazine treatment are typically those in stage C or D of heart failure. Hydralazine is recommended by experts when afterload is needed in severe cases (0.5–2.0 mg/kg PO), starting at a low dose and titrating to effect.

Because of the availability of other agents, the use is not as common for routine treatment compared with several years ago. It is more common to use other vasodilator drugs, such as the ACE inhibitors, pimobendan, and calcium-channel blocking drugs.

## Precautionary Information

### Adverse Reactions and Side Effects
Adverse effects are attributed to excess vasodilation and subsequent hypotension, which results in reflex tachycardia. Hydralazine may dangerously decrease cardiac output if not monitored carefully. Allergic reactions (lupus-like syndrome) have been reported in people and are related to acetylator status but have not been reported in animals. Repeated use will activate the renin–angiotensin–aldosterone system; therefore, consider adding an ACE inhibitor, spironolactone, or both to patients that become refractory to treatment.

### Contraindications and Precautions
Do not use in hypotensive animals.

### Drug Interactions
No specific drug interactions are reported for animals. However, use cautiously with other drugs that may lower blood pressure.

## Instructions for Use

Use of hydralazine in heart failure may accompany other drugs, such as digoxin, pimobendan, ACE inhibitors, and diuretics. The optimum dosage in animals may be adjusted by monitoring blood pressure.

## Patient Monitoring and Laboratory Tests

Monitor patients for hypotension. Monitor blood pressure to adjust dose.

## Formulations

- Hydralazine is available in 10-, 25-, 50-, and 100-mg tablets and 20-mg/mL injection.

## Stability and Storage

Store in a tightly sealed container, protected from light, and at room temperature. Exposure to light may change color and cause decomposition. Hydralazine is unstable. Mixing with juices, syrups, and flavorings may cause decomposition in as little as 24 hours.

## Small Animal Dosage

**Dogs**

- IV dose: 0.5–3 mg/kg IV bolus q12h or after initial bolus; follow with CRI of 1.5–5 mcg/kg/min IV.
- Oral dose: 0.5 mg/kg (initial dose); titrate to 0.5–2 mg/kg q12h PO.

**Cats**

- 2.5 mg/cat q12–24h PO.

## Large Animal Dosage

**Horses**

- 1 mg/kg q12h PO or 0.5 mg/kg IV as needed to reduce blood pressure.

## Regulatory Information

No regulatory information is available. For extralabel use withdrawal interval estimates, contact FARAD at www.FARAD.org.

RCI Classification: 3

# Hydrochlorothiazide

hye-droe-klor-oh-thye′ah-zide

**Trade and other names:** HydroDIURIL, Hydrozide (for cattle), and generic

**Functional classification:** Diuretic

## Pharmacology and Mechanism of Action

Hydrochlorothiazide is a thiazide diuretic. Like other thiazide diuretics, it inhibits sodium reabsorption in distal renal tubules and causes urinary diuresis. Because thiazide diuretics act in the distal tubules (at the point where the most water has already been reabsorbed), their diuretic effects are not as great compared with loop diuretics such as furosemide. Thiazide diuretics are used commonly as a first-line agent in people to control hypertension, but they are not used commonly in animals. Other agents are preferred as diuretics (e.g., furosemide) or to control hypertension.

## Indications and Clinical Uses

Like other thiazide diuretics, hydrochlorothiazide is used to increase excretion of sodium, potassium, and water. It also has been used as an antihypertensive. Because thiazide diuretics decrease renal excretion of calcium, they also have been used to treat uroliths containing calcium (calcium oxalate uroliths). The use in small animals has been primarily derived from anecdotal experience or small observational studies. There are no well-controlled clinical studies or efficacy trials to document clinical effectiveness. In cattle, hydrochlorothiazide is approved for use in dairy cattle as an aid in the treatment of postparturient udder edema.

## Precautionary Information

**Adverse Reactions and Side Effects**

Hydrochlorothiazide may cause electrolyte imbalance such as hypokalemia.

**Contraindications and Precautions**

Do not use in patients with high serum calcium. Thiazide diuretics prevent calcium excretion.

**Drug Interactions**

Use carefully with other diuretics. It may enhance the effects of other diuretics and antihypertensive agents.

## Instructions for Use

Hydrochlorothiazide is not as potent as loop diuretics (e.g., furosemide). Clinical efficacy has not been established in veterinary patients.

## Patient Monitoring and Laboratory Tests

Monitor hydration status, electrolytes, and renal function. Monitor calcium in patients that may be prone to hypercalcemia. When used in cattle, animals should be regularly and carefully observed for early signs of fluid and electrolyte imbalance.

## Formulations

- Hydrochlorothiazide is available in 10- and 100-mg/mL oral solution and 25-, 50-, and 100-mg tablets. The combination of hydrochlorothiazide and spironolactone is Aldactazide. The cattle formulation is 25 mg/mL for injection.

## Stability and Storage

Store in a tightly sealed container, protected from light, and at room temperature. Stability of compounded formulations has not been evaluated.

## Small Animal Dosage

**Dogs and Cats**

- 2–4 mg/kg q12h PO.
- Antihypertensive dose: 1 mg/kg q12h PO.

## Cats

- To decrease excretion of calcium in urine: 1 mg/kg q12h PO.
- To alkalinize urine: 2 mg/kg, q12h PO.
- Congestive heart failure: 1–2 mg/kg q12–24h PO.

### Large Animal Dosage
#### Cattle

5–10 mL (125–250 mg) IV or IM once or twice a day. After onset of diuresis, treatment may be continued with an orally administered maintenance dose. For oral treatment, use chlorothiazide boluses.

### Regulatory Information

Withdrawal time for cattle: 72-hour (6 milkings) milk withdrawal; no withdrawal time for slaughter is established. For extralabel use withdrawal interval estimates, contact FARAD at www.FARAD.org.

RCI Classification: 4

# Hydrocodone Bitartrate
hye-droe-koe′done bye-tar′trate

**Trade and other names:** Hycodan, Vicodin, Lortab, and generic

**Functional classification:** Antitussive, analgesic

## Pharmacology and Mechanism of Action

Hydrocodone is an opioid agonist analgesic. Like other opioids, hydrocodone is an agonist for mu-opiate and kappa-opiate receptors on nerves and inhibits release of neurotransmitters involved with transmission of pain stimuli (e.g., substance P). Hydrocodone is metabolized to other metabolites, including hydromorphone, which has approximately six times the potency of morphine. Central sedative and euphoric effects are related to mu-receptor effects in the brain. Other opioids used in animals include hydromorphone, codeine, oxymorphone, meperidine, and fentanyl. Hycodan also contains homatropine, which is added to decrease abuse by people. Hydrocodone formulations used for antitussive action may also contain guaifenesin or acetaminophen.

*Pharmacokinetics:* Hydrocodone is metabolized in people to hydromorphone. In dogs, this conversion to a more active form is minimal but is unknown in other animals.

## Indications and Clinical Uses

Hydrocodone is an opiate agonist that has antitussive, analgesic, and sedative properties. In people, the combinations of hydrocodone and acetaminophen (e.g., Vicodin) and hydrocodone and aspirin are often prescribed as oral treatments for pain. However, in animals, the efficacy of these medications for treating pain has not been established.

The most common use of hydrocodone in dogs has been as an antitussive for symptomatic treatment of airway diseases, and many clinicians believe (anecdotally) that it is an effective antitussive. There are no antitussive preparations marketed for use in the United States that do not contain atropine. (Canadian preparations may contain only hydrocodone.) It may also contain other ingredients for treating cough.

## Precautionary Information

**Adverse Reactions and Side Effects**

Like all opiates, side effects from opioids are predictable and unavoidable. Side effects include sedation, constipation, and bradycardia. Respiratory depression occurs with high doses but is not documented from the use in animals. Paradoxical excitement may occur in some animals.

**Contraindications and Precautions**

Do not use in patients that may be sensitive to opioid effects or experience dysphoria. Because preparations for oral use contain atropine, do not use in animals in which atropine may be contraindicated. Many formulations for treating pain in people contain hydrocodone and acetaminophen or hydrocodone and aspirin. Do not administer to animals sensitive to these other ingredients. Acetaminophen-containing products should never be administered to cats. Hydrocodone is combined with atropine in the product Hycodan. Atropine can decrease respiratory secretions but probably does not exert significant clinical effects at doses in this preparation (1.5 mg homatropine per 5-mg tablet).

**Drug Interactions**

No specific drug interactions are reported for animals. However, other typical drug interactions that affect opioids should be considered.

## Instructions for Use

Hydrocodone use in animals (primarily dogs) is derived from anecdotal experience and opinions from experts. It is most often used as an antitussive in dogs.

## Patient Monitoring and Laboratory Tests

No specific monitoring is necessary.

## Formulations

- There are many oral formulations for humans to treat pain that contain hydrocodone and other analgesics such as acetaminophen (e.g., Vicodin). Typically, these preparations contain 5 mg of hydrocodone and 500 mg of acetaminophen.
- Hydrocodone is also available as an antitussive (Hycodan) in 5-mg tablets and 1-mg/mL syrup combined with homatropine in a concentration of 1.5 mg in tablets and 0.3 mg/mL in syrup, respectively. Formulations in Canada do not contain homatropine.
- The extended-release formulations for people contain 10-, 15-, 20-, 30-, 40-, 50-, 60-, 80-, 100-, and 120-mg tablets) approved for use in people for treating pain. These extended-release formulations provide extended duration for once- or twice-daily administration but have not been evaluated for animals.

## Stability and Storage

Store in a tightly sealed container, protected from light, and at room temperature.

## Small Animal Dosage

### Dogs

- Antitussive dose: 0.5 mg/kg q8 h PO. Increase the dose if needed for tracheal collapse in dogs but not above the dose of 1.5 mg/kg.
- Analgesic dose: 0.5 mg/kg q8–12 h PO. (Analgesic properties have not been established in dogs.)

### Cats

- No dose has been established. Oral doses may be effective in cats, but caution should be used because many formulations contain acetaminophen.

## Large Animal Dosage

- No large animal doses have been reported.

## Regulatory Information

Hydrocodone is a Schedule II drug controlled by the Drug Enforcement Administration (DEA).

Hydrocodone is not recommended for food-producing animals. If administered to a food animal, consult FARAD for extralabel use withdrawal interval estimates (www.FARAD.org).

RCI Classification: 1. Do not administer to racing horses.

# Hydrocortisone
hye-droe-kor′tih-sone

**Trade and other names:** Hydrocortisone, Cortef and generic brands, hydrocortisone sodium succinate, Solu-Cortef

**Functional classification:** Corticosteroid

## Pharmacology and Mechanism of Action

Hydrocortisone is a glucocorticoid anti-inflammatory and adrenal replacement drug. Hydrocortisone has weaker anti-inflammatory effects and greater mineralocorticoid effects compared with prednisolone or dexamethasone. Hydrocortisone has properties that most closely resemble natural cortisol in the body. It is about 1/5 the potency of prednisolone and 1/25 the potency of dexamethasone. The most common use is to mimic the effects of cortisol when used in patients with hypoadrenocorticism (patients with adrenal insufficiency). Anti-inflammatory effects are complex but are primarily via inhibition of inflammatory cells and suppression of expression of inflammatory mediators.

## Indications and Clinical Uses

Hydrocortisone is used most often for adrenal corticosteroid replacement treatment in patients with adrenal insufficiency. It is less often used for its anti-inflammatory effects and not used as commonly as other corticosteroids such as prednisolone or dexamethasone except when hormone replacement to mimic the effects of cortisol is needed. Hydrocortisone sodium succinate is a rapid-acting injectable product that can be used when a prompt response is needed.

## Precautionary Information

### Adverse Reactions and Side Effects

At the doses used for replacement therapy, serious adverse effects are uncommon. Other side effects from corticosteroids are many and include polyphagia, polydipsia/polyuria, and hypothalamic–pituitary–adrenal axis suppression. Adverse effects include gastrointestinal (GI) ulceration, hepatopathy, diabetes, hyperlipidemia, decreased thyroid hormone, decreased protein synthesis, delayed wound healing, and immunosuppression. Secondary infections can occur as a result of immunosuppression and include demodicosis, toxoplasmosis, fungal infections, and urinary tract infections. In horses, additional adverse effects may include risk of laminitis, but this is poorly documented in horses unless they have predisposing factors.

### Contraindications and Precautions

Use cautiously in patients prone to ulcers or infection or in animals in which wound healing is necessary. Use cautiously in diabetic animals, animals with renal failure, or pregnant animals.

### Drug Interactions

Glucocorticoids are often synergistic with other anti-inflammatory and immunosuppressive drugs. Administration of corticosteroids with nonsteroidal anti-inflammatory drugs increases the risk of GI injury.

## Instructions for Use

Because the most common use is for adrenal replacement therapy in adrenal insufficiency, the doses administered are intended to mimic the natural release of cortisol in the body. Typically for replacement therapy (e.g., in animals with hypoadrenocorticism) dosages start at 1 mg/kg/day.

## Patient Monitoring and Laboratory Tests

Monitor electrolytes (sodium and potassium) in animals being treated for hypoadrenocorticism. Monitor liver enzymes, blood glucose, and renal function during therapy. Monitor patients for signs of secondary infections. Perform adrenocorticotropic hormone (ACTH) stimulation test to monitor adrenal function.

## Formulations

- Hydrocortisone is available in 5-, 10-, and 20-mg tablets, and hydrocortisone sodium succinate is available in various size vials for injection.

## Stability and Storage

Store in a tightly sealed container, protected from light, and at room temperature. Hydrocortisone is slightly soluble in water and is soluble in alcohol. Degradation occurs at a high pH above 7–9. Compounded suspensions have been stable for 30 days. Most compounded topical ointments and lotions are stable for 30 days.

## Small Animal Dosage

### Dogs and Cats

*Hydrocortisone*
- Replacement therapy: 1–2 mg/kg q12h PO.
- Anti-inflammatory: 2.5–5 mg/kg q12h PO.

*Hydrocortisone Sodium Succinate*
- Hypoadrenocorticism (adrenal crisis): 0.625 mg/kg/h, IV CRI.
- Shock: (not a recommended use) 50–150 mg/kg IV for two doses 8 hours apart.
- Anti-inflammatory: 5 mg/kg q12h IV.

## Large Animal Dosage
**Horses**
- Hydrocortisone sodium succinate: 5 mg/kg q12h IV.

**Foals**
- Replacement therapy for critical illness: 1–3 mg/kg/day IV.

## Regulatory Information
No regulatory information is available. For extralabel use withdrawal interval estimates, contact FARAD at www.FARAD.org.
RCI Classification: 4

# Hydromorphone
hye-droe-mor'fone

**Trade and other names:** Dilaudid, Hydrostat, and generic brands

**Functional classification:** Analgesic, opiate

## Pharmacology and Mechanism of Action
Hydromorphone is an opioid agonist, analgesic. Like other opiates, it binds to mu-opiate and kappa-opiate receptors on nerves and inhibits release of neurotransmitters involved with transmission of pain stimuli (e.g., substance P). Opiates also may inhibit release of some inflammatory mediators. Central sedative and euphoric effects are related to mu-receptor effects in the brain. Hydromorphone has similar qualitative properties as morphine but is six or seven times more potent than morphine. Other opiates used in animals include morphine, codeine, oxymorphone, meperidine, and fentanyl.

*Pharmacokinetics:* In dogs, the half-life after IV administration was 70–80 minutes. When PO hydrocodone is administered to animals, it is partially metabolized to hydromorphone (hydrocodone discussed earlier).

## Indications and Clinical Uses
Hydromorphone is used in animals for analgesia and sedation and as an adjunct for anesthesia. In dogs and cats, it is used as a single agent or in combination with other agents. Hydromorphone is similar in action to morphine; however, it is more potent than morphine (6–7×) and should be used at lower doses. Hydromorphone is approximately half as potent as oxymorphone. Studies in dogs indicate that hydromorphone at equivalent doses is equal to oxymorphone for producing sedation in dogs. In cats, duration of effect (0.1 mg/kg) has been 6–7.5 hours despite a relatively short plasma half-life of 1–1.5 hours.

## Precautionary Information

### Adverse Reactions and Side Effects

Like all opioids, side effects from hydromorphone are predictable and unavoidable. Side effects from administration include sedation, panting, constipation, urinary retention, and bradycardia. Vomiting is common after initial administration but is a predicted event and does not require treatment. In dogs, hydromorphone produces less histamine release than morphine administration and therefore may produce fewer histamine-related side effects.

In cats, the most common adverse effects are dysphoria, hypersalivation, and vomiting. Hyperthermia also has been observed in cats, but the mechanism is not known.

In horses, undesirable and even dangerous behavior actions can follow rapid IV opioid administration. Horses should receive a preanesthetic of acepromazine or an alpha$_2$ agonist.

Respiratory depression occurs with high doses. As with other opiates, a slight decrease in heart rate is expected. In most cases, this decrease does not have to be treated with anticholinergic drugs (e.g., atropine) but should be monitored. Tolerance and dependence occur with chronic administration.

### Contraindications and Precautions

Cats and horses are more sensitive to excitement than other species. Monitor the body temperature in cats because hyperthermia may occur. Hydromorphone may cause bradycardia and atrioventricular block in some patients.

### Drug Interactions

There are no specific drug interactions, but hydromorphone potentiates the effects of other anesthetics and sedatives. Hydromorphone may be used with other anesthetics, but doses should be adjusted because of potentiation of the other drugs. If butorphanol is used concurrently, it may diminish the effects of hydromorphone by antagonizing mu-opiate receptors.

**H**

## Instructions for Use

Hydromorphone may be used interchangeably with morphine or oxymorphone, provided that doses are adjusted for potency differences. Administration to cats has been more effective when injected intravenously, rather than intramuscularly or subcutaneously, and resulted in faster onset with fewer adverse effects.

Oral tablets and solution are available for human use, but use has not been reported for animals. It is uncertain if oral forms are absorbed sufficiently for clinical use in animals.

In addition to sedative and analgesic uses, hydromorphone also has been used to induce vomiting by stimulating the chemoreceptor trigger zone. This has been used for the purpose of treating an animal that has ingested a toxin. It is more effective as an emetic in dogs and cats when injected subcutaneously or intramuscularly rather than intravenously.

## Patient Monitoring and Laboratory Tests

Monitor patient's heart rate and respiration. Although bradycardia rarely needs to be treated when it is caused by an opioid, atropine or glycopyrrolate can be administered if needed. If serious respiratory depression occurs, the opioid can be reversed with naloxone (0.04 mg/kg). Monitor body temperature in cats. Hyperthermia has been observed in patients after anesthesia.

## Formulations
- Hydromorphone is available in 1-mg/mL oral solution; 2-, 4-, and 8-mg tablets; and 1-, 2-, 4-, and 10-mg/mL injection.
- Exalgo is an extended-release formulation for people in 8-, 12-, and 16-mg tablets that allows for once-daily treatment. This formulation has not been evaluated in animals.

## Stability and Storage
Store in a tightly sealed container, protected from light, and at room temperature. Hydromorphone is soluble in water. Compounded solutions in fluids have been stable for 30 days. It is a Schedule II drug and should be stored in a locked compartment.

## Small Animal Dosage
### Dogs
- 0.22 mg/kg IM or SQ. Repeat q4–6h or as needed for pain treatment.
- 0.1–0.2 mg/kg IV, repeated q2h or as necessary. A dose of 0.1 mg/kg may be used with acepromazine as a preoperative sedative.
- CRI: 0.01 mg/kg/h IV.

### Cats
- 0.1–0.2 mg/kg SQ or IM or 0.05–0.1 mg/kg IV q2–6h (as needed).
- Epidural dose: 0.05 mg/kg, diluted in saline to 0.2 mL/kg (1 mL per cat).
- Dose to produce emesis (for poisoning): 0.1 mg/kg SQ once.

## Large Animal Dosage
### Horses
- Epidural: 0.04 mg/kg diluted in 0.9% saline to 20 mL.
- No systemic doses have been reported.

## Regulatory Information
Hydromorphone is a Schedule II drug controlled by the DEA. Withdrawal times have not been established for food animals, but the elimination rate is rapid, and a brief withdrawal time is suggested. For extralabel use withdrawal interval estimates, contact FARAD at www.FARAD.org.

RCI Classification: 1

# Hydroxyethyl Starch
**Trade and other names:** HES, hetastarch, Hespan, tetrastarch, and VetStarch (veterinary product)

**Functional classification:** Fluid replacement

## Pharmacology and Mechanism of Action
Hydroxyethyl starch is a synthetic colloid volume expander that is used to maintain vascular volume in animals with circulatory shock. It is a modified branched-chain glucose polymer derived from amylopectin sources such as potatoes, sorghum, or maize. The advantage of synthetic colloids such as hydroxyethyl starch is that when administered IV, they produce oncotic pressure

in the vascular compartment, which prevents migration of fluid replacement to the interstitial compartment.

Forms available:

| Formulation | Concentration (%) | Molecular Weight (kDa) | Molar Substitution[a] | C2-to-C6 Ratio[b] |
|---|---|---|---|---|
| Hetastarch | 6 | 600–670 | 0.7–0.75 | 5:1 |
| Hetastarch | 6 | 480 | 0.7 | 5:1 |
| Hexastarch | 6 | 200 | 0.62 | 9:1 |
| Pentastarch | 6 or 10 | 200 | 0.5 | 5:1 |
| Pentastarch | 6 | 70 | 0.5 | 3:1 |
| Tetrastarch | 6 or 10 | 130 | 0.42 | 6:1 |
| Tetrastarch | 6 or 10 | 130 | 0.42 | 6:1 |

[a]Molar substitution is the number of hydroxyethyl groups substituted per 100 available anhydrous glucose binding sites.
[b]C2-to-C6 ratio refers to the substitution on the C2 and C6 carbons.

H

The hydroxyethyl starch preparations include (see table) tetrastarch, hetastarch, and pentastarch. Most hetastarch (6%) products have an average molecular weight of 200 kDa (kilodaltons) and a colloid osmotic pressure of approximately 30. Pentastarch has an average molecular weight of 200 kDa and a colloid osmotic pressure of 30–60. Tetrastarch (VetStarch) has a molecular weight of 130 kDa and a colloid osmotic pressure of 36. The number of molecular substitutions determine whether it is hetastarch, pentastarch, or hexastarch (see table). Hetastarch has the most molecular substitutions and tends to remain longest in the vasculature. Higher molecular weight compounds also have longer half-lives in plasma.

Metabolism and clearance is by serum amylase activity. Hetastarch is cleared much more slowly than tetrastarch because of poor hydrolysis in the blood. Although hetastarch has slower degradation and prolonged intravascular expansion, this property also is associated with accumulation in the reticuloendothelial system, skin, liver, and kidney. Tetrastarch compounds are cleared faster than hetastarch compounds and are associated with a better safety profile because of lower plasma and tissue retention. Higher substitutions on C2 compared to C6 leads to inhibition of metabolism by amylases and increased plasma half-lives.

## Indications and Clinical Uses

The use of hydroxyethyl starch for resuscitation in veterinary patients remains controversial. If used by emergency or critical care clinicians, hydroxyethyl starch is used primarily to treat acute hypovolemia and shock. It is administered intravenously in acute situations in which rapid restoration of circulating volume is needed. Hydroxyethyl starch solutions have a duration of effective volume expansion of 12–48 hours.

The formulations available are 6%, which is isotonic, and 10%, which is hypertonic. Because of more adverse reactions with the higher concentration 10% solution, they are not used commonly. Although hydroxyethyl starch is used by many clinical experts in critically ill hypovolemic and septic patients, other experts have recommended against its use because of its expense, lack of superiority over other treatments, and potential harm. These experts argue that because there is evidence of harm in people, this should warrant caution in animals also (see Adverse Reactions and Side Effects for more details).

## Precautionary Information

### Adverse Reactions and Side Effects

Most of the serious adverse effects reported, such as kidney injury and coagulation abnormalities, have been observed in human studies. These products are no longer recommended in critically ill human patients with sepsis, burns, renal impairment, or coagulopathies. The human Surviving Sepsis Campaign recommends against the use of hydroxyethyl starch.

The high-molecular-weight hetastarch may alter coagulation and alter viscoelastic measurements and fibrinolysis. Hydroxyethyl starch solutions may affect platelet function and produce coagulation abnormalities at clinically relevant doses for up to 24 hours. Tetrastarch solutions may have less tendency to cause coagulopathies than hetastarch; therefore the current recommendation is to use tetrastarch solutions of 6% and reduced molecular weight (130 kDa) to reduce risk of adverse effects.

High-molecular-weight products with molecular weights more than 200 kDa are associated with higher risk of kidney injury. The proposed mechanism for kidney injury is through uptake by proximal epithelial tubular cells as lysosomes leading to injury to proximal tubular cells.

The use in veterinary patients has become controversial. There have been conflicting results from studies, with some demonstrating evidence of kidney injury in dogs and conflicting results showing no kidney injury. It is possible that this difference is attributed to differences in molecular weight of the products with the lower molecular weight forms less likely to cause injury.

### Contraindications and Precautions

The most recent guidelines for treating severe sepsis and septic shock in people advise not to use synthetic colloids for fluid resuscitation. Do not use in animals with bleeding problems (coagulopathies), active hemorrhage, or preexisting coagulopathies. Do not use in animals with known kidney disease.

### Drug Interactions

Hydroxyethyl starch is compatible with most fluid solutions.

## Instructions for Use

Hydroxyethyl starch solutions are used in critical care situations and infused via CRI.

Suspend in saline (0.9%) or 5% dextrose solution for use. Administer slowly in 5-mL/kg increments to small animals; then reassess and increase the dose to rates listed in the dosing section.

## Patient Monitoring and Laboratory Tests

Monitor the patient's hydration status and blood pressure during administration. Monitor heart rate and rhythm. Monitor for signs of coagulopathy or platelet dysfunction and discontinue if there are bleeding problems. Monitor kidney parameters and discontinue use if signs of kidney injury are observed. Administration of hydroxyethyl starch solutions may increase patient's amylase for 2–3 days.

## Formulations

- See earlier table for list of products. Hydroxyethyl starch is available in 6% injectable solution as an approved veterinary formulation (tetrastarch, VetStarch). Several other hydroxyethyl starch solutions (hetastarch, pentastarch, hexastarch) in concentrations of 6% and 10% are available.

## Stability and Storage

Hydroxyethyl starch is stable in the original packaging and is compatible with most fluid administration sets.

## Small Animal Dosage

**Dogs**
- Small-volume resuscitation: 5 mL/kg IV.
- Large-volume resuscitation: 5–15 mL/kg IV.
- CRI: 10–20 mL/kg/day IV (0.4–0.8 mL/kg/h). Maximum dosages are 33–50 mL/kg/day or 70 mL/kg cumulative dose over 4 days.

**Cats**
- Resuscitation: 2–5 mL/kg IV.
- CRI: 5–10 mL/kg/day IV (0.2–0.4 mL/kg/h).

## Large Animal Dosage

**Horses**
- 8–10 mL/kg bolus dose or CRI 0.5–1 mL/kg/h.

## Regulatory Information

No regulatory information is available for food animals. Because of low risk of residues, no withdrawal times are suggested.

# Hydroxyurea

hye-droks′ih-yoo-ree-ah

**Trade and other names:** Droxia and Hydrea (Canada)

**Functional classification:** Anticancer agent

## Pharmacology and Mechanism of Action

Hydroxyurea is an antineoplastic agent. Hydroxyurea is a cell cycle–dependent agent, acting primarily at the S-phase of mitosis. The exact mechanism of action is uncertain, but it may interfere with DNA synthesis in cancer cells. The specific effects on red blood cells occur because of the activity on hemoglobin.

## Indications and Clinical Uses

In people, hydroxyurea is used for treatment of sickle cell anemia and occasionally various carcinomas. In animals, it has been used in combination with other anticancer modalities for treatment of certain tumors. In animals, the use is uncommon but one of the uses has been treatment of polycythemia vera.

## Precautionary Information

**Adverse Reactions and Side Effects**

Because of only limited use in veterinary medicine, no adverse effects have been reported. In people, hydroxyurea causes leukopenia, anemia, and thrombocytopenia.

**Contraindications and Precautions**

Avoid use in pregnant animals.

**Drug Interactions**

No specific drug interactions are reported for animals, but the use is uncommon, and the full range of drug interactions are not known.

## Instructions for Use

Hydroxyurea has been used on a limited basis in veterinary medicine. Most of the use is empirical from small observational studies or extrapolated from human medicine.

## Patient Monitoring and Laboratory Tests

Monitor complete blood count in treated animals.

## Formulations

- Hydroxyurea is available in 200-, 300-, 400-, and 500-mg capsules.

## Stability and Storage

Store in a tightly sealed container, protected from light, and at room temperature.

## Small Animal Dosage

**Dogs**

- 50 mg/kg PO once daily 3 days/wk.

**Cats**

- 25 mg/kg PO once daily 3 days/wk.

## Large Animal Dosage

- No large animal doses have been reported.

## Regulatory Information

Withdrawal times are not established for animals that produce food. This drug should not be used in animals intended for food because it is an anticancer agent.

# Hydroxyzine Hydrochloride
hye-droks′ih-zeen

**Trade and other names:** Atarax and Vistaril

**Functional classification:** Antihistamine

## Pharmacology and Mechanism of Action

Hydroxyzine is an antihistamine ($H_1$ blocker) of the piperazine class. Like other antihistamines, hydroxyzine acts by blocking the $H_1$ receptor and suppresses inflammatory reactions caused by histamine. The $H_1$ blockers have been used to control pruritus and skin inflammation, rhinorrhea, and airway inflammation.

Hydroxyzine also has sedative properties and other calming effects on the CNS that are not related to the antihistamine effects.

*Pharmacokinetics:* Another antihistamine, cetirizine, is an active metabolite of hydroxyzine. In dogs, most of the antihistamine effect of the administration of hydroxyzine is from the formation of cetirizine, which occurs readily after IV and oral administration. See Cetirizine for details. In horses, it is also metabolized to cetirizine. In horses, the half-life of hydroxyzine is 7.4 hours, and a long withdrawal time is necessary if it is used in performance horses.

## Indications and Clinical Uses

In animals, hydroxyzine has been used to treat pruritus. Efficacy in animals for treating pruritus is low and not recommended by most dermatologists as the sole agent. Although it has been shown in experimental animals to suppress histamine response, it has not been consistently effective relieving pruritus in dogs with atopic dermatitis. Other uses include allergic airway disease and rhinitis. However, efficacy is not established for these uses. Hydroxyzine is sometimes prescribed for performance horses for treatment of hypersensitivity reactions and for the production of sedation. However, the efficacy is not established for these indications in horses. In people, additional uses include treatment of anxiety and psychoneurosis and as a sedative before and after general anesthesia.

## Precautionary Information

### Adverse Reactions and Side Effects

Sedation is the most common side effect. It is the result of inhibition of histamine N-methyltransferase in the CNS. Sedation may also be attributed to the blocking of other CNS receptors such as those for serotonin, acetylcholine, and alpha-receptors. Antimuscarinic effects (atropine-like effects), such as dry mouth and decreased GI secretions, also are common.

### Contraindications and Precautions

No contraindications reported in animals. It has been safe even at high doses. Discontinue administration a minimum of 7 days prior to allergen-specific allergy testing in dogs.

### Drug Interactions

No specific drug interactions are reported for animals.

## Instructions for Use

Clinical studies have shown hydroxyzine to be effective for treatment of pruritus in some dogs, but these were small observational studies. Overall, efficacy rates are low.

## Patient Monitoring and Laboratory Tests

No specific monitoring is necessary.

## Formulations

- Hydroxyzine hydrochloride is available in 10-, 25-, and 50-mg tablets; 2-mg/mL oral syrup; and 25-mg/mL injection. It is also available in a pamoate form (Vistaril) in 25- and 50-mg capsules.

## Stability and Storage

Store in a tightly sealed container, protected from light, and at room temperature. Hydroxyzine is soluble in water. Compounded formulation with syrups was stable for 14 days.

## Small Animal Dosage
**Dogs**
- 2 mg/kg q8–12h IM or PO.

**Cats**
- Effective doses have not been established (see Cetirizine for dosing information for cats).

## Large Animal Dosage
**Horses**
- Hydroxyzine pamoate 500 mg per horse PO twice daily (efficacy not established).

## Regulatory Information
No regulatory information is available for food animals. Because of low risk of residues, no withdrawal times are suggested.
RCI Classification: 2

# Hyoscyamine
hye-oh-sye'ah-meen

**Trade and other names:** Levsin

**Functional classification:** Anticholinergic

## Pharmacology and Mechanism of Action
Hyoscyamine is an anticholinergic agent (blocks acetylcholine effect at muscarinic receptor), parasympatholytic. It is used infrequently in animals.

## Indications and Clinical Uses
Hyoscyamine is an anticholinergic drug with actions similar to atropine and related drugs. The use in animals is uncommon. It can produce an antiemetic effect to decrease vomiting associated with motion sickness and some GI diseases, but these clinical effects are not established for animals. It is indicated in animals for similar conditions for which atropine is used, in which it is important to block parasympathetic responses. It has been used to decrease GI motility and secretions, decrease salivation, and increase heart rate (to treat bradycardia).

## Precautionary Information
**Adverse Reactions and Side Effects**
Side effects include xerostomia, ileus, constipation, tachycardia, and urine retention.

**Contraindications and Precautions**
Do not use in patients with glaucoma, intestinal ileus, gastroparesis, or tachycardia.

**Drug Interactions**
Do not mix with alkaline solutions. Hyoscyamine antagonizes the effects of any cholinergic drugs administered (e.g., metoclopramide).

## Instructions for Use
Hyoscyamine is used uncommonly in veterinary medicine and the use is based on anecdotal accounts in dogs and cats for some GI and cardiovascular conditions.

## Patient Monitoring and Laboratory Tests
Monitor heart rate and intestinal motility during treatment.

## Formulations
- Hyoscyamine is available in 0.125-mg tablets, 0.375-mg extended-release tablets, and 0.025-mg/mL solution.

## Stability and Storage
Store in a tightly sealed container at room temperature.

## Small Animal Dosage
**Dogs**
- 0.003–0.006 mg/kg q8h PO.

**Cats**
- No doses have been established for cats.

## Large Animal Dosage
- No large animal doses have been reported.

## Regulatory Information
Do not use in animals that produce food.
Withdrawal time: None established in the United States (manufacturer of large animal products lists zero days for milk and meat), but it is listed as 14 days for meat and 3 days for milk in the United Kingdom.

H

## Ibuprofen

eye-byoo-proe'fen

**Trade and other names:** Motrin, Advil, Nuprin, and generic

**Functional classification:** Nonsteroidal anti-inflammatory drug

### Pharmacology and Mechanism of Action

Ibuprofen is a nonsteroidal anti-inflammatory drug (NSAID) approved for use in human medicine but not available in veterinary dosage forms. Like other NSAIDs in this class, ibuprofen produces analgesic and anti-inflammatory effects by inhibiting the synthesis of prostaglandins. The enzyme inhibited by NSAIDs is the cyclo-oxygenase (COX) enzyme. The COX enzyme exists in two isoforms: COX-1 and COX-2. COX-1 is primarily responsible for synthesis of prostaglandins important for maintaining a healthy gastrointestinal (GI) tract, renal function, platelet function, and other normal physiologic functions. COX-2 is induced and responsible for synthesizing prostaglandins that are important mediators of pain, inflammation, and fever. However, it is known that there is some crossover of COX-1 and COX-2 effects in some situations, and COX-2 activity is important for some biological effects. Ibuprofen is not selective for either COX-1 or COX-2. Ibuprofen is approved for human use, and experience with this drug in veterinary medicine is limited. The adverse effects in dogs prohibit the use in canine patients.

*Pharmacokinetics:* The pharmacokinetics have been studied in a variety of animals. In horses, the half-life is approximately 60–90 minutes. Oral absorption is high in horses (80%–90%), regardless of the dose form used, including a compounded paste. Ibuprofen is 90%–100% absorbed when administered orally to dairy goats.

### Indications and Clinical Uses

Ibuprofen is not approved for any animals in veterinary medicine. There are drugs in small animals that have been safer for the GI tract and are preferred. Use of ibuprofen in dogs is discouraged because of a high risk of GI ulceration. It has been used for musculoskeletal inflammation in horses and ruminants. Administration of 25 mg/kg IV to cows reduced some systemic variables in endotoxin-induced mastitis.

In horses, doses of 10–25 mg/kg have been used, but clinical trials of efficacy have not been reported.

### Precautionary Information

#### Adverse Reactions and Side Effects

Vomiting, severe GI ulceration, and hemorrhage have been reported in dogs. Like other NSAIDs, renal injury caused by decrease in renal perfusion has occurred with ibuprofen. Ibuprofen may inhibit platelets in animals.

#### Contraindications and Precautions

Safe doses have not been established for dogs and cats. Do not administer to animals prone to GI ulcers. Do not administer with other ulcerogenic drugs such as corticosteroids.

#### Drug Interactions

No specific drug interactions are reported. However, like other NSAIDs, ulcerogenic effects are potentiated when administered with corticosteroids. Ibuprofen, like other NSAIDs, may interfere with the action of diuretics, such as furosemide and angiotensin-converting enzyme (ACE) inhibitors.

## Instructions for Use

Avoid use in dogs. Safe dosages for other species have not been established, although there has been some extralabel use in ruminants and horses. The use in horses is based on small observational studies or opinions from equine clinicians.

## Patient Monitoring and Laboratory Tests

Monitor for signs of GI ulcers. Monitor renal function during therapy.

## Formulations

- Ibuprofen is available in 200-, 400-, 600-, and 800-mg tablets. Over-the-counter (OTC) formulations are available.

## Stability and Storage

Store in a tightly sealed container, protected from light, and at room temperature. Ibuprofen has been compounded in alcohol (ethanol) and propylene glycol solutions without loss of stability. It is poorly soluble in water. Ibuprofen has been compounded as an oral paste for horses without compromising the oral absorption.

## Small Animal Dosage

**Dogs and Cats**
- Safe dose not established.

## Large Animal Dosage

**Horses**
- 25 mg/kg q8h PO for up to 6 days.

**Ruminants**
- 14–25 mg/kg/day PO.

## Regulatory Information

No withdrawal times are established for animals intended for food. For extralabel use withdrawal interval estimates, contact Food Animal Residue Avoidance Databank (FARAD) at www.FARAD.org.

Racing Commissioners International (RCI) Classification: 4

# Imepitoin
eye-mep'i-toyn

**Trade and other names:** Pexion

**Functional classification:** Anticonvulsant, behavior drug

## Pharmacology and Mechanism of Action

Imepitoin acts as an anticonvulsant and behavior-modifying drug. The mechanism of action of imepitoin is to decrease seizures by potentiating the gamma-aminobutyric acid ($GABA_A$) receptor–mediated inhibitory effects. Although it is not classified structurally as a benzodiazepine, these actions are similar to those of diazepam and other benzodiazepines. The similar action to benzodiazepines is caused by its low-affinity binding for the benzodiazepine binding site of $GABA_A$ but has 600 times less affinity for the binding site compared to diazepam. It also may have a weak calcium channel blocking effect, which may contribute to clinical effects.

*Pharmacokinetics:* The half-life of imepitoin in beagle dogs (1.5–2 hours) was relatively short compared with other anticonvulsant drugs. The peak occurs at approximately 2 hours after oral administration. Most of the elimination is by the feces. Concentration profiles are not much different in fed versus fasted dogs except for higher exposure when administered to fasted dogs (20% higher). This difference in fed versus fasted dogs may not be enough of a difference to be clinically relevant. The protein binding was 56%–57%, but no protein-binding drug interactions have been identified.

## Indications and Clinical Uses

Imepitoin is approved in the United States for treatment of noise aversion (noise phobia) associated with loud noises that cause anxiety and behavior problems in dogs. It is approved in Europe as an anticonvulsant (epilepsy treatment) but not the United States. In Europe, it is considered a first-line treatment for idiopathic epilepsy in dogs. It has not been evaluated for treatment of status epilepticus.

There have been no studies reported in cats or other animals.

## Precautionary Information

### Adverse Reactions and Side Effects

Imepitoin acts as a central nervous system (CNS) depressant. The most common adverse effects from imepitoin reported in field trials were lethargy and sedation, polyuria and polydipsia, ataxia, and increased appetite. Most reactions are mild and generally transient. Other reported effects are hyperactivity, hypersalivation, emesis, diarrhea, and sensitivity to sound. In some animals, there were signs of aggression (see Contraindications and Precautions).

An important finding in clinical studies was that it produced fewer adverse effects than primidone or phenobarbital. In clinical studies, it did not elevate liver enzymes. Although it is a partial agonist for the $GABA_A$ binding site, there is no evidence of tolerance or dependence that develop from repeated administration of imepitoin.

During safety studies in dogs, it was well-tolerated at the label dose, but at higher doses (three and five times the label dose), there were signs of sedation, tremors, and nystagmus. There were also dose-dependent salivation and vomiting.

### Contraindications and Precautions

Safe doses have not been established for cats. When administered with other CNS depressants, especially benzodiazepines, to dogs, there may be additional sedation. Anxiolytic drugs acting at the benzodiazepine receptor site, including imepitoin, may lead to disinhibition of fear-based behaviors and may therefore result in a change in aggression level. Careful observation by the owners is recommended during treatment.

### Drug Interactions

Imepitoin is metabolized by the liver enzymes; therefore, interactions with other drugs that affect cytochrome P450 enzymes are possible but have not been studied in dogs. It did not affect activity of most human P450 isoforms, but inhibition of CYP1A1 is possible. Imepitoin had no effect on enzyme induction compared with phenobarbital. It is a partial agonist for the benzodiazepine receptor, but there is no evidence that it prevents the activity of co-administered benzodiazepines used for acute treatment (e.g., status epilepticus). In a small study, there was no evidence of interaction with co-administered phenobarbital in dogs.

Imepitoin is poorly soluble and dissolves more readily at an acid pH. Therefore it is possible that suppressing acid in the stomach (e.g., with proton pump inhibitors such as omeprazole) could interfere with oral absorption.

## Instructions for Use

The use in dogs is based on the Food and Drug Administration (FDA) approval in the United States and the approval for anticonvulsant use in Europe. For anticonvulsant use, it is recommended to start with 10 mg/kg and then increase dose to obtain the desired response. There have been no guidelines thus far for plasma/serum concentration monitoring; therefore, dose adjustment should be made on the basis of clinical response. The dose can be increased by 50% to 100% increments up to a maximum dosage of 30 mg/kg administered twice daily.

When compared with primidone in dogs for treating epilepsy in a US field trial, imepitoin efficacy was lower than primidone, but it produced fewer adverse effects in dogs than primidone. In the field trials in Europe, the efficacy of imepitoin was compared with phenobarbital in dogs with idiopathic epilepsy. Although there was lower overall efficacy for imepitoin compared with phenobarbital, some dogs were well-controlled with imepitoin treatment. It may also be considered as an add-on treatment for dogs with epilepsy.

For treatment of noise aversion (noise phobia) in dogs, start treatment (30 mg/kg) 2 days prior to the anticipated noise event (e.g., fireworks).

## Patient Monitoring and Laboratory Tests

No specific monitoring is necessary. Monitor animals for signs listed in the adverse effects section.

## Formulations

- Imepitoin is available in 100- and 400 mg-tablets. Tablets can be split if necessary.

## Stability and Storage

Store in a tightly sealed container, protected from light, and at room temperature. At this time, there is no information on stability of compounded formulations.

## Small Animal Dosage

### Dogs

- Epilepsy treatment: 10–30 mg/kg PO twice daily.
- Noise treatment: 30 mg/kg PO q12h using a suitable combination of whole and half tablets. Initiate therapy starting 2 days prior to the day of the expected noise event and continue through the noise event.

### Cats

- Safe dose not established.

## Large Animal Dosage

- No doses have been established for large animals.

## Regulatory Information

No withdrawal times are established for animals intended for food. For extralabel use withdrawal interval estimates, contact FARAD at www.FARAD.org.

# Imidocarb Hydrochloride and Imidocarb Dipropionate
im-id'oh-carb hye-droe-klor'ide

**Trade and other names:** Imizol

**Functional classification:** Antiprotozoal

## Pharmacology and Mechanism of Action

Imidocarb is an aromatic diamidine. It inhibits nucleic acid metabolism in susceptible organisms and produces anticholinergic effects. It has antimicrobial activity against protozoal organisms, which accounts for its clinical use. It appears to particularly affect the erythrocyte stages of the parasite by inhibition of inositol entry into infected erythrocytes.

## Indications and Clinical Uses

Imidocarb has been used in animals to treat intracellular tick-borne pathogens. The use is based on small observational studies, anecdotal experience, or opinions from experts. It has been used to treat *Babesia* infections and has been used to treat feline hemoplasma infections caused by the organisms *Mycoplasma haemofelis* and *Mycoplasma haemominutum*. Imidocarb also has been used to treat *Cytauxzoon felis* infections in cats and ehrlichial infections in dogs and cats. In horses, it has been used to treat equine piroplasmosis caused by *Theileria equi* and *Babesia caballi*.

## Precautionary Information

### Adverse Reactions and Side Effects

No toxic reactions were observed in trials with experimental cats. Transient pain or discomfort occurs in most animals at the site of injection. Post-treatment vomiting may occur in 10%–40% of animals. Transient increase in liver enzymes (alanine aminotransferase [ALT], aspartate aminotransferase [AST]) may occur. After IM injection, it remains in tissues for a prolonged period. Adverse effects from high doses include kidney injury (tubular necrosis) and acute hepatic necrosis.

Two forms are available: dipropionate salt and hydrochloride salt. The hydrochloride salt is more irritating when injected intramuscularly.

In horses, anticholinesterase effects are common, resulting in increased endogenous acetylcholine, which causes sweating, agitation, bronchoconstriction, salivation, colic signs, intestinal spasmodic reactions, and diarrhea. These effects are transient and not life threatening, but these signs should be treated with atropine if they are severe. To prevent these signs, one may pretreat with atropine (0.02 mg/kg IV), glycopyrrolate (0.0025 mg/kg IV), or N-butylscopolammonium bromide (scopolamine).

### Contraindications and Precautions

Administer intramuscularly only. Do not administer intravenously. Donkeys and mules are more susceptible to adverse effects than are horses, and treatment should be avoided in these animals.

### Drug Interactions

No drug interactions have been reported; however, the use is uncommon, and a full range of potential drug interactions is not available.

## Instructions for Use

Use of imidocarb has been limited in animals. Most protocols are established from small clinical trials or extrapolation from human use.

## Patient Monitoring and Laboratory Tests

No specific monitoring is necessary.

## Formulations
- Imidocarb compounded formulations are available from some pharmacies. Imidocarb dipropionate is available as 12% solution (120 mg/mL).

## Stability and Storage
Store in a tightly sealed container, protected from light, and at room temperature.

## Small Animal Dosage
### Cats
- 5 mg/kg IM two doses administered 14 days apart.

### Dogs
- *Ehrlichia canis*: 6.6 mg/kg IM (0.25 mL per 10 lb), two doses administered 14 days apart.

## Large Animal Dosage
### Horses
- 4.4 mg/kg once or 2.2 mg/kg IM for with doses with 24- to 48-hour intervals between doses. Inject in different locations. To eradicate *B. caballi*, inject 4 mg/kg IM for four treatments q72h. Consider pretreating with anticholinergic drug (see Adverse Effects).

## Regulatory Information
No regulatory information is available. For extralabel use withdrawal interval estimates, contact FARAD at www.FARAD.org.

# Imipenem + Cilastatin
ih-mih-pen′em + sye-lah-stat′in
**Trade and other names:** Primaxin
**Functional classification:** Antibacterial

## Pharmacology and Mechanism of Action
Imipenem + cilastatin is a beta-lactam antibiotic of the carbapenems class with a broad spectrum of activity. The mechanism of action is similar to the other beta-lactam antibiotics, which is to inactivate the penicillin-binding proteins (PBPs) and cause cell wall lysis or interfere with cell wall formation. The carbapenems are capable of binding to a specific PBP (PBP-1) that results in more rapid lysis compared with other beta-lactams. This results in greater bactericidal activity and a longer postantibiotic effect. Carbapenems have a broad spectrum of activity and are among the most active of all antibiotics. The spectrum includes gram-negative bacilli, including Enterobacteriaceae and *Pseudomonas aeruginosa*, that are resistant to other drugs. It also is active against most gram-positive bacteria, except methicillin-resistant strains of *Staphylococcus* and *Enterococcus* spp. Compared with imipenem, meropenem and doripenem are slightly more active. Cilastatin has no antibacterial activity, but it is a specific inhibitor of renal dipeptidase (dehydropeptidase, DHP-I). Therefore cilastatin blocks renal tubular metabolism of imipenem and improves urinary recovery of imipenem.

*Pharmacokinetics:* Dosage regimens have been developed from pharmacokinetic studies in dogs, cats, and horses. In cats, it was absorbed from IM and SQ injection 90%–100%. The half-lives were 1.2, 1.4, and 1.5 hours from IV, IM, and SQ injection, respectively, and produced a peak concentration of 6.5 and 4 mcg/mL from IM and SQ, respectively.

In dogs, the half-lives were 0.8, 0.9, and 1.54 hours from IV, IM, and SQ injection, respectively. Absorption rates from IM and SQ injection were 145% and 159%, respectively, producing peak concentrations of 13.2 and 8.8 mcg/mL, respectively. Thus, in both dogs and cats, SQ administration prolongs the half-life, which is helpful for a time-dependent agent such as imipenem. In horses, the elimination half-life from IV administration was 70 minutes, with volume of distribution of 0.4–0.5 L/kg.

## Indications and Clinical Uses

Imipenem is used primarily for infections caused by bacteria resistant to other drugs. The use in animals is based on extrapolation from human uses and results from experimental animals. There are no controlled clinical studies in veterinary medicine that have evaluated imipenem.

Imipenem can be valuable for treating resistant infections caused by *P. aeruginosa*, *Escherichia coli*, and *Klebsiella pneumoniae*. Although active against gram-positive bacteria such as staphylococci (but not methicillin-resistant strains), other drugs should be used for gram-positive infections. Meropenem and doripenem are newer drugs in the class of carbapenems and have some advantages with respect to activity and convenience of administration. Meropenem is often preferred for administration to dogs and cats because it is easier to administer and more stable.

## Precautionary Information

### Adverse Reactions and Side Effects

Allergic reactions may occur with beta-lactam antibiotics. With rapid infusion or in patients with renal insufficiency, neurotoxicity may occur. Neurotoxicity in animals has included tremors, nystagmus, and seizures. Nephrotoxicity is possible, but imipenem is combined with cilastatin to decrease renal metabolism. Vomiting and nausea are possible. IM injections can cause painful reactions.

### Contraindications and Precautions

Use cautiously in patients prone to seizures. Seizures may be more likely in patients with renal failure.

### Drug Interactions

There have been no drug interactions documented in veterinary medicine. Do not mix with other drugs in the vial.

## Instructions for Use

Efficacy studies are not available for animals. Recommendations are based on extrapolation of studies performed in humans or laboratory animals. Reserve the use of this drug for resistant, refractory infections, when other drugs cannot be used. Observe manufacturer's instructions carefully for proper administration. When the vial is initially reconstituted, it should not be given intravenously. It first must be diluted in a suitable IV fluid solution (at least 100 mL). For IV administration, it may be mixed with IV fluids. After reconstitution in vial, 250 or 500 mg should be added to not less than 100 mL of fluids and given intravenously over 30–60 minutes. IV fluid solutions are stable for 48 hours if refrigerated or 8 hours at room temperature. For IM administration, 2 mL of lidocaine (1%) may be added to decrease pain from injection. The suspension intended for IM use is stable for only 1 hour. In some hospitals, the IV solution has been diluted in fluids and administered SQ without any sign of injection-site reactions (usually 8–14 mL per injection in dogs).

## Patient Monitoring and Laboratory Tests
Susceptibility testing: Clinical and Laboratory Standards Institute (CLSI) breakpoints for sensitive organisms are ≤1 mcg/mL. Most veterinary pathogens have minimum inhibitory concentration (MIC) values less than 1.0 mcg/mL.

## Formulations
- IV solution: Imipenem + cilastatin is available in 250- and 500-mg vials for injection.
- IM suspension: IM suspension is available in 500- and 750-mg vials.

## Stability and Storage
Store in a tightly sealed container, protected from light, and at room temperature. After reconstitution, it is stable for 4 hours at room temperature and 24 hours refrigerated. Do not freeze IV fluid solutions. Slight yellow discoloration is acceptable but discard it if the color turns brown.

## Small Animal Dosage
**Dogs**
- 5 mg/kg q6–8h IV, IM, or SQ.

**Cats**
- 5 mg/kg q6–8h IV or IM, or q8h for SQ.

## Large Animal Dosage
**Horses**
- 10–20 mg/kg q6h by slow IV (10-minute) infusion.

## Regulatory Information
Withdrawal times are not established for animals that produce food. For extralabel use withdrawal interval estimates, contact FARAD at www.FARAD.org.

# Imipramine Hydrochloride
im-ip′rah-meen hye-droe-klor′ide

**Trade and other names:** Tofranil and generic brands

**Functional classification:** Behavior modification

## Pharmacology and Mechanism of Action
Imipramine is one of the tricyclic antidepressant (TCA) drugs used to treat behavior disorders in animals. Imipramine, like others in the TCA class, is used in people to treat behavior problems, anxiety, and depression. Action is via inhibition of uptake of serotonin and norepinephrine at presynaptic nerve terminals. Other TCA drugs used in animals include clomipramine and amitriptyline.

## Indications and Clinical Uses
Like other TCAs, imipramine is used in animals to treat a variety of behavioral disorders, including obsessive-compulsive disorders, separation anxiety, and inappropriate urination. There have been fewer studies of efficacy with imipramine than with clomipramine or amitriptyline. Generally, other behavior-modifying drugs such as selective serotonin reuptake inhibitors (e.g., fluoxetine) or other TCAs (clomipramine) are preferred by behavior experts for treating small animals. More information is available for these medications compared with imipramine.

## Precautionary Information

**Adverse Reactions and Side Effects**

Multiple side effects are associated with TCAs, such as antimuscarinic effects (dry mouth and rapid heart rate) and antihistamine effects (sedation). Overdoses can produce life-threatening cardiotoxicity.

**Contraindications and Precautions**

Use cautiously in patients with heart disease. Overdoses can produce severe arrhythmias.

**Drug Interactions**

Do not use with other behavior-modifying drugs, such as serotonin reuptake inhibitors. Do not use with monoamine oxidase inhibitors such as selegiline.

## Instructions for Use

Doses are primarily based on empiricism, small observational studies, and opinions from behavior experts. There are few controlled efficacy trials available for animals to compare with other drugs in this class. There may be a 2- to 4-week delay after initiation of therapy before beneficial effects are seen.

### Patient Monitoring and Laboratory Tests

Monitor heart rate and rhythm in treated animals. Like other TCAs, imipramine may decrease total tetraiodothyronine ($T_4$) and free ($T_4$) concentrations in dogs.

### Formulations

* Imipramine is available in 10-, 25-, and 50-mg tablets.

### Stability and Storage

Store in a tightly sealed container, protected from light, and at room temperature. Although imipramine has been compounded for veterinary use, the potency and stability have not been evaluated for compounded products.

### Small Animal Dosage

**Dogs**

* 2–4 mg/kg q12–24h PO.

**Cats**

* 0.5–1 mg/kg q12–24h PO.

### Large Animal Dosage

* No large animal doses have been reported.

### Regulatory Information

Do not administer to animals intended for food.
RCI Classification: 2

# Indomethacin
in-doe-meth′ah-sin

**Trade and other names:** Indocin

**Functional classification:** Nonsteroidal anti-inflammatory drug

## Pharmacology and Mechanism of Action

Indomethacin is an NSAID and analgesic. It is not approved for veterinary use but has been used extralabel in some animals. Like other NSAIDs, indomethacin produces potent analgesic and anti-inflammatory effects by inhibiting the synthesis of prostaglandins. The enzyme inhibited by NSAID is the COX enzyme. The COX enzyme exists in two isoforms: COX-1 and COX-2. COX-1 is primarily responsible for synthesis of prostaglandins important for maintaining a healthy GI tract, renal function, platelet function, and other normal physiologic functions. COX-2 is induced and responsible for synthesizing prostaglandins that are important mediators of pain, inflammation, and fever. However, it is known that there is some crossover of COX-1 and COX-2 effects in some situations, and COX-2 activity is important for some biological effects. Indomethacin is considered a prototype for a nonselective drug because it inhibits equally both COX-1 and COX-2. Indomethacin is approved for human use, and experience with this drug in veterinary medicine is limited to just a few case reports. It acts to inhibit COX that synthesizes prostaglandins but may have other anti-inflammatory effects (e.g., effects on leukocytes). In people, it is used primarily for short-term treatment of moderate pain and inflammation.

## Indications and Clinical Uses

Indomethacin, like other NSAIDs, has been used to treat pain and inflammation in people. However, it has not been used often in clinical veterinary medicine because other safer, approved drugs are available. Indomethacin is used as a prototypical nonselective COX-1 and COX-2 blocker in research. In dogs, the high risk of GI ulceration prohibits its routine use.

## Precautionary Information

### Adverse Reactions and Side Effects

Indomethacin has produced severe GI ulceration and hemorrhage in dogs. Like other NSAIDs, it may cause kidney injury via inhibition of renal prostaglandins.

### Contraindications and Precautions

Do not use in dogs or cats.

### Drug Interactions

Like other NSAIDs, several drug interactions are possible. NSAIDs have the potential to interfere with the action of diuretics, such as furosemide, and ACE inhibitors, such as enalapril. Corticosteroids, when used with NSAIDs, increase the risk of ulceration.

## Instructions for Use

Use cautiously, if at all, because safe doses have not been determined for clinical use in animals.

## Patient Monitoring and Laboratory Tests

Monitor for signs of GI toxicity (hemorrhage, ulcers, and perforation).

## Formulations

- Indomethacin is available in 20-, 25-, 40-, and 50-mg capsules and 5-mg/mL oral suspension.

## Stability and Storage

Store in a tightly sealed container, protected from light, and at room temperature. Indomethacin is practically insoluble in water but is soluble in ethanol. It decomposes in alkaline conditions and is maximally stable at pH 3.75.

## Small Animal Dosage
**Dogs and Cats**
• Safe dose has not been established.

## Large Animal Dosage
• No large animal doses have been reported.

## Regulatory Information
Withdrawal times are not established for animals that produce food. For extralabel use withdrawal interval estimates, contact FARAD at www.FARAD.org.

RCI Classification: 4

# Insulin
in'syoo-lin

**Trade and other names:** ProZinc, Lente insulin, Ultralente insulin, Regular insulin, Glargine insulin, NPH insulin, Caninsulin, Protamine zinc insulin (PZI), Humulin (human insulin), Vetsulin is porcine insulin zinc suspension (veterinary), and PZI Vet (veterinary protamine zinc insulin)

**Functional classification:** Hormone

## Pharmacology and Mechanism of Action
Insulin has multiple effects associated with utilization of glucose. It is critical to the management of diabetes mellitus in dogs and cats. Oral hypoglycemic agents are used in people; however, there is no good evidence to support their use in preference to insulin therapy in cats, and the oral hypoglycemic agents are ineffective in dogs. If owners cannot give injections, glipizide is the only oral hypoglycemic agent with evidence to support the use as a sole therapy for cats (see Glipizide for more information).

Dog insulin is identical to pork insulin, but dog insulin differs from beef insulin by three amino acids. Cat insulin is similar to beef insulin with only one amino acid difference. Despite an amino acid difference in cats, there have not been problems documented from anti-insulin antibodies in treated cats. Most beef–pork insulin combinations for humans have been discontinued and are not usually available for veterinary use. Human-recombinant insulins can be used in dogs and cats with the same effects as natural insulin. Insulin is available in several preparations as listed below:

1. **Regular insulin:** Short acting. Peaks are 1–5 hours, and duration is 4–10 hours. Usually used for short-term management such as for diabetic ketoacidosis (DKA).

2. **Neutral protamine Hagedorn** (isophane, also called NPH): 100 units/mL. Novolin-N and Humulin-N are brand names for the same drug. A human-recombinant insulin of crystalline suspension with protamine zinc that is intermediate acting. The formulation promotes crystallization in tissues to prolong effect. Peaks are 2–10 hours in dogs and 2–8 hours in cats with durations of action of 4–24 hours in dogs and 4–12 hours in cats (but usually 2–3 hours in cats). It is not commonly recommended for cats because of short duration. In dogs it can be administered twice daily.

3. **Lente insulin:** Peaks are 2–10 hours in dogs and 2–8 hours in cats with durations of action of 4–24 hours in dogs and 4–12 hours in cats. The lente forms of insulin control their duration by the size of the crystal. Addition of protamine or zinc to insulin produces a crystallized insulin in suspension that has a longer absorption rate than dissolved insulin. For example, whereas semilente is practically

amorphous, ultralente has large crystals, and lente is a combination of ultralente and semilente.

4. **Ultralente insulin:** Peaks are 4–16 hours in dogs and 2–14 hours in cats, with durations of 8–28 hours in dogs and 12–24 hours in cats. It is poorly absorbed in cats and usually not recommended. Human products have been discontinued.

5. **Vetsulin:** Also known as Caninsulin. Vetsulin is a U-40 porcine insulin, identical to canine insulin in amino acid content, and is a lente insulin of aqueous zinc suspension of crystalline and noncrystalline insulins. It produces a shorter peak of activity (4 hours) and duration than PZI insulin. This product has been temporarily suspended by some sources but has returned to the market.

6. **Protamine-zinc insulin (PZI):** Developed from recombinant human insulin and longer acting. Veterinary form is called ProZinc in a 40-unit/mL form for cats. The forms used in animals are identical to the forms marketed for people. It can be used in dogs, but the response and  pharmacokinetics among dogs can be highly variable. Peaks are 4–14 hours in dogs and 5–7 hours in cats, with durations of 6–28 hours in dogs and 13 24 hours in cats. PZI insulin of animal origin (90% bovine and 10% porcine) has been unavailable, but the human recombinant PZI form of insulin has been shown in canine studies to be an effective alternative.

7. **Glargine insulin (Lantus):** A human insulin analogue made from recombinant technology. It has four amino acid differences from feline insulin. It has a slow onset of 4–18 hours and a duration of ≥24 hours. This analogue is produced by the substitution of glycine for asparagine and the addition of two arginine molecules. These changes shift the isoelectric point toward neutral. In the pH of the vial, it is soluble, but it has reduced solubility at the pH of SQ tissue (microprecipitates), which causes it to be released slowly from the injection site, without a peak. It produces consistent concentrations without large fluctuations in peak and trough seen with other insulin formulations. The glucose-lowering properties are shorter in cats than in people, with a peak at 5–16 hours and duration of 11–24 hours. However, it produces greater glycemic control in cats than other insulins. Remission rates are highest with this form of glargine insulin in cats compared with other forms. Despite the long-lasting effect, optimum control is achieved with twice-daily dosing in cats with glargine insulin. Ordinarily, it is formulated in a 100-units/mL concentration (Lantus), but there is also a more concentrated form (Toujeo) used in people that is 300 units/mL. This more concentrated form has not been evaluated for pets.

8. **Insulin detemir (Levemir):** 100 units/mL. A human insulin analogue made from recombinant technology. Long-acting insulin. Insulin detemir has a 14-carbon fatty acid chain, which is added by acetylation to lysine, and is highly bound to albumin. High affinity to albumin in the SQ space prolongs absorption. In cats, the time to onset is approximately 2 hours, time to peak is 7 hours, and duration is 13–14 hours. In cats, the dose and interval are similar as for glargine insulin. In dogs, it is more potent than other forms, which increases the hypoglycemic effects and requires lower starting doses. A once per 12-hour dose in dogs has provided good regulation.

9. **Insulin degludec (Tresiba):** Insulin degludec is available as 100 or 200 units/mL. This preparation forms multihexamers in the SQ tissue after injection, which delays absorption and prolongs the action. It also binds to circulating albumin, which slows the elimination and prolongs the duration.

10. **Insulin glulisine (Apidra), insulin lispro (Humalog), and insulin aspart (NovoLog):** Rapidly acting insulins used in people. They are analogs of human insulin with modification to reduce formation of dimers and hexamers. They

produce a rapid onset from SQ injection and short duration They are used for their rapid onset and short duration of action. In people, they are typically used with a meal and combined with a longer-acting form. Lispro insulin has been evaluated in cats and was safe and effective for ketoacidosis. Lispro insulin is an analog of human

## Indications and Clinical Uses

Insulin in its various forms is used to treat diabetes mellitus in dogs and cats. It is used to replace insulin that is deficient. In some cats (approximately 50%), some oral hypoglycemic drugs have been used to reduce use of insulin. However, diabetic dogs are more insulin dependent. Regular insulin is short acting and more useful for emergencies such as DKA and acute nonketotic syndromes.

Intermediate- and long-acting insulin preparations are used for maintenance and are available in a variety of forms (see previous section). Most of the animal sources of insulin (beef and pork) have been discontinued, and human-recombinant insulin formulations have been substituted without differences in efficacy. In cats, glargine insulin has shown better efficacy than other forms and has been associated with a better remission rate. Glargine also has been used to treat DKA in cats and shown to be effective when administered intramuscularly. In addition to diabetes mellitus, insulin is occasionally used to treat severe cases of hyperkalemia.

## Precautionary Information

### Adverse Reactions and Side Effects

Adverse effects are primarily related to overdoses that result in hypoglycemia.

Glargine insulin has a low pH (4) and may sting from injection. Other insulins are more neutral.

### Contraindications and Precautions

Do not use without the ability to monitor glucose in animals because of the risk of hypoglycemia. Mixing regular insulin and insulins containing zinc in the same syringe will prolong absorption of the regular insulin. Do not mix isophane insulin or phosphate-buffered insulin with zinc insulins (lente, ultralente, semilente). *Do not* use insulin products from compounding pharmacies. Studies to evaluate compounded insulin products for pets have shown that they are unreliable.

### Drug Interactions

Administration of corticosteroids (prednisolone, dexamethasone, etc.) interfere with the action of insulin.

## Instructions for Use

Dietary management is essential for optimal glucose control. For proper management in cats, the mainstays of treatment are a low-carbohydrate, high-protein diet and twice-daily insulin. Many cats, if properly managed, may go into remission and not require lifelong insulin treatment. When treating dogs, feed dogs a high-fiber, low-fat diet. For all diabetic patients, the doses should be carefully adjusted in each patient depending on response.

For cats with ketoacidosis, one dosing regimen has used 0.2 units/kg of regular insulin IM initially, then 0.1 units/kg IM every hour until the glucose level is less than 300, and then 0.25–0.4 units/kg q6h SQ.

For maintenance therapy in cats, for most forms of insulin (including protamine zinc insulin and glargine insulin), twice-daily dosing usually is required. However, consider once-daily dosing in cats if blood glucose nadir develops 10 hours or longer after administration.

Pet owners should be instructed to use appropriate syringe types for administration (e.g., U-40 vs. U-100).

### Patient Monitoring and Laboratory Tests

Monitor blood glucose, glycosylated hemoglobin, and fructosamine concentrations. When treating diabetes, it is desirable to maintain glucose concentrations between 100 and 300 mg/dL, with the nadir (lowest point) being 80–150 mg/dL.

Serum fructosamine concentrations also can be monitored with the following guidance: less than 350 μmol/L, excellent control or remission; ≤450 μmol/L, good control; 450–500 μmol/L, moderate control; and greater than 500, μmol/L poor control.

### Formulations

See descriptions of each form in Pharmacology and Mechanism of Action.
- Human insulin products are usually available in 100-units/mL injection (U-100), with some veterinary products available in smaller concentration of 40 units/mL (U-40, e.g., ProZinc or Vetsulin).
- Protamine zinc beef–pork (PZI VET) insulin also may be available as 40 units/mL injection (U-40). Some previously available insulin products have been discontinued, such as Iletin II Pork Insulin (regular and NPH formulations), Humulin U Ultralente, and Humulin L Lente (Humulin U and Humulin L).

### Stability and Storage

Proper storage is critical for proper action of insulin: keep refrigerated. Warm gently and roll vial prior to injection to ensure proper mixing of vial contents. *Do not* shake vigorously. *Do not* freeze vials of insulin. *Do not* allow vials of insulin to be exposed to heat. *Do not* mix types of insulin in the same vial or syringe. Veterinarians should not use formulations of insulin that are compounded in unreliable conditions. Dilution of insulin should only be done by a pharmacist because specific diluents must be used.

### Small Animal Dosage

**Dogs**
- Short-acting regular insulin. Treatment of ketoacidosis for dogs weighing less than 3 kg: 1 unit/animal initially; then 1 unit/animal q1h. For dogs 3–10 kg: 2 units/animal initially; then 1 unit/animal q1h. For dogs weighing more than 10 kg: 0.25 unit/kg initially; then 0.1 unit/kg q1h IM.
- NPH for dogs weighing less than 15 kg: 1 unit/kg q12–24h SQ (adjust dose with monitoring); for dogs weighing more than 25 kg: 0.5 unit/kg q12–24h SQ (adjust dose with monitoring).
- Vetsulin: Initial dosage is 0.5 unit/kg once or twice daily SQ. Adjust dose (increase or decrease of 25% of dose) by monitoring.
- PZI human recombinant: Can be used as an alternative to beef/pork PZI insulin. Start with 0.5 units/kg SQ q12h. Median dosage in well-controlled dogs is 0.9 units/kg (range, 0.4–1.5 units/kg) SQ q12h.
- Glargine insulin: Start with 0.3 units/kg SQ q12h. Then monitor glucose to adjust dose. The dosage range in well-regulated dogs is 0.32–0.67 units/kg q12h SQ.
- Detemir insulin: 0.12–0.25 units/kg SQ q12h (adjust dose as needed). Because of small dose in dogs, a specific diluent may be needed to obtain accurate dose in small dogs.

## Cats

- Short-acting regular insulin. Treatment of ketoacidosis: 0.2 unit/kg IM initially, then 0.1 unit/kg IM every hour until glucose level is less than 300 mg/dL, and then continue with 0.25–0.4 unit/kg SQ q6h.
- NPH insulin is not ordinarily recommended for cats but has been used at 0.25 units/kg SQ q12h or 1–3 units per cat SQ q12h.
- Protamine zinc recombinant human insulin (ProZinc): Start with 0.2–0.7 units/kg q12h SQ (average dose, 0.5 units/kg) or 1–2 units per cat SQ q12h. Adjust dose to achieve nadir of glucose of 80–150 mg/dL. If transitioning from Caninsulin to protamine zinc insulin, start with 0.5 units/kg q12h SQ initially and adjust dose with monitoring.
- PZI insulin: Initial dose is 0.5 unit/kg SQ and then once or twice daily (usually twice is needed) with subsequent doses adjusted to produce desirable glucose levels, usually no higher than 3 units per cat. Final adjusted dose for most cats is 0.9 (± 0.4) unit/kg.
- Glargine insulin: Start with 0.5 unit/kg q12h SQ. Some cats can be managed with once-daily dosing, but twice daily is preferred. Adjust dose via monitoring. If treating DKA, one may start with glargine insulin administered intramuscularly and then switch to SQ injections for maintenance.
- Detemir insulin: Use same dosage regimen as for glargine insulin.
- Regular insulin for constant-rate infusion (CRI) administration: 1.1–1.5 units/kg/day as a CRI. Mix regular insulin with 250 mL of 0.9% sodium chloride solution. Administer at a rate of 10 mL per cat per hour. Discard the first 50 mL. Discard the entire bag after 24 hours and make a fresh bag of fluids.
- Lispro insulin: For DKA in cats, start with 0.09 units/kg/h infusion. Mix with 0.9% normal saline for IV infusion by adding 2.2 units to a 250-mL bag of 0.95 saline. Consider potassium supplementation during treatment, depending on the extent of hypokalemia.

## Horses

- Treatment of hyperkalemia: Start with regular insulin (100 units/mL) and administer at a dosage of 0.1–0.2 units/kg/hour IV infusion, with 5% dextrose solution. The IV solution can be prepared by adding 0.5 mL of regular insulin to 5 L of fluids containing 500 mL of 50% dextrose. Administer 5 L over 1 hour.

### Regulatory Information

No regulatory information is available for animals intended for food. Because of a low risk of residues, no withdrawal times are suggested.

# Interferon
in-ter-feer'on

**Trade and other names:** Virbagen omega

**Functional classification:** Immunostimulant

## Pharmacology and Mechanism of Action

Interferons are polypeptide molecules with a variety of biological functions, including immune modulation and stimulation. Multiple interferons are available for human use (e.g., treatment of AIDS-related diseases and cancer-associated diseases).

They are divided into two major types: types 1 and 2. Type 1 interferon includes interferon-alpha, interferon-beta, and interferon omega. Type 2 interferon includes only interferon-gamma, produced by lymphocytes. Subtypes of interferons may be alpha-2a, alpha-2b, n-1, and n-3. These types of interferons are not interchangeable.

Recombinant omega interferon contained in Virbagen omega is produced by silkworms previously inoculated with interferon-recombinant baculovirus. It allows the production of pure interferon. Omega interferon of feline origin, produced by genetic engineering, is a type 1 interferon closely related to alpha interferon. It is available in some other countries but not the United States.

The exact mechanism of action of interferon omega is not understood, but it may enhance nonspecific immune defenses in dogs and cats. Interferon does not act directly and specifically on the pathogenic virus but exerts its effect by inhibition of the internal synthesis mechanisms of the infected cells. After injection, it is bound to receptors in cells infected by the virus and has half-lives of 1.4 hours in dogs and 1.7 hours in cats.

## Indications and Clinical Uses

Interferon is used to stimulate the immune system in patients. It has been used to stimulate immune cells in dogs with parvovirus and in cats with feline retrovirus (feline leukemia virus [FeLV] and feline immunodeficiency virus [FIV]). It has not been effective for feline infectious peritonitis in cats. It has not been effective for naturally infected FeLV in cats but has been effective in experimentally infected animals. Feline interferon is associated with clinical improvement in cats with stomatitis associated with calicivirus.

Human interferon alpha, given orally, has improved clinical signs in cats with FIV. If human interferon is used by injection in cats, it becomes ineffective after 3–7 weeks because of development of neutralizing antibodies.

## Precautionary Information

### Adverse Reactions and Side Effects

In people, injections of interferon alpha have been associated with influenza-like symptoms. Other effects, such as bone marrow suppression, also have been reported in people.

Interferon may induce vomiting and nausea in animals. In some animals, it may induce hyperthermia 3–6 hours after injection. In cats, it may produce soft feces to mild diarrhea. A slight decrease in white blood cells, platelets, and red blood cells and an increase in the concentration of ALT may be observed. These parameters usually return to normal in the week following the last injection. In cats, it may induce transient fatigue during treatment.

### Contraindications and Precautions

Do not vaccinate dogs or cats receiving interferon. If human interferon is used in cats, it may become ineffective after several weeks because of neutralizing antibodies.

### Drug Interactions

Do not mix with any other vaccine/immunologic product, except the solvent supplied for use with the product.

## Instructions for Use
Doses and indications for animals have primarily been based on extrapolation of human recommendations, experimental studies, or specific studies in cats with viral infections.

## Patient Monitoring and Laboratory Tests
Monitor complete blood count (CBC) during treatment.

## Formulations Available
- Feline origin: Interferon is available in some countries in 5 and 10 million units/vial. The freeze-dried fraction must be reconstituted with 1 mL of the specific diluent to obtain, depending on the presentation, a solution containing 5 million units or 10 million units of recombinant interferon. Feline-origin interferon is not available in the United States.
- Human interferon: Interferon-alpha.

## Stability and Storage
Interferon has a shelf life of 2 years. The product should be used immediately after reconstitution and should be stored in its original carton. Store and transport at 4°C ± 2°C. Do not freeze.

## Small Animal Dosage
### Dogs
- 2.5 million units/kg IV once daily for 3 consecutive days.

### Cats
- Feline form of interferon-omega: 1 million units/kg IV or SQ once daily for 5 consecutive days. Three separate 5-day treatments must be performed at day 0, day 14, and day 60.
- Human interferon alpha: 10,000 to 1,000,000 units/kg q24h.
- Human interferon alpha: 10–50 units/kg human interferon alpha on an alternate-week schedule PO. (Although oral products are destroyed in stomach acid and may not be absorbed, some efficacy has been demonstrated from this route. This may be caused by a local effect on the oral or pharyngeal area.)

## Large Animal Dosage
- No large animal doses have been reported.

## Regulatory Information
Do not administer to animals intended for food.

# Iodide (Potassium Iodide)
eye′oh-dyde

**Trade and other names:** Potassium iodide, EDDI, and ethylenediamine dihydriodide

**Functional classification:** Iodine supplement

## Pharmacology and Mechanism of Action
Iodide is administered as a dietary supplement. Although its action for treating disease is not well established, it is administered as an adjunctive treatment for zygomycosis, conidiobolomycosis, and fungal granuloma. The mechanism of action against fungal

organisms is not known. Iodide is also important for thyroid gland function and has been used to treat some thyroid disorders.

## Indications and Clinical Uses

Ethylenediamine dihydriodide (EDDI) is used as a nutritional source of iodine in cattle. In people, iodide has been used to treat hyperthyroidism, but effectiveness for this use in cats has not been established. Potassium iodide is also used to protect the thyroid gland from radiation injury in the event of a radiation emergency (accidental exposure to radiation) or following administration of radioactive iodide.

Because iodide may increase respiratory secretions, it has been used as an expectorant, but the efficacy has not been established. Nevertheless, in cattle, in addition to a feed supplement, EDDI is used as an expectorant. EDDI is sometimes added to the feed of cattle for the purpose of decreasing foot rot infections, lumpy jaw (*Actinomyces bovis*), woody tongue (*Actinobacillus lignieresii*), and bronchitis. There is a lack of published scientific evidence for a beneficial effect. Iodide has been used to treat fungal granulomatous disease and infections associated with zygomycetes. The antifungal treatment has been questioned for animals because the efficacy is not established. In horses, iodine is used to treat sporotrichosis and occasionally other fungal infections such as basidiobolomycosis and conidiobolomycosis (zygomycosis). For horses, treatment is initiated with doses listed in the dosing section, and to prevent relapse, treatment is continued for 4 weeks beyond resolution of clinical signs.

In cats, potassium iodide (administered as oral capsules) has been used to treat infections caused by *Sporothrix schenckii*.

## Precautionary Information

### Adverse Reactions and Side Effects

Iodide-related adverse reactions (iodism) include excess lacrimation, swelling of eyelids, nonproductive cough, increased respiratory secretions, and dermatitis. Its use may cause abortion in horses or limb deformities in foals. Adverse effects are common when used for long periods in small animals. These effects include hepatotoxicity, lethargy, anorexia (most common), vomiting, diarrhea, hypothermia, and cardiomyopathy.

### Contraindications and Precautions

Do not use in pregnant animals.

### Drug Interactions

No drug interactions have been reported for small animals.

## Instructions for Use

Iodide has been administered as a 1-g/mL potassium iodine solution (SSKI) or as a 65-mg/mL solution. It also has been administered as a 10% potassium iodide/5% iodine solution given orally with food.

In cattle, EDDI is administered in the feed or mixed with feed, salt, or mineral mixture or in the drinking water.

## Patient Monitoring and Laboratory Tests

Monitor serum thyroid concentrations with prolonged use.

## Formulations

- Available for food animals as EDDI: equivalent to 4.6% EDDI or 46 mg/g of EDDI. Also available as potassium iodide as 1 g/mL SSKI, a 65-mg/mL oral solution, or 10% potassium iodide/5% iodine solution. Inorganic potassium iodide has been used in horses orally but must be obtained as the chemical grade and compounded for horses.

## Stability and Storage

Store in a tightly sealed container, protected from light, and at room temperature. Do not freeze solutions. Inorganic potassium iodide is unstable in light, heat, and excess humidity.

## Small Animal Dosage

### Dogs and Cats

- Fungal infections: Start with 5 mg/kg q8h PO and increase gradually to 25 mg/kg q8h PO.
- Treatment of *Sporothrix* infection in cats: 15 mg/kg per day oral for 20 weeks.
- Emergency treatment after radiation exposure: 2 mg/kg PO per day.
- Expectorant: 5 mg/kg q8h PO.

## Large Animal Dosage

### Cattle

- Feed supplement: 50–217 mg EDDI per head per day (mix with feed).
- Expectorant and other indications: 650–1300 mg EDDI per head twice daily PO for 7 days.

### Horses (treatment of fungal granuloma)

- 20–40 mg/kg per day IV for 7–10 days (using 20% sodium iodide).
- 10–40 mg/kg per day PO (using inorganic potassium iodide).
- 0.86–1.72 mg/kg of EDDI or use 20–40 mg/kg per day PO of the 4.6% organic iodine dextrose base of EDDI.

## Regulatory Information

Withdrawal times in food-producing animals have not been established.

# Ipecac
ih'peh-kak

**Trade and other names:** Ipecac and syrup of ipecac
**Functional classification:** Emetic

## Pharmacology and Mechanism of Action

Ipecac is an emetic agent used to treat poisoning. Ipecac contains two alkaloids: cephalin and emetine. These alkaloids stimulate gastric receptors linked to the chemoreceptor trigger zone to stimulate vomiting.

## Indications and Clinical Uses

Ipecac is indicated for emergency treatment of poisoning. When used in animals, it should be administered promptly after poisoning. Inducing vomiting with ipecac is not effective beyond 30–60 minutes after poisoning. After successful administration, it is estimated that vomiting removes only 10%–60% of ingested toxicant. Therefore other systemic antidotes and activated charcoal should also be considered.

## Precautionary Information

### Adverse Reactions and Side Effects
No adverse effects with acute therapy for poisoning. Chronic administration can lead to myocardial toxicity.

### Contraindications and Precautions
Do not induce vomiting if the patient has ingested caustic chemicals or if there is a risk of aspiration pneumonia.

### Drug Interactions
Ipecac is not as effective if drugs that act as antiemetics have been administered. Such drugs include tranquilizers (e.g., acepromazine), anticholinergics (e.g., atropine), antihistamines, cannabinoids, and prokinetic agents (e.g., metoclopramide).

## Instructions for Use
Ipecac is available as a nonprescription drug. Onset of vomiting may require 20–30 minutes.

## Patient Monitoring and Laboratory Tests
Poisoned animals should be monitored closely because ipecac may not entirely eliminate ingested toxicant.

## Formulations
• Ipecac is available in a 30-mL/bottle oral solution.

## Stability and Storage
Store in a tightly sealed container, protected from light, and at room temperature.

## Small Animal Dosage

### Dogs
• 3–6 mL per dog PO. Dose may be increased up to 15 mL per dog for large breeds.

### Cats
• 2–6 mL per cat PO.

## Large Animal Dosage
• Not recommended for large animals.

## Regulatory Information
No regulatory information is available for animals intended for food. Because of a low risk of residues, no withdrawal times are suggested.

# Ipodate
ih'poe-date

**Trade and other names:** Calcium ipodate and, Ipodate sodium, and Iopodate

**Functional classification:** Antithyroid agent

## Pharmacology and Mechanism of Action

Ipodate is a cholecystographic agent. This drug is an iodinated biliary radiocontrast dye. Ipodate is also used for thyroid diseases because it inhibits deiodinases responsible for conversion of thyroid hormone $T_4$ to triiodothyronine ($T_3$). It also blocks $T_3$ receptors. It lowers $T_3$ levels but not $T_4$ levels.

## Indications and Clinical Uses

Ipodate is used as treatment for hyperthyroidism in cats. Reduction of $T_3$ levels should occur within 1 week, but longer term response needs more evaluation. The use is not as common as other treatments, but it has been administered as an alternative to methimazole, radiation therapy, or surgery. Initial response rate may be as high as 66% for short-term use. In cats, iopanoic acid doses of 50–100 mg PO produced some short-term benefits for acute treatment of thyrotoxicosis but was not suitable for long-term management of hyperthyroidism in cats.

Ipodate formulations are not consistently available to veterinarians. Iopanoic acid is no longer available in the United States commercially but has been compounded. When iopanoic acid (Telepaque) was used as a substitute, it was less effective.

## Precautionary Information

### Adverse Reactions and Side Effects

Ipodate can cause hypothyroidism. No significant adverse effects have been reported in cats, but compounds containing iodide have caused hypersensitivity reactions in people. In humans, chronic high doses of compounds containing iodide can cause sore mouth, swollen tissues, skin reactions, or GI upset.

### Contraindications and Precautions

Monitor for reduction of thyroid levels in animals or clinical signs. Relapses have occurred in cats after 10 weeks to 6 months of treatment.

### Drug Interactions

No drug interactions have been reported for small animals.

## Instructions for Use

Use of iopanoic acid for treatment of hyperthyroidism in cats has been evaluated in small numbers of cats in clinical studies. In one study, most treated cats responded, but it was not considered suitable for long-term treatment. More experience is needed to determine if response to treatment is transient.

## Patient Monitoring and Laboratory Tests

Monitor serum thyroid $T_3$ concentrations. Ipodate lowers $T_3$ levels, but $T_4$ levels may be unchanged or may increase because of decreased conversion of $T_4$ to $T_3$.

## Formulations

- Ipodate has been available as either calcium or sodium ipodate, but some formulations have been discontinued. Oragrafin 500-mg capsules have been formulated into 50-mg capsules by pharmacists. (These may have to be specifically formulated for cats.)
- Iopanoic acid has been used in the past but is no longer available commercially in the United States.
- Sodium ipodate is an oral agent but is no longer available in the United States.

## Stability and Storage
Store in a tightly sealed container, protected from light, and at room temperature.

## Small Animal Dosage
**Cats**
- Ipodate: 15 mg/kg q12h PO. Most common dosage has been 50 mg per cat twice daily. Dose is equivalent regardless of whether sodium or calcium ipodate is used.
- Iopanoic acid: 50 mg per cat q12h PO. If adequate response is not observed, increase dosage to 100 mg per cat q12h PO. However, this product is no longer available commercially in the United States.

## Large Animal Dosage
- No large animal doses have been reported.

## Regulatory Information
Do not administer to animals intended for food.

# Irbesartan
er-beh-sar′tan

**Trade and other names:** Avapro

**Functional classification:** Vasodilator

## Pharmacology and Mechanism of Action
Irbesartan is a vasodilator that blocks the angiotensin receptor. These drugs are considered angiotensin receptor blockers (ARBs). Irbesartan has been shown to block angiotensin II receptors and prevent the effects associated with angiotensin II on blood vessels. It has been used in people who cannot tolerate ACE inhibitors. The metabolism in dogs and cats is uncertain, and it is not known if doses extrapolated from human use have equivalent activity in dogs and cats. Losartan, another ARB, is used as an alternative in people but is reportedly not as effective in dogs because they do not produce the active metabolite. Because there is now an approved ARB for cats (Telmisartan), it is the preferred ARB for veterinary medicine.

## Indications and Clinical Uses
Angiotensin II blockers such as irbesartan are used in people as alternatives to ACE inhibitors. Animals tolerate ACE inhibitors better than humans, but ARBs are also effective (e.g., telmisartan). Initial experience with ARB in animals was derived from empirical use and studies in which 30 mg/kg of irbesartan was administered to animals with experimentally induced renal hypertension. Otherwise, there is little clinical evidence for the use of irbesartan in dogs or cats. An approved drug for cats, telmisartan, is preferred because there are clinical studies to support the safe use and efficacy.

## Precautionary Information

**Adverse Reactions and Side Effects**

No adverse effects have been reported in animals, but this drug has been used rarely. Hypotension is a potential problem from overdosing.

**Contraindications and Precautions**

Do not administer to hypotensive or dehydrated animals. No other contraindications have been reported for animals for the use of irbesartan.

**Drug Interactions**

No drug interactions have been reported for small animals. Use cautiously with other vasodilators.

## Instructions for Use

In dogs, irbesartan is preferred over losartan because losartan is not converted to active products in dogs. However, telmisartan is preferred over both agents because there are FDA-approved dose forms for animals, and clinical studies to support the use.

## Patient Monitoring and Laboratory Tests

Monitor blood pressure and heart rate in treated animals. Monitor electrolytes if it is administered long term.

## Formulations

- Irbesartan is available in 75-, 150-, and 300-mg tablets. One product (Avalide) contains irbesartan in combination with hydrochlorothiazide.

## Stability and Storage

Store in a tightly sealed container, protected from light, and at room temperature.

## Small Animal Dosage

**Dogs**

- 30–60 mg/kg q12h PO. Start with 30 mg/kg to avoid prerenal azotemia and hypotension.

## Large Animal Dosage

- No large animal doses have been reported.

## Regulatory Information

Withdrawal times are not established for animals that produce food. For extralabel use withdrawal interval estimates, contact FARAD at www.FARAD.org.

RCI Classification: 3

# Iron Dextran and Iron Sucrose

(**Note:** Oral iron supplements are listed as ferrous sulfate and ferrous gluconate)

**Trade and other names:** AmTech Iron dextran, Ferrodex, and HemaJect. Iron sucrose is Venofer.

**Functional classification:** Mineral supplement

## Pharmacology and Mechanism of Action

Iron dextran and iron sucrose are used as iron supplements. Iron dextran is injected in animals (most commonly pigs) for prevention of iron-deficiency anemia. Iron dextran injection contains either 100 mg elemental iron per milliliter or 200 mg/mL. Ferric hydroxide is complexed with a low-molecular-weight dextran in this formulation. Iron dextran is a dark brown, slightly viscous liquid complex of ferric oxide and hydrolyzed dextran. After injection, it is slowly absorbed after IM administration into the lymphatic system. It may take 3 weeks for complete absorption. Iron sucrose is injected to treat iron-deficiency anemia.

## Indications and Clinical Uses

Most of the experience with the use is in young pigs for treatment and prevention of iron-deficiency anemia. Injections are usually made intramuscularly at 1–4 days of age. Iron dextran also can be administered intramuscularly for treatment of iron deficiency in dogs and cats.

Another preparation is iron sucrose (Venofer) injection 20 mg/mL, which may be used to treat iron-deficiency anemia.

## Precautionary Information

### Adverse Reactions and Side Effects

Injections may produce transient myositis and muscle weakness. The dextran portion can cause anaphylactoid reaction. Use iron sucrose or iron gluconate if the dextran causes a reaction.

### Contraindications and Precautions

When treating patients for iron-deficiency anemia, the total cumulative dose in a 14-day period should not exceed 15 mg/kg. Do not administer solutions intended for IV use by SQ or IM route.

### Drug Interactions

No drug interactions are reported.

## Instructions for Use

Inject iron dextran in mid-portion of rear thigh muscle in pigs. For treatment of iron-deficiency anemia with iron sucrose, inject intravenously by slow infusion over 2–5 minutes in an undiluted form or diluted in 100 mL of sodium chloride 0.9% over 15 minutes.

## Patient Monitoring and Laboratory Tests

Monitor iron concentrations in treated animals and CBC to monitor effectiveness. Iron dextran can cause a brown discoloration of serum, with false elevation of bilirubin and false decrease in serum calcium.

## Formulations

- Iron dextran is 100 or 200 mg of elemental iron per milliliter. Iron sucrose is 20 mg/mL injection.

## Stability and Storage
Store in a tightly sealed container, at room temperature, protected from light. Do not mix with other solutions. Do not freeze. When using iron sucrose, use immediately after dilution in saline solutions.

## Small Animal Dosage
- IV use for treating iron-deficiency anemia: 2–3 mg/kg IV slowly over 2–5 minutes. May be repeated five times in a 14-day period. The dose may be diluted in 0.9% saline solution and infused IV.

### Dogs
- 10–20 mg/kg IM of iron dextran once followed by oral treatment with ferrous sulfate.

### Cats
- 50 mg IM of iron dextran every 3–4 weeks.

## Large Animal Dosage
### Pigs
- 100 mg (1 mL) IM to 2- to 4-day-old pigs; repeat in 10 days.
- 200 mg (1 mL of higher concentration) IM to pigs at 1–3 days of age.

## Regulatory Information
No withdrawal time is necessary.

# Isoflupredone Acetate
eye-soe-floo′preh-done ass′ih-tate
**Trade and other names:** Predef 2X
**Functional classification:** Corticosteroid

## Pharmacology and Mechanism of Action
Isoflupredone is a corticosteroid that is infrequently used in veterinary medicine compared with other agents in this class. It produces anti-inflammatory and immunosuppressive effects that are approximately 17 times more potent than cortisol and 4 times more potent than prednisolone. Anti-inflammatory effects are complex but primarily via inhibition of inflammatory cells and suppression of expression of inflammatory mediators. The most common uses are for treatment of inflammatory and immune-mediated disease.

## Indications and Clinical Uses
Isoflupredone acetate is used for treating various musculoskeletal, allergic, and systemic inflammatory diseases. Large animal uses include inflammatory disorders, especially musculoskeletal inflammation, and equine asthma syndrome characterized by recurrent airway obstruction in horses. Isoflupredone acetate, like other corticosteroids, has been used to treat ketosis in cattle. In large animals, it also has been used to treat septic shock. However, efficacy for using corticosteroids to treat septic shock is not supported by good evidence.

## Precautionary Information
### Adverse Reactions and Side Effects
Side effects from corticosteroids are many and include polyphagia, polydipsia and polyuria, and hypothalamic–pituitary–adrenal axis suppression. Adverse effects include GI ulceration, hepatopathy, diabetes, hyperlipidemia, decreased thyroid hormone, decreased protein synthesis, delayed wound healing, and immunosuppression. Secondary infections can occur as a result of immunosuppression and include demodicosis, toxoplasmosis, fungal infections, and urinary tract infections. In horses, additional adverse effects include risk of laminitis, although a clear association between laminitis and corticosteroids has not been established.

### Contraindications and Precautions
Use with caution in patients prone to infection or GI ulcers. Administration of isoflupredone may induce hepatopathy, diabetes mellitus, or hyperlipidemia. Use cautiously in pregnant animals or in young, rapidly growing animals. Use of corticosteroids may impair healing.

### Drug Interactions
Corticosteroids will increase risk of GI ulceration when administered with NSAIDs.

## Instructions for Use
When administered to treat primary ketosis in cattle, it is advised to also administer IV glucose. When administered for conditions in cattle horses, follow label instructions for injections.

## Patient Monitoring and Laboratory Tests
Monitor liver enzymes, blood glucose, and renal function during therapy. Monitor patients for signs of secondary infections. Perform adrenocorticotropic (ACTH) stimulation test to monitor adrenal function.

## Formulations
• Isoflupredone is available in a 2-mg injection in 10- and 100-mL vials.

## Stability and Storage
Store in a tightly sealed container, protected from light, and at room temperature.

## Small Animal Dosage
• No doses are listed for isoflupredone because it is generally not administered to small animals. However, based on anti-inflammatory potency, dosages of 0.125–0.25 mg/kg/day IM can be considered.

## Large Animal Dosage
### Cattle
• 10–20 mg total dose per animal q12–24h IM.
• Ketosis: 10–20 mg as a total single dose per animal q12–24h IM.

### Horses
• 5–20 mg total dose per animal q12–24h IM.
• Pulmonary disease: 0.02–0.03 mg/kg q24h.
• Intraarticular: 5–20 mg per joint.

**Pigs**
- 0.036 mg/kg/day IM.

## Regulatory Information
Cattle and pig withdrawal time (meat): 7 days.
No milk withdrawal time is listed for US labeling. In Canada, withdrawal times are listed as 5 days for meat and 72 hours for milk.
For extralabel use withdrawal interval estimates, contact FARAD at www.FARAD.org.

# Isoflurane
eye-soe-floo'rane

**Trade and other names:** Aerrane

**Functional classification:** Anesthetic

## Pharmacology and Mechanism of Action
Isoflurane is an inhalant anesthetic agent. Like other inhalant anesthetics, the mechanism of action is uncertain. Isoflurane produces a generalized, reversible depression of the CNS. Inhalant anesthetics vary in their solubility in blood, their potency, and the rate of induction and recovery. Those with low blood/gas partition coefficients are associated with the most rapid rates of induction and recovery. Isoflurane has a vapor pressure of 250 mm Hg (at 20°C), a blood/gas partition coefficient of 1.4, and a fat/blood coefficient of 45.

## Indications and Clinical Uses
Isoflurane, like other inhalant anesthetics, is used for general anesthesia in animals. It is associated with rapid induction of anesthesia and rapid recovery rates. It is metabolized to only a small percentage (less than 1%) and has minimal effects on other organs. It has a minimum alveolar concentration (MAC) values of 1.63%, 1.3%, and 1.31% in cats, dogs, and horses, respectively.

## Precautionary Information
### Adverse Reactions and Side Effects
Adverse effects are related to anesthetic effects (e.g., cardiovascular and respiratory depression).

### Contraindications and Precautions
Do not administer unless it is possible to control ventilation and monitor heart rate and rhythm.

### Drug Interactions
No drug interactions are reported. However, like other inhalant anesthetics, other anesthetic agents act synergistically and lower dose requirements.

## Instructions for Use
Use of inhalant anesthetics requires careful monitoring. Dose is determined by depth of anesthesia.

## Patient Monitoring and Laboratory Tests
Monitor respiratory rate, heart rate, and rhythm during administration.

## Formulations
- Isoflurane is available in a 100-mL bottle.

## Stability and Storage
Store in a tightly sealed container, protected from light, and at room temperature.

## Small Animal Dosage
- Induction: 5%; maintenance: 1.5%–2.5%.

## Large Animal Dosage
- MAC value: 1.5%–2%.

## Regulatory Information
Withdrawal times are not established for animals that produce food. Clearance is rapid, and short withdrawal times are suggested.

For extralabel use withdrawal interval estimates, contact FARAD at www.FARAD.org.

# Isoniazid
eye-soe-nye′a-zid

**Trade and other names:** INH and isonicotinic acid hydrazide

**Functional classification:** Antibacterial

## Pharmacology and Mechanism of Action
Isoniazid is an antibacterial agent used infrequently in animals. The mechanism of action is via interference with lipid and nucleic acid biosynthesis in actively growing tubercle bacilli. The use is for atypical bacteria and the uses have been replaced by other agents.

## Indications and Clinical Uses
Isoniazid is used in people to treat tuberculosis. In animals, it is used to treat atypical bacterial infections, such as those caused by *Mycobacterium* spp. However, there is very little clinical information to guide dosing in animals or predict efficacy. The use is extrapolated from experience in human medicine or the opinions of experts.

## Precautionary Information

### Adverse Reactions and Side Effects
The use is uncommon in animals, and adverse effects have not been well documented. Hepatic toxicity is the most serious concern when isoniazid is used in people, which is apparently caused by a metabolite and may have a delayed onset. If liver injury is recognized (elevated liver enzymes, nausea), a return to normal is possible if treatment is discontinued. Occurrence of liver injury in dogs is uncertain because it is related to acetylation of the drug in people, and dogs lack this enzyme pathway. Other reported adverse effects include rash and peripheral neuropathy.

### Contraindications and Precautions
No specific contraindications have been reported for animals. However, it should not be used in animals with evidence of hepatic disease. Do not exceed 30 mg/kg in large animals to avoid adverse effects.

### Drug Interactions
Isoniazid metabolism may be decreased by itraconazole and increased by rifampin.

## Instructions for Use

Isoniazid administration in animals is limited to indications where other drugs are not effective.

## Patient Monitoring and Laboratory Tests

Monitor liver enzymes. Monitor patients for signs of neurologic toxicity.

## Formulations

- Isoniazid is available in 100- and 300-mg tablets; 10-mg/mL syrup; or 100-mg/mL injection.

## Stability and Storage

Store in a tightly sealed container, protected from light, and at room temperature.

## Small Animal Dosage

- 5 mg/kg per day (up to 10–15 mg/kg/day) PO, IM, or IV. It also is administered as 15 mg/kg two to three times per week.

## Large Animal Dosage

- Cattle: 10–20 mg/kg per day IM.
- Johne's disease in cattle, sheep, and goats: 10–20 mg/kg per day in combination with rifampin.

## Regulatory Information

No withdrawal time has been established for large animals. For extralabel use withdrawal interval estimates, contact FARAD at www.FARAD.org.

---

# Isoproterenol Hydrochloride
eye-soe-proe-teer'eh-nole hye-droe-klor'ide

**Trade and other names:** Isuprel and isoprenaline hydrochloride

**Functional classification:** Beta-agonist

## Pharmacology and Mechanism of Action

Isoproterenol is a potent adrenergic agonist. Isoproterenol stimulates both $beta_1$- and $beta_2$-adrenergic receptors, with little effect on alpha receptors. Like other beta agonists, it stimulates activity of adenyl cyclase. In cardiac tissue, isoproterenol is one of the most potent agonists and increases rate, conduction, and contractility. Beta agonists also relax bronchial smooth muscle and arterial smooth muscle. Isoproterenol has a rapid onset of activity, with rapid systemic clearance and short duration of action.

## Indications and Clinical Uses

Isoproterenol is administered when it is necessary for prompt stimulation of the heart (inotropic and chronotropic) or to relieve acute bronchoconstriction. It is short acting and must be administered intravenously or via inhalation. Because of availability of other agents and rare need for a rapid-onset adrenergic agent, isoproterenol is infrequently used in animals.

## Precautionary Information

### Adverse Reactions and Side Effects

Isoproterenol causes adverse effects related to excessive adrenergic stimulation, seen primarily as tachycardia and tachyarrhythmias. High doses can cause calcium accumulation in myocardium and tissue injury. Adrenergic agonists can produce potassium imbalance in animals.

### Contraindications and Precautions

Do not use if formulation turns pink or a dark color. The formulation can be unstable when mixed with other solutions. Follow the guidelines on the package insert for potential problems.

### Drug Interactions

Isoproterenol potentiates other adrenergic agonists. Treatment potentiates cardiac arrhythmias and should be used cautiously with other arrhythmogenic drugs.

## Instructions for Use

Because of a short half-life, isoproterenol must be infused via CRI or repeated if administered IM or SQ. It is recommended for short-term use only because repeated treatment causes cardiac injury.

## Patient Monitoring and Laboratory Tests

Monitor heart rate and rhythm during treatment. Monitor serum potassium with repeated use.

## Formulations

- Isoproterenol is available in 0.2-mg/mL ampules for injection.

## Stability and Storage

Store in a tightly sealed container, protected from light, and at room temperature. It is soluble in water with good aqueous stability. It is susceptible to light, and if a dark color is observed, it should be discarded (pink to brownish color). Solutions above a pH of 6.0 may decompose more rapidly. In 5% dextrose solutions, it is stable for 24 hours. It has been added to ultrasonic nebulizers in distilled water for respiratory therapy and is stable in solution for 24 hours. It also is stable if mixed with cromolyn sodium.

## Small Animal Dosage

### Dogs and Cats

- 10 mcg/kg q6h IM or SQ.
- Dilute 1 mg in 500 mL of 5% dextrose or lactated Ringer's solution and infuse IV 0.5–1 mL/min (1–2 mcg/min) or to effect.
- CRI: Administer to effect at 0.01–0.1 mcg/kg/min.

## Large Animal Dosage

- 1 mcg/kg every 15 minutes IV until desired response.

## Regulatory Information

No regulatory information is available for animals intended for food. Because of a low risk of residues, no withdrawal times are suggested.

RCI Classification: 2

# Isosorbide Dinitrate and Isosorbide Mononitrate
eye-soe-sor′bide dye-nye′trate and eye-soe-sor′bide mahn-oh-neye′trate

**Trade and other names:** Isosorbide dinitrate (Isordil) and Isosorbide mononitrate (Monoket)

**Functional classification:** Vasodilator

## Pharmacology and Mechanism of Action
Isosorbide is a nitrate vasodilator. Like other nitrovasodilators, it produces vasodilation via generation of nitric oxide. It is short acting and relaxes vascular smooth muscle, especially venous vessels. Consequently, it decreases atrial pressure, as well as afterload and preload. Isosorbide mononitrate is a biologically active form of isosorbide dinitrate. Compared with isosorbide dinitrate, it does not undergo first-pass metabolism and is completely absorbed orally.

## Indications and Clinical Uses
Isosorbide dinitrate is used to reduce preload in patients with congestive heart failure. In people, it is primarily used to treat angina. The use in animals has not been established through clinical studies but is extrapolated from the human use. Nitroglycerin is used more frequently (topically), or infusions of nitroprusside IV are used in critical care situations. Use in animals has been primarily derived from empirical use or the opinions from experts. There are no well-controlled clinical studies or efficacy trials to document clinical effectiveness.

## Precautionary Information
### Adverse Reactions and Side Effects
Adverse effects are primarily related to overdoses that produce excess vasodilation and hypotension. Tolerance may develop with repeated doses.

### Contraindications and Precautions
Do not administer to patients with hypovolemia. Use cautiously in animals with low cardiac reserve.

### Drug Interactions
No drug interactions are reported, but interactions are possible when used with other adrenergic agonists.

## Instructions for Use
Generally, doses are titrated to individuals depending on response. Isosorbide mononitrate is absorbed better than isosorbide dinitrate and may be preferred in clinical situations.

## Patient Monitoring and Laboratory Tests
Monitor patient's cardiovascular status during treatment.

## Formulations
- Isosorbide dinitrate is available in 5-, 10-, 20-, and 40-mg tablets and 40-mg capsules.
- Isosorbide mononitrate is available in 10- and 20-mg tablets.

## Stability and Storage
Store in a tightly sealed container, protected from light, and at room temperature.

## Small Animal Dosage
**Dogs and Cats**
- Isosorbide dinitrate: 2.5–5 mg/animal q12h PO or 0.22–1.1 mg/kg q12h PO.
- Isosorbide mononitrate: 5 mg/dog; administer two doses per day 7 hours apart PO.

## Large Animal Dosage
- No large animal doses have been reported.

## Regulatory Information
No regulatory information is available. For extralabel use withdrawal interval estimates, contact FARAD at www.FARAD.org.
There is a low risk of residue potential.
RCI Classification: 4

# Isotretinoin
eye-soe-tret′ih-noe-in

**Trade and other names:** Accutane and Absorica

**Functional classification:** Dermatologic agent

## Pharmacology and Mechanism of Action
Isotretinoin is a keratinization-stabilizing drug. Isotretinoin reduces sebaceous gland size, inhibits sebaceous gland activity, and decreases sebum secretion. Use in animals has been primarily derived from empirical use and experiences from human medicine. There are no well-controlled clinical studies or efficacy trials to document clinical effectiveness in animals.

## Indications and Clinical Uses
In people, it is primarily used to treat acne. In animals, dermatologists have used it to treat sebaceous adenitis, with apparent success.

### Precautionary Information
**Adverse Reactions and Side Effects**
Adverse effects are not reported for animals, although experimental studies have demonstrated that it can cause focal calcification (e.g., in myocardium and vessels).

**Contraindications and Precautions**
Isotretinoin is absolutely contraindicated in pregnant animals because of fetal abnormalities.

**Drug Interactions**
No drug interactions are reported.

## Instructions for Use

Use in veterinary medicine is confined to limited clinical experience, recommendations from experts, and extrapolation from human reports. High expense of this medication has limited veterinary use. There is a restricted distribution for humans, and it may not be available for veterinary use because of prescribing restrictions.

## Patient Monitoring and Laboratory Tests

No monitoring is necessary for animal use.

## Formulations

• Isotretinoin is available in 10-, 20-, and 40-mg capsules. Capsules may not be available for veterinary use.

## Stability and Storage

Store in a tightly sealed container, protected from light, and at room temperature.

## Small Animal Dosage

**Dogs**

• 1–3 mg/kg/day (up to a maximum recommended dosage of 3–4 mg/kg/day PO).

## Large Animal Dosage

• No large animal doses have been reported.

## Regulatory Information

Do not use in animals intended for food.

# Isoxsuprine

eye-soks′yoo-preen

**Trade and other names:** Vasodilan and generic brands

**Functional classification:** Vasodilator

## Pharmacology and Mechanism of Action

Isoxsuprine is an older vasodilator that has gone out of favor in human medicine but is sometimes used in horses. The mechanism of action for isoxsuprine has not been identified. It has been suggested to act as a $beta_2$ agonist (for which experimental evidence is not supportive) or by increasing concentrations of nitric oxide. It also may inhibit mechanisms that are calcium dependent. There is some evidence that it relaxes vessels in digits of horses.

## Indications and Clinical Uses

Isoxsuprine is used in horses for navicular disease and other diseases of the foot, such as laminitis. The efficacy has not been established for these indications even though the use has persisted for many years. There are no reports of its use in other animals.

## Precautionary Information

**Adverse Reactions and Side Effects**

Hypotension is the primary adverse effect. It lowers arterial pressure. In horses, side effects may also include rubbing noses on objects, hyperexcitability, sweating, tachycardia, and restlessness.

**Contraindications and Precautions**

Do not use in hypotensive or dehydrated animals.

**Drug Interactions**

No drug interactions are reported.

## Instructions for Use

When used in horses, it often is used with other vasodilators and anti-inflammatory drugs. It is not known if it acts synergistically with these other medications.

## Patient Monitoring and Laboratory Tests

Monitor heart rate in treated animals.

## Formulations

• Isoxsuprine is available in 10- and 20-mg tablets.

## Stability and Storage

Store in a tightly sealed container, protected from light, and at room temperature. Although isoxsuprine is compounded for equine use, stability of compounded formulations has not been evaluated.

## Small Animal Dosage

• No small animal doses are reported.

## Large Animal Dosage

**Horses**

• Navicular disease and laminitis: 0.6 mg/kg q12h PO for 6–14 weeks. In some dosing protocols, if 0.6 mg/kg q12h has not improved the horse's condition within 3 weeks, the dose is doubled.

## Regulatory Information

No regulatory information is available. For extralabel use withdrawal interval estimates, contact FARAD at www.FARAD.org.

# Itraconazole

it-rah-kahn′ah-zole

**Trade and other names:** Sporanox and Itrafungol (available for cats)

**Functional classification:** Antifungal

## Pharmacology and Mechanism of Action

Itraconazole is a widely used azole (triazole) antifungal drug. Itraconazole inhibits ergosterol synthesis in fungal cell membrane to inhibit fungal cell growth in a fungistatic manner. Itraconazole can be incorporated into sebum and stratum corneum and can be detected in skin for 3–4 weeks after treatment. It is active against dermatophytes and systemic fungi, such as *Blastomyces, Histoplasma,* and *Coccidioides* spp. It is more potent against these fungi than ketoconazole or fluconazole. There are two formulations: an oral capsule and oral solution. The oral capsule is relatively insoluble and requires food for optimum absorption. The oral solution is solubilized by hydroxypropyl-beta-cyclodextrin as a molecular inclusion complex to maintain solubility. Cyclodextrin is an oligosaccharide in the form of a cylindrical structure, which is hydrophilic on the outside and hydrophobic on the inside. As a result, absorption does not require acidity, resulting in increased bioavailability of the solution in comparison to the capsular formulation.

*Pharmacokinetics:* Experience in dogs and cats has shown it to be absorbed orally, and doses have been established for treating systemic fungal infections and dermatophytes. In horses, the oral solution is better absorbed than the capsules (65% vs. 12%). The half-life in dogs has varied among studies. In one study, the half-life from the oral capsule was approximately 7 hours, but in another study, it was approximately 33 hours for both the oral capsule and oral solution, with a peak concentration of 1.25–1.5 mcg/mL at 1.5–3 hours. The capsule is absorbed about 85% as well as the oral solution in dogs. Human-label generic, but not compounded, formulations produce similar concentrations in dogs. In cats, the oral solution is absorbed approximately five times higher than the oral capsule. After absorption in cats, the half-lives are approximately 18 hours for the capsule and 25 hours for the oral solution. This produces a prolonged effect that allows for intermittent dosing (see dosing section).

## Indications and Clinical Uses

Itraconazole is often considered the first choice for dermatophyte infections in cats. Itraconazole has regulatory approval for treating dermatophytes in cats but is also used for this treatment in dogs. In addition to treating dermatophytes, it is also used to treat systemic fungi, such as *Blastomyces, Histoplasma,* and *Coccidioides* spp., in a variety of species, including exotic and zoo animals. It also has been shown effective for treatment of *Malassezia* dermatitis, but *Malassezia* doses are lower than for other infections (see dosing section). Although it has been used to treat infections caused by *Aspergillosis* spp., efficacy has not been as good as with other antifungal drugs such as voriconazole or amphotericin B.

## Precautionary Information

### Adverse Reactions and Side Effects

Itraconazole is better tolerated than ketoconazole. Ketoconazole inhibits hormone synthesis and can lower concentrations of cortisol, testosterone, and other hormones in animals. However, itraconazole has less effect on these enzymes and does not produce endocrine effects. However, vomiting and hepatotoxicity are possible with itraconazole administration, especially at high doses. Approximately 10%–15% of dogs develop high liver enzyme levels. Itraconazole has produced skin lesions in dogs, consisting of vasculitis, sterile suppurative skin lesions, and ulcerative skin lesions. High doses in cats caused vomiting and anorexia.

**Contraindications and Precautions**
Administer with food for best oral absorption. Compounded formulations are not bioequivalent to proprietary forms and should be avoided for use in animals. Use itraconazole cautiously in any animal with signs of liver disease. Use cautiously in pregnant animals. At high doses in laboratory animals, it has caused fetal abnormalities.

**Drug Interactions**
Antacid drugs (proton pump inhibitors or $H_2$-receptor blockers) decrease oral absorption. Itraconazole is a cytochrome P450 enzyme inhibitor. It may cause drug interactions because of inhibition of P450 enzymes. This increases the concentrations of other drugs administered concurrently, such as cyclosporine. The extent of cytochrome P450 inhibition may be important for many drugs that have a narrow safety margin (see Appendixes H and I).

## Instructions for Use
Administer with food for best absorption unless the oral solution is used. The doses are based on studies in animals in which pharmacokinetics have been analyzed, as well as clinical studies to treat blastomycosis, histoplasmosis, dermatophytes, and other infections. Compared with systemic fungal diseases, lower doses may be used in cats and dogs for dermatophytes and in dogs for treating *Malassezia* dermatitis. Other less common uses or doses are based on empiricism or extrapolation from human literature. Doses in horses are based primarily on specific pharmacokinetic studies.

Ordinarily, oral formulations are administered. However, it may be administered intravenously if needed. If IV solutions are used, infuse over 30 minutes.

## Patient Monitoring and Laboratory Tests
Monitor liver enzyme concentrations. If plasma/serum drug concentrations are monitored, the trough concentration (immediately before next dose) should be in the range of 0.5–1 mcg/mL.

## Formulations Available
• Itraconazole is available in 100-mg capsules and 10-mg/mL oral liquid.
• Itrafungol for cats is a 10-mg/mL oral cherry-flavored liquid solution complexed with cyclodextrin (52-mL bottle). This product is identical in formulation and composition to the human formulation of Sporanox solution.
• Injection form (if available) is 10 mg/mL supplied in 25-mL ampules (250 mg).

## Stability and Storage
Itraconazole is practically insoluble in water but is soluble in ethanol. It is unstable and may lose potency if not maintained in manufacturer's original formulation (capsules and solution). Compounded formulations are highly unstable and insoluble. Oral absorption of compounded itraconazole suspensions and capsules is poor or barely detectable and is not recommended. Oral commercial formulation (in cyclodextrin) has a pH of approximately 2.0, and the pH should be maintained to ensure optimal absorption. Do not freeze. The 10-mg/mL injection solution can reconstituted with saline (but not dextrose or lactated Ringer's solution) and stored at either 2° C–8°C or room temperature for up to 48 hours after reconstitution. Do not mix with other drugs.

## Small Animal Dosage
### Dogs
• Regardless of formulation (oral capsule or oral solution), administer a loading dose of 20 mg/kg followed by 10 mg/kg once q24h. Alternatively, the dosage can

be split into 5 mg/kg q12h PO. Highly susceptible fungi such as some strains of *Blastomyces* spp. can be treated with lower doses of 5 mg/kg once daily.
- Dermatophytes: 3 mg/kg/day PO for 15 days.
- Cryptococcosis: 5 mg/kg q12h PO.
- *Malassezia* dermatitis: 5 mg/kg q24h PO for 2 days, repeated each week for 3 weeks.

### Cats
- General infections: 5 mg/kg PO once daily. Alternatively, 50 mg (total dose) once per day or 100 mg per cat once every other day.
- Dermatophytes: 5 mg/kg PO once daily on alternating weeks for 3 cycles. For example, treat once daily during weeks 1, 3, and 5, but not on weeks 2 and 4. Some cats may need an additional course of therapy to eliminate the infection.

### Large Animal Dosage
**Horses**
- 5 mg/kg/day (2.5 mg/kg q12h) PO. In horses, the capsules are absorbed poorly and inconsistently. Use the oral solution (Sporanox) for optimum oral absorption.

### Regulatory Information
No regulatory information is available. If itraconazole is administered to food animals, contact FARAD at www.FARAD.org for extralabel withdrawal time information.

---

# Ivermectin
eye-ver-mek′tin

**Trade and other names:** Heartgard, Ivomec, Eqvalan liquid, Equimectrin, IverEase, Zimecterin, Privermectin, Ultramectin, Ivercide, Ivercare, and Ivermax. Acarexx is a topical form for cats.

**Functional classification:** Antiparasitic

## Pharmacology and Mechanism of Action
Ivermectin is an antiparasitic drug of the avermectin class. It is a prototype for this class of antiparasitic agents, which also includes eprinomectin and milbemycins (milbemycin and moxidectin). These drugs are macrocyclic lactones and share many similarities, including mechanism of action. These drugs are neurotoxic to parasites by potentiating glutamate-gated chloride ion channels in parasites. Paralysis and death of the parasite are caused by increased permeability to chloride ions and hyperpolarization of nerve cells. These drugs also potentiate other chloride channels, including ones gated by GABA. Mammals ordinarily are not affected because they lack glutamate-gated chloride channels, and there is a lower affinity for other mammalian chloride channels. Because these drugs ordinarily do not penetrate the blood–brain barrier, GABA-gated channels in the CNS of mammals are not affected. Ivermectin is active against intestinal parasites, mites, bots, heartworm microfilaria, and developing larvae. Ivermectin can also produce heartworm adulticide effects when administered long term. Ivermectin has no effect on trematode or cestode parasites.

Ivermectin has a prolonged half-life in all the animals studied, which allows for infrequent administration to achieve clinical effects.

## Indications and Clinical Uses

Ivermectin is used in horses for the treatment and control of large strongyles (adult) (*Strongylus vulgaris, Strongylus edentatus,* and *Triodontophorus* spp.), small strongyles (adult and fourth-stage larvae) (*Cyathostomum* spp., *Cylicocyclus* spp., *Cylicostephanus* spp.), pinworms (adult and fourth-stage larvae) (*Oxyuris equi*), large roundworms (adult) (*Parascaris equorum*), hairworms (adult) (*Trichostrongylus axei*), large-mouth stomach worms (adult) (*Habronema muscae*), neck threadworms (microfilariae) (*Onchocerca* spp.), and stomach bots (*Gastrophilus* spp.).

In cattle, it is used for treatment and control of GI nematodes (adults and fourth-stage larvae) (*Haemonchus placei, Ostertagia ostertagi*) (including inhibited larvae), *Ostertagia lyrata, T. axei, T. colubriformis, Cooperia oncophora, Cooperia punctata, Cooperia pectinata, Oesophagostomum radiatum, Nematodirus helvetianus* (adults only), *Nematodirus spathiger* (adults only), *Bunostomum phlebotomum*; lungworms (adults and fourth-stage larvae) (*Dictyocaulus viviparus*); grubs (parasitic stages) (*Hypoderma bovis, H. lineatum*); sucking lice (*Linognathus vituli, Haematopinus eurysternus, Solenopotes capillatus*); and mites (scabies) (*Psoroptes ovis* [syn. *P. communis* var. *bovis*], *Sarcoptes scabiei* var. *bovis*).

In pigs, it is used for treatment and control of GI roundworms (adults and fourth-stage larvae) large roundworm, *Ascaris suum*; red stomach worm, *Hyostrongylus rubidus*; nodular worm, *Oesophagostomum* species; threadworm, *Strongyloides ransomi* (adults only); somatic roundworm larvae (threadworm, *S. ransomi* [somatic larvae]); lungworms (*Metastrongylus* spp. [adults only]); lice (*H. suis*); and mites (*Sarcoptes scabiei* var. *suis*).

In small animals (dogs and cats), it is used as a heartworm preventative (low dose) or to treat external parasites (mites) and intestinal parasites at higher doses. The benefit for heartworm prophylaxis in animals is the ability to kill young larvae, older larvae, and immature or young adults and adult filariae. Ivermectin is an effective microfilaricide after adulticide therapy. It has been recommended by the American Heartworm Society to treat heartworm-positive dogs for 2–3 months prior to adulticide therapy. This allows immature worms to reach full maturity that are more susceptible to melarsomine, as well as preventing new infection. Ivermectin can also reduce numbers of adult heartworms when administered long term at preventive doses. For optimal heartworm adulticide effect, it is often administered with oral doxycycline (10 mg/kg per day for 28 days). Treatment of *Demodex* infections is effective but requires higher doses than for any other indication. See Instructions for Use section later for instructions to treat *Demodex*.

### Precautionary Information

#### Adverse Reactions and Side Effects

Toxicity may occur at high doses and in breeds in which ivermectin crosses the blood–brain barrier. Sensitive breeds include collies, Australian shepherds, Old English sheepdogs, longhaired whippets, and Shetland sheepdogs. Toxicity is neurotoxic and signs include hypersalivation, depression, ataxia, difficulty with vision, coma, and death. Sensitivity to ivermectin occurs in certain breeds because of a mutation in the multidrug resistance gene (*ABCB1*, formerly *MDR1* gene) that codes for the membrane pump P-glycoprotein. This mutation affects the efflux pump in the blood–brain barrier. Therefore, ivermectin can accumulate in the brain of these susceptible animals. High doses in normal animals may also produce similar toxicosis. Most nonsusceptible dogs can tolerate doses of 100–400 mcg/kg. But sensitive breeds (dogs with the *ABCB1* mutation) may exhibit toxicity at doses of 150–340 mcg/kg.

Retinopathy has also been observed in dogs administered high doses. In affected animals, a sudden onset of blindness, mydriasis, or both may occur, but dogs recover if the drug is discontinued.

Ivermectin at doses of 400 mcg/kg has produced neurologic toxicosis in Siamese kittens, and doses as low as 300 mcg/kg have been lethal in kittens. In horses, adverse reactions may include itching because of effects on microfilariae.

*Treatment of intoxication:* Administer activated charcoal from excessive doses administered orally. Symptomatic treatment includes ventilation support and control of seizures. An IV administration of lipid emulsion can be used at a dose of 1.5 mL/kg bolus of a 20% emulsion.

### Contraindications and Precautions

Do not administer to animals younger than 6 weeks of age. Animals with high numbers of microfilaremia may show adverse reactions to high doses. If dogs are sensitive to ivermectin (see earlier list of breeds), they may be sensitive to other drugs in this class (other avermectins). Ivermectin at approved clinical doses for treatment of endoparasites or heartworm prevention has been safe in pregnant animals. At high doses used for treating demodicosis, safety during pregnancy is not known, but there have been no reports of teratogenic effects. In the most sensitive laboratory animal (mouse), the lowest dose that is teratogenic is 400 mcg/kg. Dogs with the *ABCB1 (MDR)* mutation may also be sensitive to other drugs such as loperamide, milbemycin, moxidectin, and anticancer drugs. Ivermectin is excreted in milk.

### Drug Interactions

Except for low doses used for heartworm prevention, do not administer with drugs that could potentially increase the penetration of ivermectin across the blood–brain barrier. Such drugs include ketoconazole, itraconazole, cyclosporine, and calcium-channel blockers. Do not administer with spinosad (Comfortis, Trifexis) because it may potentiate toxicity.

## Instructions for Use

Ivermectin is used in a wide range of animals for internal and external parasites. Dosage regimens vary, depending on the species and parasite treated. Heartworm prevention is the lowest dose; other parasites require higher doses. Products for heartworm prevention and a topical form are the only forms approved for small animals; for other indications, large-animal injectable products are often administered PO, IM, or SQ to small animals. Do not administer intravenously. Injections in pigs should be made in the neck only.

Because some dogs may be sensitive to ivermectin, if a dog has not previously received ivermectin and high doses are needed (e.g., to treat *Demodex* infection), start with a low dose (50–100 mcg/kg) and then increase by increments of 50–100 mcg/kg/day on subsequent doses every day. During this increase, the dog should be observed for signs of CNS toxicity (ataxia, tremors, sedation). When the maintenance dose is achieved (300–600 mcg/kg PO), it should be administered once daily until 4 weeks after the second consecutive negative monthly skin scraping. When using extralabel formulations to treat dogs, the aqueous formulations have better palatability than the propylene-based formulations. They can be mixed with flavorings to improve palatability.

## Patient Monitoring and Laboratory Tests

Monitor for microfilaremia prior to administration in small animals. For other parasitic infections, confirm successful treatment with fecal examinations or skin scrapings.

## Formulations

- Ivermectin is available in 1% (10 mg/mL), 2% (20 mg/mL), and 0.27% (2.7 mg/mL) injectable solution; 10-mg/mL oral solution; 5 mg/mL pour-on for cattle, 0.8-mg/mL oral sheep drench; 18.7-mg/mL oral paste; 68-, 136-, and 272-mcg tablets; and 55- and 165-mg feline tablets. A water-soluble topical product 0.01% (0.1 mg/mL) is available in ampules in foil pouches for treating ear mites in cats.
- Compounded formulations: Ivermectin is chemically unstable at certain pH ranges and after exposure to water. Unless stability and strength are documented, compounded formulations are not recommended.

## Stability and Storage

Store in a tightly sealed container, protected from light, and at room temperature. Stability of compounded formulations has not been evaluated.

## Small Animal Dosage

### Dogs

- Heartworm preventative: 6 mcg/kg every 30 days PO.
- Prior to adulticide treatment: Administer preventative dose for 2 months, and up to 3 months prior to adulticide treatment.
- Heartworm treatment: Ivermectin administered at preventive doses combined with doxycycline at 10 mg/kg PO per day for 28 days.
- Ectoparasite therapy: 200–400 mcg/kg (0.2–0.4 mg/kg) IM, SQ, or PO.
- Demodicosis therapy: Start with 100 mcg/kg/day (0.1 mg/kg) and increase dose by 100 mcg/kg/day to 600 mcg/kg/day (0.6 mg/kg) for 60–120 days PO. (Successful treatment is confirmed with negative skin scrapings.)
- Sarcoptic mange and cheyletiellosis therapy: 200–400 mcg/kg every 7 days PO or every 14 SQ for 4–6 weeks.

### Cats

- Heartworm preventive: 24 mcg/kg every 30 days PO.
- Ectoparasite therapy: 200–400 mcg/kg (0.2–0.4 mg/kg) IM, SQ, or PO, every 7 days or as needed based on skin scraping and clinical examination.
- Endoparasite therapy: 200–400 mcg/kg (0.2–0.4 mg/kg) weekly SQ or PO.
- Topical: 0.5 mL per ear (0.1 mg/mL) for treating ear mites.

## Large Animal Dosage

### Horses

- 200 mcg/kg (0.2 mg/kg) IM, oral paste, or oral solution. Oral solution dose is 1 mL per 50 kg (110 lb). Administer once or as needed as part of a comprehensive worming program.

### Calves

- Slow-release bolus: 5.7–13.8 mg/kg, as a single dose, which has a duration of 135 days.

### Cattle and goats

- Injection solution: 200 mcg (0.2 mg)/kg as a single dose SQ.
- Pour-on: 0.5 mg/kg or 1 mL/10 kg (22 lb) of 5 mg/mL solution.

### Pigs

- 300 mcg (0.3 mg)/kg SQ as a single dose.

### Sheep

- Injection solution: 200 mcg (0.2 mg)/kg as a single dose SQ.

- 200 mcg/kg PO.

## Regulatory Information

Pigs' withdrawal time for meat: 18 days for SQ injection.
Cattle and calves' withdrawal time (meat): 35 days for SQ injection or 180 days for slow-release bolus. Forty-eight days for topical (pour-on).
Because a withdrawal time in milk has not been established, do not use in female dairy cattle of breeding age.
Sheep withdrawal time (meat): 11 days.
Goats' withdrawal time: 11–14 days (meat) and 6–9 hours (milk). When administering SQ to goats, use 35 hours for meat and 40 hours for milk.

# Ivermectin + Praziquantel
eye-ver-mek'tin + pray-zih-kwon'tel
**Trade and other names:** Equimax
**Functional classification:** Antiparasitic

## Pharmacology and Mechanism of Action

Antiparasitic drug. Ivermectin + praziquantel is indicated for use in horses for treatment and control of tapeworms, large strongyles (including *Strongylus vulgaris, S. edentatus, Strongylus equines*) and small strongyles, pinworms, ascarids, hairworms, stomach worms, bots, *Habronema* spp., and other parasites.

## Indications and Clinical Uses

Ivermectin has properties as described in the Ivermectin monograph. Praziquantel is added to this formulation to increase the spectrum.

## Precautionary Information

### Adverse Reactions and Side Effects

Toxicity may occur at high doses. Ivermectin appears to be safe for pregnant animals.

### Contraindications and Precautions

Ivermectin can be administered to breeding, pregnant, and lactating animals without adverse effects.

### Drug Interactions

Use cautiously with other drugs that may affect penetration across the blood–brain barrier.

## Instructions for Use

Use of this drug is similar to the individual drugs ivermectin and praziquantel.

## Patient Monitoring and Laboratory Tests

Fecal samples should be examined for parasites to monitor effectiveness.

## Formulations

- Ivermectin + praziquantel is available in a paste composed of 1.87% ivermectin and 14.03% praziquantel.

## Stability and Storage
Store in a tightly sealed container, protected from light, and at room temperature.

## Small Animal Dosage
- No dose available for small animals.

## Large Animal Dosage
**Horses**
- 200 mcg/kg of ivermectin and 1 mg/kg of praziquantel PO.

## Regulatory Information
No withdrawal times are available for animals intended for food (extralabel use).

# Kanamycin Sulfate
kan-ah-mye′sin sul′fate

**Trade and other names:** Kantrim

**Functional classification:** Antibacterial

## Pharmacology and Mechanism of Action
Kanamycin is an aminoglycoside antibiotic. Like other aminoglycosides, the action is to inhibit bacteria protein synthesis via binding to 30S ribosome. Through this action, it causes a misreading of the genetic code and inhibits bacterial protein synthesis. Another mechanism important for gram-negative bacteria is to disrupt the cell surface biofilm, particularly on gram-negative bacteria, to produce disruption, loss of cell wall integrity, and a rapid bactericidal effect. Magnesium and calcium are important to cross-bridge adjacent lipopolysaccharide molecules. Positive-charged aminoglycosides competitively displace $Ca^{2+}$ and $Mg^{2+}$ and destabilize the bacteria outer membrane. Therefore death of the bacteria is caused by a cell surface effect rather than inhibition of the ribosome. This property is not as prominent for gram-positive bacteria unless administered with a cell-wall disrupting agent such as vancomycin or a beta-lactam antibiotic. Kanamycin is less active than other aminoglycosides such as gentamicin and amikacin, but the spectrum of activity includes most gram-negative bacterial isolates in animals, particularly gram-negative bacilli of the Enterobacteriaceae. It is not very active against streptococci and anaerobic bacteria. It has action on *Staphylococcus* spp. but is not a preferred treatment for these bacteria.

## Indications and Clinical Uses
Kanamycin is a broad-spectrum antibiotic used to treat gram-negative infections. It is less active than gentamicin, amikacin, or tobramycin. Therefore, there is little advantage for using kanamycin over the other drugs in this class. The use of kanamycin has greatly diminished, and gentamicin and amikacin are much more frequently used in animals.

## Precautionary Information
### Adverse Reactions and Side Effects
Nephrotoxicity is the most dose-limiting toxicity. Ensure that patients have adequate fluid and electrolyte balance during therapy. Ototoxicity and vestibulotoxicity also are possible.

### Contraindications and Precautions
Do not use in animals with kidney disease. Do not use in dehydrated animals.

### Drug Interactions
When used with anesthetic agents, neuromuscular blockade is possible with high doses. Do not mix in vial or syringe with other antibiotics. Ototoxicity and nephrotoxicity are potentiated by loop diuretics such as furosemide.

## Instructions for Use
Kanamycin is not as active as other aminoglycosides. For serious infections, consider gentamicin or amikacin.

## Patient Monitoring and Laboratory Tests

Susceptibility testing: Clinical and Laboratory Standards Institute (CLSI) minimum inhibitory concentration value breakpoint for susceptibility is ≤16 mcg/mL, but this is based on the human breakpoint and may be too high for testing bacteria isolated from animals. Monitor blood urea nitrogen, creatinine, and urine for evidence of renal toxicity.

## Formulations

• Kanamycin is available in 200- and 500-mg/mL injection.

## Stability and Storage

Store in a tightly sealed container, protected from light, and at room temperature. It is soluble in water but is not stable in compounded formulations. Do not mix with other drugs. Do not freeze.

## Small Animal Dosage

**Dogs and Cats**

• 20 mg/kg q24h IV or IM.

## Large Animal Dosage

**Horses**

• 10 mg/kg q24h IV.

## Regulatory Information

Avoid use in food-producing animals. Extended withdrawal times (as long as 18 months) may be needed for withdrawal time in cattle. For extralabel use withdrawal interval estimates, contact Food Animal Residue Avoidance Databank (FARAD) at www.FARAD.org.

# Kaolin and Pectin

kay′oh-lin + pek′tin

**Trade and other names:** Also called Kaopectate; generic brands

**Functional classification:** Antidiarrheal

## Pharmacology and Mechanism of Action

Kaolin and pectin are combined in various products as antidiarrheal treatments. Kaolin is a form of aluminum silicate, and pectin is a carbohydrate that is extracted from the rinds of citrus fruits. This product has a claim to act as a demulcent and adsorbent in the treatment of diarrhea. The action of kaolin–pectin is believed to be related to the binding of bacterial toxins (endotoxins and enterotoxins) in the gastrointestinal (GI) tract. However, experimental studies have shown that kaolin–pectin has been an ineffective binder of *Escherichia coli* enterotoxin, and clinical studies have failed to show a benefit from the administration of kaolin–pectin. This product may change the consistency of stools, but it does not decrease fluid or electrolyte loss, nor does it shorten the duration of illness. Most of the modern Kao-Pectate formulations contain salicylate as one of the active ingredients.

## Indications and Clinical Uses

Kaolin and pectin combinations are used for the symptomatic treatment of acute diarrhea. Despite the lack of clinical evidence of efficacy, some veterinarians administer this drug for short-term treatment. Commercial forms that contain salicylate (8.68 mg/mL) may have anti-inflammatory effects to decrease secretory diarrhea caused by bacteria.

## Precautionary Information

**Adverse Reactions and Side Effects**

Side effects are uncommon. There are 8.7 mg/mL of salicylate in the regular strength and 16 mg/mL in the extra-strength formulation. Because some animals may be sensitive to salicylates, this ingredient in the formulation should be considered before administering to animals.

**Contraindications and Precautions**

No specific contraindications in animals.

**Drug Interactions**

No drug interactions are reported. However, the kaolin component may prevent absorption of other drugs. Administer other oral drugs 30 minutes prior to kaolin–pectin to avoid drug interaction.

## Instructions for Use

Kaolin–pectin may not change the course of diarrhea but may change the character of the feces.

## Patient Monitoring and Laboratory Tests

No specific monitoring is necessary.

## Formulations

- Kaolin–pectin is no longer found in the product Kao-Pectate (previously available in a 12-oz oral suspension). All formulations for Kao-Pectate contain bismuth subsalicylate. Salicylate (8.68 mg/mL) is present in Kao-Pectate.
- Veterinary formulations of kaolin–pectin are available under various generic names in 1-quart and 1-gallon containers containing 5.8 g of kaolin and 0.139 g of pectin per 30 mL (1 oz).

## Stability and Storage

Store in a tightly sealed container, protected from light, and at room temperature.

## Small Animal Dosage

**Dogs and Cats**

- 1–2 mL/kg q2–6h PO.

## Large Animal Dosage

**Horses and Cattle**

- 180–300 mL q2–3h PO.

**Calves and Foals**

- 90–120 mL q2–3h PO.

## Regulatory Information
There is little risk of residues in animals that produce food. No withdrawal times are necessary.

# Ketamine Hydrochloride
ket'ah-meen hye-droe-klor'ide

**Trade and other names:** Ketalar, Ketavet, and Vetalar

**Functional classification:** Anesthetic

## Pharmacology and Mechanism of Action
Ketamine is a widely used anesthetic agent. The precise mechanism of action is not known, but most evidence supports its action as a centrally acting dissociative agent. Ketamine produces mild analgesia and modulates pain via its ability to act as a noncompetitive antagonist for N-methyl D-aspartate (NMDA) receptors. Ketamine is an equal concentration of two isomers (R-ketamine and S-ketamine). S-ketamine is more active and is eliminated faster. The S-isomer, called esketamine hydrochloride (Spravato), is an intranasal product that has been used in humans for treatment of depression. The mechanism by which it exerts its antidepressant effect is unknown. The major circulating metabolite noresketamine demonstrated activity at the same receptor with less affinity.

*Pharmacokinetics:* Ketamine is not active orally. It must be injected by IV, IM, or SQ routes. It has a short half-life in most animals (60–90 minutes) and is rapidly metabolized. The metabolite (norketamine) may produce more prolonged NMDA antagonistic effects but with less affinity for the receptor.

## Indications and Clinical Uses
Ketamine is commonly used for short-term anesthetic procedures in many animal species. Because of the short half-life, the duration of action is generally 30 minutes or less. For procedures that require a longer duration (e.g., surgical procedures) IV infusions have been used, often in combination with other anesthetic/sedative agents (referred to as *total intravenous anesthesia*).

Ketamine is often combined in use with other anesthetics and sedatives such as benzodiazepines (diazepam, midazolam), propofol, lidocaine, opiates (hydromorphone, morphine), or alpha$_2$ agonists (medetomidine, dexmedetomidine, and xylazine). Such combinations have been synergistic and allowed lower doses of each individual component. One example of a combination is MLK, which is morphine (or fentanyl), lidocaine, and ketamine, or equine "triple-drip," also known as "GKX," in which it is mixed with xylazine and guaifenesin (see dosing section for more details on these protocols). Another mixture, referred to as "MKX," is a combination of midazolam, ketamine, and xylazine used for anesthesia in horses. Ketamine has also been added to protocols for cattle and horses using xylazine and butorphanol for standing restraint. The dose used in these protocols is subanesthetic (e.g., 0.05–0.1 mg/kg IV).

Although ordinarily contraindicated in patients with epilepsy, it has been used to treat cases of refractory status epilepticus through its NMDA receptor effects.

## Precautionary Information

**Adverse Reactions and Side Effects**

Ketamine causes pain with IM injection (pH of solution is 3.5). Tremors, muscle spasticity, and convulsive seizures have been reported. Spontaneous movements, salivation, and increased body temperature are more common in dogs when high doses are used. Ketamine increases sympathetic tone, heart rate, and blood pressure. It produces an increased cardiac output compared with other anesthetic agents. Salivation, mydriasis, and regurgitation are increased in animals that receive ketamine, which may be reduced by premedication within atropine. Apnea may develop in some animals, and oxygen supplementation should be available. Prolonged infusions in horses may delay GI transit times.

**Contraindications and Precautions**

Do not use in animals with head injury because it may elevate cerebrospinal fluid pressure. Use cautiously, if at all, in animals with glaucoma (increases intraocular pressure). Do not use in animals prone to seizures (although some animals with seizures have been successfully treated with ketamine). Avoid use in animals with restrictive or hypertrophic cardiomyopathy. When used alone as a sole agent in horses, ketamine causes hyperexcitability and involuntary muscle movements. When used in horses, pretreat with a sedative (e.g., alpha$_2$ agonist).

**Drug Interactions**

Ketamine hydrochloride is maintained at an acidic pH for stability and solubility. If mixed with alkalinizing solutions, instability or precipitation can result. It can safely be mixed with other anesthetic agents in a syringe prior to injection as long as the pH of the solution remains low enough to prevent precipitation.

## Instructions for Use

Ketamine is often used in combination with other anesthetics and anesthetic adjuncts, such as xylazine, dexmedetomidine, medetomidine, acepromazine, opiates, propofol, lidocaine, and benzodiazepines (e.g., diazepam, midazolam). Because ketamine can cause behavior reactions and myoclonus, it is recommended to use with other agents such as alpha$_2$ agonists (e.g., dexmedetomidine) or benzodiazepines (e.g., midazolam). CRIs may be used to maintain a plane of anesthesia and analgesia. (See dosing section for infusion doses.) IV doses are generally less than IM doses. In cats, ketamine may be sprayed into the mouth (10 mg/kg) and produces similar effects as IM injection. Animals receiving ketamine have open eyelids, and artificial tears should be applied to prevent corneal injury.

## Patient Monitoring and Laboratory Tests

Monitor heart rate and breathing in patients anesthetized with ketamine. Although plasma concentrations are not typically monitored, the concentration of 0.22–0.37 mcg/mL is associated with analgesic properties in cats and 0.1–0.2 mcg/mL in people.

## Formulations

- Ketamine is available in 100-mg/mL injection solution.

- Esketamine hydrochloride (Spravato) is the S-isomer of ketamine (the active form). This product is used for intranasal delivery in people to treat depression. The use in animals has not been reported.

## Stability and Storage

Store in a tightly sealed container, protected from light, and at room temperature. Ketamine is soluble in water and ethanol. Ketamine hydrochloride has been successfully administered when combined in a syringe immediately prior to injection with drugs such as alpha$_2$ agonists, opiates, lidocaine, propofol, guaifenesin, benzodiazepines, and acepromazine. Ketamine has been mixed with propofol at a ratio of 1:1 in the same syringe and administered intravenously. Ketamine hydrochloride mixed with midazolam retained potency for 97 hours.

## Small Animal Dosage

- For all animals: Lower doses listed for IV use; higher doses listed for IM use.

**Dogs**

- 5.5–22 mg/kg IV or IM. (Generally, the lower dose range is given IV compared with IM.) It is recommended to use adjunctive sedative or tranquilizer treatment.
- CRI for peri-operative use: Administer a loading dose of 0.3–0.5 mg/kg IV followed by 0.3–0.6 mg/kg/h (5–10 mcg/kg/min) during surgery. The rate during surgery may be increased to 1 mg/kg/h if needed. After surgery, treatment can be continued to provide analgesia at a low rate of 0.12 mg/kg/h for up to 18 hours. To administer a rate of 0.3–0.6 mg/kg/h, mix 0.6 mL (60 mg) with 1 L of fluids and infuse at a rate of 5–10 mL/kg/h.
- CRI for light sedation: 1–2 mg/kg/h, which may be combined with other sedatives.
- Combination of morphine, lidocaine, and ketamine (MLK): Mixed as 100 mg/mL of ketamine (1.6 mL/500 mL fluids) + 20 mg/mL of lidocaine (30 mL/500 mL fluids) and 15 mg/mL of morphine (1.6 mL/500 mL fluids) and infused at a rate of morphine, 0.24 mg/kg h; lidocaine, 3 mg/kg/h; and ketamine, 0.6 mg/kg/h, administered as CRI for perioperative analgesia.

**Cats**

- 2–25 mg/kg IV or IM. (Generally, the lower dose range is given IV compared with IM.) Note: When used in cats, a sedative such as acepromazine (0.1 mg/kg) or a benzodiazepine is recommended prior to or combined in same syringe with administration of ketamine. When combined in same syringe, inject immediately after mixing. (In cats, it also can be sprayed into the mouth and produces similar effect as IM 10 mg/kg.)
- Short-term procedures: 3–5 mg/kg ketamine + 25 mcg/kg dexmedetomidine, mixed together and administered IM (an opiate also may be included).
- Mix with propofol combined 1:1 in the same syringe at a dose of 2 mg/kg ketamine and 2 mg/kg propofol administered IV followed by an infusion (CRI) of 10 mg/kg/h (both drugs combined).
- CRI: Loading dose of 0.3–0.5 mg/kg IV followed by 0.3–0.6 mg/kg/h (5–10 mcg/kg/min). This rate may be increased to 1 mg/kg/h (15 mcg/kg/min) if needed or lowered to 2–5 mcg/kg/min when combined with other drugs (e.g., opiates).

K

## Large Animal Dosage

### Horses, Cattle, Sheep, and Swine

- 2 mg/kg IV (in horses, pretreat with a sedative).
- Ketamine at 1.1 mg/kg mixed with xylazine at 0.5 mg/kg may be combined in the same syringe and administered IV.
- CRI for analgesia: Loading dose of 0.6 mg/kg IV followed by CRI of 0.4–0.8 mg/kg/h and increased to 1.2 mg/kg/h if needed. To prepare CRI solution for analgesia, add 30 mL of ketamine to a 1-L bag of fluids (3 mg/mL) and administer IV over a duration of 8 hours at a rate of 125 mL/h for average size horse.
- Total IV anesthesia: 2 mg/kg/h up to 6 mg/kg/h delivered IV. This may be added to fluids in a concentration of 2 mg/mL of ketamine with other agents (e.g., guaifenesin, 100 mg/mL; or detomidine, 0.02 mg/mL) and infused IV at a rate of 1–3 mL/kg/h (to effect).
- Equine "triple drip" consists of 500 mg xylazine plus 2000 mg of ketamine added to 1 L of 5% guaifenesin in dextrose. Infused at a rate of 1.1 mL/kg for induction; then 2.4 mL/kg/h for maintenance.
- 10 mg/kg IM. Often used in combination with other agents, such as xylazine.
- Foals, treatment of seizures: 0.02 mg/kg/min CRI.

## Regulatory Information

Extralabel use: Withdrawal time of at least 3 days for meat and 48 hours for milk.
Schedule III controlled drug
Racing Commissioners International (RCI) Classification: 2

## Ketoconazole
kee-toe-kah′nah-zole

**Trade and other names:** Nizoral

**Functional classification:** Antifungal

## Pharmacology and Mechanism of Action

Ketoconazole is an oral azole (imidazole) antifungal drug. Ketoconazole has a similar mechanism of action as other azole antifungal agents (itraconazole and fluconazole). It inhibits a P450 enzyme in fungi and inhibits ergosterol synthesis in the fungal cell membrane to produce a fungistatic effect. It has antifungal activity against dermatophytes and a variety of systemic fungi, such as *Histoplasma*, *Blastomyces*, and *Coccidioides* spp. and *Malassezia* yeast. Other azole antifungal drugs include voriconazole, itraconazole, posaconazole, and fluconazole. Ketoconazole is less active and has more adverse effects than the other azole antifungal agents and the use has declined. In people, it is rarely used because of availability of other agents.

For treatment of canine hypercortisolemia (Cushing's disease), it inhibits cortisol synthesis through the inhibition of cytochrome P450 enzymes involved in steroid synthesis.

*Pharmacokinetics:* It is moderately absorbed orally in dogs, with food and an acid medium required for oral absorption. After absorption of a single dose in dogs, the half-life is 2.1–5.8 hours (mean 3.6 hours), with a peak of 4.5–15.2 mcg/mL. But after multiple doses, it inhibits its own metabolism, and the half-life increases to 4.9–9.4 hours (mean, 6.8 hours). Oral absorption in horses is too low to be therapeutically effective.

## Indications and Clinical Uses
Ketoconazole is used in dogs, cats, and some exotic animals to treat dermatophytes and systemic fungi, such as *Blastomyces, Histoplasma,* and *Coccidioides* spp. It also has been shown effective for treatment of *Malassezia* dermatitis. It does not have good activity against *Aspergillus* spp. Ketoconazole should not be used in horses because oral absorption is poor unless administered with a highly acidic vehicle.

In dogs, it has a profound effect on cytochrome P450 enzymes, which affects metabolism of other drugs. It is also via the inhibition of steroid P450 biosynthesis that ketoconazole has been used as a short-term treatment for canine hyperadrenocorticism (canine Cushing's disease). However, for canine Cushing's disease, many animals do not respond adequately, and there are more adverse effects than with trilostane. Because of the availability of other drugs for treating hyperadrenocorticism (e.g., trilostane), ketoconazole has fallen out of use for this indication.

## Precautionary Information

### Adverse Reactions and Side Effects
Adverse effects in animals include dose-related vomiting (most common), diarrhea, hepatic injury, and rare thrombocytopenia in dogs. Liver enzyme elevations are common. Ketoconazole inhibits hormone synthesis and can lower concentrations of cortisol, testosterone, and other hormones in animals. Ketoconazole may produce a lighter hair coat color in some animals. It has been associated with cataract formation in dogs.

### Contraindications and Precautions
Do not administer to pregnant animals. At high doses in laboratory animals, it caused embryotoxicity and fetal abnormalities. Some of these effects on pregnancy may be because of the inhibition of estrogen synthesis by ketoconazole.

### Drug Interactions
It is a potent inhibitor of CYP3A12 and inhibits the metabolism of many drugs. Ketoconazole also inhibits the transporter P-glycoprotein. These properties inhibit metabolism and clearance of other drugs (anticonvulsants, cyclosporine, warfarin, and cisapride). This property has been used to reduce doses of cyclosporine (ketoconazole dose of 5–10 mg/kg). Particular caution should be exercised when administering ketoconazole with ivermectin. This combination may produce ivermectin toxicity by decreasing clearance and enhancing penetration across the blood–brain barrier. Antacid drugs (proton pump inhibitors, $H_2$-receptor antagonists) will inhibit oral absorption of ketoconazole.

## Instructions for Use
Oral absorption depends on acidity in the stomach. Do not administer with drugs that decrease stomach acid, such as proton pump inhibitors (omeprazole), histamine $H_2$ blockers (famotidine), or antacids. Because of endocrine effects, ketoconazole has been used for short-term treatment of hyperadrenocorticism. However, many experts believe that ketoconazole is not an effective long-term treatment for canine Cushing's disease, and this use is no longer common. Trilostane is the preferred treatment for canine hyperadrenocorticism.

## Patient Monitoring and Laboratory Tests

Monitor liver enzymes (alanine aminotransferase, alkaline phosphatase) for evidence of toxicity. Ketoconazole lowers serum cortisol levels.

## Formulations

- Ketoconazole is available in 200-mg tablets and 100-mg/mL oral suspension (Canada).

## Stability and Storage

Store in a tightly sealed container, protected from light, and at room temperature. Ketoconazole is practically insoluble in water but is soluble in ethanol. When ketoconazole was compounded extemporaneously from tablets with syrups and flavorings, it was stable for 60 days. However, ketoconazole requires acidity for solubility and may not be absorbed from these formulations. If compounded in alkaline conditions, it may precipitate.

## Small Animal Dosage

### Dogs

- 10–15 mg/kg q8–12h PO.
- *Malassezia* infection: 5 mg/kg q24h PO every 3 weeks.
- Hyperadrenocorticism: Start with 5 mg/kg q12h initially; then increase after 7 days to 12–15 mg/kg q12h PO.

### Cats

- 5–10 mg/kg q8–12h PO.

## Large Animal Dosage

### Horses

Poorly absorbed. Fluconazole, itraconazole, and voriconazole are more completely absorbed.

## Regulatory Information

Withdrawal times are not established for animals that produce food. For extralabel use withdrawal interval estimates, contact FARAD at www.FARAD.org.

# Ketoprofen

kee-toe-proe′fen

**Trade and other names:** Orudis-KT (human over-the-counter tablet), Ketofen (veterinary injection), and Anafen (outside the United States)

**Functional classification:** Nonsteroidal anti-inflammatory drug

## Pharmacology and Mechanism of Action

Ketoprofen is a nonsteroidal anti-inflammatory drug (NSAID) used in people and animals. Like other NSAIDs, produces analgesic and anti-inflammatory effects by inhibiting the synthesis of prostaglandins. The enzyme inhibited by NSAID is the cyclo-oxygenase (COX) enzyme. The COX enzyme exists in two isoforms: COX-1 and COX-2. COX-1 is primarily responsible for synthesis of prostaglandins important for maintaining a healthy GI tract, renal function, platelet function, and other normal physiologic functions. COX-2 is induced and is responsible for synthesizing prostaglandins that are important mediators of pain, inflammation, and fever. However, it is known that there is some crossover of COX-1 and COX-2 effects in some situations, and COX-2 activity is important for some biological effects. Ketoprofen is a nonselective inhibitor of COX-1 and COX-2. There is weak evidence of its ability to inhibit lipoxygenase.

*Pharmacokinetics:* Ketoprofen exists as a chiral isomer with R- and S-isomers present in the racemic formulation. In animals, the S-form is more active and there is interconversion between the R- and S-forms. The half-lives are relatively short in most animals with values of 1, 0.4, 3.5, and 1.5 hours (S-isomer) in horses, cattle, dogs, and cats, respectively.

## Indications and Clinical Uses

Ketoprofen is an NSAID that is used for treatment of moderate pain and inflammation. It has a half-life in most animals of less than 2 hours, but it has a duration of action for up to 24 hours. In the United States, if it is used in small animals, either the large-animal injectable formulation or the human oral OTC tablets are used. It is approved for treating horses using the injectable formulation. This form also has been administered to other large animals (cattle, sheep, pigs, and zoo animal hoofstock).

Although ketoprofen is not approved in the United States for small animals, it has been approved for treatment dogs and cats in other countries. It has been given by injection for short-term treatment and by tablet for long-term use. In dogs and cats, it has been shown effective for treating pyrexia. In horses, ketoprofen is used for musculoskeletal inflammation and pain, abdominal pain, and other inflammatory conditions. Ketoprofen also has been used in cattle, goats, sheep, and pigs. In cattle, it has been effective for fever, pain, and inflammation associated with mastitis.

**K**

### Precautionary Information

#### Adverse Reactions and Side Effects

All NSAIDs share the similar adverse effect of GI injury. The most common side effect is vomiting. GI ulceration is possible in some animals. Ketoprofen has been administered for 5 consecutive days in dogs without serious adverse effects, but longer treatment should be avoided. Dogs that received ketoprofen for 30 consecutive days (0.25 mg/kg/day) induced pyloric lesions and fecal occult blood. In horses, ketoprofen has been less ulcerogenic than phenylbutazone or flunixin meglumine in one study. Bleeding problems can occur if ketoprofen is administered before or after surgery.

#### Contraindications and Precautions

Do not administer to animals prone to GI ulcers. Do not administer with other ulcerogenic drugs such as corticosteroids.

#### Drug Interactions

Do not administer with other NSAIDs or with corticosteroids because these agents may exacerbate adverse GI effects. Some NSAIDs may interfere with the action of diuretic drugs and angiotensin-converting enzyme inhibitors.

## Instructions for Use

Although not approved in the United States, ketoprofen is approved for small animals in other countries. It is approved for use in cattle in Canada but is not approved in the United States. Doses listed are based on approved use in those countries. It is available as an OTC drug for humans in the United States, and these forms have been administered to dogs and cats.

## Patient Monitoring and Laboratory Tests

Monitor patient for signs of GI intoxication (vomiting and diarrhea). Monitor renal function during chronic treatment.

## Formulations

• Ketoprofen is available in 12.5-mg tablets (over the counter); 25, 50, and 75 mg (human preparation); and 100-mg/mL injection for horses. It is available in 10-mg/mL injection outside the United States.

## Stability and Storage

Store in a tightly sealed container, protected from light, and at room temperature. Ketoprofen is insoluble in water, but it is soluble in ethanol. Stability of oral compounded formulations has not been evaluated.

## Small Animal Dosage

### Dogs and Cats

• Single dose: 2 mg/kg SQ, IM, or IV.
• Multiple dose: 1 mg/kg q24h PO for up to 5 days. If longer-term treatment is needed, lower the dosage to 0.25 mg/kg once daily because it provides a better safety profile.

## Large Animal Dosage

### Horses

• 2.2–3.3 mg/kg/day IV or IM.

### Pigs

• 3 mg/kg/day PO, IV, or IM.

### Cattle and small ruminants

• 3 mg/kg/day IV or IM for up to 3 days.

## Regulatory Information

Extralabel use in the United States: Withdrawal time of at least 7 days for meat and 24–48 hours for milk at a dose of 3.3 mg/kg q24h IM or IV. However, in other countries, the withdrawal times are shorter. For example, it is approved in Canada. For swine and cattle with a meat withdrawal time of 1 day.

RCI Classification: 4

# Ketorolac Tromethamine
kee-toe′role-ak troe-meth′eh-meen

**Trade and other names:** Toradol

**Functional classification:** Nonsteroidal anti-inflammatory drug

## Pharmacology and Mechanism of Action

Ketorolac is an NSAID that is a derivative of heteroaryl acetic acid. Ketorolac, like other NSAIDs, produces analgesic and anti-inflammatory effects by inhibiting the synthesis of prostaglandins. The enzyme inhibited by NSAIDs is the COX enzyme. The COX enzyme exists in two isoforms: COX-1 and COX-2. COX-1 is primarily responsible for synthesis of prostaglandins important for maintaining a healthy GI tract, renal function, platelet function, and other normal physiologic functions. COX-2 is induced and is responsible for synthesizing prostaglandins that are important mediators of pain, inflammation, and fever. However, it is known that there is some crossover of COX-1 and COX-2 effects in some situations, and COX-2 activity is important for some biological effects. Ketorolac is a nonselective inhibitor of COX. There is some evidence that ketorolac also may affect opioid receptors centrally to produce analgesia, but it does not directly bind to opioid receptors. In some human studies, it has had comparable efficacy to morphine for postoperative pain.

*Pharmacokinetics:* The pharmacokinetics have been studied in dogs but not in other species. In dogs, it has a half-life of approximately 4.5 or 10 hours (depending on the study) and a variable volume of distribution of 0.3 to 1 L/kg, depending on the study with protein binding of 99%.

## Indications and Clinical Uses

Ketorolac is infrequently used in veterinary medicine. The use is based on limited clinical experience and extrapolation from the use in people. There are only limited data on safety and efficacy for veterinary uses. It has occasionally been used to treat pain and inflammation in dogs, with the most common use for treatment of pain associated with surgery. Ketorolac also has been used in exotic and zoo animal species for treating pain.

## Precautionary Information

### Adverse Reactions and Side Effects

Like other NSAIDs, it may cause GI ulceration and renal ischemia. Ketorolac may cause GI lesions if administered more frequently than q8h.

### Contraindications and Precautions

Do not administer more than two doses. Do not administer to animals prone to GI ulcers. Do not administer with other ulcerogenic drugs such as corticosteroids.

### Drug Interactions

Do not administer with other NSAIDs or with corticosteroids. Corticosteroids have been shown to exacerbate the GI adverse effects. Some NSAIDs may interfere with the action of diuretic drugs and ACE inhibitors.

## Instructions for Use

Limited clinical studies in dogs have been conducted. However, it may be effective in some patients for short-term use. Long-term administration is discouraged.

## Patient Monitoring and Laboratory Tests

Monitor for signs of GI ulceration. Plasma concentrations are not generally monitored but levels of 0.1–0.3 mcg/mL in people are considered in the analgesic range.

## Formulations

- Ketorolac is available in 10-mg tablets and 15- and 30-mg/mL injection in 10% alcohol.

## Stability and Storage

Store in a tightly sealed container, protected from light and humidity, and at room temperature. Ketorolac tromethamine is soluble in water and slightly soluble in ethanol. Stability of oral compounded formulations has not been evaluated.

## Small Animal Dosage

**Dogs**

- 0.5 mg/kg q8–12h PO, IM, or IV.

**Cats**

- No safe dose is established.

## Large Animal Dosage

- No large animal doses are reported.

## Regulatory Information

Withdrawal times are not established for animals that produce food. For extralabel use withdrawal interval estimates, contact FARAD at www.FARAD.org.

# Lactated Ringer's Solution
**Trade and other names:** LRS

**Functional classification:** Fluid replacement

## Pharmacology and Mechanism of Action
Lactated Ringer's solution is a common fluid solution for replacement intended for IV administration. Lactated Ringer's solution contains a balanced combination of electrolytes and an alkalinizing buffer.

| | | | Composition of Lactated Ringer's Solution | | | | | |
|---|---|---|---|---|---|---|---|---|
| Glucose (g/L) | Sodium (mmol/L) | Chloride (mmol/L) | Potassium (mmol/L) | Lactate (mmol/L) | Calcium (mmol/L) | Magnesium (mmol/L) | pH | Osmolarity (mOsm/L) |
| 0 | 130 | 112 | 4 | 28 | 1.36 | 0 | 6–7.4 | 273 |

## Indications and Clinical Uses
Lactated Ringer's solution is indicated as a replacement or maintenance fluid. It also is used as a vehicle to deliver IV medications via constant-rate infusion (CRI). It has been administered subcutaneously, intraosseously (in bone medullary cavity), and intraperitoneally (IP) in animals when IV access is not possible. It contains lactate, a metabolizable base but does not correct acidosis as quickly as bicarbonate. Severely acidemic animals may already have high lactate serum levels.

## Precautionary Information
### Adverse Reactions and Side Effects
No significant adverse effects.

### Contraindications and Precautions
Administer IV fluids only in patients monitored carefully.

### Drug Interactions
Lactated Ringer's solution has a pH of 6–7.4. Do not add medications to this solution if they are unstable at this pH. Lactated Ringer's solution contains calcium. Do not add drugs to this solution that may bind (chelate) to calcium.

## Instructions for Use
Fluid requirements vary depending on animal's needs (replacement vs. maintenance). For shock therapy, administer half the calculated dose in the first 30 minutes and in 10-mL/kg increments every 15 minutes followed by a CRI. For severe acidemia, consider fluids supplemented with bicarbonate instead of lactate. Fluid rates used in dogs and cats during anesthesia have previously been 10 mL/kg/h, IV, but some experts have lowered these recommendations to 3 mL/kg/h in cats and 5 mL/kg/h in dogs. See dosing section for calculation of maintenance rates.

## Patient Monitoring and Laboratory Tests
Monitor patient's hydration status and electrolyte balance (especially potassium, chloride, and sodium). With high administration rates, monitor patient for signs of pulmonary edema.

## Formulations
• Lactated Ringer's solution is available in 250-, 500-, and 1000-mL fluid bags.

## Stability and Storage
Store in a tightly sealed container. If container has been punctured or transferred to another container, sterility cannot be assured.

## Small Animal Dosage
**Dogs and Cats**
- Moderate dehydration: 15–30 mL/kg/h IV.
- Severe dehydration: 50 mL/kg/h IV.
- Maintenance rates:
  - Cat: 2–3 mL/kg/h.
  - Dog: 2–6 mL/kg/h.
- Maintenance (per day): 55–65 mL/kg/day IV, SQ, or IP (2.5 mL/kg/h).
- During anesthesia: Initial rate 3 mL/kg/h for cats and 5 mL/kg/h for dogs IV. If necessary to replace losses, increase to 10 mL/kg/h IV.
- Shock therapy: 90 mL/kg IV for dogs and 60–70 mL/kg IV for cats.

## Large Animal Dosage
**Cattle, Horses, and Pigs**
- Maintenance: 40–50 mL/kg/day IV.
- Moderate dehydration: 15–30 mL/kg/h IV.
- Severe dehydration: 50 mL/kg/h IV.

**Calves and Foals**
- Moderate dehydration: 45 mL/kg at a rate of 30–40 mL/kg/h IV.
- Severe dehydration: 80–90 mL/kg at a rate of 30–40 mL/kg/h IV. In severe cases, it may be given as rapidly as 80 mL/kg/h.

## Regulatory Information
There is no risk of harmful residues in animals intended for food. No withdrawal times are necessary.

# Lactulose
lak′tyoo-lose

**Trade and other names:** Chronulac and generic brands

**Functional classification:** Laxative

## Pharmacology and Mechanism of Action
Lactulose is a laxative that is sometimes used to alter the pH of the intestine. Lactulose is a disaccharide sugar containing one molecule of fructose and one molecule of galactose. Lactulose produces a laxative effect by osmotic effect in the colon. It is a nonabsorbed sugar and retains water in the intestine after oral administration via an osmotic effect. Lactulose will decreases the pH of the intestinal lumen.

## Indications and Clinical Uses
Lactulose is administered orally for treatment of hyperammonemia (hepatic encephalopathy) because it decreases blood ammonia concentrations via lowering the pH of the colon; thus, ammonia in the colon is not as readily absorbed. Lactulose also is administered orally to produce a laxative effect for treatment of constipation. The uses of lactulose in small animals are based on anecdotal observations and recommendations by experts. There are no clinical studies available to evaluate efficacy.

### Precautionary Information

**Adverse Reactions and Side Effects**

Excessive use may cause fluid and electrolyte loss.

**Contraindications and Precautions**

Use lactulose with caution in animals with diabetes because it contains lactose and galactose.

**Drug Interactions**

No drug interactions are reported for animals. It potentially could change the oral absorption of some drugs by changing the intestinal pH.

### Instructions for Use

In veterinary medicine, clinical studies to establish efficacy are not available. In addition to doses cited, 20–30 mL/kg of 30% solution retention enema has been used in cats.

### Patient Monitoring and Laboratory Tests

When used for treating hepatic encephalopathy, monitor the patient's hepatic status.

### Formulations

• Lactulose is available in 10-g/15 mL liquid solution (3.3 g per 5 mL).

### Stability and Storage

Store in a tightly sealed container, protected from light, and at room temperature. It is soluble in water. Darkening of the solution may occur without affecting stability. Avoid freezing.

### Small Animal Dosage

**Dogs**

• Constipation: 1 mL/4.5 kg q8h (to effect) PO.
• Hepatic encephalopathy: 0.5 mL/kg q8h PO.

**Cats**

• Constipation: 1 mL/4.5 kg q8h (to effect) PO.
• Hepatic encephalopathy: 2.5–5 mL/cat q8h PO.

### Large Animal Dosage

**Horses and Cattle**

• 0.25–0.5 mL/kg/day PO.

### Regulatory Information

There is little risk of residues in animals intended for food. No withdrawal times are necessary.

# Leflunomide

le-floo′noe-mide or leh-flew′nah-mide

**Trade and other names:** Arava and generic

**Functional classification:** Immunosuppressive drug

## Pharmacology and Mechanism of Action

Leflunomide is an isoxazole immunosuppressive drug. Leflunomide is not active as the parent drug, but it is converted to an active metabolite A77 1726 (also known as M1 and teriflunomide), which inhibits T-cell and B-cell proliferation and is responsible for clinical immunosuppressive effects. It inhibits the synthesis of pyrimidine via inhibition of the enzyme dihydroorotate dehydrogenase. This enzyme is important for the de novo pyrimidine synthesis, which is critical for function of activated and stimulated lymphocytes. It also may produce anti-inflammatory effects by inhibiting proinflammatory cytokines.

*Pharmacokinetics:* After oral absorption, the plasma levels of leflunomide are low or undetectable. Therapeutic effects are produced from the metabolite A77 1726 (M1) for the immunosuppressive action. If monitoring is performed, the measurement should focus on the metabolite concentrations. In people, the metabolite M1 has a very long half-life of approximately 2 weeks. But in studies performed in experimental dogs, the half-life was only 21–25 hours, and the peak concentrations were much lower than in people. In people, the long half-life requires several days to accumulate to steady-state levels and to decline from a peak level. Loading doses are often administered in people. However, because of the shorter half-life, loading doses are not needed in dogs, and steady-state concentrations are attained in approximately 5 days. In cats, the half-life is 60 hours with complete oral absorption.

## Indications and Clinical Uses

This drug is used in people primarily for rheumatoid arthritis. In dogs, it has been used for a variety of immune-mediated diseases as a substitute for other drugs such as azathioprine or mycophenolate. These diseases include myasthenia gravis, Evan syndrome, immune-mediated hemolytic anemia and thrombocytopenia, and polymyositis/polyarthritis. Efficacy has not been studied in controlled clinical studies. Dosing recommendations have been reported in small observational studies or from uncontrolled retrospective studies. In most reports, it was administered with corticosteroids. In one case report, there was a positive response in most dogs with immune-mediated polyarthritis treated at 3–4 mg/kg once daily.

## Precautionary Information

### Adverse Reactions and Side Effects

The most common adverse effects in dogs have been decreased appetite, lethargy, and diarrhea. Liver enzymes were elevated in some animals. Adverse gastrointestinal (GI) effects are more common with higher doses. Because of the GI effects, many clinicians start with a low dose and gradually titrate up to higher doses. Mild anemia and lethargy also have been observed. Although rare, leukopenia, anemia, and anorexia are possible with doses greater than 4 mg/kg. Periodic complete blood count (CBC) is recommended to monitor patients during treatment. In cats, the most common adverse effects have been intermittent vomiting, which is mild and transient.

### Contraindications and Precautions

Do not administer to pregnant animals. This drug can be toxic to a developing fetus.

### Drug Interactions

No interactions are reported.

## Instructions for Use

Leflunomide is used most often in dogs for immunosuppressive treatment when other drugs have failed or when the patient has become refractory to other drugs and a substitute is considered. The dosing protocols used currently are derived from extrapolation and some anecdotal reports. Most veterinarians start with 4 mg/kg per day and then lower the dose as the patient responds. Pharmacokinetic studies in dogs suggest that the dosage of 4 mg/kg per day may not produce drug levels that are considered therapeutic. Therefore, in patients that have not responded, there should be consideration for higher doses if it is tolerated by the patient.

## Patient Monitoring and Laboratory Tests

Monitor CBC and platelet counts in treated animals. Anemia has been reported as a consequence of treatment. If blood monitoring is pursued, plasma samples may be collected and measured for A77 1726 (the active metabolite). This metabolite is stable in serum for up to 5 months under refrigerated conditions. Drug concentrations at 12 hours (trough) are considered effective if greater than 20 mcg/mL.

## Formulations

- Available in 5-, 10-, and 20-mg tablets.

## Stability and Storage

Store in a tightly sealed container, protected from light, and at room temperature.

## Small Animal Dosage

### Dogs

- Start with 2 mg/kg per day to avoid adverse effects. It this dosage is well tolerated, increase to 4 mg/kg per day, usually in divided doses of 2 mg/kg q12h; then taper the dosage to 2 mg/kg q24h PO. After an initial induction period, the dose may be decreased by 25% increments until the patient is stabilized or until the disease resolves. Some patients may require higher starting doses.

### Cats

- 2 mg/kg per day for 2 days PO; then 2 mg/kg q48h PO.

## Large Animal Dosage

- No large animal doses are available.

## Regulatory Information

Withdrawal times are not established for animals that produce food. This drug should be avoided in food-producing animals.

# Leucovorin Calcium
loo-koe-vor′in kal′see-um

**Trade and other names:** Wellcovorin and generic brands

**Functional classification:** Antidote

## Pharmacology and Mechanism of Action

Leucovorin is a reduced form of folic acid that is converted to active folic acid derivatives for purine and thymidine synthesis. The only use in veterinary medicine is as an antidote.

## Indications and Clinical Uses

Use of leucovorin is uncommon in animals. It may be used as an antidote for folic acid antagonists. In humans, it is primarily used as rescue for overdoses of folic acid antagonists such as methotrexate and treatment of adverse reactions from methotrexate, but it also may be considered for reactions caused by pyrimethamine and trimethoprim. Because methotrexate use is uncommon in animals, the use of leucovorin is rare.

## Precautionary Information

### Adverse Reactions and Side Effects
No adverse reactions reported for animals, but allergic reactions have been reported in people.

### Contraindications and Precautions
No contraindications reported for animals.

### Drug Interactions
Leucovorin interferes with the action of trimethoprim and pyrimethamine.

## Instructions for Use
Clinical studies have not been reported in veterinary medicine. Although leucovorin may prevent toxicity from trimethoprim, it does not prevent toxic reactions that may be caused by sulfonamides in animals.

## Patient Monitoring and Laboratory Tests
Monitor CBC if this drug is used to treat overdose of folic acid antagonists.

## Formulations Available
- Leucovorin is available in 5-, 10-, 15-, and 25-mg tablets and 3- and 5-mg/mL injection.

## Stability and Storage
Store in a tightly sealed container, protected from light, and at room temperature. It is soluble in water but is insoluble in ethanol. Reconstituted solutions have stability for 7 days at room temperature or refrigerated.

## Small Animal Dosage
### Dogs and Cats
- With methotrexate administration: 3 mg/m$^2$ IV, IM, or PO.
- Treatment of methotrexate intoxication: 25–200 mg/m$^2$ q6h. As a general guideline, administer 15 mg/m$^2$ for mild toxicity, 30 mg/m$^2$ for mild toxicity, and 100 mg/m$^2$ for severe toxicity. An alternative approach is to administer the same dose as methotrexate.
- As antidote for pyrimethamine toxicosis: 1 mg/kg q24h PO.

## Large Animal Dosage
- No large animal doses are reported. However, if pyrimethamine toxicosis is suspected in horses, doses listed for small animals may be considered.

## Regulatory Information
Withdrawal times are not established for animals that produce food. If this drug is administered to food animals, contact Food Animal Residue Avoidance Databank (FARAD) at www.FARAD.org for extralabel use information.

# Levamisole Hydrochloride
leh-vam′ih-sole hye-droe-klor′ide

**Trade and other names:** Levasole, Ripercol, Tramisol, and Ergamisol

**Functional classification:** Antiparasitic

## Pharmacology and Mechanism of Action
Levamisole is an antiparasitic drug of the imidazothiazole class. It eliminates a variety of parasites via neuromuscular toxicity. Levamisole has an immunorestorative effect in animals, but the mechanism of action on the immune system is unknown. It may activate and stimulate proliferation of T cells; augment monocyte activation; and stimulate macrophages, including phagocytosis and chemotaxis. It may increase neutrophil mobility. However, it is not cytotoxic to neutrophils or immune cells.

## Indications and Clinical Uses
In cattle and sheep, levamisole is used to treat a variety of nematodes, including stomach worms (*Haemonchus, Trichostrongylus,* and *Ostertagia* spp.), intestinal worms (*Trichostrongylus, Cooperia, Nematodirus, Bunostomum, Oesophagostomum,* and *Chabertia* spp.), and lungworms (*Dictyocaulus* spp.). In pigs, it is used to treat nematodes such as large roundworms (*Ascaris suum*), nodular worms (*Oesophagostomum* spp.), intestinal thread worms (*Strongyloides ransomi*), and lungworms (*Metastrongylus* spp.). Levamisole has been used for treatment of endoparasites in dogs and as a microfilaricide. Macrocyclic lactones (e.g., milbemycin oxime or ivermectin) are considered a preferred heartworm microfilaricide. In people, levamisole has been used as an immunostimulant to aid in treatment of colorectal carcinoma and malignant melanoma. In animals, levamisole also is used as an immunostimulant, but reports of efficacy are lacking.

## Precautionary Information

### Adverse Reactions and Side Effects
Levamisole may produce cholinergic toxicity. It has produced vomiting in some dogs. The injectable formulation has caused some swelling at the site of injection. In humans, when used as an immunostimulant, it has caused stomatitis, agranulocytosis, and thrombocytopenia.

### Contraindications and Precautions
Use cautiously in animals with high heartworm microfilaria burdens. Reactions are possible from the heavy kill rate of microfilaria. There are no adverse reactions on fertility and no effects on pregnancy. In rats and rabbits, there was no evidence of teratogenicity or embryotoxicity at doses of 180 mg/kg. Levamisole is abused in people and often mixed with cocaine to either potentiate the effects to produce additional central nervous system (CNS) stimulation or is added as a marker compound. When used in this form in people, it has produced agranulocytosis in some individuals. Levamisole may potentially be converted to aminorex, a CNS stimulant in horses with amphetamine properties, which may affect performance.

### Drug Interactions
Do not use with pyrantel because they share the same mechanism of toxicity.

## Instructions for Use
In heartworm-positive dogs, it may sterilize female adult heartworms. Levamisole has also been used as an immunostimulant; however, clinical reports of its efficacy are not

available. Because of the possibility of contamination at the injection site, use a clean needle with each animal and clean the injection site.

## Patient Monitoring and Laboratory Tests
Monitor for microfilaria before treatment because of risk of reaction with a high heartworm burden.

## Formulations
- Levamisole is available in 0.184-g bolus; 2.19-g bolus; 9-, 11.7-, and 18.15-g per packet; 136.5-mg/mL and 182-mg/mL injection (levamisole phosphate); and 50-mg tablet.
- Levamisole is also available in the United States as a 46.8-g packet for cattle and sheep and an 18.15-g bottle for pigs.

## Stability and Storage
Store in a tightly sealed container, protected from light, and at room temperature. Stability of compounded formulations has not been evaluated.

## Small Animal Dosage
### Dogs
- Endoparasites: 5–8 mg/kg once PO (up to 10 mg/kg PO for 2 days).
- Hookworms: 10 mg/kg/day for 2 days.
- Microfilaricide: 10 mg/kg q24h PO for 6–10 days (recommended to use macrocyclic lactones instead).
- Immunostimulant: 0.5–2 mg/kg three times per week PO. (In humans, the immunostimulant dose is given q8h for 3 days.)

### Cats
- Endoparasites: 4.4 mg/kg once PO.
- Lungworms: 20–40 mg/kg q48h for five treatments PO.

## Large Animal Dosage
### Cattle and Sheep
- 8 mg/kg once PO or approximately one 2.19-g bolus per 450–750 lb (200–340 kg).
- Levamisole injection (for cattle): 8 mg/kg SQ into the midneck area once or approximately 2 mL per 100 lb (45 kg).

### Pigs
- 8 mg/kg in drinking water.

## Regulatory Information
Cattle withdrawal time for meat: 2 days (PO) and 7 days (SQ injection).
Sheep withdrawal time for meat: 3 days.
Pig withdrawal time (meat): 3 days.
Horses: There are some reports that levamisole can be converted to aminorex in horses, which is a CNS stimulant and a banned substance in racing horses.

# Levetiracetam
lee-ve-tye-ra'se-tam
**Trade and other names:** Keppra, Spritam, and generic
**Functional classification:** Anticonvulsant

## Pharmacology and Mechanism of Action
Levetiracetam is an anticonvulsant that has grown in popularity for managing epileptic patients in veterinary medicine. The mechanism of action does not involve inhibitory

neurotransmitters. It likely inhibits burst firing of neurons without affecting normal neuronal excitement by binding to synaptic vesicles in brain that modulate neurotransmitter release. It does not undergo hepatic metabolism but may undergo metabolism that does not include cytochrome P450 enzymes. Elimination relies on renal clearance.

Brivaracetam (Briviact) is an analog of levetiracetam with 10- to 30-fold higher activity. However, this form has not been evaluated in animals.

*Pharmacokinetics:* In dogs, the oral absorption of immediate-release levetiracetam is 100%, the half-life is 3–4 hours, and the volume of distribution (VD) is 0.4–0.5 L/kg. The short half-life requires frequent administration (q8h) when using the conventional tablets. Administration of the extended-release (XR) formulation in dogs at doses of 20–30 mg/kg produced concentration in the therapeutic range (above 12 mcg/mL) in most dogs for a duration of 12 hours, allowing for twice-daily dosing. The XR oral absorption was not affected by feeding, but it extended the peak by 3 hours in most dogs.

In cats, the oral absorption is also 100%, with a half-life of 3 hours and a VD similar to dogs. Administration of the XR tablets in cats (500 mg per cat) produced concentrations in the therapeutic range for 24 hours, with a peak of 90 mcg/mL and a half-life of 3–4 hours.

## Indications and Clinical Uses

In dogs, levetiracetam has been used to treat seizures, especially those refractory to other anticonvulsants. In dogs, it has been considered a drug of choice as an add-on medication when patients are refractory to phenobarbital and bromide therapy. It often is used in combination with other anticonvulsants. Clinical efficacy as an add-on medication with phenobarbital and bromide is uncertain, and this use is based on anecdotal experiences and opinions from veterinary neurology experts. Levetiracetam has been used to treat seizure disorders in cats at a dosage of 20 mg/kg q8h and found to be effective in some cases. Because dosing q8h can be difficult for some owners, the XR tablets have been examined. These may be administered q12h to dogs, and the 500-mg tablet may be administered once daily to cats. Clinical use in horses is uncommon, but there have been pharmacokinetic studies to guide dosing (see dosing section for horses).

### Precautionary Information

**Adverse Reactions and Side Effects**

Weakness, lethargy, and dizziness have been reported in people. Adverse effects have been rare in animals, except for occasional lethargy and decreased appetite. Oral administration can produce hypersalivation in cats, but otherwise it has been well tolerated in cats.

Changes on behavior in people are frequently reported. In dogs, behavior changes are uncommon but may occur. These include increased anxiety and aggression, and other behavioral abnormalities.

**Contraindications and Precautions**

No known contraindications.

**Drug Interactions**

Ordinarily, there are no direct interactions with drugs that inhibit or induce cytochrome P450 enzymes. However, studies in dogs and people have confirmed that phenobarbital can enhance the clearance of levetiracetam. For example, the half-life is shorter, and clearance is more rapid when dogs are administered phenobarbital simultaneously. The mechanism for the interaction is unknown but may warrant higher doses or more careful monitoring when levetiracetam is used with phenobarbital. Interactions with other concurrently used anticonvulsants have not been reported.

## Instructions for Use

Levetiracetam is rapidly and completely absorbed, and absorption is not affected by feeding. An injectable formulation is available but not used often in veterinary medicine. However, the injectable solution has been administered at a dose of 20-mg/kg IV bolus increments to a maximum of 60 mg/kg in emergency situations. Levetiracetam ordinarily should be administered q8h to maintain effective concentrations. Higher doses may be needed if administered with phenobarbital because phenobarbital significantly increases clearance in dogs. The XR tablets may have longer effects and can be administered q12h to dogs or every 24 hours in cats. If there is difficulty administering tablets to dogs or cats, the rapidly disintegrating tablets can be considered after testing the palatability in animals. (See Formulations.)

## Patient Monitoring and Laboratory Tests

Monitor seizure frequency. Currently no clinical monitoring test for serum exists in routine laboratories. However, some laboratories have this capability. Therapeutic plasma/serum concentrations in people are in the range of 10–40 mcg/mL.

## Formulations

- Levetiracetam immediate-release: 250-, 500-, 750-, and 1000-mg tablets.
- Rapidly disintegrating tablet (Spritam): 250-, 500-, 750-, and 1000-mg spearmint-flavored tablets. These tablets disintegrate in the mouth when administered with a small volume of liquid. Alternately, the tablet can be added to a small volume of liquid (one spoonful) and allow the tablet to disperse prior to administration to a pet.
- XR formulation available in 500- and 750-mg-tablets. There are several XR brands available, but differences among the brands were not demonstrated in canine studies.
- 100-mg/mL oral solution and 100-mg/mL solution for injection.
- Compounded formulation for transdermal administration to cats: Formulated in Lipoderm at 350–400 mg/mL. Plasma levels from this application are low and variable.

## Stability and Storage

Store in a tightly sealed container, protected from light, and at room temperature. Stability of compounded formulations has not been evaluated. It is soluble in water, and it may be acceptable to mix with other foods, syrups, or flavorings immediately prior to oral administration.

## Small Animal Dosage

### Dogs

- 20 mg/kg q8h PO. More frequent administration or higher doses may be necessary with concurrent phenobarbital treatment.
- Oral XR tablets: 30 mg/kg q12h PO.
- IV use (emergency situations): 20 mg/kg IV bolus, repeated if necessary, up to 60 mg/kg. Duration of injection is approximately 3 hours.
- Rectal administration: 40 mg/kg rectal administration (100-mg/mL solution) has produced effective concentrations. However, in many dogs, the volume of the administered dose is too large to be practical.

### Cats

- 20-mg/kg q8h PO.
- XR formulation: 500 mg per cat once daily or approximately 94 mg/kg once daily. (Do not split tablets.)

- Transdermal formulations: Transdermal administration, using Lipoderm as a vehicle, has been administered using a formulation of 350–400 mg/mL. This form is administered at 60 mg/kg q8h (three times the oral dose). Systemic concentrations are low and highly variable.

## Large Animal Dosage

**Horses**

- 30 mg/kg IV for short-term treatment or 30 mg/kg q24h PO.

## Regulatory Information

No regulatory information is available. For extralabel use withdrawal interval estimates, contact FARAD at www.FARAD.org.

# Levodopa
lee′voe-doe′pah

**Trade and other names:** Larodopa and L-dopa

**Functional classification:** Dopamine agonist

## Pharmacology and Mechanism of Action

Levodopa is a form of dopamine that is used infrequently in animals. When levodopa is administered systemically, it does not cross the blood–brain barrier. However, levodopa crosses more easily via a carrier-mediated process and is converted to dopamine after crossing the blood–brain barrier. Dopamine is used in neurodegenerative disorders to stimulate CNS dopamine receptors.

## Indications and Clinical Uses

In people, levodopa is used for treating Parkinson disease, and it is used in combination with carbidopa (a peripheral decarboxylase inhibitor) and entacapone (an o-methyltransferase inhibitor) to potentiate therapy. In animals, it has been used for treating hepatic encephalopathy, but there is very limited experience to confirm efficacy.

### Precautionary Information

**Adverse Reactions and Side Effects**

Adverse effects in animals have not been reported. In people, dizziness, mental changes, difficult urination, and hypotension are among the reported adverse effects.

**Contraindications and Precautions**

There are no specific contraindications for use in animals.

**Drug Interactions**

Antidopamine drugs interfere with the action of levodopa. Such drugs include metoclopramide, phenothiazines (e.g., acepromazine), and risperidone.

## Instructions for Use

Clinical studies have not been reported in veterinary medicine, and the use has been uncommon to understand the efficacy and optimum doses. The use and doses have been extrapolated from human use; therefore, titrate the dose for each individual patient based on clinical response.

## Patient Monitoring and Laboratory Tests
No specific monitoring is necessary.

## Formulations
• Levodopa is available in 100-, 250-, and 500-mg tablets or capsules.

## Stability and Storage
Store in a tightly sealed container, protected from light, and at room temperature. Levodopa is slightly soluble in water but more soluble in acid solutions. It is rapidly oxidized with exposure to air, which is indicated by a darkening of the formulation. Injectable solutions have been prepared extemporaneously and found to be stable for 96 hours.

## Small Animal Dosage
### Dogs and Cats
• Hepatic encephalopathy: 6.8 mg/kg initially PO; then 1.4 mg/kg q6h PO.

## Large Animal Dosage
• No dose has been reported for large animals.

## Regulatory Information
No regulatory information is available for animals intended for food. Because of a low risk of residues, no withdrawal times are suggested.

# Levofloxacin
lee-voe-flox′a-sin

**Trade and other names:** Levaquin and generic brands
**Functional classification:** Antibacterial

## Pharmacology and Mechanism of Action
Levofloxacin is a fluoroquinolone antibacterial. Like other fluoroquinolones, levofloxacin acts to inhibit DNA gyrase and cell DNA and RNA synthesis. It is the L-isomer (S-enantiomer) of ofloxacin and is more active in vitro against gram-positive bacteria and anaerobes than some other fluoroquinolones. Levofloxacin is a human-labeled antibiotic but has been used in veterinary medicine to treat various bacterial infections. Its spectrum of activity includes gram-negative bacilli of the Enterobacteriaceae and fluoroquinolone-susceptible *Pseudomonas aeruginosa*. It also has activity against some gram-positive cocci, including *Staphylococcus* spp. Multi-drug–resistant bacteria, including gram-negative bacilli of the Enterobacteriaceae and methicillin-resistant strains of *Staphylococcus*, are likely to be resistant to levofloxacin and other fluoroquinolones. It also has activity against some anaerobic bacteria and other organisms (e.g., *Chlamydia, Mycoplasma,* and *Mycobacterium* spp.). In human medicine, it is considered one of the "respiratory fluoroquinolones" because of its broad-spectrum activity against gram-positive, gram-negative, and anaerobic bacteria.

Levofloxacin is available as inexpensive, generic tablets, which has facilitated its use in veterinary medicine. According to the manufacturer's information for use of the drug in humans, the drug undergoes limited metabolism and is not metabolized by cytochrome P450 enzymes. It is almost entirely eliminated in the urine, and the pharmacokinetics are not affected by liver disease. The tablets can be taken with or without food.

*Pharmacokinetics:* Oral absorption of levofloxacin in dogs is nearly complete, with approximately 100% bioavailability. In dogs, the half-life is 5.6 hours, with a clearance of 0.18 L/kg/h and a VD of 1.5 L/kg. The peak concentration was 15.5 mcg/mL after a dose of 24 mg/kg PO. Protein binding in dogs is 22%–27%. In cats, after a dose of 10 mg/kg, it has a half-life of 7–8 hours with high oral bioavailability of 86% and a peak concentration of 4.7 mcg/mL. The VD in cats is 1.75 L/kg, and clearance is 0.14 L/kg/h.

## Indications and Clinical Uses

Levofloxacin is a human drug without an approved label indication for dogs or cats. However, it has been used to treat a variety of infections, including skin infections, pneumonia, and soft tissue infections. Although not approved for animals, it can be prescribed by veterinarians as long as it is not administered to animals that produce food or are intended for food. Other fluoroquinolones that can be considered for treatment include enrofloxacin, marbofloxacin, and orbifloxacin.

## Precautionary Information

### Adverse Reactions and Side Effects

High concentrations may cause CNS toxicity, especially in animals with renal failure. Levofloxacin can produce occasional vomiting. IV solution should be given slowly (over 30 minutes) because rapid injections IV can produce an anaphylactoid reaction, histamine release, and hypotension. Safety studies have not been performed in cats, but blindness in cats has not been reported for levofloxacin. All of the fluoroquinolones, including levofloxacin, have the potential to produce arthropathy in young animals. Dogs are most susceptible to quinolone-induced arthropathy in the age group of 4–28 weeks of age. Large, rapidly growing dogs are the most susceptible. Levofloxacin has not been tested in horses, but arthropathy in young animals is a concern as well as enteritis and colic from oral administration. Tendinitis and tendon rupture are described as a warning for use in people, but this effect has not been observed in animals.

### Contraindications and Precautions

Avoid use in young animals because of risk of cartilage injury. Use cautiously in animals that may be prone to seizures, such as epileptics. Do not administer IV solution rapidly.

### Drug Interactions

Coadministration with divalent and trivalent cations, such as products containing aluminum (e.g., sucralfate), magnesium, iron, zinc, and calcium, may decrease absorption. Do not mix in solutions or in vials with aluminum, calcium, iron, or zinc because chelation may occur.

## Instructions for Use

Doses are based on plasma concentrations needed to achieve sufficient plasma concentration above the minimum inhibitory concentration (MIC). Efficacy studies have not been performed in dogs or cats, and clinical use is based primarily on anecdotal experience.

## Patient Monitoring and Laboratory Tests

Susceptibility testing: CLSI breakpoint for susceptible organisms in dogs is identical to the breakpoint established for humans. The breakpoint for susceptible bacteria is ≤0.5 mcg/mL for Enterobacteriaceae and ≤1 mcg/mL for *P. aeruginosa*.

## Formulations Available

- Levofloxacin is available in 250-, 500-, and 750-mg tablets, 25 mg/mL oral solution.
- Injection solution: 5-mg/mL solution in vials of 50, 100, or 150 mL.

## Stability and Storage

Store in a tightly sealed container, protected from light, and at room temperature. Aqueous solutions of 0.5 to 2 mg/mL retain potency up to 14 days when stored. Do not mix with products that contain ions (e.g., iron, aluminum, magnesium, and calcium).

## Small Animal Dosage

### Dogs

- 25 mg/kg q24h PO.
- 25 mg/kg q24h IV (slow infusion).

### Cats

- 20 mg/kg q24h PO.
- 10 mg/kg q24h IV.

## Large Animal Dosage

- No dosing data are available.

## Regulatory Information

There are no withdrawal times established because this drug should not be administered to animals that produce food. The extralabel administration of fluoroquinolones to food-producing animals in the United States is a violation of Food and Drug Administration (FDA) regulations. Withdrawal times are not established for levofloxacin in animals that produce food.

# Levothyroxine Sodium

lee-voe-thye-roks'een soe'dee-um

**Trade and other names:** T4, L-thyroxine, Thyro-Tabs (veterinary form), and Synthroid (human form). Equine powders include Equisyn-T4, Levo-Powder, Thyroid Powder, and Thyro-L.

**Functional classification:** Hormone

## Pharmacology and Mechanism of Action

Levothyroxine is a thyroid hormone that mimics the effects of tetraiodothyronine ($T_4$). Levothyroxine is used as replacement therapy for treating patients with hypothyroidism. Levothyroxine is $T_4$, which is converted in most patients to the active triiodothyronine ($T_3$). Patient requirements, pharmacokinetics, oral absorption, and protein binding vary among animals, and doses are adjusted on the basis of thyroid monitoring.

*Pharmacokinetics:* The pharmacokinetics can be highly variable from dog to dog. Bioavailability of the oral tablet ranges from 10% to 20% and is decreased when administered with food. Levothyroxine has a half-life of approximately 10–14 hours in most dogs but can be as high as 20 hours.

## Indications and Clinical Uses

Levothyroxine is used for replacement therapy in animals with thyroid hormone deficiency (hypothyroidism). It has been used in many species, including dogs, cats, and horses.

Although it has been suggested for use in treating dogs with von Willebrand disease, clinical studies failed to show an effect on clotting factors, bleeding times, or von Willebrand factor from levothyroxine treatment (0.04 mg/kg).

Intravenous levothyroxine sodium may be used in dogs for acute treatment of hypothyroid dogs with myxedema coma (4–5 mcg/kg IV).

## Precautionary Information

### Adverse Reactions and Side Effects

High doses may produce thyrotoxicosis, but this is uncommon. Potential adverse effects from IV treatment include arrhythmias and pneumonia.

### Contraindications and Precautions

No specific contraindications are reported for small animals. When switching from one brand to another, it is advised to follow up by testing to ensure that brands are therapeutically equivalent.

### Drug Interactions

Patients receiving corticosteroids may have decreased ability to convert $T_4$ to the active $T_3$. The following drugs may lower thyroid concentrations when administered to otherwise healthy animals: nonsteroidal anti-inflammatory drugs (NSAIDs), sulfonamides, and phenobarbital, although these changes in many dogs may not be clinically significant. Although not reported in animals, in people, administration of estrogens increases thyroid-binding globulin and may decrease the active form of thyroid hormone ($T_4$) in patients receiving thyroid supplementation. Monitor $T_4$ levels in these patients and increase dose of thyroxine if necessary. Feeding may decrease oral absorption.

Levothyroxine requires acid for dissolution in the GI tract and oral absorption. Acid-suppressing drugs (e.g., proton pump inhibitors) can decrease acid secretion and can interfere with oral absorption. Other drugs known to inhibit oral absorption of levothyroxine in people but not confirmed in animals include ferrous sulfate, calcium carbonate, aluminum hydroxide, sucralfate, and raloxifene.

These foods interact with thyroid medications: walnuts, liver, albumin, and soybeans. Patients receiving these in their diets should have thyroid levels checked to ensure proper concentrations are achieved.

## Instructions for Use

Thyroid supplementation should be guided by testing to confirm diagnosis and post-medication monitoring to adjust dose. In 2016, the FDA announced that because there is only one FDA-approved canine form of levothyroxine (Thyro-Tabs), other marketed brands are unapproved and therefore, in violation of FDA regulations.

Once-daily dosing is adequate for most dogs, but many dogs require twice-daily administration. Studies with the FDA approved formulation (Thyro-Tabs) was administered at a dose of 0.22 mcg/kg once daily and had equivalent results as twice-daily dosing. The total daily dose may be split into twice-daily increments. Some dogs may require different doses and intervals; therefore, monitoring is recommended to adjust dose appropriately. Other oral tablets may not be equivalent to the

FDA-approved tablets for dogs, and post-pill testing is needed to ensure the proper dose is delivered. When prescribing human formulations, it is recommended to advise pharmacists that canine doses are much higher than human doses.

## Patient Monitoring and Laboratory Tests

Monitor serum total thyroxine ($T_4$) concentrations to guide therapy. Normal thyroxine ($T_4$) baseline levels are 20–55 nmol/L (1.5–4.3 mcg/dL). Thyrotropin-releasing hormone injection should result in at least a 1.5-fold increase in $T_4$. To monitor post-pill adequacy of therapy, it is best performed 4–6 hours after the dose is administered. When collecting a peak concentration blood sample 4–6 hours after administering the pill, the $T_4$ concentration should be between 30 and 60 nmol/L (2.3 and 4.6 mcg/dL). If administering the oral liquid, the peak concentration occurs at 2–2.5 hours. In horses, post-pill peak occurs at 1–2 hours.

## Formulations

- Levothyroxine is available as FDA-approved tablets for dogs in nine strengths from 0.1- to 1-mg tablets (in 0.1-mg increments). These tablets are scored and color coded for easy administration and dose recognition. There have been other non-FDA approved tablets available in other sizes for dogs, but the FDA has taken action to remove these products from the market. There is also a formulation of 1-g of thyroxine per 453.6 of oral powder (1 g/lb of the oral powder) used for horses.
- There are also human generic formulations. Note that levothyroxine products for animals are not bioequivalent to the human-label tablets.
- Human formulations: 25-, 50-, 75-, 88-, 112-, 125-, 137-, 150-, 175-, 200-, and 300-mcg tablets.
- Liotrix (human form) is a combination of $T_4$ and $T_3$ in a ratio: Available as ($T_4/T_3$): 12.5/3.1-, 25/6.25-, 50/12.5-, 100/25-, and 150/37.5-mcg tablets.
- Do not assume that all levothyroxine products are bioequivalent and produce the same response. When switching from one brand to another, follow-up testing is recommended to ensure the same response.

## Stability and Storage

Levothyroxine is inherently unstable and can be markedly affected by heat, light, and humidity. Store in a tightly sealed container, protected from light, and at room temperature. Thyroxine is only slightly soluble in water or ethanol. It is more soluble at pH of less than 2 or greater than 8. It has been unstable in some compounded formulations. However, it may be added to food products if administered immediately. Powder may be mixed with water and added to horse's grain every day. When it was mixed with ethanol followed by mixing with a syrup, it was stable for 15 days at room temperature and 47 days refrigerated. However, other compounded preparations have been stable for only 15 days (refrigerated) or 11 days (room temperature). Therefore, use of compounded formulations should probably be limited to a storage time of 10–15 days.

## Small Animal Dosage

### Dogs

- 18–26 mcg/kg (0.018–0.026 mg/kg) per day PO (adjust dose via monitoring). The average starting dosage is 22 mcg/kg once daily PO, which is approximately 0.1 mg per 10 lb. The entire daily dosage may be administered once per 24 hours or divided into two 12-hour treatments. It may be administered with or without food, but food decreases oral absorption by as much as 50%. To minimize the day-to-day variation in serum $T_4$ concentrations, the timing of administration and feeding should be consistent from day to day.
- IV therapy for acute treatment: 4–5 mcg/kg IV administered once or as needed q12h.

## Cats

- 10–20 mcg/kg/day (0.01–0.02 mg/kg) PO (adjust dose via monitoring).

### Large Animal Dosage

**Horses**

- 10–60 mcg/kg (0.01–0.06 mg/kg) q24h or 5–30 mcg/kg (0.005–0.03 mg/kg) q12h PO. When using the oral powder for dosing in horses, 1 level teaspoon contains 12 mg of $T_4$, and 1 tablespoon contains 36 mg of $T_4$. This powder may be mixed in with daily ration of grain (e.g., 4 level teaspoons mixed with 30 mL water and added to oats per day).
- Horses with pituitary pars intermedia dysfunction: 0.1 mg/kg (48 mg per horse) per day.

### Regulatory Information

No regulatory information is available for animals intended for food. Because of a low risk of residues, no withdrawal times are suggested.

# Lidocaine Hydrochloride

lye′doe-kane hye-droe-klor′ide

**Trade and other names:** Xylocaine and generic brands

**Functional classification:** Local anesthetic, antiarrhythmic

### Pharmacology and Mechanism of Action

Lidocaine is a common local anesthetic. Lidocaine inhibits nerve conduction via sodium channel blockade. Lidocaine is also a Class 1 antiarrhythmic and decreases phase 0 depolarization without affecting conduction. After systemic administration, lidocaine is metabolized to monoethylglycinexylidide (MEGX), which also has antiarrhythmic properties. Lidocaine also has analgesic properties after systemic administration. During IV infusion, it may decrease pain response. In horses, infusions of lidocaine have decreased postoperative ileus either through a direct effect, via suppression of painful stimuli, or through anti-inflammatory effects on neutrophils. In dogs with GI compromise caused by gastric dilatation volvulus, it improved recovery by reducing the severity of ischemic reperfusion injury and inflammatory response.

*Pharmacokinetics:* The pharmacokinetics in dogs and cats are similar; however, cats have increased sensitivity to the cardiac effects. In dogs, the half-life is approximately 1 hour with a high clearance rate (30–40 mL/kg/min). In cats, the pharmacokinetics are different than dogs with a longer half-life and slower clearance, making cats more susceptible to adverse effects than dogs. In cattle, the half-life is approximately 1 hour. In horses, the half-life ranges from 40 to 80 minutes with a high, but variable, clearance rate.

### Indications and Clinical Uses

Lidocaine is used commonly as a local anesthetic and for treatment and conversion of ventricular arrhythmias. Lidocaine should be used cautiously for treating supraventricular arrhythmias because it may increase cardiac conduction. Lidocaine has been used on a limited basis to treat seizures that are refractory to other drugs. Lidocaine also is used for pain management. It has been administered as a CRI in animals, especially in postsurgical patients to improve recovery after intestinal or gastric surgery. Lidocaine has been combined with other analgesics, which may be synergistic and allow lower doses of each individual component. One example of a combination is MLK, which is morphine (or fentanyl), lidocaine, and ketamine (see dosing section for formula).

In horses, lidocaine infusions delivered by CRI may help to restore intestinal motility and are used to treat intestinal ileus. In dogs, when it was delivered as a CRI, there was no change in gastric emptying, and there were modest effects to increase intestinal motility.

Lidocaine has been applied to animals as a transdermal patch. The patch (designed for people) is 5% strength and used primarily for neuropathic pain (postherpetic neuralgia). This patch also has been applied for some conditions in dogs and cats with anecdotal accounts of some success. Absorption from the patch is low (less than 5%), which is far below the threshold for toxic effects.

## Precautionary Information

### Adverse Reactions and Side Effects

High doses of lidocaine cause CNS effects (tremors, twitches, and seizures) and vomiting, but the risk of lidocaine-induced seizures is low. IV use and CRIs in horses have caused muscle fasciculations, rapid eye blinking, anxiety, ataxia, weakness, and seizures. Lidocaine can produce cardiac arrhythmias, but it has greater effect on abnormal cardiac tissue than normal tissue.

Use lidocaine cautiously in cats. IV doses of lidocaine in cats have resulted in death. In cats under anesthesia, lidocaine administration has caused decreased cardiac output, cardiovascular depression, and decreased oxygen delivery to tissues. In cats, lidocaine has also produced methemoglobinemia and hemolysis.

### Contraindications and Precautions

Cats are more susceptible to adverse effects, and lower doses should be used. For example, the CRI in cats is lower than the rate in dogs. Absorption from lidocaine patches in cats is only 6.3% and is not expected to present a problem. In animals with decreased blood flow to the liver (e.g., animals under anesthesia), clearance may be reduced and the risk of adverse effects increased.

### Drug Interactions

Lidocaine hydrochloride is maintained as an acidic solution for solubility. Although short-term mixing with alkaline solutions may not interfere with stability (i.e., immediately prior to administration), storage in alkalinizing solutions can cause precipitation. If mixed with alkalinizing solutions, it should be administered promptly.

## Instructions for Use

When used for local infiltration, many formulations contain epinephrine to prolong activity at the injection site. Avoid using formulations that contain epinephrine in patients with cardiac arrhythmias. Note that human formulations may contain epinephrine, but no veterinary formulations contain epinephrine. To increase pH, speed onset of action, and decrease pain from injection, one may add 1 mEq of sodium bicarbonate to 10 mL of lidocaine (use immediately after mixing). To prepare solutions for infusion in horses, mix 10 g of 2% lidocaine in 3 L of lactated Ringer's solution (0.33% solution).

For treating ventricular arrhythmia in horses, consider adding magnesium sulfate to the infusion. See dosing instructions below for the magnesium sulfate dose.

## Patient Monitoring and Laboratory Tests

Monitor for signs of neurotoxicity (e.g., depression, muscle twitching, and seizures). Monitor the electrocardiogram during treatment for cardiac rate and rhythm in treated animals.

## Formulations
- Lidocaine is available in 5-, 10-, 15-, and 20-mg/mL injection.

## Stability and Storage
Store in a tightly sealed container, protected from light, and at room temperature. Topical preparations have been prepared and found to be stable for several weeks.

## Small Animal Dosage
### Dogs
- Antiarrhythmic IV dose: 2–4 mg/kg IV (to a maximum dose of 8 mg/kg over a 10-minute period).
- Antiarrhythmic CRI dosage: 1 mg/kg initially followed by 50–75 mcg/kg/min IV CRI.
- Antiarrhythmic IM dosage: 6 mg/kg q1.5h IM.
- Epidural: 4.4 mg/kg of 2% solution.
- Adjunct to control pain and inflammation associated with surgery: 2-mg/kg IV bolus followed by 0.05 mg/kg/min CRI for 24 hours (added to patient's fluids).
- MLK: Mixed as 100 mg/mL ketamine (1.6 mL per 500 mL of fluids), 20 mg/mL lidocaine (30 mL per 500 mL of fluids), and 15 mg/mL morphine (1.6 mL per 500 mL of fluids) and infused at a rate of morphine, 0.24 mg/kg/h; lidocaine, 3 mg/kg/h; and ketamine, 0.6 mg/kg/h, administered as CRI for peri-operative analgesia.

### Cats
- Antiarrhythmic IV dose: Start with 0.1–0.4 mg/kg initially and then increase to 0.25–0.75 mg/kg IV slowly if there has been no response.
- Antiarrhythmic CRI dose: Loading dose of 0.5–1 mg/kg IV followed by 10–20 mcg/kg/min (0.6–1.2 mg/kg/h) IV CRI.
- Epidural: 4.4 mg/kg of 2% solution.

## Large Animal Dosage
### Horses
- Ventricular tachycardia: Start with 0.25–0.5 mg/kg IV injection over 5–10 minutes, up to 1.3–1.5 mg/kg for refractory cases. Follow with 0.03–0.05 mg/kg/min (30–50 mcg/kg/min) CRI. Consider adding magnesium sulfate to the infusion to enhance the efficacy. Add 2.7 g of magnesium sulfate to 1 L of 0.9% sodium chloride solution and administer over 10 minutes IV for a dose of 2–6 mg/kg.
- Postoperative ileus: 1.3-mg/kg IV bolus administered over 15 min followed by 0.05 mg/kg/min (50 mcg/kg/min) CRI.
- Analgesia: 2 mg/kg IV followed by 50 mcg/kg/min CRI.

## Regulatory Information
Extralabel use withdrawal time: 1 day for meat and 24 hours for milk.
Horses: Clearance prior to racing: approximately 2.5 days.
Racing Commissioners International (RCI) Classification: 2

# Lincomycin Hydrochloride, Lincomycin Hydrochloride Monohydrate
lin-koe-mye′sin hye-droe-klor′ide and lin-koe-mye′sin hye-droe-klor′ide mono-hye′drate

**Trade and other names:** Lincocin and Lincomix

**Functional classification:** Antibacterial

## Pharmacology and Mechanism of Action

Lincomycin is a lincosamide antibiotic. There are only two antibiotics in this group used in veterinary medicine, lincomycin and clindamycin. Lincomycin is similar in mechanism to clindamycin. The mechanism of action is also similar to macrolides, such as erythromycin, and there may be cross-resistance among these drugs. The site of action is the 50S ribosomal subunit. By inhibiting this ribosome, it decreases protein synthesis. In most bacteria, it is bacteriostatic. Lincomycin has a narrow spectrum of action. The spectrum includes primarily gram-positive bacteria (*Streptococcus* spp. and *Staphylococcus* spp.) and includes *Erysipelothrix* spp., *Leptospira* spp., and atypical bacteria such as *Mycoplasma* spp. Gram-negative bacteria of the Enterobacteriaceae and *P. aeruginosa* are inherently resistant.

## Indications and Clinical Uses

Lincomycin has a gram-positive spectrum with limited use for other infections. In small animals, it has been used for pyoderma and other soft tissue infections caused by susceptible gram-positive bacteria, but commercial availability of products for dogs and cats is limited. In pigs and birds, it is used primarily for the treatment of infections caused by *Mycoplasma* spp. In pigs, it is approved for IM use to treat infectious arthritis and pneumonia caused by *Mycoplasma* spp. and added to feed and water to control swine dysentery caused by *Brachyspira hyodysenteriae*, porcine proliferative enteropathies (ileitis) caused by *Lawsonia intracellularis*, and respiratory disease caused by *Mycoplasma hyopneumoniae*. Although it has been injected IM in cattle and sheep for treatment of septic arthritis, laryngeal abscesses, and mastitis, this treatment is not currently recommended. Compared with lincomycin, clindamycin has better activity against anaerobic bacteria. Because of more frequent use and available dose forms, clindamycin is preferred over lincomycin for administration to small animals.

## Precautionary Information

### Adverse Reactions and Side Effects

Adverse effects are uncommon in dogs, cats, and pigs. Lincomycin has caused vomiting and diarrhea in animals. Severe and even fatal enteritis can be caused by PO administration to ruminants, horses, and small rodents.

### Contraindications and Precautions

Do not administer orally to rodents, horses, ruminants, or rabbits. PO administration to ruminants and horses can cause severe enteritis.

### Drug Interactions

No drug interactions reported for animals.

## Instructions for Use

Actions of lincomycin and clindamycin are similar enough that clindamycin can be substituted for lincomycin for most indications.

## Patient Monitoring and Laboratory Tests

Susceptibility testing: Clinical and Laboratory Standards Institute (CLSI) breakpoints for sensitive organisms are $\leq 0.25$ mcg/mL for streptococci and $\leq 0.5$ mcg/mL for other organisms.

## Formulations

- Lincomycin has been available in 100-, 200-, and 500-mg tablets, but availability can vary from country to country.
- 25-, 50-, 100-, and 300-mg/mL solution for injection.

- Poultry and swine forms include: 50-g powder for mixing with water; 20 and 50 g/lb of lincomycin for chickens and pigs.
- There are several forms for poultry and swine with lincomycin combined with coccidiostats or ionophores for administration in feed or water.

## Stability and Storage
Store in a tightly sealed container, protected from light, and at room temperature. Stability of compounded formulations has not been evaluated.

## Small Animal Dosage
### Dogs and Cats
- 22 mg/kg q12h PO.
- Injection (100 mg/mL): 22 mg/kg q24h or 11 mg/kg q12h IV slowly.

## Large Animal Dosage
### Pigs
- Swine dysentery: 250 mg per gallon of drinking water, which is approximately 8.4 mg/kg/day if given as the only source of drinking water for 5–10 days.
- *Mycoplasma* infections: 11 mg/kg q24h IM injection for 3–5 days.

### Cattle
- Septic arthritis, mastitis, and abscesses: 5 mg/kg q24h IM for 5–7 days.
- Refractory infections: 10 mg/kg q12h IM.

### Sheep
- Septic arthritis: 5 mg/kg q24h for 3–5 days IM.

## Regulatory Information
Withdrawal time for pigs: 0, 1, 2, or 6 days, depending on product and route of administration. (For most products, allow 6 days for oral administration and 2 days for IM administration.) For extralabel use in cattle, FARAD recommends 7 days for meat and 96 hours for milk at a dose of 5 mg/kg.

L

# Linezolid
lih-neh-zoe'lide

**Trade and other names:** Zyvox, Zyvoxam (Canada), and generic

**Functional classification:** Antibacterial

## Pharmacology and Mechanism of Action
Linezolid is an antibiotic in the oxazolidinone class (synthetic drugs). Tedizolid (Sivextro) is a related drug but has not been used in animals. Linezolid is bacteriostatic with a unique mechanism of action. It inhibits protein synthesis by binding to a site on the bacterial 23S ribosomal RNA of the 50S subunit. This prevents formation of the 70S ribosomal unit; therefore, protein synthesis is inhibited. Because it is a synthetic drug, there are no natural reservoirs of resistance genes. The mechanism of action is different from other protein synthesis inhibitors, which may explain the lack of cross-resistance with other agents (i.e., it is not affected by ribosomal methylases, which produce resistance to macrolides and lincosamides). However, there may be cross-resistance among linezolid, chloramphenicol, and florfenicol, mediated by the *cfr* gene. The effect on protein synthesis is relevant because linezolid also inhibits the synthesis of important virulence factors in bacteria. Linezolid has good penetration into cells, extracellular fluid, and respiratory fluid. Urine concentrations are high enough to inhibit urinary tract pathogens.

*Pharmacokinetics:* In dogs, the oral absorption is almost 100%, and the half-life is slightly faster than humans. Linezolid does not undergo hepatic P450 metabolism, and one third of the total clearance relies on the kidneys. The pharmacokinetic–pharmacodynamic parameter that best predicts efficacy is the time above MIC (T>MIC) or the area-under-the-curve (AUC)/MIC ratio. MIC values range from 0.5–4 mcg/mL for staphylococci, streptococci, and enterococci.

## Indications and Clinical Uses

Linezolid is active against streptococci and staphylococci and is indicated for treatment of infections that are resistant to other drugs, particularly when there is resistance to the beta-lactam antibiotics (penicillins, ampicillin derivatives, and cephalosporins). It is not indicated for gram-negative infections. Linezolid is indicated for treatment of methicillin-resistant and oxacillin-resistant strains of *Staphylococcus* (e.g., methicillin-resistant *Staphylococcus aureus* [MRSA] and methicillin-resistant *Staphylococcus pseudintermedius* [MRSP]) and penicillin-resistant *Enterococcus* spp. It should not be used in companion animals unless there is culture and susceptibility testing confirmation. Linezolid is the only agent with activity against all species of *Nocardia* spp.

## Precautionary Information

### Adverse Reactions and Side Effects

Adverse effects include diarrhea and nausea. Rarely, anemia and leukopenia have been observed in people. The risk of bone marrow suppression, including thrombocytopenia, is most evident after 2 weeks of treatment but is reversible after treatment is discontinued. Thrombocytopenia has been rare based on limited experience with the use of linezolid in dogs and cats. Longer treatment courses should be accompanied by periodic CBC measurements. The mechanism of myelosuppression is likely caused by effects on mitochondria. Linezolid was originally investigated as an antidepressant medication for people. Therefore, some CNS changes are possible when administered to animals, but these are not well documented.

### Contraindications and Precautions

No contraindications reported. The use in animals has been uncommon; therefore the full extent of precautions and potential adverse effects are not known.

### Drug Interactions

Linezolid is a type A monoamine oxidase inhibitor. Possible interactions occur with serotonin reuptake inhibitors such as fluoxetine and selegiline to produce serotonin syndrome. Interactions are also possible if administered with adrenergic drugs such as phenylpropanolamine. However, this effect has not been reported from the limited use in animals. Linezolid is not expected to affect metabolism of other drugs. Rifampin may decrease plasma concentrations. The IV formulation is physically incompatible with other drugs in the IV line. If administered with other drugs intravenously, flush out the administration line first.

## Instructions for Use

Linezolid is reserved for infections that are resistant to other drugs, such as *Enterococcus* spp. and MRSA infections.

## Patient Monitoring and Laboratory Tests

Choice of drug should be selected on the basis of susceptibility monitoring. CLSI lists the breakpoint for susceptibility as ≤4.0 mcg/mL for *Staphylococcus* spp. and ≤2.0 mcg/mL for *Enterococcus* spp. Ideal plasma drug concentrations are 2–7 mcg/mL.

## Formulations
- Linezolid is available in 600-mg tablets, 20-mg/mL oral suspension powder (orange flavor), and 2-mg/mL injection for IV use.

## Stability and Storage
Store in a tightly sealed container, protected from light, and at room temperature. Do not mix with other drugs. Oral suspension is stable for 21 days after reconstitution at room temperature.

## Small Animal Dosage
### Dogs and Cats
- 10 mg/kg q12h PO or IV.

## Large Animal Dosage
- No large animal dose is available.

## Regulatory Information
This drug should not be administered to food-producing animals. If administered to a food animal, consult FARAD at www.FARAD.org for extralabel use guidelines.

L

# Liothyronine Sodium
lye-oh-thye'roe-neen soe'dee-um

**Trade and other names:** Cytomel

**Functional classification:** Hormone

## Pharmacology and Mechanism of Action
Liothyronine is a thyroid supplement that is used to mimic the effects of $T_3$. Liothyronine is equivalent to $T_3$. $T_3$ is more active than $T_4$, but ordinarily $T_4$ is converted in animals to the active form of $T_3$.

## Indications and Clinical Uses
Liothyronine is used for similar indications as $T_4$, except that in this instance, the active $T_3$ hormone is administered instead of relying on conversion from $T_4$ to $T_3$. It may be indicated in cases in which there is failure to convert $T_4$ to the active $T_3$ hormone; however, this is a rare occurrence. In most cases, it is preferred to administer levothyroxine instead of liothyronine.

## Precautionary Information
### Adverse Reactions and Side Effects
Adverse effects have not been reported.

### Contraindications and Precautions
No contraindications reported.

### Drug Interactions
No drug interactions reported for animals.

## Instructions for Use

Doses of liothyronine should be adjusted on the basis of monitoring $T_3$ concentrations in patients. It is rarely necessary to administer $T_3$ alone for treatment of hypothyroidism. In most patients, drugs that contain $T_4$ should be used (e.g., levothyroxine) and converted to $T_3$. Liothyronine has been used as a diagnostic test for cats.

## Patient Monitoring and Laboratory Tests

Monitor serum $T_3$ concentrations. Used for $T_3$-suppressing test in cats.

## Formulations

- Liothyronine (human formulation) is available in 5-, 25-, and 50-mcg tablets.
- Liotrix is a combination of $T_4$ and $T_3$ in a ratio: Available as ($T_4/T_3$): 12.5/3.1-, 25/6.25-, 50/12.5-, 100/25-, and 150/37.5-mcg tablets.

## Stability and Storage

Store in a tightly sealed container, protected from light, and at room temperature. Stability of compounded formulations has not been evaluated.

## Small Animal Dosage

### Dogs and Cats

- 4.4 mcg/kg q8h PO.
- $T_3$ suppression test in cats: Collect presample for $T_4$ and $T_3$, administer 25 mcg q8h for seven doses, and then collect postsamples for $T_3$ and $T_4$ after last dose.

## Large Animal Dosage

- No large animal dose is available.

## Regulatory Information

Withdrawal times are not established for animals that produce food. For extralabel use withdrawal interval estimates, contact FARAD at www.FARAD.org.

---

# Lisinopril
lye-sin′oh-pril

**Trade and other names:** Prinivil and Zestril

**Functional classification:** Vasodilator, angiotensin-converting enzyme inhibitor

## Pharmacology and Mechanism of Action

Lisinopril is an angiotensin-converting enzyme (ACE) inhibitor used infrequently in animals compared with enalapril or benazepril. Like other ACE inhibitors, lisinopril inhibits conversion of angiotensin I to angiotensin II. Angiotensin II is a potent vasoconstrictor and also stimulates sympathetic stimulation, renal hypertension, and synthesis of aldosterone. The ability of aldosterone to cause sodium and water retention contributes to congestion. Lisinopril, like other ACE inhibitors, causes vasodilation and decreases aldosterone-induced congestion and aldosterone-induced cardiac remodeling. Lisinopril also contributes to vasodilation by increasing concentrations of some vasodilating kinins and prostaglandins. Like other ACE inhibitors, lisinopril can reduce renal hypertension and improve renal perfusion, decrease glomerular pressure, and lead to improvement in some patients with renal disease.

## Indications and Clinical Uses

Lisinopril, like other ACE inhibitors, is used to treat hypertension and congestive heart failure. Enalapril and benazepril have been used more often in animals, and there is much less experience using lisinopril. The use of lisinopril is based on extrapolation from the uses of other ACE inhibitors (enalapril, benazepril) or the uses in people. Lisinopril also may be used to treat some forms of kidney disease in animals. When glomerular filtration pressures are high, lisinopril may improve some patients with kidney disease, but effects on survival have not been established.

## Precautionary Information

### Adverse Reactions and Side Effects

Like other ACE inhibitors, lisinopril may cause azotemia in some patients, but this effect has been uncommon. It can be exacerbated with administration of diuretics (e.g., furosemide); therefore, carefully monitor patients receiving high doses of diuretics.

### Contraindications and Precautions

Discontinue ACE inhibitors in pregnant animals; they cross the placenta and have caused fetal malformations and death of the fetus.

### Drug Interactions

Use lisinopril cautiously with other hypotensive drugs and diuretics. NSAIDs may decrease vasodilating effects.

**L**

## Instructions for Use

Clinical studies using lisinopril in animals have not been reported. The doses and clinical use have been extrapolated from human studies or limited anecdotal experience in animals.

## Patient Monitoring and Laboratory Tests

Monitor patients carefully to avoid hypotension. With all ACE inhibitors, monitor electrolytes and renal function 3–7 days after initiating therapy and periodically thereafter.

## Formulations

• Lisinopril is available in 2.5-, 5-, 10-, 20-, and 40-mg tablets.

## Stability and Storage

Store in a tightly sealed container, protected from light, and at room temperature. Lisinopril has been mixed with syrup for oral administration and found to be stable for 30 days at either room temperature or refrigerated.

## Small Animal Dosage

**Dogs**
• 0.5 mg/kg q24h PO.

**Cats**
• No dose established.

## Large Animal Dosage

• No large animal dose is available.

## Regulatory Information

Withdrawal times are not established for animals that produce food. For extralabel use withdrawal interval estimates, contact FARAD at www.FARAD.org.

# Lithium Carbonate

lih'thee-um kar'boe-nate

**Trade and other names:** Lithotabs

**Functional classification:** Immunostimulant

## Pharmacology and Mechanism of Action

Lithium stimulates granulopoiesis and elevates the neutrophil pool in animals. It also affects the CNS because it affects the balance of CNS neurotransmitters. The use in animals has been very uncommon.

## Indications and Clinical Uses

In people, lithium is used for treatment of depression. It has not been used for this purpose in animals. It has also been used experimentally to increase neutrophil counts after cancer therapy and to prevent cytotoxicity caused from anticancer drugs. This is also an uncommon use in animals and has not been studied with well-controlled clinical trials.

## Precautionary Information

**Adverse Reactions and Side Effects**

Adverse effects include nephrogenic diabetes insipidus, ptyalism, lethargy, and seizures. In people, cardiovascular problems, drowsiness, and diarrhea are among the adverse effects.

**Contraindications and Precautions**

Not recommended in cats.

**Drug Interactions**

No drug interactions are reported.

## Instructions for Use

Use in animals is uncommon, and little dosing information is available. The doses and intervals listed are extrapolated from the human use or limited clinical observations.

## Patient Monitoring and Laboratory Tests

Monitor neutrophil count.

## Formulations

- Lithium is available in 150-, 300-, and 600-mg capsules; 300-mg tablets; and 300-mg/5 mL syrup.

## Stability and Storage

Store in a tightly sealed container, protected from light, and at room temperature. Stability of compounded formulations has not been evaluated.

## Small Animal Dosage

**Dogs**

- 10 mg/kg q12h PO.

**Cats**

- Not recommended.

## Large Animal Dosage

- No large animal dose is available.

## Regulatory Information

Withdrawal times are not established for animals that produce food. For extralabel use withdrawal interval estimates, contact FARAD at www.FARAD.org.

# Lomustine
loe-mus'teen

**Trade and other names:** CeeNU and CCNU

**Functional classification:** Anticancer agent

## Pharmacology and Mechanism of Action

Lomustine is an anticancer agent of the nitrosourea class, used occasionally in animals for various forms of cancer. It is one of two nitrosoureas used: lomustine (1-[2-chloroethyl]-3-cyclohexyl-1-chloroethylnitrosourea), known by the abbreviation of CCNU, and carmustine (1,3-bis-2-chloroethyl-1-nitrosourea), known by the abbreviation BCNU. Both of the nitrosoureas are metabolized spontaneously to alkylating and carbamylating compounds. Lomustine transfers the chloroethyl group of the nitrosourea to the O-6 methyl of guanine on DNA. This causes interstrand and intrastrand cross-linking of DNA, which inactivates DNA synthesis and cell death. Therefore bifunctional interstrand cross-links are responsible for the cytotoxicity of nitrosoureas. Lomustine has high lipophilicity and penetrates the CNS, which can be useful for some CNS tumors.

*Pharmacokinetics:* Oral absorption and high membrane penetration are attributed to high lipophilicity. Because oral absorption is high, lomustine can be administered effectively as oral tablets. After absorption, lomustine is metabolized to antitumor metabolites. Both the parent drug and the metabolites are lipid soluble. The CNS penetration of lomustine has been determined from the plasma:cerebrospinal fluid ratio, which is 1:3.

## Indications and Clinical Uses

Lomustine (CCNU) is used to treat tumors of the CNS (brain tumors), round cell tumors, mast cell tumors, sarcomas, and lymphoma in dogs and cats. It has occasionally been used to treat other forms of cancer, such as mast cell tumors. Lomustine has been used more often than carmustine. The use is based primarily on empirical evidence and small observational studies. It has the advantage of good oral absorption, and in dogs, it is used as an oral treatment for various cancers. It has also been well tolerated in cats. At dosages of approximately 10 mg per cat every 3 weeks, it produces minimal myelosuppression. The commercial formulations of Lomustine made for people may be unavailable. Therefore, veterinarians have resorted to using compounded formulations for use in animals.

## Precautionary Information

### Adverse Reactions and Side Effects

Bone marrow effects are the most serious. In people, lomustine has a delayed nadir of bone marrow toxicity, which is as long as 4–6 weeks with slow recovery, but in dogs, the nadir of bone marrow effects generally is seen 6–7 days after dosing. The maximum tolerated dose in dogs is 90 mg/m$^2$. At higher doses (100 mg/m$^2$), myelosuppression has been reported. Thrombocytopenia also has been reported from lomustine administration as a cumulative effect. If severe neutropenia is observed in dogs, lower the dose to 40–50 mg/m$^2$.

In cats, neutropenia is the most dose-limiting effect of treatment. Thrombocytopenia also is possible. Cats resemble people in that bone marrow nadir of toxicity occurs at 3–4 weeks. Nitrosoureas also can be toxic to the rapidly dividing cells of mucosal tissues.

In people, nitrosoureas also have caused pulmonary fibrosis and hepatotoxicity, but this has not been a reported problem in dogs or cats. Hepatotoxicity can occur as a delayed reaction. In people, carmustine (BCNU) has been associated with a higher rate of hepatic injury than lomustine, but hepatic injury has been observed in dogs from lomustine and has been irreversible.

### Contraindications and Precautions
Consider the risks to bone marrow with use in small animals. Commercial forms may no longer be available, and veterinarians may need to rely on compounded forms. However, compounded formulations have been known to be highly variable in potency compared with brand name formulations, and one should select a reputable compounding pharmacy to ensure high quality of the formulation.

### Drug Interactions
Use with caution with any drugs that may cause bone marrow suppression.

## Instructions for Use
The nitrosourea drugs are used to treat CNS tumors and other forms of cancer. Protocols used in small animals are different from those given to people, which are as high as 150–200 mg/m$^2$. Oral treatment should be given on an empty stomach if possible.

## Patient Monitoring and Laboratory Tests
Monitor CBC and liver enzymes in treated patients.

## Formulations
- Lomustine was available in 10-, 40-, and 100-mg capsules. However, commercial forms may be unavailable, and veterinarians have used compounded formulations. Caution is advised when using compounded forms because they have varied greatly in potency, with some (5-mg capsules) as low as 50% of the stated strength and may not produce the desired therapeutic effects.

## Stability and Storage
Store in a tightly sealed container, protected from light, and at room temperature.

## Small Animal Dosage
### Dogs
- 70–90 mg/m$^2$ every 4 weeks PO.
- Lymphoma: 60 mg/m$^2$ every 4 weeks for four treatments.
- Brain tumors: 60–80 mg/m$^2$ every 6–8 weeks PO.
- Where liver injury is a concern in dogs, use a lower and safer dose of 40 mg/m$^2$.

### Cats
- 50–60 mg/m$^2$ every 3–6 weeks PO. Alternatively, administer 10–20 mg/cat every 3–6 weeks.

## Large Animal Dosage
- No large animal doses have been reported.

## Regulatory Information
Do not administer to animals that produce food.

# Loperamide Hydrochloride
loe-pare′ah-mide hye-droe-klor′ide
**Trade and other names:** Imodium and generic brands
**Functional classification:** Analgesic, opioid

## Pharmacology and Mechanism of Action
Loperamide is an opiate agonist, but its effects are limited to peripheral receptors, particularly those on the GI tract. Like other opiates, loperamide acts on the mu-opiate receptors of the GI tract, where it decreases propulsive intestinal contractions and increases segmentation (an overall constipating effect). It also increases the tone of GI sphincters. In addition to affecting motility, opiates have an antisecretory effect and stimulate absorption of fluid, electrolytes, and glucose. Their effects on secretory diarrhea are probably related to inhibition of calcium influx and decreased calmodulin activity. The difference between loperamide and other opioids is that the action of loperamide is limited to the intestine. CNS effects do not occur because it does not cross the blood–brain barrier, or if it penetrates the blood-brain barrier, it is removed by drug transporters (P-glycoprotein).

## Indications and Clinical Uses
Loperamide is used for symptomatic treatment of acute nonspecific diarrhea. It has been administered orally to dogs and cats. There are no clinical studies in animals, and the use is based on extrapolation from the human uses or anecdotal evidence in animals. Long-term use is discouraged because it may lead to constipation. It has been administered to large animals, but this is generally not recommended.

## Precautionary Information
### Adverse Reactions and Side Effects
Loperamide can cause severe constipation with repeated use. In some dogs that have a mutation in the *ABCB1* gene (previously known as the *MDR* gene), they may lack P-glycoprotein in the blood–brain barrier. In these susceptible animals, loperamide crosses the blood–brain barrier and causes profound sedation. Such cases may be reversed with naloxone. Dogs most susceptible include collie breeds, Australian shepherds, Old English sheepdogs, longhaired whippets, and Shetland sheepdogs.

### Contraindications and Precautions
Small dogs and collie-type dogs may be at higher risk of adverse effects.

### Drug Interactions
Do not administer with drugs that may act as MDR1 (p-glycoprotein) membrane inhibitors, such as ketoconazole. (Other inhibitors are listed in Appendix J.) These inhibitors may increase blood–brain barrier penetration and cause depression.

## Instructions for Use

Doses are based primarily on empiricism or extrapolation of human doses. Clinical studies have not been performed in animals.

## Patient Monitoring and Laboratory Tests

No specific monitoring is necessary.

## Formulations

- Loperamide is available in 2-mg tablets, 2-mg capsules, and 0.2-mg/mL oral liquid (over the counter).

## Stability and Storage

Store in a tightly sealed container, protected from light, and at room temperature. Loperamide is slightly soluble in water but only at low pH. Stability of compounded formulations has not been evaluated.

## Small Animal Dosage

Dogs
- 0.12 mg/kg q8–12h PO.

Cats
- 0.08–0.16 mg/kg q12h PO.

## Large Animal Dosage

- No large animal doses have been reported. If administered to horses or ruminants, it may induce problems associated with decreased intestinal motility.

## Regulatory Information

Withdrawal times are not established for animals that produce food. If administered to food animals, consult FARAD for extralabel use withdrawal interval estimates, at www.FARAD.org.

RCI Classification: 4

# Lorazepam
lor-ay'zeh-pam

**Trade and other names:** Ativan and generic brands

**Functional classification:** Anticonvulsant

## Pharmacology and Mechanism of Action

Lorazepam is a benzodiazepine sedative and CNS depressant. As a central-acting CNS depressant, it has actions similar to diazepam and other benzodiazepines. The mechanism of action appears to be via potentiation of gamma aminobutyric acid (GABA) receptor–mediated effects in the CNS.

*Pharmacokinetics:* In animals, lorazepam does not undergo extensive hepatic metabolism, but it is glucuronidated before excretion. Therefore, it is not subject to the same effects from cytochrome P450 enzymes as other benzodiazepines. In dogs, lorazepam has a half-life of 0.9 hours, with systemic clearance less than half that of diazepam. Oral absorption is 60%. Therefore the oral formulation may be suitable in dogs for some conditions.

## Indications and Clinical Uses

Lorazepam acts as a traditional benzodiazepine and may be considered for anxiety disorders in animals, but it has not been used as commonly as other drugs such as diazepam, alprazolam, or midazolam. Lorazepam also is effective for treating seizures, but it is not used as often in animals as other anticonvulsants. In controlled studies, it has been equally as effective as an anticonvulsant as diazepam in dogs, but the use for other indications is limited to anecdotal evidence and recommendations from clinical experts.

## Precautionary Information

### Adverse Reactions and Side Effects

Sedation is the most common side effect. Lorazepam causes polyphagia. Some animals may experience paradoxical excitement. Chronic administration may lead to dependence and a withdrawal syndrome if discontinued.

### Contraindications and Precautions

If animals have been receiving lorazepam or any other benzodiazepine for a prolonged time, dependence can occur, and if discontinued, it should be done gradually to avoid withdrawal signs. Oral administration of another benzodiazepine, diazepam, has caused idiosyncratic liver injury in cats, but this is unlikely for lorazepam because of a different route of metabolism. Use of benzodiazepines in early pregnancy has been associated with an increased risk of spontaneous abortions and fetal malformations in people. This incidence in animals is unknown.

### Drug Interactions

Use cautiously with other drugs that may cause sedation. Do not mix with buprenorphine.

**L**

## Instructions for Use

Doses are based on empiricism and limited observations in animals. There have been no clinical trials in veterinary medicine, although it is expected to produce effects similar to other benzodiazepines. For IV use, dilute 50/50 with 0.9% saline or 5% dextrose prior to use.

## Patient Monitoring and Laboratory Tests

No specific monitoring is necessary.

## Formulations Available

- Lorazepam is available in 0.5-, 1-, and 2-mg tablets and 2- and 4-mg/mL injection.

## Stability and Storage

Store in a tightly sealed container, protected from light, and at room temperature. Lorazepam is practically insoluble in water. It is slightly soluble in some infusion solutions (e.g., 0.054 mg/mL in 5% dextrose). Solutions should be discarded if they turn a dark color.

## Small Animal Dosage

### Dogs

- 0.05 mg/kg q12h PO.
- Seizures: 0.2 mg/kg IV. Repeat every 3–4 hours for seizure control if necessary or a 0.2-mg/kg bolus followed by 0.2–0.4 mg/kg/h IV CRI.

### Cats

- 0.05 mg/kg q12–24h PO.

## Large Animal Dosage

- No large animal doses have been reported.

## Regulatory Information

Do not administer to animals intended for food.
Schedule IV controlled drug.
RCI Classification: 2

## Losartan
loe-zar′tan

**Trade and other names:** Cozaar

**Functional classification:** Vasodilator

## Pharmacology and Mechanism of Action
Losartan is a vasodilator that blocks the angiotensin receptor. These drugs are considered angiotensin receptor blockers (ARBs). Losartan (or metabolite) blocks angiotensin II receptors and prevents the effects associated with angiotensin II on blood vessels. It has high affinity and selectivity for the AT1 receptor. The vasodilating action is similar to that of ACE inhibitors except that it directly blocks the receptor rather than inhibits synthesis of angiotensin II. Angiotensin II receptor blockers have the advantage of being less likely to induce hyperkalemia and are more easily tolerated in people. Losartan and other ARBs have been used in people who cannot tolerate ACE inhibitors.

*Pharmacokinetics:* In people, losartan is metabolized to the active carboxylic acid metabolite (E-3174), which is 10–40 times more potent than the parent drug and with a longer half-life than the parent drug, and is believed to be responsible for most clinical effects. In dogs, oral absorption of the parent drug is low (23%–33%), and the half-life is short (1.8–2.5 hours) with high clearance producing a short duration of activity. Dogs do not form the E-3174 metabolite, which is responsible for therapeutic effects in people. Because of this difference, dogs may require higher doses than used in people to produce therapeutic effects.

## Indications and Clinical Uses
Dogs do not convert losartan to the active metabolite, so it has little activity in dogs unless high doses are used. A related drug, irbesartan (30 mg/kg q12h) or telmisartan (see later), is more effective in dogs for blocking angiotensin II receptors. Losartan's effects in cats (2.5 mg/kg/day) for lowering blood pressure were not different than placebo. Telmisartan is in a veterinary formulation for cats and has received greater interest in dogs because of a longer half-life and higher lipophilicity. Therefore it may be more effective in dogs compared with losartan.

## Precautionary Information
### Adverse Reactions and Side Effects
No adverse reactions have been reported in animals. In people, hypotension may occur.

### Contraindications and Precautions
No specific contraindications have been reported for animals. Do not use in pregnant animals.

### Drug Interactions
Combined use of ARB and ACE inhibitor may increase risk of kidney injury.

## Instructions for Use

In dogs, losartan is not converted to the active metabolite. Therefore, it has little bioactivity (*J Pharmacol Exp Ther.* 1999;268:1199–1205), and high doses are needed to produce clinical effects. It is suggested instead to consider irbesartan at a dosage of 30 mg/kg q12h PO or telmisartan instead (see Telmisartan for more information).

## Patient Monitoring and Laboratory Tests

Monitor blood pressure in treated animals.

## Formulations

• Losartan is available in 25-, 50-, and 100-mg tablets.

## Stability and Storage

Store in a tightly sealed container, protected from light, and at room temperature. Stability of compounded formulations has not been evaluated.

## Small Animal Dosage

### Dogs

• 0.125 mg/kg per day in azotemic patients; 0.5 mg/kg/day in nonazotemic patients.

### Cats

• Not effective in cats. If an ARB drug is indicated for cats, use telmisartan.

## Large Animal Dosage

• No large animal doses have been reported.

## Regulatory Information

Do not administer to animals intended for food.
RCI Classification: 3

# Lotilaner
lote′ah lan′er

**Trade and other names:** Credelio

**Functional classification:** Antiparasitic, ectoparasiticide

## Pharmacology and Mechanism of Action

Lotilaner belongs to the isooxazolines class of ectoparasiticides. It is effective for treating and preventing infections from fleas, mites, and ticks. It produces selective inhibition of the GABA receptor and glutamate-gated chloride channels. This inhibition of the receptor produces changes in chloride channels and hyperexcitement, leading to death of the parasite. Mammals are not affected because of a lack of binding to mammalian GABA receptors.

Efficacy has been demonstrated against a wide range of ectoparasites, including fleas, various mites (including *Demodex* and *Sarcoptes* spp.), and ticks. The parasite must bite the animal for exposure to the agent. Activity of the isooxazolines has been superior to other ectoparasiticides, including fipronil and imidacloprid.

Other drugs in this class with similar activity, but different pharmacokinetics include afoxolaner, fluralaner, and sarolaner.

## Indications and Clinical Uses

Lotilaner, like the other isooxazolines is active against fleas, mites, and ticks. After oral administration or topical application, it can kill fleas rapidly. The chew tablet for dogs has an approved indication for killing adult fleas and to prevent flea infestations (*Ctenocephalides felis*). It is also approved for treatment and control of tick infestations caused by *Amblyomma americanum* (Lone Star tick), *Dermacentor variabilis* (American dog tick), *Ixodes scapularis* (black-legged tick), and *Rhipicephalus sanguineus* (brown dog tick) for 1 month in dogs.

Because of this action, lotilaner can reduce the risk that these vectors may pose for disease transmission. For example, it may prevent infections caused by *Borrelia burgdorferi* (Lyme disease) and *Babesia canis*.

The approved label indication for lotilaner is treatment of fleas and ticks, but extralabel uses, using the approved label dose, have included treatment of generalized demodicosis caused by *Demodex canis*.

The proper use of lotilaner involves administration of oral chew tablets, administered with food.

---

## Precautionary Information

### Adverse Reactions and Side Effects

Adverse effects have been rare from administration of lotilaner. In the field studies, there were rare incidences of weight loss, elevated blood urea nitrogen, polyuria, and diarrhea.

In safety studies, at up to five times the approved label dose, there were no clinically relevant treatment-related adverse effects.

There is a concern about neurologic adverse effects, including seizures, from administration of isooxazolines in dogs. This has been reported primarily with sarolaner, but the manufacturer of lotilaner warns that it should be used cautiously in dogs with a history of seizures.

### Contraindications and Precautions

There are no known contraindications for use of lotilaner in dogs, except possibly a history of seizures. The manufacturer recommends that it should not be used in dogs younger than 8 weeks of age. The safety in breeding animals has not been evaluated. The use and safety in cats have not been evaluated.

### Drug Interactions

There are no known drug interactions with lotilaner. It has been used safely with vaccines, anthelmintics, antibiotics, corticosteroids, NSAIDs, anesthetics, and antihistamines. It should not be used concurrently with other drugs in the isooxazoline class as this may increase the risk of neurologic problems.

---

## Instructions for Use

Doses for lotilaner are established from the approved label dosing. Interval of dosing is based on efficacy studies. It is effective for treatment of fleas (*C. felis*) and most ticks, including the American dog tick (*D. variabilis*), the Lone Star tick (*A. americanum*), and brown dog tick (*R. sanguineus*) for 1 month after treatment.

There is reduced oral absorption on an empty stomach; therefore, administer with a meal or within 30 minutes after feeding.

## Patient Monitoring and Laboratory Tests

There is no routine monitoring required. Monitor response to treatment through clinical examination of skin at regular check-ups.

## Formulations
- Lotilaner is available in a beef-flavored chew tablet for dogs in sizes of 56.25-, 112.5- 225-, 450-, and 900-mg tablets.

## Stability and Storage
Lotilaner should be stored in a dry place at controlled temperatures less than 25°C.

## Small Animal Dosage
**Dogs**
- 20 mg/kg once every month. Administer with food or within 30 minutes after feeding.

**Cats**
- A dose for cats has not been established.

## Large Animal Dosage
No large animal doses have been established.

## Regulatory Information
No withdrawal times are established for animals intended for food (extralabel use).

# Lufenuron
loo-fen′yoo-rahn
**Trade and other names:** Program
**Functional classification:** Antiparasitic

## Pharmacology and Mechanism of Action
Lufenuron is an antiparasitic drug that inhibits the development of fleas. Lufenuron is a benzoylurea insecticide. This class of insecticides was previously used on fruits to decrease damage by insects. Lufenuron (Program) has been used for prevention of flea infections in dogs and cats because it inhibits chitin synthesis. For this use, it has been given to dogs at a dosage of 10 mg/kg every 30 days and to cats at a dosage of 30 mg/kg every 30 days. It may also have some inhibition on fungal cell membranes because it inhibits the cell wall of fungi, which contain chitin, and other complex polysaccharides. However, the use as an antifungal agent is not well established in animals (see later).

*Pharmacokinetics:* The pharmacokinetics are characterized by an initial rapid decline in plasma drug concentrations, followed by a slow decline and clearance. Systemic clearance is 0.56 L/kg/day and 0.54 L/kg/day, with a volume of distribution of 44.8 and 48.3 L/kg and a half-life of 60.7 and 65.2 days in cats and dogs, respectively.

## Indications and Clinical Uses
Lufenuron is used to control flea infestations by preventing hatching of eggs. It has been used as part of flea control, often with other drugs that kill adult fleas. Lufenuron has been combined with milbemycin in formulations for small animals, and additional details may be found in the section on milbemycin.

There are isolated clinical reports of the use of lufenuron for treating dermatophyte infections in small animals, particularly cats, at high dosages of 80–100 mg/kg PO. However, endorsement of this use has diminished, and dermatologists have observed a high incidence of recurrence and disputed the reports of efficacy. In horses, lufenuron was not absorbed orally and is not effective for treating fungal infections. It does not have any in vitro effect on *Aspergillus fumigatus* or *Coccidioides immitis.*

## Precautionary Information

**Adverse Reactions and Side Effects**

Lufenuron has been well tolerated in animals. Refer to the section on lufenuron or milbemycin for details regarding this combination.

**Contraindications and Precautions**

No contraindications are reported for animals. Some animals may be sensitive to milbemycin, and additional details are found in that section.

**Drug Interactions**

No drug interactions reported for animals, except those that may pertain to milbemycin, when used in combination.

## Instructions for Use

Lufenuron is a highly lipophilic drug and is absorbed best with a meal. If cats have free access to their food, withhold their food until such time that a meal will be consumed readily before administering the lufenuron oral dose. Lufenuron may control flea development with administration once every 30 days in animals.

## Patient Monitoring and Laboratory Tests

No specific monitoring is necessary.

## Formulations

- Lufenuron is available in 45-, 90- 135-, 204.9-, and 409.8-mg tablets and 135- and 270-mg suspension per unit pack.

## Stability and Storage

Store in a tightly sealed container, protected from light, and at room temperature. Stability of compounded formulations has not been evaluated.

## Small Animal Dosage

**Dogs**

- Flea control: 10 mg/kg every 30 days PO.
- Dermatophytes: 80 mg/kg every 2 weeks PO (but the efficacy of this use is questionable and not recommended).

**Cats**

- Flea control: 30 mg/kg every 30 days PO or injection of 10 mg/kg SQ every 6 months.
- Dermatophytes: 80 mg/kg; 100 mg/kg PO is the minimum dose for treating cats in a cattery. These doses should be repeated initially after the first 2 weeks and possibly once per month in animals that may be re-exposed. However, as stated earlier, the efficacy of this treatment is questionable and not generally recommended.

## Large Animal Dosage

**Horses**

- Not effective.

## Regulatory Information

Withdrawal times are not established for animals that produce food. For extralabel use withdrawal interval estimates, contact FARAD at www.FARAD.org.

# Lufenuron + Milbemycin Oxime
loo-fen′yoo-rahn + mil-beh-mye′sin oks′eem

**Trade and other names:** Sentinel tablets and Flavor Tabs

**Functional classification:** Antiparasitic

## Pharmacology and Mechanism of Action
Combination of two antiparasitic drugs. Refer to sections on lufenuron or milbemycin for details.

## Indications and Clinical Uses
Lufenuron + milbemycin is used to protect against fleas, heartworms, roundworms, hookworms, and whipworms.

## Precautionary Information

**Adverse Reactions and Side Effects**

There is a high margin of safety at doses used for flea control or treatment of dermatophytes. Adverse effects have not been reported. Lufenuron appears to be relatively safe in pregnant and young animals.

**Contraindications and Precautions**

No contraindications are reported for animals.

**Drug Interactions**

No drug interactions are reported for animals.

## Instructions for Use
See Lufenuron or Milbemycin for details.

## Patient Monitoring and Laboratory Tests
Monitor for heartworm status in dogs before initiating treatment with milbemycin.

## Formulations
- The milbemycin/lufenuron ratio is as follows: 2.3/46-mg tablets and 5.75/115-, 11.5/230-, and 23/460-mg Flavor Tabs.

## Stability and Storage
Store in a tightly sealed container, protected from light, and at room temperature. Stability of compounded formulations has not been evaluated.

## Small Animal Dosage

**Dogs**
- Administer one tablet every 30 days based on tablet size and weight range listed on product label.
- Each tablet is formulated for the size of the dog.

**Cats**
- No dose is reported.

## Large Animal Dosage
- No large animal doses have been reported.

## Regulatory Information

Withdrawal times are not established for animals that produce food. For extralabel use withdrawal interval estimates, contact FARAD at www.FARAD.org.

# Lysine (L-Lysine)
lye′seen

**Trade and other names:** Enisyl-F

**Functional classification:** Antiviral

## Pharmacology and Mechanism of Action

Lysine is an amino acid–based dietary supplement. It has been recommended for treating herpes virus infection because of some accounts that it helps people with herpes virus infection. In particular, it has been used to treat feline herpes virus type 1 (FHV-1). The proposed action is through antagonism of the growth-promoting effect of arginine, which is an essential amino acid of FHV-1. In theory, it competitively interferes with arginine incorporation into viral DNA; however, this has not been supported with clinical studies.

## Indications and Clinical Uses

Lysine is a nutritional supplement that has been used for treating FHV-1 in cats. It is intended to reduce viral shedding in infected cats and may improve some clinical signs associated with FHV.

The use in cats has been controversial, but experts conclude that it is not helpful and may actually be harmful to cats with infections. In experimental cats, administration was associated with less severe conjunctivitis and reduced viral shedding. But in shelter cats, administration of an oral supplement at 250–500 mg twice daily had no positive effects compared to placebo. In other studies in which the diet was supplemented with L-lysine, there was more severe disease and viral shedding in treated cats compared with a diet not supplemented with L-lysine. For these reasons, routine use for viral infections in cats is not recommended.

## Precautionary Information

**Adverse Reactions and Side Effects**

No adverse effects have been reported in cats, except for accounts of worsening of herpes virus infections.

**Contraindications and Precautions**

No contraindications have been reported.

**Drug Interactions**

No drug interactions have been reported for animals.

## Instructions for Use

L-Lysine monohydrate can be supplied as a powder and mixed with a small amount of food.

## Patient Monitoring and Laboratory Tests

Monitor patient's CBC during treatment.

## Formulations

Paste (Enisyl-F) is distributed in syringes in which each mark on the syringe represents 1 mL (250 mg/mL). It has also been available for cats as a metered-dose pump to add to food, 100-g powder (to be mixed with food), 5-oz oral gel (Viralys), 600-mL oral paste, and flavored treats.

## Stability and Storage

Store in a tightly sealed container, protected from light, and at room temperature.

## Small Animal Dosage

### Cats

Use in cats for FHV-1 infections is not recommended.
- 400 mg/cat/day PO daily supplement added to cat food.
- Paste formulation: 1–2 mL to adult cats and 1 mL to kittens.

## Large Animal Dosage
- No large animal doses have been reported.

## Regulatory Information

No regulatory information is available. Because of a low risk of residues, no withdrawal times are suggested.

L

# Magnesium Citrate

**Trade and other names:** Citroma, CitroNesia, and Citro-Mag (Canada)

**Functional classification:** Laxative

## Pharmacology and Mechanism of Action

Magnesium citrate is a saline cathartic. It acts to draw water into the small intestine via an osmotic effect. Fluid accumulation produces distension, which promotes bowel evacuation. It is not used often in veterinary medicine.

## Indications and Clinical Uses

Magnesium citrate is administered orally for constipation and bowel evacuation prior to certain procedures. It also may be used to promote intestinal clearance of an ingested toxin. It is prompt in its cathartic action. In the formulation Pronefra (in combination with calcium carbonate), it is used as a phosphate binder to patients with kidney disease.

## Precautionary Information

### Adverse Reactions and Side Effects

Adverse effects have not been reported in animals. However, fluid and electrolyte loss can occur with overuse.

### Contraindications and Precautions

Magnesium accumulation may occur in patients with renal impairment. Cathartics containing magnesium decrease oral absorption of ciprofloxacin and other fluoroquinolones.

### Drug Interactions

No drug interactions have been reported for animals. However, it may increase clearance of some drugs administered orally.

## Instructions for Use

Magnesium citrate is commonly used to evacuate the bowel prior to surgery or diagnostic procedures. Doses are empirical and extrapolated from other species. Onset of action is rapid.

## Patient Monitoring and Laboratory Tests

No specific monitoring is necessary. However, monitor magnesium concentrations in patients if repeated treatments or high doses are administered.

## Formulations

- Magnesium citrate is available in a 6% oral suspension. The formulation Pronefra also is available as calcium carbonate and magnesium carbonate. It is an oral syrup that may be administered as a phosphate binder in cats and dogs. Pronefra is a palatable liquid suspension with poultry liver flavoring.

## Stability and Storage

Store in a tightly sealed container, protected from light, and at room temperature.

## Small Animal Dosage
**Dogs and Cats**
- 2–4 mL/kg/day PO. For the Pronefra product (in combination with calcium carbonate), administer twice daily at mealtimes. 1 mL per cat or 1 mL per dog twice daily PO, preferably at mealtimes.

## Large Animal Dosage
**Horses and Cattle**
- 2–4 mL/kg once PO.

## Regulatory Information
No regulatory information is available. Because of a low risk of residues, no withdrawal times are suggested.

# Magnesium Hydroxide
**Trade and other names:** Milk of Magnesia, Carmilax, and Magnalax

**Functional classification:** Laxative

## Pharmacology and Mechanism of Action
Magnesium hydroxide is a saline cathartic. Magnesium hydroxide acts to draw water into the small intestine via an osmotic effect. Fluid accumulation produces distension, which promotes bowel evacuation.

**M**

## Indications and Clinical Uses
Magnesium hydroxide is used for constipation and bowel evacuation prior to certain procedures. It is commonly used to evacuate the bowel prior to surgery or diagnostic procedures. The onset of action is rapid after oral administration. Magnesium hydroxide also is used as an oral antacid to neutralize stomach acid. In large animals, it is used as an antacid and mild cathartic. In cattle, approximately 1 g/kg as a single dose significantly increases rumen pH and decreases rumen microbial activity.

## Precautionary Information
**Adverse Reactions and Side Effects**
Adverse effects have not been reported in animals. However, fluid and electrolyte loss can occur with overuse.

**Contraindications and Precautions**
Magnesium accumulation may occur in patients with renal impairment.

**Drug Interactions**
Cathartics containing magnesium decrease oral absorption of ciprofloxacin and other fluoroquinolones.

## Instructions for Use
Administer to patients only if they are properly hydrated.

## Patient Monitoring and Laboratory Tests
Monitor electrolytes with chronic use.

## Formulations

- Magnesium hydroxide is available as an oral liquid 400 mg/5 mL, or 400 mg per teaspoon (Milk of Magnesia) over the counter. It is also available as a 27- or 90-g bolus for cattle and sheep and as a powder 310–360 g/lb (approximately 745 g/kg). As a powder, 1 lb of powder is equivalent to 1 gallon of Milk of Magnesia, and three 27-g boluses are equal to 1 quart of Milk of Magnesia.

## Stability and Storage

Store in a tightly sealed container, protected from light, and at room temperature.

## Small Animal Dosage
### Dogs

- Antacid: 5–10 mL/dog q4–6h PO.
- Cathartic: 15–50 mL/dog q24h PO.

### Cats

- Antacid: 5–10 mL/cat q4–6h PO.
- Cathartic: 2–6 mL/cat q24h.

## Large Animal Dosage
### Sheep and Cattle

- 1 g/kg or 1 bolus per 27 kg (60 lb) PO once (three or four boluses for adult cattle).
- For the powder, mix 1 lb (0.45 kg) with 1 gallon of water and administer 500 mL/45 kg (500 mL per 100 lb). For the product Polyox, administer 180 mL for animals weighing less than 225 kg and 360 mL for animals weighing greater than 225 kg body weight.

## Regulatory Information

Withdrawal time for animals intended for food: 12–24 hours (milk) depending on the product.

# Magnesium Sulfate

**Trade and other names:** Epsom salts

**Functional classification:** Laxative, antiarrhythmic

## Pharmacology and Mechanism of Action

Magnesium sulfate is a saline cathartic but also is the preferred magnesium source to treat cardiac arrhythmias and to treat magnesium deficiency. When administered orally, magnesium sulfate acts to draw water into the small intestine via an osmotic effect. Fluid accumulation produces distension, which promotes bowel evacuation. Magnesium sulfate is administered intravenously to patients who are magnesium deficient and is used as an antiarrhythmic. When used as an antiarrhythmic, it serves as a source of magnesium for treating refractory arrhythmias because in animals with hypomagnesemia, it acts as a cofactor for the sodium/potassium (Na/K) ATPase pump. It also may block calcium channels.

## Indications and Clinical Uses

Magnesium sulfate is used for constipation and bowel evacuation prior to certain procedures. An injectable solution of magnesium sulfate is used to treat magnesium deficiency and refractory arrhythmias in patients who are critically ill. (Magnesium chloride also has been used.) A dose of 1–2 mEq/kg of magnesium sulfate produced plasma concentrations of 8.5–12.2 mEq/L and can increase heart rate, inotropy, and cardiac output.

In horses, magnesium sulfate is administered for ventricular tachycardia, often with lidocaine infusions (see Lidocaine), that is not responsive to other drugs. In cattle, magnesium sulfate is used to treat hypomagnesemia, especially in dairy cattle.

## Precautionary Information

### Adverse Reactions and Side Effects

High doses may cause muscle weakness and respiratory paralysis. Mild signs of toxicity during magnesium treatment include vomiting, diarrhea, hypotension, and weakness. With repeated administration, fluid and electrolyte loss can occur with overuse. When treating arrhythmias, it has been administered at doses of 0.1–0.2 mEq/kg safely. At doses higher than 1.0 mmol/kg (2.0 mEq/kg), deterioration of hemodynamic parameters may occur.

### Contraindications and Precautions

Magnesium accumulation may occur in patients with renal impairment.

### Drug Interactions

Magnesium sulfate can be added to fluids containing sodium chloride (0.9%), dextrose (5%), and water. Do not mix with calcium-, bicarbonate-, and lactate-containing solutions. Cathartics containing magnesium decrease oral absorption of ciprofloxacin and other fluoroquinolones. Magnesium sulfate is incompatible with alkaline solutions. Some metal ions (e.g., calcium) may form insoluble sulfates.

M

## Instructions for Use

When used as a laxative, magnesium sulfate is administered for its prompt action to evacuate the bowel prior to surgery or diagnostic procedures. Onset of action is rapid. For use in cattle (hypomagnesemia), an initial dose can be administered IV followed by an SQ dose to produce a sustained effect. Monitor animals for hypocalcemia, which can occur simultaneously.

## Patient Monitoring and Laboratory Tests

When treating magnesium deficiency or arrhythmias with IV magnesium sulfate, monitor the electrocardiogram (ECG) during infusion and observe for bradycardia, QT interval prolongation, and QRS complex widening. Monitor magnesium, potassium, sodium, chloride, and calcium concentrations during treatment. Normal magnesium concentrations in animals are 1.32–2.46 mEq/L. Many cattle also have hypocalcemia, which should be addressed with separate treatment using calcium-containing solutions.

## Formulations

- Magnesium sulfate is available as solid crystals in generic preparations. Solution for injection is 12.5%–50%. When administering IV, dilute to concentration below 20% using sodium chloride (0.9%), 5% dextrose, or water as a diluent. IV and SQ solutions for cattle are usually 1.5–4 g/L.

## Stability and Storage

Crystals are stable if stored in a dry container. Store injectable solutions at room temperature, in a tightly sealed vial, protected from light.

## Small Animal Dosage
### Dogs
- 1–2 mEq/kg/day PO, equivalent to 0.5–1.0 mmol/kg PO (or 8–25 g/dog q24h PO).

### Cats
- 2–5 g/cat q24h PO.

### Dogs and Cats
- IV dose for magnesium deficiency or arrhythmias: 0.2–0.3 mEq/kg (0.1–0.15 mmol/kg) IV at a rate of 0.12 mEq/kg/min (0.06 mmol/kg/min).
- Constant-rate infusion (CRI) for treating arrhythmias or ongoing deficiency: 0.2–1.0 mEq/kg/day IV (0.1–0.5 mmol/kg/day).
- Use during fluid therapy: Supplement fluid solutions with 0.75–1 mEq/kg/day.

## Large Animal Dosage
### Cattle
- 2–3 g per cow IV over 10 minutes. This may be followed by 200–400 mL per cow of 25% magnesium sulfate SQ to supply 50–100 g per cow.

### Horses
- 1 g/horse q12–24h PO or 2–4 mg/kg IV. For ventricular tachycardia, an infusion of 1 g/min, up to a maximum of 25 g, can be administered intravenously. Also see Lidocaine for instructions on combining lidocaine infusions with magnesium infusions to treat refractory ventricular arrhythmias.

## Regulatory Information
No regulatory information is available. Because of a low risk of residues, no withdrawal times are suggested.

# Mannitol
man′ih-tole

**Trade and other names:** Osmitrol
**Functional classification:** Diuretic

## Pharmacology and Mechanism of Action
Mannitol is used as a hyperosmotic diuretic. Mannitol occurs naturally as a sugar in fruits and vegetables. As an osmotic diuretic, mannitol is freely filtered by the glomerulus, but it is not reabsorbed by the renal tubule. Therefore, it increases osmolality of the urine. The osmotic effect inhibits reabsorption of fluid from the renal tubules, and this produces a natriuretic effect and strong diuresis. Reabsorption of sodium chloride and solutes also is inhibited. Mannitol, compared with other diuretic drugs, produces a more profound diuretic effect, which can potentially cause excessive fluid loss in a patient. After IV administration, mannitol increases the plasma osmolality, which draws fluid from tissues to plasma, and is helpful for treating tissue edema. It reduces intracranial pressure for treating cerebral edema. It is also used as an antiglaucoma agent because it lowers intraocular pressure when administered intravenously.

## Indications and Clinical Uses

Mannitol is administered intravenously for treatment of cerebral edema, acute glaucoma, and conditions associated with tissue edema. Other agents are preferred for management of glaucoma, but mannitol can be administered in refractory cases. Mannitol also has been used to promote urinary excretion of certain toxins and in the management of anuric or oliguric renal failure.

### Precautionary Information

#### Adverse Reactions and Side Effects

Mannitol produces a profound diuresis and can cause significant fluid loss and electrolyte imbalance. An administration rate that is too rapid may expand the extracellular volume excessively.

#### Contraindications and Precautions

Do not use in patients who are dehydrated. Use cautiously when intracranial bleeding is suspected because it may increase bleeding. (This effect is controversial when dealing with intracranial hemorrhage.)

#### Drug Interactions

Do not administer simultaneously with blood replacements. If blood is administered simultaneously, sodium chloride must be added to each liter of mannitol (20 mEq/L). Mannitol may increase renal clearance of some drugs.

M

## Instructions for Use

Use only in animals in which fluid and electrolyte balance can be monitored.

## Patient Monitoring and Laboratory Tests

Monitor hydration and electrolyte balance in treated animals. Monitor intraocular pressure when treating acute glaucoma.

## Formulations

- Mannitol is available in a 5%, 10%, 15%, 20%, and 25% solution for injection. The 25% solution is equivalent to 1 g in 4-mL vials.

## Stability and Storage

Once solutions are prepared, discard unused portions. If solutions are chilled, crystals may form.

## Small Animal Dosage

### Dogs

- Diuretic: 1 g/kg of 5%–25% solution IV to maintain urine flow.
- Fluid expansion: 0.5–2 g/kg IV (or 0.1 g/kg/h).
- Glaucoma or central nervous system (CNS) edema: 0.25–2 g/kg of 15%–25% solution over 30–60 min IV (repeat in 6 hours if necessary).

### Cats

- Fluid expansion: 0.5 g/kg to 0.8 g/kg IV over 5 minutes followed by a CRI of 1 mg/kg/min.

## Large Animal Dosage

- 0.25–1 g/kg (20% solution) IV administered over 1 hour.
- Foals: 0.25–1 g/kg IV administered as 20% solution over 15–20 minutes.

## Regulatory Information

No regulatory information is available. Because of a low risk of residues, no withdrawal times are suggested.

# Marbofloxacin

mar-boe-floks'ah-sin

**Trade and other names:** Zeniquin and Marbocyl (European name)

**Functional classification:** Antibacterial

## Pharmacology and Mechanism of Action

Marbofloxacin is a veterinary fluoroquinolone antimicrobial. Marbofloxacin acts via inhibition of DNA gyrase in bacteria to inhibit DNA and RNA synthesis. Marbofloxacin is a bactericidal with a broad spectrum of activity. Susceptible bacteria include *Staphylococcus* spp., *Escherichia coli, Proteus mirabilis, Klebsiella pneumoniae,* and *Pasteurella* spp. *Pseudomonas aeruginosa* is moderately susceptible but requires higher concentrations. Some methicillin-resistant *Staphylococcus* species also may be resistant to fluoroquinolones. Marbofloxacin has poor activity against streptococci and anaerobic bacteria.

*Pharmacokinetics:* In dogs, the half-life is 7–14 hours (overall oral average is 12.4 hours), with a volume of distribution (VD) of 1.5–2 L/kg. In horses, the half-life has varied from 4.7–7.6 hours, depending on the study, with a VD of 1.5–2.8 L/kg. Oral absorption is close to 100% in small animals and approximately 60% in horses. In cattle, the half-lives are 5–9 hours in calves and 4–7 hours in ruminants. In preruminant calves, oral absorption is approximately 100%. In pigs, the half-life is 13–18 hours, with a VD of 1.6–1.75 L/kg, and oral absorption is 80%. In young pigs, the half-life is 13 hours.

## Indications and Clinical Uses

Marbofloxacin, like other fluoroquinolones, is used to treat susceptible bacteria in a variety of species. It is approved for use in dogs and cats in the United States and in other species outside the United States. Infections treated with marbofloxacin include skin and soft tissue infections, bone infections, urinary tract infections (UTIs), pneumonia, and infections caused by intracellular organisms. Marbofloxacin has been effective for some blood-borne pathogens such as *Mycoplasma haemofelis* in cats at a dosage of 2.75 mg/kg q24h PO for 14 days. Marbofloxacin also has been used in horses to treat infections caused by susceptible bacteria. In calves, it has been used to treat respiratory infections (bovine respiratory disease) at 2 mg/kg for 3–5 days or a single dose administered once at 8–10 mg/kg. In sows it is used to treat mastitis–metritis–agalactia (MMA) syndrome. In pigs, doses of 2 mg/kg and higher reached the therapeutic targets for swine respiratory disease pathogens. (See Regulatory Information regarding limitations for use in food animals in the United States.)

## Precautionary Information

### Adverse Reactions and Side Effects

High concentrations may cause CNS toxicity. Like other fluoroquinolones, it may cause some nausea, vomiting, weight loss, and diarrhea at high doses. When administered intravenously to anesthetized patients, it did not alter cardiovascular parameters. All of the fluoroquinolones may cause arthropathy in young animals. Dogs are most sensitive at 4–28 weeks of age. Large, rapidly growing dogs are the most susceptible. Marbofloxacin at a dose of twice the upper limit caused articular damage in dogs that were 4–5 months old. In cats 8 months old at dosages of 17 and 28 mg/kg for 42 days, articular cartilage injury was observed. Blindness in cats has been reported from some quinolones such as enrofloxacin and nalidixic acid. There are no known clinical reports of this reaction with marbofloxacin, and toxicity studies by the manufacturer showed that it does not cause ocular lesions or vision problems in cats. At doses of 17 and 28 mg/kg (three times and five times the upper limit of dosing, respectively), it did not produce ocular changes. Marbofloxacin has been administered to horses orally without producing adverse effects in the gastrointestinal (GI) tract.

**Contraindications and Precautions**

Avoid use in young animals because of risk of cartilage injury. Use cautiously in animals that may be prone to seizures.

**Drug Interactions**

Fluoroquinolones may increase concentrations of theophylline if used concurrently; there may be interactions with other drugs, but this is not well documented in animals. Co-administration with divalent and trivalent cations, such as products containing aluminum (e.g., sucralfate), iron, and calcium, may decrease oral absorption. Do not mix in solutions or in vials with aluminum, calcium, iron, or zinc because chelation may occur. Marbofloxacin may be administered with other antibiotics and anesthetic agents without evidence of drug interaction.

## Instructions for Use

Within the dose range listed for the approved products in the United States, generally, a dose of 5 mg/kg once daily PO is used for most indications. Doses published for European use are lower than US-approved doses, but there is no evidence that this has affected efficacy. For example, successful treatment of pyoderma in European studies has been accomplished with dosages of 2.0 mg/kg once daily, but in the United States, the lowest dosage is 2.75 mg/kg once daily.

## Patient Monitoring and Laboratory Tests

Susceptibility testing: Clinical and Laboratory Standards Institute (CLSI) breakpoints for susceptible organisms is ≤1 mcg/mL. If other fluoroquinolones are used to test susceptibility to marbofloxacin, the breakpoints may be different. When testing marbofloxacin activity against *P. aeruginosa*, a susceptible breakpoint of ≤0.25 mcg/mL should be used.

## Formulations

- Marbofloxacin is available in 25-, 50-, 100-, and 200-mg tablets.
- Injectable marbofloxacin (Marbocyl 10%, 100 mg/mL) is approved in other countries but not in the United States. Another formulation in Europe is Forcyl, which is a 16% solution for IM or IV injection.

## Stability and Storage

Store in a tightly sealed container, protected from light, and at room temperature. Do not compound with ingredients that may chelate with quinolones, such as iron or calcium.

## Small Animal Dosage

**Dogs**

- 2.75–5.5 mg/kg once daily PO.

**Cats**

- 2.75–5.5 mg/kg once daily PO.

## Large Animal Dosage

**Horses**

- 2 mg/kg once daily IV or PO for treatment of susceptible gram-negative bacteria (IV formulation not available in the United States). Because of the low oral absorption in horses, a dose of 2 mg/kg may not be sufficient for treating other bacteria that cause infections in horses, including gram-positive cocci. However, higher doses have not been tested.

**Calves**
- 2 mg/kg, IV, SQ, or IM in the neck once daily for 3–5 days or 8–10 mg/kg once IM.

**Pigs**
- 2 mg/kg once per day IM (neck) for 3–5 days or 8 mg/kg once.

### Regulatory Information
Marbofloxacin is prohibited from use in animals intended for food in the United States. There are no withdrawal times established because it should not be administered to animals that produce food. In the United States, it is illegal to administer fluoroquinolones to food animals in an extralabel manner. Outside the United States, withdrawal times have been established: 6 days withdrawal for meat in cattle at 2 mg/kg and 3 days at 8 mg/kg. Milk withdrawal is 36 hours at 2 mg/kg and 72 hours at 8 mg/kg. Withdrawal time for pigs is 4 days.

---

# Maropitant Citrate
mar-op′i-tent

**Trade and other names:** Cerenia

**Functional classification:** Antiemetic

---

### Pharmacology and Mechanism of Action
Maropitant is an antiemetic from the same group as the human drug aprepitant (Emend). These drugs act as antiemetics by blocking the neurokinin-1 (NK1) receptor (also known as substance P). NK1 is a neurotransmitter to simulate vomiting from the emetic center. It has less affinity for other neurokinin receptors (NK2 and NK3). Although NK1 receptors are involved in other physiologic and behavioral responses, at doses used to control vomiting, there were no adverse effects associated with blockade of other receptors. Maropitant can inhibit vomiting that is stimulated from both central and peripheral sources mediated by other neurotransmitters such as acetylcholine, histamine, dopamine, and serotonin. The NK1 receptor is also involved in transmission of pain (via substance P), and blockers of this receptor may have potential as adjunctive treatments for painful conditions.

Other drugs in this class used in people include aprepitant (Emend) and rolapitant (Varubi).

*Pharmacokinetics:* In dogs, the peak concentration is achieved approximately 45 minutes after SQ administration. The half-life was 4–8 hours, depending on the dose. Dose-dependent pharmacokinetics occur, with the clearance decreasing and half-life increasing with doses above 2 mg/kg. Because of nonlinear pharmacokinetics, accumulation is possible with repeated dosing. Oral absorption is 24% at 2 mg/kg and 37% at 8 mg/kg in dogs. Pharmacokinetics are not affected by feeding. In cats, the clearance is much lower than in dogs, and the half-life is longer than in dogs, at 13–17 hours. In cats, it has nearly complete SQ absorption and 50% oral absorption. In horses, oral doses produced similar concentrations as in dogs, with a half-life of approximately 11.6 hours.

### Indications and Clinical Uses
Maropitant is approved for use as an antiemetic in dogs to inhibit vomiting from both central and peripheral sources. It has been effective to inhibit vomiting from chemotherapy, GI disease, toxins, renal disease, vestibular stimuli (motion sickness), and circulating stimuli via the chemoreceptor trigger zone (CRTZ). After SQ injection, it has

a rapid onset with a peak concentration 45 minutes after injection and a duration of 24 hours. Maropitant also is approved for use in cats and has been used safely and effectively in cats to treat vomiting from a variety of sources, such as motion sickness and stimulation by emetogenic agents (alpha$_2$ agonists, opioids), with a duration of action of 24 hours.

Maropitant can be administered oral, SQ, or IV route. A recent change in labeling allows for administration IV. For dogs and cats with nausea and vomiting, other antiemetic agents can safely be added to the treatment. These agents include ondansetron, metoclopramide, and dopamine antagonists. In people, for highly emetogenic cancer chemotherapeutic agents, an NK1 receptor blocker is combined with a serotonin blocker (e.g., ondansetron) and dexamethasone. Although maropitant is an effective antiemetic agent, there are no studies to support the use for gastroesophageal reflux.

Blockade of the NK1 receptor may have potential as an adjunctive treatment for some types of pain (e.g., visceral pain). Experimental studies have shown effects, but at this time, there are no clinical studies to demonstrate analgesic effects from maropitant. Maropitant may have some antitussive properties. It has been examined in horses at an oral dose of 4 mg/kg, but clinical effects have not been reported. At a dosage of 2 mg/kg q48h, it can decrease coughing severity and frequency of coughing in dogs with chronic bronchitis but does not decrease airway inflammation.

## Precautionary Information

### Adverse Reactions and Side Effects

Maropitant may cause slight pain or irritation from SQ injection. It has been recognized that the pain is caused by alteration of the formulation, which may occur when the injectable formulation is stored at room temperature. The cyclodextrin complex of maropitant is preserved at cold temperatures and is more stable and intact when the formulation is refrigerated. Therefore, the adverse event associated with a painful injection can be reduced if injectable maropitant is stored in the refrigerator before use.

Safety studies have been conducted with maropitant in both preclinical and clinical trials. In experimental dogs, it was safe at three and five times the labeled dose. Adverse effects observed in trials included excess salivation and muscle tremors. In cats, it has been well tolerated at high doses (of a factor of 10 times) and is safe at 5 mg/kg for 15 consecutive days.

In horses, a dose of 4 mg/kg oral for 5 days produced bradycardia and heart block in some horses.

### Contraindications and Precautions

Decreased clearance and accumulation occur after repeated doses with higher doses. Therefore, because of risk of accumulation, the original label stated that it should not be administered for more than 5 consecutive days, and one should allow a 2-day washout period before instituting another course of treatment. However, follow-up studies and a new revised label indicate that it may be safely administered to dogs at 8 mg/kg for 14 consecutive days, and the label has been extended to indicate that it may be administered until the condition has been resolved in dogs 7 months of age and older. When treating protracted vomiting, veterinarians should attempt to identify any underlying disease whenever possible instead of relying on maropitant to control the clinical signs. Maropitant effects and pharmacokinetics are not affected by kidney disease.

### Drug Interactions

Single doses have been administered in an IV line, but precipitation may be observed if mixed with alkalinizing solutions. Maropitant is an NK1 inhibitor, and

M

other neurokinin receptors are affected to a lesser degree. Therefore, because of this unique mechanism of action, drug interactions have not been identified. Maropitant has been used safely with other drugs, including anesthetics, anticancer agents, and other antiemetic agents. Maropitant is highly protein bound, but it is not known if there are protein-binding interactions with other drugs.

## Instructions for Use

Clinical trials in dogs have outlined the appropriate protocols for the use of maropitant. It has been effective for a wide range of causes of vomiting in dogs. In dogs, it was more effective to prevent opiate-induced vomiting if administered at least 30 minutes prior to the opiate administration, but to prevent nausea, 60 minutes prior is suggested.

It is also approved in cats for prevention of vomiting. It has been effective for a variety of causes of vomiting, including motion sickness and stimulation from emetogenic agents. The effective dose in cats is 1 mg/kg, regardless of cause. Maropitant can be administered the day before a scheduled anesthetic procedure to reduce anesthetic-induced vomiting (see dosing section for protocol).

If maropitant alone is not sufficient to control nausea and vomiting, consider adding other antinausea agents such as ondansetron, metoclopramide, or dopamine antagonists.

## Patient Monitoring and Laboratory Tests

Monitor for clinical signs and disease that may be a cause for the vomiting. Other specific monitoring and tests are not needed to use maropitant safely.

## Formulations

- Maropitant is available in 16-, 24-, 60-, or 160-mg tablets and a 10-mg/mL injectable solution. The pH of the solution is 4.1–4.7.

## Stability and Storage

Store in a tightly sealed container, protected from light. The injectable formulation can be stored at room temperature and in the refrigerator, but as noted earlier, pain from injection can be reduced if the formulation is stored in the refrigerator. Discard vial after 28 days of first use.

## Small Animal Dosage

### Dogs

- 1 mg/kg SQ or IV or 2 mg/kg PO once daily for up to 5 days in dogs 2–7 months of age and until the problem is resolved for dogs older than 7 months.
- Motion sickness: 8 mg/kg PO once daily for up to 2 consecutive days.
- To prevent opioid-induced vomiting: 2–4 mg/kg PO or 1 mg/kg SQ or IV prior to anesthetic procedure.

### Cats

- 1 mg/kg once daily IV, SQ, or PO (same dose for all causes of vomiting, including motion sickness).
- To decrease vomiting from highly emetic agents in cats, administer at least 2–2.5 hours prior to the administration of another emetic drug.
- To decrease vomiting and nausea from kidney disease: 4 mg per cat per day PO.
- Prior to anesthesia: Administer 8 mg per cat (2.5 mg/kg) oral 18 hours prior to a scheduled anesthetic procedure to reduce anesthesia-induced vomiting. Alternatively, administer an SQ injection 20 hours prior to the scheduled anesthetic procedure.

## Large Animal Dosage
• No large animal doses have been identified.

## Regulatory Information
No regulatory information is available for food animals. There are no withdrawal times established, and it is not recommended to be administered to animals that produce food.

# Masitinib Mesylate

**Note:** Masitinib has been withdrawn from the market and is no longer available. Consult previous editions of this book for information on the pharmacology, clinical use, and dosing.

# MCT Oil
**Trade and other names:** Medium-chain triglycerides (MCT) oil
**Functional classification:** Nutritional supplement

M

## Pharmacology and Mechanism of Action
Medium-chain triglyceride (MCT) oil is an oil supplement used for animals. Specifically, MCT oil supplements triglycerides in animals.

## Indications and Clinical Uses
Medium-chain triglyceride oil is used to treat lymphangiectasia and as a component of enteral feeding formulas.

### Precautionary Information
**Adverse Reactions and Side Effects**
Adverse effects not reported in veterinary medicine. It may cause diarrhea in some patients.

**Contraindications and Precautions**
No contraindications reported.

**Drug Interactions**
No drug interactions reported.

## Instructions for Use
Results of clinical trials using MCT oil have not been reported. Many enteral feeding formulas contain MCT oil (many polymeric formulations).

## Patient Monitoring and Laboratory Tests
No specific monitoring is necessary.

## Formulations
• MCT oil is available as an oral liquid.

## Stability and Storage

Store in a tightly sealed container, protected from light, at room temperature, and in a cool place. Do not store in a plastic container. It may be mixed with fruit juices or food products prior to administration.

## Small Animal Dosage

• 1–2 mL/kg/day in food.

## Large Animal Dosage

• No large animal doses have been reported.

## Regulatory Information

No regulatory information is available. Because of a low risk of residues, no withdrawal times are suggested.

# Mebendazole
meh-ben′dah-zole

**Trade and other names:** Telmintic, Telmin, Vermox (human preparation), and generic brands

**Functional classification:** Antiparasitic

## Pharmacology and Mechanism of Action

Mebendazole is a benzimidazole antiparasitic drug used in veterinary medicine for many years. Like other benzimidazoles, mebendazole produces a degeneration of the parasite microtubule and irreversibly blocks glucose uptake in parasites. Inhibition of glucose uptake causes depletion of energy stores in the parasite, eventually resulting in death. However, there is no effect on glucose metabolism in mammals.

## Indications and Clinical Uses

Mebendazole is used in horses for treatment of infections caused by large roundworms (*Parascaris equorum*), large strongyles (*Strongylus edentatus, Strongylus equinus,* and *Strongylus vulgaris*), small strongyles, and mature and immature (fourth larval stage pinworms [*Oxyuris equi*]). In dogs, it has been used for treatment of infections of roundworms (*Toxocara canis*), hookworms (*Ancylostoma caninum* and *Uncinaria stenocephala*), whipworms (*Trichuris vulpis*), and tapeworms (*Taenia pisiformis*).

## Precautionary Information

### Adverse Reactions and Side Effects

Adverse effects are rare. It has been used for many years and has a high margin of safety. Mebendazole causes occasional vomiting and diarrhea in dogs. Some reports suggest idiosyncratic hepatic reactions in dogs, but it is not known if this is a significant risk.

### Contraindications and Precautions

No contraindications have been reported.

### Drug Interactions

No drug interactions have been reported for animals.

## Instructions for Use

The powder for horses may be sprinkled directly on the horse's grain or dissolved in 1 L of water and administered via stomach tube. For dogs, it may be added directly to food.

## Patient Monitoring and Laboratory Tests

No specific monitoring is necessary.

## Formulations

- Mebendazole is available in 40- or 166.7-mg/g powder, 200-mg/g equine paste, 33.3-mg/mL solution, and 100-mg chewable tablets (human preparation). Equine formulations contain either 83.3 mg of mebendazole plus 375 mg of trichlorfon or 100 mg of mebendazole plus 454 mg of trichlorfon in each gram of powder. The combination (Telmin) is a 33-mg/mL liquid suspension.

## Stability and Storage

Store in a tightly sealed container, protected from light, and at room temperature. Stability of compounded formulations has not been evaluated.

## Small Animal Dosage

**Dogs**

- 22 mg/kg (mixed with food) q24h for 3 days. May be repeated in 3 weeks.

## Large Animal Dosage

**Horses**

- 8.8 mg/kg PO.

## Regulatory Information

Do not administer to horses intended for food.

Withdrawal times are not established for animals that produce food. For extralabel use withdrawal interval estimates, contact Food Animal Residue Avoidance Databank (FARAD) at www.FARAD.org.

M

# Meclizine

mek'lih-zeen

**Trade and other names:** Antivert, Bonine, Meclozine (British name), and generic brands

**Functional classification:** Antiemetic, antihistamine

## Pharmacology and Mechanism of Action

Meclizine is an antiemetic from the antihistamine class. Like other antihistamines, it blocks the effect of histamine on the $H_1$ receptor. However, it also has central anticholinergic actions, which may be responsible for the central-acting antiemetic properties. The use in people is primarily for treating and preventing motion sickness, but the efficacy for this use is not established for animals.

## Indications and Clinical Uses

Meclizine is used to treat vomiting, particularly central-induced vomiting, such as motion sickness. It may suppress the CRTZ. The most common use in people is for treatment of motion sickness, but the use in animals has been primarily derived from empirical use and extrapolation of the use from human medicine. There are no well-controlled clinical studies or efficacy trials to document clinical effectiveness. The efficacy in dogs is not known, and antihistamines are not effective in cats for inhibiting vomiting. Other drugs with proven efficacy (e.g., maropitant) are often used instead of meclizine for vomiting.

## Precautionary Information

### Adverse Reactions and Side Effects
Adverse effects have not been reported in animals. Anticholinergic (atropine-like) effects may cause side effects, but these are not serious.

### Contraindications and Precautions
Use cautiously in animals with GI obstruction or glaucoma.

### Drug Interactions
No drug interactions have been reported for animals.

## Instructions for Use
Results of clinical studies in animals have not been reported. Use in animals is based on experience in people or anecdotal experiences in animals.

## Patient Monitoring and Laboratory Tests
No specific monitoring is necessary.

## Formulations
• Meclizine is available in 12.5-, 25-, and 50-mg tablets.

## Stability and Storage
Store in a tightly sealed container, protected from light, and at room temperature. Stability of compounded formulations has not been evaluated.

## Small Animal Dosage
### Dogs
• 25 mg per dog q24h PO (for motion sickness, administer 1 hour prior to traveling).

### Cats
• 12.5 mg per cat q24h PO (for motion sickness, administer 1 hour prior to traveling, but other agents are recommended because antihistamines are not effective in cats).

## Large Animal Dosage
• No large animal doses have been reported.

## Regulatory Information
Withdrawal times are not established for animals that produce food. For extralabel use withdrawal interval estimates, contact FARAD at www.FARAD.org.

# Meclofenamate Sodium and Meclofenamic Acid
mek′loe-fen′am-ate soe-dee′um and mek′loe-fen-am′ik ass′id

**Trade and other names:** Arquel and Meclofen

**Functional classification:** Nonsteroidal anti-inflammatory drug

## Pharmacology and Mechanism of Action
Meclofenamate is a nonsteroidal anti-inflammatory drug (NSAID) also known as meclofenamic acid. It is related to tolfenamic acid, which is approved in some

countries for animals. Meclofenamate and other NSAIDs have produced analgesic and anti-inflammatory effects by inhibiting the synthesis of prostaglandins. The enzyme inhibited by NSAIDs is the cyclooxygenase (COX) enzyme. The COX enzyme exists in two isoforms: COX-1 and COX-2. COX-1 is primarily responsible for synthesis of prostaglandins important for maintaining a healthy GI tract, renal function, platelet function, and other normal functions. COX-2 is induced and responsible for synthesizing prostaglandins that are important mediators of pain, inflammation, and fever. However, there may be some crossover of these properties. Meclofenamic acid is a balanced, nonselective COX-1–COX-2 inhibitor.

## Indications and Clinical Uses

Meclofenamate has been used in animals for treatment of pain and inflammation. The most common use has been musculoskeletal inflammation. This is an older NSAID and is no longer marketed in many countries. Therefore, the use in animals has diminished because of decreased availability and increased popularity of other drugs.

### Precautionary Information

**Adverse Reactions and Side Effects**

Adverse effects are not well known in animals because of infrequent use, but adverse effects common to other NSAIDs are possible. These side effects are generally GI in nature (e.g., gastritis, gastric ulcers).

**Contraindications and Precautions**

Do not administer to animals prone to GI ulcers. Do not administer with other ulcerogenic drugs such as corticosteroids. The original approved labeling for animals limited the duration of treatment to 5–7 days.

**Drug Interactions**

Like other NSAIDs, ulcerogenic effects are potentiated when administered with corticosteroids. Meclofenamic acid, like other NSAIDs, may interfere with the action of diuretics, such as furosemide, and angiotensin-converting enzyme inhibitors.

M

## Instructions for Use

Most of the experience with meclofenamate has been with horses. Commercial formulations are no longer marketed for animals in the United States. If it is available, administer with food.

## Patient Monitoring and Laboratory Tests

Monitor for signs of GI ulceration during use.

## Formulations

- Meclofenamate has been available in 50- and 100-mg capsules, but these are rarely available commercially any longer.
- 10- and 20-mg tablets (formulation for dogs) and granules for horses (5% meclofenamic acid). Neither of these forms may be available in most countries.

## Stability and Storage

Store in a tightly sealed container, protected from light, and at room temperature. Stability of compounded formulations has not been evaluated.

## Small Animal Dosage
**Dogs**
- 1.1 mg/kg/day for up to 5 days PO.

## Large Animal Dosage
**Horses**
- 2.2 mg/kg q24h PO.

## Regulatory Information
Withdrawal times are not established for animals that produce food. For extralabel use withdrawal interval estimates, contact FARAD at www.FARAD.org.
Racing Commissioners International (RCI) Classification: 4

---

# Medetomidine Hydrochloride
meh-deh-toe′mih-deen hye-droe-klor′ide

**Trade and other names:** Domitor

**Functional classification:** Analgesic, alpha$_2$ agonist

---

**Note:** The marketing of medetomidine has been discontinued in most countries and this product is no longer available. It has been replaced by dexmedetomidine (Dexdomitor), which consists of the active D-isomer. Consult section on dexmedetomidine for more information.

## Pharmacology and Mechanism of Action
Medetomidine is an alpha$_2$-adrenergic agonist. Alpha$_2$ agonists decrease the release of neurotransmitters from the neurons to inhibit pain pathways and suppress the CNS. Medetomidine is a racemic mixture containing 50% dexmedetomidine and 50% levomedetomidine. Dexmedetomidine is the active enantiomer of the mixture (D-isomer); therefore, on a milligram-per-milligram basis, dexmedetomidine is twice the potency of medetomidine but with the same pharmacologic activity and equivalent analgesic and sedative effects.

The proposed mechanism whereby the alpha$_2$ agonists decrease transmission is via binding to presynaptic alpha$_2$ receptors (negative feedback receptors). The result is decreased sympathetic outflow, analgesia, sedation, and anesthesia. Other drugs in this class include xylazine, detomidine, and clonidine. Receptor-binding studies indicate that alpha$_2$-/alpha$_1$-adrenergic receptor selectivity for medetomidine was more than 1000-fold greater than xylazine.

## Indications and Clinical Uses
Because of potency and availability, dexmedetomidine has replaced medetomidine for most indications in small animals. Medetomidine, like other alpha$_2$ agonists, is used as a sedative, anesthetic adjunct, and analgesic. Duration of effect is 0.5–1.5 hours at the low dose and up to 3 hours for the high dose. Compared with xylazine, medetomidine has produced better sedation and analgesia than xylazine in dogs. Medetomidine has been used with combinations of ketamine, butorphanol, or opioids in dogs for sedation and short-term procedures. Medetomidine combined with an opiate (butorphanol or hydromorphone) has produced a longer duration of sedation and more desirable degree of sedation than medetomidine used alone. It has been used to sedate animals for intradermal skin testing without affecting results.

## Precautionary Information
### Adverse Reactions and Side Effects
In small animals, vomiting is the most common initial effect. Alpha$_2$ agonists decrease sympathetic output. Cardiovascular depression may occur. A CRI of 1.5 mcg/kg/h has caused decreased heart rate and sinus arrhythmia in dogs. Doses as low as 1 mcg/kg IV can reduce cardiac output to less than 40% of resting value. Although medetomidine causes initial bradycardia and hypertension, the bradycardia usually does not require intervention with anticholinergic drugs (e.g., atropine). If adverse reactions are observed, reverse with atipamezole. If atipamezole is not available, yohimbine also can reverse medetomidine.

### Contraindications and Precautions
Use cautiously in animals with heart disease. The use may be contraindicated in older animals with pre-existing cardiac disease. Xylazine causes problems in pregnant animals, and this also should be considered for other alpha$_2$ agonists. Use cautiously in animals that are pregnant because it may induce labor. In addition, it may decrease oxygen delivery to the fetus in late gestation.

### Drug Interactions
Do not use with other drugs that may cause cardiac depression. Do not mix in a vial or syringe with other anesthetics, except as listed under the dosing section. Reverse with atipamezole at a dose of 25–300 mcg/kg IM. Use with opioid analgesic drugs greatly enhances the CNS depression, so consider lowering doses if administered with opioids.

M

## Instructions for Use
Medetomidine, dexmedetomidine, and detomidine are more specific for the alpha$_2$ receptor than xylazine. Dexmedetomidine has twice the potency of medetomidine. Therefore these drugs should not be used interchangeably without consulting the dose recommendations. The alpha$_2$ agonists may be used for sedation, analgesia, and minor surgical procedures. Many veterinarians use doses that are much less than the doses listed on the sponsor's label. For example, lower doses are sometimes used for short-term sedation and analgesia, particularly when combined with other drugs such as opioids. Reverse with atipamezole at a dose of 25–300 mcg/kg (equal to volume of medetomidine used) IM.

## Patient Monitoring and Laboratory Tests
Monitor vital signs during anesthesia. Monitor heart rate, blood pressure, and ECG if possible during anesthesia.

## Formulations
- Medetomidine has been available in a 1.0-mg/mL injection, but the commercial form has been discontinued in many countries and replaced by dexmedetomidine.

## Stability and Storage
Store in a tightly sealed container, protected from light, and at room temperature. Stability of compounded formulations has not been evaluated.

## Small Animal Dosage
### Dogs
- 750 mcg/m$^2$ IV or 1000 mcg/m$^2$ IM. The IV dose is equivalent to 18–71 mcg/kg IV.
- Lower doses are often used for short-term sedation and analgesia of 5–15 mcg/kg (0.005–0.015 mg/kg) IV, IM, or SQ. These doses may be increased up to

60 mcg/kg when severe pain is involved. 20 mcg/kg has been used in combination with butorphanol (0.2 mg/kg), hydromorphone (0.1 mg/kg), or ketamine for short-term procedures.

- CRI: Loading dose of 1 mcg/kg IV followed by 0.0015 mg/kg/h (1.5 mcg/kg/h). CRI may produce adverse cardiovascular effects and should be monitored closely.

**Cats**

- 750 mcg/m² IV or 1000 mcg/m² IM. The IV dose is equivalent to 18–71 mcg/kg IV. Doses in the lower range are used for short-term sedation and analgesia (e.g., 10–20 mcg/kg), but higher doses (up to 80 mcg/kg) have been used for more severe pain. Medetomidine may be administered IM or IV.
- Combination with ketamine: 5 mg/kg ketamine + 5 mcg/kg medetomidine mixed in one syringe and administered IM.

## Large Animal Dosage
**Lambs**

- 30 mcg/kg (0.03 mg/kg) IV.

**Horses**

- 10 mcg/kg IM as a sedative prior to induction for anesthesia. Some horses may need an additional dose of 4 mcg/kg IV. In horses, guaifenesin (5% solution) and ketamine (2.2 mg/kg) have been used in combination.

## Regulatory Information
Withdrawal times are not established for animals that produce food. For extralabel use withdrawal interval estimates, contact FARAD at www.FARAD.org.
RCI Classification: 3

# Medroxyprogesterone Acetate
meh-droks'ee-proe-jess'teh-rone ass'ih-tate
**Trade and other names:** Depo-Provera (injection), Provera (tablets), and Cycrin (tablets)
**Functional classification:** Hormone

## Pharmacology and Mechanism of Action
Medroxyprogesterone is a progestin hormone. Progestins are synthetic forms of the endogenous hormone progesterone. Medroxyprogesterone is a derivative of acetoxyprogesterone. Medroxyprogesterone acetate binds to the endogenous progesterone receptor and mimics progesterone's hormone effects. Medroxyprogesterone is more potent than progesterone and acts as an agonist for androgen and glucocorticoid receptors. In the Depo-Provera formulation, a single injection can produce long-acting effects. The half-life in cats is 12–17 hours following an oral dose but much longer (40–50 days) after an IM dose.

## Indications and Clinical Uses
Medroxyprogesterone acetate is used to replace progesterone in animals. Most often it is used as progesterone hormone treatment to control the estrus cycle, which is one of the uses in horses. It also is used for management of some behavioral and dermatologic disorders (e.g., urine spraying in cats and alopecia). However, its use for behavioral therapy in animals is discouraged because of high relapse rates and incidence of hormone-related adverse effects.

## Precautionary Information

### Adverse Reactions and Side Effects

Adverse effects include polyphagia, polydipsia, adrenal suppression (cats), increased risk of diabetes mellitus, pyometra, diarrhea, and increased risk of neoplasia. In cats, a single injection of medroxyprogesterone acetate has produced feline mammary fibroepithelial hyperplasia.

### Contraindications and Precautions

Do not use in animals at a high risk for diabetes. In humans, it increases the risk of thromboembolic problems. When used to suppress estrus in cats, it was effective but had negative after-effects on fertility and viability of kittens. Do not use in pregnant animals. Do not use in male cats for dermatologic problems or behavior treatment because of the risk of adverse effects.

### Drug Interactions

No drug interactions are reported. However, clearance of medroxyprogesterone is increased with drugs known to induce hepatic P450 enzymes (see Appendix H).

## Instructions for Use

Intervals of administration vary with condition. Intervals may range from once a week to once a month.

Clinical studies in animals have studied primarily the reproductive use. The effects on behavior and the dermatologic uses are based on anecdotal evidence or small observational studies. A similar drug is megestrol acetate and medroxyprogesterone acetate may have fewer side effects.

## Patient Monitoring and Laboratory Tests

It may increase concentrations of serum cholesterol and some liver enzymes.

## Formulations

- Medroxyprogesterone is available in 150- and 400-mg/mL suspension injection and 2.5-, 5-, and 10-mg tablets.

## Stability and Storage

Store in a tightly sealed container, protected from light, and at room temperature. Stability of compounded formulations has not been evaluated.

## Small Animal Dosage

### Dogs and Cats

- 1.1–2.2 mg/kg every 7 days IM.
- Suppression of estrus in cats: 0.05 mg/kg oral once daily. This dose may have a negative effect on fertility and newborn kittens when treatment is discontinued. To suppress estrus with the IM form, 2–2.5 mg/kg is injected and repeated once every 4–6 months.
- Behavior problems: 5 mg per dog once daily as needed.
- Prostatic disease (dogs): 3–5 mg/kg IM or SQ every 3–4 weeks.

## Large Animal Dosage

### Horses

- Prevent estrus: 250–500 mg/horse IM.

## Regulatory Information

There are no withdrawal times established because this drug should not be administered to animals that produce food.

# Megestrol Acetate
meh-jess'trole ass'ih-tate

**Trade and other names:** Ovaban and Megace

**Functional classification:** Hormone

## Pharmacology and Mechanism of Action

Megestrol acetate is a progestin, which is a synthetic form of progesterone. It binds to the same receptor as endogenous progesterone. Megestrol acetate is several times greater potency than endogenous progesterone. In addition, it has binding affinity for the androgen and glucocorticoid receptors, which is responsible for other effects. Megestrol acetate mimics the effects of progesterone in animals, which is used to regulate the reproductive cycle.

## Indications and Clinical Uses

Megestrol is used in animals as a progesterone hormone treatment to control the estrus cycle, which is most often to postpone the estrus cycle. It suppresses the ovulatory process by affecting secretion of estradiol by ovaries. It inhibits secretion of follicle-stimulating hormone and luteinizing hormone from the pituitary. It is also used in female dogs for the alleviation of false pregnancy. It also has been used for management of some behavioral and dermatologic disorders (e.g., urine spraying in cats and alopecia). However, its use for behavioral therapy in animals is discouraged because of high relapse rates and the incidence of hormone-related adverse effects.

In horses, it has been used to prevent estrus, but efficacy for this indication has not been good at doses of 10–20 mg/day per horse.

## Precautionary Information

### Adverse Reactions and Side Effects

Adverse effects include polyphagia, polydipsia, adrenal suppression (cats), increased risk of diabetes, pyometra, diarrhea, and increased risk of neoplasia. Adverse effects in cats are dose related. Low doses of 2.5 mg/wk can be tolerated for 30 weeks. Dosages greater than 0.625 mg/kg once daily can predispose to development of diabetes mellitus. High dosages in cats (0.625–1.25 mg/kg once daily or 2.5–5 mg/kg/wk) can lead to mammary gland lesions, uterine lesions, and more severe endocrine adverse effects.

### Contraindications and Precautions

Do not use in diabetic animals or animals that may be at risk for developing diabetes. Do not use in pregnant animals. Do not use prior to or during first estrus cycle in young animals. Do not use in the presence of a disease of the reproductive system or with mammary tumors. If estrus occurs within 30 days after cessation of treatment, mating should be prevented. Avoid use in cats for dermatologic problems or behavior treatment because of risk of adverse effects.

### Drug Interactions

No drug interactions are reported. However, clearance of medroxyprogesterone is increased with drugs known to induce hepatic P450 enzymes, and this may occur with megestrol acetate (see Appendix H).

## Instructions for Use

Clinical studies in animals have studied primarily the reproductive use. Effects on behavior and the dermatologic uses are based on anecdotal evidence or small observational studies. Medroxyprogesterone acetate, an alternate progestin, may have fewer side effects than megestrol acetate.

When used for proestrus treatment, administer 2.2 mg/kg for 8 days administered orally. For anestrus treatment, administer 0.55 mg/kg/day for 32 days. Tablets can be administered intact or crushed and mixed with food. When therapy is started, the animal should be confined for 3–8 days or until cessation of bleeding because dogs in proestrus accept a male.

## Patient Monitoring and Laboratory Tests

Because of risk of diabetes mellitus, monitor glucose concentrations during treatment periodically. Examination of vaginal smears is recommended to confirm detection of proestrus.

## Formulations

- Megestrol acetate is available in 5- and 20-mg tablets (veterinary preparation) and 20- and 40-mg tablets (human preparation).

## Stability and Storage

Store in a tightly sealed container, protected from light, and at room temperature. Stability of compounded formulations has not been evaluated.

## Small Animal Dosage

### Dogs

- Proestrus: 2 mg/kg q24h PO for 8 days (early proestrus).
- Anestrus: 0.5 mg/kg q24h PO for 32 days.
- Treatment of behavior problems: 2–4 mg/kg q24h for 8 days (reduce dose for maintenance).

### Cats

(See precautions listed above.)

- Dermatologic therapy or urine spraying: 2.5–5 mg/cat q24h PO for 1 week; then reduce to 5 mg once or twice a week per cat.
- Suppress estrus: 5 mg/day per cat for 3 days; then 2.5–5 mg once a week for 10 weeks (0.02 mg/kg). For long-term use (30 weeks), a lower dosage of 2.5 mg once per week should be used for greater safety.

## Large Animal Dosage

### Horses

- Suppress estrus: 0.5 mg/kg q24h PO.

## Regulatory Information

There are no withdrawal times established because this drug should not be administered to animals that produce food.

## Melarsomine Dihydrochloride

mel-ar′soe-meen

**Trade and other names:** Immiticide

**Functional classification:** Antiparasitic

## Pharmacology and Mechanism of Action

Melarsomine is an organic arsenical compound, primarily for treating heartworm disease in animals. Arsenicals alter glucose uptake and metabolism to eliminate heartworms. Melarsomine has replaced older arsenicals such as thiacetarsamide (Caparsolate) for treating heartworm disease.

## Indications and Clinical Uses

Melarsomine is used for heartworm adulticide therapy. See Instructions for Use for proper administration. Melarsomine is highly effective for eliminating heartworms in dogs. Efficacy in cats is only 36% and not recommended. Usually, cats are not treated because it is a self-limiting disease, and only supportive treatment is administered (corticosteroids, bronchodilators, and antiemetics).

## Precautionary Information

### Adverse Reactions and Side Effects

Melarsomine administration may lead to pulmonary thromboembolism 7–20 days after therapy, anorexia (13% incidence), injection-site reaction (32% incidence of myositis), or lethargy or depression (15% incidence). It causes elevations of hepatic enzymes. To prevent adverse reactions of adulticide therapy, the American Heartworm Society recommends a three-dose protocol, whereby the first dose is administered after 2 months of a macrocyclic lactone (e.g., ivermectin) and doxycycline. To limit lung injury, administer prednisolone or prednisone at a dosage of 0.5 mg/kg q12h for the first week after adulticide treatment and 0.5 mg/kg q24h for the second week followed by 0.5 mg/kg every other day for 1–2 weeks.

High doses (three times the dose) can cause pulmonary inflammation and death. If high doses are administered, dimercaprol (3 mg/kg IM) may be used as antidote.

Killing adult heartworms in cats with adulticide treatment can cause anaphylactic reactions, thromboembolism, and fatal reactions in cats.

### Contraindications and Precautions

Use cautiously in animals with high heartworm burden and use the three-dose protocol to reduce lung injury. Melarsomine may be contraindicated in dogs with class 4 (very severe) heartworm disease until the worm burden is reduced.

Melarsomine is not recommended for cats because adulticide treatment can produce severe and even fatal reactions.

### Drug Interactions

No drug interactions are reported. Administration of prednisolone does not affect efficacy of melarsomine.

## Instructions for Use

The most accurate and up-to-date treatment protocol is available from the American Heartworm Society (https://www.heartwormsociety.org). Follow the product insert carefully for instructions on proper injection technique. Also evaluate patient to determine class of heartworm disease (class 1–4) before initiating treatment. Class 1 and 2 are least severe. Class 3 is severe, and class 4 is the most severe and should not be treated with an adulticide before decreasing the heartworm burden.

The current three-dose protocol includes starting pretreatment with a macrocyclic lactone (e.g., ivermectin) and doxycycline (or minocycline) for 2 months and then allowing a 1-month waiting period starting on day 60. After this waiting period, administer melarsomine on day 60, wait another month, and administer the second and third doses of melarsomine on days 90 and 91. Each melarsomine dose is

2.5 mg/kg. This protocol will reduce lung and pulmonary vessel reaction associated with heartworm treatment.

Avoid human exposure by either washing hands after handling or wearing gloves. There should be strict exercise restriction in dogs during adulticide treatment.

### Patient Monitoring and Laboratory Tests
Monitor heartworm status and microfilaria after treatment. Monitor treated patients carefully for signs of pulmonary thromboembolism.

### Formulations
• Melarsomine is available in a 25-mg/mL injection.

### Stability and Storage
After reconstitution, solution retains potency for 24 hours. Do not freeze solutions after they are prepared.

### Small Animal Dosage
**Dogs**
• Administer via deep IM injection. Follow guidelines from the American Heartworm Society for the safest and most effective use of melarsomine.
• Three-dose protocol: One injection on days 60, 90, and 91 after the initial diagnosis.

**Cats**
• Not recommended because of adverse reactions.

### Large Animal Dosage
• No large animal doses have been reported.

### Regulatory Information
There are no withdrawal times established because this drug should not be administered to animals that produce food.

M

## Meloxicam
mel-oks'ih-kam

**Trade and other names:** Metacam, OroCAM, Meloxidyl, Loxicom (veterinary preparations), Mobic and Vivlodex (human preparation), Metacam suspension (equine preparation, Europe), and Mobicox (human formulation in Canada)

**Functional classification:** Anti-inflammatory

### Pharmacology and Mechanism of Action
Meloxicam is an NSAID of the oxicam class. Like other NSAIDs, meloxicam has analgesic and anti-inflammatory effects by inhibiting the synthesis of prostaglandins. The enzyme inhibited by NSAID is the COX enzyme. The COX enzyme exists in two isoforms: COX-1 and COX-2. COX-1 is primarily responsible for synthesis of prostaglandins important for maintaining a healthy

GI tract, renal function, platelet function, and other normal functions. COX-2 is induced and responsible for synthesizing prostaglandins that are important mediators of pain, inflammation, and fever. However, it is known that there is some crossover of COX-1 and COX-2 effects, and COX-2 activity is important for some biological effects. Meloxicam is relatively COX-1 sparing compared with older NSAIDs, but it is not known if the specificity for COX-1 or COX-2 is related to efficacy or safety.

*Pharmacokinetics:* Meloxicam has a half-lives of 23–24 hours in dogs, 30–40 hours in calves, and 8.5 (range, 5–14.5) in horses. In cats, it had a half-life of 15 hours in experimental cats, but in a larger population pharmacokinetic study, the half-life was 26 hours, with VD of 0.24 L/kg. Meloxicam is highly protein bound. Oral absorption is almost complete in dogs when administered with food.

Absorption is high in horses and is not affected significantly by feeding. Various oral dose forms (tablets, paste, suspension, granules) can be used interchangeably in horses because of similar pharmacokinetics. Protein binding in horses is 97%. The half-life in horses is 12.4 hours from IV injection, 24–34 hours from oral granules, varies from 6.4–13 hours for the oral suspension and varies from 5.2–12 hours for the oral tablets. The oral absorption rates were 100% from the oral granules, 75%–98% from the oral suspension, and 80%–90% from oral tablets.

Oral absorption rates were 100% in ruminant calves, with a half-life of 20–43 hours, and 79% and 72% in goats and sheep, respectively.

## Indications and Clinical Uses

Meloxicam is used to decrease pain, inflammation, and fever. It has been used for the acute and chronic treatment of pain and inflammation in dogs and cats. One of the most common uses is osteoarthritis, but it has also been used for pain associated with surgery. Both acute and long-term safety and efficacy have been established for dogs. In studies performed in dogs, higher doses (up to 0.5 mg/kg) were more effective than lower doses but also were associated with a higher incidence of GI adverse effects.

The initial labeling in the United States is limited to either short-term use, but long-term use at low doses has been established through approval in other countries and consensus guidelines from feline medicine experts. In cats, meloxicam has comparable, and even superior, effectiveness compared with butorphanol for treating pain associated with surgery. Acute response to treating fever in cats also has been demonstrated.

In European countries, it is registered for use in horses, pigs, and cattle, but in the United States, this is an extralabel use. In pigs, meloxicam is effective for MMA syndrome. In horses, meloxicam is effective for treating pain and inflammation associated with surgery. A dosage of 0.6 mg/kg per day to horses for long periods (6 weeks) is well tolerated and produces plasma drug concentrations in the therapeutic range. In the countries where it is approved, the accepted use is adjunctive therapy of acute respiratory disease, diarrhea, and acute mastitis. It has also been effective to decrease discomfort associated with dehorning procedures in cattle. Meloxicam also is used extralabel in many exotic and zoo animals, including reptiles and birds, for treatment of pain and inflammation.

## Precautionary Information

### Adverse Reactions and Side Effects

Major adverse effects are GI, including vomiting, diarrhea, and ulceration. Because meloxicam appears to be relatively COX-1 sparing, adverse effects are expected to be less than other NSAIDs that are not as selective. However, this property has not been demonstrated on controlled clinical trials and may be dependent on dose and species. Kidney injury, especially in dehydrated animals or animals with pre-existing renal disease, has been shown for some NSAIDs. Kidney injury has been reported in dogs from doses of 0.3–0.5 mg/kg and higher. GI ulceration has been observed when dogs were administered doses higher than approved doses. In cats at high doses (five times the dose), vomiting and other GI problems were reported. With repeated doses (9 days) of 0.3 mg/kg/day to cats, inflamed GI mucosa and ulceration were observed. At a lower dose of 0.05 mg/kg in cats, there were not changes on platelet aggregation. Kidney injury has been observed in cats, particularly when high doses were administered repeatedly or when administered at lower doses to dehydrated cats. However, there is no evidence that well-hydrated cats with kidney disease are more dependent on renal prostaglandins to maintain kidney perfusion; therefore, meloxicam may be administered to these cats at low doses if hydration is maintained.

At the recommended dose of 0.6 mg/kg to horses, it has been well tolerated, but at high doses to horses (3–5 times the recommended dose), there were decreased protein, GI injury, and kidney injury.

### Contraindications and Precautions

Dogs and cats with pre-existing GI problems or kidney disease may be at a greater risk of adverse effects from NSAIDs. However, at a dosage of 0.02 mg/kg/day, long-term use in cats did not cause deterioration of renal disease in cats with pre-existing kidney disease. Safety in pregnant animals is not known, but adverse effects have not been reported. The oral meloxicam solution of meloxicam contains xylitol. Xylitol is an artificial sweetener that can be toxic to dogs and can produce hypoglycemia and liver injury with high doses exceeding 0.1 g/kg. With approved doses of meloxicam oral solution, the toxic level of xylitol is not likely to be exceeded, but one should be cautious about adding other drugs that also contain xylitol.

### Drug Interactions

Do not administer with other NSAIDs or with corticosteroids. Corticosteroids have been shown to exacerbate the GI adverse effects. Some NSAIDs may interfere with the action of diuretic drugs and ACE inhibitors.

## Instructions for Use

The liquid medication may be added to food for dosing. When using the veterinary liquid formulation, the dropper bottle for the 1.5-mg/mL suspension is designed to deliver 0.05 mg per drop or 1 drop per pound body weight (2 drops per kilogram body weight). Observe the manufacturer's instructions when using dosing syringes supplied with products.

Some veterinarians have used the human generic tablets for administration to horses and dogs. The human formulation has been shown to be absorbed to the same extent as the veterinary formulations. However, caution is advised when administering the oral human tablets to dogs. The tablet size (7.5 mg) is much larger than the highest dose that should be administered to most dogs.

Administration to cats in the United States is only approved as a single dose of 0.3 mg/kg. However, long-term use at 0.05 mg/kg q24h PO has been approved for cats in other countries for prolonged use, and low doses of 0.01–0.03 mg/kg q24h have been administered safely to older cats with kidney disease.

## Patient Monitoring and Laboratory Tests

Monitor GI signs for evidence of diarrhea, GI bleeding, or ulcers. Because of the risk of renal injury, monitor renal parameters (water consumption, blood urea nitrogen, creatinine, and urine-specific gravity) periodically during treatment. Plasma concentration are usually not measured during treatment, but effective concentrations are in the range of 0.13–0.27 mcg/mL.

## Formulations

- Meloxicam is available in 0.5-mg/mL (0.02 mg per drop) oral suspension, 1.5-mg/mL (0.05 mg per drop) oral suspension, and 0.5% (5-mg/mL) injection.
- An oral transmucosal is available as a spray using the Promist technology. The spray is available in three sizes: 0.25 mg, 0.5 mg, and 1.075 mg per spray.
- In Europe, 1.0- and 2.5-mg/kg tablets are available for dogs, and a 15-mg/mL oral suspension is available for horses.
- Large animals: In countries other than the United States, there is a 50-mg/g oral paste available for horses, a 20-mg/mL injectable solution, and granules for horses in a 330 mg per sachet for oral administration.
- Human-label tablets: 7.5- and 15-mg tablets (generic) and 5- and 10- mg capsules (Vivlodex).

## Stability and Storage

Meloxicam has been compounded with water, 1% methylcellulose gel, and simple syrup or a suspending and flavoring vehicle in a ratio of 1:1 at concentrations of 0.25, 0.5, and 1.0 mg/mL. These formulations were stable for 28 days at room temperature or under refrigeration.

## Small Animal Dosage

### Dogs

- 0.2 mg/kg initial loading dose PO, SQ, or IV and then 0.1 mg/kg q24h thereafter PO, SQ, or IV.
- Oral transmucosal spray (bioequivalent to oral suspension): 0.1 mg/kg sprayed in the dog's mouth once per day.

### Cats

- 0.05 mg/kg q24h PO, with a reduction in dose if chronic treatment is pursued. Long-term treatment may be reduced to 0.03 mg/kg q24h or 0.05 mg/kg q48h to 0.05 mg/kg q72h PO.
- Single doses of 0.15–0.3 mg/kg SQ may be administered for short-term use. The manufacturer does not recommend a second dose of meloxicam injection to cats.

## Large Animal Dosage

### Pigs

- 0.4 mg/kg IM, which may be repeated in 24 hours.

### Cattle

- 0.5 mg/kg q24h IV, IM, or SQ.

### Sheep and Small Ruminants

- 1 mg/kg, single dose, IV, IM, SQ, or PO.

### Horses

- 0.6 mg/kg q24h IV or PO. In foals younger than 7 weeks of age, the frequency may be increased to 0.6 mg/kg q12h because of more rapid clearance. The various oral dose forms for horses (tablets, suspension, granules, paste) can be used interchangeably with similar results The oral dose for horses may be administered with or without food or with molasses without affecting oral absorption.

## Regulatory Information

Recommended withdrawal time for racing horses is 3 days for urine testing. In countries where meloxicam is approved for food animals, the withdrawal times are 15 days for meat and 5 days for milk at a dose of 0.5 mg/kg IM, SQ, or IV. The Canadian withdrawal times are 20 days for meat, and 96 hours for milk.

In the United States, FARAD (www.FARAD.org) recommends a 21-day withdrawal time after oral administration (single dose) and 30 days when multiple doses are administered. Withdrawal time for milk is 3.5–6 days, depending on the study and country of approval.

RCI Classification: 3

# Melphalan
mel′fah-lan

**Trade and other names:** Alkeran

**Functional classification:** Anticancer agent

## Pharmacology and Mechanism of Action

Melphalan is an anticancer agent used infrequently in veterinary medicine. Melphalan is an alkylating agent, similar in action to cyclophosphamide. It alkylates base pairs in DNA and produces a cytotoxic effect. It is absorbed orally, which is an advantage for treating animals in some protocols.

## Indications and Clinical Uses

Melphalan is not used as an anticancer agent as frequently as other alkylating agents. In animals, the most common use is to treat multiple myeloma and certain carcinomas. It has been used in dogs for refractory cases of lymphoma, in combination with prednisone. For canine multiple myeloma, the treatment of choice is a combination of melphalan and prednisone. For cats, the treatment is a combination of melphalan and prednisolone.

## Precautionary Information

### Adverse Reactions and Side Effects

Adverse effects are related to its action as an anticancer agent. Melphalan causes myelosuppression, with neutropenia being the most common.

### Contraindications and Precautions

Do not use in animals with bone marrow suppression.

### Drug Interactions

No drug interactions are reported. It has been used with other anticancer drug protocols.

## Instructions for Use

Consult specific anticancer drug protocols for more dosing information.

M

## Patient Monitoring and Laboratory Tests
Monitor complete blood count (CBC) for evidence of bone marrow toxicity.

## Formulations Available
• Melphalan is available in 2-mg tablets and 50-mg vials for injection.

## Stability and Storage
Store in a tightly sealed container, protected from light, and at room temperature. It is insoluble in water but is soluble in ethanol. After reconstitution, decomposition occurs rapidly and may precipitate. Use within 1 hour of reconstitution. When prepared in a compounded formulation for oral use, it was unstable with rapid decomposition (80% loss in 24 hours).

## Small Animal Dosage
### Dogs
• 1.5 mg/m² (or 0.1–0.2 mg/kg) q24h PO for 7–10 days (repeat every 3 weeks) or administer 7 mg/m² q24h PO for 5 days. Repeat this cycle every 21 days.
• Injectable forms have not been used in animals, but in humans, 16 mg/m² IV over 15–20 minutes has been used at 2-week intervals for multiple myeloma.

### Cats
• 2 mg per cat PO (equivalent to 0.1 mg/kg per day). The interval used has varied for treatment of multiple myeloma from every 2 days, up to every 7 days.

## Large Animal Dosage
• No large animal doses have been reported.

## Regulatory Information
Withdrawal times are not established for animals that produce food. This drug should not be used in animals intended for food because it is an anticancer agent.

---

# Meperidine Hydrochloride
meh-pare'ih-deen hye-droe-klor'ide

**Trade and other names:** Demerol and Pethidine (European name)

**Functional classification:** Analgesic, opioid

## Pharmacology and Mechanism of Action
Meperidine is a synthetic opioid agonist with activity primarily at the mu-opiate receptor. It is called pethidine in Europe. It is similar in action to morphine, except with approximately one seventh of the potency. An IM injection of 75 mg or an oral dose of 300 mg of meperidine has similar potency to 10 mg of morphine. Clearance is rapid in small animals after meperidine administration, and duration of effect is short.

## Indications and Clinical Uses
Meperidine has been used for short-term sedative effects, often used with other sedatives or anesthetics. For analgesic use, it is short acting, usually less than 2 hours and often much shorter. Therefore, its use for treating pain has not been popular and has been replaced by other opioid drugs. Meperidine may produce fewer GI motility problems compared with other opioids, but this has not been enough of an advantage

to justify common use. The use of meperidine in human medicine has declined because toxic effects have been observed from accumulation of metabolites.

## Precautionary Information

### Adverse Reactions and Side Effects

Like all opiates, some side effects are predictable and unavoidable. Side effects include sedation, urine retention, constipation, and bradycardia. Respiratory depression occurs with high doses. Tolerance and dependence occur with chronic administration. Repeated doses in humans may cause toxicity from accumulation of metabolite. One of the metabolites, normeperidine, accumulates with repeated administration because it has a half-life much longer than meperidine. The accumulation of the metabolite causes excitatory effects that may be related to serotonergic properties. Similar reactions have not been reported from clinical use in animals (see Drug Interactions for other precautions), but the use has been infrequent in animals, and these reactions may not have been reported.

### Contraindications and Precautions

Meperidine is a Schedule II controlled substance. Cats are more sensitive to excitement than other species, although they have tolerated meperidine relatively well. Avoid repeated doses because accumulation of metabolites may be toxic.

### Drug Interactions

Meperidine should not be administered with monoamine oxidase inhibitors (MAOIs), such as selegiline. Meperidine and metabolites may inhibit reuptake of serotonin and cause excess serotonin effect, especially if combined with other drugs that produce similar action, such as selective serotonin reuptake inhibitors (SSRIs; e.g., fluoxetine), tricyclic antidepressants (e.g., clomipramine), or other analgesics such as tramadol.

M

## Instructions for Use

Although comparative clinical studies have not been conducted in animals, meperidine may be effective for short duration but has not been used for long-term pain management.

## Patient Monitoring and Laboratory Tests

Monitor patient's heart rate and respiration. Although bradycardia rarely needs to be treated when it is caused by an opioid, atropine can be administered if necessary. If serious respiratory depression occurs, the opioid can be reversed with naloxone.

## Formulations

- Meperidine is available in 50- and 100-mg tablets; 10-mg/mL syrup; and 25-, 50-, 75-, and 100-mg/mL injection.

## Stability and Storage

Store in a tightly sealed container, protected from light, and at room temperature. It is soluble in water. It may be mixed with 0.9% saline or 5% dextrose for 28 days without loss of potency or stability. It is stable in syrup formulation. Protect from freezing.

## Small Animal Dosage

### Dogs

- 5–10 mg/kg IV or IM as often as every 2–3 hours (or as needed).

### Cats

- 3–5 mg/kg IV or IM every 2–4 hours (or as needed).

## Large Animal Dosage

- No large animal doses have been reported.

## Regulatory Information

Schedule II controlled drug.

Withdrawal times are not established for animals that produce food. For extralabel use withdrawal interval estimates, contact FARAD at www.FARAD.org.

RCI Classification: 1

# Mepivacaine
meh-piv'ah-kane

**Trade and other names:** Carbocaine-V

**Functional classification:** Local anesthetic

## Pharmacology and Mechanism of Action

Mepivacaine is a local anesthetic of the amide class. It inhibits nerve conduction via sodium channel blockade. It has medium potency and duration of action compared with bupivacaine. Compared with lidocaine, it is longer acting but has equal potency.

## Indications and Clinical Uses

Mepivacaine is used as a local anesthetic for local infiltration epidural analgesia/anesthesia. The use in animals is not as common as with lidocaine or bupivacaine.

## Precautionary Information

### Adverse Reactions and Side Effects

Adverse effects are rare with local infiltration. High doses absorbed systemically can cause nervous system signs (tremors and convulsions), but this rarely occurs. After epidural administration, respiratory paralysis is possible with high doses. Mepivacaine may cause less irritation to tissues than lidocaine.

### Contraindications and Precautions

No contraindications have been reported for animals.

### Drug Interactions

No drug interactions have been reported.

## Instructions for Use

For epidural use, do not exceed 8 mg/kg total dose. Duration of epidural analgesia is 2.5–3 hours.

## Patient Monitoring and Laboratory Tests

No specific monitoring is necessary.

## Formulations

Mepivacaine is available in a 2% (20-mg/mL) injection.

## Stability and Storage

Store in a tightly sealed container, protected from light, and at room temperature. Stability of compounded formulations has not been evaluated.

## Small Animal Dosage
### Dogs and Cats
- Local infiltration dose varies depending on site. Generally, 0.5–3 mL of 2% solution is used.
- Epidural: 0.5 mL of 2% solution every 30 seconds until reflexes are absent.

## Large Animal Dosage
### Horses
- Intraarticular: 150 mg (7.5 mL) injected into horse joint. Other doses are variable doses used for local infiltration, depending on the need.

## Regulatory Information
No regulatory information is available. Because of a low risk of residues when used for local infiltration, no withdrawal times are suggested.
Horses: Clearance prior to racing is approximately 2 days.
RCI Classification: 2

---

# Mercaptopurine
mer-kap-toe-pyoo′reen

**Trade and other names:** Purinethol

**Functional classification:** Anticancer agent

M

## Pharmacology and Mechanism of Action
Mercaptopurine is an anticancer agent used infrequently in veterinary medicine. Mercaptopurine is an antimetabolite agent that inhibits synthesis of purines in cancer cells. It is cell-cycle specific and acts at the S-phase of cell division. A related drug is azathioprine. Administration of azathioprine is metabolized to 6 mercaptopurine, which is further metabolized to cytotoxic products.

## Indications and Clinical Uses
Mercaptopurine has been used for various forms of cancer, including leukemia and lymphoma. Because of availability of other agents and lack of studies to evaluate protocols using mercaptopurine, it is infrequently used in veterinary medicine.

## Precautionary Information
### Adverse Reactions and Side Effects
Many side effects are possible that are common to anticancer therapy (many of which are unavoidable), including bone marrow suppression and anemia.

### Contraindications and Precautions
Do not use in animals with known sensitivity to azathioprine. Do not administer to cats.

### Drug Interactions
No drug interactions are reported. It has been used with other anticancer drug protocols.

## Instructions for Use
Consult the specific anticancer protocol for specific regimen.

## Patient Monitoring and Laboratory Tests
Monitor CBC for evidence of bone marrow toxicity.

## Formulations
• Mercaptopurine is available in 50-mg tablets.

## Stability and Storage
Store in a tightly sealed container, protected from light, and at room temperature. It is prone to oxidation if mixed with alkaline solutions. pH of solutions should be below 8. If mixed with oral vehicles, such as syrups, it is stable for 14 days.

## Small Animal Dosage
**Dogs**
• 50 mg/m$^2$ q24h PO.

**Cats**
• Contraindicated.

## Large Animal Dosage
• No large animal doses have been reported.

## Regulatory Information
Withdrawal times are not established for animals that produce food. This drug should not be used in animals intended for food because it is an anticancer agent.

# Meropenem
meer-oh-pen'em

**Trade and other names:** Merrem

**Functional classification:** Antibacterial

## Pharmacology and Mechanism of Action
Meropenem is a beta-lactam antibiotic of the carbapenem class (also known as penems) with broad spectrum of activity similar to or greater than imipenem. Action on the cell wall is similar to other beta-lactams, which is to bind penicillin-binding proteins (PBPs) that weaken or interfere with cell wall formation. The carbapenems bind to a specific PBP (PBP-1) that results in more rapid lysis compared with other beta-lactams. This results in greater bactericidal activity and a longer postantibiotic effect. Meropenem is the most active of all beta-lactams and active against aerobic and anaerobic gram-positive and gram-negative bacteria. The spectrum of activity includes gram-negative bacilli, including Enterobacteriaceae, *P. aeruginosa*, and *Acinetobacter* spp. It also is active against most gram-positive bacteria, except methicillin-resistant strains of *Staphylococcus* spp. It is not active against *Enterococcus* spp. Other related carbapenems are doripenem, imipenem, and ertapenem.

*Pharmacokinetics:* In dogs, the average from multiple studies is a half-life of 0.75 hour (± 0.9), and a volume of distribution of 0.29 L/kg (± 0.056). Systemic clearance is 0.335 L/kg/h (± 0.05). In cats the half-life for IV, IM, and SQ administration is 1.35, 2.10, and 2.26 hours, respectively. The volume of distribution in cats is 0.2 L/kg. Absorption from IM and SC in cats is near 100%.

## Indications and Clinical Uses
Meropenem is indicated primarily for infections caused by bacteria resistant to other drugs. It is especially valuable for treating resistant infections caused by *P. aeruginosa,*

*E. coli,* and *K. pneumoniae.* It is active against these strains that produce extended-spectrum beta-lactamase that are resistant to penicillins, cephalosporins, and other agents. Meropenem is slightly more active against some bacteria than imipenem and more active against *P. aeruginosa* than ertapenem. The use of meropenem in animals should be reserved for cases that have infections resistant to other antibiotics and when the infection is confirmed with a culture and susceptibility test.

---

### Precautionary Information

**Adverse Reactions and Side Effects**

Carbapenems pose similar risks as other beta-lactam antibiotics, but adverse effects are rare. Meropenem does not cause seizures as frequently as imipenem and has been well tolerated even in critically ill patients. SQ injections may cause slight hair loss at the injection site but otherwise is well tolerated.

**Contraindications and Precautions**

Some slight yellowish discoloration may occur after reconstitution. Slight discoloration will not affect potency. However, a darker amber or brown discoloration may indicate oxidation and loss of potency.

**Drug Interactions**

Do not mix in a vial or syringe with other antibiotics.

---

### Instructions for Use

Doses in animals have been based on pharmacokinetic studies rather than efficacy trials. Meropenem is more soluble than imipenem and can be injected via bolus rather than administered in fluid solutions. Meropenem has been injected SQ in dogs and cats with little pain or discomfort and no evidence of tissue reaction except for some slight hair changes at the injection site in cats.

### Patient Monitoring and Laboratory Tests

Susceptibility testing: CLSI breakpoint for susceptible bacteria is ≤1 mcg/mL for Enterobacteriaceae (*E. coli, Klebsiella pneumoniae*), and ≤2 mcg/mL for *P. aeruginosa* and *Acinetobacter* spp. If bacteria are susceptible to imipenem, they are also susceptible to meropenem.

### Formulations

• Meropenem is available in a 500-mg or 1-g vial; both produce 50 mg/mL after reconstitution for injection. Reconstitute with sodium chloride, Ringer's solution, or lactated Ringer's solution.

### Stability and Storage

Stable if stored in manufacturer's original vial. In heat and alkaline conditions, the drug may hydrolyze to meropenemic acid. At room temperature, IV solutions are stable for 12 hours. After reconstitution to a concentration of 50 mg/mL, it is stable in the refrigerator for 3 days. After 3 days, the potency declines to below 90%. Slight yellow discoloration may occur without loss of potency but observe for a darker color change as an indication that potency may be compromised during storage. Discard if particulates form in vial.

### Small Animal Dosage

**Dogs**

• Enterobacteriaceae (*E. coli, K. pneumoniae*): 10 mg/kg q8h, IV, IM, or SQ.
• *Pseudomonas aeruginosa:* 30 mg/kg, q8h, IV, IM, or SQ.
• CRI: 1 mg/kg IV; follow with a 1-mg/kg/h infusion.

**Cats**
- 10 mg/kg IM, SQ, or IV q12h.

### Large Animal Dosage
- No large animal doses have been reported. However, doses similar to the range used in small animals are suggested for foals.

### Regulatory Information
Withdrawal times are not established for animals that produce food. For extralabel use withdrawal interval estimates, contact FARAD at www.FARAD.org.

# Mesalamine
mez-ahl'ah-meen

**Trade and other names:** 5-aminosalicylic acid, Asacol, Mesasal, Pentasa, and Mesalazine

**Functional classification:** Antidiarrheal

### Pharmacology and Mechanism of Action
Mesalamine is also known as 5-aminosalicylic acid. It is the active component of sulfasalazine, which is commonly administered for treatment of colitis. (See Sulfasalazine and Olsalazine for additional information.) The action of mesalamine is not precisely known, but it appears to suppress the metabolism of arachidonic acid in the intestine. It inhibits both COX- and lipoxygenase-mediated mucosal inflammation. Systemic absorption is low; most of the action is believed to be local. Four formulations of mesalamine have been used:

1. Asacol. Asacol is a tablet coated with an acrylic-based resin. The resin dissolves at a pH of 7.0 and is designed to release 5-aminosalicylic acid in the colon.
2. Mesasal. Mesasal is a tablet coated with an acrylic-based resin that dissolves at a pH greater than 6.0. It is designed to release 5-aminosalicylic acid in the terminal ileum and colon. Approximately 35% of the salicylate is absorbed systemically. The dosage in people is 1–1.5 g/day.
3. Olsalazine sodium (Dipentum). Olsalazine is a dimer of two molecules of 5-aminosalicylic acid linked by an azo bond that is released by bacterial digestion in the colon. It is used in people who cannot tolerate sulfasalazine. Only 2% of the salicylate from this compound is absorbed systemically. The most common adverse effect in people from this preparation has been watery diarrhea.
4. Pentasa. Pentasa contains microgranules of mesalamine coated with ethyl cellulose, which releases 5-aminosalicylic acid into the small and large intestine gradually, regardless of pH.

### Indications and Clinical Uses
Mesalamine is used for treatment of inflammatory bowel disease, including colitis, in animals. Most often sulfasalazine is used; however, in some animals, especially those sensitive to sulfonamides, mesalamine may be indicated. Use in animals has been primarily derived from empirical use, anecdotal experience, and recommendations from clinical experts. There are no well-controlled clinical studies or efficacy trials to document clinical effectiveness.

## Precautionary Information

### Adverse Reactions and Side Effects

Mesalamine alone has not been associated with side effects in animals. Adverse effects associated with sulfasalazine are caused by the sulfonamide component. (See Sulfasalazine for more information.)

### Contraindications and Precautions

Drug interactions are possible, but they have not been reported in animals, probably because low systemic drug levels are achieved. Mesalamine, if absorbed sufficiently, can potentially interfere with thiopurine methyltransferase and therefore increase the risk of toxicity from azathioprine.

### Drug Interactions

No drug interactions are reported in animals. Omeprazole can potentially increase absorption by increasing intestinal pH.

## Instructions for Use

Mesalamine usually is used as a substitute for sulfasalazine in animals that cannot tolerate sulfonamides.

## Patient Monitoring and Laboratory Tests

No specific monitoring is necessary.

## Formulations

- Mesalamine is available in 400-mg tablets and 250-mg capsules. Delayed-release tablets are 400 mg (Asacol) and 1.2 g (film-coated Lialda). Controlled-release capsules are 250 and 500 mg (ethylcellulose-coated Pentasa).

## Stability and Storage

Store in a tightly sealed container, protected from light, and at room temperature. It is slightly soluble in water and ethanol. It should be protected from air and moisture. Darkening may occur after exposure to air. Do not crush coated tablets.

## Small Animal Dosage

- Veterinary doses have not been established. The usual human dosage is 400–500 mg q6–8h PO, and it has been used to extrapolate an animal dosage (e.g., 5–10 mg/kg q8h PO).

## Large Animal Dosage

- No large animal doses have been reported.

## Regulatory Information

No regulatory information is available. Because of a low risk of residues, no withdrawal times are suggested.

RCI Classification: 5

# Metaflumizone

met-ah′floo-mah-zone

**Trade and other names:** ProMeris

**Functional classification:** Antiparasitic

This product has been removed from the market. Consult previous editions of this handbook for information on pharmacology and clinical use.

# Metaproterenol Sulfate

met-ha-proe-teer′eh-nole sul′fate

**Trade and other names:** Alupent, Metaprel, and Orciprenaline sulphate

**Functional classification:** Bronchodilator, beta-agonist

## Pharmacology and Mechanism of Action

Metaproterenol is a $beta_2$-adrenergic agonist. It is most often used as a bronchodilator because of its stimulation of respiratory $beta_2$ receptors. Like other $beta_2$ agonists, it stimulates $beta_2$ receptors, activates adenyl cyclase, and relaxes bronchial smooth muscle. It also may inhibit release of inflammatory mediators, especially from mast cells.

*Pharmacokinetics:* The pharmacokinetics have not been well studied in the veterinary species, except for small studies in laboratory animals. In people, it is well absorbed from oral administration, but information on oral absorption in animals is incomplete.

## Indications and Clinical Uses

Metaproterenol has been used in animals to relax bronchial smooth muscle to treat bronchitis, obstructive pulmonary disease, airway obstruction caused by inflammation, and other airway diseases. It is indicated in animals with reversible bronchoconstriction, such as cats with bronchial asthma. Use in animals has been primarily derived from empirical use and anecdotal experiences. There are no well-controlled clinical studies or efficacy trials to document clinical effectiveness. Other selective $beta_2$ agonists are used more often in animals, such as albuterol, delivered with an inhaler, or oral forms. Beta$_2$ agonists also have been used in people to delay labor (inhibit uterine contractions), but this use has not been explored in animals.

## Precautionary Information

### Adverse Reactions and Side Effects

Metaproterenol causes excessive beta-adrenergic stimulation at high doses (tachycardia and tremors) because of excessive $beta_1$-adrenergic stimulation. Arrhythmias occur at high doses or in sensitive individuals. Beta agonists inhibit uterine contractions in animals in labor.

### Contraindications and Precautions

Use cautiously in animals with cardiac disease that may be prone to rapid heart rates or arrhythmias.

### Drug Interactions

Do not administer with MAOIs. Use cautiously with other drugs that may cause cardiac arrhythmias in animals. It may be mixed with cromolyn sodium for nebulization if used within 60–90 minutes. It also has been combined with dexamethasone without loss of stability.

## Instructions for Use

Results of clinical studies in animals have not been reported. Use in animals (and doses) is based on experience in people or anecdotal experience in animals.

## Patient Monitoring and Laboratory Tests

Monitor heart rate and rhythm of animals during treatment.

## Formulations
- Metaproterenol is available in 10- and 20-mg tablets, 5-mg/mL syrup, and inhalers.

## Stability and Storage
Store in a tightly sealed container, protected from light, and at room temperature. Avoid exposure to air and moisture. Do not freeze. Do not use if formulation turns dark color.

## Small Animal Dosage
**Dogs and Cats**
- 0.325–0.65 mg/kg q4–6h PO.

## Large Animal Dosage
- No large animal doses have been reported. There is no evidence of oral absorption in large animals.

## Regulatory Information
Do not administer to animals that produce food. Other beta agonists (clenbuterol) are banned for use in food animals.
RCI Classification: 3

---

# Metformin
met-for′min

M

**Trade and other names:** Glucophage

**Functional classification:** Antihyperglycemic

## Pharmacology and Mechanism of Action
Metformin is an oral antihyperglycemic agent used to treat non–insulin-dependent diabetes (type 2 diabetes in people). It is in the biguanide class of oral drugs for diabetes. Metformin does not have a direct effect on pancreatic beta cells, but it lowers blood glucose by reducing hepatic glucose production and improving peripheral utilization of glucose (e.g., in muscle). It increases muscle sensitivity to insulin and increases muscle glucose metabolism. Metformin is used to decrease hepatic glucose production, decrease intestinal absorption of glucose, and improve insulin sensitivity by increasing peripheral glucose uptake and utilization. It thus lowers insulin requirements without any direct effect to increase insulin secretion. It may also increase the insulin receptors on tissues. At therapeutic doses, metformin does not cause hypoglycemia.

*Pharmacokinetics:* The half-life in cats is 2.75 hours with 48% oral absorption. Oral absorption in dogs is 31% with a half-life of 12.6 hours. In insulin-resistant ponies, the half-life is 11.7 hours, with a peak after oral administration occurring at approximately 1 hour, but bioavailability is low ($\approx$4%–7%).

## Indications and Clinical Uses
In people, metformin is one of the most common drugs used to treat type 2 diabetes, or for early stages of prediabetes. It has been used in people when the sulfonylurea drugs fail. It has been used in cats to treat diabetes. However, in cats treated with 50 mg/cat q12h PO, it showed significant adverse effects and was effective in

only one fifth of treated cats. In cats, it has been more common to administer the sulfonylurea class of drugs if oral treatments are used instead of insulin injection. Sulfonylurea drugs include glipizide (Glucotrol) and glyburide (DiaBeta, Micronase). Dogs with diabetes rarely respond to oral hypoglycemic agents, and metformin is not recommended for dogs. Metformin has been considered for treatment of insulin resistance in horses and ponies, but the bioavailability is very low in horses compared with that of humans. It may have shown temporary effects in some horses, but overall efficacy is low, probably because of poor oral bioavailability. Therefore, the use in horses is not recommended.

## Precautionary Information

### Adverse Reactions and Side Effects

Metformin has caused lethargy, appetite loss, vomiting, and weight loss in cats. Use has not been common enough to document other effects. However, in people, it has caused lactic acidosis in some patients, which was serious. Metformin also has caused megaloblastic anemia by affecting vitamin $B_{12}$ absorption.

### Contraindications and Precautions

Metformin is cleared by the kidneys, so doses need to be adjusted in patients with renal failure.

### Drug Interactions

Use cautiously with drugs that may affect glycemic control such as glucocorticoids.

## Instructions for Use

Doses published for cats are based on pharmacokinetic studies that demonstrated oral absorption in cats to be 35%–70%. The half-life was 11.5 hours, which is the basis for the q12h dosage recommendation. Consistently effective doses for horses have not been established.

## Patient Monitoring and Laboratory Tests

Blood glucose should be monitored carefully. Doses should be adjusted on the basis of glucose monitoring. Some animals may require insulin injections to control hyperglycemia.

## Formulations Available

• Metformin is available in 500- and 850-mg tablets.

## Stability and Storage

Stable if maintained in original formulation.

## Small Animal Dosage

### Cats

• 25 or 50 mg/cat q12h PO (5–10 mg/kg q12h). (Efficacy is limited.)

## Large Animal Dosage

• Because of high clearance and poor bioavailability in horses (4%–7%), its use is not recommended.

## Regulatory Information

Do not administer to animals intended for food.

# Methadone Hydrochloride
meth′ah-done hye-droe-klor′ide

**Trade and other names:** Dolophine, Methadose, and generic brands

**Functional classification:** Analgesic, opioid

## Pharmacology and Mechanism of Action

Methadone is an opioid agonist and analgesic. The action of methadone is to bind to mu-opiate and kappa-opiate receptors on nerves and inhibit release of neurotransmitters involved with transmission of pain stimuli (e.g., substance P). Methadone also may antagonize n-methyl D-aspartate (NMDA) receptors, which may contribute to the analgesic effect, decrease adverse CNS effects, and inhibit tolerance. Methadone exists in two forms as Levo- and Dextro-chiral isomers: levomethadone and dextromethadone. Levomethadone, which is available in some countries, has higher affinity for mu-opiate receptors and has been available in a 2.5-mg/mL solution combined with 0.125 mg/mL of fenpipramide (an anticholinergic agent). The D-isomer is considered the active portion that antagonizes the NMDA receptors to produce additional analgesic effects. Other opiates used in animals include morphine, hydromorphone, codeine, oxymorphone, meperidine, and fentanyl.

*Pharmacokinetics:* Like other opioids, methadone is highly lipophilic (log P, 3.9) and is a weak base (pKa, 8.9). The pharmacokinetics have been studied in horses, cats, and dogs. In all species studied, oral absorption is either too low or variable to use this as a method of administration. In horses, the oral absorption was 30% from intragastric administration but three times higher from direct oral administration. (Absorption may occur from the oral mucosa in horses.) Oral absorption in dogs is negligible. The half-life in all species is short. In horses, it is approximately 1–2 hours. In dogs, the half-life is 2–4 hours with clearance of 30 mL/kg/min. The short half-life requires frequent administration to maintain effective concentrations.

## Indications and Clinical Uses

Most of the use in veterinary medicine to document the efficacy and safety of methadone is based on anecdotal experience, small observational efficacy studies, and pharmacokinetic studies. However, there is an approved formulation in Europe with controlled studies to support efficacy.

Methadone is indicated for short-term analgesia, for sedation, and as an adjunct to anesthesia. It is compatible with most anesthetics and can be used as part of a multimodal approach to analgesia and anesthesia. Administration of methadone may lower dose requirements for other anesthetics and analgesics used. Methadone IM (0.6 mg/kg) provides antinociceptive effects for up to 4 hours. It has also been administered to cats (0.5 mg/kg) in combination with alpha$_2$ agonists and administered IM for analgesia effects for 4–6 hours.

Oral doses to dogs are not absorbed systemically, and this route is not recommended. Oral mucosal (buccal) administration to dogs is not practical, but oral mucosal administration to cats may be considered (absorption, 44%). Duration of analgesia in cats is 2–4 hours and as long as 6–8 hours.

M

## Precautionary Information

### Adverse Reactions and Side Effects

Like all opiates, side effects from methadone are predictable and unavoidable. However, some side effects such as excitement and dysphoria seen with other opiates have not been as common with methadone in dogs and cats. Side effects from methadone administration may include sedation, vomiting, constipation, urinary retention, and bradycardia. Panting may occur in dogs as a result of changes in thermoregulation. Effects such as excitement and dysphoria have not been observed with administration of methadone as much as some of the other opiates. In dogs, IV administration produced less dysphoria and excitement compared with other opiates. In horses, IV administration did not produce behavior changes, sedation, increased locomotion, or decreased intestinal motility that is typical with administration of opioid mu-agonists in horses. Oral doses up to 0.4 mg/kg in horses did not produce adverse reactions.

### Contraindications and Precautions

Methadone is a Schedule II controlled substance. Cats may be more sensitive to excitement than other species, but this has not been examined for methadone. Availability of methadone in some regions may be difficult because it is used in people to treat opioid use disorder.

### Drug Interactions

Chloramphenicol, and possibly other drugs such as antifungal agents, decrease clearance and increase plasma concentrations of methadone in dogs.

## Instructions for Use

The dose in dogs is based on small clinical studies and pharmacokinetic results. Effective dose has not been established for horses, but oral administration of 0.1–0.4 mg/kg has been administered without adverse effects and produces drug concentrations in the effective range. Doses used in cats are based on pharmacokinetics and small research studies.

## Patient Monitoring and Laboratory Tests

Monitor the patient's heart rate and respiration. Although bradycardia rarely needs to be treated when it is caused by an opioid, atropine can be administered if necessary. If serious respiratory depression occurs, the opioid can be reversed with naloxone. Although plasma concentrations are not typically monitored, the range of concentrations considered therapeutic in people is 33–60 ng/mL.

## Formulations

- Methadone is available in 1- and 2-mg/mL oral solution; 5-, 10-, and 40-mg tablets; and 10-mg/mL injectable solution. There is a licensed formulation of methadone for cats available in some European countries.

## Stability and Storage

Store in a tightly sealed container, protected from light, and at room temperature. It is soluble in water and ethanol. It is a weak base, with a pKa of 8.9, and may precipitate from a solution if the pH is higher than 6. Although oral forms are not well absorbed in animals, methadone has been combined in oral mixtures with juices and syrups and remained stable for at least 14 days.

## Small Animal Dosage

**Dogs**

- 0.1–0.5 mg/kg IV or 0.5–2.2 mg/kg q3–4h SQ or IM.

**Cats**

- 0.3–0.6 mg/kg q3–4h IV, SQ, or IM. Cats have tolerated doses up to 0.6 mg/kg IM, with a 4-hour duration of activity.
- Oral mucosal administration is approximately two times the IV dose because of less than 50% absorption.

## Large Animal Dosage

**Horses**

- 0.15 mg/kg IV or IM q6–8h. Oral administration also has been used, with some evidence of adequate oral absorption.

## Regulatory Information

Do not administer to animals intended for food.
Methadone is a Schedule II controlled drug.
RCI Classification: 1

# Methazolamide
meth-ah-zole′ah-mide

**Trade and other names:** Neptazane

**Functional classification:** Diuretic

M

## Pharmacology and Mechanism of Action

Methazolamide is a carbonic anhydrase inhibitor. Methazolamide, like other carbonic anhydrase inhibitors, produces diuresis through inhibition of the uptake of bicarbonate in proximal renal tubules via enzyme inhibition. This action results in loss of bicarbonate in the urine and diuresis. The action of carbonic anhydrase inhibitors results in urine loss of bicarbonate, alkaline urine, and water loss. Methazolamide, like other carbonic anhydrase inhibitors, also decreases formation of cerebrospinal fluid by the choroid plexus and decreases the ocular fluid formation by decreasing bicarbonate secretion by the ocular ciliary body. This effect on aqueous humor formation decreases ocular pressure.

## Indications and Clinical Uses

Methazolamide is rarely used as a diuretic any longer. More potent and effective diuretic drugs are available, such as the loop diuretics (furosemide). Methazolamide, like other carbonic anhydrase inhibitors, is used primarily to lower intraocular pressure in animals with glaucoma. Its duration is relatively short in dogs; therefore, frequent administration may be required to maintain low ocular pressure. However, if a carbonic anhydrase inhibitor is needed, methazolamide is used more often than acetazolamide for this purpose because it is more effective and easily available. Nevertheless, other regimens are commonly used for the treatment of glaucoma compared with the carbonic anhydrase inhibitors. Methazolamide, like other carbonic anhydrase inhibitors, is sometimes used to produce more alkaline urine for management of some urinary calculi.

## Precautionary Information

### Adverse Reactions and Side Effects

Methazolamide may produce hypokalemia in some patients. Like other carbonic anhydrase inhibitors, it can produce significant bicarbonate loss, and patients should be supplemented with bicarbonate if repeated doses are administered.

### Contraindications and Precautions

Do not use in patients with acidemia. Use cautiously in any animal sensitive to sulfonamides. Do not use in patients with hepatic encephalopathy.

### Drug Interactions

Use cautiously with other treatments that could cause metabolic acidosis.

## Instructions for Use

Methazolamide may be used with other glaucoma agents, such as topical drugs, to decrease intraocular pressure, and it may be used to produce alkaline urine to prevent some calculi from forming. However, use in animals has been primarily derived from empirical use. There are no well-controlled clinical studies or efficacy trials to document clinical effectiveness.

## Patient Monitoring and Laboratory Tests

Monitor ocular pressure in treated patients. Monitor urine pH if it is used to produce alkaline urine. Monitor electrolyte and acid–base status if multiple doses are administered.

## Formulations Available

• Methazolamide is available in 25- and 50-mg tablets.

## Stability and Storage

Store in a tightly sealed container, protected from light, and at room temperature. Stability of compounded formulations has not been evaluated.

## Small Animal Dosage

### Dogs and Cats

• 2–3 mg/kg q8–12h PO. There does not seem to be any benefit for increasing the dose to a maximum dose of 4–6 mg/kg, but more frequent administration (q8h) may be beneficial.

## Large Animal Dosage

• No large animal doses have been reported.

## Regulatory Information

Withdrawal times are not established for animals that produce food. For extralabel use withdrawal interval estimates, contact FARAD at www.FARAD.org.

RCI Classification: 4

# Methenamine

meth-en′ah-meen

**Trade and other names:** Methenamine hippurate: Hiprex and Urex; Methenamine mandelate: Mandelamine and generic brands

**Functional classification:** Antibacterial

## Pharmacology and Mechanism of Action

Methenamine is a urinary antiseptic, which is sometimes used to prevent or manage lower UTIs. In the acid environment of the urine, methenamine is hydrolyzed to formaldehyde and ammonia to produce an antibacterial and antifungal effect. A low urine pH of 5.5 or less is needed for optimal effect. If this can be achieved, it is active against a wide range of bacteria, and resistance does not develop. It is less effective against *Proteus* spp. that produce an alkaline urine pH. Because there is no systemic absorption, it is not effective for infections other than in the lower urinary tract. Absorption is rapid and produces a peak effect in urine at 0.5–1.5 hours and has a half-life of 3–6 hours.

## Indications and Clinical Uses

Methenamine is used as a urinary antiseptic, but there is a lack of well-controlled clinical trials to show its effectiveness. The use is based on extrapolation of uses in people and clinical observations. It has been used in animals to prevent recurrences of lower UTIs, but it is probably less effective for treating ongoing infections. It is critical that the urine pH be low for conversion to formaldehyde.

M

## Precautionary Information

### Adverse Reactions and Side Effects

Although formaldehyde formation in bladder may be irritating, in people, high doses are required (greater than 8 g/day). In animals, no adverse effects have been reported.

### Contraindications and Precautions

High doses may irritate the bladder mucosa. Do not administer with sulfonamides because it may form formaldehyde–sulfonamide complexes. Do not use the mandelate formulation in patients with renal insufficiency.

### Drug Interactions

Do not administer with medications that may cause alkaline urine. Because methenamine is often administered with urine acidifiers, acid urine decreases the activity of some antibiotics administered for UTIs such as fluoroquinolone and aminoglycoside antibiotics. Methenamine can combine in the urine with sulfonamide drugs to produce antagonism.

## Instructions for Use

Results of clinical studies in animals have not been reported. Use in animals is based on experience in people or anecdotal experience in animals. Urine must be acidic for methenamine to convert to formaldehyde (monitor pH periodically). A pH less than 5.5 is optimal. Supplement with ascorbic acid or ammonium chloride to lower pH. The tablets should be enteric coated to protect from hydrolysis in the acid of the stomach and should be administered on an empty stomach.

## Patient Monitoring and Laboratory Tests

No specific monitoring is necessary. Monitor urinalysis or culture of urine to guide therapy of UTI.

## Formulations

- Methenamine hippurate is available in 0.6- and 1-g tablets. Methenamine mandelate is no longer available (previous formulations included 1-g tablets, granules for oral solution, and 50- and 100-mg/mL oral suspension).

## Stability and Storage

Store in a tightly sealed container, protected from light, and at room temperature. Methenamine is soluble in water and ethanol. In an acidic environment, it is hydrolyzed to form formaldehyde and ammonia. It has been physically incompatible when mixed with some foods and suspensions.

## Small Animal Dosage

**Dogs**

- Methenamine hippurate: 500 mg/dog q12h PO.
- Methenamine mandelate (if available): 10–20 mg/kg q8–12h PO.

**Cats**

- Methenamine hippurate: 250 mg/cat q12h PO.
- Methenamine mandelate (if available): 10–20 mg/kg q8–12h PO.

## Large Animal Dosage

- No large animal doses have been reported. It is unlikely to be effective in large animals because their urine is more alkaline.

## Regulatory Information

No regulatory information is available. Because of a low risk of residues, no withdrawal times are suggested.

# Methimazole

meth-im′ah-zole

**Trade and other names:** Tapazole, Felimazole, Thiamazole, and generic

**Functional classification:** Antithyroid agent

## Pharmacology and Mechanism of Action

Methimazole is an important antithyroid drug used mostly in cats. The action of methimazole is to serve as substrate for thyroid peroxidase and decrease incorporation of iodide into tyrosine molecules for the formation of thyroxine ($T_4$) and triiodothyronine ($T_3$). Methimazole inhibits coupling of mono- and di-iodinated residues to form $T_4$ and $T_3$. Methimazole does not inhibit release of preformed thyroid hormone. It does not affect existing thyroid hormones already circulating or stored in the thyroid gland and does not inhibit the peripheral conversion of $T_4$ to $T_3$. It generally takes 2–4 weeks for serum $T_4$ to reach the normal range in hyperthyroid cats treated with methimazole. Carbimazole is a similar drug used in Europe that is converted to methimazole in animals. Methimazole also may have immunosuppressive effects. Treatment may decrease antithyrotropin-receptor antibodies.

*Pharmacokinetics:* The pharmacokinetics have been limited to studies in cats. Methimazole has a half-life of 2.3–3.1 hours in hyperthyroid cats and 4.7 hours in normal cats. Oral absorption in cats is high (93%).

## Indications and Clinical Uses

Methimazole is used to treat hyperthyroidism in animals, especially cats. There is good evidence for efficacy, based on clinical studies, when administered to cats at recommended doses. Methimazole is preferred in cats instead of an older drug, propylthiouracil (PTU), because methimazole has a lower incidence of adverse effects. Many cats are controlled with once-daily dosing of methimazole, but there is evidence that supports twice-daily dosing in cats as more effective than once daily.

Methimazole has been formulated for use in cats as a transdermal gel for skin absorption. Transdermal gels for cats use either a gel compounded in pluronic organogel (PLO) or other vehicles (e.g., Lipoderm) to enhance transdermal penetration. (See Formulations.) These formulations are generally available through compounding pharmacies. One commercial product is available in New Zealand as Hyper-T Ear Spot. Published data indicate that transdermal methimazole is not as rapidly acting or as effective as oral dosing, but it can be effective to reduce $T_4$ concentrations in many cats. In the available studies, a dose of 10 mg per cat transdermal was more effective than 5 mg per cat transdermal and was as effective as oral treatments.

An alternative oral drug that has been used is carbimazole, which is converted to the active drug methimazole. It may produce less frequent GI problems. However, experience with carbimazole is limited in the United States (see Carbimazole for more details). If switching from methimazole to carbimazole, they are not equivalent. Six mg of methimazole is equal to 10 mg of carbimazole.

### Precautionary Information

M

#### Adverse Reactions and Side Effects

In cats, GI problems are the most common adverse effect and can include anorexia and vomiting. Most adverse effects caused by methimazole are dose related and can be decreased by lowering the dose. In cats, polyarthritis, alopecia, and scaling and crusting of the head and face have been observed, which may be manifestations of an allergic reaction. In cats, lupus-like reactions are possible, such as vasculitis and bone marrow changes, but this was more common with older drugs such as PTU. In cats, abnormal platelet counts and low blood counts can develop after 1–3 months of treatment. Bleeding abnormalities may be related to thrombocytopenia, but tests conducted in cats did not demonstrate prolongation of bleeding times (prothrombin time and activated partial antithromboplastin time). There were fewer adverse GI effects when methimazole was applied as a transdermal gel compared with administration as an oral tablet. But transdermal methimazole can produce skin irritation in some cats. Methimazole treatment may unmask hypothyroidism and renal failure in some cats. Monitor renal function with continued treatment.

#### Contraindications and Precautions

Do not administer to animals with thrombocytopenia or bleeding problems. Other drugs, such as beta blockers, are safe to administer with methimazole. Warn pet owners that transdermal methimazole can be absorbed through human skin. If an animal has had previous adverse reactions to PTU, there may also be cross-sensitivity to methimazole. Methimazole has caused fetal abnormalities and should not be used in pregnant animals.

#### Drug Interactions

There are no drug interactions reported from the use in animals. It has been used safely with beta-blockers, calcium-channel blockers, antihypertensive drugs, and other cardiovascular drugs.

## Instructions for Use

The use in cats is based on clinical studies in hyperthyroid cats and information from the feline drug sponsor. Methimazole has, for the most part, replaced PTU for use in cats. Adjust the maintenance dose of methimazole by monitoring thyroid ($T_4$) concentrations in plasma. Because it does not inhibit release of preformed thyroid, it may take 2–4 weeks to achieve maximum effect. Although once the patient is stabilized, the $T_4$ concentrations are suppressed for 24 hours, one study that evaluated dosing frequency found that 5 mg/kg q12h PO was more effective than 5 mg/kg q24h PO.

Transdermal gel use in cats: Methimazole has been prepared as a transdermal gel by compounding pharmacies. The compounded vehicle contains solvents and penetration enhancers. (See Formulations.) The Lipoderm formulation is compounded in a lipid vehicle, instead of previously used PLO gel, which may be more effective. One of the compounded formulations is compounded as a 10% concentration. The most common dose administered is 10 mg per cat (0.1 mL of the compounded product) of transdermal gel applied to the inner ear. Transdermal gel may be less effective and more variable than oral tablets, and thyroid monitoring should be performed to assess efficacy to ensure that $T_4$ is consistently within the reference range.

## Patient Monitoring and Laboratory Tests

Monitor serum $T_4$ levels. Recheck $T_4$ levels after first month of treatment. Whether the concentration was measured before dosing or during the dose interval did not affect the $T_4$ concentration. After methimazole treatment is stabilized, $T_3$ and $T_4$ are suppressed for 24 hours after each dose of methimazole. Therefore, the timing of blood sample after oral methimazole in cats does not appear to be a significant factor when assessing response to treatment. Thyroid-stimulating hormone (TSH) concentrations in cats may also be used to test effectiveness of treatment. (Feline TSH has 96% homology with canine TSH.) Monitor CBC and platelet count in cats every week or 14 days for the first 30 days of treatment. Monitor tests of renal function because of concern about increased risk of renal disease in some cats. Monitor liver enzymes before and during treatment. Some cats with hyperthyroidism also have elevated liver enzymes. Methimazole may affect thyroid scintigraphy tests because after treatment, there may be a stimulation from TSH for tissues to have enhanced uptake of 99mTcO4 by the thyroid gland.

## Formulations

- Methimazole is available in 2.5- and 5-mg coated tablets (veterinary form) and 5- and 10-mg tablets (human form).
- Transdermal: There are no approved transdermal formulations for cats in the United States. However, a 10% transdermal gel has been prepared by compounding pharmacies. For consideration of a transdermal gel, the pharmacist should consult US Patent number US2010/0137389 A1 (June 3, 2010), which lists the ingredients and process for preparing the formulation.
- Transdermal: There is a transdermal form approved in some countries (New Zealand) for cats. This product (Hyper-T Earspot) is available in a 1-mL applicator at a concentration of 100 mg/mL and applied as 0.1 mL (10 mg) once daily the pinna of the ear. Dose adjustments are recommended based on measurement of $T_4$ concentrations.

## Stability and Storage

Methimazole is stable if maintained in its original formulation. However, if prepared in compounded formulations for cats, potency and stability may be less if not prepared according to the instructions listed in the US Patent. (See Formulations.) This product was stable for 12 months after preparation and dispensed in 1-mL syringes at a 10% concentration (100 mg/mL). Carbimazole is not stable in transdermal gel formulations.

## Small Animal Dosage

### Cats

- 2.5 mg/cat q12h PO for 7–14 days; then adjust dosage up to 5–10 mg/cat PO q12h if needed. Monitor $T_4$ concentrations and adjust dosage accordingly. Some cats can be maintained on once-daily treatment.
- Transdermal dosage: 10 mg per cat transdermally once daily. After a period of adjustment, modification of dosage should be done by monitoring thyroid concentrations in cats. Some cats may require twice-daily dosing, and some cats can be maintained on a dosage of 5 mg per cat once daily. Alternate ears with each dose and wear gloves when applying.

## Large Animal Dosage

- No large animal doses have been reported.

## Regulatory Information

Withdrawal times are not established for animals that produce food. This drug should not be used in animals intended for food.

# Methionine (DL-Methionine)

meth-eye-o-nine

**Trade and other names:** DL-methionine and Racemethionine

**Functional classification:** Urine acidifier, nutritional supplement

**M**

**Note:** The proper name for this drug is Racemethionine. See the Racemethionine section for more complete information.

# Methocarbamol

meth-oh-kar'bah-mole

**Trade and other names:** Robaxin-V

**Functional classification:** Muscle relaxant

## Pharmacology and Mechanism of Action

Methocarbamol is a skeletal muscle relaxant. Methocarbamol depresses polysynaptic reflexes to cause muscle relaxation. It has been used for conditions that need muscle relaxation or for diseases that induce muscle spasms. Methocarbamol has a long history of use, but clinical us in veterinary medicine is uncommon.

## Indications and Clinical Uses

Methocarbamol has been used for the treatment of skeletal muscle spasms and increased muscle tone. Methocarbamol (Robaxin) has US Food and Drug Administration (FDA) approval for treating dogs, cats, and horses. The labeling indication lists for all three species lists "As an adjunct for treating acute inflammatory and traumatic conditions of the skeletal muscles and to reduce muscular spasms."

Methocarbamol has also been used to treat pain that is associated with increased muscle spasms or myositis, but it does not have direct analgesic effects. The highest dose listed in the dosing section are only recommended if it is used for treating tetanus or strychnine poisoning. For some indications (e.g., muscle spasms), methocarbamol has been replaced by other muscle relaxants such as orphenadrine (Norflex) or benzodiazepines. In horses, the half-life is only 60–90 minutes and may need frequent administration for effectiveness.

## Precautionary Information

### Adverse Reactions and Side Effects

Methocarbamol may cause depression and sedation of the CNS. Excess salivation, emesis, weakness, and ataxia have been observed from methocarbamol administration. Adverse effects are usually short in duration because of rapid elimination.

### Contraindications and Precautions

Use cautiously with other drugs that depress the CNS. Do not rely on methocarbamol as a treatment for pain because it has no direct analgesic properties.

### Drug Interactions

No drug interactions reported for animals.

## Instructions for Use

Results of recent clinical studies in animals have not been reported. Use in animals (and doses) is based on label recommendations on the FDA approval that was established many years ago, before substantial evidence of efficacy was required.

## Patient Monitoring and Laboratory Tests

No specific monitoring is necessary.

## Formulations

- Methocarbamol is available in 500-mg tablets and 100-mg/mL injection.

## Stability and Storage

Store in a tightly sealed container, protected from light, and at room temperature. Stability of compounded formulations has not been evaluated.

## Small Animal Dosage

### Dogs and Cats

- 44 mg/kg IV (moderate conditions) or 55 mg/kg and up to 222 mg/kg for severe conditions such as tetanus or strychnine poisoning. The total cumulative dose should not exceed 333 mg/kg. (These dose regimens are based on the FDA-approved label.)
- Oral dosage: 44 mg/kg q8h PO followed by 22–44 mg/kg q8h PO, not to exceed 14–21 days. (These dosage regimens are based on the FDA-approved label.)

## Large Animal Dosage

- 4.4–22 mg/kg q8h IV for moderate conditions and 22–55 for more severe conditions. (These dosage regimens are based on the FDA-approved label.) In horses, higher doses above 30 mg/kg IV and 50–100 mg/kg PO have been administered but are more likely to produce mild to moderate depression.

## Regulatory Information

Withdrawal times are not established for animals that produce food. For extralabel use withdrawal interval estimates, contact FARAD at www.FARAD.org.

RCI Classification: 4

# Methohexital Sodium

meth-oe-heks′ih-tahl soe′dee-um

**Trade and other names:** Brevital

**Functional classification:** Anesthetic, barbiturate

## Pharmacology and Mechanism of Action

Methohexital is a barbiturate anesthetic used infrequently in animals. Methohexital is an oxybarbiturate that it is ultra-short acting. Methohexital is twice as potent as thiopental but has a higher incidence of CNS excitatory effects. Anesthesia is produced by CNS depression, but it does not produce significant analgesia. Anesthesia is terminated by rapid redistribution of the drug in the body.

M

## Indications and Clinical Uses

Methohexital is used as an IV anesthetic in animals, given either as a bolus or CRI. It can be administered with other anesthetic adjuncts, such as tranquilizers, prior to methohexital infusion. The use of methohexital has declined because of availability of other short-term anesthetics.

## Precautionary Information

### Adverse Reactions and Side Effects

Adverse effects are related to the anesthetic effects of the drug. Severe adverse effects are caused by respiratory and cardiovascular depression. Respiratory apnea is possible after an IV bolus.

### Contraindications and Precautions

Overdoses can be caused by rapid or repeated injections. Avoid extravasation outside of the vein.

### Drug Interactions

No drug interactions have been reported for animals. Drugs that affect cytochrome P450 enzymes (see Appendixes H and I) can affect barbiturate metabolism.

## Instructions for Use

The therapeutic index is low. Use this agent only when it is possible to monitor cardiovascular and respiratory functions. Methohexital is often administered with other anesthetic adjuncts.

## Patient Monitoring and Laboratory Tests
Monitor heart rate and breathing in patients anesthetized with barbiturates.

## Formulations
• Methohexital is available in 0.5-, 2.5-, and 5-g vials for injection.

## Stability and Storage
Store in a tightly sealed container, protected from light, and at room temperature. Stability of compounded formulations has not been evaluated.

## Small Animal Dosage
### Dogs and Cats
• 3–6 mg/kg IV (give slowly to effect). Doses as high as 15 mg/kg IV have been administered to dogs over 30 seconds.
• CRI: 0.25 mg/kg/min for 30 minutes; then 0.125 mg/kg/min.

## Large Animal Dosage
• Horses: 5 mg/kg IV (to effect).
• Pigs: 5–8 mg/kg IV (to effect).

## Regulatory Information
Withdrawal times are not established for animals that produce food. For extralabel use withdrawal interval estimates, contact FARAD at www.FARAD.org.
Schedule III controlled drug.
RCI Classification: 2

# Methotrexate
meth-oh-treks′ate

**Trade and other names:** MTX, Mexate, Folex, Rheumatrex, and generic brands

**Functional classification:** Anticancer agent

## Pharmacology and Mechanism of Action
Methotrexate is an anticancer and anti-inflammatory agent. The action of methotrexate is to interfere with synthesis of biomolecules that are important for RNA, DNA, and protein synthesis. The structure of methotrexate is similar to folic acid, and methotrexate binds and inhibits the dihydrofolate reductase (DHFR) enzyme. The DHFR enzyme is a reducing enzyme necessary for purine synthesis. The reduced form of folic acid (tetrahydrofolate [FH4]) acts as an important coenzyme for biochemical reactions, particularly DNA, RNA, and protein synthesis.

## Indications and Clinical Uses
Methotrexate is used for various carcinomas, leukemia, and lymphomas. In people, methotrexate is also commonly used for autoimmune diseases, particularly rheumatoid arthritis. Use in animals has been primarily derived from empirical use and experiences in people. There are no well-controlled clinical studies or efficacy trials to document clinical effectiveness. It is rarely used to treat arthritis in animals.

## Precautionary Information

### Adverse Reactions and Side Effects

The important adverse effects in animals are anorexia, nausea, myelosuppression, and vomiting. Anticancer drugs cause predictable (and sometimes unavoidable) side effects that include bone marrow suppression, leukopenia, and immunosuppression. Hepatotoxicity has been reported in people from methotrexate therapy, but this has not been documented in veterinary medicine. In people, higher doses are often used compared to veterinary doses. In people, risk of systemic toxicity is high, and rescue therapy with leucovorin (tetrahydrofolic acid) is often used (also called calcium folinate). Leucovorin rescue therapy is used because it is an antagonist of the action of methotrexate on the DHFR enzyme. (See Leucovorin for more information.) Dose range of leucovorin in dogs is 25–200 mg/m$^2$ every 6 hours, depending on plasma methotrexate concentration. Another approach is to administer a dose of leucovorin that is equal to the dose of methotrexate.

### Contraindications and Precautions

Do not administer to pregnant animals. It has been used to induce abortion.

### Drug Interactions

Concurrent use with NSAIDs may cause severe methotrexate toxicity. Do not administer with penicillins, fluoroquinolones, pyrimethamine, trimethoprim, sulfonamides, or other drugs that may affect folic acid synthesis.

M

## Instructions for Use

Use in animals has been based primarily on experience in research animals or extrapolation of the use in people. Only limited veterinary clinical information is available. Consult specific anticancer protocols for the precise dosage and regimen.

## Patient Monitoring and Laboratory Tests

Monitor CBC for evidence of bone marrow toxicity.

## Formulations

• Methotrexate is available in 2.5-mg tablets and 2.5- and 25-mg/mL injection.

## Stability and Storage

Store in a tightly sealed container, protected from light, and at room temperature. Stability of compounded formulations has not been evaluated.

## Small Animal Dosage

### Dogs and Cats

• 2.5–5 mg/m$^2$ q48h PO (dose depends on specific cancer protocol).
• 0.3–0.5 mg/kg every week IV.

### Cats

• 0.8 mg/kg IV every 2–3 weeks.

## Large Animal Dosage

• No large animal doses have been reported.

## Regulatory Information

Withdrawal times are not established for animals that produce food. This drug should not be used in animals intended for food because it is an anticancer agent.

RCI Classification: 4

# Methoxamine
meh-thahk'seh-meen

**Trade and other names:** Vasoxyl

**Functional classification:** Vasopressor

## Pharmacology and Mechanism of Action
Methoxamine is an alpha$_1$-adrenergic agonist. Methoxamine stimulates alpha$_1$ receptors on vascular smooth muscle to produce vasoconstriction in vascular beds. The primary use of methoxamine is to produce vasoconstriction when it is necessary to increase an animal's blood pressure.

## Indications and Clinical Uses
Methoxamine is used primarily in patients in need of critical care or during anesthesia to increase peripheral resistance and blood pressure. There is little experience with this drug in veterinary medicine. Aggressive fluid administration is the first measure considered when it is necessary to increase the patient's blood pressure. Other vasopressor agents are often used if necessary.

## Precautionary Information
### Adverse Reactions and Side Effects
Adverse effects are related to excessive stimulation of alpha$_1$ receptors (prolonged peripheral vasoconstriction). Reflex bradycardia may occur.

### Contraindications and Precautions
Use cautiously in animals with heart disease.

### Drug Interactions
Do not use with MAOIs, such as selegiline.

## Instructions for Use
Methoxamine has a rapid onset and short duration of action.

## Patient Monitoring and Laboratory Tests
Monitor heart rate and blood pressure in treated patients.

## Formulations
• Methoxamine is no longer available on the US market. Some solutions have been compounded. It was previously available as a 20-mg/mL injection.

## Stability and Storage
Store in a tightly sealed container, protected from light, and at room temperature. Stability of compounded formulations has not been evaluated.

## Small Animal Dosage
### Dogs and Cats
• 200–250 mcg/kg (0.2–0.25 mg/kg) IM or 40–80 mcg/kg IV; repeat dose as needed.

## Large Animal Dosage
### Cattle and Horses
• 100–200 mcg/kg (0.1–0.2 mg/kg) IM once or as needed.

## Regulatory Information

No regulatory information is available. Because of a low risk of residues, no withdrawal times are suggested.

# Methoxyflurane
meh-thahk'seh-floo'rane

**Trade and other names:** Metofane

**Functional classification:** Anesthetic, inhalant

## Pharmacology and Mechanism of Action

Methoxyflurane is one of the older inhalant anesthetic agents. Like other inhalant anesthetics, the mechanism of action is uncertain. They produce generalized, reversible depression of the CNS. The inhalant anesthetics vary in their solubility in blood, their potency, and the rate of induction and recovery. Those with low blood/gas partition coefficients are associated with the most rapid rates of induction and recovery.

## Indications and Clinical Uses

Methoxyflurane is not used often as an inhalant anesthetic. In the past 20 years, use has declined and been replaced by other agents.

### Precautionary Information

**Adverse Reactions and Side Effects**

Adverse effects are related to anesthetic effects (e.g., cardiovascular and respiratory depression). Methoxyflurane has been reported to cause hepatic injury in animals.

**Contraindications and Precautions**

Use cautiously in animals with cardiac disease.

**Drug Interactions**

Labeling recommendations in some countries state that flunixin should not be administered to animals receiving methoxyflurane anesthesia.

M

## Instructions for Use

Use of inhalant anesthetics requires careful monitoring. Dose is determined by depth of anesthesia.

## Patient Monitoring and Laboratory Tests

Monitor heart rate and breathing in patients undergoing anesthesia with inhalant anesthetics. Monitor hepatic enzymes.

## Formulations

- Methoxyflurane is currently not available through commercial sources. It was previously available as a 4-oz bottle for inhalation.

## Stability and Storage

Store in a tightly sealed container, protected from light, and at room temperature.

## Small Animal Dosage

- Induction: 3%; maintenance: 0.5%–1.5%.

## Large Animal Dosage

- Minimum alveolar concentration value is 0.2%–0.3%.

## Regulatory Information

No withdrawal times are established for animals intended for food. Clearance is rapid, and short withdrawal times are suggested. For extralabel use withdrawal interval estimates, contact FARAD at www.FARAD.org.

# Methylene Blue 0.1%

meth'ih-leen bloo

**Trade and other names:** New Methylene Blue and generic brands

**Functional classification:** Antidote

## Pharmacology and Mechanism of Action

Methylene blue acts as a reducing agent to reduce methemoglobin to hemoglobin, which is particularly important when it is used to convert methemoglobin to hemoglobin in erythrocytes. It is reduced to leucomethylene blue in the body by combining with reduced nicotinamide adenine dinucleotide phosphate (NADPH) in the presence of NADPH reductase. Leucomethylene blue then transfers an electron to reduce methemoglobin to hemoglobin. Methemoglobin occurs as the result of oxidative damage to hemoglobin, and methylene blue has been used as an antidote for this intoxication. Sources of intoxication in animals that cause methemoglobinemia include exposure to nitrate, nitrite, or chlorate in ruminants; acetaminophen and naphthalene (mothballs) in cats (and occasionally dogs); and local anesthetics, such as benzocaine, in cats. For acetaminophen toxicity in cats, acetylcysteine may provide a better response.

## Indications and Clinical Uses

Methylene blue is used to treat methemoglobinemia caused by chlorate and nitrate toxicosis. It also has been used to treat cyanide toxicosis.

## Precautionary Information

### Adverse Reactions and Side Effects

In cats and dogs, administration of methylene blue to treat methemoglobinemia can cause oxidative damage to erythrocytes, including Heinz bodies, limiting the dose that can be used therapeutically. At the doses listed later, it has been safe, but monitoring of red blood cell effects is recommended. Heinz bodies can increase in cats from methylene blue treatment without producing anemia.

### Contraindications and Precautions

The administration for treating intoxication may produce some oxidative damage to erythrocytes (Heinz bodies and other morphologic changes) that is typically subclinical, but a risk of red cell damage and subsequent anemia increases with repeated or higher dosing. Use cautiously in cats.

### Drug Interactions

Methylene blue is a reversible MAOI. If administered with drugs that affect serotonergic mechanisms or increase serotonin, it can lead to serotonin syndrome (muscle twitching, sweating, increased temperature, shivering).

## Instructions for Use

For administration to large animals, the formulations must be compounded by a pharmacy. Consult a reliable pharmacy for instructions. For treating acetaminophen intoxication in cats, use acetylcysteine first because it will produce the most reliable response, but methylene blue also was helpful.

### Patient Monitoring and Laboratory Tests

Monitor CBC in patients treated with methylene blue. Monitor mucous membrane color (methemoglobinemia turns the blood and membranes a chocolate color).

### Formulations

- There are no commercial veterinary methylene blue products for systemic use. The human product (1% solution, 10 mg/mL) may be appropriate for use in some species, but treatment in large animals may require a compounded formulation.

### Stability and Storage

Store in a tightly sealed container, protected from light, and at room temperature.

### Small Animal Dosage

**Dogs and Cats**
- 1.5 mg/kg IV once slowly.

### Large Animal Dosage

**Cattle, Goats, and Sheep**
- 4–10 mg/kg IV as needed. This dose of methylene blue should be administered over 15 minutes. After the initial dose, lower doses may be repeated to titrate to clinical response. Higher doses may be repeated every 6–8 hours if needed. Higher doses are used for severe toxicity (15–20 mg/kg).

### Regulatory Information

Cattle withdrawal time (meat): 14 days.
  Cattle withdrawal time (milk): 4 days.

M

---

## Methylnaltrexone Bromide
meth′ihl nal-trex-own broe′mide

**Trade and other names:** Relistor

**Functional classification:** Prokinetic agent, intestinal stimulant

### Pharmacology and Mechanism of Action

Methylnaltrexone is a modified quaternary form of naltrexone that has opiate-antagonist properties. Because it is modified from naltrexone and charged, it does not cross the blood–brain barrier, and it has no centrally acting opiate inhibition. However, it antagonizes peripheral mu-receptors in the intestine to restore motility after postsurgical ileus. Opiate mu-receptors in the intestine ordinarily inhibit motility when stimulated because of pain or opioid drug administration. Another drug related to methylnaltrexone and used for similar purposes is alvimopan (Entereg).

Methylnaltrexone has not been studied in most animal species, but in horses, it had a short half-life of 47 minutes and a VD of 0.24 L/kg.

### Indications and Clinical Uses

Methylnaltrexone is approved for use in people to restore intestinal motility after surgery, after opiate administration, or when caused by a disorder (e.g., severe pain) that has stimulated mu-opiate receptors in the intestine. Use in animals is limited and has been primarily derived from empirical use. The only studies available are in horses in which methylnaltrexone increased fecal weight and prevented the effects of morphine on GI motility. However, at the dose studied (0.75 mg/kg), it did not fully antagonize the effects of morphine.

---

### Precautionary Information

**Adverse Reactions and Side Effects**

Adverse effects are only reported for people and include abdominal pain and diarrhea. Although it is an opiate antagonist, it has not triggered breakthrough pain.

**Contraindications and Precautions**

Do not use if there is intestinal obstruction.

**Drug Interactions**

No drug interactions have been reported for animals.

---

### Instructions for Use

The use in animals is primarily experimental and has been limited in clinical practice.

### Patient Monitoring and Laboratory Tests

No specific monitoring is necessary.

### Formulations

• Methylnaltrexone is available by injection only. It is available in 12-mg vials (0.6 mL), equivalent to 20 mg/mL in each vial.

### Stability and Storage

Store in a tightly sealed container, protected from light, and at room temperature.

### Small Animal Dosage

**Dogs and Cats**

• 0.15 mg/kg SQ injection once per 24 or 48 hours.

### Large Animal Dosage

**Horses**

• 0.75 mg/kg IV q12h every 4 days.

### Regulatory Information

No withdrawal information is available for food-producing animals.

---

## Methylprednisolone

meth-il-pred-niss'oh-lone

**Trade and other names:** Methylprednisolone: Medrol; methylprednisolone acetate: Depo-Medrol; and methylprednisolone sodium succinate: Solu-Medrol

**Functional classification:** Corticosteroid

---

### Pharmacology and Mechanism of Action

Methylprednisolone is a glucocorticoid anti-inflammatory drug. It is administered by the oral route, injection, and local delivery. The anti-inflammatory effects are complex, but they operate primarily via inhibition of inflammatory cells and suppression of inflammatory mediators. Compared with prednisolone, methylprednisolone is 1.25 times more potent.

## Indications and Clinical Uses

Methylprednisolone acetate is a long-acting depot formulation of methylprednisolone. It is slowly absorbed from the IM injection site producing glucocorticoid effects for 3–4 weeks in some animals. Methylprednisolone acetate is used for intralesional therapy, intra-articular administration for joint disease, and for treating other inflammatory conditions. Methylprednisolone sodium succinate is a water-soluble formulation intended for acute therapy when high IV doses are needed for rapid effect. It has been administered IV for treatment of shock and trauma of the CNS. Methylprednisolone oral tablets are used for treatment of conditions in animals that require short- to long-term therapy with an intermediate-acting corticosteroid. The indications for methylprednisolone tablets are similar to the use of prednisolone or prednisone tablets except that methylprednisolone is slightly more potent. Conditions treated include dermatitis, immune-mediated diseases, intestinal diseases, and neurologic and musculoskeletal diseases. Although high doses have been used to treat spinal cord trauma, this use has questionable benefit in animals. In large animals, methylprednisolone acetate is used for treatment of inflammatory conditions of the musculoskeletal system. Intra-articular administration is common in horses.

### Precautionary Information

**Adverse Reactions and Side Effects**

Side effects from corticosteroids are many and include polyphagia, polydipsia and polyuria, and hypothalamic–pituitary–adrenal axis suppression. However, the manufacturer suggests that methylprednisolone causes less polyuria and polydipsia than prednisolone. Adverse effects include GI ulceration, hepatopathy, diabetes, hyperlipidemia, decreased thyroid hormone, decreased protein synthesis, delayed wound healing, and immunosuppression. Dogs that receive high doses of methylprednisolone succinate (e.g., 30 mg/kg) have a high risk of GI bleeding. Secondary infections can occur as a result of immunosuppression and include demodicosis, toxoplasmosis, fungal infections, and UTIs.

M

In cats, injections of methylprednisolone may activate latent feline herpes virus infections in some cats. In cats, there is a concern that corticosteroids such as methylprednisolone can exacerbate congestive heart failure (CHF) through volume expansion and fluid shifts secondary to steroid-induced hyperglycemia. This has occurred in susceptible cats after injections of methylprednisolone acetate. In cats, methylprednisolone acetate injections have caused injection-site alopecia.

In horses, additional adverse effects may include risk of laminitis (although a direct link to induction of laminitis is controversial).

**Contraindications and Precautions**

Use cautiously in patients prone to GI ulcers and infection or in animals in which wound healing is necessary. Use cautiously in diabetic animals, animals with kidney disease, and pregnant animals. Use cautiously in cats because of volume expansion, especially cats at risk of CHF.

**Drug Interactions**

Like other corticosteroids, if methylprednisolone is administered with NSAIDs, there is increased risk of GI ulcers.

## Instructions for Use

The list of doses below are initial doses. If the patient responds and is stabilized, the dose may be tapered to the lowest dose possible (as low as 0.25 mg/kg/day) and possibly administered every other day.

Use of methylprednisolone is similar to other corticosteroids, such as prednisone or prednisolone. Dose adjustment should be made to account for difference in potency if interchanged with prednisone, dexamethasone, or triamcinolone acetonide. Use of methylprednisolone acetate should be evaluated carefully because one injection will cause glucocorticoid effects that persist for several days to weeks. There are no published studies that have evaluated the use of methylprednisolone sodium succinate in animals, but the use has been extrapolated from human medicine.

### Patient Monitoring and Laboratory Tests
Monitor liver enzymes, blood glucose, and kidney function during therapy. Monitor patients for signs of secondary infections. Perform an adrenocorticotropic hormone stimulation test to monitor adrenal function. Monitor cats for diabetes and heart disease when treated with methylprednisolone acetate.

### Formulations
- Methylprednisolone is available in 1-, 2-, 4-, 8-, 18-, and 32-mg tablets.
- Methylprednisolone acetate is available in 20- and 40-mg/mL suspension for injection.
- Methylprednisolone sodium succinate is available in 1- and 2-g and 125- and 500-mg vials for injection.

### Stability and Storage
Store in a tightly sealed container, protected from light, and at room temperature. Methylprednisolone is insoluble in water and slightly soluble in ethanol. Methylprednisolone acetate is slightly soluble in water. Methylprednisolone sodium succinate is highly soluble in water. When methylprednisolone sodium succinate is reconstituted, it should be used within 48 hours if kept at room temperature. Decomposition occurs with longer storage. It may be frozen at −20°C for 4 weeks with no loss of potency.

### Small Animal Dosage
#### Dogs
- Methylprednisolone oral tablets: 0.25–0.5 mg/kg q12–24h PO, with the dose dependent on the severity of the disease. The label dosage is 0.22–0.44 mg/kg q12–24h PO. After starting the initial dose, slowly taper the dose and frequency to the lowest dose possible that will control the disease condition. Long-term maintenance doses are in the range of 0.3–0.5 mg/kg every other day, PO.
- Methylprednisolone acetate: 1 mg/kg (or 20–40 mg/dog) IM every 1–3 weeks.
- Methylprednisolone sodium succinate (for emergency use): 30 mg/kg IV and repeat at 15 mg/kg in 2–6 hours IV.
- Replacement therapy for adrenal insufficiency: 0.2 mg/kg/day.

#### Cats
- Methylprednisolone oral tablets: 0.25–0.5 mg/kg q12–24h PO, with the dosage dependent on the severity of the disease. The label dosage is 0.22–0.44 mg/kg q12–24h PO. After starting the initial dose, slowly taper the dose and frequency to the lowest dose possible that will control the disease condition.
- Methylprednisolone acetate: 10–20 mg/cat IM every 1–3 weeks.
- Methylprednisolone sodium succinate (for emergency use): 30 mg/kg IV and repeat at 15 mg/kg in 2–6 hours IV.

### Large Animal Dosage
#### Horses
- 200 mg as a single total dose injected intramuscularly.
- Intra-articular dose: 40–240 mg total dose, with the average dose of 120 mg injected in the joint space using sterile technique.

## Regulatory Information
In horses, 200 mg per joint was detected in horses for 18 days; 100 mg per joint was detected for 7 days. For food animals, withdrawal times are not established. For extralabel use withdrawal interval estimates, contact FARAD at www.FARAD.org. RCI Classification: 4

# Methyltestosterone
meth-ill-tess-toss'teh-rone

**Trade and other names:** Android and generic brands

**Functional classification:** Hormone, anabolic agent

## Pharmacology and Mechanism of Action
Methyltestosterone is a form of testosterone used as an anabolic androgenic agent. Injections of methyltestosterone mimic the effects of testosterone and are used as a replacement for testosterone or for use in debilitated animals that require an anabolic agent.

## Indications and Clinical Uses
Methyltestosterone is used for anabolic actions or testosterone hormone replacement therapy (androgenic deficiency). Testosterone has been used to stimulate erythropoiesis. Other similar agents used include testosterone cypionate and testosterone propionate.

M

## Precautionary Information
### Adverse Reactions and Side Effects
Adverse effects are caused by excessive androgenic action of testosterone. Prostatic hyperplasia is possible in male dogs. Masculinization can occur in female dogs. Hepatopathy is more common with oral methylated testosterone formulations than with non-methylated forms. Therefore, monitor bilirubin and hepatic enzymes for evidence of liver reactions.

### Contraindications and Precautions
Do not administer to pregnant animals.

### Drug Interactions
No drug interactions have been reported for animals.

## Instructions for Use
Use of testosterone androgens has not been evaluated in clinical studies in veterinary medicine. The clinical use is based primarily on experimental evidence or experiences in people.

## Patient Monitoring and Laboratory Tests
Monitor hepatic enzymes and clinical signs for evidence of cholestasis and hepatotoxicity during treatment.

## Formulations
• Methyltestosterone is available in 10- and 25-mg tablets.

## Stability and Storage

Store in a tightly sealed container, protected from light, and at room temperature. Stability of compounded formulations has not been evaluated.

## Small Animal Dosage

**Dogs**
- 5–25 mg/dog q24–48h PO.

**Cats**
- 2.5–5 mg/cat q24–48h PO.

## Large Animal Dosage
- No large animal doses have been reported.

## Regulatory Information

Do not use in animals intended for food.
Methyltestosterone is a Schedule III controlled drug.
RCI Classification: 4

---

# Metoclopramide Hydrochloride
met-oh-kloe-prah′mide hye-droe-klor′ide

**Trade and other names:** Reglan and Maxolon
**Functional classification:** Antiemetic

## Pharmacology and Mechanism of Action

Metoclopramide is an antiemetic and prokinetic drug that has been used in small animals for many years to control postoperative vomiting and stimulate GI motility. Metoclopramide stimulates motility of the upper GI tract and is a centrally acting antiemetic. The mechanism of action of metoclopramide is not completely understood. Among the proposed mechanisms is stimulation of $5\text{-HT}_4$ (serotonin) receptors or an increase in the release of acetylcholine in the GI tract, possibly through a prejunctional mechanism. The affinity for $5\text{-HT}_4$ receptors is low compared with other, more effective motility-modifying drugs. It inhibits gastric relaxation induced by dopamine, thus enhancing the cholinergic responses of gastric smooth muscle to increase motility. It also increases the tone of the lower esophageal sphincter. Metoclopramide acts centrally to inhibit dopamine in the CRTZ, which is responsible for antiemetic effects. The antiemetic effects occur primarily through dopamine ($D_2$) receptor blocking action.

Through $D_2$ receptor antagonism, metoclopramide increases prolactin, which has effects on the mammary gland and lactation.

*Pharmacokinetics* The half-life in dogs has ranged from less than 1 hour to 2 hours; effects on the esophageal sphincter persisted for only 30–60 minutes.

## Indications and Clinical Uses

Metoclopramide is used primarily for gastroparesis and treatment of vomiting. It is not effective for dogs with gastric dilation and should not be used in dogs with megaesophagus. In dogs, it is not very effective for decreasing gastroesophageal reflux or for increasing stomach emptying. One study demonstrated effects for gastroesophageal reflux in surgical patients at high doses of 1 mg/kg IV followed by infusion of 1 mg/kg/h, but other studies showed no benefit. The primary effect in dogs appears to be via its antiemetic properties (dopamine antagonism in the vomiting center).

Because metoclopramide transiently increases prolactin secretion, there has been interest in using it for treating agalactia in animals. Metoclopramide increases prolactin and increases mammary gland development and lactation. In humans, it has been used as a galactagogue to increase lactation. This property also has been used in dogs to increase lactation in butches. At a dosage of 0.2 mg/kg PO q6h, it increases prolactin and milk lactose. Domperidone also has this activity and is preferred for this use in dogs and cats. (See Domperidone.)

In horses, it has been used to treat intestinal postoperative ileus, but adverse effects have limited the use. It is not effective in ruminants. In people, metoclopramide has also been used to treat hiccups and lactation deficiency.

## Precautionary Information

### Adverse Reactions and Side Effects

Adverse effects are primarily related to blockade of central dopaminergic receptors. Adverse effects similar to those that are reported for other centrally acting $D_2$-receptor antagonists such as phenothiazines. In horses, undesirable side effects have been common and limit the therapeutic use. Adverse effects in horses include behavioral changes, excitement, and abdominal discomfort. Excitement from IV infusions can be severe. In calves at doses greater than 0.1 mg/kg, it produces neurologic effects.

### Contraindications and Precautions

Do not use in patients with epilepsy or with diseases caused by GI obstruction. Use cautiously in horses because dangerous behavior changes may occur. In people, it has been safe to use in the first trimester of pregnancy, but the effects on pregnancy in animals have not been studied. When used to increase lactation, metoclopramide is excreted into milk but not at a high enough level to harm newborn animals.

### Drug Interactions

Efficacy is diminished when administered with parasympatholytic (atropine-like) drugs.

## Instructions for Use

The use in animals is based primarily on studies in research animals, experience in people, or anecdotal experience in animals. There have been small observational studies in clinical patients to evaluate efficacy for gastroesophageal reflux. The most common use is for general antiemetic purposes, for which it has shown efficacy in dogs. Doses as high as 2 mg/kg have been used to prevent vomiting during cancer chemotherapy (higher doses may produce antiserotonin effects).

In recent years, other antiemetic agents have become more popular and widely used in small animals compared to metoclopramide. These agents include maropitant and serotonin antagonists (e.g., ondansetron).

In horses, there is some increase in intestinal motility at recommended doses, but little effect on the large bowel has been seen. In calves, metoclopramide had little effect on rumen motility.

## Patient Monitoring and Laboratory Tests

Monitor for signs of behavior disturbances from treatment, especially when IV doses are administered.

## Formulations Available

- Metoclopramide is available in 5- and 10-mg tablets, 1-mg/mL oral solution, and 5-mg/mL injection in 2-, 10-, and 30-mL vials.

## Stability and Storage

Store in a tightly sealed container, protected from light, and at room temperature. It is incompatible with other drugs when mixed in solution. Do not freeze. Stability is less than 24 hours if not protected from light. The solution has a pH of 4–5 and is stable over a pH range of 2–9. Individual doses may be stored in plastic syringes and are stable for 90 days in the refrigerator and 60 days at room temperature.

## Small Animal Dosage

### Dogs and Cats

- Antiemetic dosage: 0.5 mg/kg q8h IV, IM, or PO.
- CRI: Administer a loading dose of 0.4 mg/kg followed by 0.3 mg/kg/h. In refractory cases, CRI dose may be increased up to 1.0 mg/kg/h. For antiemetic treatment with cancer chemotherapy, the dose used is up to 2 mg/kg per 24 hours.
- Dosage to stimulate lactation: 0.2 mg/kg PO q6h for 6 days.

## Large Animal Dosage

### Horses

- Infusion of metoclopramide (0.125–0.25 mg/kg/h) added to IV fluids to reduce postoperative ileus in horses (see precautions regarding use in horses).

### Calves and cattle

- Not recommended because it is not a suitable prokinetic agent in ruminants. At a dose of 0.1 mg/kg IV to cattle, it does not increase abomasal emptying. Adverse reactions develop at higher doses (0.3 mg/kg).

## Regulatory Information

Withdrawal times are not established for animals that produce food. For extralabel use withdrawal interval estimates, contact FARAD at www.FARAD.org.
RCI Classification: 4

---

# Metoprolol Tartrate
meh-toe′proe-lole tar′trate

**Trade and other names:** Lopressor

**Functional classification:** Beta blocker

## Pharmacology and Mechanism of Action

Metoprolol is a beta$_1$-adrenergic receptor blocker. Metoprolol has similar properties to propranolol except that metoprolol is specific for beta$_1$ receptors, with less effect on beta$_2$ receptors. Metoprolol is a lipophilic beta blocker and relies on the liver for clearance. Lipophilic beta blockers such as metoprolol undergo high first-pass clearance, which reduces oral bioavailability and causes high interpatient variability in plasma concentrations and effects. An alternative beta$_1$ blocker used in animals is atenolol, which is water soluble and cleared by the kidneys.

## Indications and Clinical Uses

Metoprolol is used to control tachyarrhythmias and to control the response from adrenergic stimulation in animals. Beta blockers effectively slow heart rate. Metoprolol is used in animals in which it is important to control ventricular rate, decrease conduction through the atrioventricular (AV) and sinoatrial nodes, and improve diastolic function. In animals, it has been used for tachyarrhythmias, hypertrophic cardiomyopathy, atrial fibrillation, and other cardiac diseases. Use in animals has been primarily derived from empirical use and recommendations from cardiology experts. There are no well-controlled clinical studies or efficacy trials to document clinical effectiveness. Atenolol is used more often for oral treatment in dogs and cats.

### Precautionary Information

**Adverse Reactions and Side Effects**

Adverse effects are primarily caused by excessive cardiovascular depression (decreased inotropic effects). Metoprolol may cause AV block.

**Contraindications and Precautions**

Use cautiously in animals prone to bronchoconstriction.

**Drug Interactions**

Lipophilic beta blockers such as metoprolol are subject to hepatic metabolism and may be prone to drug interactions that affect hepatic metabolizing enzymes. If administered with digoxin, it may potentiate an AV-nodal conduction block.

## Instructions for Use

Results of clinical studies in animals have not been reported. Use in animals (and doses) is based on experience in people or anecdotal experience in animals.

## Patient Monitoring and Laboratory Tests

Monitor heart rate and rhythm during treatment.

## Formulations

- Metoprolol is available in 25-, 37.5-, 50-, 75-, and 100-mg tablets and 1-mg/mL injection.

## Stability and Storage

Store in a tightly sealed container, protected from light, and at room temperature. Metoprolol tartrate is soluble in water and ethanol. Protect tablets from moisture and freezing. Suspensions have been prepared in syrups and other flavorings with no loss of stability after 60 days of storage.

## Small Animal Dosage

**Dogs**

- 5–50 mg per dog (0.5–1 mg/kg) q8h PO.

**Cats**

- 2–15 mg per cat q8h PO.

## Large Animal Dosage

- No large animal doses have been reported.

## Regulatory Information

Withdrawal times are not established for animals that produce food. For extralabel use withdrawal interval estimates, contact FARAD at www.FARAD.org.

RCI Classification: 3

# Metronidazole and Metronidazole Benzoate

meh-troe-nye′dah-zole

**Trade and other names:** Flagyl and generic brands

**Functional classification:** Antibacterial, antiparasitic

## Pharmacology and Mechanism of Action

Metronidazole is an antibacterial and antiprotozoal drug used frequently in small animals, primarily for GI problems. It is a second-generation nitroimidazole in which the activity involves generation of free nitro radicals via metabolism within protozoa and bacteria. Metronidazole disrupts DNA in the organism via reaction with intracellular metabolite. Its action is specific for anaerobic bacteria and protozoa. Resistance is rare. It is active against some protozoa, including *Trichomonas* spp., *Giardia* spp., and intestinal protozoal parasites. It also has in vitro activity against anaerobic bacteria and *Helicobacter* spp.

*Pharmacokinetics:* Metronidazole oral absorption is nearly complete in animals (75%–100% in horses and 60%–100% in dogs). Rectal absorption in horses is 30%. The half-lives are 2–4 hours in horses, 9–12 hours in foals, and 3–5 hours in dogs. Metronidazole benzoate is formulated for cats to improve palatability. In this form, the oral absorption (12.4 mg/kg of the base) is 64%, with a half-life of 5 hours.

## Indications and Clinical Uses

Metronidazole is not approved for use in animal animals, and the use is derived from small observational studies, anecdotal experience, and opinions from experts. It has been used to treat diarrhea and other intestinal problems caused by intestinal protozoa such as *Giardia, Trichomonas,* and *Entamoeba* spp. It may be used in small animals and horses for treatment of a variety of anaerobic infections. Common uses in horses include treatment of infections caused by *Clostridium* spp., and *Bacteroides fragilis.* Metronidazole has been used for immune-modulating activity in the intestine of animals and administered for inflammatory bowel disease in animals. However, evidence of a direct immune-modulating effect or immunosuppressive effect is lacking. A common use of metronidazole is for short-term treatment of acute nonspecific diarrhea in animals. Clinical results have been mixed for this use. One controlled study in dogs showed that there is no benefit from this treatment compared to placebo. In another study, the duration of diarrhea was decreased by approximately 1.5 days compared to placebo treatment in dogs. The diarrhea resolved in most dogs within several days, regardless of treatment. Metronidazole benzoate, an ester pro-drug of metronidazole, has been used in cats because it is more palatable.

## Precautionary Information

### Adverse Reactions and Side Effects

The most severe adverse effect is caused by toxicity to the CNS. It is highly lipophilic and readily crosses the blood–brain barrier. High doses have caused lethargy, CNS depression, ataxia, tremors, seizures, vomiting, and weakness. Most CNS toxicity caused from metronidazole in animals occurs at high doses (greater than 60 mg/kg/day). The CNS signs are related to inhibition of action of gamma-aminobutyric acid (GABA) and are responsive to benzodiazepines (diazepam 0.4 mg/kg q8h for 3 days).

In horses, adverse effects include peripheral neuropathy, hepatopathy, and decreased appetite, all of which are more likely with high doses. The drug has a longer half-life in foals, and foals may be more prone to adverse effects than adult horses.

Like other nitroimidazoles, metronidazole has the potential to produce mutagenic changes in cells, but the clinical significance of this effect is uncertain. There are no reports of increased rated of cancer in patients that have received metronidazole.

Like other nitroimidazoles, it has a bitter taste and can cause vomiting and anorexia. At a dose of 25 mg/kg in dogs, it may degrade the olfactory ability. This may affect the ability of working dogs (e.g., law enforcement dogs) to perform their duties to detect explosives, illegal drugs, and other agents. A total of 50% of the treated dogs had decreased olfactory ability in one study.

Metronidazole benzoate has been used in some cats safely at 25 mg/kg q12h for 7 days. However, there is a caution about the effect of benzoate salts in cats because it is a benzoic acid derivative. Benzoic acid can be toxic to cats and causes ataxia, blindness, respiratory problems, and other CNS disorders. Despite this concern, it is estimated that 500 mg/kg/day of metronidazole benzoate would be needed to provide a toxic dose of benzoic acid to cats. Nevertheless, any cat showing CNS or other signs of toxicity should have the metronidazole benzoate discontinued immediately.

### Contraindications and Precautions

Fetal abnormalities have not been demonstrated in animals with recommended doses but use cautiously during pregnancy.

### Drug Interactions

Like other nitroimidazoles, it can potentiate the effects of warfarin and cyclosporine via inhibition of drug metabolism.

M

## Instructions for Use

Metronidazole is one of the most commonly used drugs for anaerobic infections. Although it is effective for giardiasis, other drugs used for *Giardia* spp. include albendazole, fenbendazole, and quinacrine. CNS toxicity is a concern, but it is dose related. The maximum dose that should be administered is 50–65 mg/kg/day in any species.

Metronidazole is unpalatable and can produce a metallic taste. In cats, when the tablet is crushed or broken, the unpalatability is particularly a problem. Metronidazole benzoate has a bland taste and is better tolerated. Metronidazole benzoate is not commercially available in the United States. However, it may be available from compounding pharmacies. Because of the weight of metronidazole benzoate versus metronidazole hydrochloride, a factor of 1.6 times is used to convert a metronidazole hydrochloride dose to a metronidazole benzoate dose. Metronidazole benzoate is 62% metronidazole; therefore, 20 mg/kg of metronidazole benzoate delivers 12.4 mg/kg of metronidazole.

In horses, oral absorption of metronidazole is practically complete and not affected by feeding pattern (e.g., with or without food and similar with hay or concentrate). However, absorption from rectal administration to horses is low.

Metronidazole should not be injected directly; it is too acidic. See Stability and Storage section for mixing instructions.

## Patient Monitoring and Laboratory Tests

Monitor for neurologic adverse effects. MICs for anaerobic bacteria are typically 2–4 mcg/mL, or less. The CLSI breakpoint is ≤8 mcg/mL.

## Formulations

- Metronidazole is available in 250- and 500-mg tablets, 375-mg capsules, 50-mg/mL suspension, and 5-mg/mL injection.
- Metronidazole benzoate is a formulation not available in the United States but has been compounded for veterinary use. Metronidazole benzoate is 62% metronidazole. It has been formulated in Ora-Plus and Ora-Sweet (drug excipients) to a concentration of 16 mg/mL.

## Stability and Storage

The base is slightly soluble in water. The benzoate form is practically insoluble; the hydrochloride form is soluble in water. Metronidazole has been crushed and mixed with some flavorings to mask the taste. When mixed with some syrups or water, with exceptions listed here, decomposition occurs within 28 days.

Metronidazole benzoate prepared in vehicles such as Ora-Plus or Ora-Sweet was stable for 90 days. Metronidazole base (from tablets) also was mixed with these vehicles and was found to be stable for 90 days.

When reconstituted, metronidazole hydrochloride is too acidic (pH 0.5–2) for direct injection. Injection of 5 mg/mL should be further diluted with 100 mL (0.9% saline, 5% dextrose, or Ringer's solution) and neutralized with 5 mEq of sodium bicarbonate per 500 mg for a pH of 6–7. Reconstituted injectable forms are stable for 96 hours but after dilution should be discarded after 24 hours.

## Small Animal Dosage

### Dogs

- Anaerobic bacteria: 15 mg/kg q12h or 12 mg/kg q8h PO.
- Anaerobic bacteria: IV dose: 15 mg/kg IV via slow infusion over at least 30 minutes in a diluted form. Give slowly to avoid adverse CNS effects.
- *Giardia* infection: 12–15 mg/kg q12h for 5–7 days PO.

### Cats

- Anaerobic bacteria: 10–25 mg/kg q24h PO.
- *Giardia* infection: 17 mg/kg (one third tablet per cat) q24h for 8 days.
- Metronidazole benzoate (for treatment of *Giardia* infection): 25 mg/kg PO 12h for 7 days. Metronidazole benzoate is 62% metronidazole; therefore 20 mg/kg of metronidazole benzoate delivers 12.4 mg/kg of metronidazole.

## Large Animal Dosage

### Horses

- Treatment of anaerobic bacteria and protozoal infections: 10 mg/kg q12h PO. Note: Some clinicians have used higher doses (≤15–20 mg/kg q6h), but at these doses, side effects are more likely.
- Foals: 10–15 mg/kg IV or PO q12h.

### Cattle

- Treatment of trichomoniasis (bulls): 75 mg/kg q12h IV for three doses. (See Regulatory Information.)

## Regulatory Information

Do not administer to animals that produce food. Administration of nitroimidazoles to animals intended for food is prohibited. Treated cattle must not be slaughtered for food.

# Mexiletine

meks-il'eh-teen

**Trade and other names:** Mexitil

**Functional classification:** Antiarrhythmic

## Pharmacology and Mechanism of Action

Mexiletine is an antiarrhythmic drug used occasionally in dogs. Mexiletine is a Class IB antiarrhythmic agent. Mechanism of action is to block the fast sodium channel and depress Phase 0 of depolarization. Because lidocaine is not absorbed orally, mexiletine has been used when oral administration of a Class I antiarrhythmic agent is needed in dogs. It has a similar mechanism of action as lidocaine. It is absorbed approximately 90% in people without significant first-pass effects. It is presumed to have good absorption also in dogs, although this has not been studied.

An additional use of mexiletine is for treating chronic pain. It is used to treat pain caused by diabetic neuropathy and nerve injury at lower doses than the antiarrhythmic dose.

## Indications and Clinical Uses

Mexiletine has been used to treat ventricular arrhythmias. Although lidocaine is often the first Class I antiarrhythmic agent used for injection in the hospital, when longer-term treatment with an oral drug is needed, mexiletine is often the first choice.

The doses used in dogs are derived from empirical use and extrapolation from human medicine. It is often used in combination with atenolol or sotalol (Class II and Class III antiarrhythmic agents, respectively) because it may have better electrophysiological effects when used in combination. It may also counteract the adverse effects of sotalol on the action potential duration.

M

## Precautionary Information

### Adverse Reactions and Side Effects

In dogs, the most common adverse effects are GI problems. High doses may cause excitement and tremors. Mexiletine can be arrhythmogenic in some animals. In people, related drugs (flecainide and encainide) can be proarrhythmogenic and associated with excessive mortality.

### Contraindications and Precautions

Use cautiously in animals with liver disease or monitor liver parameters during use.

### Drug Interactions

Sotalol will increase plasma drug concentrations.

## Instructions for Use

Results of controlled clinical studies in animals have not been reported. Use in animals (and doses) is based on experience in people, research studies in experimental dogs, or anecdotal experience in animals. Administer with food to decrease GI problems.

## Patient Monitoring and Laboratory Tests

Monitor ECG during use. Effective plasma drug concentrations are 0.75–2.0 mcg/mL (extrapolated from people).

## Formulations

- Mexiletine is available in 150-, 200-, and 250-mg capsules.

## Stability and Storage

Store in a tightly sealed container, protected from light, and at room temperature. It is freely soluble in water and ethanol.

## Small Animal Dosage

### Dogs

- 6 mg/kg q8–12h PO.
- Chronic pain caused by nerve injury: 4–10 mg/kg PO q8h.

### Cats

No safe dose has been established.

## Large Animal Dosage

- No large animal doses have been reported.

## Regulatory Information

Withdrawal times are not established for animals that produce food. For extralabel use withdrawal interval estimates, contact FARAD at www.FARAD.org.

RCI Classification: 4

# Mibolerone
mih-bole′er-one

**Trade and other names:** Cheque Drops

**Functional classification:** Hormone

## Pharmacology and Mechanism of Action

Mibolerone is an androgenic steroid drug. Mibolerone mimics androgens in the body to produce hormone effects that suppress estrus.

## Indications and Clinical Uses

Mibolerone is used to suppress estrus in animals. The primary indication is to prevent estrus in adult female dogs. There are no other established indications.

## Precautionary Information

### Adverse Reactions and Side Effects

Many bitches show clitoral enlargement or discharge from treatment.

### Contraindications and Precautions

Do not use in Bedlington terriers. Do not administer to pregnant animals. Avoid administration in bitches before their first estrous period. Do not use with perianal adenoma or carcinoma. Do not use in cats. Mibolerone has been abused in people for use as a body-building drug. Therefore extreme caution should be used when dispensing this medication to animal owners.

### Drug Interactions

No drug interactions have been reported.

## Instructions for Use

Treatment ordinarily is initiated 30 days prior to onset of estrus. Continue treatment as long as needed, but it is not recommended to be used for more than 2 years. Mibolerone should not be used in bitches before the first estrous period. It is not intended for animals being used primarily for breeding purposes.

## Patient Monitoring and Laboratory Tests

Monitor hepatic enzymes periodically if used chronically because liver injury is possible.

## Formulations

- Mibolerone has been discontinued by the manufacturer. However, it may be available from some other sources. Originally, it was available in a 100-mcg/mL oral solution.

## Stability and Storage

Store in a tightly sealed container, protected from light, and at room temperature. Stability of compounded formulations has not been evaluated.

## Small Animal Dosage

### Dogs

- 2.6–5 mcg/kg/day PO.
- Bitches weighing 0.45–11.3 kg: 30 mcg/day PO.
- Bitches weighing 11.8–22.7 kg: 60 mcg/day PO.
- Bitches weighing 23–45.3 kg: 120 mcg/day PO.
- Bitches weighing more than 45.8 kg: 180 mcg/day PO.

### Cats

- Safe dose not established.

## Large Animal Dosage

- No large animal doses have been reported.

## Regulatory Information

Do not administer to animals that produce food.

M

## Midazolam Hydrochloride

mid-az′oe-lam hye-droe-klor′ide

**Trade and other names:** Versed

**Functional classification:** Anticonvulsant, sedative

## Pharmacology and Mechanism of Action

Midazolam is a widely used benzodiazepine. It has centrally acting effects and is a CNS depressant, anticonvulsant, and sedative. Midazolam, like other benzodiazepines, binds to a specific GABA-binding site. It may modify the GABA-binding sites and increase the action of GABA on nerve cells. Sedative effects of midazolam may be attributed to potentiation of GABA pathways that act to regulate release of monoamine neurotransmitters in the CNS. Benzodiazepines may act as muscle relaxants by inhibiting certain spinal pathways or directly depressing motor nerve and muscle function.

*Pharmacokinetics:* The pharmacokinetics of midazolam have been studied in dogs and horses. In dogs, the half-life is short (1–2 hours) with a high clearance (10–27 mL/kg/min). Absorption in dogs is variable from IM administration (50%–90%) but negligible from rectal administration. Metabolites are negligible in dogs. Peak plasma concentrations in dogs from IM injection is 7–8 minutes. In horses, the terminal half-lives are 2–5.8 hours at 0.05 mg/kg IV and 3.2–15 hours at 0.1 mg/kg IV. Clearance in horses is approximately 10 mL/kg/min.

## Indications and Clinical Uses

Midazolam has a variety of uses in veterinary medicine. Although it is not approved for any animal species, it is one of the most frequently used benzodiazepines used extralabel in animals. It is used as an anesthetic adjunct, frequently with other anesthetics. It is used for similar indications as diazepam, but because it is water soluble, midazolam can be administered in an aqueous vehicle and administered intramuscularly compared with other drugs of this class. (Drugs such as diazepam are not water soluble.) It has been mixed with other water-soluble anesthetic agents in the same syringe (e.g., ketamine and alpha$_2$ agonists) and administered intravenously. In horses, it has been administered in the same solution with ketamine and xylazine. In foals, it has been used to treat neonatal seizures (see dosing).

In many animal species, it also has been administered as an anticonvulsant, muscle relaxant, and sedative. These uses and dose regimens are based on observational clinical studies, pharmacokinetic studies, or opinions from anesthesiologists and other clinical experts. Midazolam solution has been administered intranasal to dogs and shown to produce effective levels for control of seizures (0.2 mg/kg). The FDA-approved intranasal treatment for seizures in people is Nayzilam, and administered as a single-dose 5-mg spray. Midazolam oral solution has been effective in children for sedation and hypnosis at a dose of 0.5–0.75 mg/kg with an onset of 10–30 minutes. The use of the oral midazolam solution has not been reported for animals.

## Precautionary Information

### Adverse Reactions and Side Effects

Side effects are consistent with effects of benzodiazepines and include sedation, ataxia, and lethargy. Midazolam administered intravenously can cause serious cardiorespiratory depression. Some animals may experience paradoxical excitement. Chronic administration may lead to dependence and a withdrawal syndrome if abruptly discontinued. In horses, it causes ataxia, swaying, agitation, and weakness shortly after IV administration. If severe adverse reactions occur, consider administering an antagonist (flumazenil, Romazicon).

### Contraindications and Precautions

Use cautiously when administered intravenously, especially with opiates. Administer slowly if administered IV or administer IM or in fluids. Diazepam and midazolam can increase intraocular pressure, and use in patients with some forms of glaucoma should be avoided.

### Drug Interactions

Compared with diazepam, it is water soluble and is more compatible with fluid solutions and IV anesthetics. It has been administered safely with several anesthetics, sedatives, preanesthetics, and anticonvulsants. However, midazolam is metabolized in the liver by P450 enzymes, which may be inhibited by some drugs (see Appendix I). For example, ketoconazole inhibits clearance of midazolam in dogs.

## Instructions for Use

Well-controlled clinical trials have not been reported, but the use of midazolam is reported in several anesthetic protocols for animals based on clinical experience. Unlike other benzodiazepines, midazolam can be administered intramuscularly.

## Patient Monitoring and Laboratory Tests

Samples of plasma or serum may be analyzed for concentrations of benzodiazepines, but this is not often performed. Plasma concentrations in the range of 100–250 ng/mL have been cited as the therapeutic range for people. Other references have cited this range as 150–300 ng/mL. However, there are no readily available tests for monitoring in many veterinary laboratories. Laboratories that analyze human samples may have nonspecific tests for benzodiazepines.

## Formulations
- Midazolam is available in a 5-mg/mL injection.
- Midazolam intranasal spray (Nayzilam) is available as a single-dose 5 mg/0.1 mL spray.
- Midazolam oral syrup is available in a cherry-flavored syrup for children in a concentration of 2 mg/mL.

## Stability and Storage
Store in a tightly sealed container, protected from light, and at room temperature. Solubility of midazolam in water is pH dependent. At lower pH values (pH less than 4), it becomes more soluble. It can be mixed for short-term use with other water-soluble anesthetics if administered immediately after mixing. Midazolam and ketamine hydrochloride are compatible when mixed in the same syringe.

## Small Animal Dosage
### Dogs
- 0.1–0.25 mg/kg IV or IM.
- 0.1–0.3 mg/kg/h IV infusion.
- Status epilepticus: 0.1–0.2 mg/kg IV bolus or 0.2 mg/kg administered intranasal in a 5-mg/mL solution.
- Oral administration: midazolam syrup (2 mg/mL), 0.5–0.75 mg/kg for sedation (dose extrapolated from pediatric use).

### Cats
- Sedation: 0.05 mg/kg IV.
- Induction of anesthesia: 0.3–0.6 mg/kg IV combined with 3 mg/kg of ketamine. (Additional doses of ketamine at 1–2 mg/kg can be administered as needed.)

## Large Animal Dosage
### Pigs
- Up to 0.5 mg/kg IM, usually in combination with ketamine.

### Horses
- Neonatal seizures in foals: 0.1–0.2 mg/kg (5–10 mg per foal) IV over 15–20 minutes or IM followed by 3 mg/h IV (range, 2–6 mL/h) CRI to control seizures. The infusion dose is prepared by adding 10 mL (5 mg/mL) to 100 mL of saline to make a solution of 0.5 mg/mL.
- Anesthetic adjunct in horses: 0.1 mg/kg IV administered with ketamine (2.2 mg/kg) or other anesthetics (e.g., xylazine).

### Sheep
- 0.5 mg/kg IV or IM for short-term sedation.

## Regulatory Information
Withdrawal times are not established for animals that produce food. For extralabel use withdrawal interval estimates, contact FARAD at www.FARAD.org.
Schedule IV controlled drug.
RCI Classification: 2

# Milbemycin Oxime
mil-beh-mye'sin ahk'seem

**Trade and other names:** Interceptor, Interceptor Flavor Tabs, and Safeheart

Milbemycin also is an ingredient in Sentinel. It is combined with spinosad in Trifexis

**Functional classification:** Antiparasitic

## Pharmacology and Mechanism of Action

Milbemycin is a commonly used antiparasitic drug in animals. Avermectins (ivermectin-like drugs) and milbemycins (milbemycin and moxidectin) are macrocyclic lactones and share similarities, including mechanism of action. These drugs are neurotoxic to parasites by potentiating glutamate-gated chloride ion channels in parasites. Paralysis and death of the parasite are caused by increased permeability to chloride ions and hyperpolarization of nerve cells. These drugs also potentiate other chloride channels, including ones gated by GABA. Mammals ordinarily are not affected because they lack glutamate-gated chloride channels, and there is a lower affinity for other mammalian chloride channels. Because these drugs ordinarily do not penetrate the blood–brain barrier, GABA-gated channels in the CNS of mammals are not affected. Milbemycin is active against intestinal parasites, mites, bots, heartworm microfilaria, and developing larvae. Milbemycin has no effect on trematode or cestode parasites.

## Indications and Clinical Uses

Milbemycin is used as a heartworm preventative, miticide, and microfilaricide. It is also used to control infections of hookworm, roundworms, and whipworms. It has been used in combination with flea control drugs (see Sentinel, which contains milbemycin oxime and lufenuron). At high doses, it has been used to treat infections caused by *Demodex* in dogs (see dosing section). It is sometimes preferred over other macrocyclic lactones for treating *Demodex* infection because it is better tolerated at high doses. (Note: The isooxazolines afoxolaner, fluralaner, lotilaner, and sarolaner are preferred for treating *Demodex* infection.) Milbemycin is widely used in animals, and the efficacy and dosing regimens are established through the approvals and clinical studies by the sponsors.

## Precautionary Information

### Adverse Reactions and Side Effects

At doses of 5 mg/kg, it was well tolerated in most dogs (10 times the heartworm preventative dose). At 10 mg/kg (20 times the heartworm preventative dose), it caused depression, ataxia, and salivation in some dogs. Toxicity may occur at high doses and in breeds in which milbemycin crosses the blood–brain barrier at dosages as low as 1.5 mg/kg per day. Sensitive breeds include collies, Australian shepherds, Old English sheepdogs, longhaired whippets, and Shetland sheepdogs. In susceptible animals, the effects are neurotoxic, and signs include depression, ataxia, difficulty with vision, coma, and death. Sensitivity to milbemycin occurs in certain breeds because of a mutation in the multidrug resistance gene (*ABCB1 gene*) that regulates the membrane pump P-glycoprotein. This mutation affects the efflux pump in the blood–brain barrier. Animals with a gene mutation lack a functional membrane pump, and milbemycin can accumulate in the brains of susceptible animals. High doses in normal animals may also produce similar toxicosis. However, at doses used for heartworm prevention, this effect is unlikely. At high doses used for treating *Demodex* infections, diarrhea may occur in some dogs.

### Contraindications and Precautions

Do not use in dogs that have shown sensitivity to ivermectin or other drugs in this class (see previous breed list). Treatment using three times the daily doses from mating to 1 week before weaning did not produce any adverse effects in the pregnant bitch, the fetus, or puppies. One-time doses of three times the monthly rate before or shortly after whelping caused no adverse effects on the puppies. Milbemycin is excreted in milk. Puppies given milbemycin at 19 times the regular dose showed adverse effects, but signs were transient for only 24–48 hours.

In cats, it is generally well tolerated. In cats treated for *Demodex* infection at high doses (1–2 mg/kg), some vomiting and diarrhea can be observed, but neurologic signs are rare.

**Drug Interactions**

Do not use with drugs that may increase penetration across the blood–brain barrier. Such drugs include p-glycoprotein inhibitors such as ketoconazole, cyclosporine, quinidine, and some macrolide antibiotics (see Appendix J for a list of p-glycoprotein inhibitors).

## Instructions for Use

Doses vary depending on parasite treated. Treatment of demodicosis requires a higher dose administered daily than the heartworm preventative dose. For *Demodex* infection, use a protocol of 1 mg/kg/day until clinical cure followed by 3 mg/kg/wk for a parasitological cure. Treatment can be long because it may require 4 months for a clinical cure and 8 months for a parasitologic cure.

## Patient Monitoring and Laboratory Tests

Monitor for heartworm status in dogs before initiating treatment with milbemycin.

## Formulations Available

- Milbemycin is available in 2.3-, 5.75-, 11.5-, and 23-mg tablets. It is also found in other combination products (e.g., with spinosad in Trifexis).

## Stability and Storage

Store in a tightly sealed container, protected from light, and at room temperature. Stability of compounded formulations has not been evaluated.

## Small Animal Dosage

**Dogs**

- Heartworm prevention and control of endoparasites: 0.5 mg/kg q30days PO.
- Demodicosis: 2 mg/kg q24h PO for 60–120 days or 1 mg/kg/day until a clinical cure is observed followed by 3 mg/kg once per week until a parasitologic cure (negative scraping) is observed.
- Sarcoptic mange: 2 mg/kg q7days for 3–5 weeks PO.
- Cheyletiellosis: 2 mg/kg/wk PO.

**Cats**

- Heartworm and endoparasite control: 2 mg/kg every 30 days PO.
- Demodicosis in cats: 1–2 mg/kg q24h PO.

## Large Animal Dosage

- No large animal doses have been reported.

## Regulatory Information

Withdrawal times are not established for animals that produce food. For extralabel use withdrawal interval estimates, contact FARAD at www.FARAD.org.

# Mineral Oil

**Trade and other names:** Generic brands

**Functional classification:** Laxative

## Pharmacology and Mechanism of Action

Mineral is a lubricant laxative that has been widely used for many years. Mineral oil has nonspecific effects to increase water content of stool and act as a lubricant for intestinal contents.

## Indications and Clinical Uses

Mineral oil is administered orally (via stomach tube in horses) to increase passage of feces for treatment of impaction and constipation. It is primarily used in large animals (especially horses), and small animal use is uncommon.

### Precautionary Information

**Adverse Reactions and Side Effects**

Adverse effects have not been reported. Chronic use may decrease absorption of fat-soluble vitamins.

**Contraindications and Precautions**

Use caution when administering via stomach tube. Accidental administration into the lungs has produced fatal reactions.

**Drug Interactions**

No drug interactions reported. Chronic use may inhibit absorption of fat-soluble vitamins.

## Instructions for Use

Use is empirical. No clinical results reported.

## Patient Monitoring and Laboratory Tests

No specific monitoring is necessary.

## Formulations

• Mineral oil is available in an oral liquid.

## Stability and Storage

Store in a tightly sealed container, protected from light, and at room temperature.

## Small Animal Dosage

**Dogs**

• 10–50 mL/dog q12h PO.

**Cats**

• 10–25 mL/cat q12h PO.

## Large Animal Dosage

**Horses and Cattle**

• 500–1000 mL (1 pint to 1 quart) per horse or cow PO as needed. Up to 2–4 L per adult horse or cow PO (usually administered via stomach tube).

**Sheep and Pigs**

• 500–1000 mL PO as needed.

## Regulatory Information

No regulatory information is available. Because of a low risk of residues, no withdrawal times are suggested.

# Minocycline Hydrochloride
min-oh-sye′kleen hye-droe-klor′ide

**Trade and other names:** Minocin and Solodyn

**Functional classification:** Antibacterial

## Pharmacology and Mechanism of Action

Minocycline is a commonly used oral tetracycline antibiotic. It is not licensed for use in animals but is administered extralabel in dogs, cats, horses, and other animals for a variety of infections. Like other tetracyclines, the mechanism of action of minocycline is to bind to 30S ribosomal subunits and inhibit protein synthesis. It has a broad spectrum of activity, including gram-positive and gram-negative bacteria, some protozoa, *Rickettsia* spp., and *Ehrlichia* spp. Resistance among *Staphylococcus* species and gram-negative bacilli may be common, but some methicillin-resistant *Staphylococcus* species may be susceptible to minocycline that are not susceptible to doxycycline. Resistance is mediated by genes called *tet* genes. For example, *tet(M)* prevents binding of tetracyclines to ribosomes and confers resistance to all tetracyclines. The *tet(K)* mediates resistance by preventing entry into bacteria and confers resistance to other tetracyclines but not minocycline. Minocycline also may have some anti-inflammatory properties that may benefit joint diseases.

*Pharmacokinetics:* Minocycline has a similar pharmacokinetic profile to doxycycline but less protein binding. In horses, oral minocycline at 4 mg/kg q12h produced a peak concentration of 0.6 mcg/mL and had a half-life of approximately 12.6 hours with 33% bioavailability (average); after IV administration at 2.2 mg/kg, the half-life is 7.7 hours. The half-life in dogs and cats after an oral dose is 4.1 and 6.3 hours, respectively. The oral absorption is 50% and 63% in dogs and cats, respectively. Oral absorption is better on an empty stomach. Protein binding is approximately 50% in dogs and 46%–60% in cats.

**M**

## Indications and Clinical Uses

Minocycline is used when tetracyclines are indicated for treating bacterial infections in animals that include skin and soft tissue infections, respiratory infections, and joint infections. The use should be supported by a culture and susceptibility test, if possible. It may also be effective for *Rickettsia* and *Ehrlichia* infections. It was equally effective as doxycycline for *Ehrlichia canis* administered twice daily for 28 days. Generally, the clinical use is similar to doxycycline, with anticipated similar efficacy. It may be substituted for doxycycline to treat heartworm-positive dogs because of its activity against *Wolbachia* spp.

## Precautionary Information

### Adverse Reactions and Side Effects

The most common adverse effect from administration of minocycline has been GI problems, primarily vomiting and nausea. The GI effects are more likely as the dose is increased from 5 to 10 mg/kg. Otherwise, it has been used safely in experimental animals without adverse effects, and there are no clinical reports of serious injury. As with any oral tetracycline, changes in intestinal microflora could increase risk of diarrhea in some animals. Rapid IV injection has been associated with adverse events in people, but when administered intravenously to dogs, horses, and cats, no adverse events were observed.

### Contraindications and Precautions

No specific precautions have been reported for animals. Tetracyclines are not administered for multiple doses to young children because of risk of teeth staining, and this may also apply to animals. It has been used in foals with no reported problems.

> **Drug Interactions**
> Oral absorption may be affected by oral products that contain cations, such as calcium, aluminum, iron, and magnesium. No other drug interactions have been reported in animals.

## Instructions for Use

Minocycline can be substituted for doxycycline, especially when there have been shortages of other tetracyclines such as doxycycline. Minocycline is frequently used as an oral option for treating dogs, cats, and horses. In dogs, oral absorption is higher when administered without food. If possible, administer minocycline at least 30 minutes prior to a meal in dogs.

## Patient Monitoring and Laboratory Tests

Susceptibility testing: The CLSI breakpoint for susceptible bacteria in dogs is ≤0.5 mcg/mL, which also can be applied to cats. In horses, the breakpoint for susceptible bacteria is ≤0.12 mcg/mL at a clinical dosage of 4–5 mg/kg PO twice daily. Tetracycline has been used as a marker to test susceptibility to minocycline in dogs, but this should not be done for isolates from horses.

## Formulations

- Minocycline is available in 50-, 75-, and 100-mg tablets and capsules and 10-mg/mL flavored oral suspension. Vials for injection should be reconstituted in 5 mL and then diluted in 500–1000 mL for IV infusion. Solution may be stored at room temperature for 24 hours.
- Delayed-release tablets (Solodyn): 45-, 90-, 135-mg tablets. (These are human tablets, and it is not known if these have delayed-release properties in animals.)

## Stability and Storage

Store in a tightly sealed container, protected from light, and at room temperature. Do not mix with other drugs.

## Small Animal Dosage

### Dogs

- 5 mg/kg q12h PO is sufficient in most dogs. For higher MIC values, administer 10 mg/kg twice daily, but the higher dosage is more likely to produce vomiting.
- If IV administration is used, reduce dose by half compared with the oral dose.

### Cats

- 8.8 mg/kg (or 50 mg per cat) PO once daily.

## Large Animal Dosage

### Horses

- 4–5 mg/kg q12h PO or 2.2 mg/kg q12h IV.

## Regulatory Information

Withdrawal times are not established for animals that produce food. For extralabel use withdrawal interval estimates, contact FARAD at www.FARAD.org.

# Mirtazapine
mir-taz′a-peen

**Trade and other names:** Remeron (oral tablets), Mirataz transdermal for cats

**Functional classification:** Antiemetic agent

## Pharmacology and Mechanism of Action

Mirtazapine is used as an antiemetic and appetite stimulant in animals, but in people, it also has antidepressant and anxiolytic activity. The most common use in cats is as an appetite stimulant, for which there is an approved formulation. Mirtazapine action on adrenergic and serotonin receptors is complicated. It acts on both serotonergic and adrenergic systems. The antiemetic action occurs through postsynaptic antagonism of serotonin ($5HT_3$, $5HT_{2A}$, and $5HT_{2C}$), antagonism of histamine receptors ($H_1$), and an agonist for the serotonin $5HT_1$ receptors. There is also antagonism of presynaptic alpha$_2$ receptors, which can increase release of serotonin and norepinephrine. The $5\text{-}HT_{2A}$ receptor inhibits appetite, and antagonism from mirtazapine administration may stimulate appetite. Because it is active on three serotonin receptors, it is not as selective as ondansetron and other related drugs that affect $5HT_3$ receptors.

*Pharmacokinetics:* After administration to cats, the half-life was 15 hours after a high dose (3.75 mg per cat) and 9–10 hours after a low dose (1.9 mg per cat). The metabolites 8-OH-mirtazapine and desmethylmirtazapine have 5%–10% of mirtazapine's activity. The half-life of mirtazapine is longer (15 hours) in cats with chronic kidney disease, necessitating a less frequent dosing interval in these cats if the oral dose is administered (see dosing section). However, when administering the transdermal dose, no adjustments have been necessary.

The half-life in beagle dogs is 6.2 hours. In horses, the half-life is 3–4 hours at a dose of 2 mg/kg and produced only half the concentration measured in dogs.

## Indications and Clinical Uses

Mirtazapine is used as an antiemetic and appetite stimulant, primarily in cats. The FDA-approved formulation lists the indication as "For the management of weight loss in cats." Although there also has been some use in dogs, it is primarily anecdotal. There are other drugs that may be preferred if an antiemetic agent is needed for animals (e.g., maropitant). In cats, mirtazapine administered at 1.9 mg per cat, oral, every 48 hours for 3 weeks increased appetite, activity, and weight in cats with kidney disease. The FDA-approved transdermal dose for cats is 2 mg per cat applied to the ear.

Mirtazapine can produce antinausea effects in dogs, as well as increasing gastric emptying and increased colon transit (accelerated transit). Mirtazapine has been considered for its intestinal pro-kinetic effects in horses; however, there are no clinical studies to support this use. The clinical effects in horses are unknown.

M

### Precautionary Information

#### Adverse Reactions and Side Effects

Adverse effects observed in cats include vocalization, begging behavior, and food-seeking behavior. At high doses in cats, ataxia, restlessness, tremors, twitching, vomiting, hypersalivation, vocalization, and cardiovascular effects have been observed. In people, sedation and weight gain have been reported. Some antihistaminic effects have been reported, but sedation similar to what is observed in people has not been as common in animals. Although this drug acts through serotonergic mechanisms, the risk of development of serotonin syndrome is low and not reported in dogs or cats. Cyproheptadine (a serotonin antagonist) can be considered an antagonist in the event of overdose or adverse effects. If cyproheptadine is needed, administer 2–4 mg per cat PO every 4–8 hours until adverse effects diminish.

#### Contraindications and Precautions

If the transdermal formulation is used, advise pet owners to wear disposable gloves when handling or applying mirtazapine to cats to prevent accidental topical exposure. After application, care should be taken that people or other animals in the household do not come in contact with the treated cat for 2 hours because mirtazapine can be absorbed transdermally and orally. However, there are negligible residues are present at the application site and the body of the cat at 2 hours after dosing. There are no known contraindications in animals.

**Drug Interactions**

No drug interactions have been reported for animals. However, if possible, avoid use with SSRIs and MAOIs such as selegiline.

## Instructions for Use

Doses and recommendations are based on the clinical use in cats with chronic kidney disease through published evidence from clinical studies and the FDA-approved label. Other uses are anecdotal and not well documented.

## Patient Monitoring and Laboratory Tests

No specific monitoring is necessary.

## Formulations

- Mirtazapine is available in 15-, 30-, and 45-mg tablets. There is also a rapidly disintegrating tablet in these sizes that dissolves easily in a pet's mouth.
- Transdermal formulation: Each gram of ointment contains 20 mg of mirtazapine (2%), supplied in a 5-g tube containing 100 mg (0.1 g) of mirtazapine.

## Stability and Storage

Store in a tightly sealed container, protected from light, and at room temperature. Stability of compounded formulations has not been evaluated.

## Small Animal Dosage

**Dogs**

- 0.5–1 mg/kg q12h PO. Generally in the range of 3.75–7.5 mg per dog daily PO.

**Cats**

- 1.9 mg per cat PO. Doses have ranged from 3.75–7.5 mg per cat per day PO (one fourth to one half of a 15-mg tablet). In healthy cats, it can be administered once daily. In cats with chronic kidney disease, increase the interval to q48h.
- Transdermal formulations: Apply a 1.5-inch ribbon of ointment (approximately 2 mg/cat or 0.5 mg/kg) on the inner pinna of the cat's ear once daily for 14 days.

## Large Animal Dosage

No large animal doses are available.

## Regulatory Information

No withdrawal time information is available for food-producing animals.

# Misoprostol
mee-soe-pross'tole

**Trade and other names:** Cytotec

**Functional classification:** Antiulcer agent

## Pharmacology and Mechanism of Action

Misoprostol is a synthetic prostaglandin. It is a synthetic analogue of prostaglandin $E_1$ ($PGE_1$). It is an agonist for the prostaglandin receptors $E_2$, $E_3$, and $E_4$, and produces a cytoprotective effect on the GI mucosa. It has been shown in dogs and people to decrease injury to GI mucosa caused by NSAIDs, such as aspirin. In studies in dogs, misoprostol was not effective for decreasing adverse effects caused by corticosteroids. Misoprostol also has anti-inflammatory effects and has been used to treat pruritus in dogs. Because it is a synthetic prostaglandin, it has uterotonic and cervical ripening effects. It produces these effects by increasing the activity of collagenases, elastase, glycosaminoglycan, and hyaluronic acid in the cervix and increases the calcium levels in the uterus to induce contractions. It can induce labor, interfere with pregnancy, and has been used to induce abortion (see later).

*Pharmacokinetics:* In horses after a dose of 5 mcg/kg, oral absorption was better in unfed horses compared with fed horses. The half-life was approximately 2.8 hours in the nonfed horses. Rectal administration of misoprostol to horses produced less complete absorption and a shorter half-life compared with oral administration.

## Indications and Clinical Uses

Misoprostol is used to decrease the risk of GI ulceration when administered concurrently with NSAIDs. Efficacy has been established for this indication in trials with aspirin but not with other NSAIDs in animals. There is no evidence to show that it decreases GI bleeding caused by other drugs (e.g., corticosteroids). Clinical trials also are available to show that misoprostol is effective for treating pruritus in patients with atopic dermatitis, although it is less effective than other drugs.

The GI effects in horses have been explored through small observational studies and anecdotal accounts. Misoprostol may be helpful in horses for treating right dorsal colitis. Equine GI experts consider misoprostol a valid first-line option for equine glandular gastric disease at a dose of 5 mcg/kg PO and was superior to omeprazole and sucralfate. However, it should not be used with omeprazole in horses or in pregnant mares. The optimum dose in horses has not been determined, but a dose of 5 mcg/kg oral produces plasma drug concentrations that are similar to effective doses in people.

Misoprostol has been used to induce abortion, but it is much more effective when used with other agents such as aglepristone or mifepristone. In people, it is used with mifepristone. It should not be used alone to induce abortion because high doses are needed, which can increase the risk of adverse effects.

M

### Precautionary Information

**Adverse Reactions and Side Effects**

Adverse effects are caused by effects of prostaglandins. The most common adverse effects are GI discomfort, vomiting, and diarrhea. Diarrhea and abdominal discomfort have been reported in horses, but these effects are usually mild and self-limiting. It was tolerated in experimental horses at a dose of 5 mcg/kg oral.

**Contraindications and Precautions**

Do not administer to pregnant animals; it may cause abortion. Women should handle this medication carefully because it can induce abortion.

**Drug Interactions**

Misoprostol may compromise the acid-suppressing effects of omeprazole, so these drugs should not be used together.

## Instructions for Use

Doses and recommendations are based on clinical trials in which misoprostol was administered to prevent GI mucosal injury caused by aspirin. These effects can likely be extended to other NSAIDs. The effects in horses for treating right dorsal colitis and equine glandular gastric disease are from observations from clinical experts. Careful handling of misoprostol should be observed because of its potential to induce abortion.

## Patient Monitoring and Laboratory Tests

No specific monitoring is necessary.

## Formulations

- Misoprostol is available in 0.1-mg (100-mcg) and 0.2-mg (200-mcg) tablets.

## Stability and Storage

Store in a tightly sealed container, protected from light, and at room temperature. Stability of compounded formulations has not been evaluated.

## Small Animal Dosage

### Dogs

- 2–5 mcg/kg q12h PO.
- Atopic dermatitis: 5 mcg/kg q8h PO.

### Cats

- 2–4 mcg/kg q12h PO
- Induce abortion: 200 mcg per cat q12h PO until abortion begins, administered with aglepristone or mifepristone. Higher doses can induce abortion when administered alone but with more frequent and more severed adverse effects.

## Large Animal Dosage

### Horses

- 5 mcg/kg q12h PO.

## Regulatory Information

Do not use in animals that produce food.
RCI Classification: 4

# Mitotane
mye'toe-tane

**Trade and other names:** Lysodren and op'-DDD

**Functional classification:** Adrenolytic agent

## Pharmacology and Mechanism of Action

Mitotane is a cytotoxic agent that has specific effects on the adrenal gland. It binds to adrenal proteins and is then converted to a reactive metabolite, which then destroys cells of the zona fasciculata and zona reticularis of the adrenal cortex. The precise mechanism of action is through inhibition of sterol-O-acetyl-transferase. This is an enzyme that converts cholesterol to the active esters. By inhibiting this conversion, cholesterol accumulates in the cells which leads to cell death. Destruction of the adrenal cells is relatively specific and can be complete or partial, depending on the dose used. If only partial destruction of adrenal cortical cells occurs, repeated administration or maintenance doses are needed to suppress hypercortisolemia. The dog is much more sensitive to the effects of mitotane than other animals, which explains the relatively specific use in this species.

Mitotane is a highly lipophilic drug. It is poorly absorbed without food, but oral absorption is enhanced when administered with food or oil.

## Indications and Clinical Uses

Mitotane is used primarily to treat pituitary-dependent hyperadrenocorticism (PDH) (Cushing's disease) in dogs. It also has been used to treat adrenal tumors. Treatment is initiated with a loading dose followed by weekly maintenance doses. Other drugs used to suppress cortisol in dogs include ketoconazole, selegiline, and trilostane. Treatment of dogs with mitotane has been mostly replaced by use of the FDA-approved drug trilostane, but mitotane may be preferred in some patients. Treatment with mitotane has been compared with trilostane and has shown that each drug, although acting through different mechanisms, produces similar survival times in dogs with PDH. However, in dogs with adrenal tumors, mitotane may be preferred because of its specific action to destroy adrenal cells. Mitotane is not recommended for cats, and trilostane is recommended instead.

### Precautionary Information

#### Adverse Reactions and Side Effects

Adverse effects, especially during the induction period, include lethargy, weakness, anorexia, ataxia, depression, and vomiting. Discontinue if signs of liver disease are observed. Adverse effects may occur in 25%–30% of dogs. Corticosteroid supplementation (e.g., hydrocortisone, prednisolone or prednisone) may be administered to minimize side effects (prednisone dosage, 0.25 mg/kg/day). Aldosterone secretion may be reduced in some dogs after treatment.

In some dogs, adverse neurologic signs may be observed, which include ataxia, head pressing, and blindness. CNS effects are the result of enlargement of the pituitary gland in response to suppression of the adrenal cortex and lack of feedback by cortisol. Loss of feedback control stimulates corticotropin-releasing hormone, pituitary enlargement, and adrenocorticotropic hormone (ACTH) secretion.

#### Contraindications and Precautions

Do not administer to animals unless there is an ability to monitor response with cortisol serum measurements, preferably after ACTH stimulation. Mitotane can cause cytotoxicity and inhibition of other steroid hormones. Caution pet owners about handling mitotane. Children and pregnant women should not be exposed to mitotane.

#### Drug Interactions

No specific drug interactions are reported for animals.

## Instructions for Use

Dose and frequency are often based on patient response. Typically, the induction period lasts 5–14 days in dogs. During the induction period, monitor water consumption, appetite, and behavior. Adverse effects are common during initial therapy. Administration with food increases oral absorption. The maintenance dose should be adjusted on the basis of periodic cortisol measurements and ACTH stimulation tests. Prednisolone or prednisone at 0.2–0.25 mg/kg is sometimes

M

administered as a replacement in patients with PDH during the induction treatment. When used to treat adrenal tumors (see dosing), the adrenal cells are destroyed as a goal of therapy. Therefore, in these patients, supplementation with adrenal steroids (glucocorticoids and mineralocorticoids) is important for long-term maintenance. Corticosteroid supplementation with prednisone or prednisolone is started usually on the third day of treatment.

Trilostane, an approved drug for dogs, has also been used instead of mitotane in dogs and should be considered when dogs do not respond to or tolerate mitotane.

### Patient Monitoring and Laboratory Tests

Monitor water consumption and appetite during the induction phase. Monitor ACTH response test to adjust dose. The urine cortisol/creatinine ratio can be used to measure whether or not the adrenal cells have been destroyed when treating an adrenal tumor. Successful treatment shows a very low ratio or undetectable cortisol levels. Monitor electrolytes periodically to screen for hyperkalemia that could result from adrenal destruction (iatrogenic hypoadrenocorticism).

### Formulations

- Mitotane is available in 500-mg tablets but has become unavailable in some countries.

### Stability and Storage

Store in a tightly sealed container, protected from light, and at room temperature. Mitotane is not stable in aqueous solutions and may lose potency in some compounded formulations.

### Small Animal Dosage

#### Dogs

- PDH: 50 mg/kg/day (in divided doses) PO for 5–10 days; then 50–70 mg/kg/wk PO for long-term maintenance.
- Adrenal tumor: 50–75 mg/kg/day (in divided doses) for 10 days; then every other day for 40 days. There may be follow-up maintenance treatment with 75–100 mg/kg/wk PO.

#### Cats

- 25–50 mg/kg/day induction followed by 25–50 mg/kg/wk for maintenance. However, it is not recommended by most experts because of poor response. Use trilostane instead.

### Large Animal Dosage

- No large animal doses have been reported.

### Regulatory Information

Do not use in animals that produce food.

---

# Mitoxantrone Hydrochloride

mye-toe-zan′trone hye-droe-klor′ide

**Trade and other names:** Novantrone

**Functional classification:** Anticancer agent

## Pharmacology and Mechanism of Action

Mitoxantrone is an anticancer antibiotic used for lymphoma, carcinomas, and various sarcomas. Mitoxantrone is an anticancer agent that is similar to doxorubicin in action. Like doxorubicin, it acts to intercalate between bases on DNA, disrupting DNA and RNA synthesis in tumor cells, and may have other antitumor effects described in the Doxorubicin section. Mitoxantrone may affect tumor cell membranes to increase cell death.

## Indications and Clinical Uses

Mitoxantrone has been used in anticancer drug protocols in animals for treatment of leukemia, lymphoma, and carcinomas. However, use in animals is uncommon compared with the use of doxorubicin. It has been substituted for doxorubicin in some anticancer protocols for treating lymphoma in dogs with a response that was as effective as doxorubicin-based protocols.

## Precautionary Information

### Adverse Reactions and Side Effects

As with all anticancer agents, certain adverse effects are predictable and unavoidable and related to the drug's action. Mitoxantrone produces myelosuppression, vomiting, anorexia, and GI upset, but it may be less cardiotoxic than doxorubicin.

### Contraindications and Precautions

Do not administer to animals with severe bone marrow suppression. If severe bone marrow suppression is observed, withhold treatment and resume with a 25% lower dose.

### Drug Interactions

No specific drug interactions are reported for animals, but like any anticancer agent, there are effects on multiple organs that are affected by other drugs.

M

## Instructions for Use

Proper use of mitoxantrone usually follows a specific anticancer protocol. Doses listed are based on input from reputable oncologists but consult specific protocol for dosing regimens that may deviate from these recommendations.

## Patient Monitoring and Laboratory Tests

Monitor CBC to look for evidence of bone marrow toxicity.

## Formulations

- Mitoxantrone is available in 2-mg/mL injection.

## Stability and Storage

Store in a tightly sealed container, protected from light, and at room temperature.

## Small Animal Dosage

### Dogs

- 5–5.5 mg/m$^2$ IV every 21 days and up to 6 mg/m$^2$ if dogs tolerate it well.

### Cats

- 6–6.5 mg/m$^2$ IV every 21 days.

## Large Animal Dosage

- No large animal doses have been reported.

## Regulatory Information

Withdrawal times are not established for animals that produce food. This drug should not be used in animals intended for food because it is an anticancer agent.

# Mitratapide
mi-trat′a-pyed

**Trade and other names:** Yarvitan

**Functional classification:** Weight loss medication

**Note:** Mitratapide (under the brand name Yarvitan) was approved for use in Europe by the European Medicines Agency (EMA) for helping with weight loss in dogs. But it was never approved in the United States, and it has since been withdrawn from the market in Europe.

Consult earlier editions of this book for more details.

# Morphine Sulfate
mor′feen sul′fate

**Trade and other names:** Generic brands, MS Contin extended-release tablets, Oramorph SR extended-release tablets, and generic brand extended-release tablets

**Functional classification:** Analgesic, opioid

## Pharmacology and Mechanism of Action

Morphine is an opioid agonist analgesic. Morphine is the prototype for other opioid agonists, and the action of other opioids is often compared in "morphine equivalents." The action of morphine is to bind to mu-opiate and kappa-opiate receptors on nerves and inhibit release of neurotransmitters involved with transmission of pain stimuli (e.g., substance P). Morphine also may inhibit release of some inflammatory mediators. The CNS effects and euphoric properties are related to mu-receptor effects in brain. Other opiates and opioids used in animals include hydromorphone, codeine, oxymorphone, meperidine, and fentanyl.

*Pharmacokinetics:* Like other opioids, it is highly lipophilic (log P, 3.3) and is a weak base (pKa, 8.6). The pharmacokinetics have been studied in most species. In horses, it has a short half-life (1.5–3 hours) and high clearance (30–35 mL/kg/min). In cats, it has a half-lives of 76 minutes IV and 93 minutes IM. Clearance in cats is 24 mL/kg/min. In dogs, the half-life is also short (1.2 hours) with high clearance (60 mL/kg/min). Oral morphine formulations are poorly bioavailable in dogs because of first-pass effects and may not be effective.

## Indications and Clinical Uses

Morphine is indicated for short-term analgesia, for sedation, and as an adjunct to anesthesia. It is compatible with most anesthetics and can be used as part of a multimodal approach to analgesia and anesthesia. Administration of morphine may lower dose requirements for other anesthetics and analgesics used. Morphine also has been used in animals for treatment of pulmonary edema. Presumably, this effect is attributed to vasodilation and reduction of preload in animals.

Although oral morphine (regular and sustained release) has been used in dogs, its absorption is poor and inconsistent. The oral dose formulations should not be relied on for treating severe pain in dogs.

Morphine oral administration has not been investigated in cats. Injectable forms can be used in cats, but doses are generally lower than in dogs to prevent excitement. In horses, it is rarely used alone or without other sedatives because undesirable behavior and cardiovascular effects may occur at doses that are needed for analgesia. At a dose of 0.3–0.6 mg/kg in horses, it significantly increases locomotor activity, produces excitement, and decreases GI motility. It produces colic at 1.0 mg/kg and severe ataxia and collapse at 2.4 mg/kg. At lower doses of 0.1–0.2 mg/kg, it did not produce colic or excitement or adverse GI effects, but these low doses were not adequate to produce analgesia.

## Precautionary Information
### Adverse Reactions and Side Effects
Like all opiates, side effects from morphine are predictable and unavoidable. Side effects from morphine administration include sedation, vomiting, constipation, urinary retention, and bradycardia. Panting may occur in dogs as a result of changes in thermoregulation. Histamine release occurs from administration of morphine, but it may be less likely than with other opioids such as hydromorphone. Excitement can occur in some animals, but it is more common in cats and horses. Respiratory depression occurs with high doses.

As with other opiates, a slight decrease in heart rate is expected. In most cases, this decrease does not have to be treated with anticholinergic drugs (e.g., atropine), but it should be monitored. Tolerance and dependence occur with chronic administration. In horses, there were ileus, constipation, and CNS stimulation (pawing and pacing) after 0.5 mg/kg. In horses, undesirable and even dangerous behavior actions can follow rapid IV opioid administration. Muscle twitching, fasciculations, and sweating also occur in horses. If used in horses, they should receive a preanesthetic of acepromazine or an alpha$_2$ agonist.

### Contraindications and Precautions
Morphine is a Schedule II controlled substance. Cats and horses are more sensitive to excitement than other species.

### Drug Interactions
Like other opiates, it potentiates other drugs that cause CNS depression.

## Instructions for Use
Effects from morphine administration are dose dependent. Low doses (0.1–0.25 mg/kg) produce mild analgesia. Higher doses (up to 1 mg/kg) produce greater analgesic effects and sedation. Usually morphine is administered IM, IV, or SQ. CRIs also have been used, and doses that are listed later produce morphine concentrations in a therapeutic range. PO morphine is available in sustained-release forms, but PO dosing can be highly variable and inconsistent. Epidural administration has been used for surgical procedures. Combination protocols include MMK, which is morphine (0.2 mg/kg) + medetomidine (60 mcg/kg) (or dexmedetomidine) + ketamine (5 mg/kg), which are mixed in one syringe and administered intramuscularly to produce short-term analgesia and anesthesia for approximately 120 minutes. Another mixture is MLK, which is morphine (or fentanyl), lidocaine, and ketamine (see dosing section for formula). Evaluation of the efficacy MLK protocols is based mostly on anecdotal

experience or small observational studies. One study did not find any benefit of MLK over morphine alone in an incision-induced pain model in dogs.

## Patient Monitoring and Laboratory Tests

Monitor patient's heart rate and respiration. Although bradycardia rarely needs to be treated when it is caused by an opioid, if necessary, atropine can be administered. If serious respiratory depression occurs, the opioid can be reversed with naloxone.

## Formulations

- Injection formulations: Morphine is available in 1-, 2-, 4-, 5-, 8-, 10-, 15-, 25-, and 50-mg/mL injection (most common is 15 mg/mL)
- Oral formulations: 15- and 30-mg tablets and extended-release tablets in 15, 30, 60, 100, and 200 mg (MS Contin, Oramorph SR, or generic brands). Morphine pentahydrate (Avinza) is available in 60-mg capsules.

## Stability and Storage

Store in a tightly sealed container, protected from light, and at room temperature. Protect from freezing. Morphine sulfate is slightly water soluble and soluble in ethanol. It is more stable at a pH less than 4. If mixed with high-pH vehicles, oxidation occurs, which may darken the formulation (brownish yellow). Solutions may be repackaged in plastic syringes and kept stable for 70 days. If mixed with sodium chloride (0.9%) for epidural injection, it is stable for 14 weeks. Morphine has been mixed with other analgesic and sedative agents in the same syringe and in fluids. An example of such a combination is MLK, which is morphine, lidocaine, and ketamine (concentration of each ingredient listed earlier). This combination has been when mixed prior to dosing.

## Small Animal Dosage

### Dogs

- Analgesia: 0.5 mg/kg q2h IV or IM. However, the full dose range is 0.1–1 mg/kg IV, IM, or SQ q4h, depending on the desired effect (dosage is escalated as needed to control severity of pain).
- CRI: Loading dose of 0.2 mg/kg IV followed by 0.1 mg/kg/h. This may be increased to a loading dose of 0.3 mg/kg followed by 0.17 mg/kg/h for more severe pain. Doses as high as a loading dose of 0.6 mg/kg followed by 0.34 mg/kg IV have been used in experimental dogs without producing adverse effects.
- Oral dosing: Regular tablets should not be used. Sustained-release tablets have been used at a dosage of 15 or 30 mg per dog q8–12h PO, but studies have shown these tablets to be inconsistently and poorly absorbed in dogs.
- Epidural: 0.1 mg/kg.
- Combination of MLK: mixed as 100 mg/mL of ketamine (1.6 mL per 500 mL fluids) + 20 mg/mL of lidocaine (30 mL per 500 mL fluids), and 15 mg/mL of morphine (1.6 mL per 500 mL fluids) and infused at a rate of morphine, 0.24 mg/kg h; lidocaine, 3 mg/kg/h; and ketamine, 0.6 mg/kg/h, administered as CRI for perioperative analgesia.

### Cats

- Analgesia: 0.1–0.2 mg/kg IM, IV, or SQ q3–6h (or as needed).
- CRI: loading dose of 0.2 mg/kg IV followed by 0.05–0.1 mg/kg/h IV.
- Epidural 0.1 mg/kg diluted in saline to 0.3 mL/kg.

## Large Animal Dosage

### Horses

- For light chemical restraint, use 0.3–0.5 mg/kg IV, in combination with other sedatives.

- For mild pain, start with 0.1–0.2 mg/kg IV or IM q6h. For more severe pain, gradually increase to 0.5–1 mg/kg IV or IM. Give IV doses slowly. Morphine may cause excitement in horses, and it is advised to first sedate with an alpha$_2$ agonist or another sedative.
- Intra-articular (use preservative-free solutions): 0.05 mg/kg; start with initial concentration of 20 mg/mL solution and dilute in saline to 5 mg/mL and administered at a rate of 1 mL per joint per 100 kg of body weight.

### Ruminants
- The benefits of using morphine in ruminants are controversial. However, 0.05–0.1 mg/kg IV and up to 0.4 mg/kg IV have been used to treat pain and in perioperative situations.

### Regulatory Information
Morphine is a Schedule II controlled drug.

Avoid use in animals intended for food. If used in a food producing animal, consult FARAD at www.FARAD.org, for information on withdrawal times.

RCI Classification: 1

---

# Moxidectin
moks-ih-dek′tin

**Trade and other names:** ProHeart, ProHeart 6, ProHeart 12 (canine), Coraxis, Quest (equine), and Cydectin (bovine and ovine)

**Functional classification:** Antiparasitic

**M**

## Pharmacology and Mechanism of Action
Moxidectin is an antiparasitic drug in the milbemycin class. Avermectins (ivermectin-like drugs) and milbemycins (milbemycin and moxidectin) are macrocyclic lactones and share similarities, including mechanism of action. Moxidectin is 100 times more lipophilic than ivermectin. These drugs are neurotoxic to parasites by potentiating glutamate-gated chloride ion channels in parasites. Paralysis and death of the parasite are caused by increased permeability to chloride ions and hyperpolarization of nerve cells. These drugs also potentiate other chloride channels, including ones gated by GABA. However, GABA-mediated mechanism may not be important for parasites. Mammals ordinarily are not affected because they lack glutamate-gated chloride channels, and there is a lower affinity for other mammalian chloride channels. Because these drugs ordinarily do not penetrate the blood–brain barrier, GABA-gated channels in the CNS of mammals are not affected. Moxidectin is active against intestinal parasites, mites, bots, heartworm microfilaria, and developing larvae. Moxidectin has no effect on trematode or cestode parasites. One of the equine formulations also contains praziquantel to control additional parasites.

## Indications and Clinical Uses
Moxidectin is used in dogs to prevent infection of heartworm (*Dirofilaria immitis*). In dogs, it can also be used and for the treatment and control of *A. caninum, U. stenocephala, T. canis, Toxascaris leonina,* and *T. vulpis.*

Moxidectin also has been used to treat *Demodex* infections in dogs at high doses. In cats, it is used for the prevention of heartworm disease caused by *D. immitis;* for the treatment and control of intestinal roundworms (*Toxocara cati*), and hookworms

(*Ancylostoma tubaeforme*). It is combined with fluralaner in a topical solution for cats (Bravecto Plus) to include treatment of fleas and ticks and in a combination tablet for dogs with sarolaner and pyrantel for treatment of roundworms, fleas, ticks, and heartworm prevention. In horses, it is used for treatment of a variety of parasites, including large strongyles (*Strongylus vulgaris* [adults and L4/L5 arterial stages], *S. edentatus* [adult and tissue stages], *Triodontophorus brevicauda* [adults], and *T. serratus* [adults]), and small strongyles ([adults] *Cyathostomum* spp., *Cylicocyclus* spp., *Cyliocostephanus* spp., *Coronocyclus* spp., and *Gyalocephalus capitatus*). It is also used to treat small strongyles, including larvae. It is used to treat ascarids, including *Parascaris equorum* (adults and L4 larval stages), pinworms (*Oxyuris equi* [adults and L4 larval stages]), hairworms (*Trichostrongylus axei* [adults]), large-mouth stomach worms (*Habronema muscae* [adults]), and horse stomach bots (*Gasterophilus intestinalis* [second and third instars] and *Gasterophilus nasalis* [third instars]). One dose also suppresses strongyle egg production for 84 days. Some formulations for horses also contain praziquantel. This increases the spectrum to include other intestinal parasites such as tapeworms.

In cattle, moxidectin injectable is used to treat intestinal roundworms (*Ostertagia ostertagi* [adults and inhibited fourth-stage larvae], *Haemonchus placei* [adults], *Trichostrongylus axei* [adults], *T. colubriformis* [fourth-stage larvae], *Cooperia oncophora* [adults], *C. punctata* [adults and fourth-stage larvae], *C. surnabada* [adults and fourth-stage larvae], *Oesophagostomum radiatum* [adults and fourth-stage larvae], *Trichuris* spp. [adults]), lungworms (*Dictyocaulus viviparus* [adults and fourth-stage larvae]), grubs (*Hypoderma bovis* and *H. lineatum*), mites (*Psoroptes ovis [P. communis* var. *bovis]*), and lice (*Linognathus vituli* and *Solenopotes capillatus*). One injection will protect cattle from reinfection with *D. viviparous* and *O. radiatum* for 42 days, *H. placei* for 35 days, and *O. ostertagi* and *T. axei* for 14 days after treatment. In sheep, the oral drench is used for the treatment and control of the adult and L4 larval stages of *Haemonchus contortus, Teladorsagia circumcincta, Teladorsagia trifurcata, Trichostrongylus axei, T. colubriformis, Trichostrongylus vitrinus, Cooperia curticei, C. oncophora, Oesophagostomum columbianum, Oesophagostomum venulosum, Nematodirus battus, Nematodirus filicollis,* and *Nematodirus spathiger.*

## Precautionary Information
### Adverse Reactions and Side Effects
Toxicity is the result of potentiation of glutamate-gated chloride channels and GABA channels, resulting in hyperpolarization of membranes. Toxicity may occur at high doses and in breeds in which moxidectin crosses the blood–brain barrier. Sensitive breeds may include collies, Australian shepherds, Old English sheepdogs, longhaired whippets, and Shetland sheepdogs. Toxicity is neurotoxic, and signs include depression, ataxia, vision problems, coma, and death. Sensitivity to moxidectin occurs in certain breeds because of a mutation in the *ABCB1* gene that codes for the membrane pump P-glycoprotein. Animals with this mutation lack a functional p-glycoprotein efflux pump in the blood–brain barrier. Adverse effects may occur when high doses of moxidectin are used to treat dogs for demodicosis. These effects include lethargy, depressed appetite, vomiting, and lesions at the site of an SQ injection. Toxicity is more likely at high doses in dogs. At five times

the label dose rate (15 mcg/kg) once every month, moxidectin was administered safely to collies that were ivermectin sensitive. However, at a single dose of 90 mcg/kg (30 times the label dose) administered to sensitive collies, ataxia, lethargy, and salivation occurred in one sixth of dogs. At 30, 60, and 90 mcg/kg (10 times, 20 times, and 30 times the label dose) administered to ivermectin-sensitive collies , no adverse effects were observed. Nevertheless, caution is advised when administering moxidectin to sensitive breeds listed previously.

Because of concern about adverse reactions and deaths in dogs from the 6-month injectable formulation (ProHeart 6), this product was temporarily discontinued several years ago. However, this safety concerns has been addressed by reformulating the product, which is now available in 6- and 12-month forms. In horses, moxidectin has been safe at three times the label dose. However, adverse effects (ataxia, depression, and lethargy) have been reported in young horses (younger than 6 months) or debilitated animals after treatment. Other adverse effects reported in horses include sedation, weakness, bradycardia, dyspnea, coma, and seizures.

Neurologic toxicity in animals producing seizures can be treated with diazepam, barbiturates, or propofol.

### Contraindications and Precautions
Do not use the 2.5% topical solution in cats. Do not use in dogs younger than 2 months of age. Despite the safety margin listed in the Adverse Reactions and Side Effects section, caution is advised when administering moxidectin at high doses to ivermectin-sensitive breeds. Affected breeds may include collies, Australian shepherds, Old English sheepdogs, longhaired whippets, and Shetland sheepdogs. Administration to foals younger than 6 months of age is not recommended. Do not apply the large animal pour-on formulation to small animals. It has been used safely in queens and kittens during pregnancy and lactation.

### Drug Interactions
Do not administer with drugs that could potentially increase the penetration of ivermectin across the blood–brain barrier. Such drugs include ketoconazole, itraconazole, cyclosporine, and calcium-channel blockers (see Appendix J).

M

## Instructions for Use
Caution is recommended if the bovine or equine formulation is considered for use in small animals. Toxic overdoses are likely because these formulations are highly concentrated.

When applying the 2.5% topical solutions to dogs, ensure that dogs do not lick the application site. Avoid exposure to people after applying the topical solution.

The approved formulations for dogs vary in their concentration and duration. For example, there are immediate-release products, 6-month products (ProHeart-6), and 12-month products (ProHeart-12). Pay attention to specific mixing and labeling instructions when administering each product.

## Patient Monitoring and Laboratory Tests
Animals should be checked for heartworm status prior to initiating treatment.

## Formulations

- 30-, 68-, and 136-mcg tablets for dogs, or 2.5% topical solution for dogs.
- 20-mg/mL equine oral gel (2% gel). Quest Plus gel for horses contains 20 mg/mL (2%) plus 125 mg of praziquantel (12.5%).
- 5-mg/mL cattle pour-on; 1-mg/mL oral drench for sheep; 10-mg/mL injectable solution for cattle;
- 6-month long-acting formulation: The 6-month injectable (ProHeart 6) formulation consists of two separate vials: one contains 10% moxidectin microspheres, and the other contains a vehicle for constitution of the moxidectin microspheres. Each milliliter of constituted, sustained-release suspension contains 3.4 mg of moxidectin.
- 12-month long-acting formulation: 10 mg of constituted suspension per milliliter. This product has two separate vials that require mixing prior to administration or use. One vial contains 10% moxidectin sterile microspheres and the second vial contains sterile vehicle for constitution; only this sterile diluent should be used for the constitution. The constituted suspension can be injected 30 minutes after mixing.
- Combination products: The formulation Advantage Multi for dogs 2.5% (25 mg/mL) includes 25% imidacloprid. Advantage Multi for cats 1% (10mg/mL) includes 10% imidacloprid. Moxidectin is combined with fluralaner in a topical solution for cats, with 280 mg of fluralaner and 14 mg moxidectin per milliliter. Moxidectin is combined with sarolaner and pyrantel in a chewable tablet for dogs (Simparica TRIO).

## Stability and Storage

Store in a tightly sealed container, protected from light, and at room temperature. Stability of compounded formulations has not been evaluated.

## Small Animal Dosage

### Dogs

- Heartworm prevention: 3 mcg/kg every 30 days PO. Topical heartworm prevention (Advantage Multi, or Coraxis) 2.5 mg/kg monthly.
- Moxidectin is combined with sarolaner and pyrantel in a chewable tablet for dogs (Simparica TRIO). The tablet is designed to deliver a dose of 1.2 mg/kg sarolaner, 24 mcg/kg moxidectin, and 5 mg/kg pyrantel, once a month oral.
- 6-month formulation: 0.17 mg/kg or 0.05 mL of the constituted suspension/kg (0.0227 mL/lb), administered as a single SQ injection once every 6 months. No more than 3 mL should be injected in a single site.
- 12-month formulation: 0.5 mg/kg (0.23 mg/lb) or 0.05 mL of the constituted suspension per kilogram (0.023 mL/lb) by SQ injection. This amount of suspension will provide 0.5 mg moxidectin per kilogram of body weight (0.23 mg/lb). To ensure accurate dosing, calculate each dose based on the dog's weight at the time of treatment.
- Endoparasite control: 25–300 mcg/kg.
- Sarcoptic mange: 200–250 mcg/kg (0.2–0.25 mg/kg) PO or SQ once per week for 3–6 weeks.
- Demodicosis: 200 mcg/kg SQ weekly or every other week for one to four doses; alternatively, higher doses of 400 mcg/kg/day PO. Higher doses are used for refractory *Demodex* cases, with dosages of 500 mcg/kg (0.5 mg/kg)/day PO for 21–23 weeks or 0.5–1.0 mg/kg SQ q72h for 21–22 weeks. Duration of treatment

for demodicosis is variable. Treat until two negative *Demodex* skin scrapings are achieved.

**Cats**

- Topical heartworm prevention with Advantage Multi is 1 mg/kg of moxidectin topically every 30 days.
- Topical solution for cats with fluralaner and moxidectin (Bravecto Plus): Administer as a single dose topically at a dose of 40 mg/kg fluralaner and 2 mg/kg moxidectin every 2 months.

## Large Animal Dosage

**Horses**

- GI parasites: 0.4 mg/kg PO. Avoid use in young horses, small ponies, and debilitated animals.

**Cattle**

- 0.2 mg/kg SQ once.
- Intestinal parasites, lungworms, mites, grubs, and lice: Topical treatment (pour-on): 0.5 mg/kg (0.23 mg/lb or 45 mL per 1000 lb). Apply topically along the midline from the withers to the tail head. Avoid exposure to human skin and to other animals.

**Sheep**

- 1 mL per 5 kg (1 mL per 11 lb, or 0.2 mg/kg) by mouth of the 1-mg/mL oral solution.

## Regulatory Information

Do not use in horses intended for food.
Cattle withdrawal time (meat): 21 days.
Sheep withdrawal time (meat): 7 days.
Goat withdrawal time (meat): 14 days.
No milk withholding time has been established. Do not use in female dairy cattle of breeding age. Do not use in female sheep providing milk for human consumption. Do not use in veal calves.

M

# Moxifloxacin

moks-ih-floks'ah-sin

**Trade and other names:** Avelox

**Functional classification:** Antibacterial

## Pharmacology and Mechanism of Action

Moxifloxacin is a fluoroquinolone antibacterial with broader spectrum than some of the older antibiotics in this class such as ciprofloxacin. Moxifloxacin, like other quinolones, inhibits DNA gyrase and prevents bacterial cell DNA and RNA synthesis. Moxifloxacin is bactericidal with broad antimicrobial activity. It has a chemical structure slightly different from older veterinary fluoroquinolones (8 methoxy substitution). As a result of this modification, this newer generation of drugs, such as moxifloxacin, has greater activity against gram-positive bacteria and anaerobes than the veterinary fluoroquinolones (enrofloxacin, orbifloxacin, and marbofloxacin). An approved veterinary drug with a similar spectrum is pradofloxacin. Pradofloxacin may be used in animals instead of moxifloxacin for some indications. Another human-label fluoroquinolone, levofloxacin, has a spectrum of activity similar to moxifloxacin and can be used in dogs and cats.

## Indications and Clinical Uses

Although moxifloxacin is a human-label drug and not licensed for veterinary use, it has been used in non–food-producing animals for many years. It has been used in small animals for treatment of infections refractory to other drugs, including skin infections, pneumonia, and soft tissue infections. The spectrum of activity includes gram-positive cocci and anaerobic bacteria that may be resistant to other quinolones. Because other veterinary fluoroquinolones (enrofloxacin, orbifloxacin, and marbofloxacin) are preferred for initial use, moxifloxacin use is usually not considered for empirical use. Data for use in small animals are sparse, and regimens are primarily extrapolated from the human label and pharmacokinetic studies. In horses, it has been administered at 5.8 mg/kg/day for 3 days. Although pharmacokinetics were favorable in horses, it caused diarrhea, which may be a risk for more serious problems. It has been well tolerated for oral administration to dogs and cats. However, another human-labeled fluoroquinolone, levofloxacin, has a similar spectrum of activity and availability of inexpensive generic tablets. (See Levofloxacin.) Therefore, levofloxacin is often used for conditions that can also be treated with moxifloxacin.

## Precautionary Information

### Adverse Reactions and Side Effects

High concentrations of fluoroquinolones may cause CNS toxicity, especially in animals with kidney disease. This has not been reported from moxifloxacin because of infrequent use but is possible. Moxifloxacin causes occasional vomiting. All of the fluoroquinolones may cause arthropathy in young animals. Dogs are most sensitive at 4–28 weeks of age. Large, rapidly growing dogs are the most susceptible. In horses, moxifloxacin at high doses caused diarrhea and is not recommended for routine use. Moxifloxacin at high doses has caused a dose-related prolongation of the QT interval. The clinical consequences of this observation for animals are not known.

### Contraindications and Precautions

Avoid use in young animals because of risk of cartilage injury. Use cautiously in animals that may be prone to seizures. Avoid use in horses, rodents, and rabbits because of risk of diarrhea.

### Drug Interactions

Some fluoroquinolones may increase concentrations of theophylline if used concurrently, but it is not known of this occurs with moxifloxacin or applies to other metabolized drugs. Coadministration with divalent and trivalent cations, such as products containing aluminum (e.g., sucralfate), iron, and calcium, may decrease absorption. Do not mix in solutions or in vials with aluminum, calcium, iron, or zinc because chelation may occur.

## Instructions for Use

The doses listed are based on pharmacokinetics in animals and plasma concentrations needed to achieve sufficient plasma concentration above the MIC value. Efficacy studies have not been performed in dogs or cats.

## Patient Monitoring and Laboratory Tests

Susceptibility testing: CLSI breakpoints for sensitive organisms are ≤1.0 mcg/mL, using the human breakpoint. Most sensitive gram-negative bacteria of the Enterobacteriaceae have MIC values ≤0.1 mcg/mL.

## Formulations

• Moxifloxacin is available in 400-mg tablets and 1.6-mg/mL IV solution.

## Stability and Storage

Store in a tightly sealed container, protected from light, and at room temperature. Do not mix with products that contain ions (iron, aluminum, magnesium, and calcium).

## Small Animal Dosage

**Dogs and Cats**
• 10 mg/kg q24h PO.

## Large Animal Dosage

**Horses**
• 5.8 mg/kg q24h for 3 days, but it causes diarrhea in some horses. Therefore there may be risks with long-term use.

## Regulatory Information

There are no withdrawal times established because this drug should not be administered to animals that produce food.

M

# Mycophenolate Mofetil
mye-koe-fen′oh-late

**Trade and other names:** CellCept

**Functional classification:** Immunosuppressant

## Pharmacology and Mechanism of Action

Mycophenolate is an ester prodrug metabolized to mycophenolic acid (MPA) through presystemic de-esterification in the liver. It is used to suppress immunity for transplantation and for treatment of immune-mediated diseases. Mycophenolate, when metabolized to MPA, inhibits inosine monophosphate dehydrogenase, which is an important enzyme for the de novo synthesis of purines in immune cells, especially stimulated lymphocytes. T and B lymphocytes are critically dependent on de novo synthesis of purine nucleotides. Therefore it effectively suppresses T- and B-cell lymphocyte proliferation and decreases antibody synthesis by B cells. It has little effect on T-cell cytokine expression in dogs. In people, it is used as a replacement for people who cannot tolerate azathioprine and has been primarily used for immune suppression in patients undergoing liver or kidney transplants. Other uses in people are based on only retrospective observational studies.

*Pharmacokinetics:* Mycophenolate oral absorption is variable in dogs and has been reported from 54%–87%, with highly variable plasma drug concentrations, depending on the study. It is metabolized to mycophenolic acid, which is the active component and is cleared by the kidneys. The half-life in dogs is only 45 minutes, but it is longer for the metabolite, with a half-life of 2.2–4.6 hours and as long as 8 hours for the metabolite in some dogs. The peak effect occurs in about 2–4 hours after administration. The pharmacokinetic studies with mycophenolate in dogs indicate that frequent dosing is needed to maintain effective concentrations of the active metabolites. The concentrations needed in dogs for immunosuppressive activity is higher than in people (20–30 mcg/mL in people vs. 200 mcg/mL in dogs). At a dose of 13 mg/kg to dogs, it failed to reach concentrations that are considered in the effective range. The pharmacokinetics also have been studied in cats. They have adequate conversion of mycophenolate to the active metabolite mycophenolic acid, but the pharmacokinetics are variable among cats.

## Indications and Clinical Uses

Mycophenolate is used to treat immune-mediated diseases in animals. It is usually used in veterinary medicine (primarily dogs and cats) when other agents such as azathioprine, cyclosporine, chlorambucil, or glucocorticoids alone fail to achieve remission of an immune-mediated disease. It is usually administered in combination with glucocorticoids, cyclosporine, or both. In dogs, mycophenolate has been used on a limited basis to treat some immune-mediated diseases such as aplastic anemia, immune-mediated hemolytic anemia, meningoencephalitis, and autoimmune skin disease. The use in these diseases is supported by anecdotal accounts and small retrospective observational studies. Responses in dogs has been variable, and it is difficult to determine if mycophenolate was responsible for clinical effects or if improvement was caused by co-administered corticosteroids. There has been no difference in response shown between corticosteroids administered with mycophenolate compared with corticosteroids administered with other agents. There was no benefit in dogs when it was added to treatment for immune-mediated hemolytic anemia. In dogs, the active metabolite (MPA) is produced inconsistently, which may explain the variable results observed in dogs. It has been used by neurologists for treatment of myasthenia gravis, but one clinical report indicated that it was not effective. For treatment of pemphigus foliaceous, it was given at a dosage of 22–39 mg/kg/day divided into three treatments. It was well tolerated, but only three of eight dogs completed the study and were improved. For other immune-mediated skin diseases in dogs, it was effective at an average dosage of 14.7 mg/kg twice daily but was administered with corticosteroids in most dogs.

In cats, the use is limited and based only on small case studies or anecdotal reports. In pharmacokinetic studies in cats in which investigators examined immune suppression, it did not effectively suppress immune cells in cats at doses that did not cause GI problems. There are no published data at this time on the use of mycophenolate in horses.

### Precautionary Information
#### Adverse Reactions and Side Effects

In dogs, GI problems (diarrhea, weight loss, anorexia, and vomiting) have been the most common effects reported, which may be caused by a direct effect on intestinal mucosa. The adverse GI effects may be delayed in some dogs. At the low dose of 10 mg/kg, it is well tolerated, but it may not be effective at this dose. As the dose is increased up to 20 and 30 mg/kg, adverse GI effects are more common (nausea, diarrhea, weight loss). In cats at 10 mg/kg PO q12h, it was well tolerated, but this dose did not suppress immune cells. At higher doses, it consistently produces adverse GI effects in cats.

**Contraindications and Precautions**

Mycophenolate is an immunosuppressive drug. Therefore, patients may be more prone to infection when receiving mycophenolate. When combined with other immunosuppressive drugs, there may exacerbated adverse effects.

**Drug Interactions**

Some drug interactions that affect oral bioavailability in humans have been reported (e.g., antibiotics, cyclosporine, antacid drugs), but these drug interactions have not been reported in animals. Mycophenolate requires acid for oral absorption; therefore, interference from acid-suppressing drugs is possible. Do not administer with azathioprine because it may increase the risk of adverse effects. However, it often administered with corticosteroids without any apparent adverse effects.

## Instructions for Use

Mycophenolate is used in some patients that cannot tolerate other immunosuppressive drugs, such as azathioprine or cyclophosphamide. It has been used in combination with corticosteroids and cyclosporine. The clinical effects in dogs and cats are not well established but are based on small observational studies and anecdotal experiences.

## Patient Monitoring and Laboratory Tests

Monitor for signs of infection in patients. Monitor CBC periodically when administering immunosuppressive agents.

**M**

## Formulations

- Mycophenolate is available in 250- and 500-mg capsules, 500-mg tablets; 200 mg/mL oral suspension (fruit flavor).
- For IV use, reconstitute the vial of mycophenolate powder with 5% dextrose in water to a concentration of 6 mg/mL. Administer over 2 hours slowly.
- Compounded formulation: A 50-mg/mL oral suspension may be made with mycophenolate mofetil capsules mixed with Ora-Plus and cherry syrup. Mix six 250 mg capsules with 7.5 mL of Ora-Plus and stir to a uniform paste. Add 15 mL of cherry syrup in incremental proportions and transfer to a bottle for dispensing. There should be sufficient cherry syrup added to make a total volume of 30 mL. Shake well before using. It is stable during storage for 210 days at 5°C, for 28 days at 25°C–37°C, and for 11 days at 45°C.

## Stability and Storage

Store in a tightly sealed container, protected from light, and at room temperature. It is slightly soluble in water. It is more stable at low pH values (less than 4). It may be prepared in a syrup suspension for flavoring and remains stable for 121 days. The oral liquid suspension has been stored at 25°C (room temperature) or in the refrigerator (5°C); it has a shelf-life of 28 days and 210 days, respectively. Shake the suspension before administration.

## Small Animal Dosage

**Dogs**

- 10 mg/kg q8h PO or 20 mg/kg q8–12h PO. (Higher doses may be needed for clinical effects, but as the dose is increased, adverse effects are more common.)

Cats

- No effective dose has been defined. A common dosage is 10 mg/kg q12h PO ≤15 mg/kg q8h, but it did not produce effects on immune cells at this dosage. At dosages less than 15 mg/kg q12h, it has been tolerated in cats, but at higher doses, GI problems are more common.

## Large Animal Dosage

- No large animal dose has been reported.

## Regulatory Information

There are no withdrawal times established because this drug should not be administered to animals that produce food.

## Naloxone Hydrochloride
nal-oks'one hye-droe-klor'ide

**Trade and other names:** Narcan and Trexonil

**Functional classification:** Opioid antagonist

## Pharmacology and Mechanism of Action

Naloxone is an opioid antagonist. Naloxone competes for opiate receptors and displaces opioid drugs from these receptors, thus reversing their effects. Naloxone is capable of antagonizing all opiate receptors and is used for rapid reversal of opioid effects in cases of overdose or if adverse effects are observed during treatment in animals.

*Pharmacokinetics:* Naloxone is rapidly absorbed from the IM route and also may be administered intranasal and IV. The half-life is short, which may necessitate repeat treatments for long-acting opioids. After IV administration to dogs, the half-life was less than 1 hour (30–40 minutes) in one study and 70 minutes in another study, with a peak concentration (0.04 mg/kg) of 19 ng/mL. The bioavailability from intranasal administration is 32%.

## Indications and Clinical Uses

Naloxone is used to reverse the effects of opiate agonists on receptors. Naloxone is usually the first drug of choice for reversing overdoses, toxicity, or adverse central nervous system (CNS) effects such as dysphoria or excitement. It will reverse effects of morphine, oxymorphone, butorphanol, hydromorphone, fentanyl, and other opioids. It is less effective for reversing buprenorphine because buprenorphine is a partial agonist. When administering naloxone to reverse opiates, the dose may be titrated gradually to achieve the optimum degree of reversal.

The dose for full reversal is typically 0.04 mg/kg (40 mcg/kg), but doses this high may not be needed, and smaller doses (producing partial reversal) can be used when it is necessary to reduce dysphoria or excitement, without reducing the analgesic effects. At very low doses (one fifth of the dose needed to fully reverse opiates), it has been used to treat opioid-induced side effects such as vomiting, nausea, and dysphoria. (This use has been referred to as microdosing.) A formulation for wildlife use (Trexonil) is more concentrated and used to reverse tranquilization in wild animals. Naloxone may have some temporary benefit for behavior modification (e.g., to suppress compulsive disorders), but the effects are short lived. For example, in horses, it temporarily decreases crib biting, but the duration of action is short.

## Precautionary Information

### Adverse Reactions and Side Effects

Tachycardia and hypertension have been reported in people. In animals, reversal of opioid may precipitate a severe reaction that includes high blood pressure, excitement, pain, tachycardia, and cardiac arrhythmias. Because of these reactions, less than a full reversal often is recommended unless the reversal is needed for a life-threatening problem.

### Contraindications and Precautions

Administration to an animal that is experiencing pain precipitates extreme reactions because of blockade of endogenous opioids.

### Drug Interactions

Naloxone reverses the action of several opioid drugs in all animal species.

## Instructions for Use

Administration may have to be individualized based on response in each patient. Naloxone's duration of action is short in animals (60 minutes), and the dose may have to be repeated when treating an overdose of a long-acting opioid. Start at the low end of the dosage rate and increase the dose to effect. Higher doses may be needed to reverse drugs that are mixed agonists–antagonists such as butorphanol or buprenorphine compared with reversing drugs that are pure agonists. Low doses may be used to reduce opioid-induced dysphoria in animals. For this use, start with the 0.04-mg/mL solution and administer increments of 1 mL every 30 seconds until vocalization or signs of dysphoria stop. A dose of 0.01 mg/kg IV has been given for this purpose without losing analgesic effects.

As a general guideline, a dose of 1 mL (0.4 mg) reverses 1.5 mg of oxymorphone, 15 mg of morphine, 100 mg of meperidine, and 0.4 mg of fentanyl.

## Patient Monitoring and Laboratory Tests

Naloxone is used to reverse opioid analgesic drugs. When opioids are reversed in some animals, serious reactions may occur. In some patients, changes in blood pressure, tachycardia, and discomfort may result.

## Formulations Available

- Naloxone is available in injectable vials with preservatives in 0.4 or 1 mg/mL; without preservatives in 0.02 mg (20 mcg), 0.4 mg, or 1 mg/mL; and as Trexonil in 50 mg/mL.

## Stability and Storage

When used intravenously, it may be diluted in other fluids. For IV infusion, it may be added to 0.9% sodium chloride solution or 5% dextrose solution. An amount of 2 mg of naloxone may be mixed with 500 mL of fluids to produce 4 mcg/mL. After dilution, it should be used within 24 hours. Do not mix with other drugs or solutions that are alkaline. Store in a tightly sealed container, protected from light, and at room temperature.

## Small Animal Dosage

### Dogs and Cats

- 0.01–0.04 mg/kg IV, IM, or SQ as needed to reverse opiate. A full antagonist dose is 0.04 mg/kg.
- Low dose to partially reverse dysphoric reaction: Administer 1 mL every 30 seconds (0.04 mg/mL solution) as needed.

## Large Animal Dosage

### Horses

- 0.02–0.04 mg/kg IV (duration of effect is only 20 minutes).

## Regulatory Information

No withdrawal times are established. It is anticipated that naloxone is cleared rapidly after administration. Because of a low risk of residues, short (24–48 hours) withdrawal times are suggested.

Racing Commissioners International (RCI) Classification: 3

# Naltrexone
nal-treks′one

**Trade and other names:** Trexan and Vivitrol

**Functional classification:** Opioid antagonist

## Pharmacology and Mechanism of Action
Naltrexone is an opiate antagonist. Naltrexone competes for opiate receptors and displaces opioid drugs from these receptors, thus reversing their effects. It is capable of antagonizing all opiate receptors. Its action is similar to naloxone except that it is longer acting and administered orally. A related drug that does not have central-acting effects is methylnaltrexone (used to treat intestinal ileus). For humans, there is a long-acting injection formulated in microspheres that persists for 1 month after a single injection. The long-acting form has not been used in animals.

## Indications and Clinical Uses
For treating overdoses of opioids, naloxone administered IV, IM, or intranasal is preferred over naltrexone. Naltrexone is used in people for treatment of opiate dependence and alcoholism. In animals, some obsessive-compulsive disorders are believed to be mediated by endogenous opioids. It has been used successfully for treatment of some obsessive-compulsive behavioral disorders, such as tail chasing in dogs, acral lick granuloma in dogs, and crib biting in horses. The effect for each of these disorders is short lived.

## Precautionary Information
### Adverse Reactions and Side Effects
Adverse effects have not been reported in animals. In people, it can precipitate opioid withdrawal signs.

### Contraindications and Precautions
Do not administer to animals in pain, or it may elicit a severe reaction.

### Drug Interactions
Naltrexone reverses the action of other opioid drugs.

## Instructions for Use
For acute treatment of opiate toxicity, use naloxone instead because it can be injected with a more rapid onset of effects. Treatment for obsessive-compulsive disorders (canine compulsive disorder) in animals has been reported with naltrexone. Relapse rates may be high.

## Patient Monitoring and Laboratory Tests
Monitor heart rate in treated animals.

## Formulations
- Naltrexone is available in 50-mg tablets. Vivitrol for humans is an encapsulated microsphere that can be injected to produce a long-lasting effect (one injection per month) to treat opioid use disorder. One vial contains 380 mg in microspheres in a 4-mL injection for IM use.

## Stability and Storage
Store in a tightly sealed container, protected from light, and at room temperature. Naltrexone is soluble in water. It has been mixed with juices and syrups to mask the bitter taste and is stable for 60–90 days.

## Small Animal Dosage
### Dogs
• For behavior problems: 2.2 mg/kg q12h PO.

## Large Animal Dosage
### Horses
• Crib biting: 0.04 mg/kg IV or SQ. (Because injectable formulations are not available, it must be compounded for this indication.) Duration of effect is 1–7 hours.
• For reversal of opiates: 100 mg/animal IV or SQ. (Because injectable formulations are not available, it must be compounded for this indication.)

## Regulatory Information
Withdrawal times are not established for animals that produce food. In wild animals that are captured with opiates and administered naltrexone for reversal, a 45-day withdrawal time is suggested. For additional extralabel use withdrawal interval estimates, contact Food Animal Residue Avoidance Databank (FARAD) at www.FARAD.org.
RCI Classification: 3

# Nandrolone Decanoate
nan'droe-lone dek-ah-noe'ate

**Trade and other names:** Deca-Durabolin

**Functional classification:** Hormone, anabolic agent

## Pharmacology and Mechanism of Action
Nandrolone is an anabolic steroid. Nandrolone is a derivative of testosterone used as an anabolic agent. Anabolic agents are designed to maximize anabolic effects while minimizing androgenic action.

## Indications and Clinical Uses
Anabolic agents have been used for reversing catabolic conditions, promoting weight gain, increasing muscling in animals, and stimulating erythropoiesis. There are no documented differences in efficacy among the anabolic steroids reported in animals.

## Precautionary Information
### Adverse Reactions and Side Effects
Adverse effects from anabolic steroids can be attributed to the pharmacologic action of these steroids. Increased masculine effects are common. There has been an increased incidence of some tumors in people. Some of the oral anabolic steroids that are 17-alpha methylated (oxymetholone, stanozolol, and oxandrolone) are associated with hepatic toxicity.

### Contraindications and Precautions
Use cautiously in patients with hepatic disease. Do not use in pregnant animals. These drugs are controlled substances and have been abused in people to increase athletic performance and muscle mass.

### Drug Interactions
No drug interactions have been reported.

## Instructions for Use

Results of clinical studies in animals have not been reported. Nandrolone use in animals (and doses) is based on experience in people or anecdotal experience in animals.

## Patient Monitoring and Laboratory Tests

Monitor liver enzymes in treated patients.

## Formulations

• Nandrolone decanoate is available in 50-, 100-, and 200-mg/mL injection.

## Stability and Storage

Store in a tightly sealed container, protected from light, and at room temperature. Stability of compounded formulations has not been evaluated.

## Small Animal Dosage

### Dogs

• 1–1.5 mg/kg/wk IM.

### Cats

• 1 mg/kg/wk IM.

## Large Animal Dosage

### Horses

• 1 mg/kg every 4 weeks IM.

## Regulatory Information

Nandrolone is a Schedule III controlled drug.
Do not administer to animals intended for food.
RCI Classification: 4

# Naproxen
nah-proks′en

**Trade and other names:** Naprosyn, Naxen, and Aleve (naproxen sodium)

**Functional classification:** Nonsteroidal anti-inflammatory drug

## Pharmacology and Mechanism of Action

Naproxen is a nonsteroidal anti-inflammatory drug (NSAID) that is widely used in people, but infrequently used in animals. Naproxen and other NSAIDs produce analgesic and anti-inflammatory effects by inhibiting the synthesis of prostaglandins. The enzyme inhibited by NSAIDs is the cyclooxygenase (COX) enzyme. The COX enzyme exists in two isoforms: COX-1 and COX-2. COX-1 is primarily responsible for synthesis of prostaglandins important for maintaining a healthy gastrointestinal (GI) tract, renal function, platelet function, and other normal functions. COX-2 is induced and responsible for synthesizing prostaglandins that are important mediators of pain, inflammation, and fever. However, there are overlapping functions of the mediators derived from these isoforms. Naproxen is a nonselective inhibitor of COX-1 and COX-2.

*Pharmacokinetics:* The pharmacokinetics of naproxen in dogs and horses differ substantially from people. Whereas in people the half-life is approximately 12–15 hours, the half-life in dogs is 35–74 hours and in horses is only 4–8 hours, which can lead to toxicity in dogs and brief duration of effects in horses.

## Indications and Clinical Uses

Naproxen is approved for use in people and is popular for treating osteoarthritis. It has been used rarely for treatment of musculoskeletal problems, such as myositis and osteoarthritis in dogs and horses. There are no veterinary formulations marketed. Its use has diminished because there are US Food and Drug Administration–approved drugs for these indications for horses and dogs.

### Precautionary Information

**Adverse Reactions and Side Effects**

Naproxen is a potent NSAID. Adverse effects attributed to GI toxicity are common to all NSAIDs. Naproxen has produced serious ulceration in dogs because elimination in dogs is many times slower than in people or horses. Because it is available over the counter (OTC) for people, dogs have been exposed from pet owner administration. Kidney injury caused by renal ischemia also is possible with repeated doses.

**Contraindications and Precautions**

Caution is advised when using the OTC formulation designed for people because the tablet size is much larger than the safe dose for dogs. Therefore warn pet owners about administration to dogs without consulting a veterinarian first. Dosing rates for people are not appropriate for dogs. Do not administer to animals prone to GI ulcers. Do not administer with other ulcerogenic drugs, such as corticosteroids.

**Drug Interactions**

Do not administer with other NSAIDs or with corticosteroids. Corticosteroids have been shown to exacerbate the GI adverse effects. Some NSAIDs may interfere with the action of diuretic drugs and angiotensin-converting enzyme inhibitors.

## Instructions for Use

Results of clinical studies in animals have not been reported. Use in animals (and doses) is based on pharmacokinetic studies in experimental animals.

## Patient Monitoring and Laboratory Tests

Monitor for signs of GI ulceration.

## Formulations

- Naproxen is available in 220-mg tablets (OTC). (A 220-mg dose of naproxen sodium is equivalent to 200-mg naproxen.) It is also available in 25-mg/mL oral suspension and 250-, 375-, and 500-mg tablets (prescription).

## Stability and Storage

Store in a tightly sealed container, protected from light, and at room temperature. Naproxen is practically insoluble in water at low pH, but it increases at high pH. It is soluble in ethanol.

### Small Animal Dosage
**Dogs**
- 5 mg/kg initially, then 2 mg/kg q48h PO. *(The use is not recommended for dogs.)*

### Large Animal Dosage
**Horses**
- 10 mg/kg q12h PO.

### Regulatory Information
Withdrawal times are not established for animals that produce food. For extralabel use withdrawal interval estimates, contact FARAD at www.FARAD.org.
RCI Classification: 4

---

# N-Butylscopolammonium Bromide (Butylscopolamine Bromide)
en-byoo-til-skoe-pahl'ah-moe-nee-um broe'mide

**Trade and other names:** Buscopan

**Functional classification:** Antispasmodic

### Pharmacology and Mechanism of Action
N-butylscopolammonium is an antispasmodic, antimuscarinic, anticholinergic drug. This is a quaternary ammonium compound derived from belladonna alkaloid. Butylscopolamine, like other antimuscarinic drugs (e.g., atropine), blocks cholinergic receptors and produces a parasympatholytic effect. It affects receptors throughout the body, but it is used more commonly for its GI effects. It effectively inhibits secretions and motility of the GI tract by blocking parasympathetic receptors. It has a short half-life (15–25 minutes) and short duration of action.

### Indications and Clinical Uses
Butylscopolamine bromide is indicated for treating pain associated with spasmodic colic, flatulent colic, and intestinal impactions in horses. It is also used to relax the rectum and reduce intestinal strain to facilitate diagnostic rectal palpation.

Because of effects to relax smooth muscle via anticholinergic mechanisms, it is effective for short-term treatment (usually one injection) to horses with recurrent airway obstruction (also known as "heaves").

### Precautionary Information
#### Adverse Reactions and Side Effects
Adverse reactions from anticholinergic drugs are related to their blocking of acetylcholine receptors and producing a systemic parasympatholytic response. As expected with this class of drugs, animals have an increased heart rate, decreased secretions, dry mucous membranes, decreased GI tract motility, and dilated pupils.

N

In target animal safety studies in which doses of 1, 3, and 5 times the approved dose and up to 10 times the dose were administered to horses, the clinical signs described previously were observed. However, at high doses, there were no complete blood count (CBC) or biochemical abnormalities or lesions identified at necropsy.

**Contraindications and Precautions**

N-butylscopolammonium bromide decreases intestinal motility. Use cautiously in conditions in which decreased motility is a concern.

**Drug Interactions**

N-butylscopolammonium bromide is an anticholinergic drug and therefore antagonizes all other medications that are intended to produce a cholinergic response (e.g., metoclopramide).

## Instructions for Use

Experience is limited to treating spasmodic colic, flatulent colic, and intestinal impactions in horses. It is also effective for treating bronchoconstriction in horses with airway obstruction. There is no experience in other animals.

## Patient Monitoring and Laboratory Tests

Monitor equine intestinal motility (gut sounds and fecal output) during treatment. Monitor heart rate in treated animals.

## Formulations

• N-butylscopolammonium is available in a 20-mg/mL solution.

## Stability and Storage

Store in a tightly sealed container, protected from light, and at room temperature.

## Small Animal Dosage

• No dose is reported for small animals.

## Large Animal Dosage

**Horses**

• 0.3 mg/kg slowly IV as a single dose (1.5 mL per 100 kg).

## Regulatory Information

Do not administer to animals intended for food.

# Neomycin
nee-oh-mye'sin

**Trade and other names:** Biosol

**Functional classification:** Antibacterial

## Pharmacology and Mechanism of Action

Neomycin is an aminoglycoside antibiotic administered orally with limited clinical usefulness, except treatment of some bacterial causes of diarrhea. The action of neomycin is to inhibit bacteria protein synthesis via binding to 30S ribosome.

It is bactericidal with a broad spectrum of activity except against streptococci and anaerobic bacteria. Neomycin differs from other aminoglycosides because it is only administered topically or orally. Systemic absorption is minimal from oral absorption.

## Indications and Clinical Uses

Neomycin is commonly available in topical formulations. It is often combined with other antibiotics (triple antibiotics) in ointments for topical treatment of superficial infections. It is also used for oral administration to produce a local effect in the intestine for treatment of intestinal infections (colibacillosis). It is given orally, and because it is not absorbed systemically, it produces a local effect limited to the intestinal lumen.

### Precautionary Information

**Adverse Reactions and Side Effects**

Although oral absorption is so small that systemic adverse effects are unlikely, some oral absorption has been demonstrated in young animals (calves) if intestinal integrity is compromised. Alterations in intestinal bacterial flora from therapy may cause diarrhea.

**Contraindications and Precautions**

Use neomycin cautiously in animals with kidney disease. If oral absorption occurs because of compromised mucosal integrity, absorption may occur from the intestine. Do not use longer than 14 days. Neomycin has been mixed with water and injected, but this practice is strongly discouraged.

**Drug Interactions**

Neomycin should not be mixed with other drugs before administration. Other drugs may bind and become inactivated.

## Instructions for Use

Efficacy for treatment of diarrhea, especially for nonspecific diarrhea, is questionable.

## Patient Monitoring and Laboratory Tests

Monitor for signs of diarrhea. If sufficiently absorbed systemically, it could cause kidney injury; therefore monitor blood urea nitrogen and creatinine with chronic use.

## Formulations

- Neomycin is available in 500-mg bolus, 50-mg/mL (equivalent to 35 mg/mL of neomycin base) and 200-mg/mL oral liquid (equivalent to 140 mg/mL of neomycin base), and 325-mg soluble powder (equivalent to 20.3 g/oz of neomycin base).

## Stability and Storage

It may be added to drinking water or milk. Do not add to other liquid supplements. Prepare a fresh solution daily. It is freely soluble in water and slightly soluble in ethanol. Aqueous solutions are stable over a wide pH range with optimum stability at a pH of 7. Store in a tightly sealed container, protected from light, and at room temperature.

## Small Animal Dosage
**Dogs and Cats**
- 10–20 mg/kg q6–12h PO.

## Large Animal Dosage
**Calves, Sheep, Goats, and Pigs**
- 22 mg/kg/day PO.

## Regulatory Information
Slaughter withdrawal times: cattle, 1 day; sheep, 2 days; swine and goats, 3 days. Oral administration may cause residues in animals intended for food; therefore do not administer to veal calves.

# Neostigmine
nee-oh-stig'meen

**Trade and other names:** Prostigmin, Stiglyn, Neostigmine bromide, and Neostigmine methylsulfate

**Functional classification:** Anticholinesterase

## Pharmacology and Mechanism of Action
Neostigmine is a cholinesterase inhibitor (anticholinesterase). This drug inhibits the enzyme that metabolizes acetylcholine into inactive products. Therefore it prolongs the action of acetylcholine at the synapse. The major difference between physostigmine and neostigmine or pyridostigmine is that physostigmine crosses the blood–brain barrier, and the others do not.

## Indications and Clinical Uses
Neostigmine is used as an antidote for anticholinergic intoxication. It is also used as a treatment for myasthenia gravis, treatment (antidote) for neuromuscular blockade, and treatment for ileus. It also has been used as a treatment of urinary retention—such as the retention observed in postoperative patients—by increasing the tone of bladder smooth muscle. In ruminants, it has been used to stimulate rumen and intestinal motility. In horses, it has been used to stimulate GI motility, but results have been mixed. It may increase intestinal motility and increase fecal output but may not increase stomach emptying.

For these uses, there are no clinical studies to guide the use and doses administered. The clinical use is based on anecdotal experience, studies in research animals, or clinical observations.

## Precautionary Information
### Adverse Reactions and Side Effects
Adverse effects are caused by the cholinergic action resulting from inhibition of cholinesterase. These effects are manifest in the GI tract as diarrhea, increased secretions, and smooth muscle contractions. Other adverse effects can include miosis, bradycardia, muscle twitching or weakness, and constriction of bronchi and ureters. Adverse effects can be treated with anticholinergic drugs such as atropine.

Pyridostigmine may be associated with fewer adverse effects than neostigmine and is preferred for some indications (e.g., myasthenia gravis treatment).

**Contraindications and Precautions**

Do not use in urinary obstruction, intestinal obstruction, asthma or bronchoconstriction, pneumonia, and cardiac arrhythmias. The administration to horses is discouraged because it may increase abdominal discomfort. Do not use in patients sensitive to bromide. If the patient is also receiving bromide (e.g., KBr) for treatment of seizures, this formulation may contribute to excess bromide accumulation.

**Drug Interactions**

Do not use with other cholinergic drugs. Anticholinergic drugs (atropine and glycopyrrolate) block the effects.

## Instructions for Use

Neostigmine is indicated primarily only for treatment of intoxication. For routine systemic use of an anticholinesterase drug, pyridostigmine may have fewer side effects. When neostigmine is used, the frequency of dose may be increased based on observation of effects.

## Patient Monitoring and Laboratory Tests

Monitor GI signs, heart rate, and rhythm.

## Formulations

- Neostigmine bromide is available in 15-mg tablets, and neostigmine methylsulfate is available in 0.25-, 0.5-, and 1-mg/mL injections.

## Stability and Storage

Store in a tightly sealed container, protected from light, and at room temperature.

## Small Animal Dosage

### Dogs and Cats

- 2 mg/kg per day PO in divided doses.
- Antimyasthenic treatment: 10 mcg/kg IM or SQ as needed. *(Not recommended for long-term treatment.)*
- Antidote for neuromuscular blockade: 40 mcg/kg IM or SQ.
- Diagnostic aid for myasthenia: 40 mcg/kg IM or 20 mcg/kg IV.

## Large Animal Dosage

When used as a treatment for neuromuscular blocking agents (cholinesterase inhibitor), the frequency of administration is determined by clinical response.

### Horses

- 0.02–0.04 mg/kg (20–40 mcg/kg) IV or SQ. It may be delivered by constant-rate infusion at a dosage of 0.008 mg/kg/h.

### Cattle

- 22 mcg/kg (0.022 mg/kg) SQ.

### Sheep

- 22–33 mcg/kg (0.022–0.033 mg/kg) SQ.

### Swine

- 44–66 mcg/kg (0.044–0.066 mg/kg) IM.

**Ruminants**
• Stimulate rumen motility: 0.02 mg/kg IM or SQ.

## Regulatory Information

Withdrawal times are not established for animals that produce food. When used to stimulate rumen motility, no withdrawal time has been used. For additional extralabel use withdrawal interval estimates, contact FARAD at www.FARAD.org.

RCI Classification: 3

# Niacinamide
nye′ah-sin′ah-mide

**Trade and other names:** Nicotinamide and vitamin B$_3$

**Functional classification:** Anti-inflammatory

## Pharmacology and Mechanism of Action

Niacinamide is a derivative of vitamin B and sometimes used for immune-mediated diseases. It is not a direct-acting immunosuppressant. The use is primarily to treat skin diseases, such as discoid lupus erythematosus and pemphigus erythematosus in dogs. The mechanism of action is not entirely known. Niacinamide may have some anti-inflammatory action such as suppression of inflammatory cells. Niacin and niacinamide are also used to treat vitamin B$_3$ deficiency. Do not confuse niacin with niacinamide. Niacin is converted to the active form niacinamide by intestinal bacteria.

Niacin is used in people as a lipid-regulating compound used to lower circulating blood triglycerides and reduce low-density lipoproteins. The primary treatment in people for niacin is to treat dyslipidemias.

## Indications and Clinical Uses

Niacinamide has been used to treat immune-mediated skin disease in small animals. For skin disorders, it is usually administered with tetracycline. It also has been used to treat vitamin B$_3$ deficiency. Use in animals has been primarily derived from a few clinical reports, small observational studies, and empirical use.

## Precautionary Information

### Adverse Reactions and Side Effects

Side effects are not common but have included vomiting, anorexia, lethargy, and diarrhea. In people, when niacin is administered to treat dyslipidemias, side effects are common, including flushing of skin. The flushing effect of niacin is thought to occur through skin prostaglandin induction and activation of prostaglandin-associated receptors. When activated, the niacin receptor functions by increasing prostaglandin synthesis and activation of vasodilatory prostaglandin receptors in the skin. In people, niacin also has been associated with liver injury.

### Contraindications and Precautions

No contraindications are reported for animals.

### Drug Interactions

No drug interactions are reported.

## Instructions for Use
For treatment of pemphigus skin disease, it is usually administered with a tetracycline.

## Patient Monitoring and Laboratory Tests
Monitor blood CBC periodically during treatment.

## Formulations
- Niacinamide is available in 50-, 100-, 125-, 250-, and 500-mg tablets (OTC) and 100-mg/mL injection.

## Stability and Storage
Store in a tightly sealed container, protected from light, and at room temperature.

## Small Animal Dosage
### Dogs
- 500 mg of niacinamide q8h PO plus 500 mg of tetracycline. This dosage is approximate based on a 10-kg dog. Eventually taper dosage to q12h and then to q24h. For dogs less than 10 kg, start with 250 mg of each drug.

## Large Animal Dosage
- No large animal doses are reported.

## Regulatory Information
No regulatory information is available. Because of a low risk of residues, no withdrawal times are suggested.

# Nifedipine
nye-fed'ih-peen

**Trade and other names:** Adalat and Procardia

**Functional classification:** Calcium-channel blocker, vasodilator

## Pharmacology and Mechanism of Action
Nifedipine is a calcium-channel blocking drug of the dihydropyridine class. It acts as a vasodilator, with less effect on the calcium channels affecting cardiac conduction. It is not used as much in veterinary medicine as amlodipine, which is in the same class. The action of nifedipine is similar to other calcium-channel blocking drugs, such as amlodipine. They block voltage-dependent calcium entry into smooth muscle cells. Drugs of the dihydropyridine class are more specific for vascular smooth muscle than the cardiac tissue. Therefore they have less effect on cardiac conduction than diltiazem.

## Indications and Clinical Uses
Nifedipine is used for smooth muscle relaxation and to induce vasodilation. It is indicated for treatment of systemic hypertension. Use in animals is rare because there is more experience with amlodipine. The use of nifedipine in animals has been primarily derived from empirical use or some isolated anecdotal reports. There are no well-controlled clinical studies or efficacy trials to document clinical effectiveness.

## Precautionary Information

### Adverse Reactions and Side Effects

Adverse effects have not been reported in veterinary medicine because of the infrequent use. The most common side effect anticipated is hypotension.

### Contraindications and Precautions

Do not administer to a patient with hypotension. Use cautiously with other agents that may lower blood pressure. Nifedipine may be teratogenic in pregnant laboratory animals or embryotoxic. Avoid use in pregnant animals.

### Drug Interactions

Do not administer with drugs known to inhibit drug-metabolizing enzymes (e.g., ketoconazole). Nifedipine may be subject to interactions from drugs that inhibit the membrane multidrug resistance pump, also known as P-glycoprotein, which may lead to toxicity. See Appendix J for drugs that may affect P-glycoprotein.

## Instructions for Use

Use of nifedipine is limited in veterinary medicine. Other calcium-channel blockers, such as diltiazem, are used to control heart rhythm. Amlodipine is more commonly used for control of systemic hypertension.

## Patient Monitoring and Laboratory Tests

Monitor blood pressure during therapy.

## Formulations

- Nifedipine is available in 10- and 20-mg capsules and 30-, 60-, and 90-mg extended-release tablets.

## Stability and Storage

Store in a tightly sealed container, protected from light, and at room temperature. It is decomposed more rapidly if exposed to light. In extemporaneous solutions, nifedipine is unstable. If mixed with solutions, it should be used immediately.

## Small Animal Dosage

- Animal dose not established. In people, the dosage is 10 mg per person three times a day and increased in 10-mg increments to effect.

## Large Animal Dosage

- No large animal doses are reported.

## Regulatory Information

Withdrawal times are not established for animals that produce food. For extralabel use withdrawal interval estimates, contact FARAD at www.FARAD.org.

RCI Classification: 4

# Nitazoxanide

nye-taz-oks'ah-nide

**Trade and other names:** Navigator (horse preparation) and Alinia (human preparation)

**Functional classification:** Antiprotozoal

## Pharmacology and Mechanism of Action

Nitazoxanide is an antiprotozoal drug that was once used for treating protozoa in horses but is no longer used for this indication. It has been used in other animals, including zoo and exotic species for treating protozoa infections. Nitazoxanide is a nitrothiazole derivative. Shortly after administration, it is metabolized to an active metabolite, and there is little nitazoxanide detected in the blood. The deacetylated metabolite, tizoxanide, is responsible for the antiprotozoal activity. Its action against protozoa is unknown, but it may be related to the inhibition of the pyruvate–ferredoxin oxidoreductase enzyme-dependent electron transfer reaction essential to anaerobic and protozoal energy metabolism.

Activity has been demonstrated against a variety of protozoa, including *Cryptosporidium parvum, Giardia* spp., *Isospora* spp., and *Entamoeba* spp. It also has activity against intestinal helminths, such as *Ascaris, Ancylostoma, Trichuris,* and *Taenia* spp. It also may be active against some anaerobic bacteria, including *Helicobacter* spp. It does not eradicate *Tritrichomonas foetus* in cats.

## Indications and Clinical Uses

Nitazoxanide was used to treat equine protozoal myeloencephalitis (EPM) as the equine paste Navigator (32% paste). However, because the adverse effects were common and included fatal enterocolitis at recommended doses, it was voluntarily withdrawn by the sponsor. It is still available in the human formulation (Alinia). This formulation for people is approved for treating protozoal infections, such as *Cryptosporidium parvum* and *Giardia* spp. There has been only limited use in dogs and cats for intestinal protozoal infections but no reports to document efficacy and safety. In people, it has been used to treat intestinal infections caused by *Cryptosporidium* spp. (500 mg per person q12h for 3 days) with good success, but there are no reports of its use to treat *Cryptosporidium* infection in animals.

### Precautionary Information

**N**

**Adverse Reactions and Side Effects**

When it was administered to cats at a dose of 75 mg/kg, all cats had adverse effects. At a dosage of 25 mg/kg q12h in cats, most cats had adverse GI effects, with no effect on *Cryptosporidium* spp. Because it may disrupt normal intestinal flora, administration to other animals has produced diarrhea. The use is no longer approved for horses because of adverse effects.

**Contraindications and Precautions**

No known contraindications.

**Drug Interactions**

No known drug interactions.

## Instructions for Use

Nitazoxanide was administered for horses to treat EPM, but the equine product has been withdrawn from the market. Use in small animals has been extrapolated from use in humans and includes treatment of intestinal protozoa.

## Patient Monitoring and Laboratory Tests

When treating patients for diarrhea, monitor electrolytes and fecal samples.

## Formulations

- Nitazoxanide was available in a 0.32-mg/mL oral paste for horses but has been withdrawn from the market by the sponsor.
- Human formulation is a pink-colored powder for oral dosing; 100 mg of powder is mixed with 48 mL of water to produce a 20-mg/mL strawberry flavored oral dose form.

## Stability and Storage

Stable if stored in manufacturer's original formulation. The oral solution for people can be mixed and remain stable for 7 days.

## Small Animal Dosage

- There are no small animal dosing instructions available. However, one dose that has been used is 100 mg per animal q12h PO for 3 days. The human pediatric dosage is 100 mg (5 mL) q12h for 3 days.

## Large Animal Dosage

### Horses

- 25 mg/kg q24h PO on days 1 through 5 followed by 50 mg/kg q24h PO on days 6 through 28. (The equine product was withdrawn from the market by the sponsor because of severe adverse effects.)

## Regulatory Information

Do not use in animals intended for food.

---

# Nitenpyram
nye-ten-pye′ram

**Trade and other names:** Capstar

**Functional classification:** Antiparasitic

## Pharmacology and Mechanism of Action

Nitenpyram is an antiparasitic drug used for treatment of fleas. It rapidly kills adult fleas. It is from the class of synthetic insecticides known as the neonicotinoids. It is related to imidacloprid and has the same mechanism of action, which is to inhibit postsynaptic nicotinic acetylcholine receptors, which produces influx of sodium ions.

*Pharmacokinetics:* Nitenpyram is absorbed completely from oral administration and has half-lives in dogs and cats of 2.8 and 7.7 hours, respectively. After oral absorption, it produces a rapid kill of adult fleas that has been observed as quickly as 30 minutes after drug administration and is 98.6% effective in dogs and 98.4% effective in cats.

## Indications and Clinical Uses

Nitenpyram is used to kill fleas on dogs and cats. It produces a rapid kill, with fleas killed within 1 hour of administration. It is often used with other drugs that act to prevent flea infestations as part of a comprehensive flea-control program. It may be used to produce an initial rapid kill of the fleas on the animal, then followed-up with a flea prevention program.

## Precautionary Information

### Adverse Reactions and Side Effects

No adverse reactions are reported. It was safe in studies in dogs and cats in which up to 10 times the dose was administered. It was tolerated even in young animals at 8 weeks of age. Some transient pruritus may occur shortly after administration, which coincides with the initial killing of fleas.

### Contraindications and Precautions

Do not use in dogs or cats weighing less than 1 kg (2 lb). Do not use in cats or dogs younger than 4 weeks of age.

### Drug Interactions

No drug interactions have been reported. It is safe to use with lufenuron, milbemycin, and the isooxazolines (fluralaner, afoxolaner, sarolaner).

## Instructions for Use

Nitenpyram is often used with lufenuron to kill adult fleas and prevent flea eggs from hatching. Administer with or without food. Other flea prevention medications may be used once nitenpyram has been administered for initial elimination of fleas on the dog or cat.

## Patient Monitoring and Laboratory Tests

No specific monitoring is necessary.

## Formulations

• Nitenpyram is available in 11.4- and 57-mg tablets.

## Stability and Storage

Store in a tightly sealed container, protected from light, and at room temperature.

## Small Animal Dosage

• 1 mg/kg daily PO as needed to kill fleas.

## Large Animal Dosage

• No large animal dose is reported.

## Regulatory Information

Withdrawal times are not established for animals that produce food. For extralabel use withdrawal interval estimates, contact FARAD at www.FARAD.org.

---

# Nitrofurantoin

N

nye-troe-fyoo′ran-toyn

**Trade and other names:** Macrodantin, Furalan, Furantoin, Furadantin, and generic brands

**Functional classification:** Antibacterial

## Pharmacology and Mechanism of Action

Nitrofurantoin is an antibacterial drug that acts as a urinary antiseptic. It is a weak acid with low water solubility. Therapeutic concentrations are reached only in the urine. In the urine, it is reduced by bacterial flavoproteins, and the reactive metabolites bind to bacterial ribosomes and inhibit bacterial enzymes involved in the synthesis of DNA and RNA. The spectrum includes *Escherichia coli, Staphylococcus* spp., and *Enterococcus* spp., including strains that are resistant to other antimicrobial agents. Resistance among bacteria is unusual, although *Proteus* spp. and *Pseudomonas aeruginosa* are intrinsically resistant and nitrofurantoin should not be used to treat urinary tract infections caused by these pathogens. Nitrofurantoin has time-dependent effects on *E. coli,* which may necessitate frequent administration for optimal clinical outcome.

*Pharmacokinetics:* The pharmacokinetics have been studied in laboratory animals, dogs, and people. There is no pharmacokinetic data to guide the use in cats. In people, the concentrations in urine reach 200 mcg/mL, but plasma concentrations are almost undetectable. In dogs, a similar profile is observed. The macrocrystalline form is slowly absorbed and less likely to cause gastric upset. The microcrystalline form is rapidly absorbed in the intestine. In dogs, oral absorption is not affected by feeding. Oral absorption is rapid in dogs, with an elimination half-life of approximately 30 minutes and oral bioavailability ranging from 38% to approximately 100%. Excretion in bile is high, producing a cholerectic effect, which may be responsible for some of the adverse GI effects observed. Urinary clearance is saturable; therefore, there are no advantages to administering high doses. Approximately 30% or 20% of the administered dose (depending on dose form) is eliminated in the urine of dogs, with most of the elimination occurring in the first 8 hours, necessitating frequent administration to dogs (e.g., every 8 hours).

## Indications and Clinical Uses

Nitrofurantoin has been an important drug for short-term treatment of urinary tract infections (UTIs) in people. The use in animals is not as common but has been considered for some cases of lower UTI, especially when infections are caused by bacteria resistant to other common antimicrobial agents. There are small observational studies and case reports available for dogs to show that it can be effective at a dose of approximately 4 mg/kg every 8 hours oral. However, failure rates are high, and adverse effects (GI and neurologic) may occur in dogs. It should not be used to treat infections caused by *Proteus* spp. or *P. aeruginosa* because these organisms are intrinsically resistant. It should not be used to treat infections in azotemic patients. Studies on the effects in cats are not available.

It is advised to use the macrocrystalline form to reduce GI upset and prolong effects. Although there are no well-controlled clinical studies or efficacy trials to document clinical effectiveness in veterinary medicine, the in vitro microbiologic studies demonstrate activity against a broad spectrum of bacteria, including those resistant to other antimicrobials.

## Precautionary Information

### Adverse Reactions and Side Effects

Adverse effects include nausea, vomiting, and diarrhea. It turns urine color rust-yellow brown. In people, respiratory problems (pneumonitis) and peripheral neuropathy have been reported. The polyneuropathies in people are caused by a demyelination and are more common from long-term use or in patients with renal compromise. The respiratory problems have not been reported in animals, but neuropathy has been observed in dogs; the risk may be higher if there is renal insufficiency.

### Contraindications and Precautions

Do not use in patients with azotemia. Do not administer during pregnancy, especially at term, because it may cause hemolytic anemia of the newborn. Do not administer to neonates. Do not rely on nitrofurantoin for systemic infections or infections of the kidney or prostate. It is active against lower UTIs only. Do not use nitrofurantoin to treat infections caused by *Proteus* spp., or *P. aeruginosa*.

### Drug Interactions

Do not give medications that may alkalinize the urine because this may reduce effectiveness.

## Instructions for Use

Two dosing forms exist. Microcrystalline is rapidly and completely absorbed. Macrocrystalline (Macrodantin) is more slowly absorbed and causes less GI irritation. This form can be administered with food to slow absorption and delay the effects in the intestine. Urine should be at acidic pH for maximum effect. The dosing guidelines for animals are derived from small observational studies, retrospective studies, or pharmacokinetic studies in experimental dogs. In people, there is an advantage for frequent administration q6h compared with q8h or q12h. There is no advantage for increasing the dose higher than recommended because excretion into urine is saturable.

## Patient Monitoring and Laboratory Tests
Monitor urine cultures or urinalysis. A microbiologic susceptibility test may overestimate the true activity against some bacteria. There are no approved breakpoints to predict susceptibility of bacteria isolated from animals to nitrofurantoin.

## Formulations
- Macrodantin and generic brands are available in 25-, 50-, and 100-mg capsules (macrocrystalline), and Furalan, Furantoin, and generic brands are available in 50- and 100-mg tablets (microcrystalline). Furadantin is available in 5-mg/mL oral suspension.

## Stability and Storage
Store in a tightly sealed container, protected from light, and at room temperature. It is slightly soluble at a concentration less than 1 mg/mL in water and ethanol. It decomposes if exposed to metals other than stainless steel or aluminum.

## Small Animal Dosage
### Dogs and Cats
- 4 mg/kg q8h, PO, or 2 mg/kg q6h PO. (Macrocrystalline formulation administered with food preferred.)
- For comparison, the dose used in people is 0.7 mg/kg (50 mg) q6h PO or 1.4 mg/kg (100 mg) q8h PO, for no longer than 5 days.

## Large Animal Dosage
### Horses
- 2 mg/kg q8h PO.

## Regulatory Information
It is prohibited from use in animals intended for food.

# Nitroglycerin
nye-troe-glih′ser-in

**Trade and other names:** Nitrol, Nitro-Bid, and Nitrostat

**Functional classification:** Vasodilator

## Pharmacology and Mechanism of Action
Nitroglycerin is a nitrate nitrovasodilator. Like other nitrovasodilators, it relaxes vascular smooth muscle (especially venous) through generation of nitric oxide (NO). The nitrate vasodilators are esters of nitrous acid. They are metabolized to inorganic nitrite and denitrated metabolites. Nitrites, organic nitrates, and nitroso compounds all act to activate the enzyme guanylate cyclase, which in turn produces cyclic guanosine monophosphate (GMP) in vascular smooth muscle and relaxes smooth muscle. NO is also known as the endothelium-derived relaxing factor.

Nitric oxide–generating compounds may also help decrease gastric adverse effects associated with NSAIDs, but this use has not been explored for veterinary patients.

*Pharmacokinetics:* Plasma concentrations are attained within 2 minutes of administration, but the half-life in animals is short (only 1–3 minutes) with high first-pass effects (i.e., not absorbed from oral administration).

## Indications and Clinical Uses

Nitroglycerin, like other nitrovasodilators, is used primarily in heart failure or pulmonary edema to reduce preload or decrease pulmonary hypertension. Nitrates relax smooth muscle in both arteries and veins, but they are often used clinically as preload reducers. When used as preload reducers, they decrease myocardial $O_2$ requirements (decrease workload of heart). Because of this effect, they have been commonly used to manage human patients with angina pectoris (chest pain caused by cardiovascular disease).

Use in animals has been primarily derived from empirical use, recommendations from clinical experts, and experience extrapolated from human use. There are no well-controlled clinical studies or efficacy trials to document clinical effectiveness. In small animals, primarily dogs, it has been used in the hospital to treat animals with advanced stages of heart failure. In horses, nitroglycerin has been used to improve blood flow to the feet in the management of laminitis. However, in experiments, this treatment was not effective in horses and did not increase blood flow to the feet.

### Precautionary Information

#### Adverse Reactions and Side Effects

The most significant adverse effect is hypotension. Methemoglobinemia can occur with accumulation of nitrites, but it is a rare problem.

#### Contraindications and Precautions

Do not administer to patients with hypotension. Nitroglycerin is absorbed through human skin. Warn pet owners not to apply ointment without wearing gloves.

#### Drug Interactions

No drug interactions are reported for animals.

## Instructions for Use

Tolerance can develop with repeated chronic use. Tolerance may be caused by a progressive depletion of sulfhydryl groups necessary for the formation of NO. Efficacy is improved if the drug is used intermittently instead of continuously because intermittent use allows time for regeneration of sulfhydryl groups. Optimum intermittent use is to provide a nitrate-free interval of 8 hours or more during the day. Nitroglycerin has high presystemic metabolism, and oral availability is poor. When using ointment, 1 inch of ointment is approximately 15 mg.

It is usually applied to an area on the patient that lacks hair and where the patient will not lick it off (e.g., pinnae of ears).

## Patient Monitoring and Laboratory Tests

Monitor patient's blood pressure during therapy.

## Formulations
- Nitroglycerin is available in 0.5-, 0.8-, 1-, 5-, and 10-mg/mL injection; 2% ointment; 0.3-, 0.4-, and 0.6-mg sublingual tablets; translingual spray; and transdermal systems (0.2 mg/h patch).

## Stability and Storage
Store in a tightly sealed container, protected from light, and at room temperature. Nitroglycerin tablets are very heat and light sensitive and should be stored in a tightly sealed glass bottle.

## Small Animal Dosage
### Dogs
- 4–12 mg (up to 15 mg) topically as needed. In dogs, it has been used as one-fourths to three-fourths inch of 2% ointment q6h (1 inch equals 15 mg).

### Cats
- 2–4 mg topically or typically one-eighth to one-quarter inch q4–6h.

## Large Animal Dosage
### Horses
- Treatment of laminitis: Apply 2% ointment to skin above the hoof. (Efficacy is questionable.)

## Regulatory Information
Do not administer to animals intended for food.
RCI Classification: 3

N

# Nitroprusside (Sodium Nitroprusside)
nye-troe-pruss'ide

**Trade and other names:** Nitropress

**Functional classification:** Vasodilator

## Pharmacology and Mechanism of Action
Nitroprusside is a nitrate vasodilator. Like other nitrovasodilators, it relaxes vascular smooth muscle (especially venous) via generation of NO. NO stimulates guanylate cyclase to produce GMP in smooth muscle, with a predominant effect of relaxing vascular smooth muscle. Nitroprusside is used only as an IV infusion in the hospital, and patients should be monitored carefully during administration. Nitroprusside has a rapid onset of effect (almost immediately) and a duration that lasts only minutes after discontinuation of IV administration.

## Indications and Clinical Uses
Nitroprusside is used for acute management of pulmonary edema and other hypertensive conditions. It is administered only by IV infusion, and the dose is titrated carefully by monitoring systemic blood pressure. Titrate to maintain the arterial blood pressure to 70 mm Hg. Use in animals has been primarily derived from empirical use and experience in humans or the opinions from clinical cardiology experts. There are no well-controlled clinical studies or efficacy trials to document clinical effectiveness. The cost of nitroprusside has increased tremendously in recent years to as much as $750 per vial. Therefore, the high cost has discouraged use in animals.

## Precautionary Information

### Adverse Reactions and Side Effects

Severe hypotension is possible during therapy. Reflex tachycardia can occur during treatment. Cyanide is generated via metabolism during nitroprusside treatment, especially at high infusion rates (greater than 5 mcg/kg/min). At high infusion rates (greater than 10 mcg/kg/min), seizures may occur, which are signs of cyanide toxicity. Sodium thiosulfate has been used in people to prevent cyanide toxicity. Methemoglobinemia is possible and, if necessary, treated with methylene blue.

### Contraindications and Precautions

Do not administer to patients with hypotension or who are dehydrated.

### Drug Interactions

No drug interactions are reported for animals but use cautiously with other drugs that produce vasodilation.

## Instructions for Use

Nitroprusside is administered via IV infusion. IV solution should be delivered in a 5% dextrose solution. (For example, add 20–50 mg to 250 mL of 5% dextrose to a concentration of 80–200 mcg/mL.) Protect from light with opaque wrapping. Discard solutions if color change is observed. Titrate dose carefully in each patient.

## Patient Monitoring and Laboratory Tests

Monitor blood pressure carefully during administration. Do not allow blood pressure to fall below 70 mm Hg during treatment. Monitor heart rate because reflex tachycardia is possible during infusion.

## Formulations Available

- Nitroprusside is available in a 50-mg vial for injection at 10 and 25 mg/mL. (Note: Vials can be extremely expensive.)

## Stability and Storage

Not compatible in some fluids. For IV use, dilute with 5% dextrose. Protect from light and cover infusion solution during administration. Nitroprusside decomposes quickly in alkaline solutions or with exposure to light.

## Small Animal Dosage

### Dogs and Cats

- 1–5 mcg/kg/min IV, up to a maximum of 10 mcg/kg/min. Generally, start with 2 mcg/kg/min and increase gradually by 1 mcg/kg/min until desired blood pressure is achieved.

## Large Animal Dosage

- No large animal doses are reported.

## Regulatory Information

Withdrawal times are not established for animals that produce food. For extralabel use withdrawal interval estimates, contact FARAD at www.FARAD.org.

# Nizatidine

nih-zah'tih-deen

**Trade and other names:** Axid

**Functional classification:** Antiulcer agent

## Pharmacology and Mechanism of Action

Nizatidine is a histamine $H_2$-blocking drug used to suppress stomach acid. Nizatidine blocks histamine stimulation of gastric parietal cells to decrease gastric acid secretion. It is 4–10 times more potent than cimetidine. It is primarily used to treat gastroesophageal reflux disease, gastric ulcers, and gastritis.

Nizatidine and ranitidine also have been shown to stimulate gastric emptying and colonic motility via anticholinesterase activity.

## Indications and Clinical Uses

Nizatidine, like other $H_2$-receptor blockers, is used to treat gastroesophageal reflux, gastric ulcers, and gastritis. These drugs inhibit secretion of stomach acid and have also been used to prevent ulcers caused from NSAIDs, but the efficacy for preventing NSAID-induced ulcers has not been demonstrated.

The use in animals is uncommon because there are other $H_2$-receptor blocking drugs that are used more widely (famotidine), and the use of proton pump inhibitors such as omeprazole is more effective. The use of nizatidine in animals has been primarily derived from empirical use and experience in humans. There are no well-controlled clinical studies or efficacy trials to document clinical effectiveness in animals.

## Precautionary Information

### Adverse Reactions and Side Effects

Side effects from nizatidine have not been reported for animals, but the use has been uncommon.

### Contraindications and Precautions

No contraindications have been reported for animals.

### Drug Interactions

No drug interactions are reported for animals.

## Instructions for Use

Results of clinical studies in animals have not been reported. Use in animals (and doses) is based on experience in people or anecdotal experience in animals. Nizatidine use in animals has not been as common as the use of other related drugs such as ranitidine or famotidine or the proton pump inhibitors (omeprazole).

## Patient Monitoring and Laboratory Tests

No specific monitoring is necessary.

## Formulations

- Nizatidine is available in 150- and 300-mg capsules and 15-mg/mL oral solution.

## Stability and Storage
Store in a tightly sealed container, protected from light, and at room temperature. Nizatidine is slightly soluble in water. It has been mixed with juices and syrups for oral administration and was stable for 48 hours. Avoid mixing with Maalox liquid.

## Small Animal Dosage
**Dogs**
- 2.5–5 mg/kg q24h PO.

## Large Animal Dosage
- No large animal doses are reported.

## Regulatory Information
Withdrawal times are not established for animals that produce food. For extralabel use withdrawal interval estimates, contact FARAD at www.FARAD.org.
RCI Classification: 5

# Norfloxacin
nor-floks'ah-sin

**Trade and other names:** Noroxin

**Functional classification:** Antibacterial

## Pharmacology and Mechanism of Action
Norfloxacin is one of the oldest fluoroquinolone antibacterial drugs that is used rarely in human or veterinary medicine. Norfloxacin acts via inhibition of DNA gyrase in bacteria to inhibit DNA and RNA synthesis. It is a bactericidal with a broad spectrum of activity but not as active as other newer fluoroquinolones. Susceptible bacteria include *Staphylococcus* spp., *E. coli*, *Proteus* spp., *Klebsiella* spp., and *Pasteurella* spp. *P. aeruginosa* is moderately sensitive.

## Indications and Clinical Uses
Norfloxacin has been replaced by other veterinary fluoroquinolones because they have more favorable pharmacokinetics and improved spectrum of activity. There is little justification for the use of norfloxacin in animals because of the availability of other fluoroquinolones. It has been used anecdotally to treat a variety of infections, including respiratory, urinary tract, skin, and soft tissue infections.

## Precautionary Information
### Adverse Reactions and Side Effects
High concentrations may cause CNS toxicity, especially in animals with renal failure. Norfloxacin may cause some nausea, vomiting, and diarrhea at high doses.

All of the fluoroquinolones may cause arthropathy in young animals. Dogs are most sensitive at 4–28 weeks of age. Large, rapidly growing dogs are the most susceptible.

**Contraindications and Precautions**

Avoid use in young animals because of risk of cartilage injury. Use cautiously in animals that may be prone to seizures. Coadministration with divalent and trivalent cations, such as products containing aluminum (e.g., sucralfate), may decrease absorption.

**Drug Interactions**

No drug interactions are reported for animals, but the use of norfloxacin has been uncommon. However, like other quinolones, coadministration with divalent and trivalent cations, such as products containing aluminum (e.g., sucralfate), iron, and calcium, may decrease absorption. Do not mix in solutions or in vials with aluminum, calcium, iron, or zinc because chelation may occur.

## Instructions for Use

Use in animals (and doses) is based on pharmacokinetic studies in experimental animals, experience in people, or anecdotal experience in animals.

## Patient Monitoring and Laboratory Tests

Susceptibility testing: Clinical and Laboratory Standards Institute breakpoints for sensitive organisms are ≤4 mcg/mL.

## Formulations

• Norfloxacin is available in 400-mg tablets.

## Stability and Storage

Store in a tightly sealed container, protected from light, and at room temperature.

## Small Animal Dosage

**Dogs and Cats**

• 22 mg/kg q12h PO.

## Large Animal Dosage

• No large animal doses have been reported.

## Regulatory Information

It is prohibited from use in animals intended for food.

## Oclacitinib Maleate
(okʹla syeʹti nib malʹee ate)

**Trade and other names:** Apoquel

**Functional Classification:** Anti-inflammatory, antipruritic

### Pharmacology and Mechanism of Action

Oclacitinib is a Janus kinase (JAK) inhibitor used for control of pruritus in dogs associated with allergic dermatitis and atopic dermatitis. Oclacitinib has a unique mechanism of action that acts to inhibit proinflammatory cytokines. It inhibits cytokines involved with pruritus in dogs that are dependent on the JAK enzyme. It inhibits preferentially the JAK1 enzyme activity over JAK2 or JAK3, with a 1.8-fold selectivity over JAK2 and 9.9-fold selectivity over JAK3. This preferential activity is important because JAK2 is involved with hematopoiesis and high doses of oclacitinib could suppress hematopoiesis. Of significance for atopic and allergic dermatitis treatment is that oclacitinib inhibits the interleukin (IL)-31 cytokine function and reduces IL-31–induced pruritus in dogs. It also may inhibit the function of other proinflammatory cytokines such as IL-2, IL-4, IL-6, and IL-13 that may be involved with allergy.

In studies of dogs with atopic dermatitis, the efficacy was 66% and 49% as assessed by pet owners and veterinarians, respectively, and 67% in a study with allergic dermatitis. This response was significantly better than placebo. Oclacitinib also was shown to have equal efficacy as prednisolone in dogs, with an onset of efficacy of both treatments in as little as 4 hours.

*Pharmacokinetics:* Oclacitinib is rapidly absorbed (89% bioavailability) and reaches a peak in less than 1 hour, producing rapid effects after administration. The rapid onset of action distinguishes it from some of the other products currently used for treatment of this disease. After absorption, the half-life is approximately 3–5 hours in dogs. Pharmacokinetics are not affected by feeding or breed of dog. The predominant clearance route is hepatic with small amounts of renal and biliary elimination. The pharmacokinetics have not been reported for other animals.

### Indications and Clinical Use

Oclacitinib is indicated for control of pruritus associated with allergic dermatitis and control of atopic dermatitis in dogs at least 12 months of age. Oclacitinib has been equally effective for reducing pruritus in dogs as glucocorticoids or cyclosporine. In a comparison with cyclosporine, oclacitinib had similar efficacy as cyclosporine, but with a more rapid onset and less gastrointestinal (GI) problems.

*Use in cats:* The clinical use in cats has been limited to some small observational studies. At a dosage of 0.4–0.6 mg/kg twice daily for 14 days and then tapered to once daily in small numbers of cats, it has produced good to excellent results. The dosage examined in some experimental cats has been approximately 0.5 mg/kg q12h. There may be a potential role for oclacitinib and other JAK inhibitors for treatment of feline asthma and allergic dermatitis, but further studies are necessary to establish clinical use.

### Precautionary Information

**Adverse Effects**

During field studies, there was a low rate of adverse reactions (diarrhea, 2.3%–4.6% and vomiting, 2.3%–3.9%), which were not different from the placebo and usually resolved after initial dosing. In a clinical study, there were a 9.2% incidence of vomiting and a 6% incidence of diarrhea in 283 dogs. Treated dogs had decreased leukocytes and serum globulin compared with the placebo group. In field trials there have been isolated cases of demodicosis, pyoderma, pneumonia, and mast cell tumor or other neoplasms, but it is not known if these were associated with the medication.

If administration is continued for long-term twice daily rather than lowering the frequency to once daily, more adverse effects may be anticipated. There was a mild, dose-dependent reduction in hemoglobin, hematocrit, and reticulocyte counts during the twice-daily dosing period for 60 days with decreases in the leukocyte subsets of lymphocytes, eosinophils, and basophils. High doses can potentially cause impairment of immune surveillance against tumors; therefore, high doses should be avoided.

**Contraindications and Precautions**

Safety has not been evaluated in breeding animals or during pregnancy. The manufacturer warns that oclacitinib should not be administered to dogs younger than 12 months of age or dogs with serious infections. The manufacturer warns that oclacitinib may increase susceptibility to infection, including demodicosis, and exacerbate neoplastic conditions.

When transitioning dogs from twice-daily administration to once-daily administration, approximately 30% of dogs may experience a flare-up of pruritus.

*Vaccination:* At an oclacitinib dose that represented three times the therapeutic dose, dogs mounted an adequate immune response to killed rabies vaccination, modified-live canine distemper virus vaccination, and modified-live canine parvovirus vaccination in 16-week-old vaccine-naïve dogs. Approximately 80% of the dogs had adequate response to canine parainfluenza virus.

**Drug Interactions**

Dermatologists have used oclacitinib with other medications such as corticosteroids, cyclosporine, and other systemic agents safely, but the manufacturer warns that safety with these medications has not been evaluated. Inhibition of canine cytochrome P450 enzymes by oclacitinib is minimal with the inhibitor concentrations 50 times higher than the peak concentrations produced from the therapeutic dose.

Oclacitinib does not interfere with the response from intradermal skin testing in dogs.

## Instructions for Use

Oclacitinib is indicated for dogs, and safe doses have not been established in other animals. It should not be administered to humans. Administer according to the sponsor's instructions with or without food. After the initial induction period of twice-daily dosing, it should be reduced to once-daily administration to decrease the risk of adverse effects.

There may be risks if a dosage of 0.4–0.6 mg twice daily is continued for long-term use. There is a risk of infections associated with immunosuppression, including bacterial pneumonia and infections caused by *Demodex* spp., at a high dose (three times and five times dose) with twice-daily administration.

## Patient Monitoring

If doses are continued at a twice-daily schedule for longer than the manufacturer recommends, monitor the complete blood count periodically to assess effects on bone marrow. Check dogs for skin lumps and signs of demodicosis.

## Formulations

- Oclacitinib is available as 3.6-, 5.4-, and 16-mg tablets. Do not use compounded formulations because stability and potency have not been evaluated.

## Storage Conditions

Store at room temperature between 20°C and 25°C (68°F and 77°F) in a manufacturer-recommended container. The pH can affect solubility. At a pH of 4, it is less soluble, and at a pH of 5.5, it is almost completely insoluble.

## Small Animal Dosage

### Dogs

- 0.5 mg/kg (0.4–0.6 mg/kg with or without food) initially on a twice-daily schedule for the first 14 days and then tapered to a once-daily administration.

### Cats

- Dose has not been established for cats.

## Large Animal Dosage

- No large animal doses have been established.

## Regulatory Information

No regulatory information is available. Oclacitinib should not be administered to animals intended for food.

# Olsalazine Sodium

ole-sal'ah-zeen soe'dee-um

**Trade and other names:** Dipentum

**Functional classification:** Antidiarrheal

## Pharmacology and Mechanism of Action

Olsalazine is an anti-inflammatory drug used for inflammatory bowel disease. It is composed of two molecules of aminosalicylic acid joined by an azo bond. Each component is released in the colon by bacterial enzymes. The released drug is also known as mesalamine (see Mesalamine). Mesalamine is also the active component of sulfasalazine, which is commonly administered for treatment of colitis. The action of mesalamine is not precisely known, but it appears to suppress the metabolism of arachidonic acid in the intestine. It inhibits both cyclooxygenase- and lipoxygenase-mediated mucosal inflammation. Systemic absorption is small; most of the action is believed to be local in the intestine. Olsalazine has a similar effect as sulfasalazine but without the sulfonamide component. Other formulations of mesalamine include Asacol, Mesasal, and Pentasa. The others are coated tablets designed to release the active component in the intestine.

## Indications and Clinical Uses

Olsalazine, like other forms of mesalamine, is used for treatment of inflammatory bowel disease, including colitis in animals. In small animals, most often sulfasalazine is used; however, in some animals, olsalazine may be indicated. Use in animals has been primarily derived from empirical use and experience in humans. There are no well-controlled clinical studies or efficacy trials to document clinical effectiveness.

## Precautionary Information

### Adverse Reactions and Side Effects
No adverse effects reported in animals.

### Contraindications and Precautions
Do not administer to patients sensitive to salicylate compounds.

### Drug Interactions
No drug interactions have been reported for animals.

## Instructions for Use
Olsalazine is used in patients that cannot tolerate sulfasalazine.

## Patient Monitoring and Laboratory Tests
No specific monitoring is necessary.

## Formulations
- Olsalazine is available in 500-mg tablets.

## Stability and Storage
Store in a tightly sealed container, protected from light, and at room temperature.

## Small Animal Dosage
- Dosage not established, but 5–10 mg/kg q8h has been used. (The usual human dosage is 500 mg twice daily.)

## Large Animal Dosage
- No doses are reported for large animals.

## Regulatory Information
Withdrawal times are not established for animals that produce food. For extralabel use withdrawal interval estimates, contact Food Animal Residue Avoidance Databank (FARAD) at www.FARAD.org.

Racing Commissioners International (RCI) Classification: 4

# Omeprazole
oh-mep′rah-zole

**Trade and other names:** Prilosec (formerly Losec; human preparation), Zegerid (human formulation), GastroGard, and UlcerGard (equine preparations); outside the United States, Peptizole and Gastrozol are available for horses

**Functional classification:** Antiulcer agent

## Pharmacology and Mechanism of Action
Omeprazole is the most widely used proton pump inhibitor (PPI) in animals. Omeprazole inhibits gastric acid secretion by inhibiting the $K^+/H^+$ pump (potassium pump). Omeprazole is more potent and longer acting than the histamine $H_2$ antagonists and is associated with better efficacy. There are other PPIs, including pantoprazole (Protonix), lansoprazole (Prevacid), and rabeprazole (Aciphex). They all act via similar mechanism and are equally effective. PPIs also have some effect for inhibiting *Helicobacter* organisms in the stomach when administered with antibiotics.

Omeprazole is decomposed in the acid environment of the stomach. Oral absorption is decreased if administered with food. Formulations are designed to protect from degradation by stomach acid, such as by adding a buffering agent or enteric coating, to improve oral absorption. Some human formulations also contain bicarbonate.

An equivalent drug is esomeprazole (Nexium) (see Esomeprazole), which is the S-isomer of omeprazole (the active isomer). It is expected to have equal efficacy at equivalent dosages, but there is some evidence of better efficacy with esomeprazole compared to omeprazole.

*Pharmacokinetics:* When administered orally to horses, maximum serum concentration occurs at 45–60 minutes with effective acid suppression within 1–2 hours. Half-life from oral administration to horses varies from 70 to 100 minutes, depending on the formulation. Pharmacokinetics and acid suppression have also been studied in dogs and cats, with effective acid suppression at the dosages provided in the dosing section.

## Indications and Clinical Uses

Omeprazole, like other PPIs, is used for treatment and prevention of GI ulcers and gastroesophageal reflux. It has been used in dogs, cats, and exotic species, but most efficacy data for animals have been produced in horses, in which it has been shown that omeprazole is effective for treating and preventing gastric ulcers. In foals, 4 mg/kg q24h suppresses acid secretion for 22 hours. By comparison, ranitidine suppresses acid up to 8 hours at a dose of 6.6 mg/kg. In studies performed in horses, omeprazole was more effective than ranitidine for treating gastric ulcers.

For treatment of ulcers in horses, the approved label treatment in the United States is 4 mg/kg PO once per day. However, there is evidence to indicate that a dosage of 1 mg/kg per day is equally effective. For more effective healing of gastric ulcers, consider twice-daily administration instead of once daily.

The equine formulations in the United States (GastroGard and UlcerGard) are buffered formulations. An enteric coated formulation is available for horses in some countries (Gastrozol). Plasma omeprazole concentrations after single doses are significantly higher with GastroGard than Gastrozol when each is administered at the labeled dose.

These formulations, when combined with environmental changes, promote healing of gastric ulcers in horses. The response to treatment will depend on the type of equine gastric ulcer syndrome being treated. Horses with equine squamous gastric disease (ESGD) respond much more favorably to acid suppression with omeprazole than those with equine glandular gastric disease (EGGD), reflecting the differences in pathogenesis and response between these two distinct forms of equine gastric disease. There was a 25% response rate for EGGD and a 78% response rate for ESGD at a dosage of 4 mg/kg once daily for 28–35 days. Some experts recommend oral omeprazole (4 mg/kg q24h) in combination with oral sucralfate 12 mg/kg q12h) for better healing rates for treating EGGD.

In dogs, 1 mg/kg q24h PO is as effective as pantoprazole (1 mg/kg) and famotidine (0.5 mg/kg q12h) for maintaining stomach pH greater than 3–4, which is the recommended pH range for ulcer healing. Twice-daily administration of omeprazole may be more effective than once daily. Repeated doses may be necessary (two to five doses) for complete inhibition of acid secretion. In dogs and cats, PPIs may be more effective than other drugs (e.g., histamine $H_2$ blockers) because of the long duration of effect.

In cats, the equine formulation and fractionated tablets were equally effective for suppressing acid secretion and were superior to an $H_2$ blocker (famotidine). In a similar study performed in dogs, omeprazole tablets or equine paste administered once daily provided superior acid suppression compared to famotidine twice daily.

Omeprazole, like other PPIs, may be effective for preventing nonsteroidal anti-inflammatory drug (NSAID)–induced ulcers. Omeprazole has also been used in combination with other drugs (antibiotics) for treatment of *Helicobacter* infections in animals.

## Precautionary Information

### Adverse Reactions and Side Effects

The only reported adverse effect in dogs has been diarrhea in some cases. Otherwise, adverse effects have not been reported in animals. In people, there is concern about hypergastrinemia with chronic use, but this has not been a concern in animals.

Horses have tolerated 20 mg/kg q24h for 91 days and 40 mg/kg q24h PO for 21 days. Dogs and cats also have tolerated the regimens listed in the dosing section. Overgrowth of *Clostridium* bacteria has been a concern from chronic use because of chronic gastric acid suppression, but the clinical importance of this observation in animals has not been established. In people, long-term use of PPIs has been associated with a modest risk of hip fractures because of decreased oral absorption of calcium and increased bone resorption by osteoclasts. This problem has not been reported in animals.

In cats with chronic kidney disease, omeprazole was well tolerated, but treatment increased sodium concentrations. The cause or the significance of this observation is undetermined. Although effects on bone have been a concern in people, when administered for 60 days to cats (1 mg/kg q12h), there was no change in cobalamin, calcium, magnesium, or bone mineral content or density.

### Contraindications and Precautions

One of the human formulations (Zegerid) is a packet to be mixed with water for oral administration. This formulation contains xylitol, which can be toxic to dogs if administered at high doses or with other medications that contain xylitol.

### Drug Interactions

Although omeprazole has not been associated with drug interactions in animals, PPIs may inhibit some drug-metabolizing enzymes (CYP450 enzymes). In people, metabolism of clopidogrel to the active metabolite can be inhibited by omeprazole, but this inhibition was not demonstrated in studies in dogs and has not been studied in horses or cats. Metabolism of other drugs may be inhibited by omeprazole, but this has not been studied in domestic animals.

Because all PPIs decrease stomach acid, do not administer with drugs that depend on stomach acid for absorption (e.g., ketoconazole and itraconazole). In people, there may be an increased risk of intestinal injury when PPIs are administered with NSAIDs, but this has not been studied in animals.

Omeprazole may be administered with sucralfate, which may increase efficacy for some gastric and esophageal diseases. However, in horses and perhaps other animals, the combination is more effective when sucralfate is administered 60–90 minutes after omeprazole.

## Instructions for Use

Omeprazole is the most common drug of this class used in animals. Other PPIs include pantoprazole (Protonix), lansoprazole (Prevacid), rabeprazole (Aciphex), and the S-isomer of omeprazole, esomeprazole. Less experience with these other products is reported for veterinary medicine. Pantoprazole and rabeprazole have the advantage in that they are available as tablets that can be crushed.

The equine formulations available include GastroGard and UlcerGard, which are buffered formulations to enhance oral absorption. Gastrozol is an enteric-coated formulation for horses available in Australia (see Indications and Clinical Use for comparison). Rectal administration has been studied in horses but has produced low and inconsistent response.

Treatment response varies in horses depending on the type of gastric ulcer syndrome treated. Patients with ESGD respond much more favorably to omeprazole than those with EGGD. In horses, it is recommended that at least 4 weeks of treatment is needed for full healing in addition to other changes in diet and feeding. To achieve the full extent of acid suppression, it is recommended to administer omeprazole to horses 60–90 minutes before feeding so that the peak concentration occurs at the time that the proton pumps in the stomach are maximally activated. This recommendation may also apply to treating other animals, such as dogs and cats. Twice-daily administration produces more consistent acid suppression to maintain the stomach pH above 3–4 than once-daily administration.

Because there are no small animal formulations available, the human forms have been administered to dogs and cats, and the equine formulation has been diluted in oil to 10 and 40 mg/mL (see the Formulations section) for administration to small animals. Studies with the equine formulation compounded in oil have shown that the equine formulation administered orally to dogs can be efficacious.

## Patient Monitoring and Laboratory Tests

Omeprazole and PPIs are generally considered safe. No routine tests for monitoring adverse effects are recommended. If gastrin concentrations are measured, a 7-day withdrawal from omeprazole treatment should be used; otherwise, there is a significant increase in serum gastrin concentrations from omeprazole treatment.

## Formulations

- Human formulations: 20-mg generic capsules. Zegerid is available either as 40- or 20-mg capsules with 1100 mg of sodium bicarbonate. Zegerid is also available either as 40-mg or 20-mg single-dose packets of powder for oral suspension with 1680 mg of sodium bicarbonate.
- Equine paste, GastroGard. The over-the-counter equine paste is UlcerGard. Paste for horses is 370 mg/g of paste in a buffered formulation to prevent degradation in the stomach. Gastrozol is an enteric-coated formulation in a paste for horses available in Australia but is not approved in the United States.

### Compounded Formulations

- Studies using compounded products from non–Food and Drug Administration (FDA) formulations in horses failed to produce therapeutic effects.
- Compounded formulations for dogs and cats have used the approved equine paste. The equine formulation can be diluted in corn oil, cod liver oil, or sesame oil for small animal use because otherwise, it is very concentrated. It has been diluted to 10 and 40 mg/mL by suspending the approved equine oral paste formulation in oil and stored at controlled cold temperature (7°C) and protected from light. The formulation has been stable for 6 months.
- Extemporaneously prepared omeprazole can be prepared from oral capsules. Empty the contents of five 20-mg capsules in 50 mL of 8.4% sodium bicarbonate solution for a final concentration of 2 mg/mL. This solution is stable for up to 14 days at 24°C and for up to 30 days at 5°C and –20°C.
- IV forms of omeprazole have been formulated in sterile water and administered to experimental horses, but these formulations are not commercially available.

## Stability and Storage

Omeprazole should be maintained in the manufacturer's original formulation (capsules or paste) for optimum stability and effectiveness. It is stable at pH 11 but rapidly decomposes at a pH less than 7.8.

## Small Animal Dosage

### Dogs

- 20 mg per dog q24h PO or 1–2 mg/kg q24h PO. For a more consistent acid-suppressing effect, administer q12h instead of q24h.

### Cats

- 1 mg/kg q24h PO. For a more consistent acid-suppressing effect, administer q12h instead of q24h.

## Large Animal Dosage

### Horses

- Treating ulcers: 4 mg/kg once daily for 4 weeks PO. Twice-daily administration may be more effective than once-daily administration for ulcers not responding to once-daily treatment. There is some evidence that 1–2 mg/kg is as effective for treatment as a higher dose.
- Preventing ulcers: 1–2 mg/kg q24h PO. (1 mg/kg was effective for prevention in studies performed in horses.)
- IV use (if a formulation is available): Loading dose of 1 mg/kg followed by 0.5 mg/kg per day for 14–28 days.

### Ruminants

- Oral absorption may not be high enough for effective therapy.

## Regulatory Information

Not intended for administration to animals that produce food. Oral absorption in ruminants is not established. Withdrawal times are not established for animals that produce food. For extralabel use withdrawal interval estimates, contact FARAD at www.FARAD.org.

RCI Classification: 5

O

# Ondansetron Hydrochloride
on-dan′sih-tron hye-droe-klor′ide

**Trade and other names:** Zofran

**Functional classification:** Antiemetic

## Pharmacology and Mechanism of Action

Ondansetron is an antiemetic drug from the class of drugs called *serotonin antagonists*. Like other drugs of this class, ondansetron acts by inhibiting serotonin type 3 (5-HT$_3$) receptors. It is effective as an antiemetic during chemotherapy, for which it has been effective by blocking emetic stimuli from the release of serotonin. During chemotherapy or after GI injury, 5-HT is released from the GI tract, which stimulates vomiting centrally. This stimulus is blocked by this class of drugs. These drugs also have been used to treat vomiting from gastroenteritis, pancreatitis, and inflammatory bowel disease. The use in dogs and cats is based primarily on anecdotal evidence and recommendations from clinical experts. There have not been well-controlled clinical studies with ondansetron in animals.

*Pharmacokinetics:* Most of ondansetron is metabolized by the liver (95%). In cats, the oral absorption rates were 32% from oral administration and 75% from SQ administration. The half-lives in cats are 1.8 hours from IV administration, 1.2 hours from oral administration, and more prolonged (3.2 hours) from SQ administration. Protein binding in cats is 81%–89%. It is not absorbed from transdermal application in cats. In dogs, it is much less bioavailable (less than 10%) after oral administration and has a shorter half-life of 30 minutes, raising questions about the clinical effectiveness of oral ondansetron in dogs.

Other serotonin antagonists used for antiemetic therapy include granisetron, ondansetron, dolasetron, azasetron, and tropisetron.

## Indications and Clinical Uses

Ondansetron, like other serotonin antagonists, is used to treat nausea and prevent vomiting. It can be effective for various types of vomiting that originate from injury to the GI tract. It is effective to prevent vomiting from drug chemotherapy (cancer drugs and dexmedetomidine). Only limited efficacy information is available for ondansetron's effectiveness in animals, but oncologists have found it to be effective for managing vomiting from chemotherapy in animals. It has been effective in cats at blocking vomiting caused by administration of sedative and anesthetic agents.

## Precautionary Information

### Adverse Reactions and Side Effects

Ondansetron's adverse effects have not been reported in animals. These drugs have little affinity for other 5-HT receptors. Because some severe adverse effects can occur from concurrent cancer drugs, it may be difficult to distinguish these from ondansetron effects.

### Contraindications and Precautions

Ondansetron is eliminated via metabolic pathways and relies less on kidneys for elimination. In cats with liver disease, there was increased exposure and decreased clearance; therefore, ondansetron should be administered less frequently if cats have liver disease. Cats with kidney disease have no significant changes in clearance. Do not administer as a transdermal formulation to cats because it is not absorbed. Oral absorption in dogs is low and may not be effective.

### Drug Interactions

If infused through an IV catheter, it may precipitate if mixed with other drugs (e.g., metoclopramide). Other drug interactions have not been reported for animals.

## Instructions for Use

Based on pharmacokinetic studies with ondansetron, it may be unlikely to maintain effective concentrations at a dosage of 0.5 mg/kg q12h orally or IV, but because of a longer SQ half-life, it may be better suited for administration via this route. In dogs, the oral absorption is low (less than 10%) because of high first-pass metabolism and a short-half-life, which raises questions about effectiveness of oral doses that have been recommended but not tested for efficacy. Granisetron is a similar drug that has been substituted for a similar purpose.

## Patient Monitoring and Laboratory Tests

Monitor GI signs in a vomiting patient.

## Formulations

- Ondansetron is available in 4- and 8-mg tablets, 4-mg/5-mL flavored syrup, and 2-mg/mL injection. Ondansetron is not absorbed in cats when administered as a transdermal formulation.

## Stability and Storage

Store in a tightly sealed container, protected from light, and at room temperature. Ondansetron is soluble in water. Solutions are stable, but pH should be less than 6 to prevent precipitation. Oral preparations have been mixed with syrups, juices, and other oral vehicles (e.g., Ora Sweet). It was stable for 42 days as long as pH remained low.

## Small Animal Dosage

### Dogs

- During cancer chemotherapy: 0.5–1 mg/kg IV or SQ 30 minutes prior to administration of cancer drugs intravenously.
- Vomiting from other causes: 0.1–0.2 mg/kg slow IV injection and repeated q6–12h. If this dosage is initially ineffective, it may be increased to 0.5 mg/kg.
- Oral administration: Although an oral form is available, oral absorption is low in dogs (less than 10%), which may compromise the effectiveness.

### Cats

- Cat dosages are similar to those for dogs: 0.5 mg/kg q8h SQ, IV, or PO. A dose of 2 mg per cat is common (half a tablet for the oral formulation), administered q8h. Reduce to twice daily in cats with liver disease.
- Constant-rate infusion (CRI): Administer 0.5 mg/kg IV loading dose followed by 0.5 mg/kg/h IV infusion.

## Large Animal Dosage

- No dosing information is available.

## Regulatory Information

No regulatory information is available. Because of a low risk of residues, no withdrawal times are suggested.

# Orbifloxacin
or-bih-floks′ah sin

**Trade and other names:** Orbax

**Functional classification:** Antibacterial

## Pharmacology and Mechanism of Action

Orbifloxacin is a fluoroquinolone antimicrobial used primarily in cats but occasionally in dogs. Orbifloxacin acts via inhibition of DNA gyrase in bacteria to inhibit DNA and RNA synthesis. It is a bactericidal with a broad spectrum of activity. The antimicrobial spectrum includes staphylococci, gram-negative bacilli, and some *Pseudomonas* species.

*Pharmacokinetics:* In dogs, the half-life is 5.6 hours; in cats, the half-life is 5.5 hours. In both species, the oral absorption is nearly 100%. However, oral suspension absorption in cats is not as high as tablets, which necessitates a higher dose (see Instructions for Use). In horses, it has a half-life of 5 hours and oral absorption of 68%.

## Indications and Clinical Uses

Orbifloxacin is approved for use in dogs and cats for a variety of infections. Like other fluoroquinolones, it is used to treat susceptible bacteria in a variety of species. Treatment of infections has included skin, soft tissue, and urinary tract infections (UTIs) in dogs and cats and soft tissue infections in horses.

## Precautionary Information

### Adverse Reactions and Side Effects

High concentrations may cause central nervous system (CNS) toxicity, especially in animals with kidney disease. It may cause some nausea, vomiting, and diarrhea at high doses. All of the fluoroquinolones may cause arthropathy in young animals. Dogs are most sensitive at 4–28 weeks of age. Large, rapidly growing dogs are the most susceptible. Blindness in cats has been reported from administration of some quinolones (nalidixic acid and enrofloxacin), but at doses up to 15 mg/kg (higher than approved label dose), orbifloxacin has not produced this effect.

### Contraindications and Precautions

Avoid use in young animals because of risk of cartilage injury. Use cautiously in animals that may be prone to seizures.

### Drug Interactions

Fluoroquinolones may increase concentrations of theophylline and perhaps other drugs administered concurrently because of enzyme interactions. However, interactions with other drugs have not been reported. Co-administration with divalent and trivalent cations, such as products containing aluminum (e.g., sucralfate), iron, and calcium, may decrease absorption. Do not mix in solutions or in vials with aluminum, calcium, iron, or zinc because chelation may occur.

## Instructions for Use

At the approved label dose, orbifloxacin is active against bacteria that tests "susceptible" with the current breakpoint. For isolates that test "intermediate," higher doses can be used. In cats, orbifloxacin oral suspension and orbifloxacin tablets are not bioequivalent. On a milligram-per-kilogram basis, orbifloxacin oral suspension provides lower and more variable plasma levels of orbifloxacin than the tablets. The dose of orbifloxacin oral suspension in the cat is 7.5 mg/kg of body weight administered once daily, but the tablet dose is lower. The oral suspension was designed for palatability with an ion-exchange agent that masks the taste until it reaches the pH of the stomach.

## Patient Monitoring and Laboratory Tests

Susceptibility testing: Clinical and Laboratory Standards Institute (CLSI) breakpoint for susceptible organisms in dogs and cats is ≤1 mcg/mL.

## Formulations
- Orbifloxacin is available in 5.7-, 22.7-, and 68-mg tablets. Oral suspension (malt flavor) is 30 mg/mL.

## Stability and Storage
Store in a tightly sealed container, protected from light, and at room temperature. Orbifloxacin is slightly water soluble. It has been mixed with various syrups, flavorings, and vehicles and was stable at room temperature for 7 days. Do not mix with vehicles that contain aluminum, calcium, or iron because this may decrease oral absorption via chelation.

## Small Animal Dosage
**Dogs and Cats**
- Tablets: 2.5–7.5 mg/kg q24h PO.
- Suspension in cats: 7.5 mg/kg (1 mL/kg) q24h PO.
- Suspension in dogs: 2.5–7.5 mg/kg q24h PO.

## Large Animal Dosage
**Horses**
- 5 mg/kg q24h PO.

## Regulatory Information
Do not use fluoroquinolones off label to animals that produce food. Orbifloxacin is prohibited from use in animals intended for food.

# Ormetoprim + Sulfadimethoxine
or-met′oe-prim + sul-fa-dye-meth-oks′een

**Trade and other names:** Primor

**Functional classification:** Antibacterial

## Pharmacology and Mechanism of Action
Ormetoprim is an antibacterial drug used in combination to treat infections in small animals. Ormetoprim combined with sulfadimethoxine is a synergistic combination similar to trimethoprim and sulfonamide combinations. Ormetoprim inhibits bacterial dihydrofolate reductase, and sulfonamide competes with para-aminobenzoic acid (PABA) for synthesis of nucleic acids. It can produce both bactericidal and bacteriostatic activity, depending on the organism. It has a broad antibacterial spectrum that includes common gram-positive and gram-negative bacteria. It also is active against some *Coccidia* species.

## Indications and Clinical Uses
Ormetoprim combined with sulfadimethoxine is used in small animals to treat a variety of bacterial infections caused by susceptible organisms, including pneumonia, skin, soft tissue, and UTIs in dogs and cats. In horses, it may be administered orally for infections caused by susceptible gram-positive bacteria (*Actinomyces* spp., *Streptococcus* spp., and *Staphylococcus* spp.), but higher doses may be needed for gram-negative infections.

## Precautionary Information
### Adverse Reactions and Side Effects
Adverse effects associated with sulfonamides include allergic reactions, type II and III hypersensitivity, arthropathy, anemia, thrombocytopenia, hepatopathy, hypothyroidism (with prolonged therapy), keratoconjunctivitis sicca (KCS), and skin reactions. Dogs may be more sensitive to sulfonamides than other animals because dogs lack the ability to acetylate sulfonamides to inactive metabolites. As a consequence, other more toxic metabolites may persist. Ormetoprim has been associated with some CNS effects in dogs, which include behavioral changes, anxiety, muscle tremors, and seizures. In horses, when IV doses were administered to experimental horses (IV formulation not commercially available), nervous system reactions such as tremors and muscle fasciculations were observed.

### Contraindications and Precautions
Do not administer to animals sensitive to sulfonamides. Discontinue treatment if abnormal CNS effects are observed.

### Drug Interactions
Sulfonamides may interact with other drugs, including warfarin, methenamine, and etodolac. They may potentiate adverse effects caused by methotrexate and pyrimethamine.

## Instructions for Use
Doses listed are based on manufacturer's recommendations and FDA-approved form for animals. Controlled trials have demonstrated efficacy for treatment of pyoderma in dogs on a once-daily schedule.

## Patient Monitoring and Laboratory Tests
Monitor tear production with long-term use because of risk of KCS in dogs from sulfonamides. For susceptibility testing, breakpoint ranges have not been determined for ormetoprim–sulfadimethoxine combinations. Use a test for trimethoprim–sulfamethoxazole combinations as a guide for susceptibility to ormetoprim–sulfadimethoxine combinations. CLSI breakpoint for susceptible organisms is $\leq 2/38$ mcg/mL (trimethoprim + sulfonamide).

## Formulations
- Ormetoprim–sulfadimethoxine combination is available in 120-, 240-, 600-, and 1200-mg tablets in a 5:1 ratio of sulfadimethoxine:ormetoprim.

## Stability and Storage
Store in a tightly sealed container, protected from light, and at room temperature.

## Small Animal Dosage
### Dogs
- 55 mg/kg on the first day followed by 27.5 mg/kg q24h PO. Doses can be divided into twice-daily treatments. (All doses are based on the combined milligram amount of both ormetoprim and sulfadimethoxine.)

### Cats
- Although doses are not reported by the manufacturer, doses similar to those for dogs have been administered.

## Large Animal Dosage
### Horses
- Loading dose of 55 mg/kg (of the combined drugs) followed by 27.5 mg/kg (of the combined drugs) q24h PO.

## Regulatory Information

Withdrawal times are not established for animals that produce food. Oral absorption has not been established for ruminants. For extralabel use withdrawal interval estimates, contact FARAD at www.FARAD.org.

# Oxacillin Sodium

oks-ah-sill'in soe'dee-um

**Trade and other names:** Prostaphlin and generic brands

**Functional classification:** Antibacterial

## Pharmacology and Mechanism of Action

Oxacillin is a beta-lactam antibiotic similar to others in the penicillin class. Oxacillin, like other beta-lactam antibiotics, binds penicillin-binding proteins (PBPs) that weaken or interfere with cell wall formation. After binding to PBPs, the cell wall weakens or undergoes lysis. Like other beta-lactams, this drug acts in a time-dependent manner (i.e., it is more effective when drug concentrations are maintained above the minimum inhibitory concentration [MIC] during the dose interval). Oxacillin has a limited spectrum of activity that includes primarily gram-positive bacteria. Resistance is common, especially among enteric gram-negative bacilli. Staphylococci are susceptible because oxacillin is resistant to the bacterial beta-lactamase produced by *Staphylococcus* spp.

*Pharmacokinetics:* Limited pharmacokinetic data are available for animals. Because of a short half-life and low oral absorption, there are limitations to its use in animals.

## Indications and Clinical Uses

Oxacillin has had limited use in small animals for treating soft tissue infections caused by gram-positive bacteria. The most common use has been for pyoderma in dogs, but the use has diminished because of limited pharmacokinetic information to guide oral dosing and the increased availability of other drugs, such as oral cephalosporins and amoxicillin and clavulanate combination.

Oxacillin is used as a marker to test for *mec-A*–mediated resistance of PBP2a in *Staphylococcus* spp. Methicillin-resistant *Staphylococcus* (e.g., methicillin-resistant *Staphylococcus aureus* [MRSA] or methicillin-resistant *Staphylococcus pseudintermedius* [MRSP]) spp. can be identified by using oxacillin breakpoints (see Patient Monitoring and Laboratory Tests).

## Precautionary Information

### Adverse Reactions and Side Effects

Adverse effects of penicillin-like drugs are most commonly caused by drug allergy. This can range from acute anaphylaxis when administered or other signs of allergic reaction when other routes are used. When administered orally, vomiting and diarrhea are possible, especially with high doses.

### Contraindications and Precautions

Use cautiously in animals allergic to penicillin-like drugs.

### Drug Interactions

No drug interactions are reported. Food may inhibit oral absorption.

## Instructions for Use

Oral forms are often unavailable and other agents with similar activity are used instead (e.g., cephalexin, amoxicillin–clavulanate). Doses are based on empiricism or extrapolation from human studies. No clinical efficacy studies are available for dogs or cats, but the use is extrapolated from studies in people. Administer on an empty stomach if possible.

## Patient Monitoring and Laboratory Tests

Culture and sensitivity testing: CLSI breakpoints to define *mec-A*–mediated resistance in *Staphylococcus aureus* is a MIC ≥4 mcg/mL, and the zone size is ≤10 mm. All other *Staphylococcus* spp. with *mec-A*-mediated resistance, including *S. pseudintermedius* (e.g., MRSP), are disk diffusion ≤17 mm and MIC ≥0.5 mcg/mL. If staphylococci are resistant to oxacillin, they should be interpreted as resistant to all cephalosporins and penicillins regardless of sensitivity result. Oxacillin resistance is usually interpreted as equivalent to methicillin resistance; therefore, oxacillin-resistant staphylococci are also referred to as MRSA or MRSP.

## Formulations

• Oxacillin has been available in 250- and 500-mg capsules and 50-mg/mL oral solution, but availability may be limited because other drugs with similar activity are used more often.

## Stability and Storage

Store in a tightly sealed container, protected from light, and at room temperature. Oxacillin is soluble in water and alcohol. The reconstituted oral solution is stable for 3 days at room temperature and 14 days in the refrigerator.

## Small Animal Dosage

**Dogs and Cats**
• 22–40 mg/kg q8h PO.

## Large Animal Dosage

• No doses are reported. Oral absorption has not been established for large animals.

## Regulatory Information

Withdrawal times are not established for animals that produce food. Oral absorption has not been established for ruminants. For extralabel use withdrawal interval estimates, contact FARAD at www.FARAD.org.

# Oxazepam

oks-ay′zeh-pam

**Trade and other names:** Serax

**Functional classification:** Anticonvulsant

## Pharmacology and Mechanism of Action

Oxazepam is a benzodiazepine used for sedation, behavior management, and occasionally seizure disorders. Oxazepam is a central-acting CNS depressant with action similar to diazepam. Its mechanism of action appears to be via potentiation of gamma-aminobutyric acid receptor–mediated effects in the CNS. Oxazepam is one of the active products of metabolism from diazepam. In contrast to diazepam, oxazepam does not undergo extensive hepatic metabolism in animals, but it is glucuronidated before excretion.

*Pharmacokinetics:* In dogs, oxazepam has a half-life of 5–6 hours, but these values were derived from administration of the parent drug diazepam. Oxazepam is eliminated by direct conjugation with glucuronide, without other intermediate metabolites produced, whereas diazepam and other benzodiazepines may produce other intermediate active metabolites.

## Indications and Clinical Uses
Oxazepam is used for treating behavior disorders and sedation and to stimulate appetite. The appetite-stimulating effects have been used, particularly in cats, to stimulate appetite that may be diminished because of other primary diseases. It has been more potent than diazepam as an appetite stimulant in cats and preferred because of a low risk of liver injury. Other drugs are now available for appetite stimulation (e.g., mirtazapine for cats) and may be preferred. Like other benzodiazepines, it also may be considered for behavior problems and anxiety disorders in animals, but it has not been used as commonly as other drugs.

### Precautionary Information

**Adverse Reactions and Side Effects**

Sedation is the most common side effect. It may also produce polyphagia. Some animals may experience paradoxical excitement. Chronic administration may lead to dependence and a withdrawal syndrome if discontinued.

**Contraindications and Precautions**

Oral administration of another benzodiazepine, diazepam, has caused severe idiosyncratic liver injury in cats. This does not appear to be a problem for oxazepam, which is a metabolite of diazepam.

Use of benzodiazepines in early pregnancy has been associated with an increased risk of spontaneous abortions and fetal malformations in people. This incidence in animals is unknown.

If oxazepam is administered long term, do not discontinue abruptly, or withdrawal signs may occur.

**Drug Interactions**

Use cautiously with other drugs that may cause sedation.

## Instructions for Use
Doses used in dogs and cats are based on empiricism and opinions from clinical experts. There have been no clinical trials in veterinary medicine, although it is widely believed to increase the appetite in cats.

## Patient Monitoring and Laboratory Tests
Samples of plasma or serum may be analyzed in some laboratories for concentrations of benzodiazepines. Plasma concentrations in the range of 100–250 ng/mL have been cited as the therapeutic range for people. Other references have cited this range as 150–300 ng/mL. Laboratories that analyze human samples may have nonspecific tests for benzodiazepines. With these assays, there may be cross-reactivity among benzodiazepine metabolites.

## Formulations
• Oxazepam is available in 10-, 15-, and 30-mg capsules.

## Stability and Storage
Stable if stored in manufacturer's original formulation. Although oxazepam has been compounded for veterinary use, the potency and stability have not been evaluated for compounded products.

## Small Animal Dosage
### Cats
• Behavior disorders: 0.2–0.5 mg/kg q12–24h PO or 1–2 mg/cat q12h PO.
• Appetite stimulant: 2.5 mg/cat PO. The maximum effect is from 1 mg/kg, but doses as low as 0.1 mg/kg have been effective.

### Dogs
• Behavior disorders or sedation: 0.2–1 mg/kg q12–24h PO. If an adequate response is not observed, the dose frequency has been increased to q8h and q6h.

## Large Animal Dosage
• No doses have been reported for large animals.

## Regulatory Information
Do not administer to animals intended for food.
Schedule IV controlled drug.
RCI Classification: 2

# Oxfendazole
oks-fen'dah-zole

**Trade and other names:** Benzelmin and Synanthic

**Functional classification:** Antiparasitic

## Pharmacology and Mechanism of Action
Oxfendazole is an antiparasitic drug of the benzimidazole class of antiparasitic drugs. Like other benzimidazole drugs, it produces a degeneration of the parasite microtubule and irreversibly blocks glucose uptake in parasites. Inhibition of glucose uptake causes depletion of energy stores in parasites, eventually resulting in death. However, there is no effect on glucose metabolism in mammals. It is used to treat intestinal parasites in animals.

## Indications and Clinical Uses
Oxfendazole is used in horses for treatment of large roundworms (*Parascaris equorum*), mature and immature pinworms (*Oxyuris equi*), large strongyles (*Strongylus edentatus, Strongylus vulgaris,* and *Strongylus equinus*), and small strongyles. In cattle, oxfendazole is approved for treatment of lungworms (*Dictyocaulus viviparus*), stomach worms (barberpole worms [*Haemonchus contortus* and *Haemonchus placei*, adult]), small stomach worms (*Trichostrongylus axei*, adult), brown stomach worms (*Ostertagia ostertagi*), intestinal worms, nodular worms (*Oesophagostomum radiatum*, adult), hookworms (*Bunostomum phlebotomum*, adult), small intestinal worms (*Cooperia punctata, Cooperia oncophora,* and *Cooperia momasteri*), and tapeworms (*Moniezia benedeni*, adult).

## Precautionary Information

### Adverse Reactions and Side Effects
Adverse reactions are rare.

### Contraindications and Precautions
Do not administer to sick or debilitated horses. Do not administer to female dairy cattle of breeding age.

### Drug Interactions
No drug interactions are reported.

## Instructions for Use
Administer to horses by mixing in a suspension and administering orally (e.g., via stomach tube) or mixing pellets with food. Administer to cattle orally with a dose syringe or intraruminally with a rumen injector. Treatment may be repeated in 6–8 weeks in horses or in 4–6 weeks in cattle.

## Patient Monitoring and Laboratory Tests
No specific monitoring is necessary.

## Formulations
- Oxfendazole is available in a 90.6- or 225-mg/mL suspension (cattle), 185-mg/g paste (cattle), 0.375 g/g of paste (equine), 90.6-mg/mL suspension (equine), and 6.49% pellets (equine).

## Stability and Storage
Store in a tightly sealed container, protected from light, and at room temperature. After mixing for oral administration, discard unused portion after 24 hours. Mix well before using, do not freeze suspension, and avoid excessive heat.

## Small Animal Dosage

### Dogs and Cats
- Dose has not been established.

## Large Animal Dosage

### Horses
- 10 mg/kg PO.

### Cattle
- 4.5 mg/kg PO.

## Regulatory Information
Do not use in dairy cattle.
Cattle slaughter withdrawal time: 7 days for suspension; 11 days for paste.

# Oxibendazole
oks-ih-ben′dah-zole

**Trade and other names:** Anthelcide EQ and Filaribits Plus Chewable tablets

**Functional classification:** Antiparasitic

## Pharmacology and Mechanism of Action

Oxibendazole is an antiparasitic drug of the benzimidazole class. Like other benzimidazole drugs, it produces a degeneration of the parasite microtubule and irreversibly blocks glucose uptake in parasites. Inhibition of glucose uptake causes depletion of energy stores in parasites, eventually resulting in death. However, there is no effect on glucose metabolism in mammals. It is used to treat intestinal parasites in animals.

## Indications and Clinical Uses

Oxibendazole is used in horses for treatment of large strongyles (*S. edentatus, S. equinus,* and *S. vulgaris*), small strongyles (species of the genera Cylicostephanus, Cylicocyclus, Cyathostomum, Triodontophorus, Cylicodontophorus, and Gyalocephalus), large roundworms (*P. equorum*), pinworms (*O. equi*) including various larval stages, and threadworms (*Strongyloides westeri*).

Formulations for dogs have contained both diethylcarbamazine citrate and oxibendazole for prevention of *Dirofilaria immitis* (heartworm disease) and *Ancylostoma caninum* (hookworm infection) and for treatment of *Trichuris vulpis* (whipworm infection) and intestinal *Toxocara canis* (Ascarid infection). However, diethylcarbamazine is no longer used for heartworm disease prevention in dogs because other alternate drugs are available.

## Precautionary Information

**Adverse Reactions and Side Effects**

Adverse reactions are rare. Occasional vomiting and nausea may occur in dogs.

**Contraindications and Precautions**

Do not administer to dogs that may have heartworms.

**Drug Interactions**

No drug interactions are reported.

## Instructions for Use

Administer suspension to horses by mixing with 1–2 L of water (3–4 pints) and administering orally (e.g., via stomach tube). Alternatively, mix powder with grain ration or use the paste. Horses should be retreated in 6–8 weeks if they are reexposed. For dogs, the tablets can be administered directly or mixed with food daily.

## Patient Monitoring and Laboratory Tests

No specific monitoring is necessary.

## Formulations

- Oxibendazole is available in 10% suspension; 22.7% paste for horses.
- Chewable tablets are available in 60-, 120-, and 180-mg diethylcarbamazine citrate + 45-, 91-, and 136-mg oxibendazole tablets.

## Stability and Storage

Store in a tightly sealed container, protected from light, and at room temperature. Mix well before using, do not freeze suspension, and avoid excessive heat.

## Small Animal Dosage

**Dogs**

- 5 mg/kg of oxibendazole (combined with 6.6 mg/kg of diethylcarbamazine) q24h PO. However, the product with diethylcarbamazine is no longer used for heartworm prevention.

**Cats**
- No dose established.

## Large Animal Dosage
**Horses**
- 10 mg/kg PO.
- Threadworms: 15 mg/kg PO once. Retreat in 6–8 weeks if necessary.

## Regulatory Information
No withdrawal times are established.
Withdrawal times are not established for animals that produce food. For extralabel use withdrawal interval estimates, contact FARAD at www.FARAD.org.

# Oxtriphylline
oks-trih´fih-lin

**Trade and other names:** Choledyl-SA

**Functional classification:** Bronchodilator

## Pharmacology and Mechanism of Action
Oxtriphylline is another name for choline theophyllinate. It is a methylxanthine bronchodilator that releases free theophylline after absorption. Therefore the therapeutic properties are the same as for theophylline. The effects may be related to increased cyclic adenosine monophosphate (cAMP) levels or antagonism of adenosine, and there may be additional anti-inflammatory and bronchodilating action.

## Indications and Clinical Uses
Oxtriphylline has been used for similar respiratory conditions, as is theophylline. It is indicated in patients with reversible bronchoconstriction, such as dogs with airway disease. The use of oxtriphylline has diminished considerably, and it is more convenient and preferable to administer theophylline in most cases. Large animal uses have not been reported.

## Precautionary Information
**Adverse Reactions and Side Effects**

Adverse effects are the same as for theophylline and include nausea, vomiting, and diarrhea. With high doses, tachycardia, excitement, tremors, and seizures are possible. Cardiovascular and CNS adverse effects appear to be less frequent in dogs than in people.

**Contraindications and Precautions**

Some patients may be at a higher risk for adverse effects. Such patients may include animals with cardiac disease, animals prone to arrhythmias, and animals at risk for seizures.

**Drug Interactions**

Drugs that inhibit cytochrome P450 enzymes may increase drug concentrations and cause toxicity. See Appendix I for a list of drugs that may be P450 inhibitors.

## Instructions for Use

Some formulations (Theochron) contain oxtriphylline and guaifenesin. When administering a slow-release tablet, do not crush it. Theophylline, which may be more readily available for oral administration, may be substituted for oxtriphylline.

## Patient Monitoring and Laboratory Tests

Therapeutic drug monitoring is recommended for chronic therapy. Interpretation of theophylline concentrations should be used to guide therapy. Generally, 10–20 mcg/mL is considered therapeutic.

## Formulations

- Oxtriphylline is available in 400- and 600-mg tablets. (Oral solutions and syrup are available in Canada but not in the United States.)

## Stability and Storage

Store in a tightly sealed container, protected from light, and at room temperature.

## Small Animal Dosage

**Dogs**

- 47 mg/kg (equivalent to 30 mg/kg theophylline) q12h PO.

## Large Animal Dosage

- No doses have been reported for large animals. Oral absorption has not been established for ruminants.

## Regulatory Information

Withdrawal times are not established for animals that produce food. For extralabel use withdrawal interval estimates, contact FARAD at www.FARAD.org.

# Oxybutynin Chloride
oks-ih-byoo'tih-nin klor'ide

**Trade and other names:** Ditropan

**Functional classification:** Anticholinergic

## Pharmacology and Mechanism of Action

Oxybutynin is an anticholinergic agent most often used for urinary problems. Oxybutynin produces an anticholinergic effect via blockade of muscarinic receptors. It produces a general anticholinergic effect, but the predominant effect is on the urinary bladder. It inhibits smooth muscle spasms via blocking action of acetylcholine. It does not block skeletal muscle, autonomic ganglia, or receptors on blood vessels. A related drug used in people is tolterodine (Detrol).

## Indications and Clinical Uses

Oxybutynin chloride has been used primarily to increase bladder capacity and to decrease spasms of the urinary tract. In people, it is used to treat urinary incontinence, but the use in animals is not common and not well documented.

## Precautionary Information
### Adverse Reactions and Side Effects
Adverse effects are related to anticholinergic effects (atropine-like effects), but they are less frequent compared with other anticholinergic drugs. Constipation, dry mouth, and dry mucous membranes are possible from routine use. If an overdose occurs, administer physostigmine for treatment to reverse the anticholinergic effects.

### Contraindications and Precautions
Use cautiously in animals with heart disease or decreased intestinal motility. Use cautiously in animals with glaucoma.

### Drug Interactions
Oxybutynin will potentiate other antimuscarinic drugs.

## Instructions for Use
Results of clinical studies in animals are not available. The use in animals (and doses) is based on extrapolation from the experience in people or anecdotal experience in animals. Although oxybutynin increases urine retention by decreasing bladder spasms, it may not be effective to treat incontinence in animals with decreased sphincter tone. Other agents are preferred for treatment of animals with incontinence caused by poor sphincter tone, such as phenylpropanolamine (PPA) and estrogens (e.g., estriol or diethylstilbestrol [DES]).

## Patient Monitoring and Laboratory Tests
No specific monitoring is necessary.

## Formulations
• Oxybutynin is available in 5-mg tablets and 1-mg/mL oral syrup.

## Stability and Storage
Store in a tightly sealed container, protected from light, and at room temperature. Oxybutynin is soluble in water and ethanol.

## Small Animal Dosage
### Dogs
• 0.2 mg/kg q12h PO; for larger dogs, use 5 mg/dog q6–8h PO.

## Large Animal Dosage
• No doses have been reported for large animals.

## Regulatory Information
Withdrawal times are not established for animals that produce food. Oral absorption has not been established for ruminants. For extralabel use withdrawal interval estimates, contact FARAD at www.FARAD.org.

# Oxymetholone
oks-ih-meth'oh-lone
**Trade and other names:** Anadrol
**Functional classification:** Hormone, anabolic agent

## Pharmacology and Mechanism of Action

Oxymetholone is an anabolic steroid. Oxymetholone is a derivative of testosterone and, like other anabolic agents, is administered to maximize anabolic effects while minimizing androgenic action. Anabolic agents have been used for reversing catabolic conditions, increasing weight gain, increasing muscling in animals, and stimulating erythropoiesis. Other anabolic agents include boldenone, nandrolone, stanozolol, and methyltestosterone.

## Indications and Clinical Uses

Anabolic agents have been used for reversing catabolic conditions, increasing weight gain, increasing muscling in animals, and stimulating erythropoiesis. They also may stimulate appetite. Although other anabolic agents have been used in animals (methyltestosterone and stanozolol), there are no differences in efficacy among the anabolic steroids demonstrated in animals. The use of oxymetholone is based on anecdotal experience and extrapolation of uses from human medicine. There are no well-controlled studies using oxymetholone in animals.

## Precautionary Information

### Adverse Reactions and Side Effects

Adverse effects from anabolic steroids can be attributed to the pharmacologic action of anabolic steroids. Increased masculine effects are common. Increased incidence of some tumors has been reported in people. The 17a-methylated oral anabolic steroids (oxymetholone, stanozolol, and oxandrolone) have been associated with hepatic toxicity.

### Contraindications and Precautions

Oxymetholone and other anabolic steroids are abused in people to increase athletic performance and muscle gain. Care should be taken when prescribing multiple doses to animals and storing these agents in veterinary hospitals. Do not use in pregnant animals.

### Drug Interactions

No drug interactions are reported.

## Instructions for Use

Results of clinical studies in animals have not been reported. Use in animals (and doses) is based on experience in people or anecdotal experience in animals.

## Patient Monitoring and Laboratory Tests

Monitor hepatic enzymes for evidence of cholestasis and hepatotoxicity.

## Formulations

- Oxymetholone is available in 50-mg tablets.

## Stability and Storage

Store in a tightly sealed container, protected from light, and at room temperature.

## Small Animal Dosage

### Dogs and Cats

- 1–5 mg/kg/day PO.

## Large Animal Dosage

- No doses have been reported for large animals.

## Regulatory Information

Oxymetholone is a Schedule III controlled drug.
Do not administer to animals intended for food.
RCI Classification: 4

# Oxymorphone Hydrochloride
oks-ih-mor'fone hye-droe-klor'ide

**Trade and other names:** Numorphan

**Functional classification:** Analgesic, opioid

## Pharmacology and Mechanism of Action

Oxymorphone is an opioid agonist and analgesic. The action of oxymorphone is
similar to morphine except that oxymorphone is 10–15 times more potent than
morphine. Oxymorphone binds to mu-opiate and kappa-opiate receptors on nerves
and inhibit release of neurotransmitters involved with transmission of pain stimuli
(e.g., substance P). Central sedative and euphoric effects related to mu-receptor
effects in the brain. Other opiates used in animals include hydromorphone, codeine,
morphine, meperidine, and fentanyl.

*Pharmacokinetics:* In dogs, the half-lives are 0.8 hours (IV) and 1 hour (SQ), with
high clearance rates (greater than 50 mL/kg/min). In dogs, there is a high first-pass
effect and oral administration is not effective. In cats, the half-life is 1.7 hours, with
clearance of 26 mL/kg/min. Effective concentrations are not established for animals,
but in people, they range from 2.5–4.5 ng/mL.

## Indications and Clinical Uses

Oxymorphone is indicated for short-term analgesia, for sedation, and as an adjunct
to anesthesia. It is compatible with most anesthetics and can be used as part of a
multimodal approach to analgesia and anesthesia. Although oxymorphone is FDA
approved for dogs, other opiates, such as hydromorphone and morphine, are used
more commonly. Administration of oxymorphone may lower dose requirements
for other anesthetics and analgesics used. The duration of action in dogs is short
(2–4 hours) and requires frequent administration for effective use. The oral dose
formulations are only 10% absorbed in people but should not be relied on for treating
severe pain in dogs.

## Precautionary Information

### Adverse Reactions and Side Effects

Like all opiates, side effects from oxymorphone are predictable and unavoidable.
Side effects from opiate administration include sedation, vomiting, constipation,
urinary retention, and bradycardia. Panting may occur in dogs as a result
of changes in thermoregulation. Histamine release, known to occur from
administration of morphine, may be less likely with oxymorphone. Excitement
can occur in animals, but it is more common in cats and horses. Respiratory
depression occurs with high doses. As with other opiates, a slight decrease in
heart rate is expected. In most cases, this decrease does not have to be treated
with anticholinergic drugs (e.g., atropine), but it should be monitored. Tolerance

and dependence occur with chronic administration. In horses, undesirable and even dangerous behavior actions can follow rapid IV opioid administration. Horses should receive a preanesthetic of acepromazine or an alpha$_2$ agonist.

**Contraindications and Precautions**
Oxymorphone is a Schedule II controlled substance. Cats and horses may be more sensitive to excitement caused by opiates.

**Drug Interactions**
Like other opiates, oxymorphone potentiates other drugs that cause CNS depression.

## Instructions for Use
There is some evidence that oxymorphone may have fewer cardiovascular effects than morphine. Oxymorphone is more readily absorbed systemically from epidural administration compared with morphine. Oxymorphone can be used in combination with other anesthetics and anesthetic adjuncts in the peri-operative period and post-surgery to enhance analgesia. It has been used with sedatives such as acepromazine, benzodiazepines, and alpha$_2$-agonists.

## Patient Monitoring and Laboratory Tests
Monitor the patient's heart rate and respiration. Although bradycardia rarely needs to be treated when it is caused by an opioid, atropine can be administered if necessary. If serious respiratory depression occurs, the opioid can be reversed with naloxone.

## Formulations
- Oxymorphone is available in 1.5- and 1-mg/mL injections.
- Oral forms: 5- and 10-mg tablets are available but have not been shown to be absorbed in animals.

## Stability and Storage
The pH of solution is 2.7–4.5. Oxymorphone is compatible with most fluid solutions. Store in a tightly sealed container, protected from light, and at room temperature.

## Small Animal Dosage
### Dogs
- Analgesia: 0.1–0.2 mg/kg IV, SQ, or IM (as needed); redose with 0.05–0.1 mg/kg q1–2h. A dosage of 0.25 mg/kg SQ q6h may be used for less severe pain.
- Preanesthetic: 0.025–0.05 mg/kg IM or SQ.
- Sedation: 0.05–0.2 mg/kg (with or without acepromazine) IM or SQ.

### Cats
- 0.03 mg/kg bolus IV followed by 0.02 mg/kg q2h or CRI with a loading dose of 5 mcg/kg followed by a 5-mcg/kg/h infusion.

## Large Animal Dosage
- No doses have been reported for large animals.

## Regulatory Information
Schedule II controlled drug.
RCI Classification: 1

# Oxytetracycline
oks'ih-tet-rah-sye'kleen

**Trade and other names:** Terramycin, Terramycin Soluble Powder, Terramycin Scours Tablets, Bio-Mycin, Oxy-Tet, and Oxybiotic Oxy 500 and Oxy 1000. Long-acting formulations include Liquamycin-LA 200 and Bio-Mycin 200.

**Functional classification:** Antibacterial

## Pharmacology and Mechanism of Action

Oxytetracycline is one of the oldest tetracycline antibiotics used in animals. The mechanism of action of tetracyclines is to bind to 30S ribosomal subunit and inhibit protein synthesis. Oxytetracycline is usually bacteriostatic. It has a broad spectrum of activity, including gram-positive and gram-negative bacteria, some protozoa, *Rickettsia* spp., and *Ehrlichia* spp. The spectrum also includes *Chlamydia* spp., spirochetes, *Mycoplasma* spp., L-form bacteria, and some protozoa (*Plasmodium* spp. and *Entamoeba* spp.). Resistance is common among gram-negative bacteria of the Enterobacteriaceae (e.g., *Escherichia coli)* and *Staphylococcus* spp.

*Pharmacokinetics:* Oxytetracycline has been available in a variety of formulations to control the release rate from an injection from an IM or SQ injection. Vehicles include polyethylene glycol, propylene glycol, povidone, and pyrrolidine. Although oral preparations are available, oral absorption is poor. For example, oral absorption of 44 mg/kg in dogs was variable and too low to produce therapeutic effects. In pigs, oral absorption was only 4% (compared with chlortetracycline, which is 13%). Most pharmacokinetic studies have been performed with injectable oxytetracycline. After IM injection in cattle, the half-life is approximately 21 hours, with a maximum concentration ($C_{MAX}$) of 5.6 mcg/mL. In horses, the half-life (IV) is approximately 10–13 hours. In pigs, the half-life (IV) is approximately 4–6 hours.

## Indications and Clinical Uses

Oxytetracycline is used to treat infections of the respiratory tract (pneumonia), urinary tract, soft tissues, and skin. It is used for infections caused by a wide spectrum of bacteria except that resistance is common among gram-negative bacilli of enteric origin and staphylococci. One of the most common uses is in cattle for treatment of bovine respiratory disease caused by *Pasteurella multocida, Mannheimia haemolytica,* and *Histophilus somni.* In pigs, tetracyclines have been used to treat atrophic rhinitis, pneumonic pasteurellosis, and *Mycoplasma* infections. In small animals, doxycycline, rather than oxytetracycline, is used as a treatment for *Rickettsia* spp. and *Ehrlichia* spp. infections. In horses, oxytetracycline has been administered to treat equine piroplasmosis caused by *Theileria equi* but was not effective for *Babesia caballi.* Oxytetracycline has been used for treating Potomac fever in horses caused by *Neorickettsia risticii,* as well as respiratory and soft tissue infections. In newborn horses, oxytetracycline has been administered at high doses for the purpose of correcting angular limb deformities. The dosages have been as high as 50–70 mg/kg IV q48h. This effect may be caused by a decrease in the viscoelastic properties in the tendons of young animals. Because this produces tendon or ligament laxity, it may correct angular limb deformities in young foals.

## Precautionary Information

### Adverse Reactions and Side Effects

Tetracyclines have produced kidney injury, but this has been rare with recommended doses and current formulations. Toxicity reported in older publications was attributed to outdated formulations that produced nephrotoxic degradation products. This ingredient that caused toxicity is no longer present, and this problem has been eliminated. Azotemia can be seen with high doses, which is attributed to inhibition of protein synthesis in mammalian cells. Therefore, this is caused by inhibition of protein synthesis with high doses rather than a direct nephrotoxic effect. At very high doses, oxytetracycline can injure other organs (e.g., liver) or cause metabolic acidosis, hemoglobinemia, or myoglobinemia, and the kidneys are injured as a consequence.

Tetracyclines can affect bone and teeth formation in young animals, but this is usually not a problem with short-term administration. It was not observed when administered for two doses for treatment of angular limb deformities in young foals. Tetracyclines have caused drug fever in cats, but the mechanism is unknown. Oxytetracycline administration to horses has been associated with colic and diarrhea because of changes in the intestinal bacterial flora.

### Contraindications and Precautions

Use cautiously in young animals because teeth discoloration is possible, especially with prolonged administration. Avoid injection volumes for IM greater than 10 mL per site in cattle and greater than 5 mL in pigs because of injection-site lesions.

### Drug Interactions

Tetracyclines bind to compounds containing calcium, which decreases oral absorption. Do not mix with solutions that contain iron, calcium, aluminum, or magnesium.

## Instructions for Use

Oral dose forms are intended for large animal use and there are no tablets for small animals. Use of injectable long-acting forms has not been studied in small animals. Use of tetracyclines in small animals has primarily relied on doxycycline or minocycline.

For large animals, there is both a conventional and a long-acting formulation of oxytetracycline. The long-acting formulation contains a viscosity excipient used to prolong the absorption from the injection site. One such excipient is 2-pyrrolidone. When using long-acting formulations, the long-acting properties only apply to IM use, not IV administration. When products that are long acting are compared with conventional injectable products, the long-acting products usually allow for longer dose intervals. However, in pigs, there were no differences in duration of plasma concentrations when equivalent doses were administered.

## Patient Monitoring and Laboratory Tests

Susceptibility testing: CLSI breakpoints for susceptible respiratory pathogens are ≤2 mcg/mL and ≤0.5 mcg/mL for cattle and swine, respectively. For other organisms, the breakpoints are ≤2 mcg/mL for streptococci and ≤4 for other organisms. Tetracycline can be used as a marker to test susceptibility for oxytetracycline, provided that CLSI methods and standards are used.

## Formulations

- Oxytetracycline is available in 250-mg tablets; 500-mg bolus; 100- and 200-mg/mL injection; and 25-, 166-, and 450-g/lb of powder.
- Feed and water additive: Oxytetracycline hydrochloride soluble powder is available to be added to drinking water for poultry, cattle, and pigs in a variety of forms. Oxytetracycline is also available as a medicated feed for cattle, poultry, fish, and pigs.
- Long-acting formulations are available in a 200-mg/mL injection.

## Stability and Storage

Store in a tightly sealed container, protected from light, and at room temperature. If solutions are diluted prior to injection, they should be discarded if not used immediately. Solution may darken slightly without losing potency.

## Small Animal Dosage

### Dogs and Cats

- 7.5–10 mg/kg q12h IV or 20 mg/kg q12h PO.

## Large Animal Dosage

### Horses

- Treatment of ehrlichiosis (Potomac fever caused by *N. risticii*) and other infections: 10 mg/kg q24h IM or IV (slowly). (IM injections can cause pain and reactions at injection site.)
- Treatment of equine piroplasmosis: 5–6 mg/kg once daily IV for 7 days.

### Foals

- Treatment of flexural limb deformities: 44 mg/kg, up to 70 mg/kg (2–3 g per foal), two doses 24 hours apart, injected slowly IV.

### Calves

- 11 mg/kg/day PO.
- Treatment of pneumonia: 11 mg/kg q12h PO.

### Cattle

- Injection for treatment of anaplasmosis, enteritis, pneumonia, and other infections: 11 mg/kg q12h IV.
- Long-acting formulations: 20 mg/kg IM as a single dose.

### Pigs

- 6.6–11 mg/kg, up to 10–20 mg/kg, q24h IM or 20 mg/kg q48h IM.

## Regulatory Information

Cattle and pig withdrawal times for meat: 7 days (oral tablets). For oral soluble powder, the withdrawal times vary greatly from one product to another for cattle and pigs. Generally, they are at least 5 days for meat, but consult specific product label for withdrawal times.

Cattle withdrawal times for injection: 18–22 days, depending on the product.
Cattle withdrawal times for long-acting formulations: 28 days.

Cattle withdrawal times for milk: 96 hours at a dose of 20 mg/kg.

Cattle withdrawal times (intrauterine administration): 7 days for milk and 28 days for meat. Cattle withdrawal times (intramammary administration): 6 days for milk and 28 days for meat.

Pig withdrawal times: 28 days and up to 42 days, depending on product.

# Oxytocin
oks-ih-toe′sin

**Trade and other names:** Pitocin, Syntocinon (nasal solution), and generic brands

**Functional classification:** Labor induction

## Pharmacology and Mechanism of Action
Oxytocin mimics the natural hormone and stimulates uterine muscle contraction via action on specific oxytocin receptors. When administered around the time of luteolysis, it stimulates prostaglandin F receptor (PGF2)-alpha secretion and disrupts luteolysis. When administered prior to luteolysis, it does not induce PGF2-alpha and disrupts luteolysis and prolongs corpus luteum function. When administered late in pregnancy, it stimulates uterine contractions.

## Indications and Clinical Uses
Oxytocin is used to induce or maintain normal labor and delivery in pregnant animals. In surgery, it may be used postoperatively after cesarean section to facilitate involution and resistance to the large inflow of blood. In large animals, oxytocin is used to augment uterine contractions and stimulate lactation. Oxytocin does not increase milk production, but it stimulates contraction, leading to milk ejection. It contracts smooth muscle cells of the mammary gland for milk letdown if the udder is in a proper physiological state. It is also used to expel the placenta after delivery. However, efficacy for retained placenta is questionable, and some experts believe that estrogen should be administered in addition to oxytocin. Oxytocin administered prior to luteolysis (prior to day 10 postovulation in horses) prolongs corpus luteum function and suppresses estrus behavior in mares.

In small animals, oxytocin is used as a treatment for nonobstructive dystocia caused by uterine inertia. The efficacy for this use is mostly based on anecdotal accounts from reproduction experts. Based on the mechanism described, it does not increase milk production in bitches or queens, but it may help empty the mammary gland of previously produced milk. Small doses administered to dogs prior to puppy suckling may help with milk letdown early in the lactation period.

## Precautionary Information

### Adverse Reactions and Side Effects
Adverse effects are uncommon if used carefully. However, careful monitoring of labor is necessary during its use.

### Contraindications and Precautions
Do not administer to pregnant animals unless for induction of parturition. Do not administer unless the cervix is fully relaxed. Do not use if there is abnormal presentation of the fetus. Women, especially if pregnant, should take extra care when handling oxytocin.

### Drug Interactions
Beta-adrenergic agonists will inhibit induction of labor.

## Instructions for Use

Oxytocin is used to induce labor. In people, oxytocin is administered via injection, CRI, or intranasal solution. Animal uses are listed in the dosing section for each species.

## Patient Monitoring and Laboratory Tests

Fetal stress and progression of normal labor should be monitored closely.

## Formulations

- Oxytocin is available in 10- and 20-units/mL injection and 40-units/mL nasal solution.

## Stability and Storage

Store in a tightly sealed container, protected from light, and at room temperature.

## Small Animal Dosage

### Dogs

- 5–20 units per dog IM or SQ (repeat every 30 minutes for primary inertia). Note: The manufacturer's label lists higher doses of 5–30 units per dog.
- To facilitate milk letdown in the early stages of lactation: 2–5 units per dog IM administered 15–30 minutes prior to nursing.

### Cats

- 2.5–3 units per cat IM or IV. Repeat up to three times every 30–60 minutes. (Maximum dose is 3 units/cat.)

## Large Animal Dosage

- Note: The following doses are all on a per-animal basis rather than a per-kilogram basis, and some doses from experts may vary from the approved label dose.

### Cattle

- To stimulate uterine contractions: 30 units IM and repeat in 30 minutes if necessary. (Manufacturer lists 100 units per cow.)
- For retained placenta: 20 units IM given immediately after calving and repeated in 2–4 hours.
- For milk letdown: 10–20 units per cow IV or IM.

### Mares

- To stimulate uterine contractions: 20 units IM. (Manufacturer lists 100 units per mare.)
- For retained placenta: 30–40 units IM at 60- to 90-minute intervals or add 80–100 units to 500 mL of saline solution and give IV.
- To suppress estrus behavior in mares: 60 units per mare IM once or twice daily on days 7–14 post-ovulation.

### Small Ruminants and Sows

- 5–10 units IM. (Manufacturer lists 30–50 units per animal.)

## Regulatory Information

No withdrawal times have been reported. Because of a low risk of residues and rapid clearance after administration, a 24-hour withdrawal time is suggested.

# Paclitaxel
pak'li tax'el

**Trade and other names:** Abraxane and Taxol (human formulations)

**Functional classification:** Anticancer agent, antineoplastic

**Note:** The previously available veterinary formulation, Paccal Vet-CA1, has been withdrawn and is no longer available for veterinary use.

## Pharmacology and Mechanism of Action
Paclitaxel is an anticancer agent that has been used in dogs for some neoplasms. It is a natural product derived from the western yew tree and obtained via a semisynthetic process from *Taxus baccata*. Paclitaxel is in the class of drugs called *taxanes*, which are tubulin-protein active drugs for treating cancer.

Derived from paclitaxel, there is also the semisynthetic drug docetaxel. These drugs differ from vincristine and vinblastine on their action on tubulin proteins. They bind to a different site on the tubulin protein and promote, rather than inhibit, mitotic spindle formation. The mitotic spindles formed are aberrant and disrupt the mitotic phase of the cell cycle. These drugs promote the assembly of microtubules from tubulin dimers and stabilize microtubules by preventing depolymerization. This stability results in the inhibition of the normal dynamic reorganization of the microtubule network that is essential for vital interphase and mitotic cellular functions. These drugs may be active in other parts of the cell cycle because they induce abnormal microtubules throughout the cell cycle and multiple asters of microtubules during mitosis.

*Pharmacokinetics:* In dogs, pharmacokinetic studies demonstrate that the terminal half-life may be as long as 12 hours in some dogs, with high volume of distribution. The pharmacokinetics have not been studied in other animals.

## Indications and Clinical Uses
Paclitaxel and the related drug docetaxel are used for a variety of cancers in people (e.g., breast cancer) as part of a chemotherapy regimen. In dogs, paclitaxel has been used for mammary carcinoma and squamous cell carcinoma and mast cell tumors (MCTs). Paclitaxel is not soluble in water; therefore, it must be administered in other vehicles. The vehicle with polyoxyethylated castor oil (Cremophor EL) administered to animals produces toxicity and should not be used.

## Precautionary Information
### Adverse Reactions and Side Effects
The human formulation, which contains Cremophor EL (polyoxyethylated castor oil) as a carrier vehicle, can cause severe anaphylactoid reactions in dogs and should be avoided. Drugs in this class can produce bone marrow suppression. The most severe neutropenia usually occurs in 5–7 days after administration. Thrombocytopenia, vomiting, and constipation also are possible. As with many other anticancer agents, vomiting, diarrhea, and nausea are common.

Do not use in dogs that are pregnant, lactating, or intended for breeding. Paclitaxel is a teratogen and can affect female and male fertility. Laboratory studies in the rat have shown reduced fertility, embryotoxicity, teratogenicity, and maternal toxicity.

**Contraindications and Precautions**

Because this is an anticancer agent, standard precautions should be applied when using this agent in animals. These precautions include following manufacturer's recommendations for safe handling of the vials and syringes and disposing of infusion supplies.

Do not use in dogs that are pregnant, lactating, or intended for breeding. Paclitaxel is a teratogen and can affect female and male fertility.

**Drug Interactions**

No known drug interactions have been reported in dogs. However, paclitaxel is metabolized by cytochrome P450 isoenzymes and is a P-glycoprotein (P-gp) substrate. Therefore, interactions are possible when administered with other drugs that may inhibit these systems or in dogs that have a deficiency in P-gp. Because most anticancer agents are often administered with other agents, complications from multiple drugs are possible.

## Instructions for Use

The previously available veterinary formulation is no longer available. This form was conditionally approved, but such approval has been canceled. The only form available currently is the human form, which can produce adverse effects in dogs.

### Patient Monitoring and Laboratory Tests

The most severe adverse effect is bone marrow suppression. Monitor complete blood count (CBC) to determine if doses need adjustment to prevent severe neutropenia. If dogs develop severe neutropenia (less than 2000 cells/$\mu$L) or have a concurrent serious infection, withhold treatment.

Paclitaxel can cause gastrointestinal (GI) adverse reactions because of transient GI mucosal cell toxicity. Monitor patients carefully for vomiting, diarrhea, and dehydration. Provide supportive care as clinically indicated.

### Formulations

- The human formulation is formulated in Cremophor EL (polyoxyethylated castor oil). This vehicle is associated with significant anaphylactoid reactions in dogs and should be avoided.

### Stability and Storage

Follow the manufacturer's label carefully for the proper preparation and storage of the vials for injection.

### Small Animal Dosage

**Dogs**

- Not usually recommended because of adverse effects. There has been some experience with 150 mg/m$^2$ IV over 15–30 minutes once every 3 weeks for up to four doses. (Dose range has been 130–150 mg/m$^2$.) If adverse reactions develop, reduce dose by increments of 10 mg/m$^2$ or delay the time for administration.

P

## Cats

- There has been limited experience in cats. However, it has been administered at a dosage of 80 mg/m² (approximately 5 mg/kg) IV every 21 days for two doses.

## Large Animal Dosage

- No doses have been reported for large animals.

## Regulatory Information

Because this is an anticancer agent, it is forbidden to administer to food-producing animals.

---

# Pamidronate Disodium
pam-ih-droe′nate dye-soe′dee-um

**Trade and other names:** Aredia

**Functional classification:** Antihypercalcemic

## Pharmacology and Mechanism of Action

Pamidronate is a bisphosphonate drug used for bone disorders and hypercalcemia. Drugs in this class include pamidronate, etidronate, tiludronate, and pyrophosphate. These drugs are characterized by a germinal bisphosphonate bond, which slows the formation and dissolution of hydroxyapatite crystals. The drugs' clinical use resides in their ability to inhibit bone resorption. They decrease bone turnover by inhibiting osteoclast activity, inducing osteoclast apoptosis, retarding bone resorption, and decreasing the rate of osteoporosis. Inhibition of bone resorption is via inhibition of the mevalonate pathway. Pamidronate, like other bisphosphonates, is not metabolized by the liver. It is primarily eliminated by the kidneys in animals and preferentially remains in the bone for prolonged periods.

## Indications and Clinical Uses

Pamidronate, like other bisphosphonate drugs, is used in people to treat osteoporosis and treatment of hypercalcemia of malignancy. In animals, pamidronate is used to decrease calcium in conditions that cause hypercalcemia, such as cancer and vitamin D toxicosis. It is helpful for managing neoplastic complications and pain associated with pathologic bone resorption caused by cancer. It also may provide pain relief in patients with pathologic bone disease and may reduce glucocorticoid-induced osteoporosis. Experimental work performed in dogs has shown it to be effective for treating cholecalciferol toxicosis, but it did not prevent decreases in renal function. After treating for hypercalcemia in dogs, the duration of effect was 11 days to 9 weeks (median, 8.5 weeks). Some bisphosphonates (see Tiludronate and Clodronate) are approved to treat bone pain in horses caused by navicular disease.

## Precautionary Information

### Adverse Reactions and Side Effects

Fever, joint pain, and myalgias have been observed from pamidronate administration, but otherwise no serious adverse effects have been identified. However, the use in animals has not been common enough to identify a wider range of adverse effects. One study in dogs reported a slight decrease in food intake. In humans, acute renal necrosis after IV administration has been reported. Because pamidronate is eliminated by the kidneys in dogs, a dose-dependent nephropathy is possible, and the risk of renal injury is more likely with doses exceeding 3 mg/kg IV. In people, there is some concern that the use of bisphosphonates produces excessive mineralization and hardening of the bone, which may result in a greater risk of fractures. However, this effect has not been reported for animals.

### Contraindications and Precautions

Although SQ administration is listed in dose protocols, the IV route is preferred. Do not administer to animals with kidney disease and ensure animals are well hydrated prior to administration. Do not administer to animals with conditions that may be associated with hypocalcemia.

### Drug Interactions

Do not mix with solutions containing calcium (e.g., lactated Ringer's solution).

## Instructions for Use

For IV infusion, dilute in fluid solution (0.9% saline) and administer over 2 hours. (Dilute 30 mg pamidronate in 250 mL of fluids.) Infusion can be repeated every 7 days. Although the SQ route is listed for some veterinary applications, it is not recommended, and IV infusion is the preferred route.

## Patient Monitoring and Laboratory Tests

Monitor serum calcium and phosphorus. Treatment of vitamin D toxicosis with pamidronate may result in decreased renal function. Monitor urea nitrogen, creatinine, urine-specific gravity, and food intake in treated animals.

## Formulations

- Pamidronate is available in 30-, 60-, and 90-mg vials for injection and 1 mg/mL in single-use vials for injection.

## Stability and Storage

Store in a tightly sealed container, protected from light, and at room temperature. Vials may be diluted in fluid solutions (e.g., 250 mL 0.9% sodium chloride) and infused over 2 hours or as long as 24 hours. Diluted solutions are stable for 24 hours at room temperature.

## Small Animal Dosage

### Dogs

- Treatment for hypercalcemia: 1–2 mg/kg IV or SQ.
- Treating malignant osteolytic disease: 1–2 mg/kg IV every 28 days as a 2-hour IV infusion.
- Treatment of cholecalciferol toxicosis: 1.3–2 mg/kg IV or SQ for two treatments after toxin exposure.

### Cats

- Treatment of hypercalcemia: 1–1.5 mg/kg IV.

## Large Animal Dosage

- No doses have been reported for large animals.

## Regulatory Information

Withdrawal times are not established for animals that produce food. For extralabel use withdrawal interval estimates, contact Food Animal Residue Avoidance Databank (FARAD) at www.FARAD.org.

---

# Pancreatic Enzyme Replacement (Pancrelipase)
pan-kreh-lye′pase

**Trade and other names:** Viokase, Pancrezyme, Creon, Pancreaze, Pertzye, Zenpep, and Ultrase

**Functional classification:** Pancreatic enzyme replacement

---

## Pharmacology and Mechanism of Action

Pancrelipase is a pancreatic enzyme intended to replace natural pancreatic enzymes in animals that have a deficiency. Pancrelipase provides a source of lipase, amylase, and protease. Pancrelipase is a mixture of enzymes (lipase, amylase, and protease) obtained from the pancreas of pigs. These enzymes enhance digestion of fats, proteins, and starches in the upper duodenum and jejunum. They are more active in an alkaline environment. There are capsules that contain coated spheres and coated microtablets and uncoated tablets. The uncoated tablets are not as bioavailable because degradation may occur in the acid of the stomach. Each milligram contains 24 units of lipase, 100 units of amylase, and 100 units of protease activity.

## Indications and Clinical Uses

Pancrelipase is used to treat pancreatic exocrine insufficiency. There are no well-controlled clinical studies of efficacy in animals, but the use is supported by anecdotal evidence, and the recommendations are from clinical experts. Pancrelipase provides enzymes lacking for digestion. It should be administered before meals. It is inactivated in gastric acid, and uncoated tablets should be administered with a drug to suppress stomach acid (e.g., $H_2$-receptor blocker or proton pump inhibitor [PPI]) to improve activity. Alternatively, capsules can be administered that have enteric-coated spheres or tablets inside to protect from stomach acid.

---

## Precautionary Information

### Adverse Reactions and Side Effects

Oral bleeding has been reported from administration of tablets. The tablets contain potent enzymes, and contact with mucosal membranes may cause lesions and mucosal ulcers. Ensure that tablets are not trapped in the esophagus, or esophageal erosions may occur. Warn owners that if they handle tablets, avoid hand-to-mucosa contact (e.g., contact with eyes or rubbing eyes after handling).

### Contraindications and Precautions

Enteric-coated tablets should not be crushed or chewed.

### Drug Interactions

If antacids are used concurrently, magnesium hydroxide and calcium carbonate may reduce effectiveness.

---

## Instructions for Use

Consult the Formulations section to see the variety of products available. Capsules are designed with enteric-coated minitablets or spheres inside capsules to protect from stomach acid. It is allowed to remove spheres or minitablets from capsules to prepare smaller doses but do not crush or allow pets to chew capsules. For patients who are unable to swallow intact capsules, it is allowed to open capsules and mix with a small amount of acidic soft food with a pH of 4.5 or less, such as applesauce, or administered with applesauce via a gastrostomy tube. Enzymes can be irritating to mucosa, and if contents are crushed, it may cause irritation. Ensure that tablets or capsules are swallowed immediately and followed with water or food to ensure complete ingestion.

If mixed with food, the contents should be mixed with a small amount of food and administered approximately 20 minutes prior to feeding a full meal. After successful results are obtained, the dose may be reduced gradually to identify the minimum effective dose. Pancreatic enzymes are more effective if administered with acid-suppressing drugs ($H_2$ blockers, PPIs, bicarbonate, or some antacids). Different brands have varying activity (see list of formulations later). If switching from one brand to another, they are not interchangeable, and not all products will result in the same therapeutic results.

## Patient Monitoring and Laboratory Tests
No specific monitoring is necessary.

## Formulations
Note that some pancreatic enzyme replacement products that were previously available were removed from the market because of lack of US Food and Drug Administration (FDA) approval. Check with a pharmacy to determine which products are still available. Products listed are not interchangeable. All products contain a combination of porcine-derived lipases, proteases, and amylases in different ratios and concentrations.

- Pancrelipase has been available in a composition of 16,800 units of lipase, 70,000 units of protease, and 70,000 units of amylase per 0.7 g. It was available as a powder, capsule, and tablets but may no longer be on the market. Various other formulations contain a variety of activity (see later).
- Viokase immediate-release tablets contain 10,440 units of lipase, 39,150 units of protease, and 39,150 units of amylase per tablet. Another strength contains 20,880/78,300/78,300 units (lipase/protease/amylase) per tablet.
- Delayed-release capsules (Pancreaze) are available as contains 4200 units of lipase/10,000 units of protease and 17,500 units of amylase. Other strengths contain 10,500/25,000/43,750 or 16,800/40,000/70,000 or 21,000/37,000/61,000 units (lipase/protease/amylase) per capsule. The capsules are coated and should not be crushed or chewed to protect from stomach acid.
- Delayed-release capsules (Creon) are available as 3000 USP units of lipase/9500 USP units of protease and 15,000 USP units of amylase. Other strengths contain 6000/19,000/30,000, 12,000/38,000/60,000, 24,000/76,000/120,000, or 36,000/114,000/180,000 units (lipase/protease/amylase) per capsule. The capsules are coated and should not be crushed or chewed to protect from stomach acid.
- Delayed-release capsules (Pertzye) are available as 8000 units of lipase/28,750 units of protease and 30,250 units of amylase. Other strengths contain 16,000/57,500/60,500 units (lipase/protease/amylase) per capsule. The capsules are coated and should not be crushed or chewed to protect from stomach acid
- Delayed-release capsules (Zenpep) are available as 5,000 units of lipase/17,000 units of proteas, and 27,000 units of amylase. Other strengths contain 10,000/34,000/55,000 and 15,000/51,000/82,000, 20,000/68,000/109,000, or 25,000/85,000/136,000 units (lipase/protease/amylase) per capsule. The capsules are coated and should not be crushed or chewed to protect from stomach acid.

## Stability and Storage
Store in a tightly sealed container, protected from light, and at room temperature. It is inactivated in an acid environment.

## Small Animal Dosage

### Dogs and Cats

- The dose is adjusted individually for each patient. Start with the smallest capsule or tablet size listed under Formulations for small animals and use larger tablet or capsule sizes for proportionately larger animals. Formulations with granules in capsules may be opened and sprinkled on food as listed in dosing instructions (e.g., approximately one capsule with meals for a dog).

## Large Animal Dosage

- No doses have been reported for large animals.

## Regulatory Information

Because of a low risk of residues and rapid clearance after administration, no withdrawal time is suggested.

---

# Pancuronium Bromide

pan-kyoo-roe′nee-um bro′mide

**Trade and other names:** Pavulon

**Functional classification:** Muscle relaxant

## Pharmacology and Mechanism of Action

Pancuronium bromide is a neuromuscular blocking agent (nondepolarizing) used to paralyze animals for surgical procedures. Pancuronium, like other drugs in this class, competes with acetylcholine at the neuromuscular end plate to produce paralysis. Sensory nerves are intact; thus, animals still feel pain after administration of pancuronium.

## Indications and Clinical Uses

Pancuronium is a paralytic agent used during anesthesia or for mechanical ventilation. It is used primarily during anesthesia or other conditions in which it is necessary to inhibit muscle contractions. It is sometimes used as an alternative to atracurium because it is longer acting.

## Precautionary Information

### Adverse Reactions and Side Effects

Pancuronium produces respiratory depression and paralysis. Neuromuscular blocking drugs have no effect on analgesia.

### Contraindications and Precautions

Do not use in patients unless mechanical ventilation support can be provided. Provide additional pain relief when administered during surgery.

### Drug Interactions

Some drugs may potentiate the action (e.g., aminoglycosides) and should not be used concurrently.

## Instructions for Use

Administer only in situations in which careful control of respiration is possible. Doses may need to be individualized for optimum effect. Do not mix with alkalinizing solutions or lactated Ringer's solution.

## Patient Monitoring and Laboratory Tests

Monitor patient's respiration rate, heart rate, and rhythm during use. If possible, monitor the oxygenation status during anesthesia.

## Formulations

• Pancuronium is available in a 1- and 2-mg/mL injection.

## Stability and Storage

Stable if stored in a tightly sealed container, protected from light, and at room temperature for 24 hours.

## Small Animal Dosage

### Dogs and Cats

• 0.1 mg/kg IV or start with 0.01 mg/kg and additional 0.01-mg/kg doses every 30 minutes.
• Constant-rate infusion (CRI): 0.1 mg/kg IV followed by a 2-mcg/kg/min infusion.

## Large Animal Dosage

• No doses have been reported for large animals.

## Regulatory Information

Withdrawal times are not established for animals that produce food. For extralabel use withdrawal interval estimates, contact FARAD at www.FARAD.org.
Racing Commissioners International (RCI) Classification: 2

# Pantoprazole
pan-toe-pray′zole
**Trade and other names:** Protonix
**Functional classification:** Antiulcer agent

## Pharmacology and Mechanism of Action

Pantoprazole is a PPI with action similar to another popular drug in this class, omeprazole. Pantoprazole inhibits gastric acid secretion by inhibiting the $K^+/H^+$ pump. Pantoprazole, like other PPIs, has potent and long-acting effects and are more effective than histamine $H_2$-blocking drugs. Acid suppression may have a duration of approximately 24 hours in some animals. Pantoprazole is the first PPI that can be administered IV and is useful for treatment in a hospital setting.

## Indications and Clinical Uses

Pantoprazole is used for treatment and prevention of GI ulcers and gastroesophageal reflux. Other PPIs include omeprazole, esomeprazole, lansoprazole (Prevacid), and rabeprazole (AcipHex). All PPIs act via a similar mechanism and are equally effective. However, there has been more experience with omeprazole in animals than the other drugs of this group. In dogs, pantoprazole (1 mg/kg) maintained a stomach pH greater than 3–4 when administered IV, which is the pH necessary for ulcer prevention and healing. Pantoprazole, being the only one in an IV formulation, is often used when an IV drug is preferred for treatment.

## Precautionary Information

### Adverse Reactions and Side Effects

Side effects have not been reported in animals. However, in people, there is concern about hypergastrinemia with chronic use. This has not been a concern in animals. Overgrowth of *Clostridium* bacteria has been a concern from chronic use because of chronic gastric acid suppression, but the clinical importance of this concern in animals has not been established. In people, the PPI may increase the risk of kidney disease, but this problem has not been reported in animals.

### Contraindications and Precautions

No known contraindications.

### Drug Interactions

Do not mix IV solution with other drugs. Do not administer with drugs that depend on stomach acid for absorption (e.g., ketoconazole, itraconazole, iron supplements). PPIs may inhibit some drug-metabolizing enzymes (CYP450 enzymes), although in people, there was a low risk of drug interactions caused by enzyme inhibition. In people, there may be an increased risk of intestinal injury when PPIs are administered with nonsteroidal anti-inflammatory drugs (NSAIDs), but this has not been studied in animals.

## Instructions for Use

For treating GI ulcers, administer once per day for 7–10 days. For gastrin-secreting tumors, use higher dose (1 mg/kg) twice daily. The primary advantage with pantoprazole compared with other PPIs is that it is available in an IV dosage formulation and can be mixed with fluid solutions. For IV use, mix a 40-mg vial with 10 mL of saline and further dilute with saline, lactated Ringer's solution, or 5% dextrose to 0.4 mg/mL. Administer IV infusion over 2 minutes or 15 minutes. Follow directions below for IV infusion. If administering the enteric-coated oral tablets, do not crush. Oral tablets can be administered with or without food. PPIs may be more effective if administered 30 minutes prior to feeding.

## Patient Monitoring and Laboratory Tests

No specific monitoring is necessary. When treating ulcers, monitor hematocrit or CBC to detect bleeding. Monitor for signs of vomiting and diarrhea.

## Formulations

- Pantoprazole is available as 20- and 40-mg delayed-release tablets. There are also granules for oral suspension (40 mg), which have been mixed with apple juice or applesauce for administration in people.
- Pantoprazole for IV use: Available as a 40-mg vial (diluted to 4 mg/mL). For IV infusion, reconstitute the 40-mg/kg vial with 10 mL of normal saline. Further dilute this solution with 100 mL of 5% dextrose, normal saline, or lactated Ringer's solution to a final concentration of 0.4 mg/mL. To prepare a larger dose (80 mg), reconstitute two vials each with 10 mL of normal saline; combine the content of both vials; and further dilute with 80 mL of 5% dextrose, normal saline, or lactated Ringer's solution to a final concentration of 0.8 mg/mL.
- Pantoprazole compounded oral suspension: To prepare a 2-mg/mL pantoprazole oral suspension, mix pantoprazole tablets with sterile water and sodium bicarbonate powder. Crush 40 tablets in a mortar and reduce to a fine powder. Mix in with 340 mL of sterile water. Next, add 16.8 g of sodium bicarbonate powder and

stir (approximately 20 minutes) until the tablets are fully disintegrated. Then add another 16.8 g of sodium bicarbonate powder and stir again for 5 minutes until all the powder has dissolved. Add enough water to bring the final volume to 400 mL. Transfer the entire contents to an amber-colored bottle and store in a refrigerator. Label with a "shake well" label. This may be stable if stored in refrigerator for 62 days and administered at the doses listed.

## Stability and Storage
Store in a tightly sealed container, protected from light, and at room temperature. Keep tablets at room temperature. Once reconstituted, the vials are stable at room temperature for 6 hours. Do not freeze reconstituted solutions. When further diluted for IV use, it is stable for up to 96 hours at room temperature. The diluted (4-mg/mL) solution may be stored in refrigerator for 28 days. The oral compounded form prepared from tablets (see earlier directions) can be stored in a refrigerator for 62 days.

## Small Animal Dosage
### Dogs and Cats
- 0.5–0.6 mg/kg, up to 1 mg/kg, twice daily PO.
- IV administration (24 hours): 0.5–1 mg/kg IV infusion over 24 hours. This dose may be delivered in 2 or 15 minutes (see next section).
- IV administration (2 or 15 minutes): First flush the IV line. Administer pantoprazole via an IV line with dextrose 5% injection, sodium chloride 0.9% injection, or Ringer's lactate injection. For the 2-minute infusion, mix 40 mg of powder with 10 mL of sodium chloride 0.9% injection for a final concentration of 4 mg/mL. Infuse a 1-mg/kg dose over 2 minutes. For a 15-minute infusion, mix a 40-mg vial with 10 mL of sodium chloride 0.9% injection. Then further admix this solution with 100 mL of dextrose 5% injection, sodium chloride 0.9% injection, or Ringer's lactate injection to a total volume of 110 mL, producing a solution with a final concentration of approximately 0.4 mg/mL. Administer the final dose (1 mg/kg) over 15 minutes.

## Large Animal Dosage
- No dose is reported for large animals. Doses have been extrapolated from human use (0.5 mg/kg q24h IV), and infusion protocols listed previously for small animals have been used.

## Regulatory Information
Withdrawal times are not established for animals that produce food. For extralabel use withdrawal interval estimates, contact FARAD at www.FARAD.org.
RCI Classification: 5

# Paregoric
pare-eh-gore'ik

**Trade and other names:** Corrective mixture

**Functional classification:** Antidiarrheal

## Pharmacology and Mechanism of Action
Paregoric (opium tincture) is an old and somewhat outdated product used to treat diarrhea. Paregoric contains 2 mg of morphine in every 5 mL of paregoric. The action is via stimulation of intestinal mu-opiate receptors to cause a decrease in intestinal peristalsis.

## Indications and Clinical Uses
Paregoric decreases signs of diarrhea via opiate effects, but its use is somewhat outdated.

### Precautionary Information
**Adverse Reactions and Side Effects**

Like all opiates, side effects are predictable and unavoidable. Side effects may include sedation, constipation, and bradycardia. Respiratory depression occurs with high doses. Tolerance and dependence occur with chronic administration.

**Contraindications and Precautions**

Paregoric contains opium and may be abused by humans. Use cautiously in horses and ruminants because intestinal motility may be decreased.

**Drug Interactions**

No drug interactions have been reported in animals.

## Instructions for Use
Use of paregoric has been replaced by more specific products such as loperamide or diphenoxylate.

## Patient Monitoring and Laboratory Tests
No specific monitoring is necessary.

## Formulations
• For every 5 mL of paregoric, there is 2 mg of morphine.

## Stability and Storage
Store in a tightly sealed container, protected from light, and at room temperature.

## Small Animal Dosage
**Dogs and Cats**
• 0.05–0.06 mg/kg q12h PO.

## Large Animal Dosage
• No doses have been reported for large animals.

## Regulatory Information
Schedule III Controlled Substance.

Withdrawal times are not established for animals that produce food. For extralabel use withdrawal interval estimates, contact FARAD at www.FARAD.org.

# Paromomycin Sulfate
pare-oe-moe-mye'sin sul'fate

**Trade and other names:** Humatin; also known as aminosidine

**Functional classification:** Antiparasitic

## Pharmacology and Mechanism of Action
Paromomycin is an antibiotic drug of the aminoglycoside class, which is also known as aminosidine. The mechanism of action of paromomycin is similar to that of other

aminoglycosides: It inhibits the ribosomal 30S subunit with subsequent inhibition of bacterial protein synthesis. The difference between paromomycin and other aminoglycosides is the spectrum that includes protozoa. The antibacterial spectrum of activity is similar to that of other aminoglycosides. However, because paromomycin is administered orally and generally not absorbed systemically, its activity is limited to intestinal pathogens, primarily protozoa.

## Indications and Clinical Uses

The use of paromomycin is limited to intestinal infections. It is not absorbed systemically and should not be used for extraintestinal infections. Paromomycin has been used to treat intestinal infections, such as cryptosporidiosis. The use is based on limited accounts in animals and extrapolation from humans. Efficacy in animals has not been tested in controlled studies. Another use of paromomycin is for treatment of *Leishmania* infection, often combined with meglumine antimoniate. This treatment requires IM injection, which may not be available in many countries.

## Precautionary Information

### Adverse Reactions and Side Effects

Paromomycin has been associated with renal failure and blindness when used in cats. Although systemic absorption is not expected to be high, cats treated with high doses for intestinal organisms developed problems.

### Contraindications and Precautions

Extreme caution is recommended when administering this drug to animals that may have a compromised bowel resulting from intestinal disease. A compromised intestinal mucosa may lead to increased systemic absorption and adverse effects.

### Drug Interactions

No drug interactions have been reported in animals.

P

## Instructions for Use

In cats, doses of 125–165 mg/kg q12h have been administered for 5–7 days PO. However, there are reports in the veterinary literature that these doses have produced toxicity in cats, including kidney injury. It is suggested to use lower doses to avoid toxicity and monitor the patient's renal parameters carefully. When there is a compromised integrity of the intestinal mucosa, as may occur with diarrhea, use of paromomycin is discouraged.

For treating *Leishmania* infections in dogs, it is used IM at a dosage of 11 mg/kg once daily for 21 days as a single agent. It is also used in combination with other anti-*Leishmania* agents (e.g., 60 mg/kg of meglumine antimoniate IM q12h for 4 weeks, plus 5 mg/kg q12h, SQ of paromomycin once daily for 3 weeks).

## Patient Monitoring and Laboratory Tests

Monitor the patient's renal function, such as urine-specific gravity, serum creatinine, and blood urea nitrogen (BUN), during treatment.

### Formulations
Paromomycin is available in 250-mg capsules.

### Stability and Storage
Store in a tightly sealed container, protected from light, and at room temperature.

### Small Animal Dosage
**Cats**
- Doses of 125–165 mg/kg q12h PO for 7 days have been recommended. However, caution is recommended when using doses this high. Lower doses should be considered (see dog dosage) in animals that may be at risk of toxicity.

**Dogs**
- The dose in dogs has been extrapolated from human medicine, which is 10 mg/kg q8h PO for 5–10 days.

### Large Animal Dosage
- No doses have been reported for large animals.

### Regulatory Information
Withdrawal times are not established for animals that produce food. Although not absorbed systemically to a large extent, it is expected that concentrations may persist in the kidneys, producing long, extended withdrawal times for slaughter.

# Paroxetine
par-oks'eh-teen

**Trade and other names:** Paxil

**Functional classification:** Behavior modification

### Pharmacology and Mechanism of Action
Paroxetine is an antidepressant drug that inhibits uptake of serotonin. Paroxetine, like other drugs in this class, is classified as a selective serotonin reuptake inhibitor (SSRI). It resembles fluoxetine (Reconcile, Prozac) in action. Its mechanism of action appears to be via selective inhibition of serotonin reuptake and downregulation of 5-HT$_1$ receptors. SSRIs are more selective for inhibiting serotonin reuptake than the tricyclic antidepressants (TCAs).

### Indications and Clinical Uses
Paroxetine, like other SSRI drugs, is used to treat behavioral disorders such as compulsive disorders (canine compulsive disorder), anxiety, and dominance aggression. In cats, it has been effective for decreasing urine spraying. Because of the small tablet size, some veterinarians have found it easy to administer to cats and small dogs. The use in animals is based on small observational studies, particularly in cats. Experts in veterinary behavior have recommended paroxetine as an alternative to other SSRI agents, and TCAs.

## Precautionary Information

### Adverse Reactions and Side Effects

Paroxetine is similar to fluoxetine, but in some animals, paroxetine is better tolerated. Adverse effects observed in dogs and cats include constipation and decreased appetite. Decreased appetite in cats is more common at higher doses.

### Contraindications and Precautions

Use cautiously in patients with heart disease. Do not use in pregnant animals. There is a risk of fetal malformations if used early in pregnancy. Serotonin-reuptake inhibitors can increase the risk of bleeding by inhibiting serotonin uptake by platelets, but this has not been reported in animals.

### Drug Interactions

Do not use with monoamine oxidase inhibitors (MAOIs), such as selegiline. Do not use with other behavior-modifying drugs, such as other SSRIs or TCAs.

## Instructions for Use

Dosing recommendations are empirical. Paroxetine has been used for conditions similar to what has been treated with fluoxetine (Prozac, Reconcile). In cats, the small tablet size has made it easier to administer convenient doses compared with chewable tablets or other drugs available in capsules. Paroxetine has caused constipation in some animals, and veterinarians may administer a feline laxative for the first week of therapy to avoid problems.

Sudden discontinuation of serotonin reuptake inhibitors can produce other behavior problems, such as anxiety, signs of agitation, and nervousness. If treatment is discontinued, gradually withdraw the medication.

## Patient Monitoring and Laboratory Tests

Use in animals has been relatively safe, and one should only monitor behavior changes.

## Formulations

- Paroxetine is available in 10-, 20-, 30-, and 40-mg tablets and 2-mg/mL oral suspension.

## Stability and Storage

Stable if stored in manufacturer's original formulation. Although paroxetine has been compounded for veterinary use, the potency and stability have not been evaluated for compounded products.

## Small Animal Dosage

### Dogs

- 0.5 mg/kg/day PO. For some compulsive disorders, increase the dosage to 1 mg/kg q24h PO.

### Cats

- One eighth to one fourth of a 10-mg tablet per cat daily PO (approximately 0.5 mg/kg q24h). For urine spraying in cats, some have responded to every-other-day treatment.

## Large Animal Dosage

- No doses have been reported for large animals.

## Regulatory Information

Do not administer to animals intended for food.
RCI Classification: 2

# Penicillamine
pen-ih-sill′ah-meen

**Trade and other names:** Cuprimine and Depen

**Functional classification:** Antidote

## Pharmacology and Mechanism of Action
Penicillamine is also called 3-mercaptovaline. It is a chelating agent for lead, copper, iron, and mercury. When used to treat copper toxicity, it helps to solubilize copper in the cells to allow for more rapid urinary excretion. Treated animals should have increased copper urinary excretion. Other drugs that have been used as chelating agents include tetrathiomolybdate, trientine, and zinc. Penicillamine also has anti-inflammatory properties. It inhibits collagen cross-linking by making it more susceptible to enzyme degradation. This antifibrotic property may contribute to its positive effect for treating animals with hepatitis; however, efficacy for this indication has been questioned (see later).

## Indications and Clinical Uses
Penicillamine has been used in people to treat rheumatoid arthritis. The primary use in animals is for treatment of copper toxicity and hepatitis associated with accumulation of copper. Treatment duration for animals with copper-storage hepatic disease may require 2–4 months. It also has been used to treat cystine calculi. Although it may inhibit collagen and reduce fibrosis in patients with hepatic disease, this effect has been disappointing in clinical patients. There is no clear demonstration that it is efficacious for this indication.

Penicillamine has recently become highly expensive for use in animals, and other alternatives are being investigated. An alternative to consider, if formulations are available, is trientine (triethylenetetramine dihydrochloride), another copper chelating agent. Trientine has been administered to dogs at a dosage of 10–15 mg/kg q12h PO.

## Precautionary Information
### Adverse Reactions and Side Effects
The most common adverse effects are anorexia and vomiting. In people, allergic reactions, cutaneous reactions, agranulocytosis, and anemia have been reported. It has also produced proteinuria and hematuria and in cats has caused neutropenia. In dogs treated for liver disease, corticosteroid-like hepatopathy has been observed. Therefore it may produce steroid-like effects in the liver.

### Contraindications and Precautions
Do not use in pregnant animals. There appears to be little cross-reaction between penicillin and penicillamine in allergic animals.

### Drug Interactions
No drug interactions have been reported in animals.

## Instructions for Use
Administer on an empty stomach (at least 30–60 minutes before meals).

## Patient Monitoring and Laboratory Tests
Monitor liver biochemistry tests during treatment. Monitor metal concentrations if used to treat intoxication.

## Formulations
Penicillamine is available in 125- and 250-mg capsules and 250-mg tablets.

## Stability and Storage
Store in a tightly sealed container, protected from light, and at room temperature. Penicillamine is soluble in water. Preparations of penicillamine in a suspension for oral use have been combined with syrups and flavorings and were stable for 5 weeks.

## Small Animal Dosage
### Dogs and Cats
- 10–15 mg/kg q12h PO, best administered 30 minutes before a meal.
- Doberman pinschers: use 250 mg per dog q12h PO.

## Large Animal Dosage
### Horses and Cattle
- 10–15 mg/kg q12h PO.

## Regulatory Information
Cattle withdrawal time: 21 days for meat; 3 days for milk. For withdrawal times for doses administered extralabel, contact FARAD at www.FARAD.org.

# Penicillin G

**Trade and other names:** Penicillin G potassium or sodium, Penicillin G benzathine (BenzaPen), Penicillin G, Procaine, and generic Penicillin V (Pen-Vee)

**Functional classification:** Antibacterial

## Pharmacology and Mechanism of Action
Penicillin G is the oldest of the beta-lactam antibiotics, but it is still used in veterinary medicine. Penicillin G is also called benzyl penicillin. Its action is similar to that of other penicillins, by binding to the penicillin-binding proteins (PBPs) to weaken or cause lysis of the cell wall. Penicillin G is bactericidal with a time-dependent action. An increased bactericidal effect is observed when drug concentrations are maintained above minimum inhibitory concentration (MIC) values. The spectrum of penicillin G is limited to gram-positive bacteria, anaerobic bacteria, and a few highly susceptible gram-negative bacteria (e.g., *Pasteurella* spp.). Practically all bacteria of the Enterobacteriaceae and beta-lactamase–producing *Staphylococcus* spp. are resistant.

*Pharmacokinetics:* Penicillin sodium or penicillin potassium, when injected intravenously, has a half-life of ≤1 hour in most animals. However, the same dose of procaine penicillin given intramuscularly may produce more prolonged concentrations and a half-life of 20–24 hours because of slow absorption from the injection site.

Formulations of penicillin G are designed to control the absorption from site of injection. Formulations include:
- Sodium or potassium penicillin G (crystalline penicillin), which is water soluble and can be administered intravenously or intramuscularly. It may also be mixed with fluids for IV administration.
- Penicillin G benzathine, which is insoluble and available as a suspension. It is slowly absorbed from an injection site to produce low but prolonged (several days of) penicillin concentrations. All benzathine penicillin G forms are combined with procaine penicillin G in commercial formulation (1:1 ratio).

- Penicillin G procaine is a poorly soluble suspension for IM or SQ administration. It is absorbed slowly, producing concentrations for 12–24 hours after injections.
- Penicillin V, oral penicillin, is not highly absorbed and has a narrow spectrum in comparison with other penicillin derivatives.

## Indications and Clinical Uses

Penicillin G is administered by injection either intravenously (potassium or sodium penicillin) or intramuscularly (procaine or procaine/benzathine penicillin G). Penicillin G is indicated for treatment of gram-positive cocci that cause respiratory infections, abscesses, and urinary tract infections (UTIs). Many staphylococci are resistant because of beta-lactamase synthesis. Streptococci are usually susceptible. Other susceptible organisms include gram-positive bacilli and anaerobic bacteria. Most gram-negative bacilli, especially those of enteric origin, such as the Enterobacteriaceae, are resistant. Some gram-negative respiratory pathogens such as *Pasteurella multocida* and *Mannheimia haemolytica* are susceptible.

Penicillin concentrations in the urine are at least 100-fold higher than plasma concentrations in treated animals; therefore some urinary pathogens may be more susceptible.

---

### Precautionary Information

**Adverse Reactions and Side Effects**

Penicillin G has a high safety margin and is usually well tolerated. Allergic reactions are possible. Diarrhea is common with oral doses, but oral forms are rarely used. Pain and tissue reactions may occur with IM or SQ injections. Formulations of procaine penicillin G contain varying amounts of free procaine (depending on the formulation). Free procaine in the formulation may elicit a central nervous system (CNS) reaction after injection in some horses. Large doses of sodium penicillin IV can decrease potassium concentrations.

**Contraindications and Precautions**

Use cautiously in animals allergic to penicillin-like drugs. Avoid injection volumes greater than 30 mL per site. Administration of the long-acting benzathine form of penicillin G increases the risk of residues in food-producing animals.

**Drug Interactions**

No drug interactions have been reported in animals.

---

## Instructions for Use

The approved dose listed on the injectable product labels are outdated and do not reflect the current clinical use of penicillin. Penicillin G benzathine is not recommended for most infections because concentrations are too low to provide therapeutic drug concentrations. A possible exception is for treatment of streptococcal infections. Avoid SQ injection with procaine penicillin G because of tissue injury and food-animal residue problems. Penicillin V is not well absorbed orally and should be avoided for serious infections.

## Patient Monitoring and Laboratory Tests

Susceptibility testing: Clinical and Laboratory Standards Institute (CLSI) breakpoint for susceptible equine pathogens (*Streptococcus equi* and *Staphylococcus* spp.) is ≤0.5 mcg/mL. The breakpoint for bovine isolates causing bovine respiratory disease is ≤0.25 mcg/mL. The CLSI breakpoints for susceptible organisms isolated from people are ≤8 mcg/mL for enterococci and ≤0.12 mcg/mL for staphylococci and streptococci.

## Formulations

Note on unitage: Penicillin is one of the few antibiotics that is still measured in terms of units rather than weight in milligrams or micrograms, and the conversion depends on the formulation. One unit of procaine penicillin is approximately 1.03 mcg, or there are approximately 975 units/mg. One unit of potassium penicillin is approximately 0.64 mcg, or there are approximately 1560 units/mg. An approximate conversion is 1000 units/mg for procaine penicillin and 1500 units/mg for potassium penicillin.
- Penicillin G potassium is available in 5- to 20-million-unit vials.
- Penicillin G benzathine is available in 150,000 units/mL and is usually combined with 150,000 units/mL of procaine penicillin G suspension. Benzathine penicillin products are not recommended.
- Procaine penicillin G is available in 300,000-units/mL suspension.
- Penicillin V is available in 250- and 500-mg tablets (250 mg is equal to 400,000 units).

## Stability and Storage

Sodium and potassium forms of penicillin G retain their potency for 72 hours at room temperature, but refrigeration is recommended. It is stable for 7 days if refrigerated and retains 90% potency for 14 days. Solutions of sodium penicillin prepared in fluids for CRI infusion should be replaced q12h. Penicillin potassium and penicillin sodium are freely soluble in water. One gram of penicillin dissolves in 250 mL of water (4 mg/mL). Degradation and inactivation of penicillin solutions are accelerated at high pH (pH greater than 8), strong acids, or oxidizing agents.

## Small Animal Dosage
- Penicillin G potassium or sodium: 20,000–40,000 units/kg q6–8h IV or IM.
- Procaine penicillin G: 20,000–40,000 units/kg q12–24h IM.
- Penicillin V: 10 mg/kg q8h PO. (Not recommended because of poor oral absorption.)

## Large Animal Dosage
### Cattle and Sheep
- Procaine penicillin G: 22,000–66,000 units/kg q24h IM. SQ use is discouraged.
- Sodium or potassium penicillin G: 20,000 units/kg IM or IV q6h.

### Pigs
- Procaine penicillin G: 15,000–25,000 units/kg q24h IM.

### Horses
- Penicillin sodium or penicillin potassium: 20,000–24,000 units/kg q6–8h IV. (Dosages up to 44,000 units/kg q6h have been used for refractory cases.)
- Procaine penicillin G: 20,000–24,000 units/kg q24h IM.
- Potassium penicillin G: 20,000–24,000 units/kg q12h IM.
- CRI: sodium penicillin G loading dose of 1.3 mg/kg followed by 2.5 mcg/kg/h CRI to achieve a target of 2 mcg/mL.

## Regulatory Information

Horses: Injections of procaine penicillin may cause a positive test result for procaine prior to racing for as long as 30 days after an injection.

Withdrawal times for benzathine penicillin at label dose of 6000–7000 units/kg in cattle: 30 days for meat (14 days in Canada).

Withdrawal times for procaine penicillin at label dose of 6000–7000 units/kg in cattle: 10 days for meat, 4 days for milk; 9 days for sheep; and 7 days for swine.

Withdrawal times for procaine penicillin G at a dose of 15,000 units/kg in pigs: 8 days.

Withdrawal times for procaine penicillin G at a dose of 21,000 units/kg in cattle: 10 days for meat and 96 hours for milk.

Procaine penicillin G at a dose of 60,000 units/kg: 21 days for cattle and 15 days for pigs.

RCI Classification: 3 for procaine; penicillin is not classified

# Pentastarch
**Trade and other names:** Pentaspan
**Functional classification:** Fluid replacement

## Pharmacology and Mechanism of Action
Pentastarch is a synthetic colloid volume expander that is used to maintain vascular volume in animals with circulatory shock. There is more compete and detailed on all of the hydroxyethyl starch formulations listed separately under Hydroxyethyl Starch.

Pentastarch is prepared from hydroxyethyl starch and is derived from amylopectin. There are two hydroxyethyl starch preparations: hetastarch and pentastarch. Hetastarch (6%) has an average molecular weight of 450,000 and colloid osmotic pressure of 32.7. Pentastarch (10%) has an average molecular weight of 280,000 and colloid osmotic pressure of 40. Because hetastarch is a larger molecular weight compound than pentastarch, it tends to remain in the vasculature and prevent loss of intravascular volume and tissue edema. After administration, pentastarch is retained in the vasculature and prevents loss of intravascular volume and tissue edema. Other colloids used are dextrans (Dextran 40 and Dextran 70). Hetastarch and the dextrans are discussed in other sections.

## Indications and Clinical Uses
Pentastarch is used primarily to treat acute hypovolemia and shock. It is administered intravenously in acute situations. Pentastarch has a duration of effective volume expansion of 12–48 hours. Pentastarch is used in similar situations as hetastarch, but it is used less frequently.

## Precautionary Information
### Adverse Reactions and Side Effects
There has only been limited use in veterinary medicine; therefore, adverse effects have not been reported. However, it may cause allergic reactions and hyperosmotic renal dysfunction. Coagulopathies are possible but are rare and less likely than with hetastarch.

### Contraindications and Precautions
No contraindications are reported for animals.

### Drug Interactions
Pentastarch is compatible with most fluid solutions.

## Instructions for Use
Pentastarch is used in critical care situations and is infused via CRI. Pentastarch may be more effective and produce fewer side effects than Dextran. Because of lower molecular weight, it can be infused more quickly than hetastarch.

## Patient Monitoring and Laboratory Tests
Monitor patient's hydration status and blood pressure during administration.

## Formulations
• Pentastarch is available in a 10% injectable solution.

## Stability and Storage
Pentastarch is stable in original packaging. Compatible with most fluid administration sets.

## Small Animal Dosage
**Dogs**
- CRI: 10–25 mL/kg/day IV.

**Cats**
- CRI: 5–10 mL/kg/day IV.

## Large Animal Dosage
**Horses**
- 8–15 mL/kg or delivered as CRI 0.5–1 mL/kg/h IV.
- No doses have been reported for other large animals.

## Regulatory Information
No regulatory requirements.

---

# Pentazocine
pen-taz′oh-seen

**Trade and other names:** Talwin-V

**Functional classification:** Analgesic, opioid

## Pharmacology and Mechanism of Action
Pentazocine is an older opioid analgesic similar in action to buprenorphine and butorphanol. The action of pentazocine results from its effect as a mu-opiate receptor partial agonist and a kappa-receptor agonist. Most of the sedative and analgesic effects are believed to be caused by the kappa-receptor effects. As a partial antagonist, pentazocine may partially reverse some mu-receptor agonist effects. Its effects are believed to be similar to buprenorphine or butorphanol, but efficacy is less.

## Indications and Clinical Uses
Pentazocine has been used for sedation and analgesia, primarily in horses. However, because of the availability of other opioids with better efficacy, the use of pentazocine has declined.

**P**

## Precautionary Information
**Adverse Reactions and Side Effects**
Adverse effects are similar to those of other opioid analgesic drugs and include constipation, ileus, vomiting, and bradycardia. Sedation is common at analgesic doses. Respiratory depression can occur with high doses. Dysphoric effects are possible in some sensitive individuals and in some species (e.g., horses).

**Contraindications and Precautions**
Pentazocine has few contraindications or precautions, except that use in horses can potentially cause behavior changes and reduced intestinal motility.

**Drug Interactions**
Pentazocine may potentiate other sedative drugs such as alpha$_2$ agonists. Pentazocine may interfere with mu-opiate effects of other drugs, such as morphine or fentanyl.

## Instructions for Use

Pentazocine is a mixed agonist–antagonist. It is relatively modest to weak in efficacy for pain control, and other opioids should be considered for better pain management.

## Patient Monitoring and Laboratory Tests

Monitor the patient's heart rate and respiration. Although bradycardia rarely needs to be treated when it is caused by an opioid, atropine can be administered if necessary. If serious respiratory depression occurs, the opioid can be reversed with naloxone.

## Formulations

Pentazocine is available in a 30-mg/mL injection (availability has been limited).

## Stability and Storage

Store in a tightly sealed container, protected from light, and at room temperature.

## Small Animal Dosage

**Dogs**

• 1.65–3.3 mg/kg q4h IM or as needed.

**Cats**

• 2.2–3.3 mg/kg q4h IM, IV, or SQ or as needed.

## Large Animal Dosage

**Horses**

• 200–400 mg per horse IV.

## Regulatory Information

Pentazocine is a Schedule IV controlled drug. Withdrawal times are not established for animals that produce food. For extralabel use withdrawal interval estimates, contact FARAD at www.FARAD.org.

RCI Classification: 3

# Pentobarbital Sodium

pen-toe-bar′bih-tahl soe′dee-um

**Trade and other names:** Nembutal and generic brands

**Functional classification:** Anesthetic, barbiturate

## Pharmacology and Mechanism of Action

Pentobarbital is a short-acting barbiturate anesthetic. The action of pentobarbital, like other barbiturates, is via nonselective depression of the CNS.

The barbiturates produce sedative, anesthetic, and anticonvulsant properties. Barbiturates depress all activity in the CNS. At doses used for anesthesia, pentobarbital produces dose-dependent respiratory depression; it reduces brain metabolism and cerebral blood flow. The onset of action is rapid (within minutes), and the duration of action is usually 3–4 hours.

## Indications and Clinical Uses

Pentobarbital is usually used as an IV anesthetic. It also is used to control severe seizures in animals for treatment during status epilepticus. In some instances, pentobarbital is included in mixtures used to induce euthanasia in animals.

Pentobarbital is not used regularly as a general anesthetic compared to many years ago. There are other agents that are safer, produce smoother recoveries, and are used more often.

Another use of pentobarbital is for euthanasia at high doses IV, usually in combination with other agents, such as muscle relaxants. (See description below.)

---

## Precautionary Information

### Adverse Reactions and Side Effects

Adverse effects are related to anesthetic action. Cardiac depression and respiratory depression are common. Respiratory apnea can occur with rapid IV doses.

### Contraindications and Precautions

Rapid IV doses can be lethal. Every patient that receives IV pentobarbital should be carefully monitored. The IV dose should be carefully titrated to produce anesthesia but avoid a dose that could be fatal. Monitor respiration rate carefully after injection because respiratory depression may occur.

### Drug Interactions

Pentobarbital potentiates the sedative and cardiorespiratory-depressing effects of other anesthetics. Pentobarbital is subject to effects from other drugs that may either induce or inhibit cytochrome P450 metabolizing enzymes. (See Appendixes H and I.)

---

## Instructions for Use

Pentobarbital has a narrow therapeutic index. When administering intravenously, inject the first half of the dose initially and then the remainder of the calculated dose gradually until anesthetic effect is achieved. It should be used only by trained clinical personnel with experience using pentobarbital.

*Euthanasia use:* Most euthanasia solutions contain pentobarbital as their active ingredient. Often other ingredients to facilitate euthanasia are included such as muscle relaxants and drugs with lethal cardiac effects (e.g., edetate disodium 0.05%). The concentration of pentobarbital in most euthanasia solutions is 390 mg/mL with a lethal dose of 1 mL per 10 lb, which is equivalent to 1 mL per 4.5 kg or 87 mg/kg IV.

## Patient Monitoring and Laboratory Tests

Monitor vital signs, especially heart rate and rhythm and respiration, during anesthesia.

## Formulations

- Pentobarbital has been available in a 50- and 65-mg/mL solution for injection (contains propylene glycol). It has been available in 50 or 20 mL multiple-dose vials. Other excipients in the vial include propylene glycol and alcohol. The availability has been inconsistent from some suppliers, but it may be available from some veterinary distributors. Some manufacturers discontinued production because of objection to its use for lethal injection in a human execution protocol.

## Stability and Storage

Store at 68°F–77°F in a tightly sealed container, protected from light. The pH of solution is 9–10.5 and may affect stability of other coadministered drugs. It precipitates if combined with most hydrochloride-based drugs or drugs with low pH. If pentobarbital is used to euthanize animals, it remains stable even under rendering conditions used for disposal of the carcass.

## Small Animal Dosage

### Dogs and Cats

- General anesthesia: 25–30 mg/kg IV to effect.
- CRI: 2–15 mg/kg IV to effect followed by 0.2–1 mg/kg/h.
- Status epilepticus: 2–6 mg/kg IV (15–20 minutes may be needed to take full effect).
- Euthanasia: See Instructions for Use.

## Large Animal Dosage

### Cattle

- Standing sedation: 1–2 mg/kg IV.

### Cattle, Sheep, and Goats

- General anesthesia: 20–30 mg/kg IV given to effect.

## Regulatory Information

If used for a euthanasia agent, the carcass should not be fed to other animals or used for food. Withdrawal times are not established for animals that produce food. For extralabel use withdrawal interval estimates, contact FARAD at www.FARAD.org. Schedule II controlled drug.
RCI Classification: 2

# Pentoxifylline
pen-toks′ih-fill-in

**Trade and other names:** Trental, oxpentifylline, and generic brands

**Functional classification:** Anti-inflammatory agent

## Pharmacology and Mechanism of Action

Pentoxifylline is a methylxanthine, in the same class as theophylline. Pentoxifylline is used primarily as a rheological agent in people (increases blood flow through narrow vessels). An improved rheologic effect has also been demonstrated with equine red blood cells (RBCs) but not neutrophils. As a phosphodiesterase inhibitor (PDE IV inhibitor), it also produces anti-inflammatory effects. It may have anti-inflammatory action via inhibition of cytokine synthesis. In experimental studies, pentoxifylline suppresses synthesis of inflammatory cytokines, such as interleukin (IL)-1 beta, IL-2, IL-6, and tumor necrosis factor (TNF) alpha and may inhibit lymphocyte activation. In experimental dogs at 20 mg/kg q8h for 30 days, it failed to suppress the acute hypersensitivity reaction but produced significant inhibition of the late-phase hypersensitivity response.

*Pharmacokinetics:* In horses, the half-life is only 23 minutes, and oral absorption has been 45% (average) but variable and inconsistent. Pentoxifylline undergoes extensive hepatic metabolism in dogs, and systemic availability after oral administration is 50% but can also be highly variable and inconsistent. In other studies in dogs, the oral absorption was only 20%–30% with a short elimination half-life (less than 1 hour). Several metabolites are produced in animals, with some being biologically active.

## Indications and Clinical Uses

Most of pentoxifylline's use in animals (including doses) is based on anecdotal experience, small observational studies, or recommendations from clinical experts.

Pentoxifylline is used in dogs for some dermatoses, vasculitis, contact allergy, atopy, familial canine dermatomyositis, to improve survival of skin flaps, to improve healing from radiation injury, and erythema multiforme.

In horses, pentoxifylline is used for a variety of conditions in which suppression of inflammatory cytokines or increased blood perfusion is desired. Such conditions have included intestinal ischemia, colic, sepsis, laminitis, and navicular disease. However, the efficacy for treating these diseases has not been shown. In experimental studies of sepsis in horses, it has improved efficacy of treatment and reduced inflammatory mediators when combined with an NSAID (flunixin).

## Precautionary Information

### Adverse Reactions and Side Effects

Pentoxifylline may cause effects similar to those of other methylxanthines, such as nausea, vomiting, and diarrhea. Nausea, vomiting, dizziness, and headache have been reported in people. Vomiting is reported in dogs. Broken tablets taste unpleasant when administered to cats. If crushed tablets are used, plasma concentration increases more rapidly than with intact tablets, leading to headaches, nausea, and possible vomiting. In horses, IV doses have caused muscle fasciculations, increased heart rate, and sweating.

### Contraindications and Precautions

None reported. Broken tablets taste unpleasant when administered to cats.

### Drug Interactions

No drug interactions are reported. However, because pentoxifylline is from the methylxanthine class, adverse reactions are possible from coadministration with a cytochrome P450 inhibitor (see Appendix I).

## Instructions for Use

Although pharmacokinetic studies in dogs and horses have been reported, results of clinical studies in animals have been more limited. The doses listed in the dosing section (recommended by experts) may need to be increased based on pharmacokinetic studies that show a short half-life in dogs. For example, the most effective dosage may be as high as 30 mg/kg q8–12h in dogs to achieve effective levels. Indications for dermatology have used a regimen of q12h, but a frequency of q8h may be considered to get an optimum response in some patients.

## Patient Monitoring and Laboratory Tests

No specific monitoring is necessary.

## Formulations

• Pentoxifylline is available in 400-mg tablets. IV solution is 50 mg/mL.

## Stability and Storage

Store in a tightly sealed container, protected from light, and at room temperature. Aqueous solubility is only 77 mg/mL, which limits the amount that can be dissolved in compounded preparations. Oral suspensions may be stable for up to 90 days, but they settle, requiring resuspension (shaking) before oral administration.

## Small Animal Dosage

### Dogs

• Dermatologic use: 10 mg/kg q12h PO, up to 15 mg/kg q8h PO.
• Familial canine dermatomyositis: 25 mg/kg q12h PO.
• Other uses: 10–15 mg/kg q8 PO or 400 mg/dog for most animals.

### Cats
- One fourth of a 400-mg tablet per cat (100 mg) q8–12h PO.

### Large Animal Dosage
#### Horses
- 8.5 mg/kg q8h IV or 10 mg/kg q8h PO (oral absorption is unpredictable).
- Respiratory disease (airway obstruction): 36 mg/kg q12h PO.

### Regulatory Information
Withdrawal times are not established for animals that produce food. For extralabel use withdrawal interval estimates, contact FARAD at www.FARAD.org.

RCI Classification: 4

## Pergolide, Pergolide Mesylate
per′goe-lide

**Trade and other names:** Prascend (equine formulation) and Permax

**Functional classification:** Dopamine agonist

## Pharmacology and Mechanism of Action
Pergolide is used to treat pituitary pars intermedia dysfunction (PPID) in horses, sometimes referred to as "equine Cushing syndrome." Pergolide is a dopaminergic agonist that stimulates postsynaptic dopamine receptors ($D_1$ and $D_2$ receptors). It is a synthetic ergot derivative. In horses with PPID, pergolide stimulates dopamine receptors, resulting in decreased release of adrenocorticotropic hormone (ACTH), melanocyte-stimulating hormone, and other pro-opiomelanocortin peptides. It is capable of stimulating dopamine receptors in conditions in which dopamine is deficient, regardless of the state of the presynaptic dopamine stores. Other drugs that may share similar effects are selegiline, apomorphine, and lisuride (previously called lysuride).

*Pharmacokinetics:* The pharmacokinetics have been variable, with the manufacturer listing the half-life of 5.9 hours, but other reports listed the half-life as 27 hours. In an IV study in horses, the half-life was 5.6 hours, the mean apparent oral clearance was 1204 mL/kg/h, and the mean apparent volume of distribution was 3082 ± 1354 mL/kg. It has been rapidly absorbed from oral administration. It is rarely used in other animals, and the pharmacokinetics have not been studied in animals other than horses.

## Indications and Clinical Uses
In people, pergolide has been used for neurodegenerative disease in which dopamine is deficient, such as Parkinson disease. For these indications, pergolide is used with levodopa or carbidopa. However, pergolide has been commercially unavailable for humans, and human use has diminished because of reports of cardiac valve damage associated with pergolide.

In animals, specifically horses, it is also has been used for dopamine-deficient states. It is believed that horses and some dogs develop hyperadrenocorticism (Cushing disease)—pituitary-dependent hyperadrenocorticism (PDH)—because of a loss of dopamine antagonism of ACTH release.

In horses, there is clinical evidence that it has successfully controlled PPID (equine Cushing syndrome). It has been used horses for longer than 2 years with success. Most horses with PPID have hyperplasia or adenoma of the pars intermedia of the pituitary. This adenoma is deficient in dopamine and produces excess ACTH. Therefore, administration of dopamine agonists acts to suppress ACTH release from the pituitary and subsequently restore cortisol levels to normal states. Although pergolide is effective for controlling PPID in horses, it does not prevent laminitis in horses with PPID.

The benefits of pergolide administration have not been established for dogs or other animals. Because of the adverse effects produced and the availability of other medications (e.g., trilostane, mitotane), pergolide is not used for treating PDH in dogs.

## Precautionary Information

### Adverse Reactions and Side Effects

Pergolide is FDA approved for use in horses and has been evaluated for safety. In field trials, decreased appetite occurred but was usually transient. Weight loss, anorexia, diarrhea, colic, lethargy, and behavioral changes have been observed in some horses. CNS effects may include ataxia and dyskinesia. Worsening of laminitis from pergolide (it is theoretically a vasoconstrictive drug) has not been proved.

Because some horses may have decreased appetite with pergolide, one can start treatment with a lower dose (half the dose) for the first 2 days in these horses before starting the full dose. Pergolide was withdrawn from the human market because of evidence that drugs that activate the 2b-serotonin receptor ($5\text{-}HT_{2b}$) are associated with a distinct form of fibrotic damage to heart valves (valvulopathy). These effects have not been observed in animals.

Pergolide inhibits secretion of prolactin and increases growth hormone. It may inhibit lactation. In dogs, at doses of 100 mcg/kg, it produces significant reactions, including vomiting, tremors, anorexia, restlessness, and diarrhea.

### Contraindications and Precautions

Unlike bromocriptine, pergolide can be used in pregnant animals, but pregnant women or lactating women should avoid exposure. If tablets are broken or crushed, pergolide tablets may cause eye irritation, an irritating smell, or headache. Women in particular should avoid human exposure and skin contact when preparing tablets for horses.

### Drug Interactions

Pergolide may interact with droperidol and phenothiazines (e.g., acepromazine), and it exacerbates the effects of selegiline. Do not administer with MAOIs.

## Instructions for Use

Use in horses is often accomplished by starting with the low dose listed for 4–6 weeks and gradually increasing the dose until the desired results are obtained. Adjust the dose based on clinical response and dexamethasone suppression test or ACTH measurement. It may be possible to obtain better efficacy when pergolide is used concurrently with cyproheptadine, but ordinarily it is used alone. When treating horses, consider supplementing their diet with magnesium and chromium to avoid deficiencies in these nutrients.

## Patient Monitoring and Laboratory Tests

To monitor the clinical response in horses, observe water consumption, hair shedding, and evidence of laminitis. Adjust doses in horses by monitoring ACTH levels in animals to document pituitary function. In horses, endogenous ACTH concentrations that exceed 27–50 pcg/mL are considered abnormal. Dexamethasone suppression tests can also be performed to monitor treatment in horses. See Dexamethasone for the procedure to perform this test. If signs of excessive dosing are observed, decrease the dose by half for 3–5 days and then slowly increase in 2-mcg/kg increments every 2 weeks until the desired effect is observed.

## Formulations
• Pergolide is available for horses in 1-mg tablets. Compounded formulations should not be used because it was shown that these degrade after 14 days.

## Stability and Storage
Degradation of tablets is accelerated by light and warm temperatures. A color change in the formulation is an indication that degradation has occurred.

Store in a tightly sealed container, protected from light. The stability of compounded formulations is limited, and use of compounded formulations is discouraged.

## Small Animal Dosage
• Small animal dosages have not been established but have been extrapolated from human use, which is to start with 1 mcg/kg (0.001 mg/kg) daily PO and increase the dose gradually by 2 mcg/kg at a time until desired effects are observed.

## Large Animal Dosage
### Horses
• Starting dosage: 0.002 mg/kg (2 mcg/kg) q24h PO (1 mg/day for 500-kg horse). After the starting dose, the dosage may be adjusted as needed (e.g., by 1-mcg/kg increments) to effect, up to 4 mcg/kg daily, although a dosage of 10 mcg/kg per day has been used in some horses.

## Regulatory Information
Do not administer to animals intended for food.

# Phenobarbital, Phenobarbital Sodium
fee-noe-bar'bih-tahl and fee-noe-bar'bih-tahl soe'dee-um

**Trade and other names:** Luminal, Phenobarbitone, and generic brands

**Functional classification:** Anticonvulsant

## Pharmacology and Mechanism of Action
Phenobarbital is a long-acting barbiturate that is used primarily as an anticonvulsant. Phenobarbital has actions similar to those of other barbiturates on the CNS. However, phenobarbital produces anticonvulsant effects without significant other barbiturate effects, such as sedation and anesthesia. As an anticonvulsant, it stabilizes neurons by increased chloride conductance via gamma-aminobutyric acid (GABA)–mediated channels.

*Pharmacokinetics:* The pharmacokinetics have been studied in several animal species. Oral absorption is high in most animals. In dogs, the pharmacokinetics are complicated. The half-life is approximately 66 hours after a single dose (average from multiple studies) but 36 hours after multiple doses because of enzyme induction. The shorter half-life from multiple doses is attributed to enzyme induction and increased clearance, which occurs after 5–7 days of dosing. Many dogs may show a 100%, or greater, increase in clearance with multiple doses, although the magnitude of increase can be highly variable.

In cats, the half-life ranges from 35–56 hours (average, 43 hours) and 59–76 hours, depending on the study. In horses, the half-life is approximately 18–24 hours but 11 hours after multiple doses. In foals, the half-life is 13 hours. These values for horses indicate a more rapid clearance than in other species.

## Indications and Clinical Uses

Phenobarbital is widely used as a drug of choice for treating seizure disorders, such as idiopathic epilepsy, in dogs, cats, horses, and exotic animals. Phenobarbital has been used in foals for treating seizures associated with perinatal encephalopathy. Phenobarbital also has been used as a sedative and for the treatment of behavior disorders. Phenobarbital has been effective for the treatment of sialadenosis in dogs caused by submandibular salivary gland enlargement.

## Precautionary Information

### Adverse Reactions and Side Effects

Most adverse effects are dose related. Phenobarbital causes polyphagia, sedation, ataxia, and lethargy. Some tolerance develops to side effects after initial therapy. Liver enzyme elevations, particularly alkaline phosphatase (ALP), are common but may not be associated with liver pathology unless other changes are observed, such as other enzyme or bilirubin elevations. However, hepatotoxicity also has been reported in some dogs and is more likely with high doses. Neutropenia, anemia, and thrombocytopenia have been associated with phenobarbital therapy in dogs. These reactions are likely to be idiosyncratic, and recovery may occur if phenobarbital is discontinued. Combinations of phenobarbital and potassium bromide have increased the risk of pancreatitis in dogs through an unknown mechanism. In dogs, superficial necrolytic dermatitis has been associated with phenobarbital administration without concurrent liver pathology. Affected dogs may have high serum concentrations of phenobarbital.

### Contraindications and Precautions

Administer with caution to animals with liver disease. Phenobarbital may induce its own metabolism, which shortens the half-life. Therefore chronic administration may lower plasma concentrations, resulting in increases in the dose requirement. Pregnant animals may have an increase in seizure frequency, and an increase in dose may be necessary.

### Drug Interactions

Phenobarbital is one of the most potent drugs for inducing hepatic microsomal metabolizing enzymes. Therefore, many drugs administered concurrently have lower (and perhaps subtherapeutic) concentrations because of more rapid clearance. Drugs affected may include theophylline, digoxin and other cardiovascular drugs, corticosteroids, anesthetics, and other drugs that may be substrates for the P-450 enzymes. Phenobarbital shortens the half-life of levetiracetam (Keppra) in dogs, which may require higher doses or more frequent administration of levetiracetam. Administration of phenobarbital may lower total tetraiodothyronine ($T_4$) thyroid concentrations, but thyroid-stimulating hormone (TSH) and triiodothyronine ($T_3$) concentrations are unaffected.

The solutions for injection are alkaline (pH, 9–11); therefore avoid mixing with acidic solutions or drugs that become unstable at alkaline pH.

Diet and dietary supplements can affect phenobarbital pharmacokinetics. Low-fat diets increase clearance. Alkaline urine increases renal clearance and shortens half-life. A diet or supplement that produces alkaline urine (e.g., potassium citrate) produces a more rapid clearance and shorter half-life for phenobarbital.

## Instructions for Use

Adjust dose based on blood levels of phenobarbital, which can be measured in most laboratories. If bromide is used concurrently (sodium or potassium bromide), lower doses of phenobarbital may be used.

Transdermal administration has been examined in cats. Therapeutic concentrations have been achieved if high doses are administered (9 mg/kg q12h) of the PLO gel or Lipoderm transdermal formulation. However, monitoring is suggested because phenobarbital serum concentrations in these cats can be highly variable.

## Patient Monitoring and Laboratory Tests

Phenobarbital doses should be carefully adjusted via monitoring serum/plasma concentrations. Collect a sample at any time during the dose interval because the timing of the sample is not critical. Avoid the use of plasma separation devices if the tube is to be stored (these devices cause a false lowering of concentrations). The therapeutic range in dogs is considered 15–40 mcg/mL (65–180 mmol/L). If dogs are also receiving bromide, phenobarbital concentrations in the range of 10–36 mcg/mL have been considered therapeutic.

To convert from mmol/L to mcg/mL, use a multiplication factor of 0.232. To convert from mcg/mL to mmol/L, multiply by 4.3.

In cats, the optimum range for therapeutic effect has been reported as 23–28 mcg/mL (99–120 mmol/L) or 15–45 mcg/mL and in another study was 28–31 mcg/mL.

In horses, the optimum range for therapeutic effect is 15–20 mcg/mL (65–86 mmol/L).

Monitor liver enzymes periodically in animals receiving phenobarbital because of risk of hepatopathy. However, some liver enzyme elevations may occur, especially with ALP, without liver pathology. Other liver tests may be needed to rule out hepatotoxicity. Liver enzymes usually return to baseline levels 1–5 weeks after discontinuing treatment. Phenobarbital can increase serum triglycerides because of delayed clearance of chylomicrons from the blood and decreased lipoprotein lipase activity.

Monitor CBC periodically in animals treated with phenobarbital because of risk of neutropenia, anemia, and thrombocytopenia. Phenobarbital administration will lower other drug concentrations. Phenobarbital did not interfere with the ACTH stimulation test or low-dose dexamethasone suppression test in dogs. It lowers thyroid $T_4$ and free $T_4$ but not $T_3$ and TSH concentrations in dogs.

## Formulations

- Phenobarbital is available in 15-, 30-, 60-, and 100-mg tablets; 30-, 60-, 65-, and 130-mg/mL injection; and 4-mg/mL oral elixir solution.

### Compounded Formulations

- Because of the bitter taste and alcohol content from the elixir oral liquid formulation, it has been compounded in other vehicles for patients. To prepare this formulation, crush ten 60-mg tablets (600 mg total) and mix with 60 mL Ora Plus and Ora Sweet in a 1:1 ratio for a final concentration of 10 mg/mL. This formulation was stable for 115 days when stored in amber plastic bottles at room temperature.
- Phenobarbital has been compounded into transdermal formulations for cats. The most common transdermal formulation prepared by pharmacies for cats is a 250 mg/mL formulation prepared in a Lipoderm vehicle (a proprietary lipophilic liposomal cream). Prepared in this vehicle, phenobarbital maintained pharmaceutical strength for 8 weeks. The doses for transdermal compounded formulations are listed in the dosing section.

## Stability and Storage

Store in a tightly sealed container, protected from light, and at room temperature. Phenobarbital is slightly soluble in water (100 mg/mL), but phenobarbital sodium is more soluble (1 g/mL). Solutions prepared in water have an alkaline pH (9–11). Precipitation may occur at lower pH values (avoid mixing with acidic syrups or flavorings). It is subject to hydrolysis in aqueous solutions. However, if prepared in propylene glycol, it is stable for 56 weeks. Stability of compounded formulation is described in the Formulations section.

## Small Animal Dosage
### Dogs
- 2–8 mg/kg q12h PO.
- Status epilepticus: Administer in increments of 10–20 mg/kg IV to effect.

### Cats
- 2–4 mg/kg q12h PO. Start with 1–2 mg/kg initially to avoid adverse effects and gradually increase dose.
- Status epilepticus: Administer in increments of 10–20 mg/kg IV to effect.
- Transdermal compounded formulation: 9 mg/kg q12h of the PLO gel or Lipoderm transdermal formulation. Serum concentrations may be more variable with transdermal application; therefore, adjust doses as needed to maintain serum concentrations within the recommended range.

## Large Animal Dosage
### Horses
- 12 mg/kg q24h PO. Note that in some horses, after initial therapy, higher doses of 12 mg/kg q12h may be needed.
- 5–20 mg/kg IV over 30 minutes (may be diluted in sodium chloride).
- Foals: 2–5 mg/kg IV administered slowly over 20 minutes. Start with lower dose and monitor for effect.

## Regulatory Information
Withdrawal times are not established for animals that produce food. For extralabel use withdrawal interval estimates, contact FARAD at www.FARAD.org.
Schedule IV controlled drug.
RCI Classification: 2

P

# Phenoxybenzamine Hydrochloride
fen-oks-ih-ben′zah-meen hye-droe-klor′ide

**Trade and other names:** Dibenzyline

**Functional classification:** Vasodilator

## Pharmacology and Mechanism of Action
Phenoxybenzamine is an $alpha_1$-adrenergic antagonist. Phenoxybenzamine binds to and antagonizes $alpha_1$ receptors on smooth muscle, causing relaxation. It tends to form a permanent covalent bond with adrenergic receptors to produce a long-lasting effect. It is a nonselective alpha-receptor ($alpha_1$ and $alpha_2$) antagonist. It affects both $alpha_{1a}$ and $alpha_{1b}$ receptors. It is a potent and long-acting vasodilator. It is rarely used as a vasodilator, except when other animals are refractory to other vasodilators (e.g., animals with pheochromocytoma).

## Indications and Clinical Uses
Phenoxybenzamine is used primarily to treat peripheral vasoconstriction. In some animals, it has been used to relax urethral smooth muscle to facilitate urine flow. Urethral smooth muscle is innervated by $alpha_1$ adrenergic receptors. This property has been used to treat urethral spasm in male cats after urethral blockage.

Phenoxybenzamine also has been used for this purpose to decease recurrence of urethral obstruction in male cats. For example, it has been administered (2 mg per cat) for 2 weeks after treatment of urethral obstruction.

Phenoxybenzamine may be used as a vasodilator when animals have been refractory to other vasodilator drugs. Severe vasoconstriction, such as that observed in cases of pheochromocytoma, have been treated with phenoxybenzamine. See dosing section for protocols in dogs.

Experimentally, phenoxybenzamine has been used to relax vascular smooth muscle in horses for treating laminitis. However, this has not been a common clinical use.

## Precautionary Information

### Adverse Reactions and Side Effects

Phenoxybenzamine causes prolonged hypotension in animals. Signs of excessive hypotension may include rapid heart rate, weakness, and syncope. In horses, phenoxybenzamine has caused diarrhea.

### Contraindications and Precautions

Use carefully in animals with cardiovascular compromise. Do not use in dehydrated animals. Use carefully in animals with low cardiac output.

### Drug Interactions

Phenoxybenzamine is a potent alpha-adrenergic antagonist. It competes with other drugs that act on the alpha receptor. It causes vasodilation and should be used cautiously with drugs that may cause vasodilation or depress the heart.

## Instructions for Use

Results of clinical studies in animals have not been reported. Use in animals (and doses) is based on experience in people or limited experimental experience in animals.

## Patient Monitoring and Laboratory Tests

Phenoxybenzamine can lower blood pressure significantly. Monitor the patient's blood pressure and heart rate if possible during treatment.

## Formulations

Phenoxybenzamine is available in 10-mg capsules. Smaller-sized tablets for cats have been prepared by compounding pharmacies for the purpose of treating male cats after urethral obstruction.

## Stability and Storage

Phenoxybenzamine is only slightly soluble in water but soluble in propylene glycol and ethanol. It is not stable in aqueous solutions and undergoes rapid degradation; therefore, it may not be stable in some compounded formulations. Store in a tightly sealed container, protected from light, and at room temperature.

## Small Animal Dosage

### Dogs
- 0.25 mg/kg q8–12h or 0.5 mg/kg q24h PO.
- For presurgical treatment of pheochromocytoma: 0.6 mg/kg q12h (range is 1–2 mg/kg/day), given 2 weeks prior to surgery to stabilize blood pressure.

### Cats
- 2 or 2.5 mg per cat q8–12h or 0.5 mg/kg q12h PO. Doses as high as 0.5 mg/kg IV have been used to relax urethral smooth muscle.

## Large Animal Dosage

**Horses**

- 1 mg/kg q24h IV or 0.7 mg/kg q6h PO.

### Regulatory Information

Withdrawal times are not established for animals that produce food. For extralabel use withdrawal interval estimates, contact FARAD at www.FARAD.org.

RCI Classification: 3

# Phentolamine Mesylate

fen-tole'ah-meen mess'ih-late

**Trade and other names:** Regitine and Rogitine (in Canada)

**Functional classification:** Vasodilator

## Pharmacology and Mechanism of Action

Phentolamine is a nonselective alpha-adrenergic blocker. It is a potent vasodilator but not used often clinically. Phentolamine blocks both $alpha_1$ and $alpha_2$ receptors on smooth muscle.

## Indications and Clinical Uses

Phentolamine is a potent vasodilator and is used primarily to treat acute hypertension. It is most useful in hypertensive emergencies but not used as often as phenoxybenzamine.

## Precautionary Information

**Adverse Reactions and Side Effects**

Phentolamine may cause excess hypotension with high doses or in animals that are dehydrated and may cause tachycardia.

**Contraindications and Precautions**

Use carefully in animals with cardiovascular compromise. Do not use in dehydrated animals. Use carefully in animals with low cardiac output.

**Drug Interactions**

Phentolamine is an alpha-adrenergic antagonist. It competes with other drugs that act on the alpha receptor. It causes vasodilation and should be used cautiously with drugs that may cause vasodilation or depress the heart.

## Instructions for Use

Results of clinical studies in animals have not been reported. Use in animals (and doses) is based on experience in people or anecdotal experience in animals. Titrate dose for each patient to produce desired vasodilation.

## Patient Monitoring and Laboratory Tests

Phentolamine can lower blood pressure significantly. Monitor the patient's blood pressure and heart rate if possible during treatment.

P

## Formulations

Phentolamine has been available in 5-mg vials for injection but in the United States may only be available as a bulk powder that must be compounded into a solution.

## Stability and Storage

Store in a tightly sealed container, protected from light, and at room temperature.

## Small Animal Dosage

**Dogs and Cats**

• 0.02–0.1 mg/kg IV.

## Large Animal Dosage

• No doses have been reported for large animals.

## Regulatory Information

Withdrawal times are not established for animals that produce food. For extralabel use withdrawal interval estimates, contact FARAD at www.FARAD.org.

RCI Classification: 3

# Phenylbutazone
fen-ill-byoo′tah-zone

**Trade and other names:** Butazolidin, PBZ, "Bute," and generic brands

**Functional classification:** Nonsteroidal anti-inflammatory drug

## Pharmacology and Mechanism of Action

Phenylbutazone is the most widely used NSAID used in horses. It is also used occasionally in other animals. Phenylbutazone, like other NSAIDs, produces analgesic and anti-inflammatory effects by inhibiting the synthesis of prostaglandins. The enzyme inhibited by NSAIDs is the cyclooxygenase (COX) enzyme. The COX enzyme exists in two isoforms: COX-1 and COX-2. COX-1 is primarily responsible for synthesis of prostaglandins important for maintaining a healthy GI tract, renal function, platelet function, and other normal functions. COX-2 is induced and responsible for synthesizing prostaglandins that are important mediators of pain, inflammation, and fever. However, it is known that there is some crossover of COX-1 and COX-2 effects in some situations, and COX-2 activity is important for some biological effects. Phenylbutazone, using in vitro assays, is a nonselective inhibitor of COX-1 and COX-2.

*Pharmacokinetics:* The pharmacokinetics have been extensively studied in horses. It has a half-life of 42–65 days in cattle, 4–6 hours in horses, and 4–6 hours in dogs. It is highly absorbed orally in horses, although feed will often delay the peak oral absorption.

## Indications and Clinical Uses

Many equine experts believe that phenylbutazone is the most cost-effective treatment for osteoarthritis in horses. The major use of phenylbutazone is in horses for musculoskeletal pain and inflammation, arthritis, soft tissue injury, and racing injuries. The duration of action in horses after a single administration to horses is approximately 24 hours.

Phenylbutazone is approved for use in dogs (and cats in Europe); however, the use in small animals is not common because of the availability of other drugs.

## Precautionary Information

### Adverse Reactions and Side Effects

Although adverse effects have been documented in horses, after more than 30 years of experience, most equine clinicians have observed good safety with phenylbutazone. Earlier studies that demonstrated common adverse effects may have been exaggerated because the studies were performed in ponies, which is a breed more sensitive than horses, or high doses were used. Likewise, draft horses appear to be more sensitive to adverse effects.

Among the adverse effects in horses are GI ulcers, which may be more likely to appear in the glandular region of the equine stomach. Gastric ulcers are more likely as the dose increases and in animals undergoing extensive training. Horses may also develop right dorsal colitis and hypoproteinemia, especially at high doses.

Phenylbutazone also has been associated with kidney injury. In horses that are dehydrated or have renal compromise, phenylbutazone can cause ischemia and renal papillary necrosis. Renal injury is not common in otherwise healthy horses that are well hydrated. In experimental horses, phenylbutazone (4.4 mg/kg q12h for 14 days) decreased proteoglycan synthesis in articular cartilage. However, this effect on articular cartilage with clinical use has not been a documented problem.

Phenylbutazone is rarely used in people because it has caused bone marrow depression, including aplastic anemia. This effect also has been observed in animals.

Phenylbutazone is generally well tolerated in dogs, but there are no data for cats. In these animals, adverse effects possible are GI toxicity such as gastritis and gastric ulcers.

### Contraindications and Precautions

Do not administer injectable formulation intramuscularly. Do not administer to animals prone to GI ulcers or to animals with kidney disease that may become dehydrated. Do not administer with other ulcerogenic drugs, such as corticosteroids.

### Drug Interactions

The use with other NSAIDs or with corticosteroids should be done cautiously because of the risk of GI injury. Phenylbutazone has been used in some horses in combination with flunixin meglumine (NSAID "stacking"), but this combination may increase risk of hypoalbuminemia and decreased total serum protein. Phenylbutazone interferes with the action of furosemide in horses.

## Instructions for Use

The doses administered are based primarily on manufacturer's recommendations and many years of clinical experience in horses. Although a range of 4.4–8.8 mg/kg per day has been administered to horses, studies have not shown an advantage for the higher dose. The high dosage of 8.8 mg/kg per day is more likely to cause GI injury, hypoalbuminemia, and neutropenia. Generally, a safe starting dose in horses is 4.4 mg/kg q12h IV or PO for 2–3 days. This dose is equivalent to 2 g PO in most horses. Then the dosage should be tapered to 2.2–3.3 mg/kg q12h PO (approximately 1 g per horse). For long-term use, 2.2 mg/kg once daily can be used. Combining other NSAIDs with phenylbutazone, such as flunixin (referred to as "stacking"), may improve response when treating lameness and other musculoskeletal problems compared with phenylbutazone alone. However, this practice must be weighed against an increased risk of GI injury.

## Patient Monitoring and Laboratory Tests
Monitor CBC for signs of bone marrow toxicity with chronic use.

## Formulations
- Phenylbutazone is available in 100-mg, 200-mg, 400-mg and 1-g tablets (bolus); oral paste for horses; and 200-mg/mL (20%) solution for injection.

## Stability and Storage
Store in a tightly sealed container, protected from light, and at room temperature. Phenylbutazone is not water soluble. It should not be compounded in aqueous vehicles.

## Small Animal Dosage
### Dogs
- 15–22 mg/kg q8–12h (44 mg/kg/day; 800 mg/dog maximum) PO or IV.

### Cats
- 6–8 mg/kg q12h IV or PO.

## Large Animal Dosage
### Horses
- 4.4–8.8 mg/kg/day (generally 2–4 g per horse) PO. Typically, a dose of 4.4 mg/kg is administered q12h for the first 2–3 days followed by a tapering dose to 2.2 mg/kg q12h (1 g per horse) and eventually once daily. It is not recommended to use the highest dose for more than 48–96 hours.
- Injection: 2.2–4.4 mg/kg/day for 48–96 hours. Give injections intravenously only because IM injections cause tissue irritation.

### Cattle
- 17–25 mg/kg loading dose; then 2.5–5 mg/kg q24h or 10–14 mg/kg q48h PO or IV. (See Regulatory Information in cattle.)

### Pigs
- 4 mg/kg q24h IV.

## Regulatory Information
Phenylbutazone is prohibited from use in female dairy cattle younger than 20 months of age. Although FDA-approved withdrawal times have not been established for animals intended for food, recommended withdrawal times are 15 days in swine and 40–50 days for slaughter in cattle (PO or IV) and are extended to 55 days in cattle if administered intramuscularly.

Residue information for horses: Although it is possible that phenylbutazone residues can occur in horses slaughtered for food, in jurisdictions where horses are slaughtered for food, the risk to human health is very low. Most experts do not regard this as a public health issue.

# Phenylephrine Hydrochloride
fen-ill-ef′rin hye-droe-klor′ide

**Trade and other names:** Neo-Synephrine

**Functional classification:** Vasopressor

## Pharmacology and Mechanism of Action
Phenylephrine is an alpha$_1$-adreneric receptor agonist. It is used infrequently in veterinary medicine, except for topical use. Phenylephrine stimulates alpha$_1$ receptors and causes smooth muscle contraction, primarily in vascular smooth muscle, to cause vasoconstriction. It may be applied topically (e.g., mucous membranes) to constrict superficial blood vessels.

## Indications and Clinical Uses
If administered intravenously, phenylephrine has been used in critical care patients or during anesthesia to increase peripheral resistance and increase blood pressure. However, this use is rare. Phenylephrine is also used more commonly as topical vasoconstrictor (as in nasal decongestants or for ophthalmic use). It has been administered to horses with nephrosplenic entrapment because it causes vasoconstriction, which may produce splenic contraction and correct the entrapment. The success rate in horses with this treatment is 56%–92%. Although the incidence of severe complications from this treatment in horses is low, phenylephrine-associated hemorrhage is possible with this procedure.

## Precautionary Information

### Adverse Reactions and Side Effects
Adverse effects related to excessive stimulation of alpha$_1$ receptors (prolonged peripheral vasoconstriction). Reflex bradycardia may occur. Prolonged topical use may cause tissue inflammation. When used for treatment of nephrosplenic entrapment in horses, the rate of severe complications is low, but it may cause fatal hemorrhagic shock. The risks and benefits must be considered before this treatment is used.

### Contraindications and Precautions
Do not use in animals with compromised cardiovascular status. It causes vasoconstriction and can increases blood pressure.

### Drug Interactions
Phenylephrine potentiates other alpha$_1$ agonists. Use cautiously with alpha$_2$ agonists such as detomidine, dexmedetomidine, or xylazine.

## Instructions for Use
Phenylephrine has a rapid onset and short duration of action.

## Patient Monitoring and Laboratory Tests
When administered intravenously, monitor blood pressure and heart rate.

## Formulations
- Injection: Phenylephrine is available in 10-mg/mL injection.
- Topical: 1% nasal solution and 2.5% and 10% ophthalmic solutions.

## Stability and Storage

Phenylephrine is soluble in water and may be mixed in IV solutions. It is also soluble in ethanol. It is subject to oxidation and turns a darker color in some solutions, especially alkaline solutions. Discard formulations that turn a dark color. Store in a tightly sealed container, protected from light, and at room temperature.

## Small Animal Dosage

### Dogs and Cats
- 10 mcg/kg (0.01 mg/kg) q15min IV as needed or 0.1 mg/kg q15min IM or SQ.
- CRI: 10 mcg/kg (0.01 mg/kg) IV followed by 3 mcg/kg/min IV.

## Large Animal Dosage
- Horses: Dilute 10–20 mg in 500 mL of 0.9% saline solution and infuse over 10–15 minutes or dilute 20 mg in 1000 mL of 0.9% saline and infuse over 10 minutes. Note that this use for nephrosplenic entrapment is controversial because of the potential for adverse effects.

## Regulatory Information

Withdrawal times are not established for animals that produce food. For extralabel use withdrawal interval estimates, contact FARAD at www.FARAD.org.

RCI Classification: 3

# Phenylpropanolamine Hydrochloride
fen-ill-proe-pah-nole′ah-meen hye-droe-klor′ide

**Trade and other names:** PPA, Proin, Proin ER, UriCon, and Propalin (veterinary preparations)

**Functional classification:** Adrenergic agonist

## Pharmacology and Mechanism of Action

Phenylpropanolamine (PPA) is an adrenergic agonist that is used most often to treat urinary incontinence in dogs. PPA is a sympathomimetic and nonselectively acts as an agonist for the alpha-adrenergic and beta-adrenergic receptor. These receptors are found throughout the body, such as on sphincters, blood vessels, smooth muscle, and heart. The most profound effects observed with PPA are on vascular smooth muscle (vasoconstriction) and urethral smooth muscle (increased tone of urethra).

*Pharmacokinetics:* The half-life of the conventional immediate-release formulation in dogs is 4–7 hours, with a duration of effect may be at least 8–12 hours and as long as 24 hours in some animals. Oral absorption is 94% There is also an extended-release (ER) tablet for dogs with a duration of effectiveness of 24 hours. A longer interval of administration between doses may prevent some downregulation of alpha receptors.

## Indications and Clinical Uses

Phenylpropanolamine has been used as a decongestant, as a mild bronchodilator, and to increase tone of the urinary sphincter. Pseudoephedrine and ephedrine are related drugs that produce similar alpha-receptor and beta-receptor effects. The most common use in animals is for treating urinary incontinence. The mechanism for this action appears to be via stimulating receptors on the urethral sphincter. It has also been used to treat priapism (persistent erection) in dogs. Abuse potential and adverse effects have limited the routine use as a decongestant and appetite suppressant in human medicine.

## Precautionary Information

### Adverse Reactions and Side Effects

Adverse effects are attributed to excess stimulation of adrenergic (alpha and beta) receptors. Side effects include tachycardia (or bradycardia), cardiac effects, CNS excitement, restlessness, and appetite suppression. There are reports of adverse effects caused by PPA in people. In particular, it has caused problems with blood pressure and increased risk of strokes. Such a concern should also apply to animals, but there have been no specific reports of these problems in animals. In animals exposed to high doses (accidental ingestion from the flavored canine tablets), it produces agitation, vomiting, mydriasis, tremors, panting and cardiovascular effects. Prognosis is good after accidental exposure if supportive care is provided.

### Contraindications and Precautions

Use cautiously in any animal with cardiovascular disease. For the extended-release (ER) formulations, do not administer to dogs smaller than 4.5 kg because this will produce a dose higher than 4 mg/kg.

Phenylpropanolamine has been abused by people and used as a recreational drug. PPA and a related drug, pseudoephedrine, can be diverted to clandestine laboratories for the manufacture of amphetamines. The Drug Enforcement Administration has issued a notice to inform individuals and businesses handling PPA that this chemical is used in the illicit manufacture of amphetamine. Most of the human preparations have been removed from the market, and the only forms readily available are those marketed for veterinary medicine.

### Drug Interactions

Phenylpropanolamine and other sympathomimetic drugs can cause increased vasoconstriction and changes in heart rate. Use cautiously with other vasoactive drugs and alpha$_2$ agonists such as dexmedetomidine and xylazine. Use cautiously with other drugs that may lower the seizure threshold. Use of inhalant anesthetics with PPA may increase cardiovascular risk. Do not use with TCAs or MAOIs. However, studies in dogs have shown that although selegiline is a MAOI, it can be administered safely with PPA.

## Instructions for Use

Although frequency of administration has been every 8–12 hours with the conventional product for dogs, an interval of q24h in dogs at a dose of 1.5 mg/kg has been just as effective in some dogs. Alternatively, the ER form can be used once-daily.

In some animals, pseudoephedrine has been substituted for PPA with good success, but these tablets are more tightly regulated because of the potential to divert to the manufacture of methamphetamine.

## Patient Monitoring and Laboratory Tests

Monitor heart rate and blood pressure in animals receiving treatment. Animals with urinary incontinence should be checked periodically for presence of UTIs.

## Formulations

- PPA is available in 25-, 50-, and 75-mg flavored tablets; 25-mg vanilla-flavored liquid; and 50-mg scored tablets (veterinary preparations). Human formulations of 15-, 25-, 30-, and 50-mg tablets are no longer available.

- PPA ER tablets are available in tablets of 18-, 38-, 74-, and 145-mg. Do not split or crush the tablets
- Human formulations have been removed from the market.

## Stability and Storage
The stability and potency of compounded formulations has not been evaluated. The ER tablets should not be broken or crushed.

## Small Animal Dosage
### Dogs
- Immediate-release formulation: 1 mg/kg q8h PO. Increase dosage to 1.5–2 mg/kg q8h PO if necessary. In some animals, it may be possible to decrease frequency to q12h or q24h PO.
- ER formulation: 2–4 mg/kg PO once daily.

### Cats
- No dosage has been determined. A dosage of 1 mg/kg q12h PO has been used (extrapolated from the canine use), and the dosage has been adjusted as needed.

## Large Animal Dosage
- No large animal dosage is available.

## Regulatory Information
There are no formulations currently marketed in the United States for human use because of abuse potential and adverse cardiovascular events.
RCI Classification: 3

# Phenytoin, Phenytoin Sodium
fen′ i toyn soe′dee-um

**Trade and other names:** Dilantin

**Functional classification:** Anticonvulsant, antiarrhythmic

## Pharmacology and Mechanism of Action
Phenytoin is an older anticonvulsant agent that is used infrequently in veterinary medicine. Phenytoin depresses nerve conduction via blockade of sodium channels. Phenytoin stabilizes neuronal membranes and limits the spread of neuronal or seizure activity from the focus. It blocks inward movement of sodium and stabilizes excitable tissue. Phenytoin also decreases calcium inward flow during depolarization, thus inhibiting $Ca^{++}$-dependent release of neurotransmitters.

Phenytoin is also classified as a Class I cardiac antiarrhythmic but is not used often for this indication. In cardiac tissue, phenytoin increases the threshold for triggering ventricular arrhythmias. It also decreases conduction velocity and does not shorten the refractory period as much as lidocaine.

*Pharmacokinetics:* The elimination is very rapid in dogs. In horses, the half-life was approximately 12–13 hours, and oral absorption is variable among horses, ranging from 14% to 85%.

## Indications and Clinical Uses
Phenytoin is commonly used as an anticonvulsant in people, but it is not effective in dogs and not used in cats. In dogs, elimination is so rapid that dosing is impractical.

In horses, phenytoin has more uses than in small animals. Phenytoin has been used in horses for ventricular arrhythmias, controlling myotonia, rhabdomyolysis, hyperkalemic periodic paresis, and stringhalt. This use is more common in athletic horses on a racetrack than in other horses and is not related to the anticonvulsant property. Pharmacokinetic studies have shown that oral absorption of phenytoin is highly variable in horses. Because of this variability, it is difficult to maintain consistent plasma concentrations. Monitoring plasma concentrations may be necessary to adjust the dose to maintain an optimum level and prevent adverse effects.

## Precautionary Information

### Adverse Reactions and Side Effects

Adverse effects include sedation, gingival hyperplasia, skin reactions, and CNS toxicity. In horses, at high doses, recumbency and excitement have been observed. Sedation in horses may be an initial sign of high plasma concentrations. Monitoring plasma concentrations in horses can prevent adverse effects.

### Contraindications and Precautions

Do not administer to pregnant animals.

### Drug Interactions

Phenytoin interacts with drugs undergoing hepatic metabolism. Phenytoin is a potent cytochrome P450 enzyme inducer. When used with cytochrome P450 inhibitors, increased levels of phenytoin may occur.

## Instructions for Use

Because of short half-life and poor efficacy in dogs, other anticonvulsants are used as the first choice before phenytoin. Although there are questions of safety in cats and little documented use, there are anecdotal accounts of successful use of phenytoin in cats for some neurologic problems. If used in racing horses, consult with local regulatory authorities for restrictions.

## Patient Monitoring and Laboratory Tests

Therapeutic drug monitoring can be performed; however, therapeutic concentrations have not been established for dogs and cats. In horses, effective plasma concentrations are 5–20 mcg/mL (average, 8.8 mcg/mL). Therapy should be aimed at producing concentrations above 5 mcg/mL in horses.

## Formulations

- Phenytoin is available in 25-mg/mL oral suspension, 30- and 100-mg capsules (sodium salt), 50-mg/mL injection (sodium salt), and 50-mg chewable tablets.

## Stability and Storage

Store protected from light at room temperature. Phenytoin sodium absorbs carbon dioxide and must be kept in a tight container. Phenytoin is practically insoluble in water, but phenytoin sodium has a solubility of 15 mg/mL. It is soluble in ethanol and propylene glycol. The pH of phenytoin is 10–12, and it may not be compatible with acidic solutions. It may precipitate from solution if mixed with solutions at a lower pH. Protect from freezing.

## Small Animal Dosage

### Dogs

- Anticonvulsant: 20–35 mg/kg q8h. (Not recommended.)
- Antiarrhythmic: 30 mg/kg q8h PO or 10 mg/kg IV over 5 minutes.

**Cats**
- Safe and effective dosage has not been established in cats.

## Large Animal Dosage
**Horses**
- Initial bolus of 20 mg/kg q12h PO for four doses followed by 10–15 mg/kg q12h PO. A single IV dose in horses of 7.5–8.8 mg/kg can be used followed by oral maintenance doses.

## Regulatory Information
Withdrawal times are not established for animals that produce food. For extralabel use withdrawal interval estimates, contact FARAD at www.FARAD.org.
RCI Classification: 4

# Physostigmine
fye-zoe-stig′meen

**Trade and other names:** Antilirium

**Functional classification:** Anticholinesterase

## Pharmacology and Mechanism of Action
Physostigmine is a cholinesterase inhibitor that is used to inhibit the cholinesterase enzyme. By inhibiting this enzyme that breaks down acetylcholine, it prolongs the action of acetylcholine at the synapse. The major difference between physostigmine and neostigmine or pyridostigmine is that physostigmine crosses the blood–brain barrier, and the others do not.

## Indications and Clinical Uses
Physostigmine is used as an antidote for anticholinergic intoxication and as a treatment (antidote) for neuromuscular blockade. It has also been used as a treatment of ileus and urinary retention (e.g., postoperative urine retention) by increasing the tone of the bladder smooth muscle.

There are no well-controlled studies to measure the efficacy of physostigmine in animals. The use is based on anecdotal experience and recommendations from clinicians.

## Precautionary Information
### Adverse Reactions and Side Effects
Adverse effects caused by the cholinergic action result from inhibition of cholinesterase. These effects in the GI tract are seen as diarrhea and increased secretions (e.g., increased salivation). Other adverse effects can include miosis, bradycardia, muscle twitching or weakness, and constriction of bronchi and ureters. Adverse effects can be treated with anticholinergic drugs such as atropine.

### Contraindications and Precautions
Do not administer with choline esters such as bethanechol.

### Drug Interactions
Do not administer with other drugs that produce cholinergic effects.

## Instructions for Use

Physostigmine is indicated primarily only for treatment of intoxication. If longer-term or routine systemic use of an anticholinesterase drug is needed, neostigmine and pyridostigmine are used because they have fewer adverse effects. When used, frequency of dose may be increased based on observation of effects.

## Patient Monitoring and Laboratory Tests

Monitor heart rate and rhythm and GI signs.

## Formulations

• Physostigmine is available in a 1-mg/mL injection.

## Stability and Storage

Store in a tightly sealed container, protected from light, and at room temperature.

## Small Animal Dosage

### Dogs and Cats

• 0.02 mg/kg q12h IV.

## Large Animal Dosage

• No doses have been reported for large animals.

## Regulatory Information

Withdrawal times are not established for animals that produce food. For extralabel use withdrawal interval estimates, contact FARAD at www.FARAD.org.

RCI Classification: 3

# Phytonadione
fye-toe-nah-dye'one

**Trade and other names:** AquaMephyton, Mephyton, Veta-K1, vitamin $K_1$, phylloquinone, and phytomenadione

**Functional classification:** Vitamin

## Pharmacology and Mechanism of Action

Phytonadione is a vitamin K supplement. Phytonadione and phytomenadione are synthetic lipid-soluble forms of vitamin $K_1$. (Phytomenadione is the British spelling of phytonadione.) Menadiol is vitamin $K_4$, which is a water-soluble derivative converted in the body to vitamin $K_3$ (menadione).

Vitamin $K_1$ is a fat-soluble vitamin used to treat coagulopathies caused by anticoagulant toxicosis (warfarin or other rodenticides). These anticoagulants deplete vitamin K in the body, which is essential for synthesis of clotting factors. Administration of vitamin K in its various formulations can be used to reverse the effect of anticoagulant toxicity.

## Indications and Clinical Uses

Phytonadione is used to treat coagulopathies caused by anticoagulant toxicosis (warfarin or other rodenticides). In large animals, it is used to treat sweet clover poisoning.

## Precautionary Information

### Adverse Reactions and Side Effects
In people, a rare hypersensitivity-like reaction has been observed after rapid IV injection. Signs resemble anaphylactic shock. These signs also have been observed in animals. To avoid anaphylactic reactions, do not administer intravenously.

### Contraindications and Precautions
Accurate diagnosis to rule out other causes of bleeding is suggested. Other forms of vitamin K may not be as rapidly acting as vitamin $K_1$; therefore consider using a specific preparation. To avoid anaphylactic reactions, do not administer intravenously.

### Drug Interactions
No drug interactions are reported.

## Instructions for Use
Consult the poison control center for a specific protocol if specific rodenticide is identified. Use vitamin $K_1$ for acute therapy of toxicity because it is more highly bioavailable. Administer with food to enhance oral absorption. If an injection is used, it can be diluted in 5% dextrose or 0.9% saline but do not use other solutions. The preferred injectable route is SQ, but IM can also be used. Although vitamin $K_1$ veterinary labels have listed the IV route for administration, these labels have not been approved by the FDA. Therefore avoid IV administration of vitamin $K_1$.

## Patient Monitoring and Laboratory Tests
Monitoring bleeding times in patients is essential for accurate dosing of vitamin $K_1$ preparations and monitoring the response to treatment. When treating long-acting rodenticide poisoning, periodic monitoring of the bleeding times is suggested.

## Formulations
- Phytonadione is available in 5-mg tablets (Mephyton) and 25-mg capsules (Veta-K1).
- Phytonadione (AquaMephyton) is available in a 2- or 10-mg/mL injection.

## Stability and Storage
Store in a tightly sealed container at room temperature. It is light sensitive and should be protected from light. Phytonadione is practically insoluble in water. However, it is soluble in oils and slightly soluble in ethanol. Do not mix with aqueous solutions. If mixed as a suspension for oral use, administer soon after preparation. Do not freeze.

## Small Animal Dosage
### Dogs and Cats
- Treatment of short-acting rodenticides: 1 mg/kg/day for 10–14 days SQ or PO.
- Treatment of long-acting rodenticides: 2.5–5 mg/kg/day for 3–4 weeks IM, SQ, or PO.

### Birds
- 2.5–5 mg/kg q24h.

## Large Animal Dosage
### Cattle, Calves, Horses, Sheep, and Goats
- 0.5–2.5 mg/kg SQ or IM.

## Regulatory Information

Withdrawal times are not established for animals that produce food. It is anticipated that milk and meat withdrawal times will be short. For extralabel use withdrawal interval estimates, contact FARAD at www.FARAD.org.

# Pimobendan
pim-oh-ben′dan

**Trade and other names:** Vetmedin

**Functional classification:** Cardiac inotropic agent

## Pharmacology and Mechanism of Action

Pimobendan is both a positive inotrope and a vasodilator. The vasodilator effects occur via inhibition of PDE III. PDE III is the enzyme that degrades cyclic adenosine monophosphate (cAMP); therefore, its action is to increase intracellular concentrations of cAMP. There may be some inhibition of PDE V in the pulmonary circulation. The inotropic effects of pimobendan are attributed to its action as a calcium sensitizer rather than the PDE inhibition. By acting as a calcium sensitizer, it increases the interaction of troponin C with contractile proteins and acts as an inotropic agent. The benefits in heart failure are caused by both positive inotropic effects and vasodilating properties. Other beneficial effects may include anti-inflammatory activity, increased sensitivity of baroreceptors, increased lusitropy, and decreased platelet aggregation.

*Pharmacokinetics:* The cardiovascular effects occur after 1 hour and persist for 8–12 hours after administration. Pimobendan is absorbed best in an acidic environment. Fluctuating pH conditions in stomach and administration with food may produce inconsistent oral absorption. Pimobendan is metabolized (demethylated) to desmethylpimobendan (DMP), which is an active metabolite with greater effect on PDE III activity. In dogs, the half-life is short, reported as 30 minutes to 1 hour, depending on the study. The oral absorption is 70%.

In cats, pimobendan produces much higher blood concentrations than dogs, and the half-life is almost three times longer than in dogs. Both pimobendan and the metabolite DMP act as calcium sensitizers, but cats are less responsive to DMP than dogs.

## Indications and Clinical Uses

Pimobendan is indicated for use in dogs for treatment of congestive heart failure (CHF). It has been used in dogs with either valvular insufficiency or cardiomyopathy. It is recommended in consensus guidelines for any dog with valvular disease with stage B2 or higher and may delay onset of CHF. In dogs with heart failure caused by valvular disease, it decreased heart rate, decreased left ventricular and left atrial dimensions, reduced heart size, and reduced preload and natriuretic peptide concentrations. In dogs with stage C valvular heart disease, it has improved survival and quality of life. It is considered by many cardiologists as an essential initial treatment for dilated cardiomyopathy in dogs. When used in dogs, it has improved signs of heart failure and increased survival. When used in dogs, it may be administered with diuretics (furosemide), spironolactone, and angiotensin-converting enzyme (ACE) inhibitors. Pimobendan treatment has produced significant improvement compared with placebo in dogs treated with an ACE inhibitor and a diuretic. Pimobendan may be helpful for treating Doberman pinschers, and probably other breeds, with occult (asymptomatic) dilated cardiomyopathy by prolonging the onset of clinical signs, improving survival and overall outcome.

It has not been recommended to administer positive inotropic agents such as pimobendan to cats with hypertrophic cardiomyopathy. However, it has been associated with improvement in clinical signs and longer survival time in cats with heart failure associated with dilated cardiomyopathy as part of a therapeutic regimen that may include other drugs (e.g., furosemide). Although not FDA approved for cats, when administered at 1.25 mg/cat q12h (0.25 mg/kg), it has been well tolerated.

## Precautionary Information

### Adverse Reactions and Side Effects

Pimobendan is potentially arrhythmogenic, but this effect (e.g., atrial fibrillation or ventricular arrhythmias) has been rare and seen primarily in animals with severe underlying cardiac disease. At doses of 0.25–0.5 mg/kg in dogs, pimobendan did not activate the renin–angiotensin–aldosterone system (RAAS), but if furosemide is added to treatment, some activation of the RAAS may occur. At therapeutic doses, there has been negligible effect on platelet aggregation.

### Contraindications and Precautions

Use pimobendan cautiously in animals prone to cardiac arrhythmias. Do not use in animals with obstructive cardiomyopathy or a fixed obstruction of the outflow tract. Compounded formulations will not achieve the same absorption profile in dogs as the proprietary form. There is a critical pH at which the oral absorption is enhanced, and some compounded formulations may lack excipients to attain this effect.

### Drug Interactions

Use cautiously with other PDE inhibitors such as theophylline, pentoxifylline, and sildenafil (Viagra) and related drugs. Sildenafil is a PDE V inhibitor, and theophylline is a PDE IV inhibitor. Pimobendan is insoluble unless in an acidic environment, and it is difficult to mix pimobendan into a solution.

## Instructions for Use

Follow the approved label instruction for use. Evaluate stage of heart failure in animals before use. Consider the addition of other drugs such as ACE inhibitors, spironolactone, furosemide, and digoxin in animals as the severity of the heart disease increases. If furosemide is used concurrently with pimobendan, consider the addition of an ACE inhibitor (e.g., enalapril, benazepril) or aldosterone antagonist (e.g., spironolactone) to inhibit RAAS activation.

## Patient Monitoring and Laboratory Tests

Monitor the patient's heart rate and rhythm during use.

## Formulations

- Pimobendan is available in chewable tablets of 1.25, 2.5, and 5 mg. In Europe, pimobendan is available in 2.5- and 5-mg capsules.

## Stability and Storage

Store in a tightly sealed container, protected from light, and at room temperature. Acidic pH conditions are important for the stability of the formulation and to ensure dissolution.

## Small Animal Dosage

**Dogs**

- 0.25–0.3 mg/kg q12h PO. If administered with an ACE inhibitor, some dogs are managed on 0.125 mg/kg q12h PO.

**Cats**

- 1.25 mg/cat q12h PO (0.1–0.3 mg/kg q12h).

## Large Animal Dosage

- No doses have been reported for large animals.

## Regulatory Information

Do not administer to animals intended for food.

---

# Piperacillin Sodium and Tazobactam
pih′per-ah-sill′in soe′dee-um taze′oh-back-tam

**Trade and other names:** Zosyn and generic; also referred to as "Pip-Taz"

**Functional classification:** Antibacterial, beta-lactam

---

## Pharmacology and Mechanism of Action

Piperacillin is a beta-lactam antibiotic of the acylureidopenicillin class. Like other beta-lactams, piperacillin binds PBPs that weaken or interfere with cell wall formation. After binding to PBPs, the cell wall weakens or undergoes lysis. Like other beta-lactams, this drug acts in a time-dependent manner (i.e., it is more effective when drug concentrations are maintained above the MIC values during the dose interval). Tazobactam is a beta-lactamase inhibitor. When administered in combination with piperacillin, it increases the spectrum to include beta-lactamase–producing strains of gram-negative and gram-positive bacteria.

Compared with other beta-lactam antibiotics, piperacillin–tazobactam has good activity against *Pseudomonas aeruginosa* and bacteria of the Enterobacterales, including some extended spectrum beta-lactamases (ESBL)–producing strains. It also has good activity against streptococci but is not active against methicillin-resistant *Staphylococcus* spp.

*Pharmacokinetics:* Pharmacokinetic data for dogs indicate a half-life of 0.55 hours, a volume of distribution of 0.27 L/kg, and clearance of 5.79 mL/kg/min. Protein binding in dogs is 18%. Because piperacillin has a short half-life in animals and must be given by injection (usually IV), the use is often limited to in-hospital use.

## Indications and Clinical Uses

Piperacillin and tazobactam is one of the most popular IV antibiotics for in-hospital use in people. The use includes septicemia, UTIs, skin, soft tissue, respiratory infections, intra-abdominal infections, and gynecologic infections. Targeted organisms include bacteria of the Enterobacterales (*Escherichia coli*, *Klebsiella pneumoniae*) and *P. aeruginosa*. The activity includes some ESBL-producing strains of the Enterobacterales. The in vitro activity against some gram-negative bacteria is enhanced when administered with an aminoglycoside (e.g., gentamicin or amikacin). The addition of tazobactam further increases the spectrum to include beta-lactamase–producing strains.

In veterinary medicine, other penicillin–beta-lactamase inhibitor combinations have been ampicillin and sulbactam (Unasyn) and ticarcillin and clavulanate. However, ampicillin and sulbactam's spectrum of coverage often does not include many gram-negative bacteria. Ticarcillin and clavulanate (Timentin), once a popular injectable antibiotic in veterinary medicine, is no longer available. Therefore piperacillin and tazobactam is a logical substitute as a penicillin–beta-lactamase inhibitor combination for in-hospital veterinary use.

---

### Precautionary Information

**Adverse Reactions and Side Effects**

Allergy to penicillin is the most common adverse effect. High doses may inhibit platelet function.

**Contraindications and Precautions**

Do not use in patients allergic to penicillin drugs. High doses contribute to the sodium load in a patient.

**Drug Interactions**

Do not mix in vials or syringes with other drugs.

---

### Instructions for Use

Piperacillin is combined with tazobactam (beta-lactamase inhibitor) in Zosyn, which increases the spectrum to include beta-lactamase–producing strains of *Staphylococcus* and gram-negative bacteria. Ticarcillin–clavulanate has a similar spectrum of activity but is no longer available. Piperacillin–tazobactam has a more active spectrum of activity against gram-negative bacteria than ampicillin–sulbactam.

### Patient Monitoring and Laboratory Tests

Susceptibility testing: CLSI breakpoints for susceptible organisms are ≤8/4 mcg/mL (piperacillin/tazobactam).

### Formulations

- Piperacillin and tazobactam are typically in 8:1 ratio of piperacillin:tazobactam. It is available in vials containing 2 g of piperacillin and 0.25 g of tazobactam, 3 g of piperacillin and 0.375 g of tazobactam, or 4 g of piperacillin and 0.5 g of tazobactam. Vials are reconstituted with sterile water, 0.9% saline solution, or 5% dextrose in water and further diluted to desired volume for IV fluid administration.
- Preparation of IV infusion: To prepare the formulation for IV infusion, first remove 10 mL from a 50-mL infusion bag and use this volume to reconstitute a 2.25-g vial. Add the contents back to the 50-mL infusion bag to make a 45-mg/mL solution. Refrigerate it. This solution will expire in 7 days. Alternatively, remove 15 mL from a 100-mL bag and reconstitute a 3.375-g vial. Add the contents back to the infusion bag for a concentration of 33.75 mg/mL. Refrigerate. This expires 7 days after mixing.

### Stability and Storage

Reconstituted solution should be used within 24 hours or 7 days if refrigerated.

### Small Animal Dosage

**Dogs and Cats**

- 50 mg/kg q6h IV or IM. Alternatively, a CRI can be administered by injecting a loading dose of 4 mg/kg (bolus) followed by 3.2 mg/kg/h.

## Large Animal Dosage

- No doses have been reported for large animals, but doses similar to those cited for dogs or extrapolated from human use would likely reach the same targets in horses. Human dose is approximately 50 mg/kg IV, every 6 hours, delivered as a 30-minute infusion.

## Regulatory Information

Withdrawal times are not established for animals that produce food. However, because of rapid elimination, it is anticipated that withdrawal times will be similar to that of other beta-lactams such as ampicillin.

For extralabel use withdrawal interval estimates, contact FARAD at www.FARAD.org.

---

# Piperazine
pih-peer′e-zeen

**Trade and other names:** Pipa-Tabs and generic brands

**Functional classification:** Antiparasitic

## Pharmacology and Mechanism of Action

Piperazine is one of the oldest and still widely used antiparasitic drugs used in animals. Piperazine produces neuromuscular blockade in parasites through selective antagonism of GABA receptors, resulting in opening of chloride channels, hyperpolarization of parasite membrane, and paralysis of worms. Efficacy is limited primarily to roundworms. In horses, it is active against small strongyles and roundworms.

## Indications and Clinical Uses

Piperazine is a common antiparasitic drug and is widely available, even over the counter (OTC). It is used primarily for treatment of roundworm (ascarid) infections in animals.

## Precautionary Information

### Adverse Reactions and Side Effects

Piperazine is remarkably safe in all species but can cause ataxia, muscle tremors, and changes in behavior.

### Contraindications and Precautions

No contraindications in animals. It may be used in all ages.

### Drug Interactions

No drug interactions have been reported in animals.

## Instructions for Use

Piperazine is a widely used antiparasitic drug with a wide margin of safety. It may be used in combination with other antiparasitic drugs.

## Patient Monitoring and Laboratory Tests

No specific monitoring is necessary.

## Formulations

- Piperazine is available in an 860-mg powder; 140-mg capsules; 50- and 250-mg tablets; and 128-, 160-, 170-, 340-, 510-, and 800-mg/mL oral solution.

## Stability and Storage
Store in a tightly sealed container, protected from light, and at room temperature.

## Small Animal Dosage
### Dogs and Cats
- 44–66 mg/kg administered once PO.

## Large Animal Dosage
### Horses and Pigs
- 110 mg/kg PO in the drinking water as the sole water source.
- Oral solution (horses): 30 mL (1 ounce) of 17% piperazine solution administered PO for each 45 kg of body weight.

## Regulatory Information
Withdrawal times are not established for animals that produce food. For extralabel use withdrawal interval estimates, contact FARAD at www.FARAD.org.

# Piroxicam
peer-oks'ih-kam

**Trade and other names:** Feldene and generic brands

**Functional classification:** Nonsteroidal anti-inflammatory drug

## Pharmacology and Mechanism of Action
Piroxicam is an NSAID of the oxicam class. Clinical effects are similar to those of other NSAIDs (see Meloxicam). These drugs have analgesic and anti-inflammatory effects by inhibiting the synthesis of prostaglandins. The enzyme inhibited by NSAIDs is the COX enzyme. The COX enzyme exists in two isoforms: COX-1 and COX-2. COX-1 is primarily responsible for synthesis of prostaglandins important for maintaining a healthy GI tract, renal function, platelet function, and other normal functions. COX-2 is induced and responsible for synthesizing prostaglandins that are important mediators of pain, inflammation, and fever. However, it is known that there is some crossover of COX-1 and COX-2 effects and COX-2 activity is important for some biological effects. Piroxicam, using in vitro assays, is somewhat more selective for COX-2 than COX-1. In animals, it is not certain that the specificity for COX-1 or COX-2 is related to efficacy or safety. Piroxicam also may have some antitumor or tumor-preventative effects and is used in some anticancer protocols.

*Pharmacokinetics:* Piroxicam has a longer half-life than other NSAIDs in dogs, with a half-life of 35–40 hours and near 100% oral absorption. The half-life is shorter in other species, with a half-life in cats of 13 hours and average oral absorption of 89% and a half-life in horses of 3–4 hours.

## Indications and Clinical Uses
Although piroxicam is not FDA-approved for animals, it is has been used extralabel, primarily used to treat pain and inflammation associated with arthritis and other musculoskeletal conditions. It is not used as much for these conditions as other approved NSAIDs for animals. Another use in dogs and cats has been as an adjunct for treating cancer. This use is based on reports of its activity for treating or suppressing some tumors, including transitional cell carcinoma of the bladder,

squamous cell carcinoma, and mammary adenocarcinoma. (This effect is not unique to piroxicam because other NSAIDs also may have antitumor properties.) Piroxicam has been used in combination with cisplatin to treat oral malignant melanoma and oral squamous cell carcinoma in dogs (0.3 mg/kg).

## Precautionary Information

### Adverse Reactions and Side Effects

Elimination of piroxicam is slow. At 0.3 mg/kg q24h PO, adverse reactions have been observed in dogs, and an administration interval of q48h should be considered. Adverse effects are primarily GI toxicity (e.g., gastric ulcers). Renal toxicity also is a risk, especially in animals prone to dehydration or that have compromised renal function. Toxic epidermal necrolysis has been reported in some dogs.

In cats, vomiting is possible during initial treatment for long-term management of some cancers. Long-term treatment was not associated with hematologic, renal, or liver toxicity in cats.

### Contraindications and Precautions

Use cautiously in dogs because the long half-life may increase risk of GI ulcers if administered once daily. The human formulation is too large a dose for most dogs and should be reformulated to avoid overdose. Warn pet owners about overdoses that could produce GI ulceration. Do not administer to animals prone to GI ulcers. Do not administer to pregnant animals. Use cautiously in animals with kidney disease that may be prone to dehydration or if administered with other drugs that may injure the kidney, such as cisplatin.

### Drug Interactions

Do not administer with other NSAIDs or with corticosteroids. Corticosteroids have been shown to exacerbate the GI adverse effects. Some NSAIDs may interfere with the action of diuretic drugs and ACE inhibitors.

## Instructions for Use

Most experience with dosing has been accumulated from studies in which dogs were treated with piroxicam for transitional cell carcinoma of the bladder. Some of these dogs tolerated piroxicam better with respect to GI toxicity if the drug was administered with misoprostol. Piroxicam has also been used in dogs for treatment of squamous cell carcinoma.

## Patient Monitoring and Laboratory Tests

Piroxicam has the potential of inducing GI ulceration. Monitor for signs of vomiting, bleeding, and lethargy. If bleeding is suspected, monitor patient's hematocrit or CBC. Monitor renal function in treated animals.

## Formulations

- Piroxicam is available in 10-mg capsules. Capsules may have to be reformulated to produce oral doses for small animals.

## Stability and Storage

Exposure to light results in photodegradation. Piroxicam is only slightly soluble in water. It is soluble in basic solutions and some organic solvents. Compounded formulations made for small animals may be stable for only 48 hours. Although an IV formulation is not available commercially, a 2-mg/mL solution has been prepared from mixing the pure powder with 0.1 N of NaOH and found to be stable if stored in a glass vial, refrigerated, and protected from light.

## Small Animal Dosage

**Dogs**

- 0.3 mg/kg q48h PO.
- Cancer treatment: 0.3 mg/kg q24h PO initially; then transitioned to q48h.

**Cats**

- 0.3 mg/kg q24h PO. A common dosage is 1 mg per cat q24h PO.

## Large Animal Dosage

There is insufficient evidence to recommend doses for large animals. Single doses of 0.2 mg/kg PO have been administered to horses without any adverse effects.

## Regulatory Information

Withdrawal times are not established for animals that produce food. For extralabel use withdrawal interval estimates, contact FARAD at www.FARAD.org.
RCI Classification: 4

# Plicamycin
plye-kah-mye′sin

**Trade and other names:** Mithracin and mithramycin

**Functional classification:** Anticancer agent

## Pharmacology and Mechanism of Action

Plicamycin is an anticancer agent used infrequently in veterinary medicine. The action of plicamycin is to complex with DNA in the presence of divalent cations and inhibit DNA and RNA synthesis. It lowers serum calcium and may have direct action on osteoclasts to decrease serum calcium.

## Indications and Clinical Uses

Plicamycin is used in cancer protocols for carcinomas and treatment of hypercalcemia. Use in animals has been primarily derived from empirical use. There are no well-controlled clinical studies or efficacy trials to document clinical effectiveness.

## Precautionary Information

### Adverse Reactions and Side Effects

Adverse effects have not been reported in animals. In people, hypocalcemia and GI toxicity have been reported. Plicamycin may cause bleeding problems.

### Contraindications and Precautions

Do not use with drugs that may increase the risk of bleeding (e.g., NSAIDs, heparin, or anticoagulants).

### Drug Interactions

No drug interactions have been reported.

## Instructions for Use

Results of clinical studies in animals have not been reported. Use in animals (and doses) is based on experience in people or anecdotal experience in animals.

## Patient Monitoring and Laboratory Tests
Monitor serum calcium concentrations.

## Formulations
- Plicamycin is available in a 2.5-mg vial for injection and 0.5 mg/mL when diluted.

## Stability and Storage
Store in a tightly sealed container, protected from light, and at room temperature.

## Small Animal Dosage
### Dogs and Cats
- Antihypercalcemic: 25 mcg/kg/day IV (slow infusion) over 4 hours.
- Antineoplastic (dogs): 25–30 mcg/kg/day IV (slow infusion) for 8–10 days.

## Large Animal Dosage
- No doses have been reported for large animals.

## Regulatory Information
Withdrawal times are not established for animals that produce food. This drug should not be used in animals intended for food because it is an anticancer agent.

# Polyethylene Glycol Electrolyte Solution
pahl-ee-eth'ill-een glye'kole

**Trade and other names:** GoLYTELY, PEG, Colyte, and Co-Lav

**Functional classification:** Laxative

## Pharmacology and Mechanism of Action
This solution is a saline cathartic. Polyethylene glycol electrolyte solution is a nonabsorbable compound that increases water secretion into the bowel via osmotic effect. These isosmotic liquids pass through the bowel without absorption. Oral administration produces a profound cathartic effect.

## Indications and Clinical Uses
Polyethylene glycol electrolyte solution is a cathartic that is used primarily for evacuating the bowel and cleansing of the intestine prior to endoscopy and surgical procedures. It is administered orally and induces a rapid osmotic cathartic effect. It is effective for bowel cleansing, but it requires high volumes to be effective. In some human patients, smaller volumes can be used if it is combined with another laxative, such as bisacodyl.

### Precautionary Information
#### Adverse Reactions and Side Effects
Water and electrolyte loss with high doses or prolonged use are common. Large volumes required may cause nausea.

#### Contraindications and Precautions
Do not administer to animals that are dehydrated because it may cause fluid and electrolyte loss. It is not indicated for chronic use.

#### Drug Interactions
No specific drug interactions.

## Instructions for Use

Used for bowel evacuation prior to surgical or diagnostic procedures. Large volumes are required. In human patients, administration of only half the volume can be used if taken with bisacodyl (one to four tablets) 2 hours prior to the procedure. This combination is called HalfLytely.

## Patient Monitoring and Laboratory Tests

Monitor electrolytes if it is administered repeatedly.

## Formulations

- Polyethylene glycol electrolyte is an oral solution. Preparations contain PEG 3350, sodium chloride, potassium chloride, sodium bicarbonate, and sodium sulfate.

## Stability and Storage

Store in a tightly sealed container, protected from light, and at room temperature.

## Small Animal Dosage

**Dogs and Cats**

- 25 mL/kg PO; repeat in 2–4 hours.

## Large Animal Dosage

**Horses and Cattle**

- Via stomach tube: 500 mL to 4 L once PO.

## Regulatory Information

No withdrawal times necessary.

---

# Polymyxin B Sulfate
poly-mix-in bee

**Trade and other names:** Generic

**Functional classification:** Antibacterial agent

## Pharmacology and Mechanism of Action

Polymyxin B is one in the group of polymyxins that is used as an antibacterial agent. Polymyxin B is from a group of polypeptide antibiotics. Polymyxins are basic surface-active cationic detergents that interact with the phospholipid within the cell membrane. They are capable of penetrating the cell membrane of bacteria and disrupting the structure. This action subsequently induces permeability changes within the cell that result in cell death, giving polymyxins bactericidal properties. Polymyxin B is capable of acting as a chelating agent to bind the lipid A portion of endotoxin in a 1:1 ratio to neutralize lipopolysaccharide.

Polymyxins contain seven amino acids in a cyclic configuration and have a molecular weight of more than 1000. Other polymyxins have been named A, B, C, D, E, and M, but only B and E in their sulfate salt forms are used clinically. Polymyxin B sulfate is a mixture of polymyxin B1 and polymyxin B2. Polymyxin E is more commonly known as *colistin*, which is also used systemically for some infections that are resistant to other drugs. Polymyxin B has a pKa ranging from 8–9 derived from the organism *Bacillus polymyxa*. It is available in many topical formulations, often in formulations considered "triple antibiotics." The injectable formulation of polymyxin B sulfate is a sulfate salt of two forms: polymyxins $B_1$ and $B_2$. It is available in formulations of not less than 6000 polymyxin B units per milligram (as the anhydrous base). Polymyxins are not absorbed from the GI tract when administered orally but are rapidly absorbed when given parenterally and have 70%–90% plasma protein binding.

## Indications and Clinical Uses

Polymyxin B for injection is in powder form suitable for preparation of sterile solutions for IM, IV drip, intrathecal, or ophthalmic use. Polymyxin B is most often administered as a topical ointment for managing infections. It is one of the components of "triple antibiotic" ointments used for topical use. Systemically, polymyxin has been used to treat infections that are resistant to other drugs. Bacteria such as *P. aeruginosa* and *Acinetobacter* spp. may develop resistance to other drugs that can be treated only with drugs such as colistin and polymyxin. In people, polymyxin B is used to treat UTI, meningitis, and septicemia. There are no well-controlled clinical studies or efficacy trials to document clinical effectiveness in animals for treating bacterial infections.

In veterinary medicine, particularly horses, polymyxin has been used because of its property to bind to the lipid A portion of bacterial endotoxin in the blood and prevent signs of bacterial septicemia without producing kidney injury. Infusions ranging from 1000 to 10,000 units/kg (a common dose is 6000 units/kg, equivalent to 1 mg/kg) administered q8h. These infusions have been shown to be safe and effective for treating endotoxemia in horses. The action is attributed to the cationic portion of polymyxin B binding to the anionic lipid A portion of this endotoxin. This effectively renders the endotoxin inactive, thereby decreasing adverse effects attributed to gram-negative endotoxin. This effect also has been demonstrated in an experimental model of feline endotoxemia in which it had antiendotoxin effects in vivo.

## Precautionary Information

### Adverse Reactions and Side Effects

Intramuscular injections cause pain. Because of its ability to bind to phospholipid membranes and cause injury, the most severe adverse reaction is caused by renal injury. Kidney injury is a dose-dependent problem caused by increased membrane permeability and influx of cations, anions, and water, causing kidney cell swelling. However, at dosages that have been used for treating endotoxemia (6000 units/kg IV q8h), it has not caused kidney injury in horses. However, at higher doses (18,000–36,000 units/kg) or for longer treatment protocols, renal injury risk increases. Allergic reactions are also possible. At high doses administered intravenously to cats (3 mg/kg and higher), it produced respiratory depression.

### Contraindications and Precautions

Use cautiously, if at all, in patients with renal disease. Animals receiving polymyxin B should receive adequate fluid support to maintain hydration and renal perfusion.

### Drug Interactions

Use cautiously with other potentially nephrotoxic agents such as aminoglycosides. Do not administer with curariform muscle relaxant and other neurotoxic drugs because of risk of respiratory depression. Polymyxin antibacterial activity is decreased in the presence of pus, in tissues containing acidic phospholipids, and in the presence of anionic detergents.

## Instructions for Use

Use in veterinary medicine has been primarily confined to topical use and the use in horses to treat endotoxemia. Doses and regimens have been derived from experimental studies. Routes of administration have been topical IM, IV infusion, intrathecal, or ophthalmic.

## Patient Monitoring and Laboratory Tests

Monitor patient hydration and electrolyte status. Monitor renal parameters (e.g., creatinine and BUN) for evidence of renal disease.

## Formulations

- Polymyxin B is available in vials containing 500,000 polymyxin B units. In some dosage protocols, the dose is listed in milligrams instead of units. One milligram of polymyxin B base is equivalent to 10,000 units of polymyxin B, and each microgram of pure polymyxin B base is equivalent to 10 units of polymyxin B.

## Stability and Storage

Store at room temperature 20°C–25°C (68°F–77°F), protected from light. Polymyxin B is soluble in water at 0.5% solution with a pH of 5–7.5. Aqueous solutions of polymyxin B sulfate have been stored up to 12 months without significant loss of potency if refrigerated. Do not mix with strong acid or alkaline solutions. It is not compatible with calcium or magnesium salts.

## Small Animal Dosage

### Dogs and Cats

- Antibacterial: 15,000–25,000 units/kg q12h IV. To prepare solution, mix 500,000 polymyxin B units with 300–500 mL of 5% dextrose for CRI.
- Antibacterial: 30,000 units/kg/day IM. To prepare solution, mix 500,000 polymyxin B units in 2 mL of sterile water for injection or sodium chloride injection or 1% procaine hydrochloride. IM injections can be painful.
- Antiendotoxin: 1 mg/kg diluted in 10 mL of 0.9% saline solution given as an IV infusion. (See earlier information for converting milligrams to units.)
- Intrathecal (to treat meningitis): Mix 500,000 polymyxin B units in 10 mL of sodium chloride (50,000 units/mL). Administer 20,000 units PO daily intrathecally; then continue 25,000 units once every other day.

## Large Animal Dosage

### Horses

- Endotoxemia: 1000–10,000 units/kg (usually 6000 units/kg, equivalent to approximately 1 mg/kg) administered q8h. The repeat treatments may be necessary if there is ongoing sepsis. The infusion may be mixed in a 1-L saline solution and administered over 15 minutes q8h for five treatments.

## Regulatory Information

Cattle: Withdrawal time after intramammary administration is 7 days for milk and 2 days for meat. Other withdrawal times have not been reported for food animals. For other extralabel use withdrawal interval estimates, contact FARAD at www.FARAD.org.

# Polysulfated Glycosaminoglycan

pahl-ee-sul'fate-ed glye-koe-sah-mee-noe-glye-kan

**Trade and other names:** Adequan Canine, Adequan IA, and Adequan IM

**Functional classification:** Antiarthritic agent

## Pharmacology and Mechanism of Action

Polysulfated glycosaminoglycan (PSGAG) is a joint supplement. It provides large-molecular-weight compounds similar to normal constituents of healthy joints. It is chondroprotective by inhibiting enzymes that may degrade articular cartilage, such as metalloproteinase. It may help to upregulate glycosaminoglycan and collagen synthesis and decrease inflammatory mediators (e.g., $PGE_2$).

## Indications and Clinical Uses

Polysulfated glycosaminoglycan is injected in dogs and horses to treat or prevent degenerative joint disease. This is an FDA-approved product; therefore, there are efficacy and safety studies to support the use for treating osteoarthritis in animals. Intra-articular injections have been effective, but IM doses may be too low to be effective in some animals.

### Precautionary Information

**Adverse Reactions and Side Effects**

Adverse effects are rare. Allergic reactions are possible. PSGAG has heparin-like effects and may elicit bleeding problems in some animals, but this has not been observed clinically.

**Contraindications and Precautions**

Intra-articular injections should be done using aseptic technique only by trained individuals. Use cautiously in animals receiving heparin therapy.

**Drug Interactions**

No drug interactions are reported in animals.

## Instructions for Use

The doses used are supported by the FDA approval for animals. There has also been experience from studies in experimental animals and clinical studies. Although effective for acute arthritis, it may not be as effective for chronic arthropathy. In horses, it is sometimes combined with amikacin (125 mg) for intra-articular use to prevent infection.

## Patient Monitoring and Laboratory Tests

Observe injected joints for signs of infection after treatment.

## Formulations

- PSGAG is available in a 100-mg/mL injection in a 5-mL vial, 100 mg/mL for IM administration, and 250 mg/mL for intra-articular use in horses.

## Stability and Storage

Store in a tightly sealed container, protected from light, and at room temperature.

## Small Animal Dosage

**Dogs**

- 4.4 mg/kg IM, twice weekly for up to 4 weeks.

## Large Animal Dosage

**Horses**

- 500 mg every 4 days IM for 28 days or 250 mg per joint once weekly for 5 weeks intra-articular.

## Regulatory Information

No withdrawal times necessary.

# Ponazuril
poe-naz′yoo-ril

**Trade and other names:** Marquis

**Functional classification:** Antiprotozoal

## Pharmacology and Mechanism of Action

Ponazuril is an antiprotozoal drug used in animals to control infections caused by protozoa. It is also considered a coccidiostat. Ponazuril (also known as toltrazuril sulfone) is a metabolite of the poultry antiprotozoal drug toltrazuril. Ponazuril is a triazine-based drug that acts to inhibit enzyme systems in protozoa or decreasing pyrimidine synthesis. It is specific for apicomplexan organisms because the action attacks the apicoplast organelle in protozoa. This action produces a specific effect as an antiprotozoal agent without affecting other organisms or the treated animal. It is approved for use in horses but also has been used in puppies, kittens, exotic, and zoo animals for treatment of coccidial infections.

*Pharmacokinetics:* Ponazuril has high, but variable, oral absorption in horses. The half-life data for horses has been conflicting with different studies reporting 1.6 days, 2.5 days, and 4.5 days. Ponazuril produces concentrations in cerebrospinal fluid (CSF) of horses that are 3.5% to 4% of serum concentrations but high enough to inhibit protozoa. One week of daily dosing in horses is needed to reach steady-state concentrations. A level of 100 ng/mL is necessary to prevent and treat infections caused by *Sarcocystis neurona*. The half-lives are 2.4 hours in cattle and 5.6 days in pigs.

## Indications and Clinical Uses

Ponazuril is FDA approved for use as a treatment of equine protozoal myeloencephalitis (EPM) caused by *S. neurona*. In clinical studies in horses with EPM, 62% of 101 horses were treated successfully with dosages of 5 or 10 mg/kg for 28 days. Although successful treatment was reported after 28 days, longer treatment duration may be needed in some animals to resolve the infection and prevent relapse.

Toltrazuril, the parent drug, has been used for protozoa such as *Isospora* spp., *Coccidia* spp., *Toxoplasma gondii*, *S. neurona*, and *Eimeria* spp., which also have been considered as treatment targets for ponazuril. There is limited information available on its use in other animals, but it has been used for treating toxoplasmosis in cats, coccidia infections in dogs and cats, and protozoa in other species. The dosage is 50 mg/kg PO once daily for 3 consecutive days for treatment of coccidiosis in dogs and cats. It has been used to treat piglets with diarrhea caused by *Isospora suis*.

### Precautionary Information

**Adverse Reactions and Side Effects**

Ponazuril is highly specific and relatively safe at approved doses. Administration of 50 mg/kg to horses (10 times the recommended dose) produces minor adverse effects. There are minimal changes in the serum analysis. Soft feces may occur at high doses.

**Contraindications and Precautions**

Avoid use in pregnant or breeding mares until more information becomes available on safety.

**Drug Interactions**

No drug interactions have been reported.

## Instructions for Use

Use in horses is based on clinical studies, field trials conducted by the drug sponsor, and pharmacokinetic studies in horses. When ponazuril paste was administered orally to horses mixed with corn oil (2 ounces per dose), there was higher oral absorption and higher concentrations in the CSF (see the following dosing section).

## Patient Monitoring and Laboratory Tests

In horses treated for EPM, monitor neurologic status during treatment. The immunoglobulin G (IgG) and albumin quotient has been measured in CSF of treated horses to monitor treatment, but this may not indicate clinical cure. When treating for coccidia infections in dogs, cats, zoo, and exotic animals, perform a fecal exam (fecal flotation) periodically to be sure that the organism has been eradicated.

## Formulations
- Ponazuril is available in 15% (150-mg/mL) oral paste for horses. One tube contains 127 g or 150 mg/g or approximately 165 mg/mL.
- Compounded formulation: To administer the equine form to small animals, it may be diluted and mixed with water or oral syrup for ease of administration and still maintain stability. One such dilution formulation for small animals is: 50 mL of ponazuril equine paste + 12.5 mL of water + 12.5 mL of syrup for flavor = 75 mL containing 100-mg/mL solution for oral dosing. Or for smaller animals: 20 mL of ponazuril equine paste + 5 mL of water + 5 mL of syrup for flavor = 30 mL of 100-mg/mL solution for oral dosing. When using a compounded version, shake up the formulation prior to administration.

## Stability and Storage
Store in a tightly sealed container, protected from light, and at room temperature.

## Small Animal Dosage
### Cats
- Toxoplasmosis: 50 mg/kg once PO or 20 mg/kg once daily for 2 days PO.
- Coccidiosis: 50 mg/kg once daily for 3 consecutive days.

### Dogs
- Coccidiosis: 50–55 mg/kg once daily PO for 3–5 days.

## Large Animal Dosage
### Horses
- Treatment of EPM: 5 mg/kg q24h PO for 28 days. A loading dose of 15 mg/kg has been used initially (day 1) followed by maintenance daily doses for 28 days. When 50 mL of corn oil (approximately 2 ounces) was administered orally to horses 1–2 minutes prior to the ponazuril paste, there was greater oral absorption and higher concentrations in the CSF.

### Pigs
- 5 mg/kg PO for treatment of *I. suis*.

## Regulatory Information
Recommended withdrawal time for pigs is 33 days. Withdrawal times for other food animals is not available. For extralabel use withdrawal interval estimates, contact FARAD at www.FARAD.org.

---

# Posaconazole
poe-sa-kon′a-zole

**Trade and other names:** Noxafil

**Functional classification:** Antifungal

---

## Pharmacology and Mechanism of Action
Posaconazole is an azole antifungal drug. Posaconazole is a relatively new antifungal and is similar to itraconazole in structure but with greater activity. The mechanism of action against fungi is similar to that of other azoles, which is to inhibit ergosterol synthesis in the fungal cell membrane and produce fungistatic activity. It is active against

dermatophytes, *Histoplasma capsulatum, Blastomyces dermatitidis, Coccidioides immitis,* and *Cryptococcus neoformans.* The difference compared with other azoles is the additional activity against other fungi. The spectrum includes *Fusarium* and *Mucorales* (formerly called *Zygomycetes*), such as *Mucor* and *Rhizopus.* Posaconazole's activity is superior to that of other antifungals against many clinically important organisms. Against many strains tested, it was more active than itraconazole, fluconazole, and amphotericin B. It is active against fluconazole-resistant strains of *Candida* spp., dermatophytes, and other opportunistic fungi and more potent than fluconazole or itraconazole against *Aspergillus* spp. It has a higher safety margin, fewer drug interactions, and a narrower toxicity profile compared with characteristics of other antifungals.

*Pharmacokinetics:* In dogs, the half-life from oral administration of the liquid suspension is 24 hours and from the delayed-release tablet was 41.7 hours. After IV administration, the half-life was 29 hours, with a volume of distribution of 3.3 L/kg. Oral absorption from the liquid suspension was 26% but was much higher and with higher peak concentrations from the oral delayed-release tablet. Plasma protein binding in dogs, as in other species, was greater than 99%. Studies in research cats showed that it had a half-life of approximately 40 hours after oral dosing and oral bioavailability of 16%.

## Indications and Clinical Uses

The use of posaconazole has been limited to a few case reports and anecdotal experience. The doses in dogs and cats are based on pharmacokinetic studies in healthy animals. In cats, it has been used to treat fungal infections such as aspergillosis and *Mucor* infections that were refractory to other drugs. In dogs, it has been used to treat fungal infections that were refractory to other treatments. In humans, it is used for invasive fungal infections, including those caused by *Aspergillus* and *Candida* spp. It is also active against dermatophytes, *H. capsulatum, B. dermatitidis, C. immitis,* and *C. neoformans.* Its advantage over other azole drugs is the activity against *Fusarium* and *Mucorales* (formerly called *Zygomycetes*), such as *Mucor* and *Rhizopus* spp. The only formulations available for systemic use are the human products, except for topical ear products for dogs.

### Precautionary Information

#### Adverse Reactions and Side Effects

The use has been relatively infrequent, and information regarding the full range of adverse effects possible from clinical use is not available. In people, similar adverse effects have been observed as with other azole antifungal drugs: headache, diarrhea, nausea, and increased liver enzymes, but there is some indication that the safety profile may be better for posaconazole than other azoles. In toxicity studies, dogs have tolerated 30 mg/kg/day for 1 year without any clinical signs. However, histologically, some neuronal vacuolation was observed at this dose. It should not be used during pregnancy because of inhibition of steroidogenesis.

#### Contraindications and Precautions

No contraindications and precautions have been reported for animals.

#### Drug Interactions

Drugs that decrease stomach acid (PPIs, $H_2$ blockers) reduce oral absorption of posaconazole. Like other azole antifungal drugs, posaconazole is a strong inhibitor of cytochrome P450 enzymes (CYP3A4) and may increase concentrations of other drugs metabolized by these enzymes.

## Instructions for Use

Use in animals has been based primarily on some isolated case reports and extrapolation from human use. Dosing recommendations are based on pharmacokinetic studies in dogs and cats. No controlled clinical studies for animals have been reported. The oral absorption is enhanced when administered with food; therefore administer with a small meal. The injection can be administered as a loading dose in patients not amenable to oral treatment, but the injection formulation is very expensive.

### Patient Monitoring and Laboratory Tests
Monitor liver enzymes in treated animals. Although plasma concentrations are generally not measured, trough concentrations above 0.5–0.7 mcg/mL for mild infections or 1 mcg/mL for severe invasive infections are associated with efficacy.

### Formulations
• Posaconazole is available in a 40-mg/mL oral suspension, 100-mg delayed-release tablet, and 18-mg/mL injection.

### Stability and Storage
Store in a tightly sealed container, protected from light, and at room temperature.

### Small Animal Dosage
**Dogs**
• Oral suspension: 10 mg/kg PO q24h.
• Oral delayed-release tablet: 5 mg/kg PO, initially administered q48h. In some animals, this interval has been increased to q72h or longer if trough concentrations can be maintained above the level of 0.5 mcg/mL.

**Cats**
• For mild infections or for preventive use, administer 15 mg/kg PO followed by 8 mg/kg PO q48h of the oral liquid suspension. For more severe invasive fungal infections, administer an oral loading dose of 30 mg/kg followed by 15 mg/kg every other day PO.

### Large Animal Dosage
• No doses have been reported.

### Regulatory Information
No regulatory information is available. For extralabel use withdrawal interval estimates, contact FARAD at www.FARAD.org.

## Potassium Chloride
**Trade and other names:** Generic brands
**Functional classification:** Potassium supplement

### Pharmacology and Mechanism of Action
Potassium chloride is a potassium supplement used for treatment of hypokalemia and maintain electrolyte balance in deficient animals. A dose of 1.9 g of potassium chloride is equivalent to 1 g of potassium. One gram of potassium chloride is equal to 14 mEq of potassium. Other potassium supplements include potassium gluconate, potassium acetate, potassium bicarbonate, and potassium citrate, which are described in other sections that follow.

### Indications and Clinical Uses
Potassium supplements are indicated for treating hypokalemia. Hypokalemia may occur with some diseases or as a consequence of diuretic use. Hypokalemia may also

occur as a consequence of beta$_2$-adrenergic agonist overdose. In cattle, potassium deficiency may occur when they are off feed. In cattle, this can be important for conditions such as retained placenta, mastitis, lipidosis, and abomasal displacement.

In most patients, potassium chloride is the supplement of choice for hypokalemia. It is better absorbed than other supplements, and the chloride ion may be helpful because hypochloremia may also occur in some patients.

## Precautionary Information

### Adverse Reactions and Side Effects

Toxicity from high potassium concentrations can be dangerous. Hyperkalemia can lead to cardiovascular toxicity (bradycardia and arrest) and muscular weakness. Oral potassium supplements can cause nausea and stomach irritation. Administration that is too rapid can cause muscle tremors, diarrhea, convulsions, and even death.

### Contraindications and Precautions

Do not exceed a rate of 0.5 mEq/kg/h IV infusion. Use cautiously in animals with kidney disease. Do not use potassium chloride if metabolic acidosis and hyperchloremia are present. Use another potassium supplement instead. IV use should be done cautiously because of a risk of hyperkalemia. Use potassium cautiously in animals that are receiving digoxin for treatment of heart disease. Do not use with potassium penicillin or potassium bromide. (Use sodium salts of these drugs instead.)

### Drug Interactions

Interactions between potassium supplements and the following drugs may occur: digoxin, thiazide diuretics, spironolactone, amphotericin B, corticosteroids, penicillins, ACE inhibitors, and laxatives.

## Instructions for Use

One gram of potassium chloride provides 13.41 mEq of potassium. It is usually added to fluid solutions. When potassium is supplemented in fluids, do not administer at a rate faster than 0.5 mEq/kg/h.

## Patient Monitoring and Laboratory Tests

Monitor serum potassium levels. Monitor electrocardiogram (ECG) in patients that may be prone to arrhythmias. Normal potassium concentrations are 4–5.5 mEq/L (dogs) and 4.3–6.0 mEq/L (cats).

## Formulations

Potassium chloride is available in various concentrations for injection (usually 2 mEq/mL). It is available in an oral suspension and oral solution as 10–20 mEq of potassium per packet. Oral bolus forms are available for cattle, also containing calcium and magnesium. One gram of potassium chloride contains 14 mEq of potassium ion.

## Stability and Storage

Store in a tightly sealed container, protected from light, and at room temperature. Potassium chloride is freely soluble in water.

## Small Animal Dosage

### Dogs and Cats

- Supplement: 0.5 mEq potassium/kg/day or add 10–40 mEq/500 mL of fluids, depending on serum potassium.
- Acute treatment of hypokalemia: 0.5 mEq potassium/kg/h.

## Large Animal Dosage
### Cattle and Horses
- Supplement in IV fluids to 20–40 mEq of potassium per liter of fluids. Do not exceed a rate of 0.5 mEq/kg/h IV.
- Oral supplement to cows either as a solution or bolus: 52 g of potassium (100 g of potassium chloride) per cow per day.

## Regulatory Information
No withdrawal times necessary.

# Potassium Citrate
**Trade and other names:** Generic and Urocit-K
**Functional classification:** Alkalinizing agent

## Pharmacology and Mechanism of Action
Potassium citrate ($K_3C_6H_5O_7$) alkalinizes urine and may increase urine citric acid. An increase in urine excretion of citrate and alkaline urine may decrease urinary calcium oxalate crystallization. Citrate combined with calcium in the urine forms calcium citrate, which is more soluble in the urine and increases the urine pH. Urinary excretion of calcium also is decreased. This treatment reduces the formation of calcium oxalate calculi. Other potassium supplements include potassium gluconate, potassium acetate, potassium bicarbonate, and potassium chloride.

## Indications and Clinical Uses
Potassium citrate is used for prevention of calcium oxalate urolithiasis. It is also used for renal tubular acidosis. In dogs, after administration of 150 mg/kg (of potassium citrate) q12h PO, the urine pH does not significantly increase, but urine concentration of calcium oxalate decreases. It has been administered as a potassium supplement to cats with chronic kidney disease, which also serves as an alkalinizing agent; thus, it serves a dual purpose of treating both hypokalemia and acidosis. Administration to cats is based on serum potassium levels. If the serum potassium is less than 3.5 mmol/L (less than 3.5 mEq/L), a recommended dosage is 1–4 mEq potassium per cat q12h.

## Precautionary Information
### Adverse Reactions and Side Effects
Toxicity from high potassium concentrations can be dangerous. Hyperkalemia can lead to cardiovascular toxicity (bradycardia and arrest) and muscular weakness. Oral potassium supplements can cause nausea and stomach irritation.

### Contraindications and Precautions
Use cautiously in animals with kidney disease. Do not use with potassium penicillin or potassium bromide.

### Drug Interactions
No drug interactions are reported in animals.

## Instructions for Use
One gram of potassium citrate provides 9.26 mEq of potassium. Administer with meals.

## Patient Monitoring and Laboratory Tests

Monitor serum potassium levels in order to regulate the dose. Normal potassium concentrations are 4–5.5 mEq/L (dogs) and 4.3–6.0 mEq/L (cats). Monitor ECG in patients that may be prone to arrhythmias.

## Formulations

- Potassium citrate is available in 5-, 10- and 15-mEq tablets. Five-mEq tablets are equivalent to 540 mg, 10-mEq tablets are equivalent to 1080 mg, and 15-mEq tablets are equivalent to 1620 mg. Some formulations are in combination with potassium chloride. Potassium citrate tablets in a delayed-released tablet are also available.

## Stability and Storage

Store in a tightly sealed container, protected from light, and at room temperature.

## Small Animal Dosage

### Dogs and Cats

- 2.2 mEq/100 kcal of energy/day PO or 0.5 mEq/kg per day PO. Higher doses have been used safely in some animals. (1000 mg potassium citrate is equivalent to 9.26 mEq of potassium.)
- 50–75 mg/kg PO q12h
- For alkalinizing urine: Add 150 mg/kg per day, mixed with the animal's food.
- For cats that need potassium supplement for chronic kidney disease, start with 1–4 mEq potassium per cat q12h (equivalent to approximately 30–100 mg/kg q12h).

## Large Animal Dosage

No doses have been reported for large animals.

## Regulatory Information

No withdrawal times necessary.

## Potassium Gluconate

**Trade and other names:** Kaon, Tumil-K, and generic brands

**Functional classification:** Potassium supplement

## Pharmacology and Mechanism of Action

Potassium gluconate is a potassium supplement that is used for treatment of hypokalemia. Potassium gluconate exists in an anhydrous form and a monohydrate form. Six grams of potassium gluconate anhydrous is equivalent to 1 g potassium; 6.45 g potassium gluconate monohydrate is equivalent to 1 g potassium. One gram of potassium gluconate is equal to 4.27 mEq of potassium. Other potassium supplements include potassium chloride, potassium acetate, potassium bicarbonate, and potassium citrate.

## Indications and Clinical Uses

Potassium gluconate is one of the supplements used for the treatment of hypokalemia and renal tubular acidosis. Hypokalemia may occur with some diseases or as a consequence of diuretic use. It has been administered as a potassium supplement to cats with chronic kidney disease. The dose is based on monitoring serum potassium concentrations. If the serum potassium concentration is less than 3.5 mmol/L (less than 3.5 mEq/L), a recommended dosage is 1–4 mEq potassium per cat q12h. Despite the availability of potassium gluconate, in most patients, potassium chloride is the supplement of choice for hypokalemia.

### Precautionary Information

**Adverse Reactions and Side Effects**

Toxicity from high potassium concentrations can be dangerous. Hyperkalemia can lead to cardiovascular toxicity (bradycardia and arrest) and muscular weakness. Oral potassium supplements can cause nausea and stomach irritation.

**Contraindications and Precautions**

Use cautiously in animals with kidney disease.

**Drug Interactions**

No drug interactions are reported in animals.

## Instructions for Use

One gram of potassium gluconate provides 4.27 mEq of potassium.

## Patient Monitoring and Laboratory Tests

Monitor serum potassium levels. Normal potassium concentrations are 4–5.5 mEq/L (dogs) and 4.3–6.0 mEq/L (cats). Monitor ECG in patients that may be prone to arrhythmias.

## Formulations

- Potassium gluconate is available in a 2-mEq tablet (equivalent to 500 mg of potassium gluconate).
- Kaon elixir is a 20-mEq potassium per 15-mL elixir (containing 4.68 g of potassium gluconate).

## Stability and Storage

Store in a tightly sealed container, protected from light, and at room temperature. Potassium gluconate is soluble in water.

## Small Animal Dosage

**Dogs**

- 0.5 mEq/kg q12–24h PO.

**Cats**

- 2–8 mEq/day divided twice daily PO. For cats that need potassium supplement for chronic kidney disease, start with 1–4 mEq of potassium per cat q12h.

## Large Animal Dosage

- No doses have been reported for large animals.

## Regulatory Information

No withdrawal times are necessary.

# Potassium Iodide

**Trade and other names:** KI, SSKI, ThyroSafe, iOSAT

**Functional classification:** Iodine supplement, antifungal, expectorant

## Pharmacology and Mechanism of Action

Potassium iodide is used as an iodine supplement. It also has some antimicrobial properties, although the exact mechanism is uncertain. The antimicrobial activity has been used as an adjunctive treatment for zygomycosis, conidiobolomycosis, and fungal granuloma. Iodide is also important for thyroid gland function and has been used to treat some thyroid disorders. Potassium iodide may irritate the respiratory tract and has been used as an expectorant.

## Indications and Clinical Uses

Potassium iodide has been used to treat fungal granulomatous disease and infections associated with zygomycetes. In small animals, it has been used for sporotrichosis. The antifungal treatment has been questioned for animals because the efficacy is not established through clinical studies. Because it may increase respiratory secretions, it has been used as an expectorant, but the efficacy has not been established. In people, iodide has been used to treat hyperthyroidism, but effectiveness for this use in cats has not been established. Potassium iodide is also used to protect the thyroid gland from radiation injury in the event of a radiation emergency (accidental exposure to radiation) or after administration of radioactive iodide.

Ethylenediamine dihydroiodide (EDDI) is another source of iodide that is used as a nutritional source of iodine in cattle. Sodium iodide also is used, particularly in large animals. See Sodium Iodide and Iodide for more information.

## Precautionary Information

### Adverse Reactions and Side Effects

High doses can produce signs of iodism, which include lacrimation, irritation of mucous membranes, swelling of eyelids, cough, dry scruffy coat, and hair loss. Potassium iodide has a bitter taste and can cause nausea and salivation. Potassium iodide administration has been associated with cardiomyopathy in cats. Its use may cause abortion in horses or limb deformities in foals.

### Contraindications and Precautions

Do not administer to foals or pregnant animals (abortion is possible). Do not administer intravenously.

### Drug Interactions

No known drug interactions.

## Instructions for Use

Clinical use in animals is primarily empirical. The doses and indications listed have not been tested in clinical trials. Other, more proven drugs for these indications should be considered as alternatives, especially for treating serious fungal infections.

## Patient Monitoring and Laboratory Tests

Monitor iodine concentrations of monitoring is available.

## Formulations

- Potassium iodide solution: 65-mg/mL, or saturated 1 g/mL. The saturated solution (SSKI) (1 g/mL) yields 38 mg per drop.
- 10% potassium iodide solution. The 5% iodine solution can be administered orally with food. The 10% solution of potassium iodide (10%) yields 6.3 mg of iodine per drop.
- Tablets: 130 and 65 mg (both tablets are scored).
- Combination tablets: ephedrine, phenobarbital, potassium iodide, and theophylline are combined in one tablet (Quadrinal), but there is no evidence of use in animals.

## Compounded Formulations
- 3.25 mg/mL oral solution made with tablets. Crush one 130-mg tablet and reduce to a fine powder. Add 20 mL of water and mix until powder is dissolved. Add an additional 20 mL of milk, juice, or syrup. Stable for 7 days under refrigeration.
- 1.6 mg/mL oral solution made with tablets. Crush one 65-mg tablet and reduce to a fine powder. Add 20 mL of water and mix until powder is dissolved. Add an additional 20 mL of milk, juice, or syrup. Stable for 7 days under refrigeration.

## Stability and Storage
Store in a tightly sealed container, protected from light, and at room temperature. Do not freeze solutions. Inorganic potassium iodide is unstable in light, heat, and excess humidity.

## Small Animal Dosage
### Dogs and Cats
- Fungal infections: start with 5 mg/kg q8h PO and increase gradually to 25 mg/kg q8h PO.
- Emergency treatment after radiation exposure: 2 mg/kg PO per day. Continue for 10 to 14 days or until risk of exposure has passed.
- Expectorant: 5 mg/kg q8h PO.

## Large Animal Dosage
### Cattle
- 10–15 g/day (adult cattle) PO for 30–60 days.
- 5–10 g/day (calves) PO for 30–60 days.
- Feed supplement and other indications: (see Iodide for EDDI doses and Sodium Iodide for other doses).

### Horses
- 10–40 mg/kg per day (using inorganic potassium iodide).
- 10–15 g/day (adult horses) PO for 30–60 days.
- 5–10 g/day (ponies) PO for 30–60 days.
- See Iodide for EDDI doses and Sodium Iodide for other doses.

## Regulatory Information
No regulatory information is available. Because of a low risk of residues, no withdrawal times are suggested.

# Potassium Phosphate
**Trade and other names:** K-Phos, Neutra-Phos-K, and generic brands
**Functional classification:** Phosphate supplement

## Pharmacology and Mechanism of Action
Potassium phosphate is used as a phosphorous supplement. Potassium phosphate is used for severe hypophosphatemia associated with diabetic ketoacidosis. It also acidifies the urine.

## Indications and Clinical Uses
Potassium phosphate has been used to reduce calcium urinary secretion in patients prone to calcium urinary calculi and to promote a more acid urine. This drug should not be used to supplement potassium. Instead, potassium chloride is the supplement of choice for hypokalemia.

P

## Precautionary Information

**Adverse Reactions and Side Effects**

Intravenous administration can cause hypocalcemia.

**Contraindications and Precautions**

Use cautiously in animals with renal disease.

**Drug Interactions**

No drug interactions are reported in animals.

## Instructions for Use

Potassium phosphate use in animals is primarily as a urinary acidifier or treatment of hypophosphatemia.

## Patient Monitoring and Laboratory Tests

Monitor calcium, potassium, and phosphorus levels in treated animals.

## Formulations

- Potassium phosphate is currently not available in tablets (previously 500 mg containing 114 mg [3.7 mmol] of phosphorus). Oral solutions can be made from powdered concentrate mixed with water for oral administration.
- Potassium phosphate is available in 224 mg of monobasic potassium phosphate and 236 mg of dibasic potassium phosphate (3 mmol [93 mg] of phosphorus) per milliliter injection.

## Stability and Storage

Store in a tightly sealed container, protected from light, and at room temperature.

## Small Animal Dosage

**Dogs and Cats**

- 0.03–0.12 mmol/kg/h IV for acute treatment.
- 0.1 mmol/kg/day IV for daily supplementation.
- 4 mg/kg phosphorus (approximately 0.1 mmol/kg) PO up to four times daily.

## Large Animal Dosage

- No doses have been reported for large animals.

## Regulatory Information

No withdrawal times are necessary.

# Pradofloxacin

pray doe-floks'ah-sin

**Trade and other names:** Veraflox

**Functional classification:** Antibacterial

## Pharmacology and Mechanism of Action

Pradofloxacin is a fluoroquinolone antibacterial drug, approved only for use in animals, with no human formulations available. Pradofloxacin is of the new generation (third generation) of fluoroquinolones. This new generation of fluoroquinolones, with substitutions at the C-8 position, have as their advantage a broader spectrum that includes anaerobic bacteria and gram-positive cocci. The difference in spectrum of activity is largely caused by increased activity against the DNA gyrase of gram-positive bacteria rather than activity against topoisomerase IV, which is the target in gram-positive bacteria for the older quinolones (e.g., enrofloxacin, ciprofloxacin, marbofloxacin, and orbifloxacin). These newer fluoroquinolones also include the human drugs gatifloxacin, gemifloxacin, and moxifloxacin. Pradofloxacin is active against bacterial isolates from dogs and cats, including *E. coli, Staphylococcus* spp., and anaerobes. Pradofloxacin is approved for use in cats in the United States but for both dogs and cats in Europe and Canada. Pradofloxacin also is active against bovine and swine respiratory pathogens but, at this time, not approved for this indication.

*Pharmacokinetics:* Pradofloxacin is almost 100% absorbed in dogs and has an elimination half-life of approximately 7–8 hours with a volume of distribution of 2.2 L/kg and clearance of 0.24 L/kg/h. High concentrations of 23–254 mcg/mL are achieved in the urine. The oral absorption of the tablet in cats is 70%, but the oral suspension has bioavailability of 84% of the value for the tablets. The half-life in cats is approximately 7–9 hours with a volume of distribution of 4.45 L/kg and clearance of 0.28 L/kg/h. The urine concentrations achieved are 18–65 mcg/mL. In cats and dogs, plasma protein binding rates are 30% and 35%, respectively.

## Indications and Clinical Uses

Pradofloxacin has been evaluated in dogs and cats, with efficacy studies published on the approved label, research abstracts and clinical reports in which it has been used for treating skin and soft tissue infections in dogs and cats, oral infections (periodontal therapy), respiratory infections in cats, and UTIs. At a dose of 3 mg/kg PO, it was effective for treatment of UTIs in dogs, and at 3 or 5 mg/kg, it was effective for canine pyoderma. At a dose of 5 mg/kg in a 2.5% oral suspension, it was effective for UTIs in cats. It has been used to effectively treat infections caused by *Chlamydophila felis* or *Mycoplasma* spp. in cats (5 mg/kg q12h PO for 28 days) and was as effective as doxycycline. It has been used to treat feline rhinitis caused by *Mycoplasma* spp., *Bordetella* spp., streptococci, or staphylococci at a dosage of 5 mg/kg once daily for seven doses. It has been effective (5 mg/kg per day) for treatment of feline blood infections caused by *Mycoplasma haemofelis*.

P

## Precautionary Information

### Adverse Reactions and Side Effects

Safety studies have been completed in cats associated with approval in the United States and in dogs and cats in Europe. It has been tolerated well in cats with no adverse effects that are different from other approved fluoroquinolones. Field trials in cats in the United States showed that the most common adverse effect was diarrhea or loose stools. In cats, administration at high doses of six times the label dose did not cause ocular problems. In dogs and cats, at high doses, pradofloxacin has caused bone marrow suppression, but this has not been reported from clinical use at approved doses.

### Contraindications and Precautions

No contraindications or precautions are available. Because it is similar to other fluoroquinolones, use cautiously in young dogs that may be susceptible to articular cartilage injury. Risks during pregnancy in dogs and cats are not known, but pradofloxacin induced eye malformations at high doses in rats.

### Drug Interactions

No drug interactions have been reported from the use thus far in animals. However, some of the same drug interactions that affect other fluoroquinolones are possible with pradofloxacin, such as chelation with oral calcium, magnesium, iron, and aluminum supplements.

## Instructions for Use

Pradofloxacin may be used for a variety of infections in dogs and cats with similar indications as for other fluoroquinolones in addition to those listed in the Indications and Clinical Uses sections.

## Patient Monitoring and Laboratory Tests

The CLSI breakpoint for susceptibility is ≤0.25 mcg/mL for both dogs and cats.

## Formulations

- Formulations contain pradofloxacin in a 2.5% oral suspension in the United States and Europe and 15-, 60-, and 120-mg tablets in Europe.

## Stability and Storage

Store in a tightly sealed container, protected from light, and at room temperature.

## Small Animal Dosage

**Dogs**

- 3–5 mg/kg q24h PO.

**Cats**

- Tablets: 3–5 mg/kg q24h PO.
- Oral suspension: 5–7.5 mg/kg q24h PO.

## Large Animal Dosage

- No doses have been approved for large animals.

## Regulatory Information

Withdrawal times are not established for animals that produce food. Extralabel use of fluoroquinolones in food-producing animals is prohibited.

# Pralidoxime Chloride
prah-lih-doks′eem klor′ide

**Trade and other names:** 2-PAM and Protopam chloride

**Functional classification:** Antidote

## Pharmacology and Mechanism of Action

Pralidoxime chloride is an oxime that is used as an adjunct to atropine for treatment of intoxication. Organophosphate intoxication results in inactivation of cholinesterase enzymes and excess accumulation of acetylcholine. Pralidoxime (also known as 2-PAM) is used to reactivate acetylcholinesterase by promoting dephosphorylation. Pralidoxime is well absorbed from IM administration, but it does not cross the blood–brain barrier. After absorption, the half-life is short, necessitating repeated administrations.

## Indications and Clinical Uses

Pralidoxime chloride is used for treatment of organophosphate toxicosis. It should be administered promptly after organophosphate intoxication is recognized. It also has been used to treat overdoses of other anticholinesterase drugs such as neostigmine, pyridostigmine, and edrophonium.

## Precautionary Information
### Adverse Reactions and Side Effects
Intramuscular injections cause pain. Rapid IV injections may bind calcium and cause muscle spasms. Rapid injections also may cause heart and respiratory problems. Use during pregnancy may produce teratogenic effects.

### Contraindications and Precautions
Pralidoxime treatment should not be used for carbamate intoxication. Do not administer rapidly intravenously, or it may cause respiratory depression and other problems.

### Drug Interactions
No drug interactions have been reported. However, other drugs should be avoided when treating organophosphate poisoning. These drugs include aminoglycosides, barbiturates, phenothiazine tranquilizers (acepromazine), and neuromuscular blocking agents.

## Instructions for Use
Dilute formulation in glucose solution before IV administration. Give slowly IV. Administer atropine (0.1 mg/kg) when using pralidoxime to minimize adverse effects. Recovery from organophosphate poisoning may take 48 hours. When treating intoxication, consult a poison control center for precise guidelines.

## Patient Monitoring and Laboratory Tests
Monitor for signs of organophosphate poisoning to determine if repeated doses are necessary. Monitor heart rate and rhythm and respiratory rate. It may be possible to monitor cholinesterase activity from a blood sample to confirm organophosphate poisoning (consult local diagnostic laboratory).

## Formulations
- Pralidoxime chloride is available in a 1-g vial to be reconstituted in 20 mL of water (50-mg/mL injection). pH of solution is 3.5–4.5.

## Stability and Storage
Store powder at room temperature and protect from light. Reconstituted solution should be stored below 25°C and protected from light. Discard reconstituted solution after 3 hours.

## Small Animal Dosage
- 20 mg/kg up to 50 mg/kg q8–12h IM or IV (initial dose slow). Dilute solution in glucose and infuse slowly IV.

## Large Animal Dosage
### Cattle, Sheep, and Pigs
- 20–50 mg/kg q8h (administered as a 10% solution) IM or via slow IV infusion or as needed. Frequency can be assessed by monitoring clinical signs.

## Regulatory Information
Cattle and pig withdrawal times (extralabel): 6 days for milk and 28 days for meat.

P

# Praziquantel
pray-zih-kwon'tel

**Trade and other names:** Droncit and Drontal (combination with febantel)

**Functional classification:** Antiparasitic

## Pharmacology and Mechanism of Action

Praziquantel is a popular and widely used antiparasitic drug used for many years to eliminate tapeworms in animals. The action on parasites related to neuromuscular toxicity and paralysis via altered permeability to calcium.

## Indications and Clinical Uses

Praziquantel is widely used to treat intestinal infections caused by cestodes (tapeworms) (*Dipylidium caninum, Taenia pisiformis,* and *Echinococcus granulosus*) and removal and control of canine cestode *Echinococcus multilocularis*. In cats, it is used for removal of feline cestodes *D. caninum* and *Taenia taeniaeformis*. In horses, it is used to treat tapeworms (*Anoplocephala perfoliata*).

Although there are no products approved for treatment of *Spirometra* spp. infections in dogs and cats, praziquantel has been used successfully, but a higher dose is needed (25 mg/kg PO) and administered for 2 consecutive days. Likewise, although no products are approved to treat *Diphyllobothrium* spp. in dogs and cats, praziquantel has been used to treat pseudophyllidean tapeworms. A dosage of 25 mg/kg PO for 2 consecutive days is used. A dose of 35 mg/kg once PO also has been used in cats.

## Precautionary Information

### Adverse Reactions and Side Effects

Vomiting occurs at high doses. Anorexia and transient diarrhea have been reported. It is safe in pregnant animals and during lactation.

### Contraindications and Precautions

Avoid use in cats younger than 6 weeks and dogs younger than 4 weeks. Praziquantel has been safe in pregnancy.

### Drug Interactions

No drug interactions have been reported in animals.

## Instructions for Use

Praziquantel is one of the most common drugs used for tapeworm treatment. It has a wide margin of safety. Some formulations of praziquantel are available in combination (e.g., combination of praziquantel and febantel; combination of ivermectin and praziquantel, moxidectin, and praziquantel).

## Patient Monitoring and Laboratory Tests

No specific monitoring is necessary.

## Formulations

- Praziquantel is available in 23- and 34-mg tablets and 56.8-mg/mL injection and is also available in pastes and gels.

- In combination, it is available as 13.6 mg of praziquantel and 54.3 mg of pyrantel,18.2 mg of praziquantel and 72.6 of mg pyrantel, or 27.2 mg of praziquantel and 108.6 mg of pyrantel. It is combined with emodepside in Profender.
- Praziquantel is available in pastes and gels for horses in combination with other drugs (e.g., ivermectin, moxidectin, febantel).

## Stability and Storage

Store in a tightly sealed container, protected from light, and at room temperature.

## Small Animal Dosage

### Dogs

- Dogs weighing less than 6.8 kg: 7.5 mg/kg once PO.
- Dogs weighing more than 6.8 kg: 5 mg/kg once PO.
- Dogs weighing less than 2.3 kg: 7.5 mg/kg once IM or SQ.
- Dogs weighing more than 2.7–4.5 kg: 6.3 mg/kg once IM or SQ.
- Dogs weighing more than 5 kg: 5 mg/kg once IM or SQ.
- Paragonimus in dogs (lung worms): 23 mg/kg PO q8h for 3 days.
- *Spirometra* spp. and *Diphyllobothrium* spp. treatment: 25 mg/kg PO once daily for 2 consecutive days.

### Cats

All doses are given once.
- Cats weighing less than 1.8 kg: 11.4 mg/cat PO.
- Cats weighing 1.8–2.2 kg: 11.4 mg/cat SQ or IM.
- Cats weighing 2.3–4.5 kg: 22.7 mg/cat SQ or IM.
- Cats weighing 2.3–5 kg: 23 mg/cat PO.
- Cats weighing more than 5 kg: 34.5 mg/cat PO or 34.1 mg/cat SQ or IM.
- *Spirometra* spp. and *Diphyllobothrium* spp. treatment: 25 mg/kg PO once daily for 2 consecutive days.

## Large Animal Dosage

### Horses

- 1.5–2.5 mg/kg PO.

## Regulatory Information

Withdrawal times are not established for animals that produce food. For extralabel use withdrawal interval estimates, contact FARAD at www.FARAD.org.

# Prazosin

pray′zoe-sin

**Trade and other names:** Minipress

**Functional classification:** Vasodilator

## Pharmacology and Mechanism of Action

Prazosin is a nonselective alpha$_1$-adrenergic blocker. Prazosin is a vasodilator that is a selective blocker for the alpha$_1$-adrenergic receptor, but it is not selective for either alpha$_{1a}$ or alpha$_{1b}$. Its action is similar to phenoxybenzamine, but it produces less tachycardia than nonselective alpha-antagonist drugs. Prazosin decreases tension in both arterial and venous vascular smooth muscle to produce vasodilation. In cats, 30% of the proximal urethra is smooth muscle, and the remaining is skeletal muscle. Therefore, it has been used to relax the urethral smooth muscle to treat and prevent urethral obstruction in male cats. The alpha$_{1b}$ adrenoreceptors regulate vascular tone, and the alpha$_{1a}$ adrenoreceptors regulate urethral smooth muscle tone. For specific urinary smooth muscle relaxation, the drugs tamsulosin (Flomax) and silodosin (Rapaflo) are more specific for the alpha$_{1a}$ receptor and can produce a more specific effect on the urethra.

## Indications and Clinical Uses

Prazosin has been used in people for vasodilation and the management of hypertension that is not responsive to other drugs. Prazosin has been used to a limited extent in veterinary medicine to produce balanced vasodilation. There are no controlled studies to establish efficacy and dose, and indications are derived from anecdotal use and extrapolation from human medicine. It has been used in cats with urethral obstruction to improve urine flow. There is some evidence that in comparison with phenoxybenzamine, it produced fewer recurrence rates of urethral obstruction (0.5 mg per cat q8h PO), but at lower doses (0.25 mg per cat q12h for 30 days) there was no difference compared with placebo for recurrence rate in cats with urethral obstruction. In dogs, there are no clinical studies that have examined effectiveness to relax the urethra. It has also been used experimentally in horses to improve digital perfusion in the treatment of laminitis. Long-term administration is not common because tolerance may develop with chronic use.

## Precautionary Information

### Adverse Reactions and Side Effects

High doses cause vasodilation and hypotension. Oral treatment in cats has caused lethargy, ptyalism, and diarrhea.

### Contraindications and Precautions

Use cautiously in animals with compromised cardiac function. It may lower blood pressure and decrease cardiac output.

### Drug Interactions

No drug interactions have been reported in animals, but when combined with other vasodilators, it may produce severe lowering of blood pressure.

## Instructions for Use

Titrate dose to the needs of the individual patient. Results of clinical studies in animals have not been reported; therefore use in animals (and doses) is based on experience in people or anecdotal experience in animals. For a more specific effect on the urethra smooth muscle, consider tamsulosin (Flomax), which is more specific for the alpha$_{1a}$ receptor and can produce a more specific effect on the urethra.

## Patient Monitoring and Laboratory Tests

Monitor for hypotension and reflex tachycardia.

## Formulations
Prazosin is available in 1-, 2-, and 5-mg capsules.

## Stability and Storage
Store in a tightly sealed container, protected from light, and at room temperature.

## Small Animal Dosage
### Dogs
- 0.5–2 mg per dog q8–24h (as needed).

### Cats
- 0.25–1 mg per cat (0.07 mg/kg or approximately 1 mg per 15 kg) q8–12h PO.
- Cats with urethral obstruction: 0.5 mg per cat PO q8h initially; then 0.25–0.5 mg per cat once daily.

## Large Animal Dosage
- No doses have been reported for large animals.

## Regulatory Information
Withdrawal times are not established for animals that produce food. For extralabel use withdrawal interval estimates, contact FARAD at www.FARAD.org.
RCI Classification: 3

---

# Prednisolone, Prednisolone Acetate
**Trade and other names:** Delta-Cortef, PrednisTab, and generic brands
**Functional classification:** Corticosteroid

## Pharmacology and Mechanism of Action
Prednisolone is one of the most widely used glucocorticoids. Prednisolone is the active form of prednisone. Prednisolone, like other glucocorticoids, produces anti-inflammatory and immunosuppressive effects. Anti-inflammatory effects are complex, but via binding to cellular glucocorticoid receptors, prednisolone acts to inhibit inflammatory cells and suppresses expression of inflammatory mediators. Prednisolone is approximately four times more potent than cortisol but only one seventh as potent as dexamethasone. Prednisolone is available as the base (usually as a tablet) or as an injectable acetate form, which can be administered intramuscularly or intraarticularly.

## Indications and Clinical Uses
Prednisolone, like other corticosteroids, is used to treat a variety of inflammatory and immune-mediated disease. The accompanying dosing section lists a range of doses for replacement therapy, anti-inflammatory therapy, and immunosuppressive therapy. Large animal uses include treatment of inflammatory conditions, especially musculoskeletal disorders. In horses, prednisolone is used for treatment of equine asthma syndrome when recurrent airway obstruction (RAO) occurs. In cattle, corticosteroids have been used in the treatment of ketosis. The prednisolone and trimeprazine formulation (Temaril-P) has been effective for treating pruritus in dogs. (See Trimeprazine for further details.)

## Precautionary Information

### Adverse Reactions and Side Effects

There are many side effects from corticosteroids, which include polyphagia, polydipsia and polyuria, behavior changes, and hypothalamic–pituitary–adrenal (HPA) axis suppression. Adverse effects include GI ulceration, steroid hepatopathy, diabetes, hyperlipidemia, decreased thyroid hormone, decreased protein synthesis, delayed wound healing, increased risk of diabetes, and immunosuppression. Secondary infections can occur as a result of immunosuppression and include demodicosis, toxoplasmosis, fungal infections, and UTIs.

In cats, there is a concern that corticosteroids such as prednisolone can exacerbate CHF through volume expansion secondary to steroid-induced hyperglycemia. This has occurred in susceptible cats after injections of methylprednisolone acetate. This has not been a clinical problem in otherwise healthy cats. In dogs, there was not an expansion of plasma volume, but short-term use can increase vascular resistance, systolic blood pressure, and increase cardiac afterload. This could potentially exacerbate CHF in some dogs. The mechanism is through increased sensitivity of the alpha receptors and angiotensin II. Thus, in both cats and dogs with heart disease, prednisolone should be used carefully.

In horses, in addition to the previously listed adverse effects, there may be an increased risk of laminitis, although documentation of this effect has been controversial and not supported by clinical evidence.

### Contraindications and Precautions

Use cautiously in patients with a risk of GI ulcers or infection and in animals in which growing or healing is necessary. Use prednisolone cautiously in patients with kidney disease because it may increase azotemia. Use prednisolone cautiously in pregnant animals because fetal abnormalities have been reported in laboratory rodents. Use cautiously in dogs and cats with heart disease because in cats it can increase volume expansion in cats at risk of CHF, and in dogs, it can increase vascular resistance and blood pressure. Do not administer prednisolone acetate intravenously. In some species, particularly horses and cats, prednisolone (the active form) is preferred for oral treatment rather than prednisone.

### Drug Interactions

Administration of corticosteroids with NSAIDs will increase the risk of GI injury. Corticosteroids may inhibit conversion of $T_4$ thyroid hormone to the active form $T_3$. However, in dogs, the concentration of total $T_4$ but not free $T_4$, is decreased. Therefore the effect on thyroid status in canine patients is expected to be minimal.

## Instructions for Use

Doses for prednisolone are of a broad range and based on severity of underlying condition. Generally, after initial treatment, if the patient responds favorably, the doses for long-term maintenance treatment can be tapered to less than 0.5 mg/kg q48h PO.

## Patient Monitoring and Laboratory Tests

Monitor liver enzymes, blood glucose, and renal function during therapy. Monitor patients for signs of secondary infections. Perform an ACTH stimulation test to monitor adrenal function. Corticosteroids can increase liver enzymes, especially ALP, without inducing liver pathology. Prednisone can increase white blood cell (WBC) count and decrease lymphocyte count. It can increase serum albumin, glucose, triglycerides, and cholesterol. Corticosteroid administration may decrease conversion of thyroid hormones to active form, but free $T_4$ concentrations should be unaffected. Prednisolone and prednisone at high doses for several weeks may produce significant proteinuria and glomerular changes in some dogs.

## Formulations

- Oral prednisolone is available in 5- and 20-mg tablets and 3-mg/mL syrup.
- Injection is available as a 25-mg/mL acetate suspension injection (10 and 50 mg/mL in Canada).
- Prednisolone sodium phosphate orally disintegrating tablets are available for people but not widely used in animals. These tablets are available in sizes of 5, 10, 15, and 30 mg.
- Prednisolone is also available in combination with trimeprazine (Temaril-P). (See Trimeprazine for more information.)

## Stability and Storage

Store in a tightly sealed container, protected from light, and at room temperature. Prednisolone is slightly soluble in water, but it is more soluble in ethanol. If diluted first in ethanol, it may be compounded into oral liquid formulations with good stability for 90 days. Prednisolone acetate is insoluble in water. Do not freeze.

## Small Animal Dosage

### Dogs

- Anti-inflammatory: The induction dose is 0.5–1 mg/kg, per day, which may be split into q12h doses, IM, or PO. Then taper the dose to 0.3–0.5 mg/kg, q48h, for long-term treatment.
- Immunosuppressive: 2.2–6.6 mg/kg/day IV, IM, or PO initially; then taper to 2–4 mg/kg q48h. Initial dosages rarely need to exceed 4 mg/kg per day.
- Neurologic disease (steroid responsive): Start with 2 mg/kg q12h PO for 2 days followed by gradual tapering to 1 mg/kg, then 0.5 mg/kg, and eventually to 0.5 mg/kg every other day.
- Replacement therapy for adrenal insufficiency: 0.2–0.3 mg/kg/day PO.
- Cancer therapy (e.g., CHOP protocol): 40 mg/m² q24h for 7 days; then 20 mg/m² every other day PO.

### Cats

- Same as for dogs, except that for many conditions they require twice the dog dose.

## Large Animal Dosage

### Horses

- Prednisolone acetate suspension: 100–200 mg total dosage IM.
- Prednisolone tablets: 0.5–1 mg/kg q12–24h PO. Taper to lower dose for long-term treatment.

### Cattle

- Treatment of ketosis: 100–200 mg total dosage IM.

## Regulatory Information

Cattle withdrawal times for prednisolone acetate: 5 days for meat; 72 hours for milk (in Canada).

Withdrawal times are not established for animals that produce food in the United States. For extralabel use withdrawal interval estimates, contact FARAD at www.FARAD.org.

RCI Classification: 4

# Prednisolone Sodium Succinate
pred-niss-oh'lone soe'dee-um suk'sih-nate

**Trade and other names:** Solu-Delta-Cortef

**Functional classification:** Corticosteroid

## Pharmacology and Mechanism of Action

Prednisolone sodium succinate is the same as prednisolone except that this is a water-soluble formulation intended for acute therapy when IV doses are needed for rapid effect. Mechanism of action and other details for prednisolone are listed in the Prednisolone section.

## Indications and Clinical Uses

Prednisolone sodium succinate has similar uses as other forms of prednisolone except this is used when prompt response is needed from injection, especially at high doses. Methylprednisolone sodium succinate (Solu-Medrol) has also been used for similar indications. The uses include treatment of immune-mediated diseases (e.g., pemphigus and hemolytic anemia), spinal cord trauma, and adrenocortical insufficiency. Large animal uses include treatment of inflammatory conditions and treatment of RAO, which is a component of equine asthma syndrome. In cattle, corticosteroids have been used in the treatment of ketosis.

The use of prednisolone for treatment of shock, snakebites, and head trauma is discouraged because of lack of proven efficacy or high risk of adverse effects.

## Precautionary Information

### Adverse Reactions and Side Effects

Adverse effects are not expected from single administration. However, with repeated use, other side effects are possible. Side effects from corticosteroids are many and include polyphagia, polydipsia and polyuria, and HPA axis suppression. Adverse effects include GI ulceration, diarrhea, steroid hepatopathy, diabetes mellitus, hyperlipidemia, decreased thyroid hormone, decreased protein synthesis, impaired wound healing, and immunosuppression. In cats, polyuria is less common than in dogs, and it has not increased calcium excretion or calcium-containing calculi. With high doses of prednisolone sodium succinate, there is a risk of GI bleeding. In horses, in addition to the previously listed adverse effects, there may be an increased risk of laminitis, although documentation of this effect has been controversial.

### Contraindications and Precautions

Use cautiously in patients with a risk of GI ulcers and bleeding or infection or in animals in which growing or healing is necessary. Use prednisolone sodium succinate cautiously in patients with kidney disease because it may increase azotemia. Use cautiously in pregnant animals because fetal abnormalities have been reported in laboratory rodents.

### Drug Interactions

Administration of corticosteroids with NSAIDs increases the risk of GI injury. Do not mix prednisolone sodium succinate with solutions containing calcium.

## Instructions for Use

Use of prednisolone sodium succinate is often at high doses for acute treatment, and oral prednisolone or prednisone is used for maintenance treatment. Doses for prednisolone are based on the severity of the underlying condition.

## Patient Monitoring and Laboratory Tests

Monitor liver enzymes, blood glucose, and renal function during therapy. Monitor patients for signs of secondary infections. Perform an ACTH stimulation test to monitor adrenal function. Corticosteroids can increase liver enzymes, especially ALP, because of enzyme induction, without inducing liver pathology. Prednisolone can increase WBC count and decrease lymphocyte count. It can increase serum albumin, glucose, triglycerides, and cholesterol. Corticosteroid administration may decrease conversion of thyroid hormones to its active form. Prednisolone and prednisone at high doses for several weeks may produce significant proteinuria and glomerular changes in some dogs.

## Formulations

• Prednisolone sodium succinate is available in 100- and 500-mg vials for injection (10, 20, and 50 mg/mL). For some indications, methylprednisolone sodium succinate (Solu-Medrol) has been substituted.

## Stability and Storage

Store in a tightly sealed container, protected from light, and at room temperature. Prednisolone sodium succinate should be used immediately after reconstitution. Do not freeze. If solution becomes cloudy, do not administer intravenously.

## Small Animal Dosage
### Dogs and Cats

• Shock (effectiveness of this use is controversial): 15–30 mg/kg IV (repeat in 4–6 hours).
• CNS trauma: 15–30 mg/kg IV, taper to 1–2 mg/kg q12h.
• Anti-inflammatory: 1 mg/kg/day IV.
• Replacement therapy for adrenal insufficiency: 0.25–0.5 mg/kg/day IV.
• Intermittent treatment (pulse therapy) of pemphigus foliaceus: 10 mg/kg IV.

## Large Animal Dosage
### Horses

• 0.5–1 mg/kg q12–24h IM or IV. IV dose should be given slowly over 30–60 seconds.
• Treatment of shock (although efficacy for treating shock has not been established): 15–30 mg/kg IV; repeat dose in 4–6 hours.

## Regulatory Information

Withdrawal times are not established for animals that produce food. For extralabel use withdrawal interval estimates, contact FARAD at www.FARAD.org.
RCI Classification: 4

## Prednisone
pred′nih-sone

**Trade and other names:** Deltasone, Meticorten, and generic brands
**Functional classification:** Corticosteroid

## Pharmacology and Mechanism of Action

Prednisone is the inactive form of prednisolone. After administration in most animals (except horses and cats), prednisone is converted to prednisolone, and the effects listed for prednisolone are expected.

Prednisone is a glucocorticoid anti-inflammatory drug. The effect of prednisone is attributed to prednisolone. Anti-inflammatory effects are complex, but via binding to cellular glucocorticoid receptors, prednisolone acts to inhibit inflammatory cells and suppresses expression of inflammatory mediators. Prednisolone is approximately four times more potent than cortisol but only one seventh as potent as dexamethasone. Prednisone appears to be well absorbed and converted to active drug in dogs. However, in horses and cats, administration of prednisone results in low systemic levels of the active drug prednisolone, either because of poor absorption of prednisone or because of a deficiency in converting prednisone into prednisolone.

## Indications and Clinical Uses

Prednisone, like other corticosteroids, is used to treat a variety of inflammatory and immune-mediated diseases. In cats, prednisone may produce therapeutic failures, and prednisolone (active drug) is preferred. There is evidence of poor conversion of prednisone to prednisolone or poor absorption of prednisone in cats and horses. Prednisolone or another active drug (e.g., triamcinolone, dexamethasone) should be used instead for these animals. There are several large animal doses cited (similar to prednisolone); however, because of poor activity in horses, the use is discouraged.

## Precautionary Information

### Adverse Reactions and Side Effects

There are many side effects from corticosteroids that include polyphagia, polydipsia and polyuria, behavior changes, and HPA axis suppression. Adverse effects include GI ulceration, diarrhea hepatopathy, diabetes, hyperlipidemia, decreased thyroid hormone (but not free $T_4$), decreased protein synthesis, delayed wound healing, and immunosuppression. Secondary infections can occur as a result of immunosuppression and include demodicosis, toxoplasmosis, fungal infections, and UTIs.

In dogs, prednisolone administration increased vascular resistance, systolic blood pressure, and increase cardiac afterload. This could potentially exacerbate CHF in some dogs. Thus, in dogs with heart disease, prednisolone should be used carefully.

### Contraindications and Precautions

Use corticosteroids cautiously in patients with a risk of GI ulcers or infections and in animals in which growing or healing is necessary. Use prednisone cautiously in patients with renal disease because it may cause azotemia. Use prednisone cautiously in pregnant animals because fetal abnormalities have been reported in laboratory rodents.

### Drug Interactions

Administration of corticosteroids with NSAIDs increases the risk of GI injury. Corticosteroids may inhibit conversion of $T_4$ thyroid hormone to the active form $T_3$. However, in dogs, the concentration of total $T_4$ , but not free $T_4$, is decreased. Therefore, the effect on thyroid status in a canine patient is expected to be minimal.

## Instructions for Use

Prednisolone and prednisone can be used interchangeably in dogs. However, cats and horses may have problems converting prednisone to the active prednisolone or problems with oral absorption of prednisone, and prednisolone should be used instead. (Alternatively, methylprednisolone or triamcinolone can be used.) As for prednisolone, the doses vary across a broad range based on severity of the underlying condition. Consult the dosing section for the range of doses administered for each condition.

## Patient Monitoring and Laboratory Tests

Monitor liver enzymes, blood glucose, and renal function during therapy. Monitor patients for signs of secondary infections. Perform an ACTH stimulation test to monitor adrenal function. Corticosteroids can increase liver enzymes, especially ALP, without inducing liver pathology. Corticosteroid administration may decrease conversion of thyroid hormones to active form. However, in dogs receiving anti-inflammatory doses of prednisone, total $T_4$ concentrations, but not free$T_4$, may be decreased.

## Formulations

- Prednisone oral forms: 1-, 2.5-, 5-, 10-, 20-, 25-, and 50-mg tablets; 1-mg/mL syrup (Liquid Pred in 5% alcohol); and 1-mg/mL oral solution (in 5% alcohol)
- Prednisone for injection: 10- and 40-mg/mL prednisone suspension for injection (Meticorten; availability has been limited).

## Stability and Storage

Store in a tightly sealed container, protected from light, and at room temperature. Prednisone is slightly soluble in water, and it is soluble in ethanol. Prednisone has been prepared by first dissolving in ethanol and then mixing with syrups and flavorings. No loss occurred, but crystallization is common in aqueous vehicles. Prednisone tablets have been crushed and mixed with syrups and other flavorings, stored for 60 days, and found to produce equal bioavailability as tablets in people.

## Small Animal Dosage

### Dogs

- Anti-inflammatory: 0.5–1 mg/kg, per day, which may be divided into twice-daily treatments, IM, or PO initially; then taper to q48h at a dose of 0.3–0.5 mg/kg.
- Immunosuppressive: 2.2–6.6 mg/kg/day IV, IM, or PO initially; then taper to 2–4 mg/kg q48h. Initial doses rarely need to exceed 4 mg/kg per day.
- Replacement therapy for adrenal insufficiency: 0.2–0.3 mg/kg/day PO.
- Neurologic disease (steroid responsive): Start with 2 mg/kg q12h PO for 2 days followed by gradual tapering to 1 mg/kg, then 0.5 mg/kg, and eventually to 0.5 mg/kg every other day.
- Cancer therapy (e.g., COAP protocol): 40 mg/m² q24h for 7 days; then 20 mg/m² every other day PO.

### Cats

- Not recommended for cats because of an inability to form active metabolite. However, if use is attempted, higher doses than used in dogs are needed.

## Large Animal Dosage

### Horses

- Prednisone suspension (Meticorten) (label dosage): 100–400 mg per horse (0.22–0.88 mg/kg) as a single dose IM to be repeated every 3–4 days. No oral doses are listed for horses because of an inability of oral treatment to produce active prednisolone concentrations.

## Regulatory Information

Withdrawal times are not established for animals that produce food. For extralabel use withdrawal interval estimates, contact FARAD at www.FARAD.org.
RCI Classification: 4

## Pregabalin
pree-ga′bah-lin

**Trade and other names:** Lyrica

**Functional classification:** Analgesic, anticonvulsant

## Pharmacology and Mechanism of Action

Pregabalin is an analgesic and anticonvulsant. Pregabalin is similar in action to gabapentin, which is an analogue of the inhibitory neurotransmitter GABA. However, like gabapentin, it is not an agonist or antagonist for the GABA receptor. The anticonvulsant effect occurs via inhibition of calcium channels in neurons. Pregabalin inhibits the alpha$_2$-delta ($\alpha_2\delta$) subunit of the N-type voltage-dependent calcium channel on neurons. Through inhibition of these channels, it reduces calcium influx that is needed for release of neurotransmitters, specifically excitatory amino acids, from presynaptic neurons. Blocking the channels has little effect on normal neurons but may suppress simulated neurons involved in seizure activity and some forms of pain.

*Pharmacokinetics:* In humans, pregabalin has better oral absorption and a longer half-life than gabapentin. Better and more predictable oral absorption is attributed to higher permeability along the length of the intestine. Gabapentin must rely on specific transporters in the intestine for absorption, which can be saturated and a source of interactions. But pregabalin does not rely on transporters and is absorbed along the length of the intestine. Pregabalin relies on renal excretion for elimination.

The half-life of pregabalin in dogs is approximately 7 hours compared with 3–4 hours for gabapentin, and it remains above the estimated effective levels for 11 hours after dosing. Oral absorption in dogs is 98%. In cats, after 4 mg/kg PO, plasma concentrations are above the levels estimated to be effective for over 12 hours, with a half-life of 10 hours. In horses, the oral absorption is 98% with a half-life of 8 hours and, at a dose of 4 mg/kg PO, it produces plasma concentrations in the same therapeutic range as for people. An exception is evidence in dogs showing that pregabalin was effective for treating neuropathic pain associated with syringomyelia (5 mg/kg oral twice daily).

## Indications and Clinical Uses

In people, pregabalin is popular for treating neuropathic pain syndromes associated with diabetes, postherpetic neuralgia, and fibromyalgia. Pregabalin is also used as an anticonvulsant. As an analgesic in animals, it has been used to treat neuropathic pain that does not respond to NSAIDs or opioids. It may be combined with these agents. When used to treat epilepsy, pregabalin has reduced seizure frequency in refractory patients when combined with phenobarbital and potassium bromide. Therefore it is considered when the seizures have become refractory to other drugs in conjunction with other anticonvulsants. For treating pain in animals, there are no clinical studies available, except for a study in dogs with syringomyelia, that provide evidence of efficacy for treating neuropathic pain. The regimens used have primarily been derived from anecdotal evidence, opinions of experts, or extrapolation from human medicine.

In horses, it can produce concentrations in the therapeutic range for people, but safety and effectiveness have not been studied.

## Precautionary Information

### Adverse Reactions and Side Effects

Sedation and ataxia are reported adverse effects that can occur at doses as high as 3–4 mg/kg. As the dose increases in dogs, sedation is more likely. In people, there may be a withdrawal syndrome from abrupt discontinuation. This has not been reported in animals, but abrupt discontinuation after long-term treatment is discouraged.

### Contraindications and Precautions

There are no known contraindications in animals. Pregabalin, like gabapentin, is excreted in the urine, and liver disease or drug metabolism interactions are not expected to affect the pharmacokinetics. Protein binding is low. In people, it has been used with other anticonvulsants and anesthetics without producing a pharmacokinetic drug interaction. Fetal abnormalities have been observed in research animals given high doses of pregabalin during pregnancy, but this has not been reported with routine use.

### Drug Interactions

There are no reported drug interactions that affect the pharmacokinetics of pregabalin, but it could exacerbate sedation and lethargy when used with other drugs that depress the CNS.

## Instructions for Use

Pregabalin may be administered with or without food. Pregabalin has been used in some animals with other drugs such as phenobarbital and bromide. It also has been used to treat neuropathic pain syndromes and can be used with NSAIDs and opioids.

## Patient Monitoring and Laboratory Tests

No specific monitoring is necessary. Routine measurement of plasma concentrations is not widely available, but therapeutic concentrations in people (2.8–8.2 mcg/mL) have been used as a guideline. In some dogs, mild increases in liver enzymes may be observed during treatment.

## Formulations

- Pregabalin is available in 25-, 50-, 75-, 100-, 150-, 200-, 225-, and 300-mg capsules.

## Stability and Storage

Store in a tightly sealed container, protected from light and humidity. Stability of compounded formulations has not been evaluated.

## Small Animal Dosage

### Dogs

- Anticonvulsant dosage: 2 mg/kg q8h PO. Start with a low dose and gradually increase to the maximum tolerated dose of 3–4 mg/kg PO.
- Neuropathic pain: Start with 4–5 mg/kg q12h PO and increase dose gradually if necessary.

### Cats

- Anticonvulsant dosage or neuropathic pain dosage: Start with 2 mg/kg q12h PO and increase to 4 mg/kg q12h PO.

## Large Animal Dosage

### Horses

- 4 mg/kg PO q8h.

## Regulatory Information

Pregabalin is a Schedule V controlled substance. No withdrawal times are available for food animals. For extralabel use withdrawal interval estimates, contact FARAD at www.FARAD.org.

# Primidone
prih'mih-done

**Trade and other names:** Mylepsin, Neurosyn, and Mysoline (in Canada)

**Functional classification:** Anticonvulsant

## Pharmacology and Mechanism of Action

Primidone is one of the oldest anticonvulsants used in animals, but it is now used infrequently. Primidone is converted to phenylethylmalonamide (PEMA) and phenobarbital, both of which have anticonvulsant activity. Most of the activity (85%) is likely attributed to phenobarbital. The pharmacology of phenobarbital is discussed in more detail under Phenobarbital. Phenobarbital acts to potentiate the inhibitory effects of GABA-mediated chloride channels. See Phenobarbital for more information on pharmacology and pharmacokinetics.

## Indications and Clinical Uses

Primidone is used for treating seizure disorders in animals, including epilepsy. The effects of primidone are primarily produced by the presence of the active metabolite, phenobarbital. Although it is possible that some patients with epilepsy that are refractory to phenobarbital alone respond better to primidone, the number of such cases is low. Primidone is approved for use in dogs, but its use has declined in favor of administration of phenobarbital, levetiracetam, bromide, and other anticonvulsants. The use of primidone in cats is rare.

## Precautionary Information

### Adverse Reactions and Side Effects

Because primidone is converted to phenobarbital, adverse effects are the same as for phenobarbital. Primidone has been associated with idiosyncratic hepatotoxicity in dogs. Although the use in cats has been discouraged on the approved product label, one study in experimental cats determined that it is safe if used at recommended doses.

### Contraindications and Precautions

There may be a higher risk of hepatic toxicity with primidone compared with other anticonvulsants. Primidone should be avoided in animals with liver disease.

### Drug Interactions

Primidone is converted to phenobarbital, which is one of the most potent drugs for inducing hepatic microsomal metabolizing enzymes. Therefore, many drugs administered concurrently have lower (and perhaps subtherapeutic) concentrations because of more rapid clearance. Drugs affected may include theophylline, digoxin, corticosteroids, anesthetics, and other drugs that are substrated for cytochrome P450 enzymes.

## Instructions for Use

The recommendations for use are similar to those for phenobarbital. When monitoring therapy with primidone, phenobarbital plasma concentrations should be measured to estimate anticonvulsant effect. When converting a patient from primidone therapy to phenobarbital, the conversion is as follows: 60 mg phenobarbital is approximately 250 mg of primidone.

## Patient Monitoring and Laboratory Tests

Doses should be carefully adjusted via monitoring serum/plasma phenobarbital concentrations. Collect a sample at any time during the dose interval because the timing of the sample is not critical. Avoid the use of plasma separation devices if the tube is to be stored. The therapeutic range in dogs is considered 15–40 mcg/mL (65–180 mmol/L). The optimum range in cats for therapeutic effect is 23–28 mcg/mL. Monitor liver function with bile acid determinations.

## Formulations

- Primidone is available in 50- and 250-mg tablets.

## Stability and Storage

Store in a tightly sealed container, protected from light, and at room temperature. Stability of compounded formulations has not been evaluated.

## Small Animal Dosage

**Dogs and Cats**

- 8–10 mg/kg q8–12h as initial dose PO; then adjust via monitoring to 10–15 mg/kg q8h.

## Large Animal Dosage

- No doses have been reported for large animals.

## Regulatory Information

Withdrawal times are not established for animals that produce food. For extralabel use withdrawal interval estimates, contact FARAD at www.FARAD.org.

RCI Classification: 3

# Procainamide Hydrochloride
proe-kane-ah'mide hye-droe-klor'ide

**Trade and other names:** Pronestyl and generic brands

**Functional classification:** Antiarrhythmic

## Pharmacology and Mechanism of Action

Procainamide is a Class I antiarrhythmic drug that is rarely used in animals because approved formulations are often unavailable. Like other Class I antiarrhythmic drugs (a class that includes quinidine), procainamide inhibits sodium influx into the cardiac cell via sodium channel blockade. It suppresses cardiac automaticity and reentrant arrhythmias, primarily in the ventricle. Procainamide is metabolized in people to N-acetyl procainamide (NAPA), which produces additional antiarrhythmic actions (Class III drug: potassium channel–blocking effects). However, dogs do not form this metabolite because of an inability to acetylate some drugs.

## Indications and Clinical Uses

Procainamide has been used in small animals to suppress ventricular ectopic beats and treat ventricular arrhythmias. Studies in experimental dogs with induced arrhythmias have documented efficacy, but clinical use is based primarily on anecdotal experience. It is used primarily during acute treatment when it can be administered by injection or tablet. Rarely is long-term treatment used. Procainamide has occasionally been used in horses to suppress ventricular arrhythmias. The availability of commercial forms of procainamide has diminished, and the use has declined in favor of other antiarrhythmic agents.

## Precautionary Information

### Adverse Reactions and Side Effects

Adverse effects include cardiac arrhythmias, cardiac depression, tachycardia, and hypotension. In people, procainamide produces hypersensitivity effects (lupus-like reactions), but these have not been reported in animals.

### Contraindications and Precautions

Procainamide can suppress the heart and produce pro-arrhythmic effects. Use cautiously in animals receiving digoxin because it may potentiate arrhythmias.

### Drug Interactions

Drugs that inhibit cytochrome P450 enzymes (e.g., cimetidine) can potentially increase procainamide concentrations.

## Instructions for Use

Because dogs do not produce the active metabolite NAPA, the dosage may be higher compared with dosage for people to control some arrhythmias. In animals, there is no evidence that slow-release oral formulations produce longer duration of sustained blood concentrations.

## Patient Monitoring and Laboratory Tests

If assays are available, monitor plasma concentrations during chronic therapy. Effective plasma concentrations in experimental dogs are 20 mcg/mL. However, in some references, concentrations as low as 8–10 mcg/mL are cited to be effective. The metabolite, NAPA, is monitored in people, but dogs do not produce this metabolite. ECGs should be monitored in treated animals.

## Formulations

- Procainamide has been available in 250-, 375-, and 500-mg tablets or capsules and 100- and 500-mg/mL injections. However, because of diminished use in human medicine in favor of other alternatives, many of the human formulations are no longer available in the United States but are available in Canada. When oral doses are unavailable, procainamide can be compounded in pharmacies.

## Stability and Storage

Store in a tightly sealed container, protected from light, and at room temperature. Procainamide is soluble in water. When stored, solutions may turn yellow without losing potency. Darker coloration indicates oxidation. Storage of injectable vials in the refrigerator prevents oxidation. The pH of oral compounded products should be maintained at pH 4–6 for maximum stability. Compounded oral products in syrups and flavorings may be stable for 60 days or more, but they should be kept in the refrigerator.

## Small Animal Dosage

### Dogs

- 10–30 mg/kg q6h PO to a maximum dose of 40 mg/kg.

- 8–20 mg/kg IV or IM.
- CRI: Initial loading dose of 10 mg/kg followed by 20 mcg/kg/min IV CRI; the CRI rate can be increased to 25–50 mcg/kg/min if needed for refractory arrhythmias.

**Cats**

- 3–8 mg/kg q6–8h IM or PO.
- CRI: 1–2 mg/kg IV slowly; then 10–20 mcg/kg/min IV.

## Large Animal Dosage

**Horses**

- 25–35 mg/kg q8h PO.
- 1 mg/kg IV, in increments, up to a total maximum dose of 20 mg/kg IV.

## Regulatory Information

Withdrawal times are not established for animals that produce food. For extralabel use withdrawal interval estimates, contact FARAD at www.FARAD.org.

---

# Prochlorperazine Edisylate and Isopropamide Iodide, Prochlorperazine Maleate, and Isopropamide Iodide

**Trade and other names:** Darbazine

**Functional classification:** Antiemetic, antidiarrheal

## Pharmacology and Mechanism of Action

This is a combination product used to treat vomiting. This combination combines either prochlorperazine edisylate (injectable form) or prochlorperazine maleate (oral form) with isopropamide (isopropamide iodide). Chlorpromazine is a central-acting dopamine antagonist (antiemetic); isopropamide is an anticholinergic drug (atropine-like effects).

## Indications and Clinical Uses

Prochlorperazine is a phenothiazine used to control vomiting, in combination with isopropamide, which is an anticholinergic used to decrease intestinal motility and GI secretions. Its use is not common because of decreased availability of formulations and lack of proven efficacy compared with each ingredient alone.

## Precautionary Information

### Adverse Reactions and Side Effects

Side effects are attributed to each component. Prochlorperazine produces phenothiazine-like effects described more fully under Prochlorperazine. Isopropamide may produce effects attributed to excess anticholinergic (antimuscarinic) stimulation and include ileus, urine retention, tachycardia, xerostomia (dry mouth), and behavior changes. Treat overdoses with physostigmine.

### Contraindications and Precautions

Use of antimuscarinic drugs is contraindicated in animals with gastroparesis and should be used cautiously in animals with diarrhea. Isopropamide should not be administered to animals with gastroparesis or decreased intestinal motility.

### Drug Interactions

Isopropamide interferes with cholinergic drugs or drugs that promote motility (e.g., metoclopramide). Prochlorperazine potentiates other sedatives.

## Instructions for Use

This combination should be used with caution, especially if considered for repeated doses, in animals with intestinal disease. It can produce ileus.

## Patient Monitoring and Laboratory Tests

No specific monitoring is necessary.

## Formulations

- Prochlorperazine edisylate + isopropamide iodide is available in 3.33-mg prochlorperazine and 1.67-mg isopropamide capsules, and prochlorperazine maleate + isopropamide iodide is available in 4 mg of prochlorperazine and 0.28 mg of isopropamide per milliliter injection.
- Capsule for dogs (Neo-Darbazine Spansule Capsule) contains prochlorperazine, isopropamide, and neomycin.

## Stability and Storage

Store in a tightly sealed container, protected from light, and at room temperature. Stability of compounded formulations has not been evaluated.

## Small Animal Dosage

**Cats**

- 0.14–0.2 mL/kg q12h SQ.

**Dogs**

- 0.14–0.2 mL/kg q12h SQ.
- 2–7 kg body weight: 1 capsule q12h PO.
- 7–13 kg body weight: 1–2 capsules q12h PO.

## Large Animal Dosage

No doses have been reported for large animals. The use is discouraged because isopropamide may decrease GI motility.

## Regulatory Information

Withdrawal times are not established for animals that produce food. For extralabel use withdrawal interval estimates, contact FARAD at www.FARAD.org.

RCI Classification: 2

# Prochlorperazine Edisylate, Prochlorperazine Maleate

proe-klor-pare′ah-zeen ed-iss′ih-late and proe-klor-pare′ah-zeen mal′ee-ate

**Trade and other names:** Compazine

**Functional classification:** Antiemetic, phenothiazine

## Pharmacology and Mechanism of Action

Prochlorperazine is a phenothiazine derivative used primarily as an antiemetic. It is a central-acting dopamine ($D_2$) antagonist that can suppress vomiting at the vomiting center. Prochlorperazine is related to other phenothiazine antiemetic agents such as chlorpromazine, but prochlorperazine has higher antiemetic efficacy than chlorpromazine. Although chlorpromazine and prochlorperazine can block histamine $H_1$ and dopamine $D_2$ receptors, prochlorperazine is 10 times more selective for $D_2$ than histamine $H_1$ receptors. By antagonizing dopamine activity in the CNS, prochlorperazine produces sedation and prevents vomiting. Antiemetic action also may be related to alpha$_2$ and muscarinic blocking effects. There are two salt formulations of prochlorperazine: prochlorperazine edisylate and prochlorperazine maleate. They are therapeutically equivalent. Other phenothiazines include chlorpromazine, perphenazine, promazine, trifluoperazine, and triflupromazine.

## Indications and Clinical Uses

Prochlorperazine has been used for sedation, for tranquilization, and as an antiemetic. The antiemetic use is the most common. In people, it is also used to treat schizophrenia and nonpsychotic anxiety. Use in animals has been primarily derived from empirical use and experience in humans. There are no well-controlled clinical studies or efficacy trials to document clinical effectiveness.

## Precautionary Information

### Adverse Reactions and Side Effects

Prochlorperazine causes sedation and other side effects attributed to other phenothiazines. It also produces extrapyramidal side effects (involuntary muscle movements) in some individuals. Because of the alpha receptor–blocking properties, it can potentially produce vasodilation and hypotension.

### Contraindications and Precautions

Like other phenothiazines, it may be contraindicated in some CNS disorders. It may lower the seizure threshold in susceptible animals.

### Drug Interactions

Prochlorperazine may potentiate other sedatives.

## Instructions for Use

Prochlorperazine is used primarily as an antiemetic in animals. Clinical trials are not available; doses are based primarily on extrapolation and anecdotal experience.

## Patient Monitoring and Laboratory Tests

No specific monitoring is necessary.

## Formulations

- Prochlorperazine is available in 5-, 10-, and 25-mg tablets (prochlorperazine maleate); 1-mg/mL oral solution; and 5-mg/mL injection (prochlorperazine edisylate).

## Stability and Storage

Store in a tightly sealed container, protected from light, and at room temperature. Prochlorperazine is slightly soluble in water and soluble in ethanol. However, the maleate form is more insoluble in water. Prochlorperazine edisylate may be mixed with fluids such as water for injection. Some yellow discoloration may not affect potency. However, if milky-white precipitate forms in the vial, do not use.

## Small Animal Dosage

### Dogs and Cats

- 0.1–0.5 mg/kg q6–8h IM, IV, or SQ.
- 0.5–1 mg/kg q6–8h PO.

## Large Animal Dosage

- No doses have been reported for large animals.

## Regulatory Information

Withdrawal times are not established for animals that produce food. For extralabel use withdrawal interval estimates, contact FARAD at www.FARAD.org.

# Promethazine Hydrochloride

proe-meth'ah-zeen hye-droe-klor-ide

**Trade and other names:** Phenergan

**Functional classification:** Antiemetic, phenothiazine

## Pharmacology and Mechanism of Action

Promethazine is a phenothiazine drug with strong antihistamine effects. Promethazine is used mostly for its antiemetic effects, for which it acts either via the antihistamine receptors or by blocking dopamine receptors associated with vomiting.

## Indications and Clinical Uses

Promethazine has dual effects. It is used for treatment of allergy (antihistamine effect) and as an antiemetic (motion sickness). The efficacy for treating allergies in animals has not been established or studied in clinical trials. The uses in animals have been derived from empirical use and experience in humans. There are no well-controlled clinical studies or efficacy trials to document clinical effectiveness. Antihistamines have not been as effective for motion sickness in animals compared with other antiemetic agents.

## Precautionary Information

### Adverse Reactions and Side Effects

Promethazine has a risk of producing phenothiazine effects such as sedation and other side effects attributed to other phenothiazines. There also may be anticholinergic effects produced by the antimuscarinic properties in some individuals.

### Contraindications and Precautions

Promethazine may produce antimuscarinic side effects, but these have not been reported from clinical use in animals.

### Drug Interactions

No drug interactions have been reported in animals, but it exacerbates CNS depression when used with other sedatives, phenothiazines, or antihistamines.

## Instructions for Use

Results of clinical studies in animals have not been reported. Therefore the use in animals (and doses) is based on experience in people or anecdotal experience in animals.

## Patient Monitoring and Laboratory Tests

No specific monitoring is necessary.

## Formulations

- Promethazine is available in 6.25- and 25-mg/5 mL syrup; 12.5-, 25-, and 50-mg tablets; and 25- and 50-mg/mL injection.

## Stability and Storage

Promethazine hydrochloride is soluble in water. If oxidized, it turns a blue color and should be discarded. It is sensitive to light and should be protected from light.

## Small Animal Dosage

### Dogs and Cats

- 0.2–0.4 mg/kg q6–8h IV, IM, or PO up to a maximum dose of 1 mg/kg.

## Large Animal Dosage

• No doses have been reported for large animals.

## Regulatory Information

Withdrawal times are not established for animals that produce food. For extralabel use withdrawal interval estimates, contact FARAD at www.FARAD.org.

RCI Classification: 3

# Propantheline Bromide

proe-pan′theh-leen broe′mide

**Trade and other names:** Pro-Banthine

**Functional classification:** Antidiarrheal

## Pharmacology and Mechanism of Action

Propantheline is an anticholinergic (antimuscarinic) drug used infrequently to treat diarrhea in animals. Propantheline blocks acetylcholine receptors to produce parasympatholytic effects (atropine-like effects). It produces systemic parasympatholytic effects that include decreased GI secretions and motility.

## Indications and Clinical Uses

Propantheline is used to decrease smooth muscle contraction and secretion of the GI tract. Through these anticholinergic effects, it also has been used to treat vagal-mediated cardiovascular effects, such as bradycardia and heart block. Use in animals has been primarily derived from empirical use and experience in humans. There are no well-controlled clinical studies or efficacy trials to document clinical effectiveness. Because it produces a profound decrease in GI tract motility, its use should be carefully weighed against the potential for adverse effects.

P

## Precautionary Information

### Adverse Reactions and Side Effects

Side effects are attributed to excess anticholinergic (antimuscarinic) effects and include ileus, urine retention, tachycardia, xerostomia (dry mouth), and behavior changes. Treat overdoses with physostigmine.

### Contraindications and Precautions

Do not use in animals with decreased intestinal motility. Use cautiously in animals with heart disease because it may increase heart rate. Do not use in animals with glaucoma.

### Drug Interactions

Propantheline interferes with cholinergic drugs or drugs that promote motility (e.g., metoclopramide). Bromide concentration in the formulation should be considered for animals also receiving other sources of bromide (e.g., potassium bromide for treatment of epilepsy).

## Instructions for Use

Propantheline has not been evaluated in clinical trials in animals, but propantheline has been used for oral therapy in cases in which an anticholinergic effect is desired.

## Patient Monitoring and Laboratory Tests

No specific monitoring is necessary.

## Formulations

• Propantheline is available in 7.5- and 15-mg tablets.

## Stability and Storage

Store in a tightly sealed container, protected from light, and at room temperature.

## Small Animal Dosage

### Dogs and Cats

• 0.25–0.5 mg/kg q8–12h PO.

## Large Animal Dosage

• No doses have been reported for large animals. The use is discouraged because of adverse effect on GI motility.

## Regulatory Information

Withdrawal times are not established for animals that produce food. For extralabel use withdrawal interval estimates, contact FARAD at www.FARAD.org.

RCI Classification: 4

---

# Propiopromazine Hydrochloride (Propionylpromazine)

proe-pee-oh-prom′ah-zeen hye-droe-klor′ide

**Trade and other names:** Tranvet

**Functional classification:** Antiemetic, phenothiazine

## Pharmacology and Mechanism of Action

Propiopromazine (also spelled as propionylpromazine in some sources) is a phenothiazine with antihistamine effects. It has actions similar to those of other systemic phenothiazine drugs. Propiopromazine is used mostly for its antiemetic and sedative effects, for which it acts either via the antihistamine receptors or by blocking dopamine receptors. This drug was once registered for human use, but the only formulations currently available are veterinary forms. A related drug is propiomazine.

## Indications and Clinical Uses

Propiopromazine has been used for its antiemetic and sedative effects, for which it acts either via the antihistamine receptors or by blocking dopamine receptors. It also has sedative and tranquilizing effects and has been used in cats and dogs to facilitate handling. It has also been used as a preanesthetic. The approved label use indicates that it is "intended for administration to dogs as a tranquilizer. It is used as an aid in handling difficult, excited, and unruly dogs, and in controlling excessive kennel barking, car sickness, and severe dermatitis. It is also indicated for use in minor surgery and prior to routine examinations, laboratory procedures, and diagnostic procedures." Despite this labeling, some of these indications are outdated, and there are better treatments to manage these conditions.

### Precautionary Information

**Adverse Reactions and Side Effects**

Phenothiazines can cause sedation as a common side effect. Propiopromazine produces extrapyramidal side effects in some individuals.

**Contraindications and Precautions**

It may lower blood pressure via alpha-adrenergic blockade.

**Drug Interactions**

Do not use with other phenothiazines, organophosphates, or procaine. Use cautiously with other sedatives, tranquilizers, or CNS depressants because it may exacerbate the effects.

## Instructions for Use

Results of clinical studies in animals have not been reported despite indications listed on the product label. Use in animals (and doses) is based on anecdotal experience in animals and the product label.

### Patient Monitoring and Laboratory Tests

No specific monitoring is necessary.

### Formulations

- Propiopromazine has been available as a 20-mg chewable tablet and a 5- or 10-mg/ mL injection. Human formulations of this medication have been discontinued.

### Stability and Storage

Store in a tightly sealed container, protected from light, and at room temperature.

### Small Animal Dosage

**Dogs and Cats**

- 1.1–4.4 mg/kg q12–24h PO.
- 0.1–1.1 mg/kg IV or IM (range of injectable doses depends on level of sedation needed).

### Large Animal Dosage

- No doses have been reported for large animals. The use is discouraged in horses and ruminants because it may inhibit GI motility.

### Regulatory Information

Withdrawal times are not established for animals that produce food. For extralabel use withdrawal interval estimates, contact FARAD at www.FARAD.org.

# Propofol
proe′poe-fole

**Trade and other names:** Rapinovet, Rapanofal, PropoFlo, and PropoFlo 28 (veterinary preparations); Diprivan (human preparation)

**Functional classification:** Anesthetic

## Pharmacology and Mechanism of Action

Propofol is a widely used short-term anesthetic. The mechanism of action is not well defined, but it is likely that it produces effects via a similar mechanism as barbiturates.

Through this action, it produces depression of the CNS through its effect on the GABA receptor. Propofol decreases GABA from dissociating from its receptors, thereby increasing chloride conductance through channels, hyperpolarization of post-synaptic cell membranes, and inhibition of the postsynaptic neurons. This produces the anesthetic effects observed in animals.

The original formulation contained propofol in castor oil. The newer formulations contain soybean oil, glycerol, and purified egg phosphatide in an emulsion.

*Pharmacokinetics:* Propofol produces a short-acting (10 minutes) anesthesia followed by a rapid and smooth recovery. Propofol is rapidly metabolized to inactive glucuronide or sulfide conjugates in the liver. Systemic clearance is equal to hepatic blood flow in most animals.

## Indications and Clinical Uses

Propofol is used as a short-term injectable anesthetic. It is often used as an induction agent followed by inhalation with one of the inhalant anesthetics, or induction may be followed with maintenance doses. If repeated doses are administered for maintenance, it does not affect the recovery time. Thus, there is no cumulative effect. It has been used safely and effectively for short-term induction and surgical procedures. It is also appropriate for procedures that require repeated anesthetic episodes in dogs and cats without producing adverse effects.

A significant advantage of propofol over other agents is smooth and rapid recovery. It is also highly compatible with other anesthetic agents. It can be used with acepromazine, diazepam, alpha$_2$ agonists (e.g., dexmedetomidine), butorphanol, ketamine, and inhalant anesthetics. The use of these other agents will lower the dose requirement for propofol. Propofol also can be used as a CRI to maintain an anesthetized state for surgical procedures. (See infusion dose rates later.) An additional use of propofol is treatment of status epilepticus.

## Precautionary Information

### Adverse Reactions and Side Effects

Apnea and respiratory depression are the most common adverse effects, which are more likely at high doses. Propofol can induce a dose-dependent cardiovascular depression, but the severity of cardiac adverse events is generally low. Propofol can induce vasodilation, which can be minimized by providing sufficient IV fluids during the induction period and during anesthesia. Propofol can cause spontaneous muscle movements (paddling, tremors, muscle rigidity), panting, nystagmus, salivation, and retraction of tongue in some animals (incidence 3%–7%). Less frequent adverse reactions include vomiting during recovery and signs of pain.

Pain upon injection occurs in people but is less common in dogs. The pain from injection is caused by the free propofol in the formulation and is decreased with newer formulations. Phenolic drugs such as propofol may potentially cause oxidative damage to hemoglobin in cats because of higher concentration of oxidizable sulfhydryl groups in feline RBCs, leading to Heinz-body formation and methemoglobinemia. However, this has not been a consistent problem with routine clinical use of propofol, and repeated anesthetic episodes have been performed safely in cats. Some formulations (PropoFlo 28) contain 2% benzyl alcohol added as a preservative (20 mg/mL), which can produce hematologic abnormalities in some animals. However, this ingredient did not cause additional morbidity or problems in cats compared with other formulations.

When used alone in horses, it can cause excitement, myotonus, and problems during recovery. Therefore, when used in horses, other sedatives are recommended.

**Contraindications and Precautions**

Propofol can induce apnea, hypoxia, and cyanosis upon induction. Supplemental oxygen should be available to prevent adverse effects. Do not administer to hypotensive animals without providing fluids to correct hypotension. When propofol has been used to sedate animals for intradermal skin testing, it may produce a greater number of positive reactions. The use of propofol in pregnant and breeding animals has not been evaluated. Propofol crosses the placenta and can cause neonatal depression. Propofol has not been evaluated in dogs younger than 10 weeks of age. Propofol should not be used alone for anesthesia in horses—combine with other sedatives or premedications.

**Drug Interactions**

Propofol can be used with several other anesthetics and adjuncts safely. It has been mixed with thiopental sodium (2.5%) in a 1:1 mixture without loss of effectiveness. Propofol has been used with atropine, glycopyrrolate, acepromazine, xylazine, oxymorphone, halothane, and isoflurane without any interactions observed.

## Instructions for Use

Shake well before using. Use strict aseptic technique for administration. Propofol may be diluted in 5% dextrose, lactated Ringer's solution, and 0.9% saline but not to less than a 2-mg/mL concentration. There is a delay in penetration to brain after the initial IV injection; therefore, expect a delayed CNS effect during injection and re-evaluate the response before administering additional injections. A mixture of 1:1 thiopental (2.5%) and propofol can be used in dogs and results in a smooth induction. When using with other anesthetics and sedatives (acepromazine, barbiturates, opioids, benzodiazepines, alpha$_2$ agonists), lower doses should be administered because premedications and other sedatives greatly reduce the propofol dose requirements. The reduction in dose when used with premedications and other sedatives is approximately 16%–20% in cats and 20%–30% in dogs but may be as high as 40%–50% in dogs.

## Patient Monitoring and Laboratory Tests

Monitor respiration rate and character during anesthesia with propofol.

## Formulations

- The human formulation of propofol is available in 1% (10-mg/mL) injection in 20-mL ampules.
- The veterinary formulation is available in multidose vials containing 10 mg of propofol per milliliter. Propofol is only slightly soluble in water; therefore it is formulated in a white, oil-in-water emulsion. It also contains soybean oil (100 mg/mL), glycerol (22.5 mg/mL), egg lecithin (12 mg/mL), and oleic acid (0.6 mg/mL) with sodium hydroxide to adjust the pH. The propofol emulsion is isotonic and has a pH of 6.0–9.0. The formulation PropoFlo 28 has benzyl alcohol added as a preservative.
- Note: The formulation known as PropoClear emulsion for dogs and cats (without lipids) was associated with adverse reactions and has been removed from the market.

## Stability and Storage

The veterinary formulation (PropoFlo, Rapinovet, Rapanofal) has no preservatives and should be discarded within 6 hours after opening the vial. When formulations without a preservative are used, there should be careful handling and injection technique to prevent microbial contamination of this formulation.

The formulation with a benzyl alcohol preservative allows for a 28-day shelf-life after opening the vial (PropoFlo 28).

Propofol has been mixed with thiopental sodium in a 1:1 mixture, and they are physically and chemically compatible. However, do not mix with other drugs unless compatibility has been verified. Propofol has a pH of 7–8.5. Store at 40°F and 72°F (4°C–22°C). Do not freeze. Protect from light. Shake well before use.

## Small Animal Dosage
### Dogs
- The FDA-approved label dose for induction ranges from 5.5 to 7.6 mg/kg IV slowly over 30–60 seconds. If necessary, additional doses can be administered in increments of 0.5–1 mg/kg for the desired effect. Most inductions can be performed with lower doses of approximately 4 mg/kg. If the patient has received a premedication with alpha$_2$ agonists, opioids, or benzodiazepines, lower the dose by at least 20%–30% (e.g., a lower dose of 3 mg/kg can be used). After initial induction, maintenance doses of 1–3 mg/kg IV can be used.
- CRI: 5–6 mg/kg slowly IV followed by 100–450 mcg/kg/min (or 6–25 mg/kg/h). In some animals the rate may be as high as 600 mcg/kg/min (36 mg/kg/h) if they are not premedicated. If other agents are included in the protocol (e.g., ketamine), the dose can be decreased.
- Status epilepticus: 1–6 mg/kg IV (to effect) followed by a CRI of 0.1–0.6 mg/kg/min.

### Cats
- Anesthesia induction: 4–8 mg/kg IV slowly. The approved label lists higher doses, but most cats can be induced with approximately 6 mg/kg IV. After the initial dose, incremental doses of 1–3 mg/kg IV can be administered as needed. If other preanesthetics and sedatives are used, reduce by 16%–24%. If combined with midazolam, the propofol requirement listed can be reduced by as much as 25%.
- CRI: 6 mg/kg slowly IV followed by 200–300 mcg/kg/min (0.2–0.3 mg/kg/h) IV. For short-term procedures, the total dose is 15 mg/kg for a 30-minute protocol.
- CRI infusion with ketamine in cats: 0.025 mg/min/kg + ketamine 23–46 mcg/kg/min.
- Short-term surgery: 10-mg/kg IV dose delivered over 1 minute (duration of anesthesia, 10–20 minutes).

## Large Animal Dosage
### Horses
- 2 mg/kg IV bolus. Guaifenesin (90 mg/kg IV) or another sedative should be administered prior to propofol to prevent excitement and myotonus and other problems during recovery.

### Small Ruminants
- 4 mg/kg IV.

### Pigs
- 2–5 mg/kg IV.

## Regulatory Information
Withdrawal times are not established for animals that produce food. For extralabel use withdrawal interval estimates, contact FARAD at www.FARAD.org.
RCI Classification: 2

# Propranolol Hydrochloride
proe-pran′oh-lole hye-droe-klor′ide

**Trade and other names:** Inderal and generic brands

**Functional classification:** Beta blocker

## Pharmacology and Mechanism of Action
Propranolol is one of the oldest and widely used beta-adrenergic blockers. It is nonselective for $beta_1$- and $beta_2$-adrenergic receptors and newer drugs that are more specific are more commonly used. It is also a Class II antiarrhythmic that inhibits cardiac conduction in the atrioventricular and sinoatrial nodes to decrease heart rate and the ventricular response to atrial stimulation. Propranolol is a lipophilic beta blocker and relies on the liver for clearance. Lipophilic beta blockers such as propranolol undergo high first-pass clearance, which reduces oral bioavailability and causes high interpatient variability in plasma concentrations and effects. Drug concentrations may be higher when there is impaired liver blood flow. By contrast, atenolol is a water-soluble beta blocker and undergoes more predictable elimination.

## Indications and Clinical Uses
Propranolol is used primarily to decrease heart rate, decrease cardiac conduction, control tachyarrhythmias, and decrease blood pressure. It is effective in controlling the response from adrenergic stimulation. Beta blockers such as propranolol are among the most effective drugs for slowing heart rate, but propranolol is not used as commonly as other more specific agents such as atenolol or metoprolol. Esmolol is preferred for short-term use.

## Precautionary Information
### Adverse Reactions and Side Effects
The adverse effects from propranolol are related to $beta_1$-blocking effects on heart. Propranolol causes cardiac depression and decreases cardiac output. $Beta_2$-blocking effects can cause bronchoconstriction and decrease insulin secretion. Switch to a more specific $beta_1$-blocker (see Instructions for Use) if $beta_2$-blocking effects are undesirable and a more specific agent is needed. Weakness and fatigue can be caused by beta blockers, which can indicate that a reduction in dose is needed.

### Contraindications and Precautions
Do not administer to animals with low cardiac reserve, bradycardia, or poor systolic function. Use cautiously in animals with respiratory problems because bronchoconstriction can occur from $beta_2$ effects. Hyperthyroid cats may have reduced clearance and increased risk of toxicity.

### Drug Interactions
Lipophilic beta blockers, such as propranolol, rely on the liver for clearance. These drugs are subject to interactions from drugs that affect liver blood flow and interact with hepatic enzymes. Decreased liver blood flow reduces propranolol's clearance.

## Instructions for Use
There may be high individual variability in clinical response. The dose should be titrated according to patient's response (e.g., by monitoring the heart rate). Start with a low dose and increase gradually to desired effect. Clearance relies on hepatic blood flow; therefore, it should be administered cautiously to animals with impaired hepatic

perfusion. In cats with hyperthyroidism, consider reducing the dose to prevent adverse effects. Cats with hyperthyroidism may have decreased clearance or increased oral absorption compared with other cats.

Propranolol is a nonspecific beta-blocker. If a more specific blocker is needed (i.e., specific for the beta$_1$ receptor), consider atenolol or metoprolol, which are listed in other sections of this book.

### Patient Monitoring and Laboratory Tests
Monitor heart rate during treatment. Monitor respiratory function in patients prone to bronchoconstriction.

### Formulations
- Oral: Propranolol is available in 10-, 20-, 40-, 60-, and 80-mg tablets and 4- and 8-mg/mL oral solution.
- Injection: Propofol is available in a 1-mg/mL injection.

### Stability and Storage
Store in a tightly sealed container, protected from light, and at room temperature. Propranolol is soluble in water and ethanol. Suspensions prepared in various syrups and flavorings were stable for 4 months, but some settling may occur (shake before administration). pH of formulations should be kept at 2.8–4 for maximum stability. In alkaline solutions, it decomposes.

### Small Animal Dosage
**Dogs**
- 20–60 mcg/kg over 5–10 minutes IV (titrate dose to effect).
- 0.2–1 mg/kg q8h PO (titrate dose to effect).

**Cats**
- 0.4–1.2 mg/kg (2.5–5 mg/cat) q8h PO.

### Large Animal Dosage
**Horses**
- 0.1 mg/kg IV slowly. Repeat in 6–8 hours if necessary. If low dose is not effective, administer 0.5 mg/kg and increase the dose to 2 mg/kg IV gradually until desired response.
- 0.4–0.8 mg/kg q8h PO.

### Regulatory Information
Withdrawal times are not established for animals that produce food. For extralabel use withdrawal interval estimates, contact FARAD at www.FARAD.org.

RCI Classification: 3

# Propylthiouracil
pro-pil-thye-oh-yoo′rah-sil

**Trade and other names:** Propyl-Thyracil, PTU, and generic brands

**Functional classification:** Antithyroid

### Pharmacology and Mechanism of Action
Propylthiouracil (PTU) is an older antithyroid drug that is not used frequently because of the availability of other agents. PTU inhibits synthesis of thyroid hormones; specifically, it interferes with conversion of T$_4$ to T$_3$.

## Indications and Clinical Uses

Propylthiouracil has been used for the treatment of feline hyperthyroidism. Because of adverse effects, use of PTU in most cats has been replaced with methimazole or carbimazole. The only remaining indication for PTU in animals is to treat an acute "thyroid storm" because it rapidly inhibits conversion of T$_3$ to T$_4$, which methimazole does not.

### Precautionary Information

**Adverse Reactions and Side Effects**

Adverse effects in cats include hepatopathy, hemolytic anemia, thrombocytopenia, and other signs of immune-mediated disease. If these signs are observed, the medication should be changed to another antithyroid agent. Because of the frequency of adverse reactions, the use of PTU for long-term use is discouraged.

**Contraindications and Precautions**

Do not use in cats with low platelet counts or bleeding problems.

**Drug Interactions**

No drug interactions have been reported in animals, but the use has declined, and these may not have been reported.

## Instructions for Use

Avoid the use of PTU because of the frequency of adverse effects. Other drugs, such as methimazole or carbimazole, can be used as a replacement.

### Patient Monitoring and Laboratory Tests

Monitor CBC to look for evidence of hematologic abnormalities. Monitor T$_4$ levels to assess therapy.

### Formulations

Propylthiouracil has been available in 50- and 100-mg tablets. The availability of commercial formulations has diminished.

### Stability and Storage

Store in a tightly sealed container, protected from light, and at room temperature. PTU is slightly soluble in water and soluble in ethanol.

### Small Animal Dosage

**Cats**

- 11 mg/kg q12h PO.

### Large Animal Dosage

- No doses have been reported for large animals.

### Regulatory Information

Withdrawal times are not established for animals that produce food. For extralabel use withdrawal interval estimates, contact FARAD at www.FARAD.org.

# Prostaglandin F$_2$ Alpha

pross-teh-glan′din

**Trade and other names:** Lutalyse, Dinoprost, and PGF$_2$ alpha

**Functional classification:** Prostaglandin

## Pharmacology and Mechanism of Action

Prostaglandin F$_2$ (PGF$_2$) alpha simulates the action of endogenous PGF$_2$ alpha in animals. It induces luteolysis and terminates pregnancy. It is also called dinoprost. The synthetic form is called cloprostenol (see Cloprostenol for more information), which is often used in animals.

## Indications and Clinical Uses

Prostaglandin F$_2$ alpha has been used to treat open pyometra in animals. In cattle, dinoprost has been used for treatment of chronic endometritis. Use for inducing abortion in small animals has been questioned, and other drugs are usually used instead. For example, synthetic PGF$_2$ alpha analogs such as cloprostenol are more potent with fewer adverse effects.

Occasionally, in large animals, dinoprost is used to induce abortion in the first 100 days of gestation. It is also used for estrous synchronization in cattle and horses by causing luteolysis. In pigs, dinoprost is used to induce parturition when given within 3 days of farrowing.

## Precautionary Information

### Adverse Reactions and Side Effects

Prostaglandin F$_2$ alpha causes increased smooth muscle tone, resulting in diarrhea, abdominal discomfort, bronchoconstriction, and an increase in blood pressure. In small animals, other side effects include vomiting, which occurs within 20 minutes of injection. Induction of abortion may cause retained placenta.

### Contraindications and Precautions

Do not administer intravenously. PGF$_2$ alpha induces abortion in pregnant animals. Use caution when handling this drug. It should not be handled by pregnant women. Absorption through the intact skin is possible. People with respiratory problems also should not handle dinoprost because absorption across the skin may lead to bronchoconstriction.

### Drug Interactions

According to the label, dinoprost should not be used with NSAIDs because these drugs inhibit synthesis of prostaglandins. However, NSAIDs should not affect concentrations of PGF$_2$ alpha after administration with this product. When using oxytocin concurrently, it should be used cautiously because there is a risk of uterine rupture.

## Instructions for Use

Use in treating pyometra should be monitored carefully because adverse effects can occur as a consequence of treatment for pyometra.

## Patient Monitoring and Laboratory Tests

Monitor for signs of estrus after treatment.

## Formulations

- PGF$_2$ is available in a 5-mg/mL solution for injection.

## Stability and Storage

Store in a tightly sealed container, protected from light, and at room temperature. It should be stored in a manner to avoid skin contact with humans.

## Small Animal Dosage

### Dogs

- Pyometra: 0.1–0.2 mg/kg once daily for 5 days SQ.
- Termination of pregnancy: 0.1–0.25 mg/kg q 8–12h SQ. Fewer adverse effects are seen with 0.1 mg/kg q8h SQ for 2 days; then increase to 0.2 mg/kg q8h, SQ until abortion is complete, usually within 9 days. It may be combined with misoprostol to shorten the protocol.

### Cats

- Pyometra: 0.1–0.25 mg/kg once daily for 5 days SQ.
- Termination of pregnancy: 0.5–1 mg/kg IM for two injections. A lower dosage and longer protocol for cats is a dosage of 0.2 mg/kg q12h, SQ on day 1 and then 0.5 mg/kg q12h SQ for up to 5 days.

## Large Animal Dosage

### Cattle

- Termination of pregnancy: 25 mg total dosage administered once IM.
- Estrus synchronization: 25 mg once IM or twice at 10- to 12-day intervals.
- Pyometra: 25 mg IM administered once.

### Horses

- Estrus synchronization: 1 mg/100 lb (1 mg/45 kg) IM or 1–2 mL administered once IM. Mares should return to estrus within 2–4 days and ovulate 8–12 days after treatment.

### Pigs

- Induction of parturition: 10 mg administered once IM. Parturition occurs within 30 hours.

## Regulatory Information

No withdrawal time required for meat or milk.

**P**

# Pseudoephedrine Hydrochloride

soo-doh-eh-fed′rin hye-droe-klor′ide

**Trade and other names:** Sudafed and generic brands

**Functional classification:** Adrenergic agonist

## Pharmacology and Mechanism of Action

Pseudoephedrine is an adrenergic agonist that acts nonselectively as a sympathomimetic. It is an agonist for the alpha-adrenergic and beta-adrenergic receptors. These receptors are found throughout the body, such as on sphincters, blood vessels, smooth muscle, and heart. Therefore pseudoephedrine can have effects on multiple organs. Pseudoephedrine produces a similar effect as ephedrine and PPA. However, compared with ephedrine, it may have fewer CNS effects.

## Indications and Clinical Uses

Pseudoephedrine has been used as a decongestant, as a mild bronchodilator, and to increase tone of urinary sphincter. Pseudoephedrine, PPA, and ephedrine have similar alpha-receptor and beta-receptor effects. The most common use in animals is for treating urinary incontinence. The mechanism for this action appears to be via stimulating receptors on the sphincter.

In people, it has been used as a decongestant. However, because pseudoephedrine is easily diverted to manufacture of methamphetamine, the availability in human medicine has diminished because of restrictions for obtaining the tablets from a pharmacy. Most of the OTC forms and combination products for people have been removed. For animals, PPA produces similar effects and may be substituted.

### Precautionary Information

**Adverse Reactions and Side Effects**

Adverse effects are attributed to adrenergic effects. These include excitement, rapid heart rate, increased blood pressure, and arrhythmias.

**Contraindications and Precautions**

Pseudoephedrine may cause some effects that are similar to PPA. Use cautiously in patients with cardiovascular disease. Use cautiously with drugs that are MAOIs. Beta agonists such as pseudoephedrine may increase blood glucose. Pseudoephedrine has been used in clandestine laboratories to illegally manufacture methamphetamine. Therefore, the availability of pseudoephedrine has been restricted in most states.

**Drug Interactions**

Pseudoephedrine, like other sympathomimetic agents, is expected to potentiate other alpha- and beta-receptor agonists. It may cause increased vasoconstriction and changes in heart rate. Use cautiously with other vasoactive drugs. Use cautiously with other drugs that may lower the seizure threshold. Use of inhalant anesthetics may increase cardiovascular risk. Do not use with TCAs or MAOIs.

### Instructions for Use

Although clinical trials have not been conducted for comparison, it is believed that the action and efficacy of pseudoephedrine are similar to those of ephedrine and PPA.

### Patient Monitoring and Laboratory Tests

Monitor heart rate in patients. If possible, monitor blood pressure and ECG in patients that may be susceptible to cardiovascular problems.

### Formulations Available

Pseudoephedrine has been available in 30- and 60-mg tablets, 120-mg capsules, and 6-mg/mL syrup, but the availability of human formulations has diminished because of reasons cited earlier. (Some combination formulations have other ingredients such as antitussives or antihistamines.)

### Stability and Storage

Store in a tightly sealed container, protected from light, and at room temperature. Pseudoephedrine is soluble in water and ethanol. Keep compounded formulations at a low pH for maximum stability. Protect from freezing.

### Small Animal Dosage

**Dogs**

• 0.2–0.4 mg/kg (or 15–60 mg/dog) q8–12h PO.

## Large Animal Dosage
• No doses have been reported for large animals.

## Regulatory Information
Because of abuse in humans, many forms are now Controlled Schedule V substances. Withdrawal times are not established for animals that produce food. For extralabel use withdrawal interval estimates, contact FARAD at www.FARAD.org.
RCI Classification: 3

# Psyllium
sill'ee-um

**Trade and other names:** Metamucil and generic brands
**Functional classification:** Laxative

## Pharmacology and Mechanism of Action
Psyllium is a common OTC bulk-forming laxative. The action of psyllium is to absorb water and expand to provide increased bulk and moisture content to the stool, which encourages normal peristalsis and bowel motility. Psyllium also may have antilipidemia effects.

## Indications and Clinical Uses
Psyllium is administered orally for treatment of constipation and bowel evacuation. In horses, it has been used for treating sand colic, but the effectiveness for this indication has not been shown.

## Precautionary Information
### Adverse Reactions and Side Effects
Adverse effects have not been reported in animals. Intestinal impaction can occur with overuse or in patients with inadequate fluid intake. In horses, it may be difficult to administer via stomach tube because it is prone to forming a gel when mixed with water.

### Contraindications and Precautions
No contraindications are reported for animals.

### Drug Interactions
No drug interactions have been reported in animals.

## Instructions for Use
Results of clinical studies in animals have not been reported. Use in animals (and doses) is based on experience in people or anecdotal experience in animals.

## Patient Monitoring and Laboratory Tests
Psyllium may lower serum cholesterol measurements.

## Formulations
- Psyllium is available as powder, usually 3.4 g per teaspoon.

## Stability and Storage
Store in a tightly sealed container, protected from light, and at room temperature.

## Small Animal Dosage
### Dogs and Cats
- 1 teaspoon/5–10 kg (added to each meal).

## Large Animal Dosage
### Horses
- Up to 1000 mg/kg per day PO via stomach tube or added to feed. Note precaution above about administering by a stomach tube in horses. It may form a gel when mixed with water and plug the tube.

## Regulatory Information
No withdrawal times are necessary.

---

# Pyrantel Pamoate and Pyrantel Tartrate
pye ran′ tel

**Trade and other names:** Nemex, Strongid, Priex, Pyran, and Pyr-A-Pam

**Functional classification:** Antiparasitic

## Pharmacology and Mechanism of Action
Pyrantel is one of the oldest antiparasitic drugs but is still used in animal for common intestinal parasites. Pyrantel is in the class of tetrahydropyrimidines. Others in this class include morantel. Pyrantel acts to interfere with ganglionic neurotransmission via blocking with acetylcholine receptors and other sites. This causes paralysis of the parasites. Paralyzed worms are expelled from the intestinal lumen by peristalsis. Pyrantel is poorly water soluble and not absorbed systemically in ruminants, although some absorption occurs in monogastric animals. Most of the activity is confined to the intestinal lumen.

## Indications and Clinical Uses
Pyrantel is indicated for treatment of intestinal nematodes. In horses, it is used for treatment and prevention of nematodes, including pinworms (*Oxyuris equi*), large roundworms (*Parascaris equorum*), large strongyles (*Strongylus edentatus, Strongylus equinus,* and *Strongylus vulgaris*), and small strongyles. When added to medicated feed, it is used to control nematodes, including pinworms (*O. equi*), large roundworms (*P. equorum*), large strongyles (*S. edentatus, S. vulgaris,* and *Triodontophorus* spp.), and small strongyles. In pigs, it is used for prevention of large roundworm (*Ascaris suum*) and prevention of the nodular worm *Oesophagostomum* spp. In dogs and cats, it is used for treatment of nematodes, including hookworms (*Ancylostoma* spp.) and roundworms (*Toxocara cati, Toxocara canis,* and *Toxascaris leonina*). There is some evidence that it is effective for control of some tapeworms, but ordinarily other drugs should be used for tapeworms (see Praziquantel).

## Precautionary Information

**Adverse Reactions and Side Effects**

Pyrantel has a good safety record. No adverse effects reported with regular use.

**Contraindications and Precautions**

No contraindications in animals. It may be used in all ages and in lactating and pregnant animals.

**Drug Interactions**

Central nervous system toxicity may be more likely when co-administered with levamisole, but this is not reported from clinical use in animals. It can be safely administered with several other antiparasitic agents.

## Instructions for Use

Shake suspension prior to use. Doses listed are for single dose, but they may be repeated as part of a parasite management program. Lower doses may be added to daily feed for prevention of parasites.

## Patient Monitoring and Laboratory Tests

Monitor fecal samples for presence of intestinal parasites.

## Formulations

- Pyrantel is available in 171-, 180-, and 226-mg/mL (base) paste; 22.7- and 113.5-mg (base) tablets; and 2.27-, 4.54-, and 50-mg/mL (base) suspension. Equine paste is 19.31%. It is also available in 10.6-, 12.6-, and 21.1-g/kg of pellets for medicated feed.
- Pyrantel pamoate is a salt and contains 34.7% pyrantel base. Doses are based on the amount of pyrantel base. Pyrantel tartrate contains 57.9% pyrantel base.
- Many of the formulations contain other antiparasitic drugs (e.g., praziquantel). For example, it is available as 13.6 mg of praziquantel and 54.3 of mg pyrantel, 18.2 mg of praziquantel and 72.6 mg of pyrantel, or 27.2 mg of praziquantel and 108.6 mg of pyrantel. The product Simparica Trio contains sarolaner, moxidectin, and pyrantel in a single chewable tablet for dogs for once per month administration.

## Stability and Storage

Store in a tightly sealed container, protected from light, and at room temperature. Protect from freezing.

## Small Animal Dosage

**Dogs**

- 5 mg/kg once PO; repeat in 7–10 days. (Combination products may be dosed on a different schedule [e.g., once per month]. Consult specific labeling for dose intervals.)

**Cats**

- 20 mg/kg once PO.
- Doses may be mixed with food.

## Large Animal Dosage

**Horses**

- Nematodes: 6.6 mg/kg PO.
- Cestodes: 13.2 mg/kg.
- Medicated feed: 12.5 mg/kg as a single dose or 2.6 mg/kg/day for prevention.

**Pigs**

- 22 mg/kg administered in feed as a single treatment.

## Regulatory Information
Pigs: 1-day withdrawal (United States); 7 days (Canada).
Withdrawal times for other species are not established. For extralabel use withdrawal
interval estimates, contact FARAD at www.FARAD.org.

# Pyridostigmine Bromide
peer-id-oh-stig′meen broe′mide

**Trade and other names:** Mestinon and Regonol

**Functional classification:** Anticholinesterase, antimyasthenic

## Pharmacology and Mechanism of Action
Pyridostigmine is a cholinesterase inhibitor and antimyasthenic drug. This drug
inhibits the enzyme that breaks down acetylcholine. Therefore it prolongs the action
of acetylcholine at the synapse. The major difference between physostigmine and
neostigmine or pyridostigmine is that physostigmine crosses the blood–brain barrier,
and the others do not. Compared with neostigmine, pyridostigmine has a longer
duration of action.

## Indications and Clinical Uses
Pyridostigmine is used as an antidote for anticholinergic intoxication and treatment
(antidote) for neuromuscular blockade. It is also used as a treatment of myasthenia
gravis, ileus, and retention of urine (e.g., postoperative ileus and urine retention) by
increasing tone of bladder smooth muscle and stimulating bowel motility. The most
common regular used for pyridostigmine is the first drug of choice for myasthenia
gravis. It is preferred over neostigmine. If animals with myasthenia gravis do not
respond to pyridostigmine alone, immunosuppressive agents are added.

## Precautionary Information
### Adverse Reactions and Side Effects
Adverse effects are caused by the cholinergic action resulting from inhibition
of cholinesterase. These effects can be seen in the GI tract as diarrhea and
increased secretions. Other adverse effects can include miosis, bradycardia,
muscle twitching or weakness, and constriction of bronchi and ureters.
Pyridostigmine may be associated with fewer adverse effects than neostigmine,
but the effects of pyridostigmine may persist longer. If adverse effects are
observed, treat with anticholinergic drugs, such as 0.125 mg of hyoscyamine
sulfate. Atropine also may be used as an antagonist to reverse adverse effects or
an overdose.

### Contraindications and Precautions
Do not use in patients with urinary obstruction, intestinal obstruction, asthma or
bronchoconstriction, pneumonia, or cardiac arrhythmias. Do not use in patients
sensitive to bromide. Consider the amount of bromide in dose in any patient also
receiving bromide for treatment of seizures.

### Drug Interactions
Bromide concentration in the formulation should be considered for animals also
receiving bromide (e.g., potassium bromide) for treatment of epilepsy. (Sodium
bromide may be used as an alternative.)

## Instructions for Use

Pyridostigmine is used for treatment of myasthenia gravis. Neostigmine and pyridostigmine have fewer side effects than physostigmine. When used, the frequency of dose may be increased based on observation of effects. After administration, pyridostigmine's benefits should be observed in approximately 15–30 minutes. The duration of action may be 3–4 hours.

## Patient Monitoring and Laboratory Tests

Monitor GI effects. Monitor cardiac rate and rhythm.

## Formulations

Pyridostigmine is available in 12-mg/mL oral syrup, 60-mg tablets (scored), and 5-mg/mL injection.

## Stability and Storage

Store in a tightly sealed container, protected from light, and at room temperature. Pyridostigmine is soluble in water. Store in acid solutions; it may decompose in alkaline vehicles.

## Small Animal Dosage

### Dogs

- Antimyasthenic: 0.02–0.04 mg/kg q2h IV or 0.5–3 mg/kg q8–12h PO.
- Antidote for muscle blockade: 0.15–0.3 mg/kg IM or IV as needed.

### Cats

- 0.1–0.25 mg/kg q24h PO. CRI: 0.01–0.03 mg/kg/h IV.

## Large Animal Dosage

- No doses have been reported for large animals.

## Regulatory Information

Withdrawal times are not established for animals that produce food. For extralabel use withdrawal interval estimates, contact FARAD at www.FARAD.org.

RCI Classification: 3

# Pyrimethamine
peer-ih-meth′ah-meen

**Trade and other names:** Daraprim

**Functional classification:** Antibacterial

## Pharmacology and Mechanism of Action

Pyrimethamine is an antibacterial and antiprotozoal drug. Pyrimethamine blocks the dihydrofolate reductase enzyme, which inhibits synthesis of reduced folate and nucleic acids. Activity of pyrimethamine is more specific against protozoa than bacteria. Pyrimethamine is rarely used alone and often combined with a sulfonamide to produce a synergistic effect.

## Indications and Clinical Uses

Pyrimethamine is used to treat protozoal infections in animals. It is most often combined with a sulfonamide, either separately or in a combined formulation. See Pyrimethamine + Sulfadiazine for additional information.

### Precautionary Information

**Adverse Reactions and Side Effects**

There is a risk of folic acid anemia when pyrimethamine and sulfonamide combinations are administered for prolonged treatment. This has been observed in 12% of treated horses in a field trial. Folic or folinic acid (preferably folinic acid) has been supplemented to prevent anemia, but the benefit of this treatment is unclear. Bone marrow suppression usually resolves after discontinuation of treatment. Diarrhea may occur after oral administration.

**Contraindications and Precautions**

Use cautiously in pregnant animals because of effects of folate inhibition on the fetus.

**Drug Interactions**

Drug interactions are not reported for animals. However, a combination of pyrimethamine with trimethoprim–sulfonamides enhances the bone marrow toxicity.

## Instructions for Use

Pyrimethamine is used either alone or in combination with sulfonamides. (See Pyrimethamine + Sulfadiazine for further details.)

## Patient Monitoring and Laboratory Tests

Monitor CBC periodically in animals receiving treatment.

## Formulations

- Pyrimethamine is available in 25-mg tablets. (Human-labeled tablets may be very expensive.)

## Stability and Storage

Store in a tightly sealed container, protected from light, and at room temperature. Pyrimethamine is poorly soluble in water, but it is more soluble in ethanol. Tablets have been crushed to make extemporaneous suspensions in syrups and other flavorings. These formulations have been stable for 7 days and up to 90 days, depending on the formulation.

## Small Animal Dosage

**Dogs**

- 1 mg/kg q24h PO for 14–21 days (5 days for *Neospora caninum*).

**Cats**

- 0.5–1 mg/kg q24h PO for 14–28 days.

## Large Animal Dosage

- Horses, EPM caused by *S. neurona*: 1 mg/kg q24h PO in combination with a sulfonamide (see details under Pyrimethamine + Sulfadiazine).

## Regulatory Information

Withdrawal times are not established for animals that produce food. For extralabel use withdrawal interval estimates, contact FARAD at www.FARAD.org.

# Pyrimethamine and Sulfadiazine
peer-ih-meth′ah-meen and sul-fa-dye′ah-zeen

**Trade and other names:** ReBalance

**Functional classification:** Antiprotozoal

## Pharmacology and Mechanism of Action

Pyrimethamine, in combination with sulfadiazine is an antibacterial and antiprotozoal drug that produce synergistic effects when used in combination. Pyrimethamine blocks dihydrofolate reductase enzyme, which inhibits synthesis of reduced folate and nucleic acids. Activity of pyrimethamine is more specific against protozoa than bacteria. Sulfadiazine provides a false substrate for para-aminobenzoic acid (PABA), which is required for synthesis of dihydrofolic acid by bacteria and protozoa. Together the combination is synergistic against protozoa.

## Indications and Clinical Uses

Pyrimethamine + sulfadiazine is used to treat horses with EPM. Although not approved for use to treat other animals, the equine formulation has been administered to small animals to treat protozoal infections caused by *Toxoplasma*, *Neospora*, and *Sarcocystis* spp. The equine formulation has extensive clinical studies to support safety and efficacy through the FDA approval. The uses in other animals are based on anecdotal experience and recommendations from experts.

P

## Precautionary Information

### Adverse Reactions and Side Effects

In horses, at high doses, decreased blood count has been observed but without evidence of anemia. Although anemia is possible, it resolves after discontinuing medication. Folic or folinic acid has been supplemented to prevent anemia, but the benefit of this treatment is unclear. Because this combination contains a sulfonamide, adverse effects are possible. Multiple adverse effects have been documented from administration of sulfonamides, particularly in dogs. These include allergic reactions, type II and III hypersensitivity, arthropathy, anemia, thrombocytopenia, hepatopathy, hypothyroidism (with prolonged therapy), keratoconjunctivitis sicca, and skin reactions. Dogs may be more sensitive to sulfonamides than other animals because dogs lack the ability to acetylate sulfonamides to metabolites.

### Contraindications and Precautions

Do not administer to animals that may be prone to anemia or in which a CBC cannot be monitored. Do not administer to animals with a history of sensitivity to sulfonamides.

### Drug Interactions

Drug interactions are not reported for animals. However, a combination of pyrimethamine with trimethoprim–sulfonamides enhances the bone marrow toxicity.

## Instructions for Use

Use of pyrimethamine–sulfadiazine has been primarily for treatment of protozoal infections in horses. However, there is anecdotal evidence that pyrimethamine + sulfadiazine may be indicated for treatment of some protozoa (e.g., *Toxoplasma, Neospora,* or *Sarcocystis* spp.) in small animals.

## Patient Monitoring and Laboratory Tests

Monitor CBC periodically in animals receiving treatment. A CBC should be performed at least monthly in treated animals.

## Formulations

- Pyrimethamine + sulfadiazine is available in an oral suspension for horses that is 250 mg of sulfadiazine and 12.5 mg of pyrimethamine per milliliter. This formulation may be diluted if necessary for small animals.

## Stability and Storage

Store in a tightly sealed container, protected from light, and at room temperature. Do not freeze.

## Small Animal Dosage

### Dogs and Cats

- 1 mg/kg of pyrimethamine and 20 mg/kg of sulfadiazine once daily PO. (Equivalent to one third a milliliter [0.33 mL] of the equine formulation per 4 kg of body weight.)

## Large Animal Dosage

- EPM caused by *S. neurona*: 1 mg/kg of pyrimethamine and 20 mg/kg of sulfadiazine q24h PO (4 mL per 110 lb). Treatment duration in horses varies from 90–270 days.

## Regulatory Information

Do not administer to animals intended for food.

# Quinacrine Hydrochloride
kwin′eh-krin hye-droe-klor′ide

**Trade and other names:** Atabrine (no longer available in the United States)

**Functional classification:** Antiparasitic

## Pharmacology and Mechanism of Action
Quinacrine is an older and somewhat outdated antimalarial drug that is rarely used in human or veterinary medicine. It inhibits nucleic acid synthesis in parasites.

## Indications and Clinical Uses
Quinacrine is used occasionally for treatment of protozoa (*Giardia* spp.), but other drugs (e.g., metronidazole and tinidazole) are preferred and used more often. Although it is not commercially available, veterinarians have obtained quinacrine through compounding pharmacies.

## Precautionary Information
### Adverse Reactions and Side Effects
Side effects are common. Vomiting occurs after oral administration.

### Contraindications and Precautions
No contraindications are reported for animals.

### Drug Interactions
No drug interactions have been reported in animals.

## Instructions for Use
Doses listed are for treatment of giardiasis. Effects for other organisms are not reported.

## Patient Monitoring and Laboratory Tests
No specific monitoring is necessary.

## Formulations
• Quinacrine has been available in 100-mg tablets. Quinacrine may no longer be marketed in the United States, but it may be available from some pharmacies in a compounded formulation.

## Stability and Storage
Store in a tightly closed container, protected from light, and at room temperature. Stability of compounded formulations has not been evaluated.

## Small Animal Dosage
**Dogs**
• 6.6 mg/kg q12h PO for 5 days.

**Cats**
• 11 mg/kg q24h PO for 5 days.

## Large Animal Dosage
• No doses have been reported for large animals.

Q

## Regulatory Information

Withdrawal times are not established for animals that produce food. For extralabel use withdrawal interval estimates, contact Food Animal Residue Avoidance Databank (FARAD) at www.FARAD.org.

---

# Quinidine, Quinidine Sulfate
kwin-ih-deen

**Trade and other names:** Quinidine gluconate (Duraquin), quinidine polygalacturonate (Cardioquin), and quinidine sulfate (Cin-Quin and Quinora)

**Functional classification:** Antiarrhythmic

## Pharmacology and Mechanism of Action

Quinidine is an older antiarrhythmic drug of the Class I antiarrhythmics. It is rarely used in animals except for some occasional use in horses and small animals. It is considered the prototype for Class I antiarrhythmic agents. Like other Class I antiarrhythmic drugs, its action is to inhibit sodium influx via blockade of sodium channels. Therefore it suppresses cardiac phase 0 action potential and decreases ectopic arrhythmic foci.

## Indications and Clinical Uses

Quinidine is used to treat ventricular arrhythmias and occasionally to convert atrial fibrillation to sinus rhythm. In small animals, it is rarely used because other more effective and safer alternatives are available. For example, an oral alternative for dogs is mexiletine. In horses and cattle, quinidine has been the drug of choice to treat atrial fibrillation. However, other alternatives are considered because of the frequency of adverse effects in horses and the decreased availability of commercial forms of quinidine. Alternatives include diltiazem and electrical cardioversion.

## Precautionary Information

### Adverse Reactions and Side Effects

Side effects with quinidine are more common than procainamide and include nausea and vomiting. Adverse effects include hypotension and tachycardia (because of vagolytic effect). With IV dosing, adverse effects such as hypotension and tachyarrhythmias are common in cattle. In horses, adverse effects are common, which include hypotension, gastrointestinal problems, and supraventricular tachycardia. Sudden cardiac death is possible but uncommon in horses.

### Contraindications and Precautions

Quinidine may increase the heart rate. Use cautiously in animals with heart disease.

### Drug Interactions

Quinidine is a well-known multidrug resistance (*ABCB1*, also known as *MDR1*) membrane pump (P-glycoprotein) inhibitor. It interferes with membrane channels and increases concentrations of some coadministered drugs. Coadministration with digoxin may increase digoxin concentrations. See Appendix K for a list of potential P-glycoprotein substrates.

Quinidine, Quinidine Sulfate 805

## Instructions for Use

Quinidine has a rapid clearance in cattle (half-life, 2.25 hours), which results in the need for frequent administration. Equine doses are usually administered orally via a stomach tube. Because of decreased availability of commercial forms and frequency of adverse effects, quinidine is not used as commonly as other Class I antiarrhythmic drugs. If quinidine is administered, calculate the dose to the amount of quinidine base in each formulation: 324 mg of quinidine gluconate has a 202-mg quinidine base; 275 of mg quinidine polygalacturonate has a 167-mg quinidine base; and 300 mg of quinidine sulfate has a 250-mg quinidine base.

## Patient Monitoring and Laboratory Tests

Quinidine can be hypotensive and vagolytic. Monitor patient's electrocardiogram for arrhythmias and monitor blood pressure.

## Formulations

- In some countries, quinidine is being discontinued and may be difficult to obtain. Older formulations include quinidine gluconate 324-mg tablets and 80-mg/mL injection; quinidine polygalacturonate in 275-mg tablets; and quinidine sulfate in 100-, 200-, and 300-mg tablets, 200- and 300-mg capsules, and 200-mg/mL injection.

## Stability and Storage

Store in a tightly sealed container, protected from light, and at room temperature. Quinidine is slightly soluble in water. Quinidine salts may form a dark color when exposed to light and should not be used. Quinidine has been compounded for oral use in syrups (e.g., Ora Sweet) and is stable for 60 days.

## Small Animal Dosage

### Dogs

- Quinidine gluconate: 6–20 mg/kg q6h IM or 6–20 mg/kg q6–8h PO (of base).
- Quinidine polygalacturonate: 6–20 mg/kg q6h PO (of base).
- Quinidine sulfate: 6–20 mg/kg q68h PO (of base) or 5–10 mg/kg q6h IV.

## Large Animal Dosage

### Cattle

- Treatment of atrial fibrillation: Quinidine is poorly absorbed orally in cattle and must be given intravenously. A loading dose of 49 mg/kg (given over 4 hours) to be followed by 42 mg/kg IV maintenance dose. Or give 40 mg/kg diluted in 4 L of fluid slowly at a rate of 1 L/h until fibrillation is converted.

### Horses

- Atrial fibrillation treatment (usually orally with a stomach tube): 5 g per 450 kg of body weight (per 1000 lb) for the first treatment; thereafter give 10 g per 450 kg every 2 hours until the sinus rate is achieved. IV dosage is 1–1.5 mg/kg every 10–15 minutes to a total dose of 10 mg/kg or until sinus rate conversion.

## Regulatory Information

Withdrawal times are not established for animals that produce food. Because of rapid elimination, short withdrawal times can be used. For extralabel use withdrawal interval estimates, contact FARAD at www.FARAD.org.

Racing Commissioners International Classification: 4

# Racemethionine
rah-see′meth-eye′oh-neen

**Trade and other names:** Methio-Form, and generic brands and Pedameth, Uracid, and generic brands (human preparations); also listed as DL-methionine

**Functional classification:** Acidifier

## Pharmacology and Mechanism of Action

Racemethionine is used as a urinary acidifier. DL-methionine lowers urinary pH as a racemic mixture, and this formulation is the DL-racemic mixture, which explains the name of racemethionine. Racemethionine also has been used to protect against acetaminophen overdose in people by restoring hepatic concentrations of glutathione.

## Indications and Clinical Uses

Racemethionine is used as a urinary acidifier. In people, it also is used to treat dermatitis caused by urinary incontinence by reducing irritation to the skin (reduces urine ammonia). Another use is to administer to dogs for the purpose of acidifying dog urine to prevent urine-induced damage to lawns. The so-called "lawn-saver" products contain 133–500 mg of methionine per pill, biscuit, or chew and may be obtained over the counter (OTC). It is also used as a nutritional supplement and feed supplement for livestock. DL-methionine has been administered to cats for lowering the urine pH, but this use is no longer recommended.

## Precautionary Information

### Adverse Reactions and Side Effects

Adverse effects are reported because of the common use to acidify urine in animals and because animals can be exposed from food supplements. In dogs exposed to high doses, the most common adverse effects are gastrointestinal (GI) and neurologic. Vomiting is the most common GI sign. The most common neurologic sign is ataxia. Neurologic signs are identified when the dose is greater than 95 mg/kg. When discontinued, dogs recover from adverse effects within 48 hours. Doses of 0.5–1 mg/kg per day to cats can produce Heinz body anemia and methemoglobinemia.

### Contraindications and Precautions

Do not use in animals with metabolic acidosis. Do not use in young cats. Do not use in animals with hepatic disease.

### Drug Interactions

No drug interactions have been reported in animals.

## Instructions for Use

Use for acetaminophen toxicity has been replaced by acetylcysteine.

## Patient Monitoring and Laboratory Tests

Monitor complete blood count and hepatic enzymes if used to treat toxicity.

## Formulations

- Racemethionine is available in 500-mg tablets, 75-mg/5-mL pediatric oral solution, 200-mg capsules, and powders to add to an animal's food.

- Methionine (identified as DL-methionine) is available in several feed supplements.
- Products listed as "lawn-saver" products for dogs usually contain 133 mg of racemethionine per tablet or chew.

## Stability and Storage
Store in a tightly sealed container, protected from light, and at room temperature.

## Small Animal Dosage
**Dogs**
- 150–300 mg/kg/day PO.
- Manufacturers of "lawn-saver" products (use is described earlier) recommend 15–266 mg/kg, depending on the product. A typical dose for a large dog is 23 mg/kg.

**Cats**
- 1–1.5 g per cat PO (added to food each day).

## Large Animal Dosage
- No doses have been reported for large animals.

## Regulatory Information
Withdrawal times are not established for animals that produce food. For extralabel use withdrawal interval estimates, contact Food Animal Residue Avoidance Databank (FARAD) at www.FARAD.org.

# Ramipril
ram′ih-pril

**Trade and other names:** Vasotop

**Functional classification:** Vasodilator, angiotensin-converting enzyme inhibitor

## Pharmacology and Mechanism of Action

R

Ramipril is an angiotensin-converting enzyme (ACE) inhibitor. Like other ACE inhibitors, ramipril inhibits conversion of angiotensin I to angiotensin II. Angiotensin II is a potent vasoconstrictor and stimulates sympathetic stimulation, renal hypertension, and synthesis of aldosterone. The ability of aldosterone to cause sodium and water retention contributes to congestion. Ramipril, like other ACE inhibitors, causes vasodilation and decreases aldosterone-induced congestion. ACE inhibitors also contribute to vasodilation by increasing concentrations of some vasodilating kinins and prostaglandins. There is evidence for a cardioprotective effect when used to treat dogs with heart disease caused by cardiomyopathy or valvular disease.

## Indications and Clinical Uses
Ramipril is used to treat hypertension and congestive heart failure. It has not been studied as much as other ACE inhibitors in animals (e.g., enalapril or benazepril), but it is expected to have similar pharmacodynamic effects. Because no ACE inhibitor has been shown to be superior to another, there is little reason to use ramipril instead of enalapril or benazepril in dogs or cats. It has been primarily used in dogs. It has also been used safely in cats to control hypertension but has not been effective for treating hypertrophic cardiomyopathy.

## Precautionary Information

### Adverse Reactions and Side Effects

It has not been used as often as other drugs in this class; therefore a full range of potential adverse effects has not been reported. Ramipril was well tolerated in clinical studies in dogs, but adverse effects reported for other ACE inhibitors may be expected in dogs and cats.

### Contraindications and Precautions

Studies performed in experimental dogs indicated that dose adjustments are not necessary when administering ramipril in dogs with impaired kidney function. However, as with any ACE inhibitor, monitor patients carefully if they have renal insufficiency or decreased glomerular filtration rate that could be impaired with ACE inhibitor treatment. Discontinue use of ACE inhibitors in pregnant animals; they cross the placenta and have caused fetal malformations and death of the fetus.

### Drug Interactions

Use cautiously with other hypotensive drugs and diuretics. Nonsteroidal anti-inflammatory drugs (NSAIDs) may decrease vasodilating effects.

## Instructions for Use

Clinical efficacy has been demonstrated in dogs with dilated cardiomyopathy. Other drugs used for treatment of heart failure may be used concurrently. Dogs also may receive pimobendan, digoxin, and/or furosemide with ramipril.

## Patient Monitoring and Laboratory Tests

Monitor patients carefully to avoid hypotension. With all ACE inhibitors, monitor electrolytes and renal function 3–7 days after initiating therapy and periodically thereafter.

## Formulations

• Ramipril is available in 1.25-, 2.5-, 5-, and 10-mg capsules.

## Stability and Storage

Store in a tightly sealed container, protected from light, and at room temperature.

## Small Animal Dosage

### Dogs

• 0.125–0.25 mg/kg daily PO to a maximum of 0.5 mg/kg per day.

### Cats

• 0.125 mg/kg q24h PO.

## Large Animal Dosage

• No doses have been reported for large animals.

## Regulatory Information

Withdrawal times are not established for animals that produce food. For extralabel use withdrawal interval estimates, contact FARAD at www.FARAD.org.

# Ranitidine Hydrochloride

rah-nit′ih-deen hye-droe-klor′ide

**Trade and other names:** Zantac

**Functional classification:** Antiulcer agent

**Note:** In 2020, the US Food and Drug Administration (FDA) requested manufacturers to withdraw all ranitidine products from the market. The reason for withdrawal is that the agency found N-nitrosodimethylamine (NDMA) levels in some ranitidine products that increase with time and temperature. NDMA poses a risk to consumers because it is a human and animal carcinogen.

Ranitidine is listed here, but products containing ranitidine may no longer be available.

## Pharmacology and Mechanism of Action

Ranitidine is a histamine$_2$ antagonist (H$_2$ blocker). Ranitidine, like other H$_2$ blockers, suppresses histamine stimulation of gastric parietal cells to decrease gastric acid secretion and increase stomach pH. Ranitidine is longer acting and 4–10 times more potent than one of the older drugs, cimetidine. The half-life of ranitidine is longer than cimetidine, which results in decreased frequency of administration for ranitidine.

*Pharmacokinetics:* In horses, the half-lives after IV and oral administration are 2.8 and 1.4 hours, respectively. The oral absorption in horses is 27%. In dogs, the half-lives are 2.3 and 2.2 hours after oral and IV administration, respectively, with 95% oral absorption. When adjusting doses, ranitidine hydrochloride is 81% ranitidine.

## Indications and Clinical Uses

Ranitidine has been used to treat GI ulcers, gastritis, and reflux esophagitis. It does not produce as much of a sustained increase in stomach pH as proton pump inhibitors (omeprazole). Proton pump inhibitors such as omeprazole have been preferred in dogs, cats, and horses because they produce a more consistent and sustained suppression of gastric acid secretion for ulcer healing, preventing ulcers, and preventing reflux esophagitis. The dose requirements used clinically may not be sufficient to maintain stomach pH in the range to prevent ulcers in dogs. Ranitidine (6.6 mg/kg PO) in foals suppressed acid for 6 hours, but omeprazole is superior and suppresses acid for 22 hours at 4 mg/kg. Ranitidine has been used to prevent NSAID-induced ulcers in animals, but the efficacy has not been demonstrated for this effect. In horses, ranitidine does not improve healing of ulcers induced by NSAIDs, and it is not as effective as omeprazole for treating gastric ulcers from other causes. Ranitidine may stimulate stomach emptying and colon motility via anticholinesterase action. In horses, the effect on gastric emptying is minimal.

## Precautionary Information

**R**

### Adverse Reactions and Side Effects

See the note at the top of the page regarding removal of ranitidine products from the market. Other adverse effects are usually seen only with decreased renal clearance. In people, central nervous system (CNS) signs may occur with high doses. Ranitidine may have fewer effects on endocrine function and drug interactions compared with cimetidine.

### Contraindications and Precautions

Fewer drug interactions are possible with ranitidine compared with cimetidine because ranitidine does not inhibit cytochrome P450 enzymes.

### Drug Interactions

Ranitidine and other H$_2$-receptor blockers block secretion of stomach acid. Therefore they interfere with oral absorption of drugs dependent on acidity, such as ketoconazole, itraconazole, and iron supplements. Unlike cimetidine, ranitidine is not known to inhibit microsomal P450 enzymes.

## Instructions for Use

Pharmacokinetic information in dogs suggests that ranitidine may be administered less often than cimetidine to achieve continuous suppression of stomach acid secretion. However, ranitidine may be less effective in dogs and cats to produce effective suppression of stomach acid secretion than previously thought. Use in horses and foals is based on experimental studies and pharmacokinetic data, and these studies show that it is less effective than omeprazole.

### Patient Monitoring and Laboratory Tests
No specific monitoring is necessary.

### Formulations
• Ranitidine was available in 75-, 150-, and 300-mg tablets; 150- and 300-mg capsules; and 25-mg/mL injection. Some forms were available OTC. However, in 2020, the FDA announced a removal of ranitidine products from the market. Therefore, these formulations may not be available in the United States.

### Stability and Storage
Store in a tightly sealed container, protected from light, and at room temperature. Ranitidine hydrochloride is soluble in water. Tablets have been crushed and mixed with water and syrup and were stable for 7 days. Protect from freezing.

### Small Animal Dosage
**Dogs**
• 2 mg/kg q8h IV or PO.

**Cats**
• 2.5 mg/kg q12h IV or 3.5 mg/kg q12h PO.

### Large Animal Dosage
**Horses**
• 2.2–6.6 mg/kg q6–8h PO. The higher dose (6.6 mg/kg) is more effective at suppressing stomach acid.
• 2 mg/kg q6–8h IV.

**Calves**
• 50 mg/kg q8h PO in milk-fed calves.
• Adult cattle: 6.6 mg/kg IM (only effective for 1 hour).

### Regulatory Information
Withdrawal times are not established for animals that produce food. For extralabel use withdrawal interval estimates, contact FARAD at www.FARAD.org.

Racing Commissioners International (RCI) Classification: 5

# Remifentanil Hydrochloride
rem-i-fen′ta-nil

**Trade and other names:** Ultiva

**Functional classification:** Anesthetic, analgesic, opioid

### Pharmacology and Mechanism of Action
Remifentanil is an ultra-short opioid similar in potency and activity to fentanyl. Like fentanyl, remifentanil has activity primarily at the mu-opiate receptor. The difference between remifentanil and other opioids is that it has an ultrashort action. The rapid onset and peak effect and short duration of action are attributed to its unique disposition.

Remifentanil is quickly metabolized by hydrolysis of the propanoic acid–methyl ester by blood and tissue esterases. Therefore it is rapidly metabolized in the blood, does not depend on liver metabolism, and can be used safely in patients with liver or kidney disease. It also is rapidly delivered to tissues with a high octanol:water partition coefficient of 17.9 at a pH of 7.3. However, it does not accumulate in tissues or blood even after prolonged IV infusions.

*Pharmacokinetics:* Because of the rapid metabolism and quick equilibration between plasma and tissues, remifentanil has a fast onset of activity after IV injection. The half-life in dogs is approximately 3–6 minutes and does not change with increasing doses. Recovery occurs rapidly (within 5–10 minutes), and when using constant-rate infusions (CRIs), new steady-state concentrations can be achieved within 5–10 minutes after changes in infusion rate. Because of rapid equilibration with tissues, it can be easily titrated to the desired depth of anesthesia and analgesia by changing the continuous infusion rate or by administering an IV bolus injection.

## Indications and Clinical Uses

Remifentanil is used for induction and maintenance of anesthesia, often in combination with other agents. Because of its rapid metabolism and short half-life, it should be administered by CRI to maintain a balanced anesthetic effect. It can be administered with other drugs, including inhalant anesthetics, propofol, alpha$_2$ agonists, sedatives, and tranquilizers. Because it does not require hepatic metabolism or renal elimination, it can be administered safely to patients that have liver or kidney disease. Experience with remifentanil use in dogs is limited to a few studies and case reports. Doses in animals have been extrapolated from humans (human starting dosage is 0.1 mcg/kg/min CRI). Remifentanil has been infused safely in cats, and over a wide range of doses (0.06–16 mcg/kg/min) IV, it did not affect isoflurane's minimum alveolar concentration.

## Precautionary Information

### Adverse Reactions and Side Effects

Like other opioids and opiates, remifentanil has adverse effects that are attributed to the binding to opiate receptors. These effects include reduced heart rate and sedation. In people, at rates greater than 0.2 mcg/kg/min, respiratory depression occurs. In cats, remifentanil induced dysphoria at high infusion rates (greater than 8 mcg/kg/min). Adverse effects quickly dissipate when the infusion is discontinued because of the drug's rapid metabolism in the plasma and tissues. The opioid activity of remifentanil is antagonized by opioid antagonists such as naloxone.

### Contraindications and Precautions

Remifentanil potentiates the effects of other anesthetics. Use cautiously in animals sensitive to opioids. It is intended for IV administration only. Do not administer via epidural, intrathecal, intradermal, IM, or SQ routes.

### Drug Interactions

Other anesthetics are potentiated when used with remifentanil. Lower doses of other anesthetic agents may be used when combined with remifentanil.

R

## Instructions for Use

Administer intravenously as a CRI. A bolus dose may be administered prior to the start of the CRI.

## Patient Monitoring and Laboratory Tests

Monitor patients during anesthetic protocol. Monitor electrocardiogram (ECG), heart rate, and breathing character.

## Formulations

- Remifentanil is available in a 1-mg/mL solution and in vials of 1, 2, or 5 mg of remifentanil base. Add 1 mL of diluent per milligram of remifentanil to produce a solution of 1 mg/mL. This solution can be further diluted for IV use to a concentration of 20, 25, 50, or 250 mcg/mL.

## Stability and Storage

The vial is available in a lyophilized powder that must be reconstituted prior to use. Store powder for injection in refrigerator (36°–46°F) or at room temperature (less than 78°F). Remifentanil HCl has a pKa of 7.07, but the pH of reconstituted solutions ranges from 2.5–3.5. The pH of solutions should be considered when combining with other drugs or fluid solutions. Remifentanil is compatible with sterile water, lactated Ringer's solution, 5% dextrose, 0.9% sodium chloride, and 0.45% sodium chloride. After being mixed in solution, it is stable for 24 hours at room temperature. It can also be mixed in solution with propofol. Because of the presence of plasma esterases, it should not be mixed with blood products. Therefore administration with IV blood transfusions is not recommended.

## Small Animal Dosage

### Dogs

- CRI: 0.2 mcg/kg/min, up to 1 mcg/kg/min. The infusion rate can be adjusted to achieve the desired effect, but 0.30 mcg/kg/min is optimum to achieve desired effects in anesthetized dogs. Higher rates did not produce increased benefit. For CRI administration, it may be administered with propofol.

### Cats

- CRI: 2.5 mcg/kg bolus injection followed by 0.2–0.4 mcg/kg/min CRI. In a dose-ranging study, the optimum dosage for cats undergoing ovariohysterectomy was a CRI of 0.4 mcg/kg/min IV.

## Large Animal Dosage

- No doses have been reported for large animals.

## Regulatory Information

Remifentanil is a Schedule II controlled substance. Withdrawal times are not established for animals that produce food. For extralabel use withdrawal interval estimates, contact FARAD at www.FARAD.org.

# Riboflavin (Vitamin B₂)

rye′boe-flay-vin

**Trade and other names:** Vitamin B₂

**Functional classification:** Vitamin

## Pharmacology and Mechanism of Action

Riboflavin is a vitamin B₂ supplement. Thiamine is commonly included as an ingredient in vitamin B complex aqueous solutions for injection. In these formulations, it is available as 5′ phosphate sodium riboflavin. Vitamin B complex often contains thiamine (B₁), riboflavin, niacinamide, and cyanocobalamin B₁₂.

## Indications and Clinical Uses

Riboflavin is used as a vitamin B$_2$ supplement. It is usually administered for maintenance in patients who are vitamin B$_2$ deficient. It is often added to infusion fluids to patients that are suspected of being vitamin B deficient.

### Precautionary Information

**Adverse Reactions and Side Effects**

Adverse effects are rare because water-soluble vitamins are easily excreted. Riboflavin may discolor the urine.

**Contraindications and Precautions**

Do not administer injectable solution by IV rapidly if it contains thiamine (vitamin B$_{12}$) because this may cause an anaphylactic reaction.

**Drug Interactions**

No drug interactions have been reported in animals.

## Instructions for Use

It is not necessary to supplement in animals with well-balanced diets.

## Patient Monitoring and Laboratory Tests

No specific monitoring is necessary.

## Formulations

- Riboflavin is available in various-sized tablets in increments from 10–250 mg. Riboflavin is most commonly formulated with other vitamins in a "vitamin B complex" aqueous solution for injection (2 and 5 mg/mL of riboflavin).

## Stability and Storage

Store in a tightly sealed container, protected from light, and at room temperature.

## Small Animal Dosage

**Dogs**

- 10–20 mg/day PO.
- 1–4 mg/dog q24h SQ.

**Cats**

- 5–10 mg/day PO.
- 1–2 mg/cat q24h SQ.

## Large Animal Dosage

**Lambs**

- 2–4 mg q24h IM or SQ.

**Calves and Foals**

- 6–10 mg q24h IM or SQ.

**Cattle and Horses**

- 20–40 mg q24h IM or SQ.

**Sheep and Pigs**

- 10–20 mg q24h IM or SQ.

## Regulatory Information

Because of a low risk of harmful residues in animals intended for food, no withdrawal time is necessary.

R

## Rifampin

rih-fam′pin

**Trade and other names:** Rifadin, Rimactane, and rifampicin

**Functional classification:** Antibacterial

### Pharmacology and Mechanism of Action

Rifampin is an antibacterial used in people but also has been administered extralabel in animals for treatment of atypical bacterial infections or bacteria resistant to other antibacterial agents. Rifampin is known in some countries as rifampicin. Rifamycin and rifabutin are structurally similar antibiotics—all in the group of rifamycins—but are not identical.

The action of rifampin is to inhibit bacterial RNA synthesis. Rifampin is a semisynthetic antibiotic derived from rifamycin B to produce rifampin. Rifampin has a high activity against gram-positive bacteria (*Staphylococcus* spp.), *Mycobacterium* spp., *Haemophilus* spp., *Neisseria* spp., and *Chlamydia* spp. but more limited activity against the gram-negative bacteria because it penetrates gram-positive organisms more easily than gram-negative organisms. Rifampin is highly lipid soluble and is capable of diffusing into cells to concentrate in leukocytes to inhibit intracellular bacteria. This is a therapeutic advantage for treating intracellular organisms (*Brucella, Mycobacterium, Rhodococcus, Chlamydia* spp.) and chronic granulomatous diseases. Rifampin enters the microbial cell and forms stable complexes with the beta subunit of DNA-dependent RNA polymerases of microorganisms. This binding results in inactive enzymes and inhibition of RNA synthesis by preventing chain initiation. Resistance occurs via a single mutation of the amino acid sequence of the beta subunit of the DNA-dependent RNA polymerase enzyme.

*Pharmacokinetics:* Rifampin is rapidly absorbed from the GI tract after oral administration in humans, dogs, calves, horses, and foals. Pharmacokinetics in adult horses shows rapid oral absorption of rifampin, a half-life of approximately 5–7 hours, and a volume of distribution of 0.7 L/kg, but the half-life is longer in foals, at approximately 18 hours. The half-life in dogs is approximately 8 hours.

### Indications and Clinical Uses

Rifampin is used in people primarily for treatment of tuberculosis. In veterinary medicine, rifampin has been used to treat susceptible gram-positive and intracellular bacteria, including *Staphylococcus* spp. (including methicillin-resistant strains); *Streptococcus* spp.; *Rhodococcus equi*; *Corynebacterium pseudotuberculosis*; and most strains of *Bacteroides* spp., *Clostridium* spp., *Neisseria* spp., and *Listeria* spp. Gram-negative organisms are not affected at typical doses. In small animals, the most common use is to treat staphylococcal infections, particularly methicillin-resistant strains. Resistance among bacteria (e.g. *Staphylococcus* spp.) may develop, but this occurrence is generally not common and should not prevent its use in animals. One of the most common uses of rifampin is for treating infections caused by *R. equi* in horses. For this treatment, it is frequently combined with erythromycin, azithromycin, or clarithromycin. Rifampin also may have activity against bacteria in biofilms. This effect may assist treatment of staphylococcal infections on orthopedic implants. However, there are insufficient reports to confirm the clinical effectiveness for treating biofilm bacteria in animals.

## Precautionary Information

### Adverse Reactions and Side Effects

In people, hypersensitivity and flulike symptoms are reported. Hepatotoxicity is seen more commonly in dogs than other animals. It is more common when high doses are administered (10 mg/kg and higher). In one study, adverse effects occurred in 16% of treated dogs (vomiting, anorexia, diarrhea), and 27% had reversible elevations of liver enzymes. When treating dogs, clinicians are advised to check liver enzymes and bilirubin periodically during rifampin treatment. If elevations occur, rifampin should be discontinued, and most animals are expected to recover. Urine is colored orange to reddish-orange in treated patients. It also discolors saliva, tears, feces, sclera, and mucous membranes to a reddish-orange color. The discoloration is not pathogenic and is a normal occurrence. Rifampin is unpalatable and may be difficult to administer to some animals. Pancreatitis has been associated with rifampin administration but not well documented in dogs or cats.

### Contraindications and Precautions

Use cautiously in animals that are at risk for pancreatitis. Because of a risk of hepatitis, use cautiously with any other drug that may be potentially hepatotoxic (e.g., sulfonamides, anticonvulsants, acetaminophen). Avoid use in pregnant animals.

### Drug Interactions

Multiple drug interactions are possible. Rifampin is one of the most potent inducers of cytochrome P450 hepatic enzymes. Elevation of cytochrome P450 enzyme activity may persist for 4 days but returns to baseline by 8 days in people. The duration of this activity is not known in animals. Drugs that may have decreased levels because of rapid metabolism when administered with rifampin include barbiturates, chloramphenicol, progestins, digitalis, warfarin, corticosteroids (prednisolone), and potentially many other drugs concurrently administered with rifampin. Rifampin has decreased clarithromycin by 90% in horses because of increased clearance. Rifampin is also an inducer of membrane efflux pump (P-glycoprotein), which may have the consequence of decreasing oral absorption of other drugs.

R

## Instructions for Use

Most of the documented clinical experience has been for treating *R. equi* infections in horses, primarily foals. In these protocols, it is often combined with a macrolide antibiotic (erythromycin, clarithromycin, or azithromycin), but it is not known if combination therapy is more effective than single-drug treatment. When selecting a dose, the 10-mg/kg PO dose was adequate for susceptible gram-positive infections in the adult horse. Use in small animals (and doses) is based on experience, primarily in dogs in which rifampin was used to treat methicillin-resistant *Staphylococcus* infections. It is often recommended to administer rifampin in small animals in combination with other drugs to decrease emergence of resistance. However, there is no clinical evidence in animals or analysis of studies from people that addition of other antibiotics is necessary when treating infections caused by *Staphylococcus* spp. Rifampin may be used as monotherapy in these cases. Administer on an empty stomach whenever possible.

## Patient Monitoring and Laboratory Tests

Susceptibility testing: Clinical and Laboratory Standards Institute (CLSI) breakpoint for susceptible organisms isolated from people is ≤1.0 mcg/mL, but a breakpoint is not available for isolates from animals. Whereas minimum inhibitory concentrations (MICs) for gram-positive organisms generally occur at 0.1 mcg/mL, gram-negative organisms have MIC values ranging from 8–32 mcg/mL and are considered resistant. Because of the risk of liver injury in dogs, it is advised to periodically, initially after the first 7 days and then regularly every 10–14 days. During monitoring, check the liver enzymes and serum bilirubin to monitor for signs of liver injury.

## Formulations

- Rifampin is available in 150-mg and 300-mg capsules and 600-mg Rifadin IV injectable solution.

## Stability and Storage

Store in a tightly sealed container, protected from light, and at room temperature. Rifampin is slightly soluble in water and ethanol. It is more soluble at acidic pH. Acid should be added to solutions (e.g., ascorbic acid) to prevent oxidation and improve solubility. Rifampin has been mixed with syrups and flavorings for oral administration and is stable for 4–6 weeks. The injectable solution is prepared by adding 10 mL of saline to a 600-mg vial and mixing (60 mg/mL). It may be infused with 0.9% saline or 5% dextrose solution. Reconstituted injectable solution is stable for 24 hours.

## Small Animal Dosage

### Dogs and Cats

- 5 mg/kg q12h PO or 10 mg/kg q24h PO. (Low dose; twice daily is preferred.)

## Large Animal Dosage

### Horses

- 10 mg/kg q24h PO.
- Foals for treatment of *R. equi:* 5 mg/kg q12h PO. In some protocols, rifampin is combined with erythromycin (25 mg/kg q8h PO) or other macrolides (e.g., azithromycin), but it is not established if combination treatment is more effective than monotherapy.

### Cattle, Sheep, and Goats

- 20 mg/kg q24h PO. For treatment of Johne's disease combine with isoniazid.

## Regulatory Information

Avoid administration in food-producing animals. Withdrawal times have not been established for animals that produce food. For extralabel use withdrawal interval estimates, contact FARAD at www.FARAD.org.

# Ringer's Solution

**Trade and other names:** Generic brands

**Functional classification:** Fluid replacement

## Pharmacology and Mechanism of Action

Ringer's solution is an IV solution for fluid replacement. Ringer's solution contains 147 of mEq/L sodium, 4 mEq/L of potassium, 155 mEq/L of chloride, and 4 mEq/L of calcium. Ringer's lactate (lactated Ringer's) and Ringer's acetate may contain different amounts of these electrolytes in addition to lactate or acetate.

## Indications and Clinical Uses

Ringer's solution is used as a fluid replacement and for maintenance. It has a balanced electrolyte concentration, but it does not contain any bases (see Lactated Ringer's Solution for solutions that contain bases).

## Precautionary Information

### Adverse Reactions and Side Effects

Ringer's solution is considered an acidifying solution because with prolonged administration, the chloride increases renal excretion of bicarbonate. Fluid overload occurs at high infusion rates.

### Contraindications and Precautions

Do not exceed fluid rates of 80 mL/kg/h. Consider supplementing with potassium because this fluid will not meet maintenance potassium needs.

### Drug Interactions

Ringer's solution contains calcium; do not mix with drugs that may bind to calcium.

## Instructions for Use

When administering IV fluid solution, monitor rate and electrolyte concentrations carefully. Add bicarbonate to fluids, if necessary, based on the calculation of the base deficit.

Fluid administration rates are as follows: normal maintenance rates: 40–65 mL/kg/24 h ($\approx$2–2.5 mL/kg/h). For replacement fluid, use the following calculation:

$$\text{Liters needed} = \% \ \text{dehydration} \times \text{body weight (kg)}$$

or

$$\text{Milliliters needed} = \% \ \text{dehydration} \times \text{body weight (kg)} \times 1000$$

## Patient Monitoring and Laboratory Tests

Monitor pulmonary pressure when infusing high doses. Monitor electrolyte balance, especially potassium, during treatment.

## Formulations

Ringer's solution is available in 250-, 500-, and 1000-mL bags for infusion.

## Stability and Storage

Store in a tightly sealed container, protected from light, and at room temperature.

## Small Animal Dosage

### Dogs and Cats

- 55–65 mL/kg day (2.5 mL/kg/h) IV, SQ, or intraperitoneal (IP) for maintenance.
- 15–30 mL/kg/h IV for moderate dehydration.
- 50 mL/kg/h IV for severe dehydration.

## Large Animal Dosage

### Large Animals

- 40–50 mL/kg day IV, SQ, or IP for maintenance.
- 15–30 mL/kg/h IV for moderate dehydration.
- 50 mL/kg/h IV for severe dehydration.

### Calves

- Moderate dehydration: 45 mL/kg given at a rate of 30–40 mL/kg/h.
- Severe dehydration: 80–90 mL/kg given at a rate of 30–40 mL/kg/h or as fast as 80 mL/kg/h if necessary.

## Regulatory Information

Because of low risk of harmful residues in animals intended for food, no withdrawal time is suggested.

---

# Rivaroxaban

riv-a-rox'a-ban

**Trade and other names:** Xarelto

**Functional classification:** Anticoagulant

---

## Pharmacology and Mechanism of Action

Rivaroxaban is a direct-acting anticoagulant developed for human use but is gaining more use in companion animals. Rivaroxaban has direct antagonist effects on the active form of factor X in the coagulation cascade (antifactor Xa). By inactivating factor Xa, rivaroxaban inhibits platelet activation and fibrin clot formation via direct, selective, and reversible inhibition of factor Xa (FXa) in both the intrinsic and extrinsic coagulation pathways. FXa, as part of the prothrombinase complex consisting also of factor Va, calcium ions, factor II, and phospholipid, catalyzes the conversion of prothrombin to thrombin. Thrombin activates platelets and catalyzes the conversion of fibrinogen to fibrin.

The other agents in this class that has the same mechanism of action is apixaban (Eliquis) and edoxaban (Savaysa), for which there has been much less attention in veterinary medicine compared with rivaroxaban.

## Indications and Clinical Uses

Rivaroxaban is approved in people for treatment of venous thrombosis and pulmonary embolism and prevention of venous thrombosis. It is also used in patients with atrial fibrillation. It is used in situations when the alternatives may include vitamin K antagonists (warfarin) or low-molecular weight heparin (enoxaparin). The advantage of rivaroxaban is that it can be administered orally and does not require the monitoring (international normalized ratio monitoring) that is needed to optimize the dose of warfarin.

In animals, the uses identified at this time are based on small studies or anecdotal observations. Compared with warfarin, rivaroxaban is easier to use because the pharmacokinetics are more predictable, and a fixed dose may be administered to produce results without routine monitoring as required for warfarin. Rivaroxaban has been administered to dogs at an average dosage of 0.89 mg/kg once daily and was well tolerated, but the therapeutic benefits compared with traditional drugs are not known. In cats that received a range of doses from 1.25–5 mg per cat q12h PO, all doses were effective with a peak effect at 3 hours and a duration of 12 hours.

## Precautionary Information

### Adverse Reactions and Side Effects

Rivaroxaban has not been used to a large extent at this time in veterinary medicine to know all the possible adverse effects. Obviously, excessive bleeding is the major concern when administering any agents from this group.

Adverse effects reported in people but not reported during animal use include abdominal pain, fatigue, muscle spasms, dizziness, anxiety, pruritus, and increased liver enzymes.

If a reversal of the antifactor Xa effect is required because of an overdose, there is a human product (*Andexanet alfa*), which is a genetically modified variant of human factor Xa (alanine is substituted for serine) that acts as a decoy, binding to factor Xa inhibitors and neutralizing their anticoagulant effect. This agent is very expensive and has not been tested in animals.

### Contraindications and Precautions

The most important concern and precaution is any existing bleeding abnormality that exists in a patient prior to administration. Do not use in patients with hepatic impairment.

### Drug Interactions

No specific drug interactions have been identified in animals, but the use has been infrequent at this time and rarely reported to understand the full scope of possible drug interactions. In people, rivaroxaban is a substrate for cytochrome P450 enzymes and P-glycoprotein. Potentially, other drugs that inhibit (e.g., ketoconazole) or induce (e.g., rifampin, phenobarbital) these enzymes and the P-glycoprotein transporter could affect response to rivaroxaban. Administration with antiplatelet drugs (aspirin, clopidogrel) could increase the risk of bleeding.

## Instructions for Use

Administration of human rivaroxaban tablets may require modification. If whole tablets cannot be used, the tablets may be crushed and mixed with food (in people, applesauce is used) immediately prior to oral administration.

## Patient Monitoring and Laboratory Tests

Monitor for signs of bleeding. Routine coagulation testing is not recommended or necessary for direct oral anticoagulants such as rivaroxaban. If antifactor Xa activity is measured, it must be specifically calibrated for rivaroxaban.

If coagulation tests are performed, it will prolong the activated partial thromboplastin time.

## Formulations

Oral tablets: 2.5-, 10-, 15-, and 20 mg tablets.

## Stability and Storage

Store in a tightly sealed container, protected from light, and at room temperature.

## Small Animal Dosage

### Dogs

- 1–2 mg/kg PO q24h.
- Human dosage (listed here as a comparison): 0.2 mg/kg q12h PO initially for 3 weeks; then 0.3 mg/kg once-daily PO thereafter. For prophylaxis, the dosage is 0.14 mg/kg PO q24h.

## Cats

- 0.5–1 mg/kg q24h PO. Cats can also be administered tablets of 1.25-, 2.5-, and 5 mg per cat, oral.

## Large Animal Dosage

- No large animal doses have been identified.

## Regulatory Information

No withdrawal information or regulatory requirements are available. Avoid use in food-producing animals.

# Robenacoxib
Roe-ben-A-cocks-ib

**Trade and other names:** Onsior (veterinary preparation)

**Functional classification:** Anti-inflammatory

## Pharmacology and Mechanism of Action

Robenacoxib is an NSAID approved for use in dogs and cats but not available for people. Like other drugs in this class, robenacoxib has analgesic and anti-inflammatory effects by inhibiting the synthesis of prostaglandins. The enzyme inhibited by NSAIDs is the cyclooxygenase (COX) enzyme. The COX enzyme exists in two isoforms: COX-1 and COX-2. COX-1 is primarily responsible for synthesis of prostaglandins important for maintaining a healthy GI tract, kidney function, platelet function, and other normal functions. COX-2 is induced and responsible for synthesizing prostaglandins that are important mediators of pain, inflammation, and fever. However, it is known that there is some crossover of COX-1 and COX-2 effects and that COX-2 activity is important for some biological effects. For example, COX-1 and COX-2 are constitutively expressed in the kidneys, and their products are important for renal perfusion and tubular function.

Robenacoxib is more selective for COX-2 using in vitro assays compared with older nonselective NSAIDs, but it is not known if the specificity for COX-1 or COX-2 is associated with improved efficacy or safety.

*Pharmacokinetics:* Robenacoxib has a short half-life in both dogs and cats, but tissue concentrations persist for much longer, which may explain the efficacy with once-daily dosing despite a short half-life. The half-lives are 0.6–1.1 hours in dogs and 1.49, 1.87, 0.84, and 0.78 hours in cats (depending on the study). The volume of distributions re 0.24 L/kg in dogs and 0.13 and 0.19 L/kg in cats, depending on the study. Oral absorption rates are 84% in dogs (nonfed) or 62% (fed) and 49% in cats(nonfed) and 10% (fed). Protein binding rates are 98% and 99.9% in dogs and cats, respectively. Thus, it appears that feeding greatly influences oral absorption. Therefore, it is recommended in cats that it should be administered without food to maximize oral absorption.

## Indications and Clinical Uses

Robenacoxib is used to decrease pain, inflammation, and fever. The FDA-approved dosage in dogs and cats in the United States is once per day PO for 3 days to treat pain associated with surgery and other conditions. The injectable formulation is intended to be administered prior to surgery (30 minutes) and continued for 2 more days to treat pain and inflammation associated with surgery.

It is also approved in Europe for dogs and cats to treat acute pain and inflammation associated with musculoskeletal disorders and has been administered for longer than 3 days. Outside the United States, tablets are approved for long-term treatment of pain and inflammation in dogs associated with chronic osteoarthritis. It has also been administered for long-term treatment in cats without safety problems.

Robenacoxib has not been investigated for use in large animals.

## Precautionary Information

### Adverse Reactions and Side Effects

Major adverse effects are GI, including vomiting, diarrhea, and ulceration. In field trials, the most common adverse effects associated with robenacoxib administration in cats and dogs are GI adverse events (vomiting, soft feces). In dogs, after long-term oral treatment, an increase in liver enzyme activities may occur but is not necessarily associated with liver pathology. The solution for injection might cause pain on injection, apparently because of the excipient in the solution.

Because robenacoxib appears to be relatively COX-2 specific and has a short half-life, adverse effects are expected to be less than other NSAIDs that are not as selective. However, veterinarians should consider the potential for NSAID-induced adverse effects as with any other drug in this class. Kidney injury, especially in dehydrated animals or animals with preexisting renal disease, has been shown for some NSAIDs, including those with COX-2 selectivity.

In safety studies in cats, robenacoxib was well tolerated even in cats with kidney disease and even when treatment was for longer and at higher doses than approved.

### Contraindications and Precautions

Dogs and cats with preexisting GI problems or kidney disease may be at a greater risk of adverse effects from NSAIDs. However, in cats with chronic kidney disease, robenacoxib did not cause any changes in kidney parameters during clinical studies. Safety in pregnant animals is not known, but adverse effects have not been reported. Do not use the dog tablets in cats because accurate dosing may be difficult. Administer the injection by the SQ route and avoid IM or IV injections.

### Drug Interactions

Do not administer with other NSAIDs or with corticosteroids. Corticosteroids have been shown to exacerbate the GI adverse effects. Some NSAIDs may interfere with the action of diuretic drugs and ACE inhibitors. Robenacoxib has been administered prior to surgery with other agents such as sedatives, anesthetic agents, and antibiotics without producing any adverse reactions.

R

## Instructions for Use

The oral tablet may be administered once daily for up to 3 days in the United States and for 6 days in Europe. Studies in cats have shown that it is safe for cats for much longer periods for conditions such as osteoarthritis without adverse events. It was safe in cats for multiple doses even in animals with chronic kidney disease. Dogs also have been treated once daily chronically with safety.

When used to decrease postoperative pain, it can be administered prior to surgery. The injection is administered subcutaneously to cats or dogs approximately 30–45 minutes before the start of surgery at 2 mg/kg. After surgery, it may be continued for an additional 2 days.

The oral absorption is greatly diminished with food in cats, and it is recommended to administer without food or with just one third of the daily ration (small meal).

## Patient Monitoring and Laboratory Tests

Monitor GI signs for evidence of diarrhea, GI bleeding, or ulcers. Because of risk of kidney injury, monitor renal parameters (water consumption, blood urea nitrogen, creatinine, and urine-specific gravity) periodically during treatment. Safety has been evaluated in dogs and cats prior to approval in the respective countries. In safety studies, young healthy cats have tolerated 10 mg/kg q12h for 42 days.

## Formulations

- Tablets for cats: 6 mg.
- Tablets for dogs: 10, 20, and 40 mg.
- Cats and dogs: 20-mg/mL injectable solution in a 20-mL vial.

## Stability and Storage

Store protected from excessive heat and in dry conditions. Stability of compounded formulations has not been evaluated.

## Small Animal Dosage

### Dogs

- Oral: 2 mg/kg q24h PO.
- Injection: 2 mg/kg q24h SQ.

### Cats

- Oral: 1 mg/kg PO once per day.
- Injection: 2 mg/kg q24h SQ for 3 days. Administer 30 minutes prior to surgery if used to decrease surgical pain.

## Large Animal Dosage

- No large animal doses have been reported.

## Regulatory Information

Withdrawal times or regulatory information for food-producing animals is not available. If administered to food-producing animals, contact FARAD at www.FARAD.org to identify the appropriate milk and meat slaughter withdrawal times.

# Romifidine Hydrochloride

roe-mif'ih-deen hye-droe-klor'ide

**Trade and other names:** Sedivet

**Functional classification:** Analgesic, alpha$_2$ agonist

## Pharmacology and Mechanism of Action

Romifidine is an alpha$_2$-adrenergic agonist. Alpha$_2$ agonists decrease release of neurotransmitters from the neuron. The proposed mechanism whereby they decrease transmission is via binding to presynaptic alpha$_2$ receptors (negative feedback receptors). The result is decreased sympathetic outflow, analgesia, sedation, and anesthesia. Romifidine is structurally similar to clonidine. Other drugs in this class include xylazine, detomidine, dexmedetomidine, and medetomidine. The alpha$_2$-specific effects are measured by comparing the alpha$_1$/alpha$_2$-receptor affinity ratio. The ratios are 1:160 for xylazine, 1:260 for detomidine; 1:360 for romifidine, and 1:1620 for dexmedetomidine. Thus, receptor-binding studies indicate that alpha$_2$/alpha$_1$-adrenergic receptor selectivity for romifidine is approximately twice as much higher than that of xylazine. Romifidine has been studied in horses more than other animals.

*Pharmacokinetics:* In horses, at 80 mcg/kg, it has a half-life of 2.3 hours and high clearance of 25–38 mL/kg/min. Romifidine has an onset of effect of 2 minutes and a duration of 1–1.5 hours.

## Indications and Clinical Uses

Romifidine, like other alpha$_2$ agonists, is used as a sedative and anesthetic adjunct and for analgesia. It produces the longest duration of sedative effects compared with other agents followed by detomidine, medetomidine, and xylazine. A dose of 80 mcg/kg of romifidine IV is equipotent to 1 mg/kg of xylazine IV and 20 mcg/kg detomidine IV. Its use is primarily limited to horses in which it is used as a sedative and analgesic to facilitate handling, clinical examinations, clinical procedures, and minor surgical procedures and for use as a preanesthetic prior to the induction of general anesthesia.

## Precautionary Information

### Adverse Reactions and Side Effects

Romifidine, like other alpha$_2$ agonists, decreases sympathetic output. Bradycardia is common, and cardiovascular depression may occur. Cardiac effects can include sinoatrial block, first-degree and second-degree AV block, bradycardia, and sinus arrhythmia. In horses, it causes effects similar to other alpha$_2$ agonists, including ataxia, head drooping, sweating, and bradycardia. Facial edema is common, especially with higher doses. Even at high doses in experimental horses (up to 600 mcg/kg), there were no deaths.

### Contraindications and Precautions

Romifidine, like other alpha$_2$ agonists, should be used cautiously in animals with heart disease. The use may be contraindicated in older animals with preexisting cardiac disease. Xylazine causes problems in pregnant animals, and this also should be considered for other alpha$_2$ agonists. Use cautiously in animals that are pregnant; it may induce labor. In addition, it may decrease oxygen delivery to fetuses in late gestation. In case of overdose, reverse with atipamezole or yohimbine.

### Drug Interactions

Do not use with other drugs that may cause cardiac depression. It may be used in horses with other sedatives and anesthetics such as benzodiazepines or ketamine. Do not mix in vial or syringe with other anesthetics. Use with opioid analgesic drugs greatly enhances CNS depression. Consider lowering doses if administered with opioids. Romifidine can interfere with conversion of thyroid hormone (T$_4$) to the active form of triiodothyronine (T$_3$).

## Instructions for Use

Romifidine, like other alpha$_2$ agonists, can be administered with ketamine or benzodiazepines. It can be reversed with alpha$_2$ antagonists such as atipamezole or yohimbine. The doses administered to horses has ranged from 40 to 120 mcg/kg IV. The most common dose is 80 mcg/kg. These doses produce sedation, cardiac effects, and analgesia that are dose-dependent effects. At a dose of 80 mcg/kg, strong

R

sedation is produced in horses that lasts for approximately 45–60 minutes. Deeper sedation occurs with higher doses. Each dose produced effects for at least 60 minutes, and some are observed for 180 minutes. A duration of 180 minutes is more likely with higher doses.

### Patient Monitoring and Laboratory Tests
Monitor vital signs during anesthesia. Monitor heart rate, blood pressure, and ECG if possible during anesthesia.

### Formulations
• Romifidine is available in a 1% injection (10 mg/mL).

### Stability and Storage
Store in a tightly sealed container, protected from light, and at room temperature.

### Small Animal Dosage
#### Dogs and Cats
• Doses not established for small animals.

### Large Animal Dosage
#### Horses
• Sedation and analgesia: 40–120 mcg/kg IV. (A dose-dependent degree of sedation is observed.)
• Preanesthetic: 100 mcg/kg IV.

### Regulatory Information
Do not administer in animals intended for food.

---

# Ronidazole
roe-nid'ah-zole

**Trade and other names:** Generic

**Functional classification:** Antibacterial, antiparasitic

---

### Pharmacology and Mechanism of Action
Ronidazole is an antibacterial and antiprotozoal drug. It is a nitroimidazole in which the activity involves generation of free nitroradicals via metabolism within protozoa and bacteria. Ronidazole disrupts DNA in an organism via reaction with intracellular metabolites. Its action is specific for anaerobic bacteria and protozoa. Like other nitroimidazoles, it is active against some protozoa, including *Trichomonas* spp., *Giardia* spp., and intestinal protozoal parasites.

*Pharmacokinetics:* After oral administration in cats, it is rapidly and completely absorbed. The half-life in cats is approximately 10 hours.

### Indications and Clinical Uses
Ronidazole is currently not an FDA-approved drug, but it has been used in cats to treat intestinal protozoal parasites. Studies for treatment of other organisms are not available. For treatment of feline *Tritrichomonas foetus* intestinal infections, it has been administered orally at a dosage of 30 mg/kg twice daily for 2 weeks. However, twice-daily administration is more likely to produce CNS adverse reactions, and pharmacokinetic data indicate that 30 mg/kg once daily may be equally effective.

Efficacy for long-term remission has not been established, but temporary resolution of feline *T. foetus* intestinal infections has been observed.

## Precautionary Information

### Adverse Reactions and Side Effects

Like other nitroimidazoles, the most severe adverse effect is caused by toxicity to the CNS. High doses may cause lethargy, CNS depression, ataxia, tremors, hyperesthesia, seizures, vomiting, and weakness. The CNS signs are related to inhibition of action of gamma-aminobutyric acid (GABA) and are responsive to benzodiazepines (diazepam). Dogs show neurotoxicity at doses of 50–200 mg/kg (seizures, tremors, and ataxia). Avoid dosages that exceed 60 mg/kg per day in cats. Like other nitroimidazoles, it has the potential to produce mutagenic changes in cells, but this has not been demonstrated in animals. Like other nitroimidazoles, it has a bitter taste and can cause vomiting and anorexia.

### Contraindications and Precautions

Fetal abnormalities have not been demonstrated in animals with recommended doses, but use cautiously during pregnancy.

### Drug Interactions

Like other nitroimidazoles, it may potentiate the effects of warfarin and cyclosporine via inhibition of drug metabolism.

## Instructions for Use

Ronidazole is currently not a marketed drug but has been prepared from bulk powder in compounding pharmacies.

## Patient Monitoring and Laboratory Tests

Monitor for neurologic adverse effects.

## Formulations

- No available formulation exists; it is compounded from bulk chemicals. IV formulations have been prepared by dissolving ronidazole pure powder in 5% dextrose in water (D5W) to a concentration of 3.2 mg/mL. This formulation has been safely administered to research animals.

## Stability and Storage

Store in a tightly sealed container, protected from light, and at room temperature. Stability of compounded formulations has not been evaluated.

## Small Animal Dosage

### Dogs

- No dose has been reported.

### Cats

- 30 mg/kg q24h PO for 2 weeks. Early clinical studies were performed with 30 mg/kg q12h, but twice-daily administration is more likely to produce CNS toxicity, and an interval of q24h may be equally effective.

## Large Animal Dosage

- No doses have been reported for large animals.

## Regulatory Information

Do not administer to animals that produce food. Administration of nitroimidazoles to animals intended for food is prohibited. Treated cattle must not be slaughtered for food.

# S-Adenosylmethionine (SAMe)
ess'ah-den'oh-sill-meh-thye'oh-neen

**Trade and other names:** Denosyl, Denamarin, and SAMe

**Functional classification:** Nutritional supplement

## Pharmacology and Mechanism of Action
S-Adenosylmethionine is a dietary supplement, usually abbreviated as SAMe. This compound is found naturally in tissues and is formed from methionine and adenosine triphosphate (ATP). It is used for a variety of clinical problems, but as a dietary supplement, there are no therapeutic claims. In veterinary medicine, it is primarily used as a liver supplement. It has been associated with improvement in acetaminophen-induced hepatotoxicity in humans and has been beneficial for some conditions that affect the liver according to isolated reports in veterinary medicine. It serves as a methyl donor, catalyzed by methyltransferase. It also is a substrate for a transsulfuration reaction in which demethylated SAMe is metabolized to glutathione (GSH). GSH may conjugate certain drug metabolites to enhance excretion. Cats and dogs have low levels of GSH, and SAMe may help restore GSH in animals that have been intoxicated or may help to supplement animals that have liver disease. It is a methyl donor for neurotransmitter metabolism in the synthesis and turnover of biogenic monoamines (central nervous system [CNS] neurotransmitters such as serotonin, dopamine, and norepinephrine). There is very little pharmacokinetic information available, but in dogs, the half-life after oral administration is approximately 2 hours.

## Indications and Clinical Uses
SAMe has been used as a dietary supplement, primarily to support patients with hepatic disease. It may help restore hepatic GSH concentrations in deficient animals. It also has been administered to treat liver injury caused by intoxication of acetaminophen and other drugs that produce hepatotoxic oxidative drug injury. Another dietary supplement, silymarin (see Silymarin), also known as *milk thistle* and *silybin*, has hepatic antioxidant properties and has been combined with SAMe for treatment in dogs and cats (Denamarin). Via the effect on neurotransmitter synthesis, SAMe has been used to improve cognitive function in dogs. In dogs older than 8 years, SAMe (18 mg/kg/day) improved age-related mental impairment compared with placebo. It has been used to treat arthritis in dogs, but no studies have demonstrated effectiveness.

Most of the benefits from SAMe in dogs and cats are based on small observational studies, clinical observations, and opinions from experts. There are no well-controlled studies that have supported therapeutic claims or confirmed the optimum dose through dose-ranging studies.

## Precautionary Information
### Adverse Reactions and Side Effects
As with most dietary supplements, there is a wide margin of safety. It may produce a self-limiting transient gastric upset. No other adverse effects are reported.

### Contraindications and Precautions
No contraindications are reported for animals.

### Drug Interactions
Reactions of SAMe with tricyclic antidepressants (TCAs) have been reported, although the mechanism is not known. In laboratory animals, administration with clomipramine has caused serotonin syndrome.

## Instructions for Use

SAMe is a dietary supplement widely available without a prescription (over the counter [OTC]). The potency of formulations may vary. Absorption is decreased when given with a meal. Administer 30 minutes to 1 hour before feeding. To ensure passage into the stomach of cats, administer with water. Coated tablets (e.g., Denosyl) protect the active ingredient from moisture during storage and destruction by stomach acid. Do not break tablets or disrupt coating.

## Patient Monitoring and Laboratory Tests

Monitor liver enzymes in animals being treated for toxicity.

## Formulations

- SAMe is widely available OTC in tablets and powder. The brand Denosyl is available in 90-, 225-, and 425-mg tablets. Veterinary formulations (e.g., Denamarin) may also contain silymarin (silybin) and vitamin E.

## Stability and Storage

Store in a tightly sealed container, protected from light, and at room temperature. Do not disrupt coating on tablet.

## Small Animal Dosage

### Dogs

- 20 mg/kg per day PO or 90 mg (small dogs), 225 mg (medium dogs), and 425 mg (large dogs).
- For dogs with acetaminophen toxicity, administer 40 mg/kg PO followed by 20 mg/kg q24h for 7 days. (Note: Acetylcysteine is a more reliable antidote.)

### Cats

- 90 mg/cat/day PO up to 5 kg body weight.
- For cats exposed to acetaminophen, administer 180 mg per cat SAMe q12h PO daily for 3 days and then 90 mg per cat q12h for 11 days. (Note: Acetylcysteine is a more reliable antidote.)

## Large Animal Dosage

- No dose has been reported for large animals.

## Regulatory Information

Because of a low risk of harmful residues in food animals, no withdrawal time is suggested.

# Sarolaner

sar′ oh lan′ er

**Trade and other names:** Simparica

**Functional classification:** Antiparasitic agent (flea and tick insecticide)

## Pharmacology and Mechanism of Action

Sarolaner belongs to the isooxazolines class of ectoparasiticides. It is effective for treating and preventing infections from fleas, mites, and ticks. It produces selective inhibition of the gamma-aminobutyric acid (GABA) receptor and glutamate-gated chloride channels. Inhibition of this receptor produces changes in chloride channels, or hyperexcitement of the parasite. As a GABA antagonist, the effects on chloride transmission in nerve and muscle cells in fleas and ticks produces paralysis and death. Mammals are not affected because of a lack of binding to mammalian GABA receptors.

Efficacy has been demonstrated against a wide range of ectoparasites, including fleas, various mites (including *Demodex* and *Sarcoptes* spp.), and ticks. Fleas, ticks, and mites are exposed and killed during their blood meal. Therefore, the parasite must bite the animal for exposure to the agent. Activity of the isooxazolines has been superior to those of other ectoparasiticides, including fipronil and imidacloprid. Other drugs in this class with similar activity, but different pharmacokinetics, include fluralaner, lotilaner, and afoxolaner.

*Pharmacokinetics:* In dogs, the oral dose is almost completely absorbed, and the half-life is 10–12 days. It is more than 99% bound to plasma proteins. The route of excretion is via bile and feces.

## Indications and Clinical Uses

Sarolaner is indicated to kill adult fleas and is indicated for the treatment and prevention of flea infestations (*Ctenocephalides felis*) and the treatment and control of the Lone Star tick (*Amblyomma americanum*), Gulf Coast tick (*Amblyomma maculatum*), American dog tick (*Dermacentor variabilis*), black-legged tick (*Ixodes scapularis*), and brown dog tick (*Rhipicephalus sanguineus*) infestations in dogs and puppies 6 months of age and older, weighing 4 lb of body weight or greater, for 1 month. It is also effective for treatment of demodicosis caused by *Demodex* mites. Combination products contain moxidectin and pyrantel to prevent heartworms and intestinal roundworms.

Because of this action, sarolaner can reduce the risk that these vectors may pose for disease transmission. For example, it may prevent infections caused by *Borrelia burgdorferi* (Lyme disease) and *Babesia canis*.

The approved label indication for sarolaner is treatment of fleas and ticks, but extralabel uses, using the approved label dose, have included treatment of generalized demodicosis caused by *Demodex canis*. Dogs with *Demodex* infection treated with sarolaner once a month had significant mite reduction after treatment. Sarolaner can eliminate sarcoptic mange (*Sarcoptes scabiei*) and ear mites (*Otodectes cynotis*) in dogs.

## Precautionary Information

### Adverse Reactions and Side Effects

Sarolaner has been safe for use in dogs at least 6 months of age. Adverse effects reported from field studies include vomiting, diarrhea, and lethargy. Other reported adverse effects include tremors, seizures, and hyperactivity. Target animal safety studies performed in dogs indicate good tolerance at the therapeutic dose, but beagles treated at three or five times the therapeutic dose have demonstrated tremors at three times the dose and other neurologic signs, including seizures at five times the dose. In clinical field studies with the isooxazoline group of insecticides, adverse effects reported include vomiting, diarrhea, anorexia, and lethargy.

Based on clinical experience, there is a concern about neurologic adverse effects, including seizures, from administration of isooxazolines in dogs. This has been reported with the use of sarolaner, and the manufacturer warns that it should be used cautiously in animals with a history of seizures. Other neurologic signs possible include tremors and ataxia.

### Contraindications and Precautions

There are no known contraindications for use of sarolaner. The isooxazoline group of insecticides have been associated with seizures in animals. Use cautiously in animals that may be prone to seizures. Safety in breeding or lactating animals has not been established. Safety and use in cats have not been established.

### Drug Interactions

No drug interactions are reported in animals.

## Instructions for Use

Administer oral once per month with appropriate tablets for the dog's body weight. Other measures for flea and tick control in the pet's environment also may be used.

## Patient Monitoring and Laboratory Tests

No specific monitoring is needed.

## Formulations

- Sarolaner is available in chewable tablets containing 5-, 10-, 20-, 40-, 80-, and 120-mg sarolaner.
- Sarolaner is also available in a combination product with moxidectin and pyrantel.

## Stability and Storage

Store at room temperature (below 30°C) protected from light in the manufacturer's packaging.

## Small Animal Dosage

### Dogs

- 2 mg/kg PO (one tablet, according to dog weight) once per month during flea and tick season. For treatment of *Demodex* infection, it has been administered once per month.
- The combination product is administered at a dose of 1.2 mg/kg once per month (with moxidectin and pyrantel).

### Cats

- No dose for cats has been established.

## Large Animal Dosage

- No large animal doses are available.

## Regulatory Information

- Although the risk of harmful residues is low, do not administer to food-producing animals.

---

# Selamectin
sel-ah-mek′tin

**Trade and other names:** Selarid, Revolution

**Functional classification:** Antiparasitic

**S**

## Pharmacology and Mechanism of Action

Selamectin is an antiparasitic agent with action similar to ivermectin. It is a microfilaricide for heartworm prevention in dogs and cats. Selamectin is a semisynthetic avermectin. Avermectins (ivermectin-like drugs) and milbemycins (milbemycin, doramectin, and moxidectin) are macrocyclic lactones. Avermectins and milbemycins share similarities, including mechanism of action. These drugs are neurotoxic to parasites by potentiating glutamate-gated chloride ion channels in parasites. Paralysis and death of the parasite are caused by increased permeability to chloride ions and hyperpolarization of nerve cells. These drugs also potentiate other chloride channels, including ones gated by GABA. Mammals ordinarily are not affected because they lack glutamate-gated chloride channels, and there is a lower affinity for other mammalian chloride channels. Because these drugs ordinarily do not penetrate the blood–brain barrier, GABA-gated channels in the CNS of mammals are not affected.

*Pharmacokinetics:* After topical application, selamectin has high affinity for sebaceous glands and skin. The terminal half-lives of selamectin are 11 days in dogs and 8 days in cats.

## Indications and Clinical Uses

Selamectin is approved for prevention of heartworms; control of fleas, mites, and ticks in dogs; and prevention of heartworms, control of fleas, mites, hookworms, and roundworms in cats. Selamectin also can be used to treat scabies (*Sarcoptes* spp.) and is sometimes preferred over ivermectin.

### Precautionary Information

#### Adverse Reactions and Side Effects

Transient, localized alopecia, with or without inflammation, at or near the site of application is observed in approximately 1% of treated cats. Other adverse effects include nausea, lethargy, salivation, tachypnea, and muscle tremors.

#### Contraindications and Precautions

Do not use in dogs younger than 6 weeks of age. Do not use in cats younger than 8 weeks of age.

#### Drug Interactions

No drug interactions have been reported in animals.

## Instructions for Use

Apply as indicated on product label to skin of dogs and cats.

### Patient Monitoring and Laboratory Tests

Monitor heartworm status in animals.

### Formulations

• Selamectin is available in 60- and 120-mg/mL transdermal solution.

### Stability and Storage

Store in a tightly sealed container, protected from light, and at room temperature.

## Small Animal Dosage

### Dogs and Cats

• Heartworm prevention: 6–12 mg/kg applied topically every 30 days.
• Other parasites: The same dose as for heartworm prevention may be applied for treatment and prevention of ear mites and fleas. In cats, the preferred dosage is 6 mg/kg every 30 days.
• Sarcoptic mange treatment: 6–12 mg/kg twice 30 days apart. (However, many dermatologists administer it at 2- to 3-week intervals.)

## Large Animal Dosage

• No dose has been reported for large animals.

## Regulatory Information

Withdrawal times are not established for animals that produce food. For extralabel use withdrawal interval estimates, contact Food Animal Residue Avoidance Databank (FARAD) at www.FARAD.org.

# Selegiline Hydrochloride

se-leh′jeh-leen hye-droe-klor′ide

**Trade and other names:** Anipryl (also known as deprenyl and ʟ-deprenyl), Eldepryl (human preparation), and Emsam transdermal patch

**Functional classification:** Dopamine agonist

## Pharmacology and Mechanism of Action

Selegiline is a dopamine agonist. Selegiline has been known by many names. Selegiline hydrochloride is the official United States Pharmacopeia (USP) drug name, but many clinicians know it by the older name, L-deprenyl. (L-Deprenyl is distinguished from its stereoisomer D-deprenyl.) A related drug is rasagiline. Selegiline has been used in humans for treatment of Parkinson disease and occasionally for Alzheimer disease with the trade name Eldepryl. (Efficacy for Alzheimer disease has not been established.)

The veterinary formulation is approved for treatment of pituitary-dependent hyperadrenocorticism (PDH) (Cushing's disease) in dogs and canine cognitive dysfunction. The action of selegiline is to inhibit monoamine oxidase (MAO) type B (and other MAO inhibitors [MAOIs] at higher doses). By inhibiting MAO type B, it inhibits the metabolism of dopamine in the CNS. The action for PDH may be through increased dopamine levels in the brain, which decreases adrenocorticotrophic hormone (ACTH) release, resulting in lower cortisol levels. Secondary effects are related to inhibition of the metabolism of phenylethylamine. (Phenylethylamine in laboratory animals produces amphetamine-like effects.) Two active metabolites are L-amphetamine and L-methamphetamine, but it is not known to what extent these contribute to pharmacologic effects. In horses, the metabolism to amphetamine-like metabolites is low.

## Indications and Clinical Uses

In dogs, selegiline is approved to control clinical signs of PDH (Cushing's disease) and to treat cognitive dysfunction in older dogs. However, the efficacy for Cushing's disease is not as high as for other drugs such as mitotane or trilostane. Selegiline effects may be limited to PDH caused by lesions of the pars intermedia and may not be effective for other forms of PDH. (Most cases of canine PDH have lesions of the pars distalis.) It may improve some clinical signs without lowering cortisol levels in dogs with PDH when administered at 1.0 mg/kg once daily.

For canine cognitive dysfunction (dementia) in aged dogs, treatment with selegiline inhibits MAO type B and increases dopamine concentrations in the brain, which restores dopamine balance and may improve cognitive ability. It has been administered to some older cats with age-related behavior problems, but clinical results in cats have not been reported, and doses are based on limited anecdotal experiences. It does not appear to produce any clinical effects in horses from oral administration.

### Precautionary Information

#### Adverse Reactions and Side Effects

Adverse effects are rare in dogs but have included vomiting, diarrhea, and hyperactive and restless behavior. Amphetamine-like signs can be produced in experimental animals. At high doses in dogs, hyperactivity has been observed (doses greater than 3 mg/kg), which include salivation, panting, repetitive movements, decreased weight, and changes in activity level. At doses of 30 mg per horse IV or PO, there were no behavior effects.

Two active metabolites are L-amphetamine and L-methamphetamine. Even though there were increases in amphetamine concentrations in dogs, they were not high enough to produce adverse effects at the approved label dose. However, at high doses (greater than 3 mg/kg), it may produce behavioral changes attributed to CNS stimulation. The L-isomer metabolites are not as active as their D forms, and studies have not supported a potential for amphetamine-like abuse or dependency from selegiline compared with other amphetamine-like drugs.

#### Contraindications and Precautions

Selegiline is not indicated for adrenal tumors. Use cautiously with other drugs. (See the following list of interactions.)

S

> **Drug Interactions**
>
> Do not use with other MAOIs. Do not use with TCAs, such as clomipramine and amitriptyline, or with selective serotonin reuptake inhibitors, such as fluoxetine. Do not administer with meperidine, dobutamine, or amitraz. Use cautiously with sympathetic amines and other drugs that may produce interactions such as linezolid and tramadol. However, one clinical study showed that there were no adverse effects in dogs when selegiline was administered in combination with phenylpropanolamine.

## Instructions for Use

Titrate the dose in each patient to achieve the desired effect without inducing excess CNS excitement. Start with low dose and increase gradually until clinical effect is observed. The transdermal patch for humans has not been evaluated for animals.

## Patient Monitoring and Laboratory Tests

No specific monitoring is required. Serum cortisol testing is not valuable for evaluating efficacy.

## Formulations

- Selegiline is available in 2-, 5-, 10-, 15-, and 30-mg tablets for animals; 5-mg tablets or capsules for humans; and 20-, 30-, and 40-cm$^2$ transdermal patches (EmSam) for humans.

## Stability and Storage

Stable if stored in manufacturer's original formulation.

## Small Animal Dosage

### Dogs

- Begin with 1 mg/kg q24h PO. If there is no response within 2 months, increase the dosage to a maximum of 2 mg/kg q24h PO.

### Cats

- 0.25–0.5 mg/kg q12h PO. In some cats, once-daily treatment may be sufficient.

## Large Animal Dosage

- No dose has been reported for large animals. In preliminary studies in which selegiline was administered at a dose of 30 mg/horse PO or IV, there were no observed effects on behavior or locomotor activity.

## Regulatory Information

Do not administer to animals intended for food.
Racing Commissioners International (RCI) Classification: 2

# Senna
sen′na

**Trade and other names:** Senokot

**Functional classification:** Laxative

## Pharmacology and Mechanism of Action

Senna is one of the older laxative agents. It is rarely used in veterinary medicine but may be effective for some types of constipation. Senna acts via local stimulation or via contact with intestinal mucosa.

## Indications and Clinical Uses

Senna has been used for management of constipation. The clinical use in veterinary medicine has been limited. The efficacy and doses listed are based on limited empirical evidence.

## Precautionary Information

### Adverse Reactions and Side Effects
Adverse effects not reported for animals. However, excessive doses are expected to cause fluid and electrolyte loss.

### Contraindications and Precautions
Do not administer to animals with gastrointestinal (GI) obstruction. Do not administer to dehydrated animals.

### Drug Interactions
No drug interactions have been reported in animals.

## Instructions for Use
Doses and indications are not well established for veterinary medicine. Use is strictly based on anecdotal experience.

## Patient Monitoring and Laboratory Tests
No specific monitoring is necessary.

## Formulations
- Senna is available in granules in concentrate or syrup.

## Stability and Storage
Store in a tightly sealed container, protected from light, and at room temperature.

### Small Animal Dosage
#### Dogs
- Syrup: 5–10 mL/dog/day PO.
- Granules: ½–1 tsp/dog/day PO.

#### Cats
- Syrup: 5 mL/cat q24h.
- Granules: ½ tsp/cat q24h (with food).

## Large Animal Dosage
- No doses have been reported for large animals.

## Regulatory Information
Because of a low risk of harmful residues in animals intended for food, no withdrawal time is suggested.

S

# Sevelamer Carbonate
se-vel′a-mer

**Trade and other names:** generic

**Functional classification:** Phosphate binder

## Pharmacology and Mechanism of Action
Sevelamer is a non-absorbed oral phosphate binder. It is a polymeric amine, anion exchange resin that binds directly to phosphorous. It contains multiple amines in a protonated form in the intestine. These amines bind to phosphate molecules in the intestine and decrease absorption. Sevelamer effectively lowers the phosphate levels in the serum. Phosphate binding capacity: Sevelamer HCl 400 mg binds approximately 32 mg of phosphate, and 800 mg binds approximately 64 mg of phosphate.

Sevelamer also may bind to bile acids in research animals. This effect may lower serum cholesterol.

## Indications and Clinical Uses

Sevelamer is used as an oral treatment to bind phosphate in patients with chronic kidney disease. There are two forms, sevelamer carbonate and sevelamer hydrochloride salt. The two forms react similarly and are interchangeable.

## Precautionary Information

### Adverse Reactions and Side Effects

Adverse effects are not reported for animals. In people, it has had a good safety margin with constipation being the major adverse effect. There is no systemic absorption. Long-term administration can potentially decrease fat-soluble vitamins such as vitamins A, D, and K because of the effect on bile acids and normal fat absorption.

### Contraindications and Precautions

There are no specific contraindications or precautions.

### Drug Interactions

No drug interactions have been reported for animals. However, it may potentially interfere with oral absorption of other drugs. In people, it decreased oral absorption of fluoroquinolones by 50%.

## Instructions for Use

Administer only by the oral route with food. When using the powder form, empty the entire contents of a 0.8- or 2.4-g packet into a container and add 30 mL of water (for the 0.8-g packet) or 60 mL of water (for the 2.4-g packet). If switching from sevelamer hydrochloride to sevelamer carbonate, use the same dose and frequency. Phosphate levels in the blood are better controlled with frequent administration during the day with each meal rather than with one single dose.

## Patient Monitoring and Laboratory Tests

Adjust dose based on measuring serum phosphorous.

## Formulations

- Sevelamer is available in a film-coated tablet, 800 mg, and sevelamer carbonate powder (citrus flavor).

## Stability and Storage

Sevelamer should be stored in a dry place in a tightly sealed container at room temperature.

## Small Animal Dosage

- 80–100 mg/kg (approximately) per day. This dose should be divided up equally for each meal fed to the pet (e.g., 25–30 mg/kg PO three times daily).

## Large Animal Dosage

- No large animal doses have been identified.

## Regulatory Information

No withdrawal times are established for animals intended for food. Because the effects are limited to the intestine, no withdrawal times are anticipated.

# Sevoflurane

see-voe-floo'rane

**Trade and other names:** Ultane

**Functional classification:** Anesthetic

## Pharmacology and Mechanism of Action

Sevoflurane is one of the inhalant anesthetics. Like other inhalant anesthetics, the mechanism of action is uncertain. Sevoflurane produces a generalized, reversible depression of the CNS. The inhalant anesthetics vary in their solubility in blood, their potency, and the rate of induction and recovery. Those with low blood/gas partition coefficients are associated with the most rapid rates of induction and recovery. Sevoflurane has a vapor pressure of 160 mm Hg (at 20°C), a blood/gas partition coefficient of 0.65, and a fat/blood coefficient of 48. Sevoflurane is similar to isoflurane in many respects except that it has lower solubility, resulting in faster induction and recovery times.

## Indications and Clinical Uses

Sevoflurane is used as an inhalant anesthetic. There are not any significant advantages over the use of isoflurane, and it is more expensive than isoflurane. It has minimum alveolar concentration (MAC) values of 2.58%, 2.36%, and 2.31% in cats, dogs, and horses, respectively. Sevoflurane, like other inhalant anesthetics, can be used with preanesthetics, opioids, alpha$_2$-agonists, and tranquilizers.

## Precautionary Information

### Adverse Reactions and Side Effects

Adverse effects are related to anesthetic effects (e.g., cardiovascular and respiratory depression). Sevoflurane can produce byproducts of fluoride ions and compound A, which can be toxic to the kidneys, but this is a rare problem.

### Contraindications and Precautions

Do not use unless there is an adequate facility to monitor patients. Use only with approved anesthetic vaporizer delivery systems.

### Drug Interactions

No drug interactions have been reported for animals.

## Instructions for Use

Use of inhalant anesthetics requires careful monitoring. Dose is determined by depth of anesthesia.

## Patient Monitoring and Laboratory Tests

Carefully monitor patient's heart rate and rhythm and respiratory rate during use.

## Formulations

• Sevoflurane is available in a 100-mL bottle.

## Stability and Storage

Sevoflurane is highly volatile and should only be stored in approved containers.

## Small Animal Dosage

• Induction: 8%; maintenance: 3%–6%.

## Large Animal Dosage

### Horses

• MAC value: 2.31.

## Regulatory Information

No withdrawal times are established for animals intended for food. Clearance is rapid, and short withdrawal times are suggested. For extralabel use withdrawal interval estimates, contact FARAD at www.FARAD.org.

# Sildenafil Citrate
sill-den′-ah-fil

**Trade and other names:** Viagra and Revatio

**Functional classification:** Vasodilator

## Pharmacology and Mechanism of Action
Sildenafil is used as a vasodilator. Sildenafil's vasodilator effects are specific for phosphodiesterase V. Sildenafil and similar drugs act to increase cyclic guanosine monophosphate (GMP) by inhibiting its breakdown by phosphodiesterase V (PDE V). Relaxation of smooth muscle occurs from generation of nitric oxide. There are two important locations of PDE V, (1) vascular smooth muscle of the lungs and (2) corpus cavernosum. The effects on the corpus cavernosum produce the desired clinical effects for treating erectile dysfunction in people. The effect on vascular smooth muscle of the lungs produces vasodilation of the pulmonary vascular bed in patients with pulmonary hypertension. Other drugs that have been used for this effect are tadalafil (Cialis) at a dosage of 1–2 mg/kg q12h PO in dogs.

Sildenafil also relaxes smooth muscle in other sites, including portions of the GI tract, uterus, and gallbladder. Relaxation of the esophageal muscle may improve some dogs with clinical megaesophagus. Most of the esophagus in dogs is comprised of striated muscle, but the lower esophageal sphincter is made of smooth muscle, which can be relaxed by some agents.

*Pharmacokinetics:* In dogs, the half-life is approximately 5 hours.

## Indications and Clinical Uses
Sildenafil and related drugs are used in people for treating erectile dysfunction via the effect on the corpus cavernosum. This effect has not been explored in veterinary medicine. The use in veterinary medicine has been limited to the treatment of pulmonary arterial hypertension and megaesophagus. In dogs, there is clinical evidence for the beneficial effects of sildenafil in patients with pulmonary hypertension. Results of prospective studies in dogs show that the response may be inconsistent but that many dogs have lower pulmonary artery pressure after treatment with sildenafil. On the other hand, some dogs do not respond. Sildenafil has been used to improve clinical signs in dogs with congenital idiopathic megaesophagus. This improvement occurs through relaxation of the lower esophageal sphincter muscle to facilitate emptying of the esophagus to the stomach.

## Precautionary Information

### Adverse Reactions and Side Effects
Cutaneous flushing of the inguinal area has been observed in dogs. Otherwise, adverse effects have not been reported with clinical use in dogs. Potential effects are attributed to the vasodilator action. If high doses or other vasodilators are administered, especially those that increase cyclic GMP levels, hypotension can occur.

### Contraindications and Precautions
Use cautiously in conjunction with other vasodilator drugs.

### Drug Interactions
No drug interactions reported for animals, but in people, there are precautions about use with other vasodilators such as alpha blockers and nitrates. When used for treating megaesophagus in dogs, it should not be used with cisapride or metoclopramide because they antagonize the effect.

## Instructions for Use
The use in veterinary medicine has been based on studies in dogs with pulmonary hypertension and in dogs with megaesophagus. The dosages and clinical use are based on these limited reports.

## Patient Monitoring and Laboratory Tests
No specific monitoring is necessary but monitor the patient's cardiovascular function (blood pressure and heart rate) in animals at risk for cardiovascular complications.

## Formulations
• Sildenafil is available as 20-, 25-, 50-, and 100-mg tablets.

## Stability and Storage
Store in a tightly sealed container, protected from light, and at room temperature.

## Small Animal Dosage
### Dogs
• Pulmonary hypertension: 2 mg/kg q12h PO. Dose interval may range from 8–24 hours, and doses as high as 3 mg/kg have been administered to some dogs. There are variations in the dose range because of limitation in tablet sizes.
• Megaesophagus: 1 mg/kg PO q12h.

### Cats
• 1 mg/kg q8h PO.

## Large Animal Dosage
• No dose has been reported for large animals.

## Regulatory Information
No withdrawal times are established for animals intended for food. For extralabel use withdrawal interval estimates, contact FARAD at www.FARAD.org.

# Silymarin
sill-ih-mare′in

**Trade and other names:** Silybin, Marin, milk thistle, and generic brands
**Functional classification:** Hepatic protectant

## Pharmacology and Mechanism of Action
Silymarin is a dietary supplement that contains silybin as the most active ingredient. It is also known as milk thistle, the plant from which it is derived. Silymarin is a mixture of antihepatotoxic flavonolignans (derived from the plant Silybum). Silymarin has three components that are considered flavonolignans: silidianin, silcristin, and silybin (which is the major component and also called *silymarin* and *silibinin*). Silymarin has been used for the treatment of a variety of liver disorders in humans. The mechanism of silymarin's action is thought to be an antioxidant effect, in which it inhibits both peroxidation of lipid membranes and GSH oxidation. Experimental data have supported the hepatoprotective properties of silymarin as an antioxidant and a free radical scavenger.

*Pharmacokinetics:* One product (Marin) is complexed with phosphatidylcholine, which may increase oral bioavailability. The combination products contain vitamin E (aqueous alpha tocopherol, 10–100 IU/kg/day), which has also been advocated for its antioxidant effects.

The pharmacokinetics of silymarin have been studied in dogs, cats, and horses. After oral administration to cats, the half-life is 3.2 hours (±1.74) but the oral absorption is low (e.g., 7% in cats). However, the bile concentrations are much higher than serum levels, which may indicate that higher levels occur in the liver. In horses, the oral absorption is low (0.6%) when administered in feed and 2.9% when administered with a nasogastric tube.

## Indications and Clinical Uses

As a dietary supplement, the manufacturer is not obligated to make therapeutic claims for marketing. Silymarin has been used to treat hepatic disease, including those caused by hepatotoxic reactions in people and animals. It has been administered to animals for the hepatoprotective effects after hepatotoxic drug injury caused by carbon tetrachloride, mushrooms, arsenic, and acetaminophen. It has also been recommended for dogs, cats, and horses with liver disease, but there are no well-controlled clinical studies documenting effectiveness for this use. In one observational study, the combination product with silymarin and SAMe reduced liver enzyme elevations associated with chemotherapy in tumor-bearing dogs. Studies in humans produced mixed results, and studies in dogs, cats, and horses are limited to small observational studies.

Silymarin is used as a complementary treatment in canine and feline liver disease through antioxidant effects. However, there is no specific information on the optimum dose or evidence of efficacy of silymarin treatment based on well-controlled studies. Silymarin can be used with SAMe, and there are preparations that include both silymarin and SAMe (Denamarin).

When administered to horses, it produced only minor changes in antioxidant capacity of blood.

## Precautionary Information

### Adverse Reactions and Side Effects

This is a natural chemical and no adverse reactions have been reported.

### Contraindications and Precautions

No contraindications have been reported for animals.

### Drug Interactions

No drug interactions have been reported.

## Instructions for Use

SAMe, silymarin, and vitamin E are considered dietary supplements and, as such, are not subject to regulation as drugs by the US Food and Drug Administration (FDA). Products available OTC and through various outlets are not regulated by the FDA and may differ considerably in purity and potency.

## Patient Monitoring and Laboratory Tests

Monitor liver enzymes in animals being treated for toxicity.

## Formulations

- Silymarin tablets are widely available OTC. Commercial veterinary formulations (Marin) also contain zinc and vitamin E in a phosphatidylcholine complex in tablets for dogs and cats. The combination of Denamarin contains both silymarin and SAMe.

## Stability and Storage

Store in a tightly sealed container, protected from light, and at room temperature.

## Small Animal Dosage

### Dogs and Cats

- 5–15 mg/kg PO once daily. Some sources recommend a higher dosage with a minimum of 30 mg/kg PO per day.

## Large Animal Dosage

### Horses

- No clinically effective dosages have been reported for large animals. At dosages of 6.5, 13, and 26 mg/kg q12h for 7 days, only minor antioxidant effects were observed.

### Regulatory Information

Because of a low risk of harmful residues in animals intended for food, no withdrawal time is suggested.

---

# Sodium Bicarbonate

**Trade and other names:** Baking soda, soda mint, Citrocarbonate, and Arm & Hammer pure baking soda

**Functional classification:** Alkalinizing agent

---

## Pharmacology and Mechanism of Action

Sodium bicarbonate ($NaHCO_3$) is an old and widely available alkalizing agent and is commonly called baking soda. When administered orally, it acts as a gastric antacid. After absorption, it increases plasma and urinary concentrations of bicarbonate. When administered IV it produces systemic alkalinizing effects for treating acidemia. One gram of sodium bicarbonate is equal to 12 mEq sodium and bicarbonate ions; 3.65 g sodium bicarbonate is equal to 1 g sodium.

## Indications and Clinical Uses

Sodium bicarbonate is an alkalinizing solution, once used commonly as a gastric antacid, but other agents are more commonly used for suppressing stomach acid. It is the most frequent alkalinizing solution used for IV therapy of systemic acidosis and to treat severe hyperkalemia. When adding to fluid therapy, the goal is to maintain $PaCO_2$ within 37–43 mm Hg. It also has been administered to alkalize urine.

## Precautionary Information

### Adverse Reactions and Side Effects

Adverse effects have been attributed to alkalizing activity. Hypokalemia may occur with excessive administration. Hyperosmolality, hypernatremia, paradoxical CNS, and intracellular acidosis may occur.

### Contraindications and Precautions

Do not administer to animals with hypocalcemia (may exacerbate tetany). Do not administer to animals with excessive chloride loss because of vomiting. Do not administer to animals with alkalosis. Administration of sodium bicarbonate may increase risk of hypernatremia, paradoxical CNS acidosis, and hyperosmolality. When used during cardiac resuscitation, caution is advised because of a risk of hyperosmolality, hypernatremia, and paradoxical CNS acidosis.

### Drug Interactions

Sodium bicarbonate should not be mixed with drugs that require an acidic medium for stability and solubility. Such drugs may include solutions containing hydrochloride (HCl) salts. When mixing IV solutions, do not mix bicarbonate with solutions containing calcium. (Chelation may result.) When administered orally, interaction may occur to decrease absorption of other drugs. (A partial list includes anticholinergic drugs, ketoconazole, fluoroquinolones, and tetracyclines.)

S

## Instructions for Use

When used for systemic acidosis, the dose should be adjusted on the basis of blood gas measurements or assessment of acidosis. The following equation may be used to estimate requirement:

$$\text{mEq Bicarbonate needed} = \text{body weight (kg)} \times \text{base deficit (mEq/L)} \times 0.3$$

Initially, administer 25%–50% of this dose in IV fluids over 20–30 minutes.

In calves or neonates, use a factor of 0.5 instead of 0.3 in the equation above because of higher water content in these animals.

## Patient Monitoring and Laboratory Tests

Monitor acid–base status.

## Formulations

- Sodium bicarbonate is available in 325-, 520-, and 650-mg tablets.
- In each teaspoonful (3.9 g) of citrocarbonate, there are 780 mg of sodium bicarbonate and 1.82 g of sodium citrate.
- Injection solutions: 4.2% is 0.5 mEq/mL (11.5 mg/mL of sodium), and 8.4% is 1 mEq/mL (23 mg/mL of sodium).

Note on strength of formulations:

- 1.4% solution = 0.17 mEq/mL and provides 13 g/L of bicarbonate.
- 8.5% solution = 1 mEq/mL of $NaHCO_3$.
- One teaspoon of baking soda is approximately 2 g of $NaHCO_3$.
- 12 mEq of bicarbonate is equivalent to 1 g of sodium bicarbonate.

## Stability and Storage

Store in a tightly sealed container at room temperature. Alkaline solution with pH of 7–8.5. Do not mix with acid solutions. Sodium bicarbonate is soluble in water. If exposed to air, it may decompose to sodium carbonate, which is more alkaline.

## Small Animal Dosage

### Dogs and Cats

- Metabolic acidosis: 0.5–1 mEq/kg IV.
- Alkalinization of urine: 50 mg/kg q8–12h PO.
- Oral antacid: 2–5 g mixed with water PO. (Other agents are more effective to suppress gastric acid.)
- Cardiopulmonary resuscitation: 1 mEq/kg with additional doses of 0.5 mEq/kg at 10-minute intervals.

## Large Animal Dosage

- Metabolic acidosis: 0.5–1 mEq/kg IV slowly. Other doses should be calculated based on base deficits. Oral doses vary; 10–12 g of sodium bicarbonate may be given orally to adult large animals (horses and cattle) and 2–5 g to calves, foals, and pigs.

## Regulatory Information

Because of a low risk of harmful residues in animals intended for food, no withdrawal time is suggested.

# Sodium Chloride 0.9%

**Trade and other names:** Normal saline and generic brands

**Functional classification:** Fluid replacement

## Pharmacology and Mechanism of Action
Sodium chloride is a common fluid used for IV infusion and as a replacement fluid. It is not a suitable maintenance solution. Sodium chloride (0.9%) contains 154 mEq/L of sodium and 154 mEq/L of chloride. See Appendix L for comparison with other fluid solutions.

## Indications and Clinical Uses
Sodium chloride is used for IV fluid supplementation. However, it is not a balanced electrolyte solution and should not be used for maintenance. It also is frequently used as a vehicle to deliver IV medications via constant-rate infusion.

## Precautionary Information
### Adverse Reactions and Side Effects
It is not a balanced electrolyte solution. Long-term infusion may cause electrolyte imbalance. Because saline solution is not balanced, it may cause acidemia because it increases renal elimination of bicarbonate. Prolonged use may cause hypokalemia.

### Contraindications and Precautions
Do not exceed the maximum dose rate of 80 mL/kg/h. This solution does not contain electrolyte balance for maintenance.

### Drug Interactions
No drug interactions have been reported in animals.

## Instructions for Use
When administering IV fluid solution, monitor the rate and electrolyte concentrations carefully.

Fluid administration rates are as follows:

Replacement fluid: calculate as liters needed = % dehydration × body weight (kg)

or

Milliliters needed = % dehydration × body weight (kg) × 1000

Add bicarbonate to fluids if necessary based on calculation of base deficit.

## Patient Monitoring and Laboratory Tests
Monitor hydration status and serum electrolytes, particularly potassium.

## Formulations
- Sodium chloride 0.9% is available in a 500- and 1000-mL infusion.

## Stability and Storage
Store in a tightly sealed container at room temperature.

## Small Animal Dosage
### Dogs and Cats
- Maintenance administration (no deficits): 1.5–2.5 mL/kg/h. (Caution: this is not a balanced maintenance solution.)
- Moderate dehydration: 15–30 mL/kg/h IV.
- Severe dehydration: 50 mL/kg/h IV.

## Large Animal Dosage
- 40–50 mL/kg day IV, intraperitoneal, or SQ maintenance.
- Moderate dehydration: 15–30 mL/kg/h IV.
- Severe dehydration: 50 mL/kg/h IV.

**Calves**
- Moderate dehydration: 45 mL/kg given at a rate of 30–40 mL/kg/h.
- Severe dehydration: 80–90 mL/kg given at a rate of 30–40 mL/kg/h or as fast as 80 mL/kg/h if necessary.

### Regulatory Information

Because of a low risk of harmful residues in animals intended for food, no withdrawal time is suggested.

## Sodium Chloride 7.2% and 7.5%

**Trade and other names:** Hypertonic saline solution and HSS

**Functional classification:** Fluid replacement

### Pharmacology and Mechanism of Action

Sodium chloride 7.2% (also available as a 7.5% solution) is a concentrated sodium chloride solution used for special situations instead of 0.9% sodium chloride solution. This concentrated solution is used for acute treatment of hypovolemia when a rapid response is needed. Hypertonic saline solution causes rapid expansion of plasma volume and may improve microvascular blood flow. Hypertonic saline solution contains 2566 mOsm/L, 1232 mEq/L sodium, and 1232 mEq/L of chloride.

### Indications and Clinical Uses

Hypertonic saline is used to treat hypovolemic shock in animals. The duration of its benefit is short lived because it quickly dissipates from the blood vessels. There may be benefits for combination with colloids such as Dextran 70 to maintain vascular pressure. It has been used at doses of 4 mL/kg IV to dogs during a 5-minute infusion to be effective for treatment of septic shock.

### Precautionary Information

**Adverse Reactions and Side Effects**

This is not a balanced electrolyte solution. Long-term infusion may cause electrolyte imbalance.

**Contraindications and Precautions**

Do not administer to hypernatremic animals. Do not administer solutions high in sodium to animals with renal insufficiency.

**Drug Interactions**

No drug interactions have been reported in animals.

### Instructions for Use

Hypertonic saline is used for short-term infusion for rapid replacement of vascular volume.

### Patient Monitoring and Laboratory Tests

Monitor hematocrit and blood pressure in treated animals.

### Formulations

- Sodium chloride is available in either 7.2% or 7.5% concentrated solution as an IV infusion.

## Stability and Storage
Store in a tightly sealed container at room temperature.

## Small Animal Dosage
### Dogs and Cats
- 3–8 mL/kg IV of 7.2% solution. (The rate of administration should not exceed 1 mL/kg/min.)
- Hemorrhagic shock: 4–5 mL/kg IV over 10 minutes.

## Large Animal Dosage
- 4–8 mL/kg of 7.2% solution IV at a rate of 1 mL/kg/min.

## Regulatory Information
Because of a low risk of harmful residues in animals intended for food, no withdrawal time is suggested.

# Sodium Iodide (20%)
**Trade and other names:** Iodopen and generic brands

**Functional classification:** Iodine replacement

## Pharmacology and Mechanism of Action
Sodium iodide is a concentrated iodide solution used to treat iodine deficiency. Occasionally, it is used for treating fungal infections, but this is an outdated treatment.

## Indications and Clinical Uses
Sodium iodide is used to treat fungal infections and is preferred over potassium iodide. It has been used for bacterial, actinomycete, and fungal infections, primarily in horses and cattle. In cattle, it has been used for actinomycosis (lumpy jaw) and actinobacillosis (wooden tongue and necrotic stomatitis). In small animals, it has been used for sporotrichosis. Proof of efficacy for these indications has not been established. This is an old product and there are no recent clinical reports to document efficacy. See Iodide and Potassium Iodide for additional information on use and formulations available.

S

## Precautionary Information
### Adverse Reactions and Side Effects
High doses can produce signs of iodism, which include lacrimation, irritation of mucous membranes, swelling of eyelids, cough, dry and scruffy coat, and hair loss. Potassium iodide has a bitter taste and can cause nausea and salivation.

### Contraindications and Precautions
Do not use in pregnant animals; it may cause abortion.

### Drug Interactions
No drug interactions have been reported.

## Instructions for Use
For treatment in cattle, administer slowly IV. Be careful not to inject outside the vein or tissue necrosis may occur. Clinical use in animals is primarily empirical. The doses

and indications listed have not been tested in clinical trials. Other, more proven drugs for these indications should be considered as alternatives.

## Patient Monitoring and Laboratory Tests

No specific monitoring is necessary.

## Formulations

- Sodium iodide is available in a 20-g/100 mL (20%) injection, which contains 100-mcg elemental iodide (118 mcg of sodium iodide) per milliliter injection.

## Stability and Storage

Store in a tightly sealed container, protected from light, and at room temperature.

## Small Animal Dosage

### Dogs and Cats

- Consult oral dose for potassium iodide in another section of this book.

## Large Animal Dosage

### Horses

- 125 mL of a 20% solution IV daily for 3 days; then 30 g/horse daily injection for 30 days.

### Cattle

- 67 mg/kg IV (15 mL per 100 lb) slowly; repeat weekly.

## Regulatory Information

Because of a low risk of harmful residues in animals intended for food, no withdrawal time is suggested.

# Sotalol Hydrochloride

soe'tah-lole hye-droe-klor'ide

**Trade and other names:** Betapace

**Functional classification:** Beta blocker, antiarrhythmic

## Pharmacology and Mechanism of Action

Sotalol is an antiarrhythmic agent that has effects as a nonselective beta-receptor (beta$_1$ and beta$_2$) adrenergic blocker (Class II antiarrhythmic). The action as a Class II antiarrhythmic is similar to propranolol (one-third potency); however, it has beneficial effects through additional antiarrhythmic effects. In addition to being a Class II antiarrhythmic drug, sotalol may have some Class III (potassium channel–blocking) activity. The Class III activity prolongs the refractory period by decreasing potassium conduction in delayed rectifier currents. The benefit during treatment with sotalol is that the negative inotropic effects from beta-receptor antagonism is balanced by increased action potential duration, leading to a prolonged time for calcium reentry.

Sotalol is a water-soluble beta blocker and relies less on the liver for clearance than other beta blockers. Plasma levels and interindividual differences in clearance are expected to be less than other beta blockers.

## Indications and Clinical Uses

Sotalol is indicated for control of refractory ventricular arrhythmias. It has also been used for refractory atrial fibrillation. Although sotalol has been used as a preferred oral antiarrhythmic agent administered to small animals, particularly dogs, there are no controlled studies to establish efficacy over other agents. The use and doses are derived primarily from small observational studies or anecdotal and clinical experience.

In horses, sotalol (2 mg/kg q12h) produces lower peak concentrations than comparable doses in people. However, it has decreased heart rate and increased the QT interval, which facilitates cardioversion in horses with atrial fibrillation.

## Precautionary Information

### Adverse Reactions and Side Effects

Adverse effects have not been reported for animals but are expected to be similar to those of propranolol. In people, reported adverse effects include atrioventricular (AV) block, hypotension, dyspnea, bronchospasm, bradycardia, and QT interval prolongation. These effects are possible but not reported from the use in animals. Like many antiarrhythmic agents, sotalol may have some proarrhythmic activity. Negative inotropic effects may cause concern in some animals with poor cardiac contractility.

### Contraindications and Precautions

Sotalol should be administered cautiously to patients with heart failure or AV block. Use cautiously in patients with poor cardiac reserve because it may decrease cardiac contractility. In dogs with ventricular arrhythmias, it produces a mild decrease in left ventricular function; otherwise, it has been well tolerated in dogs with atrial enlargement and systolic dysfunction.

### Drug Interactions

Use cautiously with other cardiovascular drugs that may depress the heart. A full range of drug interactions is not known for dogs because the use is extralabel, and such records are not kept. However, drug interactions are possible from other medications that interfere with drug metabolism.

## Instructions for Use

The beta-blocking effects occur at low doses; Class III antiarrhythmic effects occur at higher doses. In people, sotalol has been a more effective maintenance agent for controlling arrhythmias than other drugs, and this may be true in animals also.

## Patient Monitoring and Laboratory Tests

Monitor heart rate during treatment. Monitor the electrocardiogram for response to treatment.

## Formulations

- Sotalol is available in 80-, 120-, 160-, and 240-mg tablets.

## Stability and Storage

Store in a tightly sealed container, protected from light, and at room temperature. Sotalol is soluble in both water and ethanol. It has been mixed with syrups and flavorings and is stable for 12 weeks, but it should be stored in the refrigerator.

## Small Animal Dosage

### Dogs

- 2 mg/kg q12h PO. (For medium- to large-breed dogs, begin with 40 mg per dog q12h; then increase to 80 mg per dog if no response.)

### Cats

- 1–2 mg/kg q12h PO. A dosage of 10–20 mg per cat q12h also has been used.

## Large Animal Dosage

### Horses

- Treatment of atrial fibrillation: 2 mg/kg PO q12h for 3 days.
- Ventricular tachycardia: 1 mg/kg PO q12h up to 2–3 mg/kg PO q12h. (Increase dose as needed to control the response.)

## Regulatory Information

Withdrawal times are not established for animals that produce food. For extralabel use withdrawal interval estimates, contact FARAD at www.FARAD.org.

RCI Classification: 3

# Spectinomycin and Spectinomycin Dihydrochloride Pentahydrate

spek-tih-noe-mye'sin

**Trade and other names:** Spectam, Spectogard, Prospec, Linco-Spectin, and Adspec

**Functional classification:** Antibiotic, aminocyclitol

## Pharmacology and Mechanism of Action

Spectinomycin is an aminocyclitol antibiotic that shares similar features with the aminoglycoside class of antibiotics. However, it differs in that it does not contain amino sugars or glycosidic bonds. It is highly water soluble and is easily mixed in aqueous solutions. Spectinomycin, like aminoglycosides, inhibits protein synthesis via a 30S ribosomal target. It is a broad-spectrum drug with activity against gram-positive and some gram-negative bacteria and *Mycoplasma* spp. but with little anaerobic activity. It is not absorbed orally but is administered either in drinking water for treatment of enteritis or by injection for other infections. After injection, the half-life in animals is 1–2 hours.

## Indications and Clinical Uses

Spectinomycin has in vitro activity against some gram-negative bacteria and has also been administered orally for treatment of bacteria enteritis caused by *Escherichia coli* and as an injection for treatment of respiratory infections. Spectinomycin has been used in cattle to treat bovine respiratory disease infections caused by *Pasteurella* spp., *Mannheimia* spp., and *Histophilus somni*. It also has activity against *Mycoplasma* spp. It has been used in dogs, but this use is uncommon.

The approved indication for dogs is oral treatment "of infectious diarrhea and gastroenteritis caused by organisms susceptible to spectinomycin." The injectable or oral formulation is for "treatment of infections caused by gram-negative and gram-positive organisms susceptible to spectinomycin." However, these are outdated indications, and the use in small animals is uncommon. It is approved for pigs for treatment and control of infectious bacterial enteritis associated with *E. coli* in pigs younger than 4 weeks of age. It is also approved for poultry to be added to drinking water.

## Precautionary Information

### Adverse Reactions and Side Effects

Injection-site lesions may occur from administration to cattle.

### Contraindications and Precautions

The powder intended to be used in drinking water should not be formulated with water or saline for IV injection. This solution has produced severe pulmonary edema and death.

### Drug Interactions

No drug interactions are reported.

## Instructions for Use
Injections in cattle should be made in the neck muscle.

## Patient Monitoring and Laboratory Tests
The Clinical and Laboratory Standards Institute (CLSI) approved breakpoint for susceptible bacteria is ≤32 mcg/mL.

## Formulations
- Injectable solution: 100-mg spectinomycin sulfate per milliliter of solution.
- The lincomycin–spectinomycin combination contains 50 mg of lincomycin with 100 mg of spectinomycin *(Linco-Spectin)* per milliliter. Formulations for poultry include 500 mg/g of water-soluble powder.
- Oral solution for pigs: 50 mg/mL.
- Injection for dogs: 50- or 100-mg/mL solution.
- Tablets for dogs: 100-mg tablet.

## Stability and Storage
Store at room temperature. Protect from freezing. Stability of compounded formulations has not been evaluated.

## Small Animal Dosage
### Dogs
- 22 mg/kg q12h PO for 4 days.
- 5.5–11 mg/kg q12h IM for 4 days.

## Large Animal Dosage
### Pigs
- 6.6–22 mg/kg q12–24h IM or 50–100 mg per pig PO.

### Cattle
- 10–15 mg/kg q24h SQ (in neck) for 3–5 days.

## Regulatory Information
Cattle withdrawal time for meat: 11 days. Discoloration of meat at site of injection may persist for 15 days.

Pig withdrawal time for meat: 21 days. At doses of 20 mg/kg, the withdrawal time is 30 days.

Do not administer to calves to be slaughtered for veal. A milk discard time has not been established. Do not administer to dairy cattle 20 months of age or older.

# Spinosad
spin-oh′sad

**Trade and other names:** Comfortis and Trifexis (with milbemycin)

**Functional classification:** Antiparasitic

## Pharmacology and Mechanism of Action
Spinosad is used as an antiparasitic agent to treat fleas. It is a member of the spinosyns class of insecticides. These resemble tetracycline macrolides but are not antibacterial. Spinosad is a combination of spinosyn A and spinosyn D derived from bacteria (*Saccharopolyspora spinosa*). The action of spinosad in fleas is activation of nicotinic acetylcholine receptors but not other nicotinic receptors or GABA receptors. The

actions in insects treated with spinosad are muscle contractions and tremors in motor neurons, paralysis, and flea death. It does not affect mammals because of differences in the susceptibility of nicotinic acetylcholine receptors.

## Indications and Clinical Uses

Spinosad is used as a monthly treatment for flea infestations. After administration, spinosad can kill fleas within 30 minutes and has complete kill within 4 hours. Efficacy may decline after the initial 2 weeks of treatment in areas with heavy flea populations, and efficacy for treating fleas may be better if administered every 2 weeks than once per month in some dogs.

Spinosad plus milbemycin is indicated for prevention of heartworm disease (*Dirofilaria immitis*), as well as for killing fleas (*Ctenocephalides felis*) and the treatment and control of adult hookworm (*Ancylostoma caninum*), adult roundworm (*Toxocara canis* and *Toxascaris leonina*), and adult whipworm (*Trichuris vulpis*) infections in dogs and puppies 8 weeks of age or older and 2.5 kg of body weight or greater.

## Precautionary Information

### Adverse Reactions and Side Effects

In safety studies, administration of high dosages (100 mg/kg once daily for 10 days) did not produce any serious adverse effects other than vomiting and mild elevation of liver enzymes. Oral administration of spinosad (300 mg/kg) to collie dogs with the multidrug resistant (*MDR*) gene mutation (p-glycoprotein deficient) did not cause signs of toxicosis. Occasional vomiting may be observed with routine use. (See Instructions for Use about dosing after vomiting.)

In cats, the most common adverse event is vomiting.

### Contraindications and Precautions

It can be used safely with heartworm preventatives, including ivermectin but do not administer with high-dose ivermectin for treatment of *Demodex* infection. Use cautiously in pregnant and breeding animals. Some adverse effects on puppies have been reported from safety studies on pregnant dogs. Adverse effects in puppies nursing from dams administered spinosad also have been reported.

### Drug Interactions

Spinosad significantly increased ivermectin concentrations when both drugs were administered together. The proposed interaction is caused by inhibition of P-glycoprotein membrane transporter, which may increase the risk of adverse effects caused by ivermectin. Therefore, do not administer this agent with ivermectin. Spinosad has been used safely with other drugs, including heartworm preventatives.

## Instructions for Use

Spinosad should be administered with food for maximum absorption. If vomiting occurs within an hour of administration, redose with another full dose. If a dose is missed, administer Comfortis chewable tablets with food and resume a monthly dosing schedule. Treatment with spinosad may begin at any season of the year, preferably started before fleas emerge. It can also be used year round.

Although not approved for cats in the United States (but approved in some countries), spinosad has been used safely with once-monthly treatment to control fleas.

## Patient Monitoring and Laboratory Tests

No specific monitoring is necessary.

## Formulations

- Spinosad is available in five chewable tablet sizes containing 140, 270, 560, 810, or 1620 mg.
- Spinosad + milbemycin chewable tablets are available as 140 mg of spinosad and 2.3 mg of milbemycin oxime, 270 mg of spinosad and 4.5 mg of milbemycin oxime, 560 mg of spinosad and 9.3 mg of milbemycin oxime, 810 mg of spinosad and 13.5 mg of milbemycin oxime, and 1620 mg of spinosad and 27 mg of milbemycin oxime.

## Stability and Storage

Store in blister packs and at room temperature.

## Small Animal Dosage

### Dogs

- 30 mg/kg (13.5 mg/lb) PO administered once per month.

### Cats

- 50–100 mg/kg PO once per month. (The approved dosage in some countries for cats is 50 mg/kg once per month.)

## Large Animal Dosage

- No dose has been reported for large animals.

## Regulatory Information

Withdrawal times are not established for animals that produce food. For extralabel use withdrawal interval estimates, contact FARAD at www.FARAD.org.

# Spironolactone
speer-one-oh-lak′tone

**Trade and other names:** Aldactone and Prilactone (Europe)

**Functional classification:** Diuretic

## Pharmacology and Mechanism of Action

Spironolactone is considered a potassium-sparing diuretic, but it also acts as an aldosterone antagonist. The action of spironolactone is to interfere with sodium reabsorption in distal renal tubules by competitively inhibiting the action of aldosterone. Aldosterone mediates retention of water and sodium. Spironolactone binds directly to the aldosterone receptor, but at usual doses, it does not block the action of other steroid receptors. It is more properly referred to as an *aldosterone antagonist* rather than a diuretic because it does not produce a significant diuretic action. Because aldosterone may have direct effects on remodeling of cardiac muscle cells and vascular endothelium, spironolactone may act by blunting aldosterone-induced myocardial remodeling and myocardial fibrosis. There are minor antiandrogenic effects produced; therefore, a related drug, eplerenone (Inspra), has been used in people because it produces fewer antiandrogenic effects compared with aldosterone. But the endocrine effects and antiandrogenic effects are not as much of a problem in dogs compared with people, and spironolactone is still the preferred agent in this class.

*Pharmacokinetics:* In dogs, the oral absorption is 50% but is increased to 80%–90% when administered with food. At the currently recommended dose in dogs (2 mg/kg), it produces approximately 88% inhibition of aldosterone.

## Indications and Clinical Uses

Spironolactone is used for treating high blood pressure and congestion caused by heart failure. It is approved in Europe (Prilactone) for dogs to be used with standard therapy for the treatment of congestive heart failure (CHF) caused by valvular disease. (Other treatments can include pimobendan, digoxin, angiotensin-converting enzyme [ACE] inhibitors, and furosemide.) Spironolactone is not recommended for routine use to delay the onset of heart failure in patients with valvular disease (stage B2). Spironolactone may also be used with angiotensin-converting enzyme (ACE) inhibitors to achieve a synergistic effect for treatment of heart failure in animals. The addition of spironolactone to traditional cardiac therapy can reduce the risk of cardiac morbidity and mortality in dogs with valvular disease. The proposed benefit of spironolactone treatment is via aldosterone antagonism and can be used to inhibit the renin–angiotensin–aldosterone system (RAAS) activation that occurs from diuretic administration (e.g., furosemide) or with some diseases that produce congestion. Despite treatment with ACE inhibitors, some animals may still exhibit aldosterone synthesis, which has been known as *aldosterone breakthrough*. Spironolactone may be effective to decrease the effects caused by aldosterone breakthrough.

Spironolactone has also been used for managing hepatic cirrhosis because it inhibits ascites formation caused by excess aldosterone. It has not been beneficial for treatment in cats with hypertrophic cardiomyopathy (see also Adverse Reactions and Side Effects for more information on cats).

### Precautionary Information

#### Adverse Reactions and Side Effects

Spironolactone can produce hyperkalemia in some patients. Facial dermatitis has been reported from administration of spironolactone to cats, which may limit its clinical use in these animals. The mechanism of these reactions is not known. High doses and long-term use may produce some steroid-like side effects, but this has not been a significant clinical problem in dogs. However, in people, these endocrine effects have been associated with antiandrogenic effects such as gynecomastia, hirsutism, and impotence. The only antiandrogenic effects reported from its use in animals is prostatic atrophy, which has been observed in some male dogs.

#### Contraindications and Precautions

Do not use in patients that are dehydrated. Nonsteroidal anti-inflammatory drugs (NSAIDs) may interfere with action. Avoid concurrent use of supplements that are high in potassium. Do not administer to patients with gastric ulcers or who may be prone to GI disease such as gastritis or diarrhea.

#### Drug Interactions

Spironolactone is often used together with ACE inhibitors, such as enalapril. It acts synergistically with ACE inhibitors and does not ordinarily produce adverse changes in potassium concentrations. However, in some animals, the dual treatment with spironolactone and an ACE inhibitor may increase the risk of kidney injury and may increase the risk of hyperkalemia. Therefore, some monitoring is advised to avoid this problem. Use cautiously with other drugs that can increase potassium concentrations such as trimethoprim and NSAIDs. Other cardiac treatments have been safely administered with spironolactone such as pimobendan, digoxin, and furosemide.

## Instructions for Use

Spironolactone usually is administered with other drugs (e.g., ACE inhibitors, inotropic agents, vasodilators) for treating CHF.

## Patient Monitoring and Laboratory Tests

Monitor serum potassium concentration when administering with an ACE inhibitor (e.g., enalapril maleate). Administration of spironolactone may cause a slightly false-positive result for digoxin assay.

## Formulations

- Spironolactone is available in 25-, 50-, and 100-mg tablets. Tablets can be split easily. In Europe, there is an approved formulation for animals. In the United States, the human generic formulation is used.
- Oral suspension: 5 mg/mL.

## Stability and Storage

Store in a tightly sealed container, protected from light, and at room temperature. Spironolactone is insoluble in water, but it is slightly more soluble in ethanol. It has been mixed with syrups for an oral suspension (after first mixing with ethanol) and found to be stable for 90–160 days.

## Small Animal Dosage

### Dogs

- 2–4 mg/kg/day (or 1–2 mg/kg q12h) PO. In dogs, start with 2 mg/kg/day and increase gradually, not to exceed 4 mg/kg/day. In Europe, the approved dosage for dogs is 2 mg/kg/day.

### Cats

- Use in cats is controversial because it may produce dermatitis and because the efficacy is questionable. However, dosages in the range of 2–4 mg/kg/day (or 1–2 mg/kg q12h) PO have been administered for some conditions.

## Large Animal Dosage

- No dose has been reported for large animals.

## Regulatory Information

Withdrawal times are not established for animals that produce food. For extralabel use withdrawal interval estimates, contact FARAD at www.FARAD.org. RCI Classification: 4

S

# Stanozolol
stan-oh'zoe-lole

**Trade and other names:** Winstrol-V

**Functional classification:** Hormone, anabolic agent

## Pharmacology and Mechanism of Action

Stanozolol is an anabolic steroid. Stanozolol is a derivative of testosterone. These anabolic agents are designed to maximize anabolic effects while minimizing androgenic action. Other anabolic agents include boldenone, nandrolone, oxymetholone, and methyltestosterone.

## Indications and Clinical Uses

Anabolic agents, such as stanozolol, have been used for reversing catabolic conditions, increasing weight gain, increasing muscling in animals, and stimulating erythropoiesis. It has been used in horses during training. Stanozolol has been used in animals with chronic kidney disease, and there is some evidence of an improvement in the nitrogen balance in dogs with renal disease treated with stanozolol. Use in cats is associated with toxicity.

## Precautionary Information

### Adverse Reactions and Side Effects

Adverse effects from these agents are attributed to the pharmacologic action of androgens on various body systems. Increased masculine effects are common. Increased incidence of some tumors has been reported in people. Some 17-alpha–methylated oral anabolic steroids (oxymetholone, stanozolol, and oxandrolone) are associated with hepatic toxicity. Stanozolol administration in cats with kidney disease has been shown to consistently produce increased hepatic enzymes and hepatic toxicosis.

### Contraindications and Precautions

Do not administer to cats with kidney disease. Use cautiously in dogs that have other pre-existing disease such as liver failure. Do not administer to pregnant animals. Stanozolol, like other anabolic steroids, has a high potential for abuse in humans. This drug is abused by humans to enhance athletic performance and increase muscle development.

### Drug Interactions

No drug interactions have been reported in animals.

## Instructions for Use

For many indications, use in animals (and doses) is based on experience in people or anecdotal experience in animals. There is an approved formulation, but the indication is limited to treating debilitated animals when weight gain and appetite stimulation is needed. Other uses are considered extralabel.

## Patient Monitoring and Laboratory Tests

Monitor liver enzymes for signs of hepatic injury (cholestatic) during treatment.

## Formulations

- Oral: 2-mg tablets, regular and chewable for dogs.
- Stanozolol is available in a 50-mg/mL injection as a sterile suspension. However, there has been limited availability of veterinary injectable formulations. Commercial forms have been withdrawn from the market, but some compounding sources still persist.

## Stability and Storage

Store in a tightly sealed container, protected from light, and at room temperature. Stability of compounded formulations has not been evaluated.

## Small Animal Dosage

### Dogs

- 2 mg/dog (or range of 1–4 mg/dog) q12h PO. The FDA-approved dosages are 1–2 mg per dog (small breeds) q12h and 2–4 mg per dog q12h for large breeds. The tablets may be crushed and administered in food.
- 25 (small breeds) to 50 mg/dog (large breeds) per week IM.

### Cats

- Oral: 1–2 mg/cat q12h PO. The tablets may be crushed and administered in food.
- Injection: 25 mg/cat/wk IM (use cautiously in cats).

## Large Animal Dosage

### Horses

- 0.55 mg/kg (5 mL per 1000 lb) or 25 mg per 100 lb IM once a week for up to 4 weeks.

## Regulatory Information

Stanozolol is a Schedule III controlled drug and should not be administered to animals that produce food.

RCI Classification: 4

# Streptozocin
strep-toe-zoe′sin

**Trade and other names:** Streptozotocin and Zanosar

**Functional classification:** Antihyperglycemic agent

## Pharmacology and Mechanism of Action

Streptozocin (also known as streptozotocin) is an agent with specific effects on pancreatic beta cells. Because pancreatic beta cells have high concentrations of glucose transporter 2 (GLUT2), streptozocin is selectively toxic to these cells. It is a nitrosourea alkylating agent with selective uptake into pancreatic beta cells because of similarity to glucose in structure. It can produce diabetes mellitus in normal animals, but it is used primarily for treating insulinoma tumors in animals. Occasionally, it has been used as a cytotoxic agent for treating other tumors in humans (e.g., lymphoma, sarcomas), but these uses are not reported for animals. Streptozocin has a rapid half-life in animals, but metabolites may be active.

## Indications and Clinical Uses

In animals, streptozocin is used primarily for treating insulin-secreting tumors (insulinoma). It has been used in experimental animals to create models of diabetes mellitus.

## Precautionary Information

### Adverse Reactions and Side Effects

Diabetes mellitus is anticipated in treated animals. In humans, the major adverse effect is kidney injury caused by tubular necrosis. Kidney injury has been reported in dogs at doses greater than 700 mg/m$^2$. Other adverse effects include vomiting, nausea, and diarrhea. The GI toxicity occurs immediately or within 4 hours of administration but usually resolves within 24 hours. Increases in hepatic enzymes and hepatic injury have been reported in dogs; however, hepatotoxicity appears to be reversible. Bone marrow suppression is rare in animals. Local phlebitis may occur from IV administration.

### Contraindications and Precautions

Streptozocin may produce diabetes mellitus in treated animals. In addition, there may be a sudden release of insulin after IV administration, and IV dextrose should be available to treat acute hypoglycemia. Monitor animals for evidence of renal and hepatic injury. Do not administer to pregnant animals.

### Drug Interactions

No specific drug interactions are reported for animals; however, use with any other nephrotoxic, hepatotoxic, or myelotoxic drug exacerbates toxicity.

S

## Instructions for Use

Risk of renal toxicosis caused by streptozocin may be decreased with administration of fluid diuresis. The diuresis should consist of administration of fluids (e.g., 0.9% saline) intravenously prior to drug administration. Antiemetics should be administered with each infusion because vomiting is common. Treatment with streptozocin is continued every 3 weeks until signs of tumor recurrence occur or until toxicosis limits the continuation of treatments.

Reconstitute the injection vial prior to use by adding 9.5 mL of 5% dextrose or 0.9% saline to vial. Resulting solution is 100 mg/mL. Further dilute this vial with 5% dextrose or 0.9% saline for IV infusion.

## Patient Monitoring and Laboratory Tests

Monitor serum glucose in treated animals. Monitor serum creatinine, urea nitrogen, and hepatic enzymes for evidence of hepatotoxicity and renal injury. Although myelotoxicity is unusual, monitor complete blood count before each treatment.

## Formulations

- Streptozocin is available in 1-g vials for injection.

## Stability and Storage

Store vial between 2°C and 8°C. After preparation, use the vial within 12 hours after reconstitution at room temperature. The approved formulation also contains citric acid. Do not use if color changes from pale yellow to a darker brown because this indicates degradation.

## Small Animal Dosage

### Dogs

- 500 mg/m$^2$ IV infused over 2 hours every 3 weeks (use with a saline diuresis).

### Cats

- A safe dose has not been reported for cats.

## Large Animal Dosage

- No dose has been reported for large animals.

## Regulatory Information

Do not administer to animals that produce food.

---

# Succimer
suks′ih-mer

**Trade and other names:** Chemet

**Functional classification:** Antidote

---

## Pharmacology and Mechanism of Action

Succimer is a chelating agent used to treat toxic exposure to heavy metals in animals. Succimer chelates lead and other heavy metals such as mercury and arsenic and increases their elimination from the body. Succimer is an analogue to British anti-Lewisite (BAL).

## Indications and Clinical Uses

Succimer is used for treatment of heavy metal toxicosis, primarily toxicosis caused by lead. Other chelators that have been used for lead toxicity include calcium-EDTA (ethylenediaminetetraacetic acid), BAL, and penicillamine. Calcium-EDTA is often the preferred drug for initial treatment. The advantages of succimer over other chelators are that it is better tolerated with fewer GI adverse effects, and it is not associated with nephrotoxicosis. It also does not bind other minerals such as copper, zinc, calcium, and iron.

## Precautionary Information

### Adverse Reactions and Side Effects

No adverse effects have been reported in dogs. However, kidney injury has been associated with succimer treatment in cats. Succimer should not be used as a phosphate binder in cats. When administered to cats, it did not decrease phosphorous, and caused vomiting and clinical decompensation.

### Contraindications and Precautions

Do not use in cats with kidney disease. (See Adverse Effects and Side Effects.)

### Drug Interactions

No drug interactions have been reported in animals.

## Instructions for Use

Doses cited are based on studies in dogs. In cats, succimer has been used at 10 mg/kg q8h PO for 2 weeks. Treatment response and duration of treatment is monitored by measuring the blood levels of the toxin (e.g., lead). A poison control center may be contacted for specific protocols to treat toxicity in animals.

## Patient Monitoring and Laboratory Tests

Monitor the patient's blood lead levels during treatment. Monitor renal function during treatment because renal failure has been associated with succimer administration in cats.

## Formulations

• Succimer is available in 100-mg capsules.

## Stability and Storage

Store in a tightly sealed container, protected from light, and at room temperature. Stability of compounded formulations has not been evaluated.

## Small Animal Dosage

### Dogs

• 10 mg/kg q8h PO for 5 days; then 10 mg/kg q12h PO for 2 more weeks. It has also been administered rectally in vomiting dogs.

### Cats

• 10 mg/kg q8h PO for 2 weeks.

## Large Animal Dosage

• No dose has been reported for large animals.

## Regulatory Information

Withdrawal times are not established for animals that produce food. For extralabel use withdrawal interval estimates, contact FARAD at www.FARAD.org.

# Sucralfate

soo-krahl'fate

**Trade and other names:** Carafate and Sulcrate (in Canada)

**Functional classification:** Antiulcer agent

## Pharmacology and Mechanism of Action

Sucralfate is a gastric mucosa protectant that has both antiulcer effects and some esophageal protectant effects. Sucralfate dissociates in the stomach to form sucrose octasulfate and aluminum hydroxide. Sucrose octasulfate polymerizes to a viscous, sticky substance that creates a protective effect by binding to ulcerated mucosa in the upper GI tract. It has an affinity for negatively charged injured tissue. It protects the stomach mucosa by preventing back-diffusion of hydrogen ions and inactivates pepsin and adsorbs bile acid. The aluminum hydroxide released from sucralfate acts as a buffering agent to reduce injury to the stomach and esophagus from stomach acid. There is some evidence that sucralfate may act as a cytoprotectant by increasing prostaglandin synthesis in the gastric epithelium. This property may enhance the protective effect of prostaglandins in the mucosa and prevent stomach and esophageal injury.

## Indications and Clinical Uses

Sucralfate is used to prevent and treat gastric ulcers and prevent injury from gastroesophageal reflux. Sucralfate is administered orally and may protect ulcerated tissue and promote healing. There is little evidence that it prevents ulcers from NSAIDs in small animals, but experimental evidence demonstrates protective effects in horses. Prevention of esophageal injury from acid reflux is based on studies in people and laboratory animals. Dosage regimens for sucralfate have been extrapolated from human dosages but have been examined in observational studies in small animals and horses.

### Precautionary Information

#### Adverse Reactions and Side Effects

Because sucralfate is not absorbed, it is virtually free of systemic adverse effects. The most common side effect associated with its use in people has been constipation.

#### Contraindications and Precautions

No contraindications have been listed for animals. Administration of intact tablets may not be effective (see Instructions for Use).

#### Drug Interactions

Sucralfate may decrease absorption of other drugs administered orally via chelation with aluminum (e.g., fluoroquinolones, digoxin, theophylline, and tetracyclines). Administer these other drugs at least 30 minutes to 2 hours before sucralfate.

## Instructions for Use

Dosing recommendations are based largely on empiricism and extrapolation from the human dose. There are no studies to demonstrate clinical efficacy of sucralfate in animals, but some evidence is available from studies in research animals. Sucralfate may be administered concurrently with histamine type 2 inhibitors ($H_2$ blockers) without causing an interaction, but this combination is rarely necessary. There is evidence that when intact sucralfate tablets are administered to animals, they may not undergo dissolution in the stomach and pass through the intestine intact. Therefore it is recommended to crush up tablets and prepare a liquid suspension prior to administration to small animals.

## Patient Monitoring and Laboratory Tests

No specific monitoring is necessary.

## Formulations

- Sucralfate is available in 1-g tablets and a 200-mg/mL oral suspension.

## Stability and Storage

Store in a tightly sealed container, protected from light, and at room temperature. Sucralfate is insoluble in water unless it is exposed to strong acid or alkaline conditions.

The tablets may be crushed and suspended in water to a concentration of 200 mg/mL and stored in the refrigerator for 14 days. Shake this suspension before using.

## Small Animal Dosage

### Dogs

- 0.5–1 g q8–12h PO.
- If tablets are used in dogs, it is advised to crush up tablets to form a liquid suspension prior to administration.

### Cats

- 0.25 g (one-fourth tablet) q8–12h PO.

## Large Animal Dosage

### Foals

- 1 g q8h PO.

## Regulatory Information

Because of a low risk of harmful residues in animals intended for food, no withdrawal time is suggested.

# Sufentanil Citrate

soo-fen′tah-nil sih′trate

**Trade and other names:** Sufenta

**Functional classification:** Analgesic, opioid

## Pharmacology and Mechanism of Action

Sufentanil is a synthetic opioid agonist related to fentanyl. The action of fentanyl derivatives is via mu-opiate receptor. Sufentanil is 5–7 times more potent than fentanyl, and in some studies, it is as much as 10 times more potent than fentanyl. Doses of 13–20 mcg of sufentanil produce analgesia equal to 10 mg of morphine.

## Indications and Clinical Uses

Sufentanil, like other opiate derivatives, is used for sedation, general anesthesia, and analgesia. It can be used as part of a regimen for balanced general anesthesia. It can be used with other agents or as a primary agent in patients intubated and delivered oxygen. Sufentanil has a rapid onset of effect and rapid recovery. It does not accumulate in tissues; therefore recovery is rapid after an anesthetic procedure. It can also be administered by the epidural route. Compared with other opioids, such as fentanyl, the use of sufentanil has been uncommon in animals. The use is derived from limited clinical observations and extrapolation of the uses from human medicine.

## Precautionary Information

### Adverse Reactions and Side Effects

Adverse effects are similar to those of morphine. Like all opiates, side effects are predictable and unavoidable. Side effects include sedation, constipation, and bradycardia. Respiratory depression occurs with high doses.

### Contraindications and Precautions

Use cautiously in animals with respiratory disease. Because of its high potency compared with morphine and other opiates, calculate dose carefully.

### Drug Interactions

Like other opiates, sufentanil may potentiate other sedatives and anesthetics.

## Instructions for Use
When used for anesthesia, animals are often premedicated with acepromazine or a benzodiazepine.

## Patient Monitoring and Laboratory Tests
Monitor the patient's heart rate and respiration. Although bradycardia rarely needs to be treated when it is caused by an opioid, atropine can be administered if necessary. If serious respiratory depression occurs, the opioid can be reversed with naloxone.

## Formulations
- Sufentanil is available in a 50-mcg/mL injection in ampules of 1, 2, and 5 mL.

## Stability and Storage
Store in a tightly sealed container, protected from light, and at room temperature. Stability of compounded formulations has not been evaluated. Sufentanil is a Schedule II drug and should be stored in a locked compartment.

## Small Animal Dosage
### Dogs and Cats
- 2 mcg/kg IV (0.002 mg/kg) up to a maximum dose of 5 mcg/kg (0.005 mg/kg).

## Large Animal Dosage
- No doses have been reported for large animals.

## Regulatory Information
Schedule II controlled drug.
Avoid use in animals intended for food. Withdrawal times are not established. However, for extralabel use withdrawal interval estimates, contact FARAD at www.FARAD.org.
RCI Classification: 1

# Sulfachlorpyridazine
sul-fah-klor-peer-id'ah-zeen

**Trade and other names:** Vetisulid. (Name previously used was Sulphachlorpyridazine.)
**Functional classification:** Antibacterial

## Pharmacology and Mechanism of Action
Sulfachlorpyridazine is a sulfonamide antibacterial agent. Sulfonamides compete with para-aminobenzoic acid (PABA) for an enzyme that synthesizes dihydrofolic acid in bacteria. It is synergistic with trimethoprim. Like other sulfonamides, it has a broad spectrum of activity, including gram-positive bacteria, gram-negative bacteria, and some protozoa. However, when used alone, resistance is common.

## Indications and Clinical Uses
Sulfachlorpyridazine is used as a broad-spectrum antimicrobial to treat or prevent infections caused by susceptible organisms. Infections treated may include pneumonia, intestinal infections (especially coccidia), soft tissue infections, and urinary tract infections (UTIs). However, resistance is common. The use of sulfachlorpyridazine has not been reported for small animals. It is used primarily for pigs and cattle and not used as frequently as other agents for these infections.

## Precautionary Information

### Adverse Reactions and Side Effects

Adverse effects associated with sulfonamides (primarily in dogs) include allergic reactions, type II and III hypersensitivity, hepatotoxicity, hypothyroidism (with prolonged therapy), keratoconjunctivitis sicca (KCS), and skin reactions.

### Contraindications and Precautions

Do not administer in animals with sensitivity to sulfonamides.

### Drug Interactions

Several interactions have been reported for sulfonamide administration in small animals. (See Sulfonamide.) However, these interactions have not been relevant for its use in cattle and pigs.

## Instructions for Use

The most common use of sulfachlorpyridazine is for treatment of enteritis in pigs and calves. Indications and dosages are based on the approved labeling.

## Patient Monitoring and Laboratory Tests

Sulfonamides are known to decrease thyroxine ($T_4$) concentrations in dogs after 6 weeks of treatment. Susceptibility testing: CLSI breakpoint for susceptible organisms is ≤256 mcg/mL, but according to CLSI, susceptibility tests for sulfonamides should only be used to interpret urinary bacteria isolates. The susceptibility test results should not be applied to testing of bovine or swine pathogens.

## Formulations

- Sulfachlorpyridazine is available in a 2-g bolus and a 200-mg/mL injection.

## Stability and Storage

Store in a tightly sealed container, protected from light, and at room temperature. Stability of compounded formulations has not been evaluated.

## Small Animal Dosage

- No doses reported for dogs and cats.

## Large Animal Dosage

### Cattle

- 33–50 mg/kg q12h PO or IV.

### Pigs

- 22–39 mg/kg q12h PO or 44–77 mg/kg/day PO in the drinking water.

## Regulatory Information

Extralabel use of sulfonamides is prohibited from use in lactating dairy cattle older than 20 months of age.
Cattle withdrawal time for meat: 7 days.
Pig withdrawal time for meat: 4 days.

# Sulfadiazine

sul-fa-dye′a-zeen

**Trade and other names:** Generic brands and combined with trimethoprim as Tribrissen and Equisul-SDT

**Functional classification:** Antibacterial

## Pharmacology and Mechanism of Action

Sulfadiazine is a common sulfonamide antibacterial, usually administered in combination with trimethoprim. Sulfonamides compete with PABA for an enzyme that synthesizes dihydrofolic acid in bacteria. It is synergistic with trimethoprim, which is usually administered in combination. Like other sulfonamides, it has a broad spectrum of activity, including gram-positive bacteria, gram-negative bacteria, and some protozoa. However, when used alone, resistance is common.

*Pharmacokinetics:* Sulfadiazine has been studied in horses more than other animals. After a dosage of 25 mg/kg PO to horses, the half-life is 8.5 hours (average from all studies), with a volume of distribution of 1.3 L/kg and a peak concentration of 18 mcg/mL. Oral absorption is 64%. Protein binding has ranged from 20%–63%, depending on the study. In dogs, there is less information. After a dose of 25 mg/kg, the average half-life is approximately 10 hours with an average plasma concentration of 50 mcg/mL. Concentrations were high in the urine (above the minimum inhibitory concentration of susceptible bacteria) for 24 hours. In pigs, the half-life has ranged from 4–11 hours, depending on the study. In calves and cattle, the half-life is considerably shorter than other animals, ranging from 3–6 hours, depending on the study.

## Indications and Clinical Uses

Sulfadiazine is used alone occasionally; however, efficacy is not established for many infections. Most often, it is used with trimethoprim to treat a variety of infections, including UTIs and skin infections. (See Trimethoprim–Sulfonamides for a more complete description.)

## Precautionary Information

### Adverse Reactions and Side Effects

Adverse effects associated with sulfonamides include allergic reactions, type II and III hypersensitivity, arthropathy, anemia, thrombocytopenia, hepatopathy, hypothyroidism (with prolonged therapy), KCS, and skin reactions. Dogs may be more sensitive to sulfonamides than other animals because dogs lack the ability to acetylate sulfonamides to metabolites. Other more toxic metabolites may persist.

### Contraindications and Precautions

Do not administer to animals with sensitivity to sulfonamides. Doberman pinschers may be more sensitive than other canine breeds to reactions from sulfonamides. Use cautiously in this breed.

### Drug Interactions

Sulfonamides may interact with other drugs, including warfarin, methenamine, dapsone, and etodolac. They may potentiate adverse effects caused by methotrexate and pyrimethamine. Sulfonamides increases the metabolism of cyclosporine, resulting in decreased plasma concentrations. Methenamine is metabolized to formaldehyde that may form a complex and precipitate with sulfonamides. Sulfonamides administered to horses that are receiving detomidine may develop cardiac arrhythmias. This precaution for horses is only listed for IV forms of trimethoprim–sulfonamides.

## Instructions for Use

Usually, sulfonamides are combined with trimethoprim or ormetoprim in a 5:1 ratio, and sulfonamides are rarely used alone in small animals and horses. There is no clinical evidence that one sulfonamide is more or less toxic or efficacious than another sulfonamide.

## Patient Monitoring and Laboratory Tests

Sulfonamides are known to decrease $T_4$ concentrations in dogs after 6 weeks of treatment. Susceptibility testing: CLSI breakpoint for susceptible organisms is ≤256 mcg/mL, but according to CLSI, susceptibility tests for sulfonamides should only be used to interpret urinary bacteria isolates.

## Formulations

- Sulfadiazine is available in 500-mg tablets. See Trimethoprim–Sulfadiazine for information on those formulations.

## Stability and Storage

Store in a tightly sealed container, protected from light, and at room temperature. Stability of compounded formulations has not been evaluated.

## Small Animal Dosage

### Dogs and Cats

- 100 mg/kg IV PO (loading dose) followed by 50 mg/kg q12h IV or PO. In the combination with trimethoprim, it is administered at a dose of 25 mg/kg (see Trimethoprim for more information).

## Large Animal Dosage

- For horses, see dosing for trimethoprim combinations. In the combination, it is administered at a dose of 25 mg/kg.

## Regulatory Information

Extralabel use of sulfonamides is prohibited from use in lactating dairy cattle older than 20 months of age. No withdrawal times are established. However, for extralabel use withdrawal interval estimates, contact FARAD at www.FARAD.org.

# Sulfadimethoxine
sul-fah-dye-meth-oks′een

**Trade and other names:** Albon, Bactrovet, and generic brands
**Functional classification:** Antibacterial

S

## Pharmacology and Mechanism of Action

Sulfadimethoxine is a sulfonamide antibacterial. Sulfonamides compete with PABA for an enzyme that synthesizes dihydrofolic acid in bacteria. It is synergistic with ormetoprim and used in combination in formulations for small animals. Like other sulfonamides, it has a broad spectrum of activity, including gram-positive bacteria, gram-negative bacteria, and some protozoa. However, when used alone, resistance is common.

## Indications and Clinical Uses

Sulfadimethoxine is used as a broad-spectrum antimicrobial to treat or prevent infections caused by susceptible organisms, usually in livestock. Infections treated may include pneumonia, intestinal infections (especially coccidia), soft tissue infections, and UTIs. It is also approved for treatment of calf diphtheria and foot rot associated with *Fusobacterium necrophorum* susceptible to sulfadimethoxine. However, resistance is common unless combined with ormetoprim (see Primor).

## Precautionary Information
### Adverse Reactions and Side Effects
Adverse effects associated with sulfonamides include allergic reactions, type II and III hypersensitivity, arthropathy, anemia, thrombocytopenia, hepatopathy, hypothyroidism (with prolonged therapy), KCS, and skin reactions. Dogs may be more sensitive to sulfonamides than other animals because dogs lack the ability to acetylate sulfonamides to metabolites. Other more toxic metabolites may persist.

### Contraindications and Precautions
Do not administer in animals with sensitivity to sulfonamides. Doberman pinschers may be more sensitive than other canine breeds to reactions from sulfonamides. Use cautiously in this breed.

### Drug Interactions
Sulfonamides may interact with other drugs, including warfarin, methenamine, dapsone, and etodolac. They may potentiate adverse effects caused by methotrexate and pyrimethamine. Sulfonamides increase the metabolism of cyclosporine, resulting in decreased plasma concentrations. Methenamine is metabolized to formaldehyde, which may form a complex and precipitate with sulfonamides. When sulfonamides are administered to horses that are receiving detomidine, these horses may develop cardiac arrhythmias. This precaution is only listed for IV forms of trimethoprim–sulfonamides.

## Instructions for Use
Usually, sulfonamides such as sulfadimethoxine are rarely used alone in small animals and horses. There is no clinical evidence that one sulfonamide is more or less toxic or efficacious than another sulfonamide. Sulfadimethoxine has been combined with ormetoprim in Primor.

## Patient Monitoring and Laboratory Tests
Sulfonamides are known to decrease $T_4$ concentrations in dogs after 6 weeks of treatment. Susceptibility testing: CLSI breakpoint for susceptible organisms is ≤256 mcg/mL, but according to CLSI, susceptibility tests for sulfonamides should only be used to interpret urinary bacteria isolates.

## Formulations
• Sulfadimethoxine is available in 125-, 250-, and 500-mg tablets; 400-mg/mL injection; and 50-mg/mL suspension.

## Stability and Storage
Store in a tightly sealed container, protected from light, and at room temperature. Stability of compounded formulations has not been evaluated.

## Small Animal Dosage
### Dogs and Cats
• 55 mg/kg PO (loading dose) followed by 27.5 mg/kg q12h PO. (For doses of combination with ormetoprim, see Primor.)

## Large Animal Dosage
### Cattle
• Treatment of pneumonia and other infections: 55 mg/kg as the initial dose followed by 27 mg/kg q24h PO for 5 days.
• Sustained-release bolus (Albon-SR): 137.5 mg/kg PO as a single dose.

## Regulatory Information

Cattle withdrawal time for meat: 7 days.
Cattle withdrawal time for milk: 60 hours.
Withdrawal time for sustained-released bolus: 21 days.
Extralabel use of sulfonamides is prohibited from use in lactating dairy cattle older than 20 months of age. Currently, sulfadimethoxine is the only sulfonamide with approved indications in dairy cattle.

# Sulfamethazine
sul-fah-meth′ah-zeen

**Trade and other names:** Sulmet and generic brands

**Functional classification:** Antibacterial

## Pharmacology and Mechanism of Action

Sulfamethazine is a sulfonamide antibacterial. Sulfonamides compete with PABA for an enzyme that synthesizes dihydrofolic acid in bacteria. Like other sulfonamides, it has a broad spectrum of activity, including gram-positive bacteria, gram-negative bacteria, and some protozoa. However, when used alone, resistance is common.

*Pharmacokinetics:* There have been several pharmacokinetic studies, mostly in food animals and horses. In cattle, the half-life is approximately 3.5–6.5 hours, depending on the study. In pigs, it is longer at 10–16 hours. In horses, the half-life has varied, depending on the study, between 6 and 14 hours.

## Indications and Clinical Uses

Sulfamethazine is used as a broad-spectrum antimicrobial to treat or prevent infections caused by susceptible organisms. Infections treated may include pneumonia, intestinal infections (especially coccidia caused by *Eimeria bovis* and *Eimeria zuernii*), soft tissue infections, calf diptheria, foot rot, and UTIs. However, resistance is common, and this agent should not be considered a first-line agent for these infections.

### Precautionary Information

**Adverse Reactions and Side Effects**

Adverse effects associated with sulfonamides include allergic reactions, type II and III hypersensitivity, arthropathy, anemia, thrombocytopenia, hepatopathy, hypothyroidism (with prolonged therapy), KCS, and skin reactions. Dogs may be more sensitive to sulfonamides than other animals because dogs lack the ability to acetylate sulfonamides to metabolites. Other more toxic metabolites may persist.

**Contraindications and Precautions**

Do not administer in animals with sensitivity to sulfonamides. Doberman pinschers may be more sensitive than other canine breeds to reactions from sulfonamides. Use cautiously in this breed.

**Drug Interactions**

Sulfonamides may interact with other drugs, including warfarin, methenamine, dapsone, and etodolac. They may potentiate adverse effects caused by methotrexate and pyrimethamine. Sulfonamides increase metabolism of cyclosporine, resulting in decreased plasma concentrations. Methenamine is metabolized to formaldehyde, which may form a complex and precipitate with sulfonamides. Sulfonamides administered to horses that are receiving detomidine may develop cardiac arrhythmias. This precaution is only listed for IV forms of trimethoprim–sulfonamides.

S

## Instructions for Use

Usually sulfonamides are combined with trimethoprim or ormetoprim in a 5:1 ratio. Sulfonamides such as sulfamethazine are not as effective as other agents that are used to treat infections in livestock. There is no clinical evidence that one sulfonamide is more or less toxic or efficacious than another sulfonamide.

## Patient Monitoring and Laboratory Tests

Sulfonamides are known to decrease $T_4$ concentrations in dogs after 6 weeks of treatment. Susceptibility testing: CLSI breakpoint for sensitive organisms is ≤256 mcg/mL, but according to CLSI, susceptibility tests for sulfonamides should only be used to interpret urinary bacteria isolates.

## Formulations
• Sulfamethazine is available in a 30-g bolus.
• Injectable solution: 250 mg/mL.

## Stability and Storage

Store in a tightly sealed container, protected from light, and at room temperature. Stability of compounded formulations has not been evaluated.

## Small Animal Dosage
### Dogs and Cats
• 100 mg/kg PO (loading dose) followed by 50 mg/kg q12h PO. *(The use is rare in small animals.)*

## Large Animal Dosage
### Cattle
• Treatment of pneumonia and other infections: 220 mg/kg as the initial dose followed by 110 mg/kg q24h IV.
• Use of soluble powder as a drench or in drinking water: 237 mg/kg as the initial dose followed by 119 mg/kg q24h PO.
• Sustained-release bolus: 350–400 mg/kg PO as a single dose.
• Calves: 180 mg/kg, PO per day.

### Pigs
• Use of soluble powder as a drench or in drinking water: 237 mg/kg as the initial dose followed by 119 mg/kg q24h PO.

### Horses
• 222 mg/kg PO per day, on day 1, and 111 mg/kg PO per day thereafter.

## Regulatory Information

Extralabel use of sulfonamides is prohibited from use in lactating dairy cattle older than 20 months of age.
Cattle withdrawal time for meat: 10 or 11 days.
Cattle withdrawal time for meat (soluble powder): 10 days.
Pig withdrawal time for meat (soluble powder): 15 days.
Cattle withdrawal time for meat (sustained-release bolus): 8–18 days, depending on the product.

# Sulfamethoxazole
sul-fah-meth-oks'ah-zole

**Trade and other names:** Gantanol

**Functional classification:** Antibacterial

**Note:** This drug has been discontinued and is no longer available. Consult earlier editions of this book for information on the pharmacology, mechanism of action, and clinical use.

# Sulfaquinoxaline
sul-fah-kwin-oks′ah-leen

**Trade and other names:** Sulfa-Nox

**Functional classification:** Antibacterial

## Pharmacology and Mechanism of Action

Sulfaquinoxaline is a sulfonamide antibacterial. Sulfonamides compete with PABA for an enzyme that synthesizes dihydrofolic acid in bacteria. It is also effective against protozoa, and the most common use is for treatment of intestinal disease caused by coccidia. Like other sulfonamides, it has a broad spectrum of activity, including gram-positive bacteria, gram-negative bacteria, and some protozoa. However, when used alone, resistance is common.

## Indications and Clinical Uses

Sulfaquinoxaline is used as a broad-spectrum antimicrobial to treat or prevent infections caused by susceptible organisms. This agent is used primarily in food animals but is not used frequently because of availability of other more effective antimicrobial agents. The approved indication for cattle is coccidiosis caused by *Eimeria bovis* or *E. zurnii*. Treatment of other infections may include pneumonia, intestinal infections, soft tissue infections, and UTIs. However, resistance is common.

## Precautionary Information

### Adverse Reactions and Side Effects

Adverse effects associated with sulfonamides include allergic reactions, type II and III hypersensitivity, arthropathy, anemia, thrombocytopenia, hepatopathy, hypothyroidism (with prolonged therapy), KCS, and skin reactions. Dogs may be more sensitive to sulfonamides than other animals because dogs lack the ability to acetylate sulfonamides to metabolites. Other more toxic metabolites may persist.

### Contraindications and Precautions

Do not administer in animals with sensitivity to sulfonamides. Avoid contact with skin or mucous membranes when mixing in water.

### Drug Interactions

Sulfonamides may interact with other drugs, including warfarin, methenamine, dapsone, and etodolac. They may potentiate adverse effects caused by methotrexate and pyrimethamine. Sulfonamides increase the metabolism of cyclosporine, resulting in decreased plasma concentrations. Sulfonamides administered to horses that are receiving detomidine may develop cardiac arrhythmias. This precaution is only listed for IV forms of trimethoprim–sulfonamides.

## Instructions for Use

Mix in the drinking water. Make fresh solutions daily. The most common use of sulfaquinoxaline is for treatment of enteritis caused by coccidia in calves, sheep, and poultry.

## Patient Monitoring and Laboratory Tests

Sulfonamides are known to decrease $T_4$ concentrations in dogs after 6 weeks of treatment. Susceptibility testing: CLSI breakpoint for sensitive organisms is ≤256 mcg/mL, but according to CLSI, susceptibility tests for sulfonamides should only be used to interpret urinary bacteria isolates.

## Formulations

- Sulfaquinoxaline is available in 34.4-, 128.5-, 192-, 200-, 286.2-, and 340-mg/mL solution. Some formulations have been voluntarily withdrawn by the sponsor.

## Stability and Storage

Store in a tightly sealed container, protected from light, and at room temperature. Stability of compounded formulations has not been evaluated.

## Small Animal Dosage

- No doses reported for dogs and cats.

## Large Animal Dosage

**Calves**

- 13.2 mg/kg/day PO (usually administered in the drinking water as a 0.015% solution for 5 days).

## Regulatory Information

Extralabel use of sulfonamides is prohibited from use in lactating dairy cattle older than 20 months of age.
Cattle withdrawal time: 10 days.
Sheep withdrawal time: 10 days.
Poultry withdrawal time: 10 days.
Rabbit withdrawal time: 10 days.

# Sulfasalazine
sul-fah-sal′ah-zeen

**Trade and other names:** Azulfidine and Salazopyrin (in Canada)
**Functional classification:** Antibacterial, antidiarrheal

## Pharmacology and Mechanism of Action

Sulfasalazine is a sulfonamide combined with an anti-inflammatory drug for oral treatment of intestinal diseases. Sulfasalazine has little effect on its own, and salicylic acid (mesalamine) has anti-inflammatory effects. (See Mesalamine for more details on its use.) When administered as the combination of salicylic acid and the sulfonamide sulfapyridine, the salicylic acid is released by colonic bacteria to produce an anti-inflammatory effect in the intestinal epithelium. The anti-inflammatory effect is believed to be through antiprostaglandin action, antileukotriene activity, or both.

## Indications and Clinical Uses

Sulfasalazine is used in small animals for the treatment of idiopathic colitis and other inflammatory intestinal diseases. It is often used for treatment when dietary therapy has been unsuccessful. Although sulfasalazine has been commonly used in small animals, use in animals has been primarily derived from empirical use and opinions from gastroenterologist specialists. There are no well-controlled clinical studies or efficacy trials to document clinical effectiveness. The section on mesalamine has additional information on clinical use.

## Precautionary Information

### Adverse Reactions and Side Effects

Adverse effects are attributed to the sulfonamide component. Adverse effects are associated with sulfonamides and include allergic reactions, type II and III hypersensitivity, hypothyroidism (with prolonged therapy), KCS, and skin reactions. KCS has been reported in dogs that received sulfasalazine for chronic treatment. The amount of salicylate absorbed appears to be small in cats; therefore, adverse effects from salicylate in cats are unlikely.

### Contraindications and Precautions

Do not administer to animals that are sensitive to sulfonamides. Drug interactions are possible but have not been reported in animals, probably because low systemic drug concentrations are achieved. Mesalamine can potentially interfere with thiopurine methyltransferase and therefore increase the risk of toxicity from azathioprine.

### Drug Interactions

Sulfonamides may interact with other drugs, including warfarin, methenamine, dapsone, and etodolac. They may potentiate adverse effects caused by methotrexate and pyrimethamine. Sulfonamides increase metabolism of cyclosporine, resulting in decreased plasma concentrations.

## Instructions for Use

Sulfasalazine is usually used for treatment of idiopathic colitis, often in combination with dietary therapy. For animals sensitive to sulfonamides, consider other forms of mesalamine (see Mesalamine for more details).

## Patient Monitoring and Laboratory Tests

Monitor tear production in dogs that receive chronic therapy.

## Formulations

- Sulfasalazine is available in 500-mg tablets and has been compounded as an oral suspension for smaller animals.

## Stability and Storage

Store in a tightly sealed container, protected from light, and at room temperature. Stability of compounded formulations has not been evaluated.

## Small Animal Dosage

### Dogs

- 10–30 mg/kg q8–12h PO.

### Cats

- 20 mg/kg q12h PO.

## Large Animal Dosage

- No doses have been reported for large animals.

## Regulatory Information

Extralabel use of sulfonamides is prohibited from use in lactating dairy cattle older than 20 months of age.

RCI Classification: 4

# Tacrolimus
tak-roe-lih'mus

**Trade and other names:** Protopic, FK506

**Functional classification:** Immunosuppressant

## Pharmacology and Mechanism of Action
Tacrolimus is a microbial product isolated from the organism *Streptomyces tsukubaensis*. It binds to an intracellular receptor and subsequently binds to calcineurin and inhibits the calcineurin pathway that stimulates the nuclear factor of activated T cells (NFAT). The action resembles that of cyclosporine (both drugs are calcineurin inhibitors), although the cellular receptors differ. By inhibiting the action of NFAT, tacrolimus decreases synthesis of inflammatory cytokines. In particular, synthesis of interleukin-2 (IL-2) is inhibited, which results in decreased activation of T lymphocytes. It is 10–100 times more potent than cyclosporine. Tacrolimus also inhibits release of mast cell and basophil mediators and decreases inflammatory mediator expression.

## Indications and Clinical Uses
Tacrolimus is used as an immunosuppressive drug to treat autoimmune disease, prevent organ transplant rejection, and treat atopic dermatitis. Most use in animals is with a topical formulation. It has been applied topically (ointment) for localized areas of atopic dermatitis or on skin areas of dogs where local immunosuppressive treatment is needed (e.g., on the bridge of the nose). In some cases, after resolution of lesions with systemic treatment with cyclosporine, isolated skin lesions are managed topically with tacrolimus ointment. There has been limited use for preventing renal transplant rejection in cats because the pharmacokinetics have been highly variable. A related drug, pimecrolimus, also has been used topically.

### Precautionary Information

#### Adverse Reactions and Side Effects
There may be a slight burning or pruritic sensation with initial topical application. These reactions are mild and decrease as the skin heals. With systemic administration, dogs may show gastrointestinal (GI) signs, which include diarrhea, intestinal discomfort, vomiting, intestinal intussusception, and intestinal injury. Tacrolimus is minimally absorbed systemically from topical application.

#### Contraindications and Precautions
Tacrolimus is a potent immunosuppressant. Use cautiously in animals prone to infection. Pet owners should be cautioned about skin contact when handling the medication for their pets. Safety from systemic treatment with tacrolimus has not been established in animals.

#### Drug Interactions
No drug interactions have been identified from topical administration.

## Instructions for Use
There are no reports of safe systemic doses used in dogs. Most use is topical. It can be used topically for immune-mediated skin lesions where local treatment can be used

(e.g., on the bridge of the nose). It has also been applied topically for perianal fistula in addition to systemic prednisolone.

## Patient Monitoring and Laboratory Tests
No specific monitoring is necessary with topical use.

## Formulations Available
- Tacrolimus is available in 0.1% and 0.03% topical ointment in 30-, 60-, and 100-g tubes.

## Stability and Storage
Ointment is stable if stored in manufacturer's original formulation. Compounded formulations of tacrolimus have been available from pharmacists. It is practically insoluble in water and usually formulated in lipid-soluble bases (e.g., ointments). When prepared in a suspension, it was stable for several weeks, but the stability of other formulations has not been evaluated.

## Small Animal Dosage
### Dogs and Cats
- Apply topical ointment (0.1%) to localized lesions on affected areas of skin. It has been used in dogs twice daily. For perianal fistula, it has been applied twice daily.

## Large Animal Dosage
- No doses have been reported for large animals.

## Regulatory Information
Do not administer to animals intended for food.

---

# Tadalafil
tah-da'la-fil

**Trade and other names:** Cialis

**Functional classification:** Vasodilator

---

## Pharmacology and Mechanism of Action
Tadalafil has been used on a limited basis as a vasodilator in animals. Tadalafil's vasodilator effects are specific for phosphodiesterase (PDE) V. Tadalafil and similar drugs, such as sildenafil, act to increase cyclic-GMP by inhibiting its breakdown by PDE V. Tadalafil is more specific for PDE V, but it is not known if this translates to improved clinical effects.

Relaxation of smooth muscle occurs from generation of nitric oxide (NO). There are two important locations of PDE V: (1) vascular smooth muscle of the lungs and (2) the corpus cavernosum. The effects on the corpus cavernosum produces the desired clinical effects that is responsible for the use in human medicine. The effect on vascular smooth muscle of the lungs produces vasodilation of the pulmonary vascular bed in patients with pulmonary hypertension. Other drugs that have been used for this effect are sildenafil (Viagra) in dogs.

Tadalafil can potentially relax smooth muscle in other sites, including portions of the GI tract, uterus, and gallbladder. Relaxation of the esophageal muscle may improve some dogs with clinical megaesophagus. This property has been studied for sildenafil in dogs but not for tadalafil.

T

*Pharmacokinetics:* In beagles, after an administration of a 5-mg tablet, the half-life was 4.17 hours, with a peak concentration of 59.5 ng/mL at 1.7 hours. By comparison, in people, the half-life is much longer at 17 hours.

## Indications and Clinical Uses

Tadalafil and related drugs are used in people for treating erectile dysfunction via the effect on the corpus cavernosum. This effect has not been explored in veterinary medicine. The use in veterinary medicine has been limited to the treatment of pulmonary arterial hypertension. In dogs, a comparison with sildenafil showed that both drugs were equally effective in patients with pulmonary hypertension. Sildenafil has been used to improve clinical signs in dogs with congenital idiopathic megaesophagus, but this use has not been explored for tadalafil.

### Precautionary Information

**Adverse Reactions and Side Effects**

Clinical use has been in only small observational studies and not sufficient to document the full range of potential adverse effects. Adverse effects observed in dogs have included decreased appetite, hindlimb weakness, and increased sexual behavior.

Potential effects are attributed to the vasodilator action. If high doses or other vasodilators are administered, especially those that increase cyclic-GMP levels, hypotension can occur.

**Contraindications and Precautions**

Use cautiously in conjunction with other vasodilator drugs.

**Drug Interactions**

No drug interactions reported for animals, but in people, there are precautions about use with other vasodilators such as alpha blockers and nitrates.

## Instructions for Use

The use in veterinary medicine has been based on small observational studies in dogs with pulmonary hypertension and extrapolation of the use in people. Although sildenafil has been used in dogs with megaesophagus, this has not been studied for tadalafil.

Administer tablets with or without food. Do not split tablets.

## Patient Monitoring and Laboratory Tests

No specific monitoring is necessary but monitor the patient's cardiovascular function (blood pressure and heart rate) in animals at risk for cardiovascular complications.

## Formulations

• Tadalafil is available as 2.5-, 5-, 10-, and 20-mg tablets.

## Stability and Storage

Store in a tightly sealed container, protected from light, and at room temperature.

## Small Animal Dosage

**Dogs**

• Pulmonary hypertension: 2 mg/kg q24h PO. Dose interval may be variable, depending on response.
• Megaesophagus: dose not established

**Cats**
- Dose not established

## Large Animal Dosage
- No dose has been reported for large animals.

## Regulatory Information
No withdrawal times are established for animals intended for food.

---

# Tamsulosin Hydrochloride
tam-soo′loe-sin

**Trade and other names:** Flomax

**Functional classification:** Smooth muscle relaxant

## Pharmacology and Mechanism of Action
Tamsulosin is a selective alpha$_{1A}$-adrenergic receptor antagonist. The effects of tamsulosin are targeted for the smooth muscle receptors of the prostate and urethra. Blocking this receptor relaxes the smooth muscle of the bladder and urethra to improve urine flow. It is primarily used when an enlarged prostate impedes normal urine flow and bladder emptying.

The alpha-1 adrenergic receptors are divided into alpha$_{1B}$ adrenoreceptors, which regulate vascular tone, and the alpha-$_{1A}$ adrenoreceptors, which regulate urethral smooth muscle tone. Blocking of the alpha-$_{1A}$ adrenoreceptors produces relaxation of smooth muscle in the bladder neck and prostate to improve urine flow. In men, approximately 75% of the alpha$_1$ receptors in the prostate are of the alpha$_{1A}$ subtype. The drugs tamsulosin (Flomax) and silodosin (Rapaflo) are more specific for the alpha$_{1A}$ receptor and can produce a more specific effect on the urethra.

*Pharmacokinetics:* The pharmacokinetics have not been well-studied in animals. In people, it is highly absorbed, and the half-life is approximately 12 hours with a peak effect of 5–6 hours. In dogs, it is 40%–50% absorbed orally and has a half-life of 1.5 hours.

## Indications and Clinical Uses
The major use of tamsulosin in people is treatment of benign prostate enlargement that is responsible for interfering with urine flow. It is often used with other drugs, such as finasteride, that interfere with the action of testosterone on the prostate. It is highly effective in men and studied in multiple clinical trials.

The use in dogs and cats has been anecdotal and based on extrapolation of the use and doses from human medicine. It has been used to improve the outcome posturethral blockage in male cats and to improve urine flow in dogs after surgery or calculi removal. It has improved urine flow in dogs with neurogenic bladders (0.4 mg per dog). In experimental dogs, it was more effective than prazosin for relaxing the urethral smooth muscle.

The use in cats extends from the use of other alpha$_1$ antagonists such as phenoxybenzamine and prazosin in cats with urethral obstruction to improve urine flow.

## Precautionary Information

### Adverse Reactions and Side Effects

High doses cause vasodilation and hypotension, but this has been unusual. No other treatment-related effects have been reported.

### Contraindications and Precautions

It may lower blood pressure and decrease cardiac output, but this likely would require high doses.

### Drug Interactions

No drug interactions have been reported in animals, but the use has been rare, and a full range of potential drug interactions is not known. In people, it is highly metabolized by cytochrome P450 enzymes, and the metabolites undergo extensive conjugation to glucuronide or sulfate for elimination.

## Instructions for Use

The dose form for people is a 0.4-mg capsule (approved dose is 0.8 mg per person), which is difficult to administer to some animals. A pharmacist may be able to divide up the capsule into smaller doses for animals.

## Patient Monitoring and Laboratory Tests

Monitor urine flow and evidence for hypotension and reflex tachycardia.

## Formulations

Tamsulosin is available as 0.4-mg capsules.

## Stability and Storage

Store in a tightly sealed container, protected from light, and at room temperature.

## Small Animal Dosage

### Dogs

- 0.1–0.4 mg per dog. Often a full capsule (0.4 mg per dog) is administered q24h PO. It is effective at 10–30 mcg/kg, but such a precise dose may be difficult because of the capsule size.

### Cats

- 0.1–0.4 mg per cat q24h PO.

## Large Animal Dosage

- No doses have been reported for large animals.

## Regulatory Information

Withdrawal times are not established for animals that produce food.

# Tamoxifen Citrate

tah-moks′ih-fen sih′trate

**Trade and other names:** Nolvadex

**Functional classification:** Antiestrogen

## Pharmacology and Mechanism of Action

Tamoxifen is a nonsteroidal estrogen receptor blocker. Tamoxifen also has weak estrogenic effects. It also increases release of gonadotropin-releasing hormone (GnRH). It is used primarily in women for treating complications from breast cancer. The use in veterinary medicine has been limited.

## Indications and Clinical Uses

Tamoxifen is used as adjunctive treatment for certain tumors, especially estrogen-responsive tumors. The most common use in animals is adjunctive treatment for mammary neoplasia. In women, the most common use is as an adjunct for the treatment of breast cancer. It also has been used to induce ovulation by stimulating release of GnRH from the hypothalamus.

### Precautionary Information

#### Adverse Reactions and Side Effects

Adverse effects have not been thoroughly documented in animals. However, in people, tamoxifen has been reported to cause increased tumor pain. There are several adverse effects reported in women because of the effect on estrogen blockade, but it is not known if these effects occur in animals.

#### Contraindications and Precautions

Do not use in pregnant animals.

#### Drug Interactions

Tamoxifen is a potent cytochrome P450 enzyme inhibitor. It may interact with other drugs that are cytochrome P450 substrates.

## Instructions for Use

Tamoxifen is often used with other anticancer drug protocols. Consult specific protocols from oncology sources for optimum use and doses.

## Patient Monitoring and Laboratory Tests

No specific monitoring is necessary.

## Formulations Available

- Tamoxifen is available in 10- and 20-mg tablets.

## Stability and Storage

Store in a tightly sealed container, protected from light, and at room temperature.

## Small Animal Dosage

- Veterinary dosage not established but has been extrapolated from the human dose. Human dosage is 10 mg q12h PO ($\approx$0.14 mg/kg q12h).

## Large Animal Dosage

- No doses have been reported for large animals.

## Regulatory Information

Do not administer to animals intended for food.

# Taurine

tore'een

**Trade and other names:** Generic brands

**Functional classification:** Nutritional supplement

## Pharmacology and Mechanism of Action

Taurine is a naturally occurring amino acid used as a nutritional supplement. Taurine is an amino acid considered essential for cats. If diets are deficient in animals, it can lead to blindness and heart disease. Taurine may have some cardiac inotropic effects.

## Indications and Clinical Uses

Taurine is used in the prevention and treatment of ocular and cardiac disease (dilated cardiomyopathy) caused by taurine deficiency. Although current commercial diets have adequate amounts of taurine, it has been supplemented in dogs and cats with heart disease.

## Precautionary Information

**Adverse Reactions and Side Effects**

Adverse effects have not been reported. This is a naturally occurring amino acid.

**Contraindications and Precautions**

No contraindications are reported for animals.

**Drug Interactions**

No drug interactions have been reported in animals.

## Instructions for Use

Routine supplementation with taurine may not be necessary in animals that are receiving a balanced diet. However, supplementation may be necessary in animals with diseases associated with taurine deficiency.

## Patient Monitoring and Laboratory Tests

Taurine concentrations can be measured in some laboratories to detect deficiencies. Normal levels in plasma are 60–120 nmol/mL in dogs and cats or 200–350 nmol/mL in whole blood. Levels below 40 nmol/mL in plasma and 150 nmol/mL in whole blood are considered deficient.

## Formulations Available

- Taurine is available in powder or supplemented in some diets. Consult a compounding pharmacy for availability.

## Stability and Storage

Store in a tightly sealed container, protected from light, and at room temperature.

## Small Animal Dosage

**Dogs**

- 500 mg/dog q12h PO.

**Cats**

- 250 mg/cat q12h PO.

## Large Animal Dosage
No doses have been reported for large animals.

## Regulatory Information
Because of a low risk of harmful residues in animals intended for food, no withdrawal time is suggested.

---

# Tegaserod Maleate
teg-ah-ser'odd mal'ee-ate

**Trade and other names:** Zelnorm

**Functional classification:** Gastrointestinal stimulant

---

**Note:** In 2007, tegaserod was removed from the US market and was made available to physicians only through a restricted distribution program from the manufacturer. Beginning in April 2008, tegaserod was no longer available through the restricted distribution program; therefore the US Food and Drug Administration (FDA) has decided to make tegaserod available only to physicians for patients in emergency situations that are life threatening or require hospitalization.

Thus this drug is no longer available to veterinarians. For information on the pharmacology, use, and dosing for tegaserod, please consult previous editions of this book.

---

# Telmisartan
tel' mi sar' tan

**Trade and other names:** Semintra (veterinary form) and Micardis (human form)

**Functional classification:** Vasodilator

---

## Pharmacology and Mechanism of Action
Telmisartan is a vasodilator that functions as an angiotensin II receptor blocker (ARB). Angiotensin II acts primarily on the type 1 and type 2 receptors, but telmisartan has high affinity and selectivity for the angiotensin II subtype 1 (AT-1) receptor and preserves the beneficial effects from the AT-2 subtype (angiotensin II, subtype 2 receptor). Compared with angiotensin-converting enzyme (ACE) inhibitors, it directly blocks the receptor, rather than inhibits synthesis of angiotensin II. Angiotensin II is produced in animals with heart disease and kidney disease and in response to an activated renin–angiotensin–aldosterone system (RAAS). Telmisartan has a long binding affinity for the angiotensin II receptor, producing long-lasting effects and is capable of blocking the AT-1 receptor, regardless of the source of angiotensin; therefore it is effective in states of *angiotensin breakthrough*. Telmisartan and other ARBs have been used in people who cannot tolerate ACE inhibitors. ARBs have the advantage of being less likely to induce hyperkalemia and are more easily tolerated in people.

In cats, telmisartan has an approved indication for treating hypertension in cats and has been shown to be superior to ACE inhibitors for this use. It was approved for use in cats by the FDA in May 2018. Hypertension in cats is a common problem that often occurs with chronic kidney disease (CKD) and hyperthyroidism. Proteinuria has been associated with renal hypertension, and telmisartan can be helpful to decrease proteinuria.

T

In dogs, telmisartan does not have an FDA-approved indication but is used to treat hypertension when other agents have been ineffective. It may produce a more complete blockade of aldosterone production than ACE inhibitors.

Telmisartan may have some anticancer properties through activation of a receptor that can induce apoptosis of cancer cells The application of this property in animals has so far been unexplored.

*Pharmacokinetics:* Telmisartan has a longer half-life and is more lipophilic than other ARBs. In dogs, the half-life is approximately 5 hours. In cats, the oral bioavailability is approximately 33%. Oral absorption is lower with feeding, but it may be administered with a small amount of food if necessary, without decrease in efficacy. Peak concentration occurs in 15–30 minutes after administration. The half-life in cats is approximately 8–8.5 hours. By comparison, the half-life in people is 20–24 hours.

## Indications and Clinical Uses

Telmisartan is the only ARB that has been rigorously tested in cats. It was more effective than ACE inhibitors, irbesartan, and losartan. Compared with placebo, it significantly lowers the systolic blood pressure in cats after 14 days of treatment. In cats, the approved indication is for treatment of hypertension and proteinuria caused by CKD. In cats, it can be considered a first choice for treating hypertension and has been preferred over ACE inhibitors such as benazepril.

The use in dogs is based on less rigorous studies, but studies in experimental animals and anecdotal experience support the use. In dogs, it is generally used for hypertension and proteinuria when other agents such as ACE inhibitors (e.g., enalapril, benazepril) are ineffective or not tolerated. In experimental dogs, telmisartan (1 mg/kg) was more effective than enalapril. It has also been administered concurrently with other antihypertensive agents in dogs. A related drug, irbesartan (30 mg/kg q12h), has also been shown to block angiotensin II receptors in dogs, but losartan is less potent because it relies mostly on an active metabolite that dogs do not produce (see Losartan for more details). Because telmisartan is more active than losartan in dogs and easily available to veterinarians, it should be a preferred if an angiotensin II blocker is needed.

## Precautionary Information

### Adverse Reactions and Side Effects

Adverse effects have been uncommon, but clinical trials in cats have shown vomiting, hypersalivation, weight loss, diarrhea, lethargy, anemia, and hypotension. Drugs that act on the RAAS can produce a decrease in red blood cell count. If hypotension is observed, a dose adjustment is appropriate. If severe hypotension is observed, treat with fluid therapy until the patient is stabilized; then re-evaluate the dose or the drug regimen.

In cats, there was no increase in creatinine even in cats with stage 2 or 3 CKD. During safety studies, up to five times the approved dose was administered to cats for 6 months, and adverse effects were not observed other than those listed earlier, which included hypotension and decreased red blood cell count.

### Contraindications and Precautions

No specific contraindications have been reported for animals. Safety in breeding, pregnant, or lactating animals has not been established.

### Drug Interactions

Combined use of an ARB and an ACE inhibitor may increase the risk of kidney injury because of dual blockade. This may be associated with increased risks of hypotension, hyperkalemia, and changes in kidney function.

## Instructions for Use

In cats, the dose protocols are based on the FDA-approved indications and label instructions for treating proteinuria in cats with CKD. The oral solution is well tolerated in cats and can be administered directly or with small amounts of food. It should not be mixed in with food but can be given simultaneously with a meal. When using the dosing syringe, rinse with water between treatments. In dogs, the use is based more on anecdotal experience and studies in research dogs but is an accepted use by most cardiologists.

## Patient Monitoring and Laboratory Tests

Monitor blood pressure in treated animals. Typically, the blood pressure should be checked within 7–10 days of initiating treatment. If the patient is stable, blood pressure measurements can be performed at the same time as regular checkups. If blood pressure is too low (defined as less than 120/60 mm Hg) with clinical signs of weakness, syncope, or tachycardia, the dose should be lowered by 0.5-mg/kg increments. Monitor the complete blood count (CBC) periodically during treatment because of a risk of lower red blood cell count.

## Formulations

- Telmisartan is available for cats as a 10-mg/mL oral solution in a 35-mL bottle.
- Tablets: formulation for people in sizes of 20-, 40-, and 80-mg tablets.

## Stability and Storage

Store in a tightly sealed container, protected from light, and at room temperature. Stability of compounded formulations has not been evaluated.

## Small Animal Dosage

### Dogs

- 1 mg/kg once per day PO as a starting dosage. Increase to 3 mg/kg once per day and then to twice daily if needed.

### Cats

- 1.5 mg/kg PO q12h initially for the first 14 days. Thereafter, 2 mg/kg PO q24h. For the oral solution, this is equivalent to 0.2 mL/kg. May be administered directly or with small amount of food, but not mixed in with food. Adjust the dose by 0.5-mg/kg increments by monitoring the blood pressure. Cats that are hypotensive from 2 mg/kg are usually adjusted down to 1 mg/kg.

## Large Animal Dosage

- No large animal doses have been reported.

## Regulatory Information

Do not administer to animals intended for food.
Racing Commissioners International (RCI) Classification: 3

# Tepoxalin
tep-oks′ah-lin

**Trade and other names:** Zubrin

**Functional classification:** Anti-inflammatory

**Note:** Although this is still an FDA-approved drug, the manufacturer has voluntarily withdrawn tepoxalin from the veterinary market in the United States. Information is included regarding pharmacology, indications, and dosing in the event that it may return to the market in the future.

If more information is needed, refer to earlier editions of this book.

---

## Terbinafine Hydrochloride
ter-bin'ah-feen hye-droe-klor'ide

**Trade and other names:** Lamisil

**Functional classification:** Antifungal

---

### Pharmacology and Mechanism of Action

Terbinafine is an antifungal drug used primarily for dermatophytes. Terbinafine belongs to the allylamine group of antifungal drugs. It acts on ergosterol biosynthesis by targeting fungal squalene epoxidase (SE). SE is a membrane-bound enzyme and is involved in the conversion of squalene into squalene 2,3-epoxide, which is subsequently converted into lanosterol and ergosterol, which is essential for the fungal cell membrane. Terbinafine produces an accumulation of squalene, which is toxic to the cell membrane, causing fungal cell death. Terbinafine is selective for fungal SE.

Terbinafine is active against yeasts and a wide range of dermatophytes with a low minimum inhibitory concentration (MIC) of ≤0.01 mcg/mL. It is fungicidal against *Trichophyton* spp., *Microsporum* spp., and *Aspergillus* spp. It is also active against *Blastomyces dermatitidis*, *Cryptococcus neoformans*, *Sporothrix schenckii*, *Histoplasma capsulatum*, *Candida* spp., and *Malassezia pachydermatis* yeast. There may be some activity against protozoa (e.g., *Toxoplasma* spp.). Despite the in vitro activity listed here, there are not enough data on clinical response from these infections to recommend terbinafine over other more traditional treatments in animals.

*Pharmacokinetics:* Oral bioavailability ranges from 31% in cats to greater than 46% in dogs. The half-lives in dogs and cats are 8.6 and 8.1 hours, respectively. Oral absorption in horses is low and inconsistent compared absorption in with dogs, and it is not recommended for oral treatment in horses. Because of its lipophilicity, high concentrations are attained in tissues such as the stratum corneum, hair follicles, sebum-rich skin, and nails. In people, after 12 days of therapy, the concentrations in the stratum corneum exceed those in plasma by a factor of 75. In cats, after a daily dose of 30–40 mg/kg, the concentrations in hair persist for 5 weeks after discontinuation of treatment at 14 days. However, dogs appear to be an exception. After administration of 30 mg/kg to dogs once daily for 21 days, it did not reach sufficient concentrations in canine stratum corneum or sebum that were high enough for treatment of *Malassezia* infection.

### Indications and Clinical Uses

Terbinafine has been used for treatment of dermatophyte infections in dogs, cats, birds, and some exotic animals. Clinical evidence of efficacy has not been established for these uses in well-controlled clinical trials. For dermatophytes in animals, the doses necessary for efficacy are much higher than those used in people. Although there has been experience with using terbinafine in animals, primarily for dermatophytes, there is no evidence that terbinafine is more effective than other oral antifungal agents. In dogs, it was partially effective for the treatment of *Malassezia* dermatitis when given at 30 mg/kg PO once a day or twice a week for at least 3 weeks. However, this treatment produced insufficient resolution and only partial remission even though there was clinical improvement. In cats (e.g., shelter cats), it has not been consistently effective for dermatophyte infections. Treatment of infections in horses with terbinafine has not been successful, probably because of poor oral absorption. Doses are listed later for horses based on limited observations, but there are no clinical efficacy studies available.

## Precautionary Information

### Adverse Reactions and Side Effects

Vomiting has been the most common adverse effect. Adverse effects, including nausea and anorexia, have been observed in dogs. Liver enzymes may be elevated in some animals. Hepatotoxicity is possible, but it has not been reported from use in animals. Facial pruritus has been observed in some treated cats. In people, a persistent taste disturbance, GI problems, and headache have been reported.

Tablets crushed and mixed with molasses for oral administration in horses produced oral mucosal irritations.

### Contraindications and Precautions

No contraindications have been reported for animals.

### Drug Interactions

No drug interactions have been reported in animals.

## Instructions for Use

Treatment of dogs and cats requires much higher doses than the doses used in people. Despite the in vitro activity of terbinafine against many fungi and the favorable pharmacokinetics in dogs and cats, the clinical results have not consistently produced clinical resolution in some patients.

## Patient Monitoring and Laboratory Tests

No specific monitoring is necessary.

## Formulations

- Terbinafine is available in 250-mg tablets, 1% topical solution, and 1% topical cream.

## Stability and Storage

Store in a tightly sealed container, protected from light, and at room temperature. Terbinafine is slightly soluble in water and alcohol. When suspensions are prepared from crushed tablets in a vehicle (Ora-Sweet), it is stable for 42 days.

## Small Animal Dosage

### Dogs

- 30–40 mg/kg q24h PO (with food) for 2–3 weeks.

### Cats

- 30–40 mg/kg/day PO for at least 2 weeks. Or administer one quarter of a tablet for small cats (62.5 mg), half a tablet for medium-size cats (125 mg), and one tablet for large cats (250 mg), all administered once daily.

## Large Animal Dosage

### Horses

- 30 mg/kg PO q12h. However, there are no studies to demonstrate efficacy in horses.

## Regulatory Information

Withdrawal times are not established for animals that produce food. For extralabel use withdrawal interval estimates, contact Food Animal Residue Avoidance Databank (FARAD) at www.FARAD.org.

---

# Terbutaline Sulfate
ter-byoo′tah-leen sul′fate

**Trade and other names:** Brethine and Bricanyl

**Functional classification:** Bronchodilator, beta agonist

---

## Pharmacology and Mechanism of Action

Terbutaline is a beta$_2$-adrenergic agonist. It is used primarily as a bronchodilator. Terbutaline stimulates beta$_2$-receptors to relax bronchial smooth muscle. Terbutaline is more beta$_2$ specific than drugs such as isoproterenol, which affect both beta$_1$- and beta$_2$-adrenergic receptors. Other beta$_2$-specific drugs include albuterol and metaproterenol. In addition to the beta$_2$ effects to relax bronchial smooth muscle and relieve bronchospasm, the beta$_2$ agonists may inhibit release of inflammatory mediators from mast cells.

## Indications and Clinical Uses

Terbutaline, like other beta$_2$-agonists, is indicated in animals with reversible bronchoconstriction, such as cats with bronchial asthma. It also has been used in dogs to relieve bronchoconstriction and in animals with bronchitis and other airway diseases. Is has been useful as an injection to rapidly relieve bronchospasm in small animals associated with inflammatory airway disease or clinical procedures.

It has been used in horses for short-term administration, by injection, to relieve bronchoconstriction associated with recurrent airway obstruction (RAO), which is a component of equine asthma syndrome. The use in animals has been primarily derived from empirical use, experience in humans, and recommendations from clinical experts. There are no well-controlled clinical studies or efficacy trials to document clinical effectiveness in animals. Albuterol injection may be used as an alternative for terbutaline injection (4 mcg/kg bolus up to 8 mcg/kg as needed). Terbutaline is not absorbed by the PO route in horses; therefore, it is not effective in horses for PO administration. Clenbuterol usually is the first drug of choice for oral administration in horses. (See Clenbuterol.)

Terbutaline (and other beta$_2$-agonists) have also been used during pregnancy to delay labor. (The dosage in people is 2.5 mg q6h PO.)

## Precautionary Information
### Adverse Reactions and Side Effects

Excessive beta-adrenergic stimulation from terbutaline at high doses can produce tachycardia and muscle tremors. Arrhythmias are possible with high doses. All beta$_2$ agonists inhibit uterine contractions at the end of gestation in pregnant animals. High doses of beta$_2$ agonists can lead to hypokalemia because they stimulate Na$^+$-K$^+$-ATPase and increase intracellular potassium while decreasing serum potassium and producing hyperglycemia. Treatment consists of potassium chloride (KCl) supplement at a rate of 0.5 mEq/kg/h.

### Contraindications and Precautions

Administer cautiously to animals with cardiac disease, particularly animals that may be susceptible to tachyarrhythmias. Do not use late in gestation unless the intended effect is to delay uterine contractions.

### Drug Interactions

Use cautiously with other drugs that may stimulate the heart and cause tachycardia.

## Instructions for Use

Terbutaline may be administered PO, IM, or SQ. Other beta$_2$ agonists used in animals for relief of bronchoconstriction include albuterol and salmeterol, and clenbuterol in horses. Animals with acute bronchoconstriction may also benefit from corticosteroid treatment and oxygen therapy. Caution should be used when administering repeated SQ doses. The maximum SQ dose in people is 500 mcg/person (0.5 mg) within a 4-hour period.

## Patient Monitoring and Laboratory Tests

Monitor heart rate in animals during treatment. Monitor potassium concentration if high doses are administered.

## Formulations

- Terbutaline is available in 2.5- and 5-mg tablets and 1-mg vials with a concentration of 1 mg/mL for injection.

## Stability and Storage

Store in a tightly sealed container, protected from light, and at room temperature. Terbutaline sulfate is soluble in water and can be diluted in sterile water prior to administration. Solutions may be subject to degradation. Observe for color change and discard if solution turns a dark color. Suspensions have been prepared from tablets in syrup and remained stable for 55 days.

## Small Animal Dosage
### Dogs

- 1.25–5 mg/dog q8h PO.
- 3–5 mcg/kg (0.003–0.005 mg/kg) SQ, usually as a single dose in an emergency. If necessary, repeat in 4–6 h.

### Cats

- 0.1 mg/kg q8h PO.
- 0.625 mg/cat (one quarter of a 2.5-mg tablet) q12h PO.
- 5–10 mcg/kg (0.005–0.01 mg/kg) q4h SQ or IM. The most common dose in cats is 0.05 mg per cat (equivalent to 0.05 mL) injected SQ.

T

## Large Animal Dosage
### Horses
• Not absorbed orally. Use IV for treatment of chronic RAO: 2–5 mcg/kg q6–8h IV or as needed.

## Regulatory Information
Terbutaline has similar properties as clenbuterol and should not be administered to animals intended for food.
RCI Classification: 3

# Testosterone
tess-toss′ter-one

**Trade and other names:** Testosterone cypionate ester: Andro-Cyp, Andronate, Depo-Testosterone, and generic brands and testosterone propionate ester: Testex and Malogen (in Canada)

**Functional classification:** Hormone

## Pharmacology and Mechanism of Action
Testosterone ester for injection is available in two forms: testosterone cypionate and testosterone propionate. Testosterone is used to supplement testosterone in deficient animals. It also produces anabolic effects in debilitated animals and increases weight gain. Testosterone esters are administered intramuscularly to avoid first-pass effects that occur from PO administration. Esters in oil are absorbed more slowly from IM injections. Esters are then hydrolyzed to free testosterone. Other agents with more specific anabolic activity include boldenone, oxymetholone, nandrolone, stanozolol, and methyltestosterone.

## Indications and Clinical Uses
Anabolic agents have been used for reversing catabolic conditions, increasing weight gain, increasing muscling in animals, and stimulating erythropoiesis. Testosterone and other anabolic agents have also been abused in people to enhance athletic performance and increase muscle development.

## Precautionary Information
### Adverse Reactions and Side Effects
Adverse effects are caused by excessive androgenic action of testosterone. Prostatic hyperplasia is possible in male dogs. Masculinization can occur in female dogs. Hepatopathy is more common with oral methylated testosterone formulations than with injected formulations. In men who take excessive testosterone supplements, there are cardiovascular risks.

### Contraindications and Precautions
Use cautiously in patients with hepatic disease. Do not administer to pregnant animals. This drug has potential for abuse in humans for anabolic uses.

### Drug Interactions
No drug interactions have been reported in animals.

## Instructions for Use

Use of testosterone androgens has not been evaluated in clinical studies in veterinary medicine. Use is based primarily on experimental evidence or experiences in people.

## Patient Monitoring and Laboratory Tests

Monitor hepatic enzymes in treated patients periodically.

## Formulations

- Testosterone cypionate ester is available in 100- and 200-mg/mL injections.
- Testosterone propionate ester is available in 100-mg/mL injections.

## Stability and Storage

Testosterone is insoluble in water but soluble in oils and ethanol. Protect from light, heat, and freezing. When mixed with oil, it has been stable for 60 days.

## Small Animal Dosage

### Dogs and Cats

- Testosterone cypionate ester: 1–2 mg/kg every 2–4 weeks IM.
- Testosterone propionate ester: 0.5–1 mg/kg two to three times per week IM.

## Large Animal Dosage

There are no large animal formulations available except for implants for calves. Do not administer injections to animals intended for food.

## Regulatory Information

Testosterone is a Schedule III controlled drug.
RCI Classification: 4

# Tetracycline, Tetracycline Hydrochloride

tet-rah-sye′kleen and tet-rah-sye′kleen hye-droe-klor′ide

**Trade and other names:** Panmycin, Duramycin powder, and Achromycin V

**Functional classification:** Antibacterial

## Pharmacology and Mechanism of Action

Tetracycline is an old antibiotic, not used systemically frequently, but related to other drugs in the tetracycline class. The mechanism of action of tetracyclines is to bind to 30S ribosomal subunit and inhibit protein synthesis. The action is time dependent and against some bacteria is bacteriostatic. Tetracycline, like other tetracyclines, has a broad spectrum of activity, including bacteria, some protozoa, *Rickettsia spp.,* and *Ehrlichia spp.* Resistance is common especially with Enterobacteriaceae bacteria.

Of the tetracyclines used in animals (oxytetracycline, doxycycline, minocycline) all have similar activity. However, minocycline may have better activity against some strains of *Staphylococcus* (see Minocycline for more details). Tigecycline is a new tetracycline that has improved activity against bacteria that are resistant to other drugs. However, there are no reports of its use in animals.

## Indications and Clinical Uses

Tetracyclines are used to treat a variety of infections, including soft tissue infections, pneumonia, and urinary tract infections (UTIs). Tetracycline is not often used for treatment in animals because there are few dosage forms (except topical), and other derivatives in this group are used more frequently in animals for treatment include oxytetracycline, minocycline, and doxycycline. Consult sections containing those drugs in this book for a more complete list of clinical use and indications.

## Precautionary Information

### Adverse Reactions and Side Effects

Tetracycline is usually used topically, and adverse reactions are rare. Tetracyclines can affect bone and teeth formation in young animals. They have been implicated in drug fever in cats. Hepatotoxicity may occur at high doses in susceptible individuals. PO administration can cause diarrhea in some animals.

### Contraindications and Precautions

Avoid repeated systemic use in young animals because it can affect bone and teeth formation.

### Drug Interactions

Tetracyclines bind to compounds that contain calcium, which decreases oral absorption. Do not mix with solutions that contain iron, calcium, aluminum, or magnesium.

## Instructions for Use

Pharmacokinetic and experimental studies have been conducted in small animals but not in clinical studies. Use of tetracyclines in small animals has primarily been replaced by doxycycline or minocycline. In cattle, pigs, and other large animals, the most commonly administered tetracycline is oxytetracycline, either in feed or water, or by injection. The most common oral tetracycline in horses is doxycycline or minocycline.

## Patient Monitoring and Laboratory Tests

Tetracycline can be tested as the class representative for susceptibility to chlortetracycline, doxycycline, minocycline, and oxytetracycline. Organisms that are susceptible to tetracycline are often susceptible to the other tetracyclines. However, some organisms that are intermediate or resistant to tetracycline may be susceptible to doxycycline or minocycline or both.

Susceptibility testing: Clinical and Laboratory Standards Institute (CLSI) breakpoints for sensitive organisms are ≤2 mcg/mL for streptococci and ≤4 mcg/mL for other organisms, based on the human breakpoint. However, on the basis of plasma concentrations achieved in animals, the human breakpoint cannot always be extrapolated to predict susceptibility of pathogens from animals. When testing *Staphylococcus* spp. from dogs, the breakpoint for susceptible isolates is ≤0.25 mcg/mL. When using tetracycline to test for susceptibility to oxytetracycline in pathogens from cattle, use a breakpoint of ≤2 mcg/mL for susceptible bacteria. When using tetracycline to test for susceptibility to oxytetracycline in pathogens from swine, use a breakpoint of ≤0.5 mcg/mL for susceptible bacteria.

## Formulations

- Tetracycline is available in 250- and 500-mg capsules, 500-mg calf bolus, 100-mg/mL oral suspension, and 25 and 324 g/lb of powder.

## Stability and Storage

Store in a tightly sealed container, protected from light, and at room temperature. Tetracycline has poor aqueous solubility. However, tetracycline hydrochloride is more soluble (100 mg/mL). The pH of tetracycline hydrochloride solution is approximately 2.0. It decomposes if kept at an alkaline pH. Tetracycline hydrochloride is unstable, and compounded preparations are better prepared from tetracycline base as a suspension. Tetracycline darkens with exposure to light. Protect from freezing.

## Small Animal Dosage
### Dogs and Cats
- 15–20 mg/kg q8h PO.
- 4.4–11 mg/kg q8h IV or IM.
- Rickettsial infection (dogs): 22 mg/kg q8h for 14 days PO.

## Large Animal Dosage
### Calves and Pigs
- For treatment of enteritis and pneumonia: 11 mg/kg q12h or 22 mg/kg once daily administered in the water or as a bolus. When administered in the water, the dose may actually vary among animals, depending on their water intake.

## Regulatory Information
Cattle and pig withdrawal times: 5 days for meat with the oral powder; 18 days for meat and 72 hours for milk when used as intrauterine bolus in cattle; and 12, 14, and 24 days when oral tablets are used for intrauterine treatment, depending on product (check label of individual products).

# Thenium Closylate
thee'nee-um kloe'sill-ate

**Trade and other names:** Canopar

**Functional classification:** Antiparasitic

## Pharmacology and Mechanism of Action
Thenium is an old antiparasitic drug. Thenium has specific action for hookworms and is used infrequently compared with other agents.

## Indications and Clinical Uses
Thenium closylate is used to treat adult forms of the species *Ancylostoma caninum* and *Uncinaria stenocephala* (hookworms).

T

## Precautionary Information
### Adverse Reactions and Side Effects
Thenium may cause occasional vomiting after oral administration.

### Contraindications and Precautions
No contraindications are reported for animals.

### Drug Interactions
No drug interactions have been reported in animals.

## Instructions for Use
Tablet is bitter if coating is broken.

## Patient Monitoring and Laboratory Tests

Monitor fecal samples for evidence of parasites.

## Formulations

- Thenium closylate is available in 500-mg tablets (veterinary preparation).

## Stability and Storage

Store in a tightly sealed container, protected from light, and at room temperature.

## Small Animal Dosage

- Dogs weighing greater than 4.5 kg: 500 mg PO once and repeat in 2–3 weeks.
- Dogs weighing 2.5–4.5 kg: 250 mg (half a tablet) twice a day PO for 1 day; repeat in 2–3 weeks.

## Large Animal Dosage

- No doses have been reported for large animals.

## Regulatory Information

Do not administer to animals intended for food.

# Theophylline
thee-off'ih-lin

**Trade and other names:** Many generic brands and theophylline sustained release

**Functional classification:** Bronchodilator

## Pharmacology and Mechanism of Action

Theophylline is a methylxanthine bronchodilator. It is a nonselective PDE inhibitor. PDE is the enzyme that converts cyclic adenosine monophosphate (cAMP) to inactive forms, and cAMP accumulates. Therapeutic effects may be caused by cAMP or antagonism of adenosine. There appears to be both anti-inflammatory action and bronchodilating action.

*Pharmacokinetics:* Oral theophylline is well absorbed orally in dogs, cats, and horses with bioavailability exceeding 90%. After absorption, theophylline has a half-lives in dogs, cats, and horses of 5–6 hours, 14–18 hours, and 12–15 hours, respectively. Some oral formulations contain aminophylline, and theophylline is the active component of aminophylline. Sustained-release preparations are intended to decrease frequency of administration, but there are few of these formulations left on the market, and they have not demonstrated a long duration of effect compared with conventional forms.

## Indications and Clinical Uses

Theophylline is administered for inflammatory airway disease in cats, dogs, and horses. Use in animals has been primarily derived from empirical use, some experimental models, and experience in humans. There are no well-controlled clinical studies or efficacy trials to document clinical effectiveness. It has been used to control clinical signs of reversible airway constriction, such as seen with feline asthma. In dogs, the uses include collapsing trachea, bronchitis, and other airway diseases. In horses, it will relieves signs of RAO (heaves) associated with equine asthma syndrome, but the IV dose may cause adverse effects in horses. Other drugs (e.g., clenbuterol, albuterol, ciclesonide) are often used for this condition in horses. It has not been effective for respiratory diseases in cattle.

Other methylxanthine drugs have been examined for treatment of dogs and cats with airway disease, but these medications are not readily available in the United States and are not widely used. These drugs include propentofylline, which is an approved veterinary drug in some countries (Karsivan or Vivitonin), as 50-mg tablets for dogs administered at a dosage of 3–5 mg/kg q12h PO (cat dose: 5 mg/kg). It has been effective for feline bronchial disease. In dogs, it is approved for treatment of cognitive dysfunction in aged dogs (e.g., lethargy, apathy, stiff gait, poor appetite).

## Precautionary Information

### Adverse Reactions and Side Effects
Adverse effects of theophylline include nausea, vomiting, and diarrhea. With high doses, tachycardia, excitement, tremors, and seizures are possible. Cardiovascular and central nervous system (CNS) adverse effects appear to be less frequent in dogs than people. Overdoses can cause hypokalemia.

### Contraindications and Precautions
Administer with caution to patients with cardiovascular disease or patients with seizure disorders. Studies in people have concluded that administration of methylxanthines increases risk of seizures in susceptible patients.

### Drug Interactions
Use cautiously with other PDE inhibitors such as pentoxifylline, sildenafil (Viagra), and pimobendan. Many drugs inhibit the metabolism of theophylline and potentially increase concentrations. Drugs responsible include cimetidine, erythromycin, fluoroquinolones, and propranolol. Some drugs decrease concentrations by increasing metabolism. Such drugs include phenobarbital and rifampin.

## Instructions for Use
Adjust the dose of theophylline to maintain therapeutic blood levels. Older slow-release and extended-release (ER) formulations are no longer available. Some ER forms are sold through compounding pharmacies, but there is no evidence that they produce extended-duration treatment effects compared with conventional forms. The doses listed later were primarily established through pharmacokinetic studies using human-labeled tablets and capsules in dogs and cats. Some of these forms may no longer be available commercially.

## Patient Monitoring and Laboratory Tests
Plasma concentrations of theophylline should be monitored in patients receiving chronic therapy to maintain plasma concentrations between 10 and 20 mcg/mL. Regularly monitor plasma concentrations in patients receiving chronic treatment.

## Formulations
- Theophylline has been available in 100-, 125-, 200-, 250-, and 300-mg tablets; 27-mg/5-mL (5.3-mg/mL) oral solution or elixir; and injection in 5% dextrose.
- Theophylline extended release was available in 100-, 200-, 300-, 400-, 450-, and 600-mg tablets. However, availability of various sizes of ER formulations may vary, and most are no longer available. Some veterinarians have relied on compounded immediate-release tablets and capsules. But there is no evidence that the compounded versions are equivalent to the proprietary formulations.
- Transdermal theophylline in Lipoderm and PLO gel has been tested but produced ineffective plasma concentrations.

## Stability and Storage

Store in a tightly sealed container, protected from light, and at room temperature. Theophylline is slightly soluble in water (8 mg/mL). It has been mixed with some oral liquids and found to be stable if administered shortly after mixing. When using the slow-release tablets or capsules in dogs and cats, do not disrupt coating on formulation.

## Small Animal Dosage

**Dogs**

- Theophylline: 9 mg/kg q8h PO (immediate-release formulations).
- Theophylline sustained release: 10 mg/kg q12h PO.

**Cats**

- 4 mg/kg q8–12h PO (immediate-release formulations).
- Theophylline sustained release: 20 mg/kg for tablets (100 mg per cat) q24h PO or 25 mg/kg for ER capsule (125 mg per cat) q24h PO. With long-term use in cats, this interval may be increased to q48h.

## Large Animal Dosage

- Horses, treatment of equine asthma syndrome, with RAO: 5 mg/kg q12h PO.
- Although theophylline has been administered to horses intravenously, this administration has caused transient excitement and restlessness. Give IV administration slowly.
- Cattle use as a bronchodilator: 20 mg/kg q12h PO. When treating diseases secondary to virus infections, decrease frequency to once every 24 hours.

## Regulatory Information

Withdrawal times are not established. However, for extralabel use withdrawal interval estimates, contact FARAD at www.FARAD.org.
RCI Classification: 3

# Thiabendazole
thye-ah-ben′dah-zole

**Trade and other names:** Omnizole, Equizole, TBZ, and Thibenzole

**Functional classification:** Antiparasitic

## Pharmacology and Mechanism of Action

Thiabendazole is a benzimidazole antiparasitic drug. Like other benzimidazoles, it produces a degeneration of the parasite microtubule and irreversibly blocks glucose uptake in parasites. Inhibition of glucose uptake causes depletion of energy stores in the parasite, eventually resulting in death. However, there is no effect on glucose metabolism in mammals.

## Indications and Clinical Uses

Availability of commercial forms of thiabendazole has been limited. Some forms are no longer available. In horses, it has been used for control of large and small strongyles; *Strongyloides*, and pinworms of the genera *Strongylus*, *Cyathostomum*, and *Cylicobrachytus* and related genera *Craterostomum*, *Oesophagodontus*, *Poteriostomum*, and *Oxyuris*. In ruminants, it has been used for infections of GI roundworms in sheep and goats (*Trichostrongylus* spp. *Haemonchus* spp., *Ostertagia* spp., *Cooperia* spp., *Nematodirus* spp., *Bunostomom* spp., *Strongyloides* spp., *Chabertia* spp., *Oesophagostomum* spp., *Trichostrongylus colubriformis, Trichostrongylus axei,* and *Ostertagia* spp.).

---

### Precautionary Information
**Adverse Reactions and Side Effects**
Adverse effects are uncommon.

**Contraindications and Precautions**
No contraindications are reported for animals.

**Drug Interactions**
No drug interactions have been reported in animals.

---

### Instructions for Use
Thiabendazole is ordinarily administered to horses and cattle. Experience in small animals is limited.

### Patient Monitoring and Laboratory Tests
Monitor fecal samples for evidence of intestinal parasites.

### Formulations Available
- Thiabendazole has been available in paste, pellets, and solution for oral administration and premix for feeds. Some formulations are no longer commercially available.

### Stability and Storage
Store in a tightly sealed container, protected from light, and at room temperature.

### Small Animal Dosage
**Dogs**
- 50 mg/kg q24h for 3 days; repeat in 1 month.
- Treating respiratory parasites: 30–70 mg/kg q12h PO.

### Cats
- *Strongyloides* spp: 125 mg/kg q24h for 3 days.

### Large Animal Dosage
**Horses**
- 44 mg/kg PO (single dose).

**Sheep and Goats**
- 44 mg/kg PO (single dose) up to 67 mg/kg PO for some infections.

### Cattle
- 67 mg/kg PO (single dose) up to 111 mg/kg PO for more severe infections.

**Pigs (baby pigs)**
- 67–90 mg/kg PO.

### Regulatory Information
Withdrawal time for milk: 96 hours.
Sheep and goat withdrawal time for meat: 30 days.
Cattle withdrawal time for meat: 3 days.
Pig withdrawal time for meat: 30 days.

# Thiacetarsamide Sodium
thye-ass-et-ars'ah-mide soe'dee-um

**Trade and other names:** Caparsolate

**Functional classification:** Antiparasitic

**Note:** Thiacetarsamide sodium is no longer recommended or available for treating heartworm infections in dogs and cats. Melarsomine dihydrochloride (Immiticide) is recommended instead for treatment of adult heartworms. The information on pharmacology and clinical use of thiacetarsamide is listed briefly here for countries where it may still be available and used for treating heartworm infections.

## Pharmacology and Mechanism of Action
Thiacetarsamide is an older organic arsenical that produces toxicity in parasites such as adult heartworms.

## Indications and Clinical Uses
Thiacetarsamide has been used for treatment of adult heartworm infections. Caparsolate is no longer recommended as an adulticide heartworm treatment by the American Heartworm Society. Caparsolate is less effective in cats than in dogs, with a higher incidence of adverse reactions. In dogs, melarsomine is considered safer and has replaced thiacetarsamide for routine treatment.

## Precautionary Information
### Adverse Reactions and Side Effects
Adverse effects are common, especially anorexia, vomiting, and hepatic injury. Pulmonary thromboembolism may occur as a consequence of heartworm kill.

### Contraindications and Precautions
Its use is not recommended in cats unless they can be carefully monitored. Cats are less susceptible to arsenical toxicity than dogs, but they are more prone to pulmonary thromboembolism. If cats are treated, they should be confined under close observation for 3–4 weeks.

### Drug Interactions
No drug interactions have been reported in animals.

## Instructions for Use
Thiacetarsamide is administered via four injections over 2 days; however, if severe adverse effects are observed, discontinue regimen. Extravasation can result in skin slough. It is recommended to substitute melarsomine for thiacetarsamide, if possible, for treating heartworm disease.

## Patient Monitoring and Laboratory Tests
Monitor renal and hepatic function.

## Formulations
- Thiacetarsamide was previously available in 10-mg/mL injections. There are no longer commercial supplies of thiacetarsamide, and its availability is uncertain.

## Stability and Storage
Store in a tightly sealed container, protected from light, and at room temperature.

## Small Animal Dosage
**Dogs**
- 2.2 mg/kg IV twice daily for 2 days.

**Cats**
- Not recommended.

## Large Animal Dosage
- No doses have been reported for large animals.

## Regulatory Information
Do not administer to animals intended for food.

# Thiamine Hydrochloride
thye′ah-min hye-droe-klor′ide

**Trade and other names:** Vitamin $B_1$, Bewon, and generic brands

**Functional classification:** Vitamin

## Pharmacology and Mechanism of Action
Vitamin $B_1$ (thiamine) is used for treatment of vitamin deficiency. Vitamin B complex often contains thiamine ($B_1$), riboflavin, niacinamide, and cyanocobalamin $B_{12}$.

## Indications and Clinical Uses
Thiamine is used to provide vitamin $B_1$ supplementation or to treat vitamin $B_1$ deficiency. It is often administered in combination with other vitamins (vitamin B complex). Vitamin B complex is often administered to patients, sometimes supplemented in IV fluids to help recovery from illness.

## Precautionary Information
### Adverse Reactions and Side Effects
Adverse effects are rare because water-soluble vitamins are easily excreted.

### Contraindications and Precautions
Administer solutions of vitamin $B_1$ very slowly intravenously if at all. Rapid IV administration has caused anaphylactic reactions.

### Drug Interactions
Thiamine hydrochloride is an acidic solution and may be susceptible in incompatibility when this hydrochloride is mixed with alkalinizing solutions.

## Instructions for Use
Vitamin B supplements are administered often in combination with other B vitamins as vitamin B complex solutions.

## Patient Monitoring and Laboratory Tests
No specific monitoring is necessary.

T

## Formulations

- Thiamine is available in 250-mcg/5-mL elixir, 5- to 500-mg tablets, and 100- and 500-mg/mL injections.
- Vitamin B complex aqueous solutions for injection usually contain 12.5 mg/mL of vitamin $B_1$.

## Stability and Storage

Store in a tightly sealed container, at room temperature, and protected from light. When mixed with other solutions (e.g., fluid solutions), incompatibility may result.

## Small Animal Dosage

### Dogs

- 10–100 mg/dog/day PO.
- 12.5–50 mg/dog/day IM or SQ.

### Cats

- 5–30 mg/cat/day PO up to a maximum dosage of 50 mg/cat/day.
- 12.5–25 mg/cat/day IM or SQ.

## Large Animal Dosage

- All dosages are listed on a per-animal basis.

### Lambs

- 12.5–25 mg/day IM.

### Sheep and Pigs

- 65–125 mg/day IM.

### Calves and Foals

- 37.5–65 mg/day IM.

### Cattle and Horses

- 125–250 mg/day IM.

## Regulatory Information

Withdrawal time for animals intended for food: 0 days.

# Thioguanine
thye-oh-gwah'neen

**Trade and other names:** Generic brands

**Functional classification:** Anticancer agent

## Pharmacology and Mechanism of Action

Thioguanine is an anticancer agent. It is infrequently used in veterinary medicine. It acts as an antimetabolite of purine analogue type and inhibits DNA synthesis in cancer cells.

## Indications and Clinical Uses

Thioguanine is used in some anticancer protocols. It is not commonly used in animals. Use in animals has been primarily derived from empirical use and experience in humans. There are no well-controlled clinical studies or efficacy trials to document clinical effectiveness.

## Precautionary Information
### Adverse Reactions and Side Effects
Adverse effects, as with any anticancer drug, are expected. Adverse effects from thioguanine may be similar to those observed from mercaptopurine. Immunosuppression and leukopenia are common.

### Contraindications and Precautions
Do not administer to patients with depressed bone marrow.

### Drug Interactions
No drug interactions have been reported in animals.

## Instructions for Use
Thioguanine may be combined with other agents for treatment of cancer.

## Patient Monitoring and Laboratory Tests
Monitor the CBC to screen for evidence of bone marrow toxicity.

## Formulations
• Thioguanine is available in 40-mg tablets.

## Stability and Storage
Store in a tightly sealed container, protected from light, and at room temperature.

## Small Animal Dosage
### Dogs
• 40 mg/m$^2$ q24h PO.

### Cats
• 25 mg/m$^2$ q24h PO for 1–5 days; then repeat every 30 days.

## Large Animal Dosage
• No dose has been reported for large animals.

## Regulatory Information
Withdrawal times are not established for animals that produce food. This drug should not be used in animals intended for food because it is an anticancer agent.

# Thiopental Sodium
thye-oh-pen′tahl soe′dee-um

**Trade and other names:** Pentothal (previously used name was Thiopentone)

**Functional classification:** Anesthetic, barbiturate

## Pharmacology and Mechanism of Action
Thiopental is an ultrashort-acting barbiturate used primarily for IV administration to induce anesthesia. Anesthesia is produced by CNS depression but does not provide analgesia. The action of thiopental is similar to that of other barbiturates. It is a gamma-aminobutyric acid (GABA$_A$) receptor agonist that enhances inhibitory neurotransmission. It increases GABA binding (inhibitory neurotransmitter) to its receptor, which increases transmembrane chloride conductance, resulting

in hyperpolarization of the postsynaptic cell membrane and inhibition of the postsynaptic neuron. Anesthesia is terminated by redistribution in the body. It is a short-acting agent, and the clearance is rapid.

## Indications and Clinical Uses

Thiopental is the most commonly used injectable barbiturate in veterinary medicine. It is used primarily for induction of anesthesia or for short duration of anesthesia (10- to 15-minute procedures). It induces a rapid, smooth, and generally excitement-free induction. It can be administered intravenously, with prior premedication of other anesthetic adjuncts such as tranquilizers and sedatives (e.g., alpha$_2$ agonists, phenothiazines, and opioids). Thiopental has been combined with propofol in a 1:1 mixture without loss of effectiveness. This mixture of 1:1 2.5% thiopental and propofol has been used to induce anesthesia in dogs.

## Precautionary Information

### Adverse Reactions and Side Effects

The most common effect is transient apnea and respiratory depression. Other adverse effects are related to the anesthetic effects of the drug (CNS depression). Thiopental may cause cardiovascular depression with a slight decrease in stroke volume and little change in cardiac output or blood pressure. Premedication reduces the risk of cardiovascular events. Supplementation with oxygen during induction also decreases cardiovascular events. Overdoses are caused by rapid or repeated injections. Avoid extravasation outside of the vein.

### Contraindications and Precautions

Use carefully in patients with respiratory or cardiac disease. Do not use unless there is an ability to monitor and maintain respiration. Because respiratory apnea can occur during induction, there should be a capability to ventilate the patient, if necessary.

### Drug Interactions

Thiopental is compatible with other anesthetics. However, use of other sedatives and anesthetics lowers the dose of thiopental.

## Instructions for Use

The therapeutic index is low. Administer to effect, by giving intermittent injections and observing the patient's response. Use only in patients in which it is possible to monitor cardiovascular and respiratory functions. Thiopental is often administered with other anesthetic adjuncts.

## Patient Monitoring and Laboratory Tests

Monitor cardiovascular and respiratory function during anesthesia with thiopental.

## Formulations

• Thiopental is available in 250-mg to 10-g vials (mix to desired concentration with sterile diluent). The concentration can vary, but generally, the 2.5% solution is used with small animals, and the 2.5% or 5% solution is used with larger animals.

## Stability and Storage

Thiopental, when prepared properly, is chemically stable and resists bacterial growth for up to 4 weeks when refrigerated. Thiopental has a pH of 10–11 and should not be mixed with acidifying solutions. If mixed with other drugs, the alkalinity of the solution may affect their stability. Propofol has been mixed with thiopental sodium in a 1:1 mixture, and they are physically and chemically compatible if used promptly.

## Small Animal Dosage
### Dogs
* 10–25 mg/kg IV (induction dose; administer to effect).

### Cats
* 5–10 mg/kg IV (induction dose; administer to effect).

## Large Animal Dosage
### Cattle
* Induction: 6–12 mg/kg IV (to effect).

### Pigs
* 10–20 mg/kg IV (to effect).

## Regulatory Information
Extralabel use: Establish a withdrawal time of at least 1 day for meat and 24 hours for milk.
Pig withdrawal time for meat: 0 days.
Schedule III controlled drug.
RCI Classification: 2

## Thiotepa
thye-oh-tep′ah

**Trade and other names:** Thioplex and generic brands

**Functional classification:** Anticancer agent

## Pharmacology and Mechanism of Action
Thiotepa is an anticancer agent that is infrequently used in veterinary medicine. Thiotepa is an alkylating agent of the nitrogen mustard type (similar to cyclophosphamide). Other alkylating agents are used more often to treat cancer in animals.

## Indications and Clinical Uses
Thiotepa has been used for various tumors, especially malignant effusions. The most common mode of administration is local infiltration of a lesion or local infusion (e.g., into the urinary bladder). For cancer of the bladder, 30 mg has been diluted in 30 mL of distilled water and instilled directly in the bladder once per week.

T

## Precautionary Information
### Adverse Reactions and Side Effects
Adverse effects are similar to other anticancer agents and alkylating drugs (many of which are unavoidable). Bone marrow suppression is the most common effect. When administered locally or by local infiltration, there is less systemic effect.

### Contraindications and Precautions
Avoid use in animals with depressed bone marrow.

### Drug Interactions
No drug interactions have been reported in animals.

## Instructions for Use

One should consult the specific cancer chemotherapy protocol for guidance on administration. Thiotepa usually is administered directly in body cavities.

## Patient Monitoring and Laboratory Tests

Monitor the CBC for evidence of bone marrow suppression.

## Formulations

Thiotepa is available in 15-mg injections (usually in a solution of 10 mg/mL).

## Stability and Storage

Store in a tightly sealed container, protected from light, and at room temperature. When mixing solution, add 1.5 mL of sterile water to each vial. This solution is stable for 5 days if refrigerated. Solutions may be clear to slightly opaque, but if cloudiness or precipitate appears, discard the vial.

## Small Animal Dosage

### Dogs and Cats

- 0.2–0.5 mg/m$^2$ weekly or daily for 5–10 days IM, intracavitary, or injected directly into the tumor.

## Large Animal Dosage

- No dose has been reported for large animals.

## Regulatory Information

Withdrawal times are not established for animals that produce food. This drug should not be used in animals intended for food because it is an anticancer agent.

# Thyroid-Releasing Hormone

**Trade and other names:** TRH, Protirelin, Thyrel

**Functional classification:** Hormone, thyroid

## Pharmacology and Mechanism of Action

Thyroid-releasing hormone (TRH) is used as a diagnostic agent. It is used to detect hyperthyroidism when tetraiodothyronine (T$_4$) is not elevated, but hyperthyroidism is suspected. It is a synthetic tripeptide that is structurally identical to the naturally occurring thyrotropin-releasing hormone produced by the hypothalamus. This agent has no place in treatment; it is only used for testing.

## Indications and Clinical Uses

Thyroid-releasing hormone has been used for diagnostic testing. See Thyrotropin for diagnostic testing for hypothyroidism. There are no specific therapeutic uses. Thyrotropin-releasing hormone has been used to test for pituitary pars intermedia dysfunction (PPID) in horses.

## Precautionary Information

### Adverse Reactions and Side Effects

No significant adverse effects have been reported. Allergic reactions are possible.

**Contraindications and Precautions**
No contraindications are reported for animals.

**Drug Interactions**
No drug interactions have been reported in animals.

## Instructions for Use
Used for diagnostic purposes. It is rarely used in small animals but has been used in protocols to test horses for PPID.

## Patient Monitoring and Laboratory Tests
Monitor thyroid concentrations. Collect post-TRH $T_4$ sample at 4 hours after the test dose. When used for testing PPID in horses, it is used in combination with the insulin sensitivity test.

## Formulations
- Thyrel TRH (Protirelin) is supplied as 1-mL ampules. Each ampule contains 500 mcg of protirelin. However, this form is currently difficult to obtain.

## Stability and Storage
Store in a tightly sealed container, protected from light, and at room temperature.

## Small Animal Dosage
- Collect baseline $T_4$ followed by 0.1 mg/kg IV. Collect the post-TRH $T_4$ sample at 4 hours.

## Large Animal Dosage
- To test for PPID in horses (equine Cushing's syndrome), administer 1 mg synthetic TRH IV and collect samples. The optimum sample time is 0 and 30 minutes.

## Regulatory Information
Because of a low risk of harmful residues in animals intended for food, no withdrawal time is suggested.

# Thyrotropin
thye-roe-troe′pin

**Trade and other names:** Thytropar, Thyrogen, and TSH

**Functional classification:** Hormone, thyroid

## Pharmacology and Mechanism of Action
Thyrotropin is a thyroid-stimulating hormone (TSH) used for diagnostic testing; it stimulates normal secretion of thyroid hormone. It is not used for treatment of any disease. This formulation (Thyrogen), also known as thyrotropin alpha for injection, is a purified recombinant form of human TSH produced by recombinant DNA technology. An older form, Thytropar, is difficult to obtain. The amino acid sequence of thyrotropin alpha is identical to that of human pituitary TSH. TSH activity is not species specific, and the human product may be used in animals to stimulate the thyroid.

Recombinant human thyrotropin (rhTSH) also has been used for the diagnosis of hypothyroidism.

## Indications and Clinical Uses

Thyroid-stimulating hormone is used to stimulate secretion of thyroid hormone for diagnostic testing. Because of the limited availability of TSH for diagnostic testing and the high cost of the human form, this test is rarely performed. Bovine TSH has been used in dogs, but anaphylactoid reactions and safety concerns led to a discontinuation of the use. Human recombinant thyrotropin can be administered intravenously and results in a total $T_4$ increase at 4 and 6 hours.

---

### Precautionary Information

**Adverse Reactions and Side Effects**

Adverse reactions are rare. In people, allergic reactions have occurred.

**Contraindications and Precautions**

No contraindications have been reported for animals.

**Drug Interactions**

No drug interactions have been reported in animals.

---

## Instructions for Use

To prepare solution, add 2 mL of sodium chloride to a 10-unit vial. Consult the testing laboratory for specific guidelines for thyroid testing.

If the patient is already receiving thyroxine supplement, withdraw treatment for 6–8 weeks before testing.

## Patient Monitoring and Laboratory Tests

After IV injection, collect post-TSH sample at 4 or 6 hours (6 hours is optimal). See dosing section for complete information on testing in dogs.

## Formulations

- Recombinant human TSH, also known as thyrotropin alpha or Thyrogen, has been available in a 1.1-mg vial containing thyrotropin alpha. After reconstitution with 1.2 mL of sterile water, the thyrotropin alpha concentration is 0.9 mg/mL. (See dosing section for specific instructions for preparing the canine dose.) The pH of the reconstituted solution is approximately 7.0. Other forms (Thytropar) are difficult to obtain. Bovine TSH caused reactions in dogs and is no longer available.

## Stability and Storage

Store in a tightly sealed container, protected from light, and at room temperature. Reconstituted solutions retain potency for 2 weeks at 2°C–8°C, for 4 weeks at 4°C, and 12 weeks if frozen (–20°C).

## Small Animal Dosage

### Dogs

- 50–150 mcg injection per dog.
- Diagnostic testing procedure for dogs: Reconstitute one vial (1.1 mg) with 6 mL of sterile water and divide into 12 aliquots. Place 0.5 mL in plastic insulin syringes and store in a freezer for future use. For each dose, thaw the syringe and administer one syringe per dog intravenously. The dose that is effective has ranged from 75–150 mcg per dog. The higher dose is reported to have better discriminating power. After injection, measure thyroid hormone ($T_4$) at 4 or 6 hours after injection (6 hours is optimal). Post-TSH response should be at least 1.9 mcg/dL over baseline.

Generally, a response of 2.5–3.1 mcg/dL is consistent with euthyroidism, less than 1.6 mcg/dL is indicative of hypothyroidism, and 1.6–2.5 mcg/mL is in the intermediate range and may require follow-up testing.

## Large Animal Dosage
• No dosage has been reported for large animals.

## Regulatory Information
Because of a low risk of harmful residues in animals intended for food, no withdrawal time is suggested.

# Ticarcillin Disodium
tye-kar-sill'in dye-soe'dee-um

**Trade and other names:** Ticar and Ticillin

**Functional classification:** Antibacterial

**Note:** The formulations of ticarcillin have been withdrawn from the human market, as well as formulations containing clavulanate. There is still an approved veterinary formulation for horses, but availability may be limited.

## Pharmacology and Mechanism of Action
Ticarcillin is a beta-lactam antibiotic derivative of penicillin. Like other beta lactam antibiotics, ticarcillin binds penicillin-binding proteins (PBPs) that weaken or interfere with cell wall formation. After binding to PBPs, the cell wall weakens or undergoes lysis. Like other beta-lactams, this drug acts in a time-dependent manner, which indicates that it is more effective when drug concentrations are maintained above the MIC values during the dose interval. Ticarcillin has action similar to ampicillin and a spectrum similar to carbenicillin, but carbenicillin is no longer available. Ticarcillin (when available) is primarily used for gram-negative infections, especially those caused by *Pseudomonas* spp.

## Indications and Clinical Uses
Ticarcillin has been used in animals for treatment of various infections, including pneumonia, soft tissue infections, and bone infections. It has similar activity as ampicillin but is extended to include many organisms that otherwise are resistant to ampicillin, such as *Pseudomonas aeruginosa* and other gram-negative bacilli. Its activity against *Pseudomonas* spp. may be enhanced when administered with an aminoglycoside. Use in animals has been primarily derived from empirical use and from pharmacokinetic–pharmacodynamic (PK–PD) information. It is administered intravenously in most animals because IM administration can be painful. Ticarcillin also has been infused directly in the uterus of horses to treat metritis.

## Precautionary Information
### Adverse Reactions and Side Effects
Adverse effects are uncommon. However, allergic reactions are possible. High doses can produce seizures and decreased platelet function.

### Contraindications and Precautions
Administer cautiously, if at all, to animals with penicillin allergies.

### Drug Interactions
Do not combine in same syringe or in vial with aminoglycosides.

## Instructions for Use

Ticarcillin may be combined with clavulanic acid (see Ticarcillin and Clavulanate for more details). Ticarcillin is synergistic with and often combined with aminoglycosides (e.g., amikacin and gentamicin). Lidocaine (1%) may be used for reconstitution to decrease pain from IM injection (see Formulations).

## Patient Monitoring and Laboratory Tests

Susceptibility testing: CLSI breakpoints for sensitive organisms are ≤64 mcg/mL for *Pseudomonas* spp. and ≤16 mcg/mL for gram-negative enteric organisms.

## Formulations

- Note: The availability of commercial formulations may be limited. Ticarcillin has been available in 3-g vials. Mix a 3-g vial with 6 mL of sterile water, sodium chloride, or 1% lidocaine hydrochloride solution (without epinephrine) to produce a final concentration of 384.6 mg/mL. Ticarcillin + clavulanate also has been used, but commercial forms have been voluntarily withdrawn from the market. (See the next section for more information.)

## Stability and Storage

Store powder for injection in original vial, protected from light, and at room temperature. Use reconstituted solution immediately. If diluted for IV administration with sodium chloride or 5% dextrose, it may be stable for up to 72 hours at room temperature or 14 days if refrigerated. IV solution prepared in lactated Ringer's solution is stable for up to 48 hours at room temperature or 14 days if refrigerated. If diluted IV solutions are frozen, they are stable for up to 30 days but should be used within 24 hours after being thawed. Do not refreeze thawed solutions.

## Small Animal Dosage

### Dogs and Cats

- 33–50 mg/kg q4–6h IV or IM.

## Large Animal Dosage

### Horses

- 44 mg/kg q6–8h IV or IM.
- Ticarcillin also has been used in horses as an intrauterine infusion at a dose of 12.4 mg/kg diluted in 60–100 mL saline.

## Regulatory Information

Withdrawal times are not established. However, excretion is similar to that of other beta-lactam antibiotics, such as ampicillin. Follow ampicillin guidelines for withdrawal times.

# Ticarcillin and Clavulanate Potassium
tye-kar-sill'in + klav'yoo-lan'ate

**Trade and other names:** Timentin

**Functional classification:** Antibacterial

**Note:** The manufacturer has voluntarily withdrawn ticarcillin and clavulanate from the market in the United States. It is an FDA-approved product but is no longer marketed. For more information regarding pharmacology, indications, and dosing, refer to earlier editions of this book.

If another injectable penicillin beta-lactamase inhibitor is indicated in a patient, the combination of piperacillin and tazobactam is a logical substitute, and there is experience with its use in veterinary medicine. Consult the section on piperacillin and tazobactam for more information on the pharmacology and clinical use.

# Tildipirosin
il'di-pir'oh-sin

**Trade and other names:** Zuprevo

**Functional classification:** Antibacterial, Macrolide

## Pharmacology and Mechanism of Action

Tildipirosin is an antibacterial of the macrolide class. It is a 16-membered ring (tilmicosin, a related drug, also is a 16-member ring molecule) macrolide antimicrobial with three charged nitrogen atoms (tulathromycin, a related drug, also has three charged nitrogen atoms). Like other macrolides, tildipirosin inhibits bacterial protein synthesis by binding to the ribosomal 50S subunit, specifically, the 23S rRNA within the 50S subunit. After binding, tildipirosin interacts with ribosomal RNA (rRNA) and ribosomal proteins adjacent to the peptidyl-transferase enzyme. Thus, like other macrolides, it inhibits protein synthesis by blocking the prolongation and release of developing polypeptides. Tildipirosin has a spectrum of activity that is limited to gram-positive bacteria and some gram-negative bacteria that cause respiratory diseases in cattle and pigs (e.g., *Mannheimia haemolytica, Mycoplasma* spp., *Pasteurella multocida, Actinobacillus pleuropneumoniae, Bordetella bronchiseptica*, and *Haemophilus parasuis*). *Escherichia coli* and *P. aeruginosa* are resistant. Some *Staphylococcus* spp. and *Streptococcus* spp. may be susceptible.

There is evidence for bactericidal activity against *M. haemolytica*, bovine *P. multocida, Histophilus somni, H. parasuis*, and *A. pleuropneumoniae* and bacteriostatic activity against *B. bronchiseptica*.

*Other properties:* Tildipirosin, like other macrolides, exerts therapeutic benefits not solely explainable by antibacterial activity. Like azithromycin, tildipirosin may have multiple immunomodulatory effects that likely contribute to the therapeutic response in respiratory infections, and perhaps other diseases. Other beneficial effects may be caused by enhanced degranulation and apoptosis of neutrophils and inhibition of inflammatory cytokine production. It also may help clear infections by enhancing macrophage functions.

*Pharmacokinetics:* The pharmacokinetic data in cattle list a long half-life (mean, 204 hours, or 8.5-day plasma half-life), with a peak concentration at the label dose of 0.64 mcg/mL and bioavailability from injection in cattle of 79%. The volume of distribution, like most macrolide antibiotics, is large, with a value in cattle of 49 L/kg. The lung concentrations in cattle are more than 150 times the plasma drug concentrations with a half-life of 10 days. Bronchial fluid concentrations are approximately 40 times the plasma drug concentrations, with a half-life of 11 days.

In pigs, the plasma half-life is 106 hours (4.4 days), with a peak concentration of 0.9 mcg/mL after IM injection of 4 mg/kg. The lung concentrations in pigs were approximately 80 times higher than plasma concentrations with a half-life of 6.8 days. The bronchial fluid concentrations were 680 times higher than plasma drug concentrations at 5 days after injection.

## Indications and Clinical Uses

Tildipirosin has been approved for the treatment and control/prevention of cattle with bovine respiratory disease (BRD) associated with *M. haemolytica, P. multocida,* and *H. somni* and in some European countries (but not the United States) for the treatment of pigs with swine respiratory disease (SRD) associated with *A. pleuropneumoniae, P. multocida, B. bronchiseptica*, and *H. parasuis.* The use in other animals for treatment of respiratory disease has not been reported.

Other long-acting macrolide antibiotics used in cattle include tilmicosin, tulathromycin, and gamithromycin.

### Precautionary Information

#### Adverse Reactions and Side Effects

Serious systemic adverse reactions have not been observed. In cattle, tildipirosin injection may cause injection-site swelling and inflammation, which may be severe. Swelling and visible lesions in edible tissue can persist at least 35 days after injection.

Adverse effects may be seen in pigs. See Contraindications and Precautions.

Because of structural similarities between tildipirosin and tilmicosin (both are 16-membered macrolides), cardiotoxic studies were performed in dogs. At 10 mg/kg IM, there was no effect, and at 20 mg/kg, there were changes in pulse pressure. In an oral dose study in dogs, there were no electrocardiogram (ECG) changes after single (300 mg/kg body weight) or repeated (150 or 200 mg/kg daily for 2 days and 200 mg/kg daily for 7 days) doses.

#### Contraindications and Precautions

The FDA-approved label in the United States lists the following precautions: For subcutaneous injection in beef and nonlactating dairy cattle only. Not for use in female dairy cattle 20 months of age or older or in calves to be processed for veal. Do not use tildipirosin (Zuprevo) in swine. Fatal adverse events have been reported after the use of tildipirosin in swine.

#### Drug Interactions

No drug interactions have been reported. Macrolide antibiotics may interfere with cytochrome P450 enzyme activity, but this has not been studied for tildipirosin. Antibacterial activity is decreased in an acidic environment.

## Instructions for Use

In cattle, administer as a single SQ injection in the neck. Do not inject more than 10 mL per injection site. In pigs (in countries where approved), administer as a single IM injection.

## Patient Monitoring and Laboratory Tests

The CLSI breakpoints for susceptible bacteria are ≤4 mcg/mL for *P. multocida* in pigs and *M. haemolytica* in cattle; ≤8 mcg/mL for *B. bronchiseptica* in pigs, *H. somni* in cattle, and *P. multocida* in cattle; and ≤16 mcg/mL for *A. pleuropneumoniae* in pigs.

## Formulations

Tildipirosin is available in a 180-mg/mL (18%) solution for injection for cattle and, in some European countries, 40-mg/mL solution for injection for pigs.

## Stability and Storage

Store in a tightly sealed container, protected from light, and at room temperature.

## Small Animal Dosage

• No small animal doses have been established.

## Large Animal Dosage

### Cattle

• 4 mg/kg (equivalent to 1 mL/100 lb) SQ (neck) as a single injection.

### Pigs

• 4 mg/kg (equivalent to 1 mL/10 kg) IM as a single injection. Check approval status in each country before considering use. It is not approved in the United States.

### Horses

• No dosing information is available for horses.

## Regulatory Information

No milk withdrawal times are established. Do not use in female dairy cattle 20 months of age or older. Do not use in veal calves.
Cattle withdrawal time for meat: 21 days.
Pig withdrawal time for meat: 7 days.

# Tiletamine and Zolazepam
till-eh'tah-meen and zole-az'eh-pam

**Trade and other names:** Telazol and Zoletil

**Functional classification:** Anesthetic

## Pharmacology and Mechanism of Action

Tiletamine and zolazepam is a combination anesthetic with both agents in the same vial for injection. The combination consists of tiletamine (a dissociative anesthetic agent similar in action to ketamine) and zolazepam (a benzodiazepine similar in action to diazepam). Tiletamine with zolazepam produces a short duration (30 minutes) of anesthesia. In cats, the effect of the zolazepam has a longer duration than tiletamine. In dogs, tiletamine has a longer duration than zolazepam. Therefore anesthesia appears to be smoother in cats than in dogs.

## Indications and Clinical Uses

Tiletamine and zolazepam is used for short-term anesthesia in animals. For longer procedures, other drugs should be used. It is usually injected IM in animals for short-term procedures or occasionally for induction when other anesthetic agents are added. The approved uses and doses are based on the FDA-approved labeling for animals, clinical experience, and recommendations from anesthesiology experts. The use in large animals is extralabel but has been tested in small observational studies. (See protocol for pigs listed later.)

## Precautionary Information

### Adverse Reactions and Side Effects

Tiletamine and zolazepam has a wide margin of safety, which is greater in cats than in dogs. The use is also reported in pigs. Side effects include excessive salivation (may be antagonized with atropine), erratic recovery, and muscle twitching. Drying of the cornea may occur unless ophthalmic ointment is applied to the eyes. IM injection in animals can be painful. Adverse reactions have been observed when administered to ferrets.

### Contraindications and Precautions

Low doses do not provide sufficient anesthesia for surgery. For surgical procedures, other anesthetic agents should be added. Do not use in patients with pancreatic disease. Avoid use in ferrets.

### Drug Interactions

No drug interactions have been reported in animals.

## Instructions for Use

Administer by deep IM injection.

## Patient Monitoring and Laboratory Tests

Monitor heart rate and rhythm during anesthesia. Monitor body temperature because of risk of hypothermia.

## Formulations

- Tiletamine and zolazepam is available in 50 mg of each component per milliliter (100 mg total per milliliter).

## Stability and Storage

Store in a tightly sealed container, protected from light, and at room temperature.

## Small Animal Dosage

(All doses listed are based on the combined milligrams of each component.)

### Dogs

- Initial IM dose is 6.6–10 mg/kg for minor procedures.
- Short-term anesthesia: 10–13 mg/kg IM.

### Cats

- 10–12 mg/kg IM for minor procedures and higher doses of 14–16 mg/kg IM for surgery.

## Large Animal Dosage

(All doses listed are based on the combined milligrams of each component.)

### Pigs

- 3.5–6 mg/kg IM. (The addition of a muscle relaxant and sedative is recommended; see later.)
- The TXK protocol for pigs: To prepare this solution, add 2.5 mL of ketamine (100 mg/mL) and 2.5 mL of xylazine (100 mg/mL) to one vial of tiletamine–zolazepam powder. This solution contains 100 mg/mL of tiletamine and ketamine plus 50 mg/mL each of xylazine and zolazepam. Administer this solution IM at a dose of 1 mL per 35–75 kg.

## Regulatory Information

No regulatory information is available. For extralabel use withdrawal interval estimates, contact FARAD at www.FARAD.org.
Schedule III controlled drug

# Tilmicosin Phosphate

til-mye'koe-sin foss'fate

**Trade and other names:** Micotil and Pulmotil AC (for water), Pulmotil tilmicosin premix

**Functional classification:** Antibacterial

## Pharmacology and Mechanism of Action

Tilmicosin is a macrolide antibiotic used in cattle and pigs for respiratory infections. Tilmicosin is a 16-membered macrolide structure (another macrolide, tildipirosin, is also a 16-member macrolide) with two charged nitrogen atoms. Like other macrolides, it inhibits bacterial protein synthesis by binding to the ribosomal 50S subunit, specifically, the 23S rRNA within the 50S subunit. After binding, tildipirosin interacts with rRNA and ribosomal proteins adjacent to the peptidyl-transferase enzyme. Thus, like other macrolides, it inhibits protein synthesis by blocking the prolongation and release of developing polypeptides. Tilmicosin has a spectrum of activity that is limited primarily to gram-positive aerobic bacteria; *Mycoplasma* spp.; and respiratory pathogens such as *P. multocida, M. haemolytica,* and *H. somni.*

*Other properties:* Tilmicosin, like other macrolides, exerts therapeutic benefits not solely explainable by antibacterial activity. Anti-inflammatory effects may include some reduced leukocyte release of inflammatory mediators in the lungs associated with tilmicosin treatment. There also may be reduced prostaglandin synthesis with tilmicosin administration in alveolar macrophages. Other beneficial effects may be caused by enhanced degranulation and apoptosis of neutrophils and inhibition of inflammatory cytokine production. It also may help clear infections by enhancing macrophage functions.

*Pharmacokinetics:* In cattle, tilmicosin has a half-life of 28 hours in plasma from IV treatment and 31 hours after SQ treatment. The volume of distribution is 28 L/kg.

## Indications and Clinical Uses

Tilmicosin is active against respiratory pathogens and is effective for prevention and treatment of BRD and ovine respiratory disease in sheep associated with *M. haemolytica.* One injection has duration of at least 72 hours, based on prolonged half-life. When used to control BRD in calves that are entering feedlots, the use of tilmicosin at the time of feedlot arrival has reduced incidence of respiratory disease in cattle. Tilmicosin can also be added to feed of cattle for the control of BRD associated with *M. haemolytica, P. multocida,* and *H. somni* in groups of beef and nonlactating dairy cattle when active BRD has been diagnosed in at least 10% of the animals in the group.

Tilmicosin (Pulmotil) is used in medicated feed and water for swine for control of SRD associated with *A. pleuropneumoniae, P. multocida,* and *H. parasuis.* It should not be injected in pigs.

Other long-acting macrolide antibiotics used in cattle include gamithromycin, tildipirosin, and tulathromycin.

## Precautionary Information

### Adverse Reactions and Side Effects

Tilmicosin may be cardiotoxic in some animals. Injections to pigs have been fatal because of cardiotoxicity. The cardiac effects are increased heart rate and decreased contractility. However, administration of tilmicosin oral premix in feed of pigs has been safe. In dogs, tilmicosin injections have caused cardiac toxicosis and may be caused by calcium-channel blockade; it was reversed by administration of calcium. In goats, injections greater than 10 mg/kg IM or SQ can cause toxicity. In horses, injections of tilmicosin IM or SQ greater than 10 mg/kg can lead to toxicity.

### Contraindications and Precautions

Do not administer intravenously to any species.

People handling tilmicosin should take precautions to prevent accidental injection. Fatal cardiac reactions caused by injections have been reported in people and accidental injection in people requires immediate treatment. People who receive an accidental injection should be taken to an emergency facility for treatment immediately. Treatment consists of beta-adrenergic agonists (e.g., dobutamine) and supportive care.

Tilmicosin reaches high concentrations in milk for up to 42 days. Do not administer to lactating dairy cattle. Do not administer to goats. Do not allow horses or other equine access to feeds containing tilmicosin. Do not administer to any animals intravenously or death can result.

### Drug Interactions

The cardiac adverse effects are exacerbated by administration of beta blockers such as propranolol. Dobutamine and administration of calcium may offset cardiac effects.

## Instructions for Use

Administer SQ. If a person handling the drug is accidentally injected, consult a physician immediately. Severe cardiac toxicity has occurred in some species of animals. Tilmicosin can also be added to feed and drinking water for pigs.

## Patient Monitoring and Laboratory Tests

Susceptibility information: CLSI breakpoints for susceptible organisms are ≤8 mcg/mL for bovine respiratory pathogens and ≤16 mcg/mL for swine respiratory pathogens.

## Formulations

- Tilmicosin is available in 300-mg/mL injection (Micotil) and 200 g/kg (90.7 g/lb) of premix (Pulmotil). For mixing with water for pigs, it is available as 250 mg/mL of tilmicosin.

## Stability and Storage

Store in a tightly sealed container, protected from light, and at room temperature.

## Small Animal Dosage

- It is not recommended for small animals.

## Large Animal Dosage

### Cattle
- 10–20 mg/kg SQ single dose. Avoid IV or IM administration.
- Added to feed: 568–757 g per ton of feed to provide 12.5 mg/kg body weight for 14 days.

### Sheep
- 10 mg/kg SQ single dose.

### Goats
- Do not use.

### Horses
Do not use. Safety not established.

### Pigs
- Pneumonia: 181–383 g per ton of feed. Feed only this ration for 21 days, beginning at the time of disease outbreak.
- Drinking water: Add 200 mg tilmicosin/L (200 ppm) for 5 consecutive days.

## Regulatory Information
Cattle withdrawal time for meat: 28 days. No withdrawal time established for milk; if injected intramammary to lactating cows, discard milk for a minimum of 82 days.
Pig withdrawal time for meat: 7 days.
Sheep withdrawal time for meat: 28 days.

# Tiludronate Disodium
til-u-droe'nate dye-soe'dee-um

**Trade and other names:** Tildren (veterinary form) and Skelid (human form)

**Functional classification:** Antihypercalcemic

## Pharmacology and Mechanism of Action
Tiludronate is a bisphosphonate drug used in horses for treatment of bone diseases. Drugs in this class also include pamidronate, etidronate, and pyrophosphate. Another equine drug from this class is clodronate. These drugs are characterized by a germinal bisphosphonate bond. Their clinical use resides in their ability to inhibit bone resorption. These drugs decrease bone turnover by inhibiting osteoclast activity, inducing osteoclast apoptosis, retarding bone resorption, and decreasing the rate of osteoporosis. Inhibition of bone resorption is via inhibition of the mevalonate pathway. Bisphosphonates are classified as nitrogen containing and nonnitrogenous based on the structure, with the nitrogen-containing drugs being more potent and associated with more adverse effects. Tiludronate and clodronate (Osphos) are non–nitrogen-containing bisphosphonates. It also may have some anti-inflammatory properties.

*Pharmacokinetics:* Tiludronate has a plasma half-life in horses of 3–7 hours, but bone levels may be retained for months to years. It is excreted by glomerular filtration and not metabolized.

T

## Indications and Clinical Uses

Tiludronate is licensed in countries in Europe and approved in the United States for treatment of palmar foot pain associated with navicular syndrome in horses. It also is used to treat distal tarsal osteoarthritis (bone spavin). Other bisphosphonate drugs are used in people to treat osteoporosis and hypercalcemia of malignancy. Like other drugs in this class, tiludronate is helpful for managing complications associated with pathologic bone resorption. It also may provide pain relief in patients with pathologic bone disease. Another bisphosphonate, clodronate (Osphos), also is approved for treating navicular disease in horses.

Efficacy studies conducted in horses have shown that at a dosage of 0.1 mg/kg for 10 days (1.0 mg total dose), it is effective for treatment of navicular disease and distal tarsal osteoarthritis. Beneficial effects for treating chronic lameness are less certain.

## Precautionary Information

### Adverse Reactions and Side Effects

Reaction to tiludronate has only been reported for horses. After IV infusion, increases in heart rate, restlessness, and transient hypocalcemia have been observed. About 30%–45% of horses administered tiludronate develop signs of colic after IV administration. However, colic signs that have been observed in horses resolved uneventfully. In people, there is some concern that it may result in excessive mineralization and hardening of the bone, which may result in a greater risk of fractures. However, this effect has not been reported for animals. No adverse effects on bone mineral density have been reported.

### Contraindications and Precautions

Do not use in horses with kidney disease because it is excreted by the kidney and could accumulate. After injection, monitor horses for signs of colic. The manufacturer warns that concurrent administration of nonsteroidal anti-inflammatory drugs (NSAIDs) with tiludronate may the increase risk of kidney injury. Use carefully in conditions associated with hypocalcemia. The manufacturer warns that horses with hyperkalemic periodic paralysis may be at an increased risk for adverse reactions, including colic signs, hyperkalemic episodes, and death. Do not use in pregnant mares because the safety in pregnancy has not been evaluated.

*Use in young horses:* The manufacturer states that the safety of tiludronate in horses younger than 4 years of age has not been evaluated. The effect of bisphosphonates on the skeleton of growing horses has not been studied; however, bisphosphonates inhibit osteoclast activity, which impacts bone turnover and may affect bone growth. It is recommended *not* to administer bisphosphonates such as tiludronate in young performance horses because the change in bone metabolism may predispose young horses to fracture. In some racing jurisdictions, these drugs are prohibited in horses younger than 4 years of age. One study that examined clodronate and tiludronate in young horses concluded that tiludronate and clodronate did not appear to significantly impact bone tissue on a structural or cellular level using standard dose and administration schedules in young horses.

### Drug Interactions

Do not mix with solutions containing calcium (e.g., lactated Ringer's solution). Do not administer with NSAIDs (see Contraindications and Precaution). If antacids are used concurrently, magnesium hydroxide and calcium carbonate may reduce effectiveness.

## Instructions for Use

Make sure horses are well hydrated prior to use to avoid kidney injury. For IV infusion, dilute in solvent and infuse slowly over 90 minutes. Observe horses for 4 hours after IV administration for signs of colic.

## Patient Monitoring and Laboratory Tests

Monitor serum calcium and phosphorus. Monitor urea nitrogen, creatinine, urine-specific gravity, and food intake in treated animals.

## Formulations

- Tiludronate is available in 50-mg vials for injection to be reconstituted with 10 mL of diluent.

## Stability and Storage

Store in a tightly sealed container, protected from light, and at room temperature.

## Small Animal Dosage

- No doses have been established for dogs or cats.

## Large Animal Dosage

### Horses

- 1 mg/kg administered as 0.1 mg/kg per day for 10 days intravenously or administer as a single 1-mg/kg IV infusion for one dose. Administer an IV infusion in 1 L of 0.9% saline solution over 30–60 minutes.

## Regulatory Information

In some racing jurisdictions, these drugs are prohibited in horses younger than 4 years of age. Withdrawal times are not established for animals that produce food. For extralabel use withdrawal interval estimates, contact FARAD at www.FARAD.org.

# Tinidazole

tih-nih′dah-zole

**Trade and other names:** Tindamax

**Functional classification:** Antiprotozoal

## Pharmacology and Mechanism of Action

Tinidazole is an antiprotozoal with action similar to metronidazole. It is a second-generation nitroimidazole in which the activity involves generation of free nitroradicals via metabolism that occurs within protozoa. It has action against *Trichomonas* spp., *Giardia* spp., and intestinal protozoal parasites. It also has in vitro activity against anaerobic bacteria and *Helicobacter* spp.

*Pharmacokinetics:* The half-lives are approximately 5.5 hours in horses, 8.5 hours in cats, and 4.5 hours in dogs. Oral absorption in dogs, cats, and horses is approximately 100%.

## Indications and Clinical Uses

Tinidazole is indicated to treat diarrhea and other intestinal problems caused by intestinal protozoa such as *Giardia*, *Trichomonas*, and *Entamoeba* spp. In people, a single dose of tinidazole has been effective for treating infections caused by *Giardia* spp.; however, the single-dose protocol has not been tested in animals. Tinidazole also is active against many anaerobic bacteria and may be used as a substitute for metronidazole in small animals and horses for treatment of a variety of anaerobic infections.

## Precautionary Information

### Adverse Reactions and Side Effects

Tinidazole has similar action as metronidazole. With high doses, it can cause neurologic problems, including ataxia, tremors, nystagmus, and seizures. The CNS signs are related to inhibition of action of GABA and are responsive to benzodiazepines (diazepam). Like other nitroimidazoles, it has the potential to produce mutagenic changes in cells, but this has not been demonstrated in vivo. Nitroimidazoles such as tinidazole have a bitter taste and can cause vomiting and anorexia. However, the bitter taste is not as bad as that of metronidazole.

### Contraindications and Precautions

Do not administer to animals that may be prone to seizures. Do not administer to animals already known to be sensitive to metronidazole. Do not administer to pregnant animals.

### Drug Interactions

Like other nitroimidazoles, it can potentiate the effects of warfarin and cyclosporine via inhibition of drug metabolism.

## Instructions for Use

Give oral dose with food to minimize the unpleasant taste and decrease nausea.

## Patient Monitoring and Laboratory Tests

No specific monitoring is necessary. Most anaerobic bacteria have MIC values below 2 mcg/mL.

## Formulations

- Tinidazole is available in 250- and 500-mg tablets.

## Stability and Storage

Tablets have been crushed and mixed with flavorings to improve palatability. These suspensions are stable for 7 days.

## Small Animal Dosage

### Dogs

- 15 mg/kg q12h PO. Duration of treatment is not known for all conditions, but *Giardia* infections can be treated with 5 days of treatment or less.

### Cats

- 15 mg/kg q24h PO. The duration of therapy depends on whether one is treating *Giardia* infection (5 days) or other anaerobic infections (longer than 5 days).

## Large Animal Dosage

### Horses

- 10–15 mg/kg q12h PO.

## Regulatory Information

Do not administer to animals that produce food. Administration of nitroimidazoles to animals intended for food is prohibited.

# Tissue Plasminogen Activator
**Trade and other names:** tPA and Retavase
**Functional classification:** Anticoagulant, fibrinolytic

## Pharmacology and Mechanism of Action
Tissue plasminogen activator, usually referred to as tPA, is a thrombolytic agent. It activates plasminogen in tissues to dissolve clot formation. It is a synthetically derived (recombinant DNA origin) form of human tissue-type plasminogen activator. The advantage of tPA over other clot dissolving drugs is that tPA acts only at the tissue site where thrombin and fibrin are present, thus preventing more systemic effects.

*Pharmacokinetics:* The pharmacokinetics have not been studied in animals. It is expected that, as in people, the half-life and duration of action is short. In people, the half-life is 40–50 minutes for elimination.

## Indications and Clinical Uses
Tissue plasminogen activator is used in people to treat acute stages of myocardial infarction. The other uses include pulmonary embolism, ischemic stroke, arterial thrombosis, to remove clots from occluded IV catheters, and occasionally for other disease in which thromboembolism occurs.

In animals, the use is infrequent, but it is used in dogs and cats to dissolve blots associated with thromboembolism. In cats, this includes aortic thromboembolism, but there has been no convincing evidence that treatment with tPA is superior to other standard care protocols. In dogs, specific uses have not been defined, but it could potentially be used for diseases that are associated with thromboembolic episodes.

The doses and protocols used in animals have not been rigorously tested. The cost is very high, which prevents more frequent use. The use in animals is based on limited clinical experience and observations from clinical experts. It is usually administered with antiplatelet drugs (e.g., clopidogrel) and anticoagulants (e.g., heparin).

## Precautionary Information
### Adverse Reactions and Side Effects
Tissue plasminogen activator is very effective at dissolving blood clots and causes serious bleeding episodes with excessive use or if proper monitoring is not performed. In cats, there is a high frequency of adverse effects, some of which have been fatal. The problems identified in cats arise because of reperfusion injury, release of cytokines after blood flow is restored, and hyperkalemia.

### Contraindications and Precautions
Do not administer to animals that have any ongoing bleeding problems. Do not administer unless the patient can be monitored carefully by clinical experts who are experienced with the use of tPA. If administered with other agents that impair clot formation, serious bleeding can result.

### Drug Interactions
The use with any other drug that inhibits coagulation and clot formation exacerbates bleeding.

T

## Instructions for Use

If tPA is selected for use, treatment should begin as promptly as possible. The vial should be reconstituted by mixing 50 mg of tPA with 50 mL of sterile water. Use water without preservatives. This provides a concentration of 1 mg/mL. If larger vials are used, reconstitute 100 mg of tPA with 100 mL of sterile water. There will be some slight foaming, which is expected during reconstitution. This solution can be injected directly IV or may be diluted further to 0.5 mg/mL with 0.9% sodium chloride solution or 5% dextrose solution. Mix the vials with gentle swirling but not vigorous agitation.

Use reconstituted or diluted solutions within 8 hours. Discard any unused solutions.

## Patient Monitoring and Laboratory Tests

Monitor carefully for any signs of bleeding. Monitor any needle puncture sites for signs of bleeding.

## Formulations

- tPA is available as in vials containing 50 or 100 mg. 100 mg is equivalent to 58 million units.

## Stability and Storage

Store the vials containing lyophilized powder at less than 30°C or refrigerate at 2°C–8°C

## Small Animal Dosage

### Dogs and Cats

- 1–1.5 mg/kg IV. Infuse the first half of the dose over 1 hour, with 10%–20% of this dose in the first 10 minutes and then the remaining dose over the next 2 hours.

## Large Animal Dosage

- No large animal doses have been investigated.

## Regulatory Information

Do not administer to animals that produce food.

## Tobramycin Sulfate

toe-brah-mye'sin sul'fate

**Trade and other names:** Nebcin and Tobi (human nebulization product)

**Functional classification:** Antibacterial

## Pharmacology and Mechanism of Action

Tobramycin is an aminoglycoside antibacterial drug. Like other aminoglycosides, tobramycin is rapidly bactericidal. It binds to the 30S ribosomal subunit in bacteria. Through this action, it causes a misreading of the genetic code and inhibits bacterial protein synthesis. Another mechanism important for gram-negative bacteria is to disrupt the cell surface biofilm, particularly on gram-negative bacteria, to produce disruption, loss of cell wall integrity, and a rapid bactericidal effect. Magnesium and calcium are important to cross-bridge adjacent lipopolysaccharide molecules.

Positive-charged aminoglycosides competitively displace $Ca^{2+}$ and $Mg^{2+}$ and destabilize the bacteria outer membrane. Therefore, death of the bacteria is caused by a cell surface effect rather than inhibition of the ribosome. This property is not as prominent for gram-positive bacteria unless administered with a cell wall–disrupting agent such as vancomycin or a beta-lactam antibiotic. It is concentration dependent in its antibacterial action. Tobramycin has similar activity (MIC in same range) as gentamicin against *Klebsiella pneumoniae* and *E. coli*. Tobramycin is usually more active against *P. aeruginosa* than gentamicin. Generally, if an organism is susceptible to tobramycin, it is also susceptible to amikacin.

*Pharmacokinetics:* Tobramycin pharmacokinetics in animals indicates that it has similar clearance and distribution as other aminoglycosides. In horses, the half-life is 4.6 hours, with a volume of distribution of 0.18 L/kg.

## Indications and Clinical Uses

Tobramycin, like other aminoglycosides, is used to treat serious systemic infections caused by gram-negative bacteria. It is often administered simultaneously with beta-lactam antibiotics to broaden the spectrum to include more gram-positive bacteria and anaerobes. It may produce a synergistic effect against some bacteria, but whether or not this translates to clinical effects is uncertain.

The infections treated with tobramycin include pneumonia, soft tissue infections, and sepsis. Like many off-label antibiotics in animals, the use in animals has been primarily derived from empirical use and from PK–PD information. Tobramycin has also been used topically. It has been used in nebulizing solutions for respiratory infections. For nebulization, there is a unique formulation used in people (Tobi) that is without preservatives and is intended to treat infections caused by *P. aeruginosa* in the airways of human cystic fibrosis patients. After administration by this route, tobramycin remains concentrated primarily in the airways, and concentrations in plasma or serum are very low and unlikely to cause toxicity. This method of administration has been used in veterinary patients, but the efficacy has not been reported.

### Precautionary Information

**Adverse Reactions and Side Effects**

Nephrotoxicity is the most dose-limiting toxicity. Ensure that patients have adequate fluid and electrolyte balance during therapy. Ototoxicity and vestibulotoxicity also are possible.

**Contraindications and Precautions**

Avoid use in patients with kidney disease. Aminoglycosides may exacerbate already-existing renal compromise. When used with anesthetic agents, neuromuscular blockade is possible. Do not mix in a vial or syringe with other antibiotics.

**Drug Interactions**

Avoid mixing in vials with other drugs. It is incompatible with other antibiotics, and inactivation occurs rapidly.

### Instructions for Use

Inject intravenously or intramuscularly. Synergistic effects with beta-lactam antibiotics have been demonstrated in vitro, but it is not known if this translates to a clinical effect. For nebulization treatment of respiratory infections, dosing guidelines for animals have not been determined. In people (including pediatric patients), the nebulization protocol uses an administration of 300 mg of tobramycin (total dose) twice daily for 28 days. The solution used for nebulization (in individual packets with no preservatives) is called Tobi, but it is more expensive than injectable formulations. Tobramycin injectable has been used instead, but it contains preservatives that could induce bronchospasm. If this form is used in animals, use diluted tobramycin with 3 mL of saline and administer albuterol before nebulization to decrease bronchospasm.

## Patient Monitoring and Laboratory Tests

Susceptibility testing: The CLSI MIC value breakpoint for susceptibility is ≤4 mcg/mL. Monitor blood urea nitrogen, creatinine, and urine for evidence of kidney injury. Blood concentrations can be monitored to detect problems with systemic clearance. When monitoring trough levels in a patient dosed once daily, the trough levels should be below the limit of detection. Alternatively, measure half-life from samples taken at 1 hour and 2–4 hours after dosing. Clearance should be above 1.0 mL/kg/min, and the half-life should be less than 2 hours.

## Formulations

• Tobramycin is available in 40-mg/mL injections. The solution for nebulization (Tobi) is 60 mg/mL contained in 5-mL ampules.

## Stability and Storage

Store in a tightly sealed container, protected from light, and at room temperature. Store powder at room temperature. Reconstituted solutions are stable for 24 hours at room temperature and 96 hours refrigerated. Do not use discolored solutions. Tobramycin sulfate diluted in fluids can be frozen and stable for 30 days. Ophthalmic solutions have been compounded and shown to be stable for 90 days. Do not mix in a vial or syringe with other antibiotics, especially beta-lactam agents (penicillins and cephalosporins) because inactivation may occur.

## Small Animal Dosage

### Dogs

• 9–14 mg/kg q24h SQ, IM, or IV.
• Nebulization therapy is sometimes used in small animals. (See Instructions for Use for details on nebulization therapy.)

### Cats

• 5–8 mg/kg q24h SQ, IM, or IV.

## Large Animal Dosage

### Horses

• 4 mg/kg attains targeted concentrations for most bacteria, but to reach the target for bacteria at the breakpoint of 4 mcg/mL, a dose of 7.2 mg/kg is needed. These doses may be administered IV or IM once daily.

## Regulatory Information

Do not administer to animals intended for food or animals that produce food. Other drugs in this class require extralabel withdrawal times of 18 months.

# Tocainide Hydrochloride
toe-kay′nide hye-droe-klor′ide

**Trade and other names:** Tonocard

**Functional classification:** Antiarrhythmic

## Pharmacology and Mechanism of Action

Tocainide is an antiarrhythmic drug used infrequently in veterinary medicine. Tocainide is a class Ib antiarrhythmic. Like other class I antiarrhythmic drugs, such as lidocaine, it blocks sodium channels in cardiac tissues and inhibits phase 0 depolarization to suppress spontaneous depolarization.

## Indications and Clinical Uses

Tocainide is an oral substitute used for treatment and control of ventricular arrhythmias when injectable class I antiarrhythmic agents cannot be used. The use in veterinary medicine has been uncommon. Use in animals has been primarily derived from empirical use and experience in humans. There are no well-controlled clinical studies or efficacy trials to document clinical effectiveness. If an oral antiarrhythmic agent is needed in animals, consider mexiletine or sotalol (depending on the underlying clinical circumstances) as an alternative.

## Precautionary Information

### Adverse Reactions and Side Effects

In dogs, anorexia and GI adverse effects have been reported. In one study, 35% of dogs showed GI adverse effects. Arrhythmias, vomiting, and ataxia also are possible.

### Contraindications and Precautions

Use cautiously in animals that are also receiving beta blockers. Do not use in patients with heart block.

### Drug Interactions

No drug interactions have been reported for animals, but the use is uncommon, and it is possible that a full range of adverse effects is not known.

## Instructions for Use

Tocainide has limited experience in animals. However, some small clinical observational studies demonstrated efficacy.

## Patient Monitoring and Laboratory Tests

If monitoring is possible, therapeutic concentrations reported for people are 6–10 mcg/mL.

## Formulations

- Tocainide is available in 400- and 600-mg tablets.

## Stability and Storage

Store in a tightly sealed container, protected from light, and at room temperature.

## Small Animal Dosage

### Dogs

- 15–20 mg/kg q8h PO.

### Cats

- No dose has been established.

## Large Animal Dosage

- No dose has been reported for large animals.

## Regulatory Information

No regulatory information is available. For extralabel use withdrawal interval estimates, contact FARAD at www.FARAD.org.

RCI Classification: 4

# Toceranib Phosphate
toe ser′ a nib

**Trade and other names:** Palladia

**Functional classification:** Anticancer agent

## Pharmacology and Mechanism of Action

Toceranib is an anticancer agent, approved for dogs for mast cell tumors, but also used for other tumors. It is approved for treatment of grade II or III cutaneous mast cell tumors in dogs. Toceranib (Palladia) is a receptor tyrosine kinase (RTK) inhibitor that kills tumor cells and decreases the blood supply to the tumor. The antiangiogenic properties occur via inhibition of RTK activity (otherwise known as vascular endothelial growth factor [VEGF]). These properties produce antiangiogenic and antiproliferative effects that limit growth of the tumor. Toceranib also produces a significant decrease in regulatory T cells in dogs with cancer, which may increase immune surveillance. An additional mechanism to explain the response to toceranib is the inhibition of signaling of $c$-KIT, which is a pro-oncogene coding RTK. This effect produces direct antitumor and anti-angiogenesis properties.

Another drug that had been used for the same indication in dogs, was known as masitinib (Kinavet-CA1, Masivet). However, this drug has been withdrawn by the FDA.

*Pharmacokinetics:* After administering toceranib to dogs, it is widely distributed (volume of distribution greater than 20 L/kg) and has a half-life of approximately 16–17 hours. It has good oral absorption (77%) and high protein binding (91%–93%). Feeding does not affect oral absorption. High concentrations appear in the bile, liver, and feces and indicate that it is primarily eliminated by metabolism, and there is little drug excreted in the urine (renal clearance is approximately 7%).

## Indications and Clinical Uses

Toceranib is an approved anticancer agent for dogs. The use and safety has been established in clinical studies for grade II or III cutaneous mast cell tumors. Many dogs are also treated with corticosteroids (prednisolone). Alternative drugs also may be used for mast cell tumors, such as vinblastine plus prednisone. During treatment of mast cell tumors, antihistamines (e.g., cetirizine) can also be used to minimize the effects of histamine.

Although toceranib is approved for mast cell tumors in dogs, some clinicians have used it to treat adenocarcinoma, melanoma, mammary carcinoma, soft tissue sarcoma, and anal gland adenocarcinoma; however, efficacy for these indications has not yet been established.

Toceranib has been used in cats to treat epithelial tumors, squamous cell carcinoma, and mast cell tumors (in combination with corticosteroids). Dosage suggestions are listed later. There is not sufficient information available to document efficacy or safety in cats, but preliminary results were a low overall response rate.

## Precautionary Information

### Adverse Reactions and Side Effects

Dogs with mast cell tumors often have GI problems associated with the tumor and treatment. Therefore many dogs are treated simultaneously with antihistamines and drugs to suppress stomach acid (e.g., $H_2$ blockers or proton pump inhibitors). The most common adverse effects are diarrhea, loss of appetite, lameness, musculoskeletal pain, weight loss, and blood in the feces. In people, tyrosine kinase inhibitors have been associated with proteinuria, thrombosis, hemorrhage, and systemic hypertension (discussed later).

Tyrosine kinase inhibitors may cause systemic hypertension in some animals. The mechanism may be related to decreased NO availability. VEGF increases production of NO by endothelial cells, which helps to regulate blood pressure. Decreased NO caused by administration of tyrosine kinase inhibitors have a potential to cause systemic hypertension. This may occur in dogs, and they should be screened and monitored for this possibility during treatment.

Toceranib can disrupt the hypothalamic–pituitary–thyroid axis in dogs by decreasing blood flow to the thyroid and altered iodine uptake. Therefore, as noted in the monitoring section, check the $T_4$ and free $T_4$ during treatment.

Adverse effects in cats are similar as in dogs. These effects include vomiting, decreased appetite, and mild increase in alanine aminotransferase and alkaline phosphatase enzymes.

### Contraindications and Precautions

Daily dosing should not be administered because of frequency of adverse events. Administration every other day is better tolerated. Toceranib should not be administered during pregnancy. People handling the drug, especially pregnant women, should receive proper instructions about the drug's adverse effects.

### Drug Interactions

No drug interactions have been reported for animals. Metabolism is primarily via flavin monooxygenase, which is not typically involved in drug–drug interactions. It is not known if toceranib may be responsible for drug–drug interactions that involve the cytochrome P450 system.

## Instructions for Use

Toceranib is approved for cutaneous mast cell tumor in dogs. There is clinical use for other tumors, but efficacy has not yet been established for other uses. Administer every other day to minimize the adverse effects. If adverse effects occur at the initial dose, a lower dose (e.g., 2.5 mg/kg) may be considered.

## Patient Monitoring and Laboratory Tests

No specific monitoring is necessary. If assays are available, the targeted plasma drug concentration is 40 ng/mL or greater for 48 hours. Because of potential effects on the thyroid, check the $T_4$ and free $T_4$ during treatment.

## Formulations

Toceranib is available in 10-, 15-, and 50-mg tablets, which are film coated and should not be split.

## Stability and Storage

Store in a tightly sealed container, protected from light, and at room temperature. Toceranib is only soluble at low pH values (pH less than 3). If mixed with other vehicles, it precipitates at higher pH values. Studies on compounded oral formulations of toceranib phosphate from compounding pharmacies found the strengths of formulations (capsules, tablets, suspensions) to be lower than the acceptable range.

## Small Animal Dosage

### Dogs

- The approved label dosage is 3.25 mg/kg PO every other day. However, medical oncologists recommend a lower dosage of 2.5–2.75 mg/kg per dose and treat on a schedule of 3 days per week (e.g., Monday, Wednesday, Friday). The minimum effective dosage is 2.2 mg/kg every other day. If adverse reactions occur, discontinue the drug (for up to 2 weeks) and reinstate treatment at a lower dose.

### Cats

- 2.5–2.75 mg/kg given three times per week or once every other day.

## Large Animal Dosage

- No dose has been reported for large animals.

## Regulatory Information

Do not administer to food-producing animals.

# Toltrazuril
tole-traz′yoo′ril

**Trade and other names:** Baycox

**Functional classification:** Antiprotozoal

## Pharmacology and Mechanism of Action

Toltrazuril is an antiprotozoal drug that is used as a coccidiostat and to treat other protozoan infections in animals. Toltrazuril is a triazinone derivative that is effective for *Isospora* spp. and coccidiosis, *Toxoplasma gondii,* and *Eimeria* spp. Toltrazuril is a derivative of another drug, ponazuril, that is also used for the same conditions. Toltrazuril sulfone (ponazuril) is found in serum and cerebrospinal fluid of treated horses. See Ponazuril for more details.

## Indications and Clinical Uses

Toltrazuril has been used as a treatment of equine protozoal myeloencephalitis (EPM) caused by *Sarcocystis neurona*. However, it is recommended to use an approved drug, ponazuril (Marquis) for treatment of horses instead of administering toltrazuril.

Toltrazuril has been used in puppies and kittens for treating intestinal protozoal infections. For treatment of coccidial infections in kittens, it has been administered at 30 mg/kg once or 15 mg/kg once daily for 3 days and then repeated again 10 days later. It has been administered successfully to puppies at 10, 20, or 30 mg/kg in 4-week-old puppies.

## Precautionary Information

### Adverse Reactions and Side Effects

Administration of 50 mg/kg to horses (5 and 10 times the recommended dose) produced minor adverse effects, according to the manufacturer. There were minimal changes in the serum analysis.

### Contraindications and Precautions

No contraindications are reported for animals.

### Drug Interactions

No drug interactions have been reported in animals.

## Instructions for Use

Although toltrazuril has been used in horses, the approved drug ponazuril is preferred for use.

## Patient Monitoring and Laboratory Tests

No specific monitoring is necessary. Fecal analysis should be performed to assess the effects for treating intestinal protozoa.

## Formulations

- Toltrazuril is not currently available in commercial formulations in the United States for horses. It is available in suspension for poultry and livestock in other countries. It has been imported to the United States after permission from the FDA.

## Stability and Storage

Store in a tightly sealed container, protected from light, and at room temperature. Stability of compounded formulations has not been evaluated.

## Small Animal Dosage

### Cats

- Treatment of toxoplasmosis: 5–10 mg/kg q24h PO for 2 days.
- Coccidia in kittens: 30 mg/kg once or 15 mg/kg once daily for 3 days; then repeated again 10 days later.

### Dogs

- Puppies, treatment of intestinal protozoa: 10–30 mg/kg q24h PO for 3 days.

## Large Animal Dosage

### Horses

- EPM caused by *S. neurona*: 5–10 mg/kg (7.5 mg/kg for most horses) q24h PO for a minimum of 30 days.

## Regulatory Information

No regulatory information is available. For extralabel use withdrawal interval estimates, contact FARAD at www.FARAD.org.

# Torsemide
tor′sem-ide

**Trade and other names:** Demadex

**Functional classification:** Diuretic

## Pharmacology and Mechanism of Action

Torsemide is a high-ceiling loop diuretic with properties and mechanism of action similar to furosemide, except that it is more potent ($10\times$) and longer-acting. Like furosemide, it inhibits the $Na^+/K^+/2Cl^-$ cotransporter in the ascending thick loop of Henle. It is considered *a high-ceiling diuretic* because it is more effective than other classes of diuretics. Torsemide decreases the sodium, chloride, and potassium reabsorption from the tubule. Subsequently, these ions are retained in the renal tubule and presented to the distal nephron. Dilute urine is produced because water is retained in the tubule when it reaches the distal tubule. In addition, there is an associated urine loss of $Mg^{2+}$ and $Ca^{2+}$. Torsemide is primarily used in place of furosemide because it has greater potency than furosemide, is longer acting, and can be used in refractory cases.

Additional properties include vasodilation, decreased cardiac remodeling, and anti-aldosterone effects, perhaps by direct effects on aldosterone.

*Pharmacokinetics:* In people, it has a half-life of 3.5 hours. It is highly absorbed orally with a peak concentration at 1 hour and 99% protein binding. In dogs, it has a long half-life of 8 hours (compared with 1–2 hours for furosemide), which contributes to a duration of action for 12 hours. Oral absorption is 80%–100%. In horses, torsemide has a half-life of approximately 8–10 hours and a peak concentration of 10 mcg/mL. Oral absorption in horses is high.

## Indications and Clinical Uses

In small animals, torsemide is used in place of furosemide for refractory cases that require a longer duration of effect. It has been used in dogs when furosemide becomes ineffective (diuretic resistance) or if the dosages of furosemide exceed 4 mg/kg per day (or according to other sources, greater than 6–8 mg/kg per day).

Torsemide is also more potent and requires less of a dose than furosemide. Conditions appropriate for torsemide are mostly in dogs with stage C or D congestive heart failure (CHF). However, it may also be considered to treat conditions that cause edema, including pulmonary edema, liver disease, heart disease, and vascular disease.

Torsemide increases potassium and calcium excretion and is used to treat hyperkalemia and hypercalcemia.

There is no established use of torsemide for acute kidney disease treatment.

Although furosemide is used to treat exercise-induced pulmonary hemorrhage in horses, torsemide is not allowed by racing authorities for this use. It has been considered for oral treatment in horses for other uses in which furosemide might be used, and doses are listed in the dosing section; however, there are no clinical trials to compare furosemide with torsemide.

## Precautionary Information

### Adverse Reactions and Side Effects

Adverse effects are primarily related to diuretic effect (loss of fluid and electrolytes). In dogs, hyponatremia can occur. In horses, there is a risk of hypokalemia and metabolic acidosis.

### Contraindications and Precautions

Administer conservatively in animals receiving ACE inhibitors to decrease the risk of azotemia. Repeated administration may increase aldosterone levels via activation of RAAS, but this may be less than with furosemide.

### Drug Interactions

There are no specific drug interactions identified for torsemide use in animals. It is assumed that similar drug interactions that affect furosemide could affect torsemide. (See Furosemide for additional details.)

## Instructions for Use

Torsemide is used in dogs when patients become refractory to furosemide, or if the dose of furosemide is greater than 4 mg/kg per day (or 6–8 mg/kg per day in some references). When switching from furosemide to torsemide, take the total daily dose of furosemide and divide by 10 and divide this into twice daily administration, PO. For example, if the total daily dose of furosemide is 100 mg, this translates to 5 mg/kg of torsemide q12h PO.

## Patient Monitoring and Laboratory Tests

Monitor electrolyte concentrations (particularly potassium) and hydration status in patients during treatment.

## Formulations

- Torsemide is available in 5-, 10-, 20-, and 100-mg tablet sizes.
- Injection: 10 mg/mL.
- Compounded formulation: 5-mg/mL suspension prepared in Ora Plus and Ora Sweet vehicles in a 1:1 ratio. If not buffered, this suspension degrades in 7 days, but at a pH of 8.3, it is stable for 90 days stored at room temperature or in a refrigerator.

## Stability and Storage

Store in a tightly sealed container, protected from light, and at room temperature. Do not mix with acidic solutions. In a compounded formulation, the buffered suspension for oral administration had a 90-day beyond-use date.

## Small Animal Dosage

**Dogs**

- 0.2 mg/kg q12h PO. When switching from furosemide to torsemide, take the total daily dose of furosemide and divide by 10 and administer twice daily PO. (See Instructions for Use, above.)

**Cats**

- No dose has been reported. The dose for dogs could be considered by referring to dosing guidelines.

## Large Animal Dosage

**Horses**

- 0.5–1 mg/kg q12h PO.

**Cattle**

- Doses for cattle have not been established.

## Regulatory Information

There are no withdrawal times available for food-producing animals. Consult FARAD at www.FARAD.org for information regarding withdrawal time after extralabel use.

# Tramadol Hydrochloride
tram′ah-dole

**Trade and other names:** Ultram, and generic brands; outside the United States, Tramadol and Altadol

**Functional classification:** Analgesic

## Pharmacology and Mechanism of Action

Tramadol is an oral analgesic used for treatment of pain in dogs, cats, horses, and occasionally zoo and exotic animals. Tramadol is a racemic mixture that has a complicated mechanism of action. It has some mu-opioid receptor action, but this effect is 10 times lower than codeine and 6000 times lower than morphine. Tramadol also inhibits the reuptake of norepinephrine (NE) and serotonin (5-HT) and produces secondary effects on alpha$_2$-adrenergic receptors in pain pathways. One isomer has greater effect on 5-HT reuptake and greater affinity for mu-opiate receptors. The other isomer is more potent for NE reuptake and less active for inhibiting 5-HT reuptake. Taken together, the effects of tramadol may be explained through inhibition of 5-HT reuptake, action on alpha$_2$ receptors and mild activity on opiate mu-receptors, but the contribution of each of these mechanisms for treatment of pain in animals is undetermined.

Tramadol has as many as 11 metabolites. One metabolite (O-desmethyl tramadol, also called M1) may have greater opiate effects than the parent drug (e.g., 200–300 times greater opiate effect than tramadol), but this activity is still lower than morphine. In animals and humans that produce this metabolite in sufficient amounts, some analgesic action may be attributed to opiate-mediated effects from the active metabolite. The other metabolites have not been shown to have active analgesic activity.

A drug with similar structure and activity as tramadol is tapentadol (Nucynta). Tapentadol is used for moderate pain in people (50–200 mg q4–6h), but, except for studies in experimental animals, its use has not been reported in animals.

*Pharmacokinetics:* The pharmacokinetics of tramadol and metabolites have been studied extensively in dogs, horses, cats, and some exotic animals. The pharmacokinetics are inconsistent among studies, with variation in clearance, oral absorption, and metabolism to the active metabolite among studies within and between species. Most studies agree that the active metabolite (M1) in dogs is a minor metabolite and contributes little, if any, to the analgesic effects. In most studies, the concentrations of this metabolite were either too low to quantify or nonexistent. Tramadol's half-life in dogs is approximately 1.0–2.7 hours with oral absorption as high as 65%, but variable, and as low as 2.6%, depending on the study.

In cats, the half-life is 3–4 hours and they produce higher and more sustained concentrations of the active metabolite (M1) than other animals, presumably because of differences in their ability to clear the metabolite. The concentration of the active metabolite in cats parallels the concentrations of tramadol. The studies in horses have produced conflicting results. Some studies in horses show that the levels of the active metabolite were low or undetectable. In horses, the oral absorption has been extremely variable, ranging from 3% to 64%, but in most studies, it has been low. The half-life also has been highly variable in horses ranging from 2–10 hours in nine studies. In most studies, the half-life in horses is short at 2–2.5 hours.

## Indications and Clinical Uses

Tramadol has been used as an analgesic in people, dogs, cats, horses, and minor species (e.g., rabbits, goats, birds). It is an alternative analgesic to pure opiate analgesics and NSAIDs in patients that require treatment for mild to moderate pain. In people, it is regarded as a mild analgesic, but the pharmacokinetics of tramadol are different in people compared with animals, and clinical effects in humans cannot necessarily be extrapolated to animals. In animal studies, both clinical and experimental, the results have been variable and inconsistent to demonstrate its effectiveness as an analgesic. The studies have varied in the dose, route, and pain stimulus evaluated. There has been some evidence of analgesia after administration for treating pain associated with elective surgery, but there is a lack of evidence for an antinociceptive effect when experimental models of pain have been used. When oral administration was tested for treating osteoarthritis in dogs, efficacy has been poor or produced only mild benefit. When tested in dogs for treating pain from orthopedic surgery, the results have been inconsistent with some studies showing little benefit and other studies showing a mild benefit. The clearance is increased with repeated administration in dogs, which makes chronic treatment less effective than short-term treatment. Some studies that have demonstrated efficacy have used injectable formulations (at 2–4 mg/kg) rather than oral forms, but injectable formulations are not available in North America. It may be more effective when used with an NSAID or other analgesics such as ketamine or alpha$_2$ agonists. Tramadol has also been administered by the epidural route (diluted in saline) in horses, dogs, and cats (1–2 mg/kg). Although some analgesic was documented in these studies, the effects and pharmacokinetics were similar to other parenteral routes of administration, and it is assumed that tramadol is rapidly distributed systemically after epidural administration.

Cats produce more of the active opiate metabolite (O-desmethyl tramadol) than other animal species. Tramadol administration may produce opiate effects in cats, and limited clinical trials suggest some efficacy. It has improved outcomes in cats with osteoarthritis at 2 mg/kg twice daily for 5 days, but higher doses were less effective. Adverse effects occurred in 70% of treated cats and included euphoria, dysphoria, sedation, decreased appetite, and diarrhea.

In horses, the efficacy of tramadol has been variable and evaluated only in small observational studies. It may produce transient analgesia, but there has been significant variation among horses. Tramadol is not a routinely used analgesic in horses. It was not effective in antinociceptive studies. However, some clinical use has been documented. When tested for treatment of laminitis in horses, it had only limited efficacy when used alone at a dosage of 5 mg/kg q12h PO but had greater efficacy when combined with a ketamine infusion (ketamine dosage, 0.6 mg/kg/h infusion).

## Precautionary Information

### Adverse Reactions and Side Effects

In cats, some vomiting, behavior changes, excitement, and mydriasis may be observed, which are dose related. Both euphoria and dysphoria have been observed in cats. In horses, there may be short-term (approximately 20–40 minutes) agitation, head nodding, decreased gut sounds, trembling, muscle fasciculation, tachycardia, sweating, and ataxia. The effects in horses are most prominent after a rapid IV injection and minimized if the injection is administered slowly over 10 minutes. In dogs, adverse effects have been rare. Some sedation has been observed, which is dose related. There have been minimal cardiovascular or GI problems in dogs. At very high doses in dogs, seizures may occur. If adverse effects occur, they are only partially antagonized by naloxone.

### Contraindications and Precautions

Use cautiously with other drugs that have CNS-depressing effects, such as opiates, alpha$_2$ agonists, or serotonin uptake inhibitors (e.g., antidepressants and behavior-modifying drugs). Tramadol may potentiate their actions. Use cautiously in animals with seizure disorders because high doses can lower the threshold for a seizure. Metabolites may be eliminated via the urine. Use with caution in animals with kidney disease.

T

**Drug Interactions**

Drug interactions are possible because of the complex metabolism of tramadol in animals. Fluconazole has been shown to inhibit the metabolism of tramadol to the inactive metabolites and increase the concentration of the active metabolite (M1) in dogs. This may occur with other drugs that have a capability to inhibit cytochrome P450 enzymes (see Appendix I). Administration of cimetidine or ketoconazole to dogs increased the oral bioavailability but did not increase the concentrations of the active metabolite, M1.

Other drug interactions have not been reported in animals, but because of multiple effects from tramadol (serotonin reuptake inhibition, adrenergic effects, and opiate effects), interactions are possible with other drugs that act via similar mechanisms. Serotonin syndrome is theoretically possible when used with other serotonin reuptake inhibitors (SSRIs), but such interactions have not been reported in animals. It has been used safely with NSAIDs. It has been administered with inhalant anesthetics without any signs of adverse drug interaction.

## Instructions for Use

Dosing information is based on experimental studies in dogs, cats, and horses and some clinical studies. In most animals the oral immediate-release tablets are administered either whole or crushed and mixed with a vehicle. In some countries an injectable formulation is available that has been injected IV, IM, SQ, and epidurally. Tramadol ER tablets have been used in people, but in dogs, these tablets show delayed absorption and plasma levels five times less than people at equivalent (mg/kg) doses. Therefore, ER tablets for people may be inequitable in dogs and cats.

## Patient Monitoring and Laboratory Tests

No specific monitoring is necessary. Tramadol is not routinely measured, but effective concentrations have been reported to be in ranges of 200–400 ng/mL for tramadol and 20–40 ng/mL for the active metabolite (M1).

## Formulations

- Tramadol immediate-release tablets are available in 50-mg tablets.
- Tramadol ER is available in 100-, 200-, or 300-mg tablets.
- Injection (not available in the United States): In Europe and other countries, an injectable formulation is available as a 50-mg/mL injection that can be diluted further in 0.9% saline solution for IV administration.
- Compounded formulations of tramadol have been prepared in sterile water at a concentration of 10 mg/mL. This solution is stable up to 1 year if stored in the refrigerator protected from light.

## Stability and Storage

Store in a tightly sealed container, protected from light, and at room temperature. Tramadol is water soluble. When mixed with aqueous vehicles, it has maintained potency and is stable for weeks. However, stability of compounded formulations that may contain flavorings and other excipients has not been evaluated.

## Small Animal Dosage

### Dogs

- 5 mg/kg q6–8h PO. If an injectable form is available at 4 mg/kg IV q6–8h.

## Cats

- Start at 2 mg/kg and increase up to 4 mg/kg q8–12h PO. When injectable forms have been available, it also has been injected at a dosage of 2 mg/kg IV and 2–4 mg/kg SQ q8h.

### Large Animal Dosage
**Horses**

- 2 mg/kg IV (slowly) and 4–5 mg/kg PO. In horses, the optimum dosing interval is not known, but because of the short half-life, every 6 hours may be appropriate and extended to q12h in patients that respond favorably. Do not exceed 2 mg/kg IV or 5 mg/kg PO in horses.

### Regulatory Information
Tramadol was moved to Drug Enforcement Administration–controlled drug status in 2015. It is now a Schedule IV controlled drug.

It is not recommended for food animals, but the half-life in most animals is short, and extended withdrawal times may not be necessary in food-producing animals. For extralabel use withdrawal interval estimates, contact FARAD at www.FARAD.org.

RCI Classification: 2

# Trandolapril
tran-doe'lah-pril

**Trade and other names:** Mavik

**Functional classification:** Vasodilator, ACE inhibitor

## Pharmacology and Mechanism of Action
Trandolapril is an ACE inhibitor. It is infrequently used in animals compared with enalapril or benazepril. Like other ACE inhibitors, it inhibits conversion of angiotensin I to angiotensin II. Angiotensin II is a potent vasoconstrictor and stimulates sympathetic stimulation, renal hypertension, and synthesis of aldosterone. The ability of aldosterone to cause sodium and water retention contributes to congestion. Trandolapril, like other ACE inhibitors, causes vasodilation and decreases aldosterone-induced congestion. ACE inhibitors also contribute to vasodilation by increasing concentrations of some vasodilating kinins and prostaglandins. Trandolapril is converted to active trandolaprilat after administration.

T

## Indications and Clinical Uses
Trandolapril, like other ACE inhibitors, is used for treatment of hypertension and for management of CHF. Compared with other ACE inhibitors, such as enalapril and benazepril, it is not used commonly in veterinary medicine, and the use has been derived from anecdotal experiences.

### Precautionary Information
#### Adverse Reactions and Side Effects
Trandolapril may cause azotemia in some patients; carefully monitor patients receiving high doses of diuretics. When administered with diuretics (furosemide), the RAAS may be activated.

**Contraindications and Precautions**

Use cautiously with other hypotensive drugs and diuretics. NSAIDs may decrease vasodilating effects. Discontinue ACE inhibitors in pregnant animals; they cross the placenta and have caused fetal malformations and death of the fetus.

**Drug Interactions**

Use cautiously with other hypotensive drugs and diuretics. NSAIDs may decrease vasodilating effects.

## Instructions for Use

Trandolapril has not been used extensively in veterinary patients. Most of the experience has been extrapolated from uses in people. Ordinarily, other ACE inhibitors, such as enalapril or benazepril, are used initially in animals. If patients cannot tolerate these drugs, consider an ARB such as telmisartan.

## Patient Monitoring and Laboratory Tests

Monitor patients carefully to avoid hypotension. With all ACE inhibitors, monitor electrolytes and renal function 3–7 days after initiating therapy and periodically thereafter.

## Formulations Available

- Trandolapril is available in 1-, 2-, and 4-mg tablets.

## Stability and Storage

Store in a tightly sealed container, protected from light, and at room temperature. Stability of compounded formulations has not been evaluated.

## Small Animal Dosage

- The dose has not been established for dogs. The dosage in people is 1 mg/person/day to start, which is then increased to 2–4 mg/day.

## Large Animal Dosage

- No dose has been reported for large animals.

## Regulatory Information

No regulatory information is available. For extralabel use withdrawal interval estimates, contact FARAD at www.FARAD.org.

# Trazodone Hydrochloride
traz'oh-done

**Trade and other names:** Desyrel and generic

**Functional classification:** Antianxiety agent, behavioral modification

## Pharmacology and Mechanism of Action

Trazodone is an antianxiety agent used in animals for anxiety problems and sedation. It is a triazolopyridine derivative and belongs to the phenylpiperazine group of centrally acting drugs. The pharmacology is complicated because it acts both as a serotonin 2A (5-HT$_{2A}$) and 2B (5-HT$_{2B}$) receptor antagonist, a partial agonist for serotonin 1A (5-HT$_{1A}$), and a (weak) SSRI, with little effect on dopamine. It has nonspecific sedating properties and is used as a sedative and hypnotic. It has an active metabolite that also may have effects on the serotonin-1 receptor. The action as an antidepressant and antianxiety agent appears to be distinct from the tricyclic antidepressants (TCAs) and SSRIs.

*Pharmacokinetics:* Trazodone is highly metabolized in people, but the metabolism and pharmacokinetics are not as well understood in animals. The half-life is 6–9 hours in people but only 2.8 hours in dogs, with 85% oral absorption. When administered with food to dogs, it has a peak at 7 hours, with high variation. There have been preliminary studies in cats in which it appears to be well absorbed orally and has a sufficiently long half-life for short-term treatment of anxiety and behavior problems. In horses, it has not been recommended for clinical use but has an oral absorption of 63% and a half-life of approximately 7 hours.

## Indications and Clinical Uses

Trazodone has been used in dogs for events that trigger anxiety and fear such as visits to the veterinarian, separation anxiety, thunderstorms, noise phobias, travel in a car, and other phobias and generalized anxiety events. It has been used to decrease stress in dogs and facilitate handling, confinement, and hospitalization. Although trazodone has been helpful to relieve anxiety in these situations, it has a delayed onset of activity and can be unpredictable. To optimize the effects, it should be administered approximately 1 hour prior to an anticipated anxiety-inducing event. It also has been used to calm anxious dogs to restrict activity after surgery in order to facilitate confinement tolerance.

In cats, it has been used for temporary sedation and to facilitate events that may produce anxiety, such as to facilitate transportation of cats and visits to the veterinarian.

## Precautionary Information

### Adverse Reactions and Side Effects

Although the experience has been mostly limited to small observational studies, there have not been serious adverse effects from oral trazodone in dogs. Uncommon but possible adverse effects in dogs have included soft feces, diarrhea, vomiting, paradoxical anxiety, agitation, vocalization, drowsiness, incontinence, and aggression. The most common effect is sedation at higher doses, which is not always an undesirable event for some of the suggested clinical uses. It has been used in some dogs safely for 28 days at dosages of 7–10 mg/kg q8–12h. It may have fewer anticholinergic effects than the TCAs. It has not produced adverse cardiac effects or seizure activity. When administered intravenously to dogs, adverse effects are more likely, which include aggression, behavior changes, and tachycardia.

In cats, clinical studies with a dose of 100 mg per cat did not produce adverse effects. There were no instances of anorexia, vomiting, diarrhea, ataxia, tremor, paradoxical excitation, or behavioral disinhibition. No laboratory test abnormalities or physical exam changes were observed in any cat. It has been used in cats to facilitate echocardiographic examination without affecting the results. It may lower the blood pressure in treated cats.

In horses, a dose of trazodone of 1.5 mg/kg caused ataxia and tremors. At high doses, trazodone caused tremors, aggression, and excitement.

T

## Contraindications and Precautions

Because of the effect of trazodone on serotonin metabolism, reuptake, and receptors, it should be used cautiously, if at all, with other drugs that affect serotonin. Serotonin syndrome effects have not been observed in dogs, but it should be used cautiously with drugs such as SSRIs (fluoxetine, paroxetine), TCAs (clomipramine), tramadol, and monoamine oxidase inhibitors (selegiline). Do not administer intravenously to dogs.

## Drug Interactions

Trazodone is highly metabolized by cytochrome P450 enzymes. Such enzymes can be inhibited or induced by co-administration with other drugs. Although specific drug interactions have not been reported for dogs, there should be caution when administering to animals receiving other drugs known to affect cytochrome P450 enzymes. (See Appendixes H and I for a list of possible drugs.) Because of the effects of trazodone on serotonin receptors, there should be caution when administering trazodone with other drugs that may affect serotonin, such as tramadol and antidepressants (e.g., fluoxetine, clomipramine). However, based on reports available, excess serotonin effects have not been observed, and it has been administered with tramadol, TCAs, and other serotoninergic drugs safely. Thus far, there have been no adverse effects reported when trazodone was administered prior to anesthesia and surgery in dogs.

## Instructions for Use

Start with a low dose in dogs (approximately 5 mg/kg) and work up gradually to higher doses as needed. In dogs, the starting dosage is generally 25 or 50 mg per dog (depending on dog's size) once or twice per day; then increase the dose gradually if desired effects are not observed and there are no signs of adverse events. Compared with other behavior-modifying drugs such as SSRIs and TCAs, trazodone has a more rapid onset of effect. It may be administered 1 hour prior to an anticipated event that elicits anxiety in an animal, such as thunderstorms, loud noises, car ride, or visit to the veterinarian. It may be administered with benzodiazepine drugs.

In cats, it may be administered up to doses of 100 mg per cat. When administered to cats, it may be mixed with food to facilitate dosing. After dosing to cats, it produces significant sedation and decreased activity. Peak sedation occurs between 2 and 2.5 hours.

## Patient Monitoring and Laboratory Tests

No specific monitoring is necessary. Trazodone concentrations are usually not measured, but in people, plasma concentrations of 0.13–2 mcg/mL were responsible for antidepression effects.

## Formulations

- It is available as 50-, 75-, 100-, 150-, and 300-mg tablets.

## Stability and Storage

Store in a tightly sealed container, protected from light, and at room temperature.

## Small Animal Dosage

### Dogs

- A typical starting dose for dogs is 5–8 mg/kg q12h; then increase the dose as needed to achieve desirable effects. Administer at least 1 hour prior to an anticipated event that may trigger anxiety. The frequency may vary from q8h to q24h, depending on the use. Alternatively, to avoid breaking tablets, give 25 or 50 mg per dog (depending on the dog's size) once daily and increase gradually to a maximum of 300 mg per dose or 900 mg per dog per day.

**Cats**
- 50–100 mg per cat PO (peak effect occurs in 2–2.5 hours) as needed to control anxiety; 50 mg per cat is usually sufficient for most cats. Time to peak sedation in cats occurs in approximately 2 hours.

## Large Animal Dosage
- Trazodone has been studied in horses, but no safe and effective dose has been established.

## Regulatory Information
Withdrawal times are not established for animals that produce food. For extralabel use withdrawal interval estimates, contact FARAD at www.FARAD.org.

---

# Triamcinolone Acetonide, Triamcinolone Hexacetonide, Triamcinolone Diacetate
trye′ am sin′ oh lone

**Trade and other names:** Vetalog, TriamTabs, Aristocort, Kenalog (human injection), and generic brands

**Functional classification:** Corticosteroid

## Pharmacology and Mechanism of Action
Triamcinolone acetonide is a glucocorticoid anti-inflammatory drug. Anti-inflammatory effects are complex, but they are primarily via inhibition of inflammatory cells and suppression of expression of inflammatory mediators. Some older references indicate that triamcinolone (not triamcinolone acetonide) has potency that is approximately equal to methylprednisolone (about 5 times cortisol and 1.25 times prednisolone). However, triamcinolone acetonide, has a different structure than triamcinolone, and is much more potent. This potency is 6–7 times that of prednisolone and slightly more potent than dexamethasone. Most veterinary dermatologists have observed that triamcinolone acetonide is approximately 6–10 times more potent than prednisolone. Thus, the oral doses listed reflect this higher potency.

*Pharmacokinetics:* The pharmacokinetics have not been well studied in small animals. After IV administration (not a recommended route), the half-life was 6 hours, the intra-articular half-life was 24 hours, and the half-life from IM administration was 150 hours. The long IM half-life was due to a prolonged absorption phase. The IM injection suppressed cortisol for 15 days.

## Indications and Clinical Uses
Triamcinolone acetonide, like other corticosteroids, is used to treat inflammatory and immune-mediated diseases in animals. It is used for similar purposes as prednisolone, except with higher potency. It is an acceptable substitute for prednisolone in cats.

Triamcinolone acetonide suspension is also used for intralesional and intra-articular injections to produce local anti-inflammatory effects. When injected IM, the suspension is absorbed slowly. Therefore, the IM injection may have a duration

T

of activity lasting 2–4 weeks. After intra-articular injection, the duration may be maintained for several weeks.

In addition to joint infections, other large animal uses include treatment of inflammatory and immune-mediated conditions and for RAO, formerly called *chronic obstructive pulmonary disease*, in horses associated with equine asthma syndrome.

## Precautionary Information

### Adverse Reactions and Side Effects

Side effects from corticosteroids are many and include polyphagia, polydipsia and polyuria, and hypothalamic–pituitary–adrenal axis suppression. Injections of triamcinolone acetonide can have long-lasting effects. In people, injections can produce adrenal suppression for 30 days.

Other adverse effects include GI ulceration, hepatopathy, diabetes, hyperlipidemia, decreased thyroid hormone, decreased protein synthesis, impaired wound healing, and immunosuppression. When triamcinolone acetonide is used for ocular injections, there is some concern that granulomas may occur at the injection site. When administered to horses at a dose of 0.05 mg/kg IM, it induces hyperglycemia for 3 days, but this does not lead to laminitis. Although adverse effects typically include increased risk of laminitis in horses, evidence for this effect has been controversial and not supported by well-controlled studies.

### Contraindications and Precautions

Do not administer injectable suspension IV. The injectable product is intended for IM, intra-articular, or intralesional injection. Use cautiously in patients prone to ulcers or infection and in animals in which wound healing is necessary. Do not use the ocular form in animals with corneal ulcers. Use cautiously in animals with diabetes or renal failure and in pregnant animals. Because of the high potency (equal to or slightly greater potency than dexamethasone), high doses should be avoided.

### Drug Interactions

Use cautiously in conjunction with NSAIDs because it may potentiate the GI adverse effects.

## Instructions for Use

Triamcinolone acetonide, like other corticosteroids such as prednisolone, is administered in a variety of doses, depending on the severity of the condition being treated. The injectable product is a suspension. Shake well before using. Note that cats may require higher doses than dogs.

## Patient Monitoring and Laboratory Tests

Monitor liver enzymes, blood glucose, and renal function during therapy. Monitor patients for signs of secondary infections. Perform an adrenocorticotropic hormone (ACTH) stimulation test to monitor adrenal function.

## Formulations

- Vetalog (veterinary preparation of triamcinolone acetonide) is available in 0.5- and 1.5-mg tablets.
- Human preparations of triamcinolone acetonide are available in 1-, 2-, 4-, 8-, and 16-mg tablets, but many tablet sizes have been discontinued. Human tablets of 4 mg (scored tablet) are usually available.

- Triamcinolone hexacetonide (Canadian product) is available in a 5- and 20-mg/mL suspension.
- Triamcinolone diacetate is available in a 25-mg/mL suspension.
- Triamcinolone acetonide for injection is available in 10- or 40-mg/mL suspension (human form) or 2- and 6-mg/mL suspension (veterinary form).

## Stability and Storage

Store in a tightly sealed container, protected from light, and at room temperature. Avoid freezing of injectable suspension. Stability of compounded formulations has not been evaluated.

## Small Animal Dosage

- Dogs: For anti-inflammatory treatment, start with 0.1–0.2 mg/kg per day PO; then gradually taper to 0.1 mg/kg every other day. Eventually, some conditions can be controlled with 0.03–0.055 mg/kg q48h PO. (The manufacturer recommends dosages of 0.11–0.22 mg/kg/day.)
- Cats: For anti-inflammatory treatment, start with 0.2 mg/kg per day PO. Gradually taper to a dosage of 0.1 mg/kg (0.5 mg per cat [one tablet] is a common dose) every other day. Some cats can be controlled with low dosages of 0.05 mg/kg q48h.
- Immune-mediated disease (dogs and cats): triamcinolone tablets at doses of 0.2–0.6 mg/kg/day, with maintenance doses of 0.1–0.2 mg/kg q48h PO.
- Triamcinolone acetonide: 0.1–0.2 mg/kg IM or SQ; repeat in 7–10 days.
- Intralesional: 1.2–1.8 mg or 1 mg for every centimeter diameter of tumor every 2 weeks or longer.
- Intra-articular: 5–15 mg per joint for large joints; 2.5–5 mg for small joints. Injections in tendon sheaths are in the range of 2.5–5 mg.

## Large Animal Dosage

### Horses

- 12–20 mg per horse IM. The maximum recommended dose is 0.05 mg/kg IM.
- Triamcinolone acetonide suspension: 0.022–0.044 mg/kg as a single dose IM.
- RAO: 0.09 mg/kg as a single dose IM.
- Intra-articular: 6–18 mg as a total dose per joint (usually 9–12 mg). Repeat in 4–13 days if necessary.

### Cattle

- Triamcinolone acetonide is not approved in cattle, and there are no established doses. If triamcinolone acetonide suspension is injected in cattle, the same dose regimens as used in horses can be used, and extralabel withdrawal times should be followed.

## Regulatory Information

No regulatory information is available. For extralabel use withdrawal interval estimates, contact FARAD at www.FARAD.org.
RCI Classification: 4

# Triamterene
trye-am′ter-een

**Trade and other names:** Dyrenium

**Functional classification:** Diuretic

## Pharmacology and Mechanism of Action

Triamterene is a potassium-sparing diuretic that also acts as an aldosterone antagonist. Triamterene is used in people as an alternative to spironolactone but is not used frequently in animals. Triamterene has similar action to spironolactone except that spironolactone has a competitive inhibiting effect on aldosterone; triamterene does not.

## Indications and Clinical Uses

Triamterene has been used infrequently in veterinary medicine. For treating congestive diseases requiring aldosterone antagonism, spironolactone is the recommended agent. The use of triamterene in animals is derived from empirical use and experience in humans. There are no well-controlled clinical studies or efficacy trials to document clinical effectiveness or compare the effects to spironolactone.

### Precautionary Information

**Adverse Reactions and Side Effects**

Triamterene can produce hyperkalemia in some patients.

**Contraindications and Precautions**

Do not use in dehydrated patients. NSAIDs may interfere with action. Avoid supplements that are high in potassium.

**Drug Interactions**

No specific drug interactions are reported for animals, but it is used infrequently, and a full range of drug interactions is not documented. It could potentially increase the effects of ACE inhibitors. Use cautiously with other drugs that may contain potassium or cause potassium retention. Such drugs include trimethoprim.

## Instructions for Use

There is little clinical experience available for triamterene. There is no convincing evidence that triamterene is more effective in animals than spironolactone.

## Patient Monitoring and Laboratory Tests

Monitor hydration status, serum potassium levels, and renal function.

## Formulations

- Triamterene is available in 50- and 100-mg capsules.

## Stability and Storage

Store in a tightly sealed container, protected from light, and at room temperature. Stability of compounded formulations has not been evaluated.

## Small Animal Dosage

**Dogs and Cats**

- 1–2 mg/kg q12h PO.

## Large Animal Dosage

- No dose has been reported for large animals.

## Regulatory Information

No regulatory information is available. For extralabel use withdrawal interval estimates, contact FARAD at www.FARAD.org.

RCI Classification: 4

# Trientine Hydrochloride
trye-en'teen hye-droe-klor'ide

**Trade and other names:** Syprine

**Functional classification:** Antidote

## Pharmacology and Mechanism of Action
Trientine is a chelating agent. Trientine chelates copper to enhance its clearance in the urine. It may be more potent than penicillamine and has replaced penicillamine in human protocols for copper chelation.

## Indications and Clinical Uses
Trientine is used to chelate copper when penicillamine cannot be tolerated in a patient. In people, it is preferred over penicillamine. Use in animals has been primarily derived from empirical use and experience in humans. It is more potent than penicillamine and may produce fewer GI problems than penicillamine.

## Precautionary Information

**Adverse Reactions and Side Effects**

Adverse effects have not been reported in animals.

**Contraindications and Precautions**

Do not administer to pregnant animals; it may be teratogenic.

**Drug Interactions**

No drug interactions have been reported in animals.

## Instructions for Use
Trientine is used for copper chelation, primarily in patients that cannot tolerate penicillamine.

## Patient Monitoring and Laboratory Tests
Monitor copper levels in treated patients.

## Formulations
- Trientine is available in 250-mg capsules.

## Stability and Storage
Store in a tightly sealed container, protected from light, and at room temperature. Stability of compounded formulations has not been evaluated.

## Small Animal Dosage
**Dogs**
- 10–15 mg/kg q12h PO 1–2 hours before feeding.

## Large Animal Dosage
- No dose has been reported for large animals.

## Regulatory Information
No regulatory information is available. For extralabel use withdrawal interval estimates, contact FARAD at www.FARAD.org.

# Trifluoperazine Hydrochloride

trye-floo-oh-pare′ah-zeen hye-droe-klor′ide

**Trade and other names:** Stelazine

**Functional classification:** Antiemetic, phenothiazine

## Pharmacology and Mechanism of Action

Trifluoperazine is a phenothiazine sedative and antiemetic. Like other phenothiazines, it is a central-acting dopamine ($D_2$) antagonist and suppresses dopamine activity in the CNS to produce sedation and prevent vomiting. Other phenothiazines include acepromazine, chlorpromazine, perphenazine, prochlorperazine, promazine, and propiopromazine (propionylpromazine).

## Indications and Clinical Uses

Trifluoperazine is used for treatment of anxiety, to produce sedation, and as an antiemetic. It is a weaker sedative than some of the other phenothiazines. In people, it is used to treat psychotic disorders. Use in animals has been primarily derived from empirical use and experience in humans. There are no well-controlled studies in animals to examine efficacy or to compare with the effects of other phenothiazines.

## Precautionary Information

### Adverse Reactions and Side Effects

Adverse effects have not been reported in animals but are expected to be similar to those of other phenothiazines. Phenothiazines can lower the seizure threshold in susceptible animals, although this is controversial for acepromazine. Phenothiazines can also cause sedation as a common side effect and extrapyramidal side effects (involuntary muscle movements) in some individuals.

### Contraindications and Precautions

Use cautiously in patients that are hypotensive because phenothiazines can cause vasodilation. If patients have been treated with multiple doses, do not stop treatment abruptly. Gradually taper the dose.

### Drug Interactions

No drug interactions have been reported in animals, but use is infrequent, and a full range of drug interactions is not known. However, these drugs are metabolized and may be subject to cytochrome P450 drug interactions.

## Instructions for Use

Results of clinical studies in animals have not been reported. Use in animals (and doses) is based on experience in people or anecdotal experience in animals.

## Patient Monitoring and Laboratory Tests

No specific monitoring is necessary.

## Formulations

- Trifluoperazine is available in a 10-mg/mL oral solution; 1-, 2-, 5-, and 10-mg tablets; and 2-mg/mL injection.

## Stability and Storage

Store in a tightly sealed container, protected from light, and at room temperature. Trifluoperazine is soluble in water and slightly soluble in ethanol. It is oxidized rapidly if exposed to air or light.

## Small Animal Dosage
### Dogs and Cats
- 0.03 mg/kg q12h IM.
- Oral treatment: Start with 0.03 mg/kg, oral, q12h. Titrate dose up to achieve the desired effect. In people, oral doses as high as 0.3–0.5 mg/kg have been used to control severe conditions.

## Large Animal Dosage
- No dose has been reported for large animals.

## Regulatory Information
No regulatory information is available. For extralabel use withdrawal interval estimates, contact FARAD at www.FARAD.org.

RCI Classification: 2

# Triflupromazine Hydrochloride
trye-floo-proe′mah-zeen hye-droe-klor′ide

**Trade and other names:** Vesprin and fluopromazine (former name)

**Functional classification:** Antiemetic, phenothiazine

## Pharmacology and Mechanism of Action
Triflupromazine is a phenothiazine sedative and antiemetic agent. It is a central-acting $D_2$ antagonist with actions similar to other phenothiazines. Triflupromazine suppresses dopamine activity in the CNS to produce sedation and prevent vomiting. Compared with other phenothiazines, triflupromazine may have stronger antimuscarinic activity. Other phenothiazines include acepromazine, chlorpromazine, perphenazine, prochlorperazine, promazine, and propiopromazine (propionylpromazine).

## Indications and Clinical Uses
Triflupromazine is used to produce sedation and as an antiemetic. In people, it is used to treat psychotic disorders. Use in animals has been primarily derived from empirical use and experience in humans. Little information on animal use is available, and the use is purely anecdotal.

## Precautionary Information
### Adverse Reactions and Side Effects
Adverse effects have not been reported in animals because of infrequent use but are expected to be similar to those of other phenothiazines. Phenothiazines can lower the seizure threshold in susceptible animals, but this is controversial and has not been a problem with acepromazine. Phenothiazines can cause sedation as a common side effect and extrapyramidal side effects (involuntary muscle movements) in some individuals.

### Contraindications and Precautions
Use cautiously in patients that are hypotensive because they can have vasodilating effects. If patients have been treated with multiple doses, do not stop treatment abruptly. Gradually taper the dose.

### Drug Interactions
No drug interactions have been reported in animals, but use is infrequent, and a full range of drug interactions is not known. However, these drugs are metabolized and may be subject to cytochrome P450 drug interactions.

T

## Instructions for Use

Results of clinical studies in animals have not been reported. Use in animals (and doses) is based on experience in people or anecdotal experience in animals.

## Patient Monitoring and Laboratory Tests

No specific monitoring is necessary.

## Formulations

• Triflupromazine is available in 10- and 20-mg/mL injections.

## Stability and Storage

Store in a tightly sealed container, protected from light, and at room temperature. Stability of compounded formulations has not been evaluated.

## Small Animal Dosage

### Dogs and Cats

• 0.1–0.3 mg/kg q8–12h IM.

## Large Animal Dosage

• No dose has been reported for large animals.

## Regulatory Information

No regulatory information is available. For extralabel use withdrawal interval estimates, contact FARAD at www.FARAD.org.
RCI Classification: 2

---

# Trilostane
trye'loe-stane

**Trade and other names:** Modrenal and Vetoryl

**Functional classification:** Adrenal suppressant

## Pharmacology and Mechanism of Action

Trilostane inhibits synthesis of cortisol in dogs. It is a competitive and reversible inhibitor of 3-beta-hydroxysteroid dehydrogenate. Inhibiting this enzyme interferes with the steps that lead to cortisol secretion from the adrenal cortex. Inhibition of cortisol is dose dependent and reversible. Compared with mitotane, which destroys adrenocortical cells, trilostane produces a transient decrease in cortisol. Ordinarily, the zona glomerulosa is spared from trilostane effects, but aldosterone production may be affected in some dogs. Therefore, other hormones also may be decreased as a consequence from treatment with trilostane, such as aldosterone, corticosterone, and androstenedione. It also affects conversion of pregnenolone to progesterone. Adrenal necrosis is possible because of loss of negative feedback during treatment, resulting in high levels of ACTH. Adrenal necrosis affects all steroid hormones.

## Indications and Clinical Uses

Trilostane is used to treat hypercortisolemia associated with pituitary-dependent hyperadrenocorticism (PDH) in dogs (Cushing's disease). Peak concentrations of trilostane occur at approximately 2–4 hours after an oral dose. Cortisol concentrations will decrease as early as 7–10 days after initiating treatment with trilostane. Trilostane improves polyuria, polydipsia, and polyphagia in 70%–80% of dogs with PDH. Treatment with mitotane has been compared with trilostane, and it has been shown that each drug, although acting through different mechanisms, produces similar survival times in dogs with PDH. Other drugs used to treat canine PDH include mitotane (Lysodren), selegiline (Anipryl), and ketoconazole, all drugs acting through different mechanisms. Treatment of alopecia X in dogs (Pomeranians and poodles) has been effective in most animals (9–12 mg/kg/day PO).

Surprisingly, some dogs do well despite high cortisol concentrations. Explanations for this observation is that it may affect glucocorticoid receptors or may convert cortisol to inactive cortisone in dogs by increasing 11-beta-hydroxysteroid dehydrogenase.

Trilostane also has been used to manage clinical signs in dogs with adrenal tumors. Trilostane reduces clinical signs by reducing synthesis of cortisol but does not affect the tumor. The use of trilostane in these cases is palliative. Mitotane may be considered a more effective treatment in these cases.

Trilostane also has been effective in cats with hyperadrenocorticism, with no reported adverse effects. Trilostane can decrease clinical signs of hyperadrenocorticism in cats but cannot produce resolution of clinical signs. It can also improve regulation of diabetes, which is often found concurrently in cats with hyperadrenocorticism.

In horses, trilostane has been used to treat PPID (equine Cushing's disease), and there is preliminary evidence of some benefit (improved clinical signs, reduced laminitis, reduced cortisol) from trilostane at a dosage of 1 mg/kg per day PO.

### Precautionary Information
#### Adverse Reactions and Side Effects
In some dogs, transient lethargy, decreased appetite, or vomiting has been observed, which may be caused by excessive cortisol suppression. If excessive cortisol suppression has occurred, oral prednisolone or prednisone can be administered, and the dog should improve within 2 hours. When trilostane is again reintroduced in these cases, the dose should be reduced. Glucocorticoid or mineralocorticoid deficiency or development of adrenal gland necrosis has been associated with trilostane treatment. Trilostane may decrease aldosterone in some dogs; therefore, dehydration, weakness, hyponatremia, and hyperkalemia are possible and may be observed in some dogs that are sensitive to the mineralocorticoid inhibition.

Although the effects of trilostane are ordinarily transient and reversible, some dogs have had irreversible adrenal gland necrosis from trilostane. These dogs must be managed for hypoadrenocorticism and treated with glucocorticoid and mineralocorticoid supplement.

Adverse effects in cats are similar to dogs and include anorexia, lethargy, weight loss, and pancreatitis.

#### Contraindications and Precautions
Trilostane may decrease synthesis of other adrenocortical hormones besides cortisol. Use cautiously in animals with low potassium concentrations. Do not administer to animals with kidney or liver disease and do not administer to animals intended for breeding.

#### Drug Interactions
Use cautiously, if at all, with aldosterone antagonists, such as spironolactone. If administered with ACE inhibitors, there is a risk of hyperkalemia.

T

## Instructions for Use

Adjust dose as needed by monitoring cortisol concentrations. Trilostane is a short-acting drug with a peak effect at approximately 4 hours and duration of 8–10 hours. Administer with food if possible because food improves oral absorption. Most dogs can be controlled with treatment at a starting dosage of 2–3 mg/kg once daily. (This is lower than the manufacturer's range of 3–6 mg/kg once a day.) Within this range, larger dogs can be maintained on lower doses (mg/kg) than smaller dogs. In many dogs, 24-hour cortisol suppression does not occur; therefore, consider administration twice daily in patients that are not adequately controlled to improve clinical response. When using twice-daily treatment, a starting dosage of 0.5–1 mg/kg q12h PO can be used and gradually increased to 1.5–3 mg/kg q12h PO. In some dogs, administration three times daily may be needed. During treatment, especially in the initial phases, dogs may show adverse effects attributable to cortisol deficiency. In these cases, it is acceptable to instruct pet owners to administer a single dose of 0.5 mg/kg prednisone to relieve adverse clinical signs.

In cats, once-daily dosing can be considered, but many cats are better controlled with twice-daily administration. If a cat is also receiving insulin twice daily, trilostane should also be given twice daily to coincide with the insulin treatment.

## Patient Monitoring and Laboratory Tests

### Monitoring Dogs

Monitor cortisol concentrations in treated animals approximately 10–14 days after starting treatment and then approximately every 3 months. Clinical signs such as the patient's thirst, urination habits, appetite, and skin condition also should be monitored during treatment. In most dogs, signs of successful treatment are observed within a few weeks, with improved activity and reduced polyuria, polydipsia, and polyphagia. Improvements in skin and hair coat may take longer.

The baseline serum cortisol, collected preferably at 4–6 hours after trilostane administration, has been used to monitor initial effectiveness of trilostane therapy. The ideal target range is 1.3–2.9 mcg/dL (35–80 nmol/L), or ≤50% of the pretreatment baseline cortisol concentration.

However, some endocrinologists have suggested that baseline measurements of cortisol are not valuable. If further evaluation is needed, use the ACTH stimulation test. Perform testing after 2 weeks of treatment at 4–6 hours after trilostane administration to coincide with peak effects. (Alternatively, some endocrinologists recommend 2–4 hours after trilostane administration.) Cortisol concentrations of 1.45–5.4 mcg/dL (40–150 nmol/L) have been considered adequate after ACTH stimulation, in addition to monitoring clinical signs. Many endocrinologists round-off these values to a desired range of between 2 and 6 mcg/dL tested after 2 weeks of treatment. If cortisol is too low, consider lowering the dose; if cortisol is too high, consider increasing the dose. Monitor sodium and potassium concentrations in treated dogs. If necessary, supplement with potassium because of aldosterone inhibition. Measurement of endogenous ACTH is not recommended for testing response to trilostane. The levels of ACTH do not correlate with clinical response.

### Monitoring Cats

In cats, start with 1–2 mg/kg per day; then monitor with ACTH stimulation testing. The test should be performed 2–4 hours after trilostane administration.

## Formulations

Veterinary formulations approved in the United States and Europe include capsules of 10, 30, 60, and 120 mg.

## Stability and Storage

Store in a tightly sealed container, protected from light, and at room temperature. The quality of compounded formulations has been highly variable. Tested products have varied from 40% to 150% in strength and the oral absorption is uncertain.

## Small Animal Dosage

### Dogs

- Manufacturer's label dosage is 2.2–6.7 mg/kg once per day PO (average, 5.9 mg/kg). However, many dogs are controlled with a lower dosage starting at 0.5–1 mg/kg q12h PO (or 2–3 mg/kg once daily) and increased to 1.5–3.8 mg/kg q12h PO as needed based on testing. Refer to previous Instructions for Use section, for more complete dosing instructions.
- Adjust dosage based on cortisol measurements.
- Large dogs (weighing greater than 25–30 kg) may require a lower dosage than small dogs (weighing less than 15 kg), which can be verified through posttreatment testing.
- Treatment of alopecia X: 9–12 mg/kg/day PO.

### Cats

- Start with 1–2 mg/kg per day PO. Gradually increase as needed to 3–6 mg/kg q24h PO. The dosage for most cats is generally 10–30 mg per cat q24h.
- Some cats are better controlled with twice-daily administration. In these cats, start with 3 mg/kg q12h PO; then reevaluate and increase the dosage to 5 mg/kg q12h PO as needed.

## Large Animal Dosage

### Horses

- 0.4–1 mg/kg/day PO (added to feed).

## Regulatory Information

Trilostane should not be used in animals that produce food.

## Trimeprazine Tartrate and Trimeprazine–Prednisolone

trye-mep'rah-zeen tar'trate

**Trade and other names:** Temaril, Panectyl (in Canada), alimemazine, and Temaril-P (with prednisolone)

**Functional classification:** Antiemetic, phenothiazine

## Pharmacology and Mechanism of Action

Trimeprazine is a phenothiazine derivative that decreases pruritus in dogs, possibly through antihistamine activity. The antihistamine effects have not been confirmed with independent study, but it may act synergistically with corticosteroids. It also produces sedation similar to other phenothiazines.

## Indications and Clinical Uses

Trimeprazine is used alone or in combination with corticosteroids for inflammatory and allergic problems. The most common use is for pruritus in dogs in combination with prednisolone (Temaril-P). It also has been used for treating motion sickness and is approved in combination with prednisolone as an antitussive in dogs. The therapeutic efficacy for treating pruritus in dogs is attributed to the combined antihistamine and sedative effect of trimeprazine and the anti-inflammatory effect of prednisolone. This combination may be more effective for pruritus than prednisolone alone and may allow lower doses of prednisolone when used in the combination.

## Precautionary Information

### Adverse Reactions and Side Effects

Adverse effects are attributed to the antihistamine and phenothiazine effects. The most common is sedation, but ataxia and behavior changes also can occur.

### Contraindications and Precautions

Phenothiazines can potentially lower seizure threshold in sensitive animals, although this has not been shown for acepromazine in animals and has not been reported for trimeprazine.

### Drug Interactions

No drug interactions have been reported for animals. However, it is metabolized by liver enzymes, which potentially could be affected by drugs that affect the cytochrome P450 enzymes.

## Instructions for Use

There is evidence that trimeprazine is more effective when combined with prednisolone for treatment of pruritus. The combination product is Temaril-P, which contains trimeprazine and prednisolone.

## Patient Monitoring and Laboratory Tests

No specific monitoring is necessary.

## Formulations

- Trimeprazine is available in 2.5-mg/5-mL syrup and 2.5-mg tablets.
- Temaril-P is available in tablets that contain 5 mg trimeprazine + 2 mg prednisolone. Capsules are available with 3.75 mg of trimeprazine + 1 mg of prednisolone and 7.5 mg of trimeprazine + 2 mg of prednisolone.

## Stability and Storage

Store in a tightly sealed container, protected from light, and at room temperature.

## Small Animal Dosage

### Dogs

- 0.5 mg/kg q12h PO.
- Prednisolone + trimeprazine: Start with 0.5 mg/kg of prednisolone + 1.25 mg/kg of trimeprazine per day. Taper the dosage to 0.3 mg/kg prednisolone + 0.75 mg/kg trimeprazine once daily or once every other day PO.
- Tablet equivalents: One-half tablet for dogs weighing less than 4.5 kg; one tablet for dogs 5–9 kg; two tablets for dogs 10–18 kg; and three tablets for dogs weighing more than 20 kg. All doses started with twice daily and eventually tapered to once daily and once every other day.

### Cats

- It is not recommended for cats. Adverse effects have been reported from administration of trimeprazine in cats.

## Large Animal Dosage
• No dose has been reported for large animals.

## Regulatory Information
No regulatory information is available. For extralabel use withdrawal interval estimates, contact FARAD at www.FARAD.org.

RCI Classification: 4

# Trimethobenzamide
trye-meth-oh-ben′zah-mide

**Trade and other names:** Tigan

**Functional classification:** Antiemetic

## Pharmacology and Mechanism of Action
Trimethobenzamide is an antiemetic used infrequently in animals. Trimethobenzamide inhibits vomiting at the chemoreceptor trigger zone (CRTZ). Other antiemetics are used more commonly in animals.

## Indications and Clinical Uses
Trimethobenzamide has been used for antiemetic treatment, especially when vomiting is induced from the CRTZ (e.g., from chemotherapeutic drugs). Use in animals has been primarily derived from empirical use and experience in humans. There are no well-controlled clinical studies or efficacy trials to document clinical effectiveness. Other antiemetics (e.g., maropitant) are more often used for these indications in dogs and cats.

### Precautionary Information

**Adverse Reactions and Side Effects**

Adverse effects not reported in animals.

**Contraindications and Precautions**

Not recommended for use in cats.

**Drug Interactions**

No drug interactions have been reported in animals, but use has been infrequent, and a full range of possible drug interactions is not known.

## Instructions for Use
Efficacy as antiemetic not reported in animals.

## Patient Monitoring and Laboratory Tests
No specific monitoring is necessary.

## Formulations
• Trimethobenzamide is available in 100-mg/mL injections and 100- and 250-mg capsules.

## Stability and Storage
Store in a tightly sealed container, protected from light, and at room temperature.

## Small Animal Dosage

**Dogs**
- 3 mg/kg q8h IM or PO.

**Cats**
- Not recommended.

## Large Animal Dosage
- No dose has been reported for large animals.

## Regulatory Information
Because of a low risk of harmful residues in animals intended for food, no withdrawal time is suggested.

# Trimethoprim and Sulfadiazine
trye-meth′oh-prim and sul-fah-dye′ah-zeen

**Trade and other names:** Tribrissen, Uniprim, Tucoprim, Equisul-SDT, and Di-Trim

**Functional classification:** Antibacterial

## Pharmacology and Mechanism of Action
Trimethoprim and sulfonamides combine the antibacterial drug action of trimethoprim and a sulfonamide. The activity is attributed to their synergistic effect in inhibiting folic acid metabolism in bacteria. Sulfonamides are competitive inhibitors of dihydrofolate synthesis. Trimethoprim inhibits the enzyme dihydrofolate reductase. When used in combination, it has a broad spectrum of activity against susceptible bacterial infections (gram-negative and gram-positive bacteria). Trimethoprim and sulfadiazine is only available as a veterinary preparation, but trimethoprim and sulfamethoxazole is a human preparation and is widely used in animals. There are no published reports of differences in efficacy between trimethoprim and sulfadiazine versus trimethoprim and sulfamethoxazole. The primary difference between sulfamethoxazole and sulfadiazine is that sulfamethoxazole is metabolized more extensively, and sulfadiazine may attain higher active urine concentrations in some patients. The pharmacokinetics vary among species and routes of administration. In most animals, trimethoprim eliminates faster than the sulfonamide component. The combination is administered as a 1:5 ratio (trimethoprim:sulfonamide), but the ratio after administration varies considerably to 1:20 or lower. A ratio of 1:20 has been suggested as optimum for antibacterial effects, but this ratio has not been confirmed in clinical studies in animals.

*Pharmacokinetics:* In horses, this combination is well absorbed, and the oral treatment is sufficient for most susceptible bacterial infections. After administration to horses, the half-life of trimethoprim is 3.7 hours, and the half-life sulfadiazine is 8.5 hours (average of all studies reported). Oral absorption is 65% for sulfadiazine and 46%–67% for trimethoprim.

## Indications and Clinical Uses
Trimethoprim and sulfadiazine is used to treat a variety of infections in dogs, cats, horses, and some exotic animals. For many indications, the use of trimethoprim–sulfadiazine and trimethoprim–sulfamethoxazole has been interchangeable. The combination has efficacy for susceptible bacterial infections (gram-negative and

gram-positive bacteria), including respiratory infections, soft tissue and skin infections, wounds, abscesses, and urogenital infections. In horses, the combination has been used for respiratory infections, joint infections, abdominal infections, prostate infections, soft tissue infections, and infections of the CNS. In horses, it is approved for treatment of respiratory infections caused by *Streptococcus equi* for 10 days. The combination also is used occasionally for infections caused by protozoa (e.g., coccidial and *Toxoplasma* infections). The combination has not been successful for treating infections in abscesses or infections caused by anaerobic bacteria, possibly because of interactions with material in necrotic tissues.

## Precautionary Information

### Adverse Reactions and Side Effects

In horses, oral administration of trimethoprim and sulfonamides may be associated with diarrhea. Other effects observed in horses include idiosyncratic neurologic reactions consisting of behavior changes, gait abnormalities, and hyperesthesia. These effects improved soon after discontinuing the medication.

Adverse effects associated with sulfonamides in dogs include allergic reactions, type II and III hypersensitivity, arthropathy, anemia, thrombocytopenia, hepatopathy, keratoconjunctivitis sicca (KCS), and skin reactions. Dogs may be more sensitive to sulfonamides than other animals because dogs lack the ability to acetylate sulfonamides to metabolites; therefore, more toxic metabolite may accumulate in some animals. Dogs should be observed for signs of adverse reactions because some of these problems may resemble other disease (e.g., arthropathy, hepatopathy, skin reactions). Trimethoprim and sulfonamides may decrease thyroid hormone after treatment in dogs. Effects on thyroid function are most apparent after 2 weeks of treatment, but they are reversible.

### Contraindications and Precautions

Do not administer in animals with sensitivity to sulfonamides. Doberman pinschers may be more sensitive than other canine breeds to reactions from sulfonamides. Use cautiously in this breed. At the first sign of potential adverse drug reaction in dogs, discontinue treatment and substitute another antibiotic and pursue appropriate diagnostic tests. If diarrhea develops in horses, discontinue treatment.

*Pregnancy precaution:* Use in pregnant mares is justified when the benefits outweigh the risk to the fetus. Use of potentiated sulfonamides during pregnancy has been associated with increased risk of congenital abnormalities that may be caused by folate deficiency. In humans, sulfonamides exposure to the newborn (via placenta and milk) can cause hyperbilirubinemia-induced neurotoxicity. However, this syndrome has not been described in animals.

### Drug Interactions

Sulfonamides may interact with other drugs, including warfarin, dapsone, and some NSAIDs (etodolac). They may potentiate adverse effects caused by methotrexate and pyrimethamine. Sulfonamides increase metabolism of cyclosporine, resulting in decreased plasma concentrations. The urinary antiseptic methenamine is metabolized to formaldehyde, which may form a complex and precipitate with sulfonamides. Sulfonamides administered to horses that are receiving detomidine may develop cardiac arrhythmias. This precaution is only listed for IV forms of trimethoprim and sulfonamides.

T

## Instructions for Use

The dose listed in the dosing section is of the combined components. Thus, 30 mg/kg = 5 mg/kg of trimethoprim and 25 mg of sulfonamide. There is evidence that 30 mg/kg once per day is efficacious for canine pyoderma, but for other infections, 30 mg/kg twice daily has been recommended. Oral trimethoprim is not absorbed in ruminants.

## Patient Monitoring and Laboratory Tests

Culture and susceptibility testing: All susceptibility testing is based on a 1:19 ratio of trimethoprim:sulfonamide. The CLSI breakpoint for susceptible organisms is ≤2/38 mcg/mL. For streptococci, this breakpoint is ≤2/38 mcg/mL. Values listed are the concentration of trimethoprim:sulfonamide ratio and are based on human breakpoints. There are no specific breakpoints established for animals.

Trimethoprim and sulfonamides may affect the monitoring of thyroid hormones. In dogs, trimethoprim and sulfadiazine may cause a functional hypothyroidism and lower total thyroid $T_4$ concentrations. Trimethoprim and sulfamethoxazole decreased thyroid function at 30 mg/kg q12h and at 15 mg/kg q12h. Trimethoprim and sulfadiazine at 15 mg/kg q12h for 4 weeks did not affect thyroid function in one study. Effects of trimethoprim and sulfonamides on thyroid function in dogs are reversible. In horses, trimethoprim and sulfadiazine did not affect assays of thyroid function. Monitor tear production in treated dogs because sulfonamides may produce KCS.

## Formulations

- Tablets: Trimethoprim and sulfadiazine has been available in 30-, 120-, 240-, 480-, and 960-mg tablets. (All formulations have a ratio of 5:1, sulfadiazine to trimethoprim.) However, some tablet sizes have become unavailable.
- Equine formulations: Available as an oral paste and suspension (333 mg of sulfadiazine and 67 mg of trimethoprim) for horses. As a powder for horses, each gram contains 67 mg of trimethoprim and 333 mg of sulfadiazine. It has also been available as a 48% injectable suspension for horses, but the availability of injectable formulations has diminished.

## Stability and Storage

Store in a tightly sealed container, protected from light, and at room temperature. Stability of compounded formulations has not been evaluated.

## Small Animal Dosage

### Dogs and Cats

Doses are listed as the combined sulfonamide and trimethoprim.
- 15 mg/kg q12h PO or 30 mg/kg q12–24h PO.
- *Toxoplasma* infection: 30 mg/kg q12h PO.

## Large Animal Dosage

### Horses

- The approved label dosage for the oral suspension is 24 mg/kg (20 mg/kg of sulfadiazine and 4 mg/kg of trimethoprim) twice daily for 10 days. Many equine clinicians use a slightly higher dosage of 25–30 mg/kg (approximately 25 mg of sulfonamide and 5 mg of trimethoprim) q12h PO for most treatments.

### Cattle

- No approved doses have been established. Trimethoprim is not absorbed orally in ruminants, but it is absorbed in calves. Trimethoprim and sulfadoxine has been used in cattle (16 mg/kg combined drug every 24 hours IV or IM), but this combination is not available in the United States.

## Regulatory Information

Withdrawal times are not available. Extralabel use of sulfonamides is prohibited from use in lactating dairy cattle. Do not use in horses intended for food.

---

# Trimethoprim and Sulfamethoxazole
trye-meth'oh-prim and sul-fah-meth-oks'ah-zole

**Trade and other names:** Bactrim, Septra, and generic brands

**Functional classification:** Antibacterial

---

## Pharmacology and Mechanism of Action

Trimethoprim and sulfonamides combine the antibacterial drug action of trimethoprim and a sulfonamide. The activity is attributed to their synergistic effect in inhibiting folic acid metabolism in bacteria. Sulfonamides are competitive inhibitors of dihydrofolate synthesis. Trimethoprim inhibits the enzyme dihydrofolate reductase. When used in combination, it has a broad spectrum of activity against susceptible bacterial infections (gram-negative and gram-positive bacteria). Trimethoprim has been combined with both sulfadiazine and sulfamethoxazole. Trimethoprim and sulfadiazine is only available as a veterinary preparation, but trimethoprim and sulfamethoxazole is a human preparation. There are no published reports of differences in efficacy between trimethoprim and sulfadiazine versus trimethoprim and sulfamethoxazole. The primary difference between sulfamethoxazole and sulfadiazine is that sulfamethoxazole is metabolized more extensively. Sulfadiazine may attain higher active urine concentrations in some patients.

The combination is administered as a 1:5 ratio (trimethoprim:sulfonamide), but the ratio after administration varies considerably to 1:20 or lower. A ratio of 1:20 has been suggested as optimum for antibacterial effects, but this ratio has not been confirmed in clinical studies in animals.

## Indications and Clinical Uses

The combination of trimethoprim and sulfamethoxazole has been used to treat a variety of infections in dogs, cats, horses, and some exotic animals. For many indications, the use of trimethoprim–sulfadiazine and trimethoprim–sulfamethoxazole has been interchangeable. Trimethoprim is used for treatment of UTIs, skin and soft tissue infections, prostate infections, pneumonia, and CNS infections. The combination also is used occasionally for infections caused by protozoa (e.g., coccidial and *Toxoplasma* infections).

In horses, trimethoprim–sulfamethoxazole has been used for respiratory infections, joint infections, abdominal infections, soft tissue infections, and infections of the CNS. However, there is more information available for the equine-approved formulation of trimethoprim–sulfadiazine.

The combination of trimethoprim–sulfonamide has not been successful for treating infections in abscesses or infections caused by anaerobic bacteria.

**T**

## Precautionary Information

### Adverse Reactions and Side Effects

In horses, oral administration of trimethoprim and sulfonamides may be associated with diarrhea. Other effects observed in horses include idiosyncratic neurologic reactions consisting of behavior changes, gait abnormalities, and hyperesthesia. These effects improved soon after discontinuing the medication. Adverse effects associated with sulfonamides administered to dogs include allergic reactions, type II and III hypersensitivity, arthropathy, anemia, thrombocytopenia, hepatopathy, KCS, and skin reactions. Dogs may be more sensitive to sulfonamides than other animals because dogs lack the ability to acetylate sulfonamides to metabolites and higher levels of more toxic metabolites. Dogs should be observed for signs of adverse reactions because some of these problems may resemble other disease (e.g., arthropathy, hepatopathy, skin reactions). Trimethoprim and sulfonamides may decrease thyroid hormone after treatment in dogs. Effects on thyroid function are most apparent after 2 weeks of treatment, but they are reversible.

### Contraindications and Precautions

Do not administer in animals with sensitivity to sulfonamides. Doberman pinschers may be more sensitive than other canine breeds to reactions from sulfonamides. Use cautiously in this breed. The injectable preparation contains benzyl alcohol, which may cause reactions in small patients. The injectable preparation should be diluted and injected slowly intravenously using instructions listed later.

At the first sign of potential adverse drug reaction, discontinue treatment and substitute another antibiotic and pursue appropriate diagnostic tests. If horses develop diarrhea, treatment should be discontinued.

### Drug Interactions

Sulfonamides may interact with other drugs, including warfarin, dapsone, and some NSAIDs (etodolac). They may potentiate the adverse effects caused by methotrexate and pyrimethamine. Sulfonamides increase metabolism of cyclosporine, resulting in decreased plasma concentrations. The urinary antiseptic methenamine is metabolized to formaldehyde, which may form a complex and precipitate with sulfonamides. Sulfonamides administered to horses that are receiving detomidine may develop cardiac arrhythmias, but this precaution is only listed for IV forms of trimethoprim and sulfonamides.

## Instructions for Use

The dosage listed is of the combined components; thus, 30 mg/kg = 5 mg/kg of trimethoprim and 25 mg of sulfonamide. There is evidence that 30 mg/kg once daily is efficacious for pyoderma, but for other infections, 30 mg/kg twice daily has been recommended. When using the injectable formulation, each 5-mL vial should be diluted in 75–125 mL of 5% dextrose. The diluted formulation should then be administered by IV infusion over 60 minutes.

## Patient Monitoring and Laboratory Tests

Culture and susceptibility testing: All susceptibility testing is based on a 1:19 ratio of trimethoprim:sulfonamide. The CLSI breakpoint for susceptible organisms is

≤2/38 mcg/mL. For streptococci, this breakpoint is ≤2/38 mcg/mL. Values listed are the concentration of trimethoprim and sulfonamide ratio and are based on human breakpoints because animal-specific breakpoints have not been established.

In dogs, trimethoprim and sulfadiazine may cause a functional hypothyroidism and lower total thyroid $T_4$ concentrations. Trimethoprim and sulfamethoxazole decreased thyroid function at 30 mg/kg q12h and at 15 mg/kg q12h. Trimethoprim and sulfadiazine at 15 mg/kg q12h for 4 weeks did not affect thyroid function in one study. Effects of trimethoprim and sulfonamides on thyroid function in dogs are reversible. In horses, trimethoprim and sulfadiazine do not affect assays of thyroid function. Monitor tear production in treated dogs because sulfonamides may produce KCS.

## Formulations
- Oral forms: Trimethoprim and sulfamethoxazole is available in 480- and 960-mg tablets and a 240-mg/5 mL (48 mg/mL) oral suspension. (All formulations have a ratio of 5:1 sulfamethoxazole to trimethoprim.)
- Injection: 80 mg of sulfamethoxazole and 16 mg of trimethoprim per milliliter in 5-mL vials or as 400 mg of sulfamethoxazole and 80 mg of trimethoprim per 5-mL injection. The solution can be further diluted; for example, the vial can be mixed by adding 5 mL to 75 mL 5% dextrose solution, or for larger dilutions, add the vial to a 125-mL 5% dextrose solution.

## Stability and Storage
Store in a tightly sealed container, protected from light, and at room temperature. Injectable formulations should be stored at room temperature and not refrigerated.

Injectable formulation contains 0.3% sodium hydroxide. After preparation of the IV solution, the 80 mg per 125 mL solution has 6-hour stability at 0.64 mg/mL, the 80 mg per 100 mL solution has a stability of 4 hours at 0.8 mg/mL, and the 80 mg per 75 mL solution has a stability of 2 hours. If upon visual inspection there is cloudiness or evidence of crystallization, the solution should be discarded.

## Small Animal Dosage
### Dogs and Cats
Doses are listed as the combined sulfonamide and trimethoprim.
- 15 mg/kg q12h PO or 30 mg/kg q12–24h PO.
- 30 mg/kg q12h IV. (See Instructions for Use for preparation of IV formulation.)

## Large Animal Dosage
### Horses
- 30 mg/kg (25 mg of sulfonamide and 5 mg of trimethoprim) q12h PO. Consult protocols for trimethoprim–sulfadiazine for more specific instructions.

### Cattle
- No dose is established. Trimethoprim is not absorbed orally in ruminants, but it is absorbed in calves. The combination of trimethoprim and sulfadoxine has been used in cattle (16 mg/kg combined drug every 24 hours IV or IM), but this drug is not available in the United States.

## Regulatory Information
Extralabel use of sulfonamides is prohibited from use in lactating dairy cattle. However, trimethoprim and sulfadoxine has a withdrawal time in Canada for cattle of 10 days for meat and 96 hours for milk.

# Tripelennamine Citrate and Tripelennamine Hydrochloride

tri-peh-len′eh-meen sih′trate

**Trade and other names:** Pelamine, Histanin, and PBZ

**Functional classification:** Antihistamine

## Pharmacology and Mechanism of Action

Antihistamine ($H_1$ blocker). Similar to other antihistamines, tripelennamine acts by blocking the histamine type 1 receptor ($H_1$) and suppresses inflammatory reactions caused by histamine. The $H_1$ blockers have been used to control pruritus and skin inflammation in dogs and cats; however, success rates in dogs have not been high. More commonly used antihistamines include clemastine, chlorpheniramine, diphenhydramine, cetirizine, and hydroxyzine.

## Indications and Clinical Uses

Tripelennamine is used to prevent allergic reactions and for pruritus therapy in dogs and cats. In large animals, tripelennamine hydrochloride is used to treat laminitis, allergy, insect bites, pulmonary edema, and urticaria in horses. In cattle, it is used to treat urticaria and allergic reactions. Use in animals has been primarily derived from empirical use and experience in humans. Success rates for treatment of pruritus are low. In addition to the antihistamine effect for treating allergies, these drugs block the effect of histamine in the vomiting center, vestibular center, and other centers that control vomiting in animals.

## Precautionary Information

### Adverse Reactions and Side Effects

Sedation is the most common side effect. Antimuscarinic effects (atropine-like effects) also are common. Members of this class (ethanolamines) have greater antimuscarinic effects than other antihistamines. GI adverse effects, such as ileus and decreased stomach emptying, may occur.

### Contraindications and Precautions

No contraindications are reported for animals.

### Drug Interactions

No drug interactions are reported for animals.

## Instructions for Use

There are no clinical reports of use in veterinary medicine and no evidence that it is more efficacious than other drugs in this class. The clinical uses listed above are based on clinician experience and recommendations from experts.

## Patient Monitoring and Laboratory Tests

No specific monitoring is necessary.

## Formulations

- Tripelennamine is available in 25- and 50-mg tablets, 20-mg/mL injections (generic), and 5-mg/mL elixir oral liquid. Tripelennamine hydrochloride (Histanin) is available as a 25-mg/mL injection.

## Stability and Storage

Store in a tightly sealed container, protected from light, and at room temperature.

## Small Animal Dosage

### Dogs and Cats

- The dosage is not clearly established. It has been listed as 1 mg/kg q12h PO. For comparison, the human dosage is 1.25 mg/kg q4–6h PO. Tripelennamine hydrochloride injection: 0.25 mL per 5 kg body weight.

## Large Animal Dosage

- Pigs, cattle, and horses: 1 mg/kg I every 6–12 hours. Equivalent to 10 mL per 250 kg or 1 mL per 25 kg body weight.

## Regulatory Information

Withdrawal time for pigs and cattle: 48 hours for meat; 48 hours for milk.
RCI Classification: 3

# Tulathromycin
too-lath-roe-mye′sin

**Trade and other names:** Draxxin and Draxxin 25

**Functional classification:** Antibacterial, macrolide

## Pharmacology and Mechanism of Action

Tulathromycin is an antibacterial of the macrolide class of drugs. It is a 15-membered macrolide structure (gamithromycin also is a 16-member molecule) and considered a triamilide macrolide with three charged nitrogens. It is derived from azalide macrolides, such as azithromycin. Like other macrolides, it inhibits bacterial protein synthesis by binding to the ribosomal 50S subunit. It is considered bacteriostatic, but it may have bactericidal properties in vitro. Because of a positively charged molecule, it may penetrate gram-negative bacteria more easily than other macrolide antibiotics. Tulathromycin has a spectrum of activity that is limited to gram-positive bacteria and some gram-negative bacteria that cause respiratory diseases in cattle and pigs (e.g., *M. haemolytica*, *Mycoplasma* spp., and *P. multocida*). Enterobacteriaceae bacteria (*E. coli*, *K. pneumoniae*, and so on) and *P. aeruginosa* are resistant.

*Other properties:* Tulathromycin, like other macrolides, exerts therapeutic benefits not solely explainable by antibacterial activity. Like azithromycin, tulathromycin may have multiple immunomodulatory effects that likely contribute to the therapeutic response in respiratory infections and perhaps other diseases. Other beneficial effects may be caused by enhanced degranulation and apoptosis of neutrophils and inhibition of inflammatory cytokine production. It also may help clear infections by enhancing macrophage functions.

*Pharmacokinetics:* The half-life is long, with 80- to 90-hour plasma half-life in pigs and cattle, and 8- and 6-day tissue half-life in cattle and pigs, respectively, which prolongs the drug concentration at the site of infection. The volume of distribution is greater than 10 L/kg. Absorption from injection is greater than 80% in cattle and pigs.

## Indications and Clinical Uses

In cattle, tulathromycin is used for treatment of BRD caused by *M. haemolytica*, *P. multocida*, and *H. somni*. It is also effective for treating infections caused by *Mycoplasma bovis*. It also may be used to prevent infections caused by these pathogens when used in high-risk calves. It is also used for the treatment of bovine foot rot (interdigital necrobacillosis) associated with *Fusobacterium necrophorum* and *Porphyromonas levii*. A single dose has been effective for bovine infectious keratoconjunctivitis (*Moraxella bovis*).

In pigs, it has been used for control and treatment of SRD associated with *A. pleuropneumoniae, P. multocida, B. bronchiseptica, Mycoplasma hyopneumoniae,* and *H. parasuis.*

In foals (extralabel use), tulathromycin has been used for treatment of pulmonary abscesses. Uses in small animals have not been explored.

Other long-acting macrolide antibiotics used in cattle include tilmicosin, tildipirosin, and gamithromycin.

## Precautionary Information

### Adverse Reactions and Side Effects

Serious adverse reactions have not been observed except in experimental animals at high doses. Injection-site reactions are possible in some animals with swelling or irritation at the injection site. High doses (five times the dose) produce myocardial lesions in some animals. However, most animals have tolerated up to 10 times the labeled dose without toxicity. In treated foals (IM injection once per week), self-limiting diarrhea and injection-site reactions (IM injection) developed in approximately one third of the foals.

It is ordinarily not administered to dogs, but in toxicity tests performed in dogs, it did not produce significant toxicity unless high doses were administered. There were no drug-related effects on heart rate, respiration rate, body temperature, blood pressure, or ECG parameters in dogs even at high doses.

### Contraindications and Precautions

In cattle, do not administer to female dairy cattle 20 months of age or older. In cattle, do not inject more than 10 mL per injection site. In pigs, do not inject more than 2.5 mL per injection site.

### Drug Interactions

No drug interactions have been reported. However, macrolide antibiotics are known to inhibit some cytochrome P450 enzymes. Therefore some drugs interactions are possible but not well documented.

## Instructions for Use

In cattle, administer as a single SQ injection in the neck. In pigs, administer as a single IM injection in the neck.

## Patient Monitoring and Laboratory Tests

CLSI breakpoint for susceptible bacteria is ≤16 mcg/mL except that swine isolates of *A. pleuropneumoniae* use a susceptible breakpoint of ≤64 mcg/mL.

## Formulations

Tulathromycin is available in a 25- and 100-mg/mL solution for injection.

## Stability and Storage

Store in a tightly sealed container, protected from light, and at room temperature.

## Small Animal Dosage

- No small animal doses have been established.

## Large Animal Dosage

### Cattle
- 2.5 mg/kg SQ (neck) as a single injection (1.1 mL per 100 lb for 100-mg/mL solution).

### Pigs
- 2.5 mg/kg IM (neck) as a single injection.

### Foals
- 2.5 mg/kg IM once per week.

## Regulatory Information

No milk withdrawal times are established.

Do not use in female dairy cattle 20 months of age or older. Do not use in veal calves.

Cattle withdrawal time for meat: 18 days when using Draxxin 100 mg/mL; when using 25 mg/mL, the withdrawal time is 22 days.

Pig withdrawal time for meat: 5 days.

# Tylosin
tye'loe-sin

**Trade and other names:** Tylocine, Tylan, and tylosin tartrate

**Functional classification:** Antibacterial, macrolide

## Pharmacology and Mechanism of Action

Tylosin is a 16-membered macrolide approved for therapy of a variety of infections in pigs, cattle, dogs, and poultry (see Indications and Clinical Uses). It is formulated as tylosin tartrate or tylosin phosphate. Like other macrolide antibiotics, tylosin inhibits bacteria by binding to the 50S ribosome and inhibiting protein synthesis. The spectrum of activity is limited primarily to gram-positive aerobic bacteria. *Clostridium* and *Campylobacter* spp. are usually susceptible. The spectrum also includes the bacteria that cause BRD. *E. coli* and *Salmonella* spp. are resistant. In pigs, *Lawsonia intracellularis* is usually susceptible.

## Indications and Clinical Uses

In cattle, tylosin is used for treatment of BRD caused by *Mannheimia* spp., *P. multocida,* and *H. somni.* It is used for interdigital necrobacillosis (foot rot) in cattle caused by *F. necrophorum* or *B. melaninogenicus.* In pigs, it is used for treatment of swine arthritis caused by *Mycoplasma hyosynoviae,* swine pneumonia caused by *Pasteurella* spp., swine erysipelas caused by *Erysipelothrix rhusiopathiae,* swine dysentery associated with *Serpulina (Treponema) hyodysenteriae,* and proliferative enteropathy caused by *L. intracellularis.* For treatment in pigs, it is also added to feed (type A–medicated feed article) or drinking water. In small animals, it is used for gram-positive soft tissue and skin infections. However, this use is uncommon, and the most frequent use in dogs is for treatment of diarrhea, referred to as *antibiotic-responsive diarrhea,* that has not responded to other treatments. The etiology of the diarrhea is not known but may be caused by *Clostridium* or *Campylobacter* spp. For this use, the powdered formulation (swine formulation) has been added to food daily for maintenance.

T

## Precautionary Information
### Adverse Reactions and Side Effects
Tylosin may cause diarrhea in some animals. However, for oral treatment for colitis in dogs, it has been administered for several months with safety. Skin reactions have been observed in pigs. Oral administration to horses has been fatal.

### Contraindications and Precautions
Do not administer orally to rodents or rabbits. Do not administer to horses. Avoid IV administration. Do not inject more than 10 mL in one IM site to avoid local reactions.

### Drug Interactions
Although other macrolides have been associated with inhibition of cytochrome P450 enzymes, no drug interactions have been reported for animals.

## Instructions for Use
Tylosin is used in pigs and cattle for controlling BRD and SRD and the other diseases listed in the Indications section. It is rarely used in small animals for uses other than intestinal disease. Powdered formulation (tylosin tartrate) has been administered on food for control of signs of colitis in dogs. Tablets are approved for treatment of colitis in Canada.

## Patient Monitoring and Laboratory Tests
No specific monitoring is necessary.

## Formulations
- Tylosin is available as tylosin phosphate and tylosin tartrate. It is available in a soluble powder of 100 g/lb of tylosin phosphate or approximately 3 g per teaspoon (Tylosin-100 type A–medicated premix).
- Tylosin tartrate is equal to 800 mcg/mg of tylosin base.
- Tylosin is available as a 50- and 200-mg/mL injection (with propylene glycol).

## Stability and Storage
Store in a tightly sealed container, protected from light, and at room temperature.

## Small Animal Dosage
### Dogs
- 7–15 mg/kg q12–24h PO.
- 8–11 mg/kg q12h IM.
- Colitis: 12–20 mg/kg q8h with food; then if there is a response, increase the interval to q12h and eventually to q24h. (20 mg/kg is approximately 1/8 teaspoon of tylosin phosphate or Tylan for a 20-kg dog.)

### Cats
- 7–15 mg/kg q12–24h PO.
- 8–11 mg/kg q12h IM.

## Large Animal Dosage
### Swine
- Treatment of arthritis, erysipelas, and swine dysentery: 8.8 mg/kg q12h IM.

### Cattle
- Pododermatitis and pneumonia: 17.6 mg/kg q24h IM.

- Swine: Medicated feed dose is administered at a dose of 22–220 g/kg (of the premix), with the dose depending on the specific product. Consult package information.

### Regulatory Information
Pig withdrawal time for meat: 14 days.
Cattle withdrawal time for meat: 21 days.
Not to be used in lactating cattle.

T

# Urofollitropin

yoo-roe-fah'lih-troe-pin

**Trade and other names:** Metrodin, FSH, and Fertinex

**Functional classification:** Hormone

## Pharmacology and Mechanism of Action

Urofollitropin contains follicle-stimulating hormone (FSH) and stimulates ovulation. In people, it is used in combination with human chorionic gonadotropin (hCG) to stimulate ovulation.

## Indications and Clinical Uses

Although urofollitropin is used in people in combination with hCG to stimulate ovulation, the use in animals is uncommon. Other than anecdotal accounts, there is little evidence of use in veterinary medicine.

## Precautionary Information

### Adverse Reactions and Side Effects

Side effects have not been reported in animals, but the use is rare. In people, thromboembolism or severe ovarian hyperstimulation syndrome has been reported. In humans, ovarian enlargement and ovarian cysts have been reported.

### Contraindications and Precautions

Do not use in pregnant animals.

### Drug Interactions

No drug interactions are reported for animals.

## Instructions for Use

Results of clinical studies in animals have not been reported. Use in animals is extrapolated from the experience in people. Use in humans is followed by administration of hCG.

## Patient Monitoring and Laboratory Tests

Monitor estrogen, or progesterone, or both with treatment.

## Formulations

- Urofollitropin is available in 75 units per vial for injection.

## Stability and Storage

Store in a tightly sealed container, protected from light, and at room temperature.

## Small Animal Dosage

- Dosages not established. However, the usual human dosage is 75 units/day IM for 7 days. This may be increased to 150 units/day IM for an additional 7 days.

## Large Animal Dosage

- Dosages not established. However, the usual human dosage is 75 units/day IM for 7 days. This may be increased to 150 units/day IM for an additional 7 days.

## Regulatory Information

It is expected to pose little risk from residues in animals intended for food, and no withdrawal times are recommended.

# Ursodiol, Ursodeoxycholic Acid
er-soe-dye′ole, er-soe-dee-oks-ih-koe-lik ass′id

**Trade and other names:** Actigall and Urso

**Functional classification:** Laxative, choleretic

## Pharmacology and Mechanism of Action
Ursodiol (ursodeoxycholic acid) is a hydrophilic bile acid. Ursodiol has anticholelithic and choleretic properties. Ursodiol is the short name for ursodeoxycholic acid. This is a naturally occurring, water-soluble bile acid. Ursodiol, like other bile acids, can act as a choleretic and increase bile flow. In dogs, it may alter the pool of circulating bile acids, displacing the more hydrophobic bile acids or enhancing their secretion in liver and bile. By modulating the composition of biliary bile salts in favor of more hydrophilic bile salts, injury to the biliary epithelium, such as the cytotoxic potential of endogenous bile acids, is less likely than with hydrophobic bile salts. There is also evidence that for treating acute liver injury, it may have antioxidant properties.

## Indications and Clinical Uses
Ursodiol is used for treatment of liver diseases. It is used to treat primary biliary cirrhosis, cholestatic liver disorders, cholangitis, and chronic liver disease. Although experimental evidence exists for its benefit in dogs, there are no well-controlled clinical trials that demonstrate efficacy. In people, it has been used as a laxative and to prevent or treat gallstones. It has also been used to treat chronic constipation because it may increase water content of feces and stimulate colonic peristalsis. In people, the use for treating cholangitis is controversial.

## Precautionary Information

### Adverse Reactions and Side Effects
Loose feces and pruritus are the most common problems in people. In animals, ursodiol may cause diarrhea. (It has been used as a laxative.) Adverse effects can be lessened by gradually increasing the dose to the target range over 1–2 weeks.

### Contraindications and Precautions
No contraindications are reported for animals.

### Drug Interactions
No drug interactions have been identified for animals. In people, it interferes with some cholesterol-lowering drugs.

## Instructions for Use
Results of clinical studies in animals have not been reported. Use in animals (and doses) is based on experience in people or anecdotal experience in animals. It has been recommended by veterinary clinical experts for treatment of gallbladder disease in dogs and cats. The optimum dosage in animals is not known, but in people, the most common dosage is 13–15 mg/kg per day PO. Once or twice daily is as effective as three to four times per day. Administer with meals.

## Patient Monitoring and Laboratory Tests
Monitor bile acids and hepatic enzymes during treatment to monitor effects.

U

## Formulations
- Ursodiol is available in 300-mg capsules and 250- or 500-mg tablets.

## Stability and Storage
Store in a tightly sealed container, protected from light, and at room temperature. Suspensions have been prepared in vehicles for oral use and found to be stable for 35–60 days.

## Small Animal Dosage
### Dogs and Cats
- 10–15 mg/kg q24h PO; the dosage used most often in animals with liver disease is 15 mg/kg PO q24h.

## Large Animal Dosage
- No large animal doses are available.

## Regulatory Information
It is expected to pose little risk from residues in animals intended for food, and no withdrawal times are recommended.

# Valacyclovir
val-a-sye′kloe-veer
**Trade and other names:** Valtrex
**Functional classification:** Antiviral

## Pharmacology and Mechanism of Action

Valacyclovir is an antiviral drug that is used in people primarily for herpes virus infections. The only use identified for veterinary medicine is in horses. Valacyclovir is acyclovir complexed with an amino acid (L-valine) by an ester. Therefore valacyclovir is a prodrug converted to the active acyclovir. Acyclovir has antiviral activity against herpes virus. The action is related to the affinity for the enzyme thymidine kinase (TK). After it is converted to acyclovir, it is phosphorylated by TK to the monophosphate form. Acyclovir monophosphate accumulates in cells infected with herpes virus and is converted by guanylate cyclase to acyclovir diphosphate and subsequently to the triphosphate form, which is an inhibitor of viral DNA polymerase. This terminates viral enzyme activity. However, resistance among some virus forms is possible because of changes in TK or in the DNA polymerase. Other drugs in this class include penciclovir and famciclovir; information can be found in other chapters.

Acyclovir is active against equine herpes virus (EHV). However, there are differences in activity among various strains of EHV. Some are more susceptible than other strains. It has poor activity against the feline herpes virus, and it is not recommended for this treatment.

*Pharmacokinetics:* After administration of oral valacyclovir to horses, the oral absorption was 26% or as high as 48% (depending on the study) with a peak concentration of 4.2 mcg/mL (20 mg/kg) or 5.26 mcg/mL (26.6 mg/kg).

## Indications and Clinical Uses

Valacyclovir is an antiviral drug converted to acyclovir; therefore it can be used for similar indications as acyclovir but with better and more consistent oral absorption. Valacyclovir has been administered orally to horses because oral absorption of acyclovir is insufficient. Acyclovir is able to inhibit replication of EHV-1 in vitro, and valacyclovir has been used for oral treatment of EHV-1. The effectiveness of valacyclovir is better when administered for prophylaxis than as a treatment. When administered as oral treatment to horses for 7 or 14 days, it improved clinical signs, reduced viral shedding, and decreased viremia, and ataxia was not as severe.

The activity against feline herpes virus is poor, and it produces adverse effects; therefore it is not recommended for cats.

**V**

## Precautionary Information
### Adverse Reactions and Side Effects

The most serious adverse effect in humans is acute renal insufficiency. This may be prevented by slow IV infusion and proper hydration. No adverse effects were identified in limited studies performed in horses. In cats, significant adverse effects have been observed, which included myelosuppression and kidney and liver injury, including fatal hepatic and renal necrosis.

**Contraindications and Precautions**
If perivascular injection occurs, immediate flushing of area with fluids is recommended.

**Drug Interactions**
No drug interactions have been reported in animals.

## Instructions for Use
The dosages listed in the dosing section are based on pharmacokinetic studies to achieve the optimal plasma drug concentration in horses. Oral administration in horses is not affected by feeding.

## Patient Monitoring and Laboratory Tests
Monitor blood urea nitrogen and creatinine during use. In horses, doses should be administered to maintain plasma concentrations above 0.3 mcg/mL.

## Formulations
- Valacyclovir is available in 500-mg and 1-g tablets. For administration to horses, the tablets have been crushed and mixed with corn syrup.

## Stability and Storage
Store tablets in a tightly sealed container, protected from light, and at room temperature.

## Small Animal Dosage
### Dogs
- Canine doses have not been determined.

### Cats
- Do not administer to cats.

## Large Animal Dosage
### Horses
- 27 mg/kg PO loading dose q8h for 2 days. This is followed by a maintenance dosage of 18 mg/kg PO q12h for 7–14 days.

## Regulatory Information
Because of mutagenicity, it should not be administered to animals intended for food.

# Valproic Acid, Valproate Sodium
val-proe′ik ass′id, val′proe-ate soe′dee-um

**Trade and other names:** Depakene (valproic acid), Depakote (divalproex), and Epival (in Canada)

**Functional classification:** Anticonvulsant

## Pharmacology and Mechanism of Action
Valproic acid and valproate sodium are used as anticonvulsants. Their use is uncommon in animals. The mechanism of action is not known, but valproate may

increase gamma-aminobutyric acid (GABA) concentrations in the central nervous system (CNS). Valproic acid and valproate sodium are slightly different chemically, but both have been used. Divalproex is composed of both valproic acid and sodium valproate. Equivalent oral doses of divalproex sodium and valproic acid deliver equivalent quantities of valproate ion.

## Indications and Clinical Uses
Valproate is used, usually in combination with phenobarbital, to treat refractory epilepsy in animals. Most of the experience has been in dogs, but the use is uncommon. The use of valproate in animals has declined because other anticonvulsants for treating refractory epilepsy have been identified such as gabapentin, pregabalin, zonisamide, and levetiracetam. The little clinical experience available is derived from small observational studies or anecdotal experience.

## Precautionary Information
### Adverse Reactions and Side Effects
Adverse effects have not been reported in animals, but hepatic failure has been reported in people. Sedation may be seen in some animals.

### Contraindications and Precautions
Do not use in pregnant animals. Birth defects have been reported in people.

### Drug Interactions
Valproate may cause bleeding if used with drugs that inhibit platelets.

## Instructions for Use
This drug is usually used as an add-on with phenobarbital. Controlled-release forms designed for people do not show the same oral absorption profile in dogs as in people.

## Patient Monitoring and Laboratory Tests
Therapeutic drug monitoring can be performed; however, therapeutic concentrations have not been established for dogs and cats, and ranges cited for people are used: 50–100 mcg/mL (desired trough concentration). Concentrations greater than 100 mcg/mL are associated with adverse effects.

## Formulations
- Valproic acid immediate-release formulations are available in 250-mg capsules and 50-mg/mL syrup. Delayed-release formulations of valproic acid and divalproex are available in 125-, 250-, and 500-mg tablets or capsules. Divalproex is also available in 125-mg capsules and 250- and 500-mg extended-release tablets. Valproate sodium (Depacon) is available in a 100-mg/mL injection.

## Stability and Storage
Store in a tightly sealed container, protected from light, and at room temperature. Valproic acid is slightly soluble in water, but valproate sodium is soluble in water. Extemporaneous emulsions have been prepared and were comparable to absorption of syrup.

## Small Animal Dosage
### Dogs
- 50–250 mg per dog (adjust the dose proportional to the size of the dog) q8h PO.
- Delayed-release formulations: Start with 250 mg per dog q12h PO and increase to 500 mg per dog q12h as needed.

## Cats
- Dose not established.

### Large Animal Dosage
- No dose has been reported for large animals.

### Regulatory Information
No regulatory information is available. For extralabel use withdrawal interval estimates, contact Food Animal Residue Avoidance Databank (FARAD) at 1-888-USFARAD (1-888-873-2723).

# Vancomycin
van-koe-mye′sin

**Trade and other names:** Vancocin and Vancoled

**Functional classification:** Antibacterial

## Pharmacology and Mechanism of Action
Vancomycin is an antibacterial drug that is usually reserved for resistant infections. Vancomycin is an older agent introduced in the 1950s. It is a glycopeptide antibiotic derived from a fungus *Amycolatopsis orientalis* (formerly *Nocardia orientalis*). Vancomycin binds to the D-alanyl-D-alanine portion of cell wall precursors. The bactericidal action occurs by activating bacterial cell wall autolysins. Vancomycin has a narrow antibacterial spectrum that includes *Streptococcus, Enterococcus,* and *Staphylococcus* spp. Strains of *Staphylococcus* treated include the methicillin-resistant *Staphylococcus* (e.g., methicillin-resistant *Staphylococcus aureus* [MRSA] or *Staphylococcus pseudintermedius* [MRSP]). Gram-negative bacteria are resistant to vancomycin.

New drugs for humans related to vancomycin are dalbavancin (Dalvance), oritavancin (Orbactiv), and telavancin (Vibativ). These drugs are lipoglycopeptides. Oritavancin and dalbavancin are unique because they have very long half-lives of 10–14 days in people and can be administered once per 7–14 days. At this time, these new agents are very expensive and have not been tested for clinical use in animals.

*Pharmacokinetics:* In dogs, the half-life of vancomycin is approximately 2.3 hours but shortens to 1.7 hours after 10 days.

## Indications and Clinical Uses
Vancomycin is used for resistant strains of *Staphylococcus* or *Enterococcus* spp. in animals. It is commonly used in people as an injectable drug to treat methicillin-resistant *Staphylococcus* spp. and drug-resistant *Enterococcus* spp. It is not effective against gram-negative bacteria. The use in animals is much less frequent than in people because it is inconvenient to administer, and some countries have placed restrictions on use in animals. However, it can be valuable for treatment of enterococci or staphylococci that are resistant to other antibiotics when other options are not available. It has been administered orally to people for diarrhea caused by *Clostridium* spp., but this use has not been explored in animals. Occasionally, it has been used in horses intravenously, or for local infiltration, such as with regional limb perfusion. It is not allowed in food animals.

## Precautionary Information

### Adverse Reactions and Side Effects

Adverse effects reported in animals have been reported from small observational or retrospective studies. Because of limited use, a full range of possible adverse effects has not been recognized. Adverse effects in people include neutropenia, kidney injury, and histamine release. Reactions, especially those associated with histamine release, are more likely with a rapid IV injection. In dogs, reactions attributed to histamine release have not been observed. Kidney injury can occur because of oxidative stress. The risk is greater after 4–8 days of treatment but resolves after treatment is discontinued. Combination with aminoglycosides may increase risk of kidney injury. Acute kidney injury (AKI) has been reported in dogs and cats, but other underlying factors (co-administered drugs, underlying disease) may have contributed to these observations. The frequency of kidney injury in people is less than in the past because the formulations used today are purer and of better quality.

### Contraindications and Precautions

Do not administer rapidly intravenously. It causes pain if injected by other routes (IM, SQ). Administer by slow infusion to avoid acute adverse reactions.

### Drug Interactions

Do not mix with other drugs in infusion solution; incompatibilities are reported for many drugs. Incompatible drugs include beta-lactam antibiotics, fluoroquinolones, aminoglycosides, macrolides, propofol, anticonvulsants, corticosteroids, and furosemide. It is incompatible with alkaline solutions.

## Instructions for Use

Vancomycin must be administered via IV infusion, although in rare instances, intraperitoneal administration has been used in people. (Oral administration is limited to intestinal infections.) Vancomycin systemic use in horses is rare. Local administration in horses via regional limb perfusion has been used for localized joint or bone infections.

Doses are derived from pharmacokinetic studies in each species. In dogs, to maintain the plasma concentration between a suggested range of 10 and 30 mcg/mL, a dosage of 15 mg/kg q8h IV is recommended. (This dosage actually produces peaks and troughs of approximately 40 and 5 mcg/mL, respectively, but it is the most convenient dosage that can be used because of the short half-life in dogs.) This dose should be infused slowly over 30–60 minutes, or at a rate of approximately 10 mg/min. The total dose to be administered can be diluted in 0.9% saline or 5% dextrose solution but not alkalinizing solutions.

## Patient Monitoring and Laboratory Tests

V

Monitoring of trough plasma concentrations is recommended to ensure proper dose. Ideally, the dose and frequency should be adjusted to maintain trough concentration above 10 mcg/mL or an area under the curve/minimum inhibitory concentration (AUC/MIC) ratio greater than 400. There may be better outcomes with serious infections when trough concentrations are 15–20 mcg/mL. The Clinical and Laboratory Standards Institute (CLSI) guidelines for susceptibility testing list breakpoints of ≤4 mcg/mL for *Enterococcus* spp., ≤1 mcg/mL for *Streptococcus* spp., and ≤2 mcg/mL for *Staphylococcus* spp.

Monitor kidney parameters during treatment because of the risk of AKI.

## Formulations
• Vancomycin is available in 500-mg and 1-, 5-, and 10-g vials for injection.

## Stability and Storage
Stability may be compromised if mixed with other drugs in infusion solutions. Store in a tightly sealed container, protected from light, and at room temperature. It is soluble in water and ethanol. After reconstitution with sterile water, it may be further diluted in 5% dextrose or saline. Solutions may have a dark color. After reconstitution, it is stable for 14 days either at room temperature or in the refrigerator. A concentrated solution of up to 83 g/L is stable for 72 hours at 37°C. Some ophthalmic compounded formulations are not stable and have a low pH that can be irritating to the eyes.

## Small Animal Dosage
### Dogs
• 15 mg/kg q6–8h IV infusion. (Start with this dose q8h, and if necessary, based on monitoring, increase interval to q6h.)
• Constant-rate infusion (CRI): Loading dose of 3.5 mg/kg followed by CRI of 1.5 mg/kg/h mixed in 5% dextrose in water.

### Cats
• 12–15 mg/kg q8h IV infusion.

## Large Animal Dosage
### Horses
• 4.3–7.5 mg/kg q8h IV given as an infusion over 1 hour.
• Regional limb perfusion: Infuse 300 mg diluted in a 0.5% solution.

## Regulatory Information
Do not administer to animals intended for food. The Food and Drug Administration (FDA) has prohibited the extralabel use of glycopeptides in food-producing animals because of a risk of producing glycopeptide-resistant bacteria.

# Vasopressin
vay-zoe-press′in

**Trade and other names:** Arginine vasopressin (AVP), antidiuretic hormone (ADH), and Pitressin

**Functional classification:** Hormone

## Pharmacology and Mechanism of Action
Vasopressin is an antidiuretic hormone (ADH). Vasopressin mimics the effect of ADH on the receptors of the renal tubule. ADH permits reabsorption of water in the renal tubule. Without ADH, more diluted urine is excreted. (See Desmopressin for additional formulations and use.) Vasopressin also has potent vasopressive activity via activation of the $V_1$ vascular receptor. The $V_1$ vascular receptors are in high density on vascular smooth muscle, whereas the $V_2$ receptors on the renal-collecting duct are responsible for increasing water reabsorption. Because of the vasopressive action, it has been used to treat vasodilatory shock. During infusion, it rapidly increases mean arterial pressure. A related drug, terlipressin, is more specific for the vascular $V_1$ receptor but has not been used in animals.

## Indications and Clinical Uses

Vasopressin is used for treatment of polyuria caused by central diabetes insipidus. It is not effective for polyuria caused by renal disease. Desmopressin is the preferred formulation used more frequently in animals for treating diabetes insipidus (see Desmopressin for more details.) Vasopressin is used to treat vasodilatory shock via CRI in addition to fluid therapy. In shock caused by cardiogenic mechanisms or vasodilatory shock, protocols vary with respect to the vasopressor used in emergency situations. Some protocols still rely on catecholamines (e.g., norepinephrine) for their vasoconstrictive properties (via alpha$_1$-adrenergic receptors), and some protocols advocate vasopressin. There are no clinical trials in veterinary medicine that establish a superiority of one treatment over another.

### Precautionary Information

**Adverse Reactions and Side Effects**

Adverse effects have not been reported for use in animals. Allergic reactions and increase in blood pressure have been reported in people.

**Contraindications and Precautions**

No contraindications are reported for animals.

**Drug Interactions**

No drug interactions have been reported in animals.

## Instructions for Use

For IV use, dilute in 0.9% saline and titrate dose to effect. For antidiuretic use, doses are adjusted on the basis of monitoring of water intake and urine output.

## Patient Monitoring and Laboratory Tests

Monitor blood pressure during infusion to maintain systolic blood pressure of 100–120 mm Hg and urine output of 0.5–1.5 mL/kg/h. Titrate the infusion rate to achieve desired blood pressure response. When used for antidiuretic effects, monitor water intake, urine output, and urine-specific gravity.

## Formulations

- Vasopressin is available in a 20-units/mL (aqueous) solution.

## Stability and Storage

Store in a tightly sealed container, protected from light, and at room temperature.

## Small Animal Dosage

**Dogs and Cats**

- Antidiuretic: 10 units IV or IM. (Desmopressin is preferred in animals for treating diabetes insipidus.)
- Vasopressor (shock): 0.01–0.04 units/min. Do not exceed 0.04 units/min (0.5–5 milliunits/kg/min).
- CPR: 0.8 units/kg IV bolus; can be repeated during cardiopulmonary resuscitation.

## Large Animal Dosage

- No dose has been reported for large animals.

## Regulatory Information

Because of a low risk of harmful residues in animals intended for food, no withdrawal time is suggested.

V

# Verapamil Hydrochloride
ver-ap′ah-mill hye-droe-klor′ide

**Trade and other names:** Calan and Isoptin

**Functional classification:** Calcium antagonist

## Pharmacology and Mechanism of Action
Verapamil is an older calcium-channel blocking drug of the nondihydropyridine group that is not used often in veterinary medicine. Verapamil blocks calcium entry into cells via blockade of the voltage-dependent slow channel. It produces vasodilation, negative chronotropic, and negative inotropic effects.

## Indications and Clinical Uses
Verapamil has been used to control supraventricular arrhythmias. However, the use of verapamil has greatly diminished because of adverse effects. It has practically become an outdated drug in veterinary medicine. The preferred drug from this class to use in animals is usually diltiazem.

## Precautionary Information
### Adverse Reactions and Side Effects
Adverse effects include hypotension, cardiac depression, bradycardia, and atrioventricular block. It may cause anorexia in some patients. Verapamil has caused sudden cardiac arrest in some patients with IV administration.

### Contraindications and Precautions
Do not use in patients with decompensated congestive heart failure or advanced heart block. It is not well tolerated in cats.

### Drug Interactions
Verapamil, like other calcium-channel-blocking drugs, is subject to interaction with drugs that interfere with the multidrug resistance (MDR) membrane pump (P-glycoprotein) and the cytochrome P450 enzymes. (See Appendixes I and J for a list of drugs that may cause interference.)

## Instructions for Use
The oral formulation of verapamil is not absorbed sufficiently (of the active stereoisomer) for adequate effects. Diltiazem is preferred over verapamil in patients with heart failure because of less myocardial depression.

## Patient Monitoring and Laboratory Tests
Monitor heart rate and rhythm during treatment.

## Formulations
- Verapamil is available in 40-, 80-, and 120-mg immediate-release tablets; 120-, 180-, and 240-mg slow-release tablets and capsules; and a 2.5-mg/mL injection.

## Stability and Storage
Store in a tightly sealed container, protected from light, and at room temperature. Verapamil is soluble in water. Aqueous solutions are stable for 3 months. Maximum stability is at a pH of 3–6. It can be mixed with infusion solutions and is compatible. Suspensions have been prepared for oral administration and found to be stable for 60 days.

## Small Animal Dosage
### Dogs
- 0.05 mg/kg every 10–30 minutes IV (maximum cumulative dose is 0.15 mg/kg).
- The PO dose is not established.

### Cats
- Not recommended.

## Large Animal Dosage
- No dose has been reported for large animals.

## Regulatory Information
Do not administer to animals intended for food.
Racing Commissioners International (RCI) Classification: 4

# Vinblastine Sulfate
vin-blast′een sul′fate

**Trade and other names:** Velban

**Functional classification:** Anticancer agent

## Pharmacology and Mechanism of Action
Vinblastine is an anticancer agent that is used occasionally in some protocols for animals. Vinblastine, like vincristine, belongs to the vinca alkaloid group of anticancer agents. Vinblastine sulfate is the salt of an alkaloid derived from the *Vinca rosea* plant, also known as the periwinkle flower. The vinca alkaloids have been called *spindle poisons* because they have an affinity for tubulin in cells. Tubulin is the protein that forms the microtubules responsible for chromosome migration during mitosis. Vinca alkaloids block polymerization of the cellular microtubules and therefore arrest mitosis in the metaphase (m-phase specific).

## Indications and Clinical Uses
Vinblastine is used in cancer chemotherapy protocols for various tumors. One of the most common uses is for canine mast cell tumors (MCTs). There does not appear to be cross-resistance from vincristine to vinblastine. Vinblastine has been used for lymphoreticular neoplasia and for canine transitional cell carcinoma and other tumors. Do not use vinblastine to increase platelet numbers as is done occasionally with vincristine. (Vinblastine may actually cause thrombocytopenia.)

The doses and protocols for vinblastine are derived from small clinical studies and observational studies by oncologists. There is a lack of well-controlled studies to examine the effects of vinblastine in animals.

**V**

## Precautionary Information
### Adverse Reactions and Side Effects
The most dose-limiting effect is bone marrow suppression, with the nadir of neutropenia occurring at 1 week after administration and recovery occurring at 2 weeks. Gastrointestinal toxicity is the second most important effect, but it is milder. Vinblastine does not produce neuropathy as vincristine does. It causes tissue necrosis if injected outside the vein.

**Contraindications and Precautions**
If perivascular injection occurs, immediate flushing of area with fluids is recommended.

**Drug Interactions**
No drug interactions have been reported in animals.

## Instructions for Use

Vinblastine may be used with other anticancer drugs or combined with prednisolone for MCTs. The most common dosage has been 2 mg/m$^2$ every 7–14 days by slow IV infusion or rapid IV bolus. However, to increase the response rate for MCTs, evidence suggests that dose intensity should be increased to a dosage of 3.5 mg/m$^2$ IV every 2 weeks. This dose produced more toxicity but higher efficacy.

## Patient Monitoring and Laboratory Tests

Monitor complete blood count during treatment.

## Formulations

• Vinblastine is available in a 1-mg/mL injection.

## Stability and Storage

Store in a tightly sealed container, protected from light, and at room temperature.

## Small Animal Dosage

**Dogs and Cats**

• 2 mg/m$^2$ IV (slow infusion) once a week. (See Instructions for Use regarding higher doses.)

## Large Animal Dosage

• No dose has been reported for large animals.

## Regulatory Information

Withdrawal times are not established for animals that produce food. This drug should not be used in animals intended for food because it is an anticancer agent.

# Vincristine Sulfate
vin-kriss'teen sul'fate

**Trade and other names:** Oncovin, Vincasar, and generic brands

**Functional classification:** Anticancer agent

## Pharmacology and Mechanism of Action

Vincristine is an anticancer agent used frequently in cancer protocols for animals. Vincristine, like vinblastine, belongs to the vinca alkaloid group of anticancer agents. Vincristine is derived from the *Vinca rosea* plant, also known as the periwinkle flower. The vinca alkaloids have been called *spindle poisons* because they have an affinity for tubulin in cells. Tubulin is the protein that forms the microtubules responsible for chromosome migration during mitosis. Vinca alkaloids block polymerization of the cellular microtubules and therefore arrest mitosis in the metaphase (m-phase specific).

Vincristine has an affinity for the tubulin of platelets. For thrombocytopenia, vincristine increases thrombopoiesis, increases fragmentation of megakaryocytes, and decreases platelet destruction. It may also decrease destruction of platelets by macrophages.

## Indications and Clinical Uses

Vincristine is used in combination chemotherapy protocols. It is included in several anticancer chemotherapy protocols, usually with corticosteroids, alkylating agents, and other drugs. It has been used in veterinary medicine for lymphoreticular tumors, transmissible venereal tumors, mammary neoplasia in cats, and other solid tumors. It is a component of several combination protocols and may also be useful as a single agent for some tumors. Vincristine is also administered to increase platelet counts in patients with immune-mediated thrombocytopenia (ITP). The protocol for treating ITP is listed later.

### Precautionary Information

**Adverse Reactions and Side Effects**

Vincristine is generally well tolerated. It is less myelosuppressive than other anticancer drugs. Peripheral neuropathy has been reported, but it is rare. Constipation can occur. Vincristine is irritating to tissues; avoid extravasation outside the vein during administration. If accidental injection is made outside the vein, prompt action is needed to avoid severe tissue injury.

**Contraindications and Precautions**

If perivascular injection occurs, immediate flushing of the area with fluids is recommended to decrease tissue injury. When handling vincristine, pharmacy and hospital staff should take appropriate precautions to prevent exposure to people. Dogs with the *ABCB1* mutation (P-glycoprotein deficient) may have an increased risk of toxicity.

**Drug Interactions**

There are no significant drug interactions reported in animals.

## Instructions for Use

Vincristine is used in cancer chemotherapy protocols for various tumors. For example, in the COAP protocol (an acronym for cyclophosphamide, Oncovin, asparaginase, and prednisolone), the Oncovin component is vincristine. Vincristine also increases numbers of functional circulating platelets and is used for thrombocytopenia. When used to treat immune-mediated thrombocytopenia, it may be administered with a corticosteroid (e.g., prednisone at 2 mg/kg) to produce a rapid increase in functional platelets. This regimen (compared with prednisone alone) has shortened the duration of hospitalization for dogs with immune-mediated thrombocytopenia.

## Patient Monitoring and Laboratory Tests

Monitor platelets during therapy if used to increase platelet numbers.

## Formulations

- Vincristine is available in a 1-mg/mL injection.

## Stability and Storage

Maintain in the injectable vial. Do not mix with other drugs in vial.

## Small Animal Dosage
### Dogs and Cats
- Antitumor: 0.5–0.75 mg/m$^2$ IV (or 0.025–0.05 mg/kg) once a week.
- Thrombocytopenia: 0.02 mg/kg IV once a week (with prednisolone).

## Large Animal Dosage
- No dose has been reported for large animals.

## Regulatory Information
Withdrawal times are not established for animals that produce food. This drug should not be used in animals intended for food because it is an anticancer agent.

---

# Vitamin A

**Trade and other names:** Retinol, Aquasol-A, vitamin AD, and vitamins A and D

**Functional classification:** Vitamin supplement

## Pharmacology and Mechanism of Action
Vitamin A is a vitamin supplement. See also Isotretinoin (Accutane) for analogues used for other conditions.

## Indications and Clinical Uses
Vitamin A is used as a supplement for animals with deficiency.

## Precautionary Information
### Adverse Reactions and Side Effects
Excessive doses can cause bone or joint pain and dermatitis. Other signs of hypervitaminosis A can be excessive bleeding, confusion, diarrhea, and peeling of skin.

### Contraindications and Precautions
Hypervitaminosis A can occur from high doses of vitamin A administered chronically. Doses needed to cause toxicity can be as high as 10,000 units/kg/day.

### Drug Interactions
No drug interactions have been reported in animals.

## Instructions for Use
Dosing of vitamin A may be expressed as units, retinol equivalents (REs), or mcg of retinol. One RE equals 1 mcg of retinol. One RE of vitamin A is equal to 3.33 units of retinol. To convert from units of vitamin A to mcg, multiply units by 0.3. To convert from mcg vitamin A to units, divide by 0.3. (For example, 5000 units of vitamin A = 1500 mcg vitamin A.) One unit of vitamin A is equal to 0.6 mcg of beta-carotene.

## Patient Monitoring and Laboratory Tests
Monitor for signs of toxicity if high doses are used.

## Formulations

- Vitamin A is available in 5000 units (1500 RE) per 0.1-mL oral solution and in 10,000-, 25,000-, and 50,000-unit tablets. These tablets are listed as 3000, 7500, and 15,000 REs, respectively. Injectable formulations used in veterinary medicine usually are included with vitamin D. These combinations contain 100,000, 200,000, or 500,000 units/mL.

## Stability and Storage

Store protected from light at room temperature. Vitamin A, like other fat-soluble vitamins, is insoluble in water but soluble in oils. It is subject to oxidation and should be kept in a tightly sealed container.

## Small Animal Dosage

### Dogs and Cats

- 625–800 units/kg q24h PO.

## Large Animal Dosage

- All doses are listed as per animal and may be repeated in 2–3 months.

### Calves

- 500,000–1 million units IM.

### Sheep and swine

- 500,000–1 million units IM.

### Cattle

- 1–2 million units IM.

## Regulatory Information

Because of a low risk of harmful residues in animals intended for food, no withdrawal time is suggested.

## Vitamin E

**Trade and other names:** Tocopherol, alpha-tocopherol, Aquasol E, and generic brands

**Functional classification:** Vitamin

## Pharmacology and Mechanism of Action

Vitamin E is also known as *alpha-tocopherol*. It should be distinguished from beta-, gamma-, and delta-tocopherol because only alpha-tocopherol meets dietary requirements. It is a fat-soluble vitamin that is considered an antioxidant. Vitamin E also is found in solutions as D-alpha-tocopherol (natural source of vitamin E). It is often a component of omega fatty acid formulations used in oral dietary supplements.

## Indications and Clinical Uses

Vitamin E is used as supplement and as treatment of some immune-mediated dermatoses and hepatobiliary disorders. Vitamin E has been used as an oral treatment for discoid lupus in dogs; however, efficacy for many skin diseases has been questioned. Vitamin E is often included in a mixture with other dietary supplements (e.g., fish oils).

## Precautionary Information

### Adverse Reactions and Side Effects

At high doses, vitamin E can cause coagulopathies. Dosages known to cause coagulopathy are 1000 units/day (15 units/kg/day) in humans. Coagulopathies are caused by a decrease in vitamin K–dependent coagulation factors.

### Contraindications and Precautions

Use carefully in animals with coagulopathies.

### Drug Interactions

Vitamin E may interact with anticoagulants. It may exacerbate the anticoagulant effect of warfarin.

## Instructions for Use

Vitamin E has been proposed as treatment for a wide range of human illnesses, but evidence for efficacy in animals is lacking. In animals, it is used as adjunctive antioxidant therapy for a variety of diseases. However, there are no well-controlled studies to document efficacy for these uses.

- To convert to vitamin E for a product labeled as alpha-tocopherol: multiply units by 0.9 to determine mg. To convert from mg to units, divide by 0.9.
- To convert to vitamin E for a product labeled as alpha-tocopherol: multiply units by 0.67 to determine mg.
- To convert from mg to units, divide by 0.67. For example, 1 unit of vitamin A is equivalent to 0.67 mg alpha-tocopherol or 0.9 mg alpha-tocopherol.

## Patient Monitoring and Laboratory Tests

Monitor for bleeding in animals treated with high doses.

## Formulations

- Oral: Vitamin E is available in capsules, tablets, and an oral solution (e.g., 1000 units/capsule). Injectable formulations for veterinary medicine may also contain vitamins A and D or selenium.
- Injection: Usually injectable combinations contain 300 units/mL.
- Solutions: Vitamin E is found in solutions as alpha-tocopherol (natural source of vitamin E). It is also often a component of omega fatty acid (fish oils) formulations.

## Stability and Storage

Vitamin E, like other fat-soluble vitamins, is insoluble in water but soluble in oils. Store in a tightly sealed container, protected from light, and at room temperature.

## Small Animal Dosage

### Dogs and Cats

- 100–400 units q12h PO (as alpha-tocopherol).
- Immune-mediated skin disease: 400–600 units q12h PO.
- Discoid lupus erythematosus (dogs): 200–400 units q12h PO.
- Liver disease: 10–15 units/kg/day, PO.

## Large Animal Dosage

All doses are listed as per animal and may be repeated in 2–3 months.

### Calves

- 1200–1800 units IM.

**Cattle**
- 2400–3000 units IM.

**Sheep and Swine**
- 1200–1800 units IM.

### Regulatory Information
Because of a low risk of harmful residues in animals intended for food, no withdrawal time is suggested.

## Vitamin K

**Trade and other names:** AquaMEPHYTON (injection), Mephyton (tablets), Veta-K1 (capsules), Veda-K1 (oral and injectable), vitamin K, phylloquinone, and phytomenadione

**Functional classification:** Vitamin supplement

### Pharmacology and Mechanism of Action
See Phytonadione for additional information. Vitamin K is a cofactor used to synthesize coagulation factors in the liver (factors II, VII, IX, and X). Vitamin $K_1$ is also known as *phytonadione* and *phylloquinone* (phytomenadione is the British spelling of phytonadione). Vitamin $K_2$ is also known as *menaquinone*. Vitamin $K_3$ is known as *menadione*. Vitamin $K_3$ is a synthetic analogue and is not equivalent to Vitamin $K_1$. Vitamin $K_3$ is not recommended for clinical use. Vitamin $K_1$ is absorbed better with meals that contain fat. See Instructions for Use for the optimum formulation for treating animals.

### Indications and Clinical Uses
Vitamin $K_1$ is a fat-soluble vitamin used to treat coagulopathies caused by anticoagulant toxicosis (warfarin or other rodenticides). Anticoagulants deplete vitamin K in the body, which is essential for synthesis of clotting factors. In large animals, it is used to treat sweet clover poisoning.

### Precautionary Information

**Adverse Reactions and Side Effects**

In people, a rare hypersensitivity-like reaction has been observed after rapid IV injection. This reaction may be caused by histamine release from the drug vehicle, polysorbate 80. Signs resemble anaphylactic shock. These signs also have been observed in animals with IV administration. To avoid anaphylactic reactions, do not administer intravenously. Reactions from IM injection, such as hematoma, may occur in animals with coagulopathies.

**Contraindications and Precautions**

Accurate diagnosis to rule out other causes of bleeding is suggested. Other forms of vitamin K may not be as rapidly acting as vitamin $K_1$; therefore consider using a specific preparation for the best outcome. To avoid anaphylactic reactions, do not administer intravenously.

**Drug Interactions**

Some drugs, such as cephalosporins, may decrease vitamin K–dependent clotting factors.

V

## Instructions for Use

Consult a poison control center for specific protocol if specific rodenticide is identified. Use vitamin $K_1$ for acute therapy because it is more highly bioavailable. Administer with food to enhance absorption. Foods with fat are better because this is a fat-soluble vitamin. Phytonadione and phytomenadione are synthetic lipid-soluble forms of vitamin $K_1$. Menadiol is vitamin $K_4$, which is a water-soluble derivative converted in the body to vitamin $K_3$ (menadione).

The injection can be diluted in 5% dextrose or 0.9% saline but not other solutions. Although vitamin $K_1$ veterinary labels have listed the IV route for administration, these labels have not been approved by the FDA. Therefore avoid IV administration of vitamin $K_1$. The preferred route is SQ, but IM also can be used. When treating for poisoning by second-generation rodenticides, which have long half-lives, 6 weeks of therapy may be necessary.

## Patient Monitoring and Laboratory Tests

Monitoring bleeding times in patients is essential for accurate dosing of vitamin $K_1$ preparations. When treating long-acting rodenticide poisoning, periodic monitoring of the bleeding times is suggested.

## Formulations

- Vitamin K is available in 2- or 10-mg/mL injection. Mephyton is a 5-mg tablet. Veta-K1 is a 25-mg capsule. Phytonadione (aqueous colloidal formulation) is a 2- or 10-mg/mL injection.

## Stability and Storage

Vitamin K, like other fat-soluble vitamins, is insoluble in water but soluble in oils. Store in a tightly sealed container, protected from light, and at room temperature.

## Small Animal Dosage

**Dogs and Cats**
- Short-acting rodenticides: 1 mg/kg/day IM, SQ, or PO for 10–14 days.
- Long-acting rodenticides: 2.5–5 mg/kg/day IM, SQ, or PO for 3–4 weeks and up to 6 weeks.

**Birds**
- 2.5–5 mg/kg q24h SQ, IM, or PO for 14–28 days.

## Large Animal Dosage

**Cattle, Calves, Horses, Sheep, and Goats**
- 0.5–2.5 mg/kg SQ or IM.

## Regulatory Information

No meat or milk withdrawal time is necessary.

# Voriconazole
vor-ih-kahn′ah-zole

**Trade and other names:** Vfend

**Functional classification:** Antifungal

## Pharmacology and Mechanism of Action

Voriconazole is an azole (triazole) antifungal drug. Voriconazole is a second-generation triazole antifungal drug and similar to the other currently available azole and triazole antifungals, except with better activity. Voriconazole inhibits the fungal cytochrome P450–dependent 14 alpha-sterol demethylase, which is essential for formation of ergosterol in the fungal cell membrane. Voriconazole is similar in structure to fluconazole; however, it is more active and potent. Voriconazole is active against dermatophytes and systemic fungi, such as *Blastomyces, Histoplasma,* and *Coccidioides* spp. It also has activity against yeast, such as *Candida* and *Malassezia* spp. Voriconazole has greater activity against *Aspergillus* and *Fusarium* spp. than other drugs of this class. Voriconazole is more lipophilic than fluconazole and more water soluble than itraconazole or ketoconazole, with intermediate protein binding. These properties provide good oral bioavailability and tissue distribution.

*Pharmacokinetics:* The pharmacokinetics may be dose dependent and variable among animals. In people, a wide variation in cytochrome P450 metabolism produces variable plasma concentrations. Experimental studies in dogs have shown rapid and complete absorption of the drug after oral administration. Pharmacokinetics have been studied in dogs, cats, and horses. Oral absorption is higher than in most other drugs in this class. In horses, voriconazole is absorbed 92% and has a half-life of 13 hours. The oral half-life is much longer than the IV half-life in cats, producing accumulation with repeated administration to cats. The IV half-life is 12.4 hours with a volume of distribution of 1.3 hours. The oral half-life in cats is 43 hours with a peak of 2.3 mcg/mL at a dose of 4–6 mg/kg. Oral tablets and oral suspension in cats are absorbed equally well. Because of the difference in half-life, the oral administration to cats produces higher blood concentrations than the IV route (by a factor of 2.6). In dogs, after oral administration of 6 mg/kg, the half-life is 3.1 hours (±0.8) with a peak concentration of 3 mcg/mL. After repeated doses, the metabolism may be induced in dogs, producing a shorter half-life.

## Indications and Clinical Uses

Voriconazole has been used to treat dermatophytes and systemic fungi, such as *Blastomyces, Histoplasma,* and *Coccidioides* spp. It has been used to treat infections caused by *Aspergillus* and *Fusarium* spp. The efficacy in humans for treating *Aspergillus* spp. is better than with other oral antifungal drugs and comparable to amphotericin B. Penetration into the CNS and eye is high enough to treat infections in these areas.

Most of the use in veterinary medicine has been empirical or extrapolated from the use in humans. The doses for small animals are listed in the dosing section that follows. Clinical experience in horses has used a dosage of 2 mg/kg once daily PO. However, research studies have showed that a dosage of 4 mg/kg once daily PO or 3 mg/kg q12h PO produces adequate in-plasma and tissue concentrations (ocular tear film, cerebrospinal fluid, urine, epithelial lining fluid of the lung, and synovial fluid) for susceptible fungi, including *Aspergillus* spp. It has also been administered topically in horses for ocular fungal infections (using the IV 1% solution every 4 hours). Voriconazole also has been used in birds to control infections caused by *Aspergillus* spp., but some birds develop toxicity from this use.

V

### Precautionary Information
#### Adverse Reactions and Side Effects

Voriconazole has been associated with neurotoxicity in cats at doses of 10 mg/kg via an unknown mechanism. Some cats administered therapeutic doses exhibited CNS signs that resolved after discontinuation of the drug. These reactions have not been reported in other animals (dogs, horses, birds) treated with voriconazole. Cats also had signs of anorexia, ataxia, paresis, arrhythmias, and hypokalemia. In a study with lower doses (4–6 mg/kg), it was generally tolerated much better, but miosis and hypersalivation were common effects observed in cats.

Although it is generally better tolerated than ketoconazole in most species, increased liver enzymes, neurologic adverse effects, and decreased appetite have been observed in some dogs. Vomiting and hepatotoxicity are more likely at high doses. In people, transient ocular problems (blurred vision, photophobia) also have been reported.

### Contraindications and Precautions

Doses of 10 mg/kg have caused neurologic problems in cats. A lower dosage of 2–3 mg/kg every other day may be safe if administered for multiple doses, but an evaluation of the long-term safety has not been conducted in cats. Use cautiously in any animal with signs of liver disease. Use cautiously in pregnant animals. At high doses in laboratory animals, drugs in this class have caused fetal abnormalities. Use the oral formulation rather than the IV form in animals with renal disease.

### Drug Interactions

Voriconazole is a potent cytochrome P450 enzyme inhibitor. It may cause drug interactions because of inhibition of P450 enzymes. Drugs affected by this inhibition can include cyclosporine, vincristine, cyclophosphamide, and perhaps others.

## Instructions for Use

The dosages listed for voriconazole are based on experimental studies in animals or clinical reports. Some uses in animals are based on empiricism, small observational studies, or extrapolation from human literature. When used intravenously, the 10-mg/mL solution should be further diluted with fluids to a concentration greater than 5 mg/mL and infused slowly. IV solutions should be used immediately or stored in a refrigerator no longer than 24 hours. If mixed with fluid solutions, it is compatible with lactated Ringer's solution, 5% dextrose, or sodium chloride 0.9%. Do not mix IV solution with blood products or concentrated electrolytes.

## Patient Monitoring and Laboratory Tests

Monitor liver enzyme concentrations during treatment. Plasma concentration monitoring can help predict clinical success. Higher treatment success has been observed in people when trough concentrations were kept above 0.5 mcg/mL and a worse outcome when the concentrations were below 0.5 mcg/mL. Concentrations greater than 3 mcg/mL are associated with a higher risk of hepatic toxicity, and concentrations above 4 mcg/mL are associated with neurotoxicity. Therefore, administer sufficient doses to maintain the trough concentration above 0.5 or 1 mcg/mL but below 3 mcg/mL. Avoid exceeding a peak plasma concentration greater than 4–6 mcg/mL.

## Formulations

- PO: Voriconazole is available in 50- and 200-mg film-coated tablets and a 40-mg/mL oral liquid suspension. The suspension has a 14-day shelf life after reconstitution.
- Injection: 200-mg (10 mg/mL) injection. The IV solution requires reconstitution to 10 mg/mL; then dilution to ≤5 mg/mL for CRI (3 mg/kg/h for 1–2 hours).
- Compounded forms: A variety of compounded forms have been prepared for animals: A drug suspension for animals has been prepared by mixing crushed tablets

(200 mg) with 20 mL of water and 60 mL of Ora-Plus to make a suspension of 2.5 mg/mL. After mixing, this suspension retained the original strength for 17 days. A compounded mixture also has been prepared by mixing two 200-mg tablets crushed to a powder and mixed with 10 mL of a suspending agent and flavoring agent (Ora Plus/Ora Sweet in a ratio of 1:1 or Ora Plus and water in a 3:1 ratio). The suspension should be stored in a brown plastic (not glass) bottle in refrigerator or room temperature. The final formulation is 40 mg/mL and is stable for 30 days. For horses, crushed tablets have been mixed with 30 mL of corn syrup to a concentration of 33 mg/mL and are stable for 48 hours at 8°C. This formulation can be administered to horses orally via syringe.

## Stability and Storage

Store in a tightly sealed container, protected from light, and at room temperature. The commercial suspension has a 14-day shelf-life after reconstitution. See the previous Formulations section for stability information on compounded preparations. Use the IV formulation immediately after mixing or store it in a refrigerator for no longer than 24 hours. Do not mix IV solutions with concentrated electrolytes or blood products.

## Small Animal Dosage

### Dogs

- 5–6 mg/kg q12h PO is the published dose based on studies in research dogs. However, a dosage of 2.5–3.3 mg/kg q12h PO in a clinical report produced adequate plasma concentrations. (The safety of repeated doses in dogs has not been confirmed.)

### Cats

- Administer a loading dose of 25 mg per cat (range, 4.2–4.6 mg/kg) PO, followed by 12.5 mg (2–2.3 mg/kg) every other day. Accumulation may occur after repeated doses; therefore observe for signs of adverse effects with multiple dosing.

### Birds

- 10 mg/kg q12h PO administered as a powder or crushed tablets mixed with water in a liquid suspension (0.5 mg/mL).

## Large Animal Dosage

### Horses

- 2–4 mg/kg q24h or 3 mg/kg q12h PO.
- 1.5 mg/kg q24h IV.

## Regulatory Information

No regulatory information is available. For extralabel use withdrawal interval estimates, contact FARAD at www.FARAD.org.

V

# Warfarin Sodium
war′far-in soe′dee-um

**Trade and other names:** Coumadin and generic brands

**Functional classification:** Anticoagulant

## Pharmacology and Mechanism of Action
Warfarin is an anticoagulant that acts on specific vitamin K–dependent clotting factors. It is used infrequently in animals because of variable response and requirement for monitoring. Warfarin sodium depletes vitamin K, which is responsible for generation of clotting factors.

*Pharmacokinetics:* The half-life of warfarin in animals is 36–42 hours (20–30 hours in cats).

## Indications and Clinical Uses
In small animals, it has been used to treat hypercoagulation disease and prevent thromboembolism. In horses, warfarin has been used to treat navicular disease, although it is no longer popular for this use. The use of warfarin has diminished in small animals because it requires monitoring to optimize the dose and because no clinical trials have shown efficacy for hypercoagulation states in animals. Instead, other anticoagulants and platelet-inhibiting drugs are used.

## Precautionary Information

### Adverse Reactions and Side Effects
Adverse effects are attributable to decreased blood clotting. Spontaneous bleeding can result in blood loss, hemoperitoneum, hemarthrosis, gastrointestinal bleeding, epistaxis, and excessive bleeding from trauma or surgery. If excessive bleeding occurs, patients should be treated with vitamin K.

### Contraindications and Precautions
Do not administer to animals that may be prone to bleeding. Administer carefully with other drugs that are known to interfere with coagulation or with antiplatelet medications (e.g., aspirin or clopidogrel).

### Drug Interactions
Multiple drugs and some foods may affect warfarin's action. Some of these that may potentiate warfarin's action include aspirin, chloramphenicol, phenylbutazone, ketoconazole, and cimetidine. Drug interactions are possible with administration with other highly protein-bound drugs, but such reactions are poorly documented in animals. Drug interactions are also possible with trimethoprim sulfonamides and metronidazole. Do not administer with some cephalosporin drugs (particularly those with N-methylthiotetrazole [NMTT]) because cephalosporins may induce bleeding through anti–vitamin K–dependent mechanisms.

## Instructions for Use
Warfarin response can be highly variable among animals. Pharmacokinetic studies have attempted to correlate plasma pharmacokinetics with clinical response (prothrombin time [PT]). However, such a correlation has been difficult to

demonstrate. A particular dose and plasma concentration that produces an effective prolongation of PT in one patient may not be effective in another individual. Because of the variation in response, adjust doses by monitoring bleeding times in treated animals. For a rapid effect, consider a loading dose of 6 mg per dog once daily for two treatments. Initial doses in cats have ranged from 0.06–0.09 mg/kg (0.25–0.5 mg/cat/day). When dividing tablets for treatment, it is best to crush up a whole tablet into a powder and divide the doses equally from the powder. When tablets are cut into halves or quarters, there may be uneven distribution of warfarin within the tablet. Some fractions of the tablet may contain a higher amount than others.

## Patient Monitoring and Laboratory Tests

Adjust the dose by monitoring clotting times because the optimum dose is highly individualistic. The best method to monitor warfarin therapy is with the one-stage PT. PTs are reported in seconds and recorded as a ratio of the PT of the patient to the mean normal PT of the laboratory and as the international normalized ratio (INR). The INR is the most reliable way to monitor the PT, but it may not be available in all laboratories. In animals, the dose is adjusted to maintain PT at 1.5–2 times normal (or an INR of 2–3).

## Formulations

• Warfarin sodium is available in 1-, 2-, 2.5-, 4-, 5-, 7.5-, and 10-mg tablets.

## Stability and Storage

Warfarin sodium is soluble in water. It is light sensitive and should be packaged in tight containers. Solutions should have a pH greater than 8 to maintain solubility. Some tablets do not have the drug distributed evenly; therefore uneven doses can result from splitting tablets.

## Small Animal Dosage

### Dogs

• 0.1–0.2 mg/kg q24h PO. Start with this dose q12h for the first 2–4 days because of a lag time before maximum effect is observed.

### Cats

• Start with 0.25–0.5 mg/cat/day (¼ to ½ of a 1-mg tablet) and adjust the dose based on bleeding time assessment. A dosage of 0.1 mg/kg per day generally prolongs the PT by 1.5–2 times.

## Large Animal Dosage

### Horses

• 0.02 mg/kg q24h PO (9 mg per 450 kg of body weight [1000 lb]). Increase this dosage gradually by increments of 20% until a 2- to 4-second increase in PT bleeding time is achieved. Allow 7 days between changes in dose.

## Regulatory Information

Do not administer to animals intended for food.
Racing Commissioners International Classification: 5

**W**

# Xylazine Hydrochloride
zye'lah-zeen hye-droe-klor'ide

**Trade and other names:** Rompun and generic brands

**Functional classification:** Alpha$_2$-adrenergic agonist, analgesic, sedative

## Pharmacology and Mechanism of Action

Xylazine is the oldest alpha$_2$-adrenergic agonists used in veterinary medicine. Alpha$_2$ agonists decrease release of neurotransmitters from the neuron. They decrease transmission via binding to presynaptic alpha$_2$ receptors (negative-feedback receptors). The results are decreased sympathetic outflow, analgesia, sedation, and anesthesia. Other drugs in this class include medetomidine, dexmedetomidine, romifidine, detomidine, and clonidine. Xylazine is not as specific as other drugs in this group. The alpha$_2$-specific effects are measured by comparing the alpha$_1$/alpha$_2$-receptor affinity ratio. The ratios are 1:160 for xylazine, 1:260 for detomidine; 1:360 for romifidine, and 1:1620 for dexmedetomidine (medetomidine). Thus, receptor-binding studies indicate that xylazine is the least specific of this class.

*Pharmacokinetics:* The pharmacokinetics have been studied in all domestic species. The pharmacokinetics are characterized by rapid (within minutes) distribution to the central nervous system and elimination half-life of 20–40 minutes from a bolus injection. In horses, after a constant rate infusion (CRI), the terminal half-life is approximately 2 hours.

## Indications and Clinical Uses

Xylazine has been used for many years for short-term sedation, anesthesia, and analgesia in horses, dogs, cats, cattle, and exotic animals. Like other alpha$_2$ agonists, it is used as an anesthetic adjunct and analgesic. The duration of effect is approximately 30 minutes after a bolus injection, but it also may be administered by a CRI for up to 6 hours. Compared with xylazine, dexmedetomidine and medetomidine produce better sedation and analgesia in dogs. Xylazine is used more commonly in large animals for sedation and analgesia than in small animals. Usually, dexmedetomidine is preferred in dogs and cats. Romifidine produces the longest duration of sedative effects followed by detomidine, medetomidine (dexmedetomidine), and xylazine.

## Precautionary Information

### Adverse Reactions and Side Effects

In small animals, vomiting is the most common acute effect, which is more prominent in cats than dogs. Xylazine produces sedation and ataxia, which is expected from all alpha$_2$ agonists. Xylazine, like other alpha$_2$ agonists, decreases sympathetic output. Cardiovascular depression may occur. Xylazine produces an initial hypertensive phase, followed by a hypotensive phase. Cardiac effects can include sinoatrial block, first- and second-degree atrioventricular block, bradycardia, and sinus arrhythmia. Like other alpha$_2$ agonists, xylazine produces transient hyperglycemia, which may increase urine flow.

In ruminants, use of xylazine may decrease gastrointestinal motility and cause bloating, salivation, and regurgitation. Note that cattle, sheep, and goats are much more sensitive to xylazine than other animals; therefore doses need to be lower than those in other animals. Among horses, draft horses are more sensitive to the effects than thoroughbred and Arab horses.

### Contraindications and Precautions

Ruminants are much more sensitive to xylazine than other species, and lower doses must be used compared with other animals. Use cautiously in animals that are pregnant. Xylazine impairs blood flow to the uterus during gestation in cows and may decrease oxygen delivery to the fetus, especially in late gestation. Use caution when using xylazine to sedate pregnant cows. It also may induce labor. Use cautiously, if at all, in patients with cardiac disease. Because of cardiac depression, it should not ordinarily be used with tranquilizers such as phenothiazines that can produce vasodilation.

### Drug Interactions

Use with opioid analgesic drugs greatly enhances the central nervous system depression. Consider lowering doses if administered with opioids. Do not administer with other drugs that cause significant cardiac depression.

## Instructions for Use

Xylazine is often used in combination with other drugs (e.g., ketamine, opioids, or butorphanol). It is combined with guaifenesin and ketamine in the equine "triple drip" combination (see dosing section, below).

Although low heart rates are anticipated with xylazine, it is not necessary to premedicate animals with atropine. For large animals, if sedation is needed without recumbency, use the lower end of the dose range. Reverse effects of xylazine with an alpha$_2$ antagonist (e.g., yohimbine, tolazoline, or atipamezole) if adverse effects are serious enough to warrant reversal. Xylazine also may be administered intraosseously to horses when it is not possible to give an IV injection. It is equally bioavailable from the intraosseous route as IV.

## Patient Monitoring and Laboratory Tests

Monitor heart rate and rhythm during anesthesia with xylazine. It may cause increased plasma glucose concentrations in animals.

## Formulations Available

* Xylazine is available in 20- and 100-mg/mL injections.

## Stability and Storage

Store in a tightly sealed container, protected from light, and at room temperature.

## Small Animal Dosage

### Dogs

* 1.1 mg/kg IV.
* 2.2 mg/kg IM.
* Short-term treatment of pain: 0.1–0.5 mg/kg IM, IV, or SQ.

### Cats

* 1.1 mg/kg IM.
* Emetic dosage: 0.4–0.5 mg/kg IM or IV.
* Short-term treatment of pain: 0.1–0.5 mg/kg IM, IV, or SQ.

## Large Animal Dosage

### Horses

* 1–2 mg/kg IM.
* Standing chemical restraint: 0.5–1.0 mg/kg IV bolus. (The IV dose also can be administered intraosseously with equal bioavailability.)

- 0.5–1.1 mg/kg IV followed by (if necessary) a 0.72–1 mg/kg/h CRI.
- For colic pain: 0.3–0.5 mg/kg IV (150–250 mg IV for an average-size horse).
- For anesthesia purposes, it is sometimes combined with other agents such as ketamine and guaifenesin in the equine "triple-drip" combination. This combination consists of 500 mg of xylazine and 2 g of ketamine added to 1 L of 5% of guaifenesin in dextrose. It is administered at a rate of 1.1 mL/kg for induction followed by 2–4 mL/kg/h for maintenance. Recovery usually occurs in 25–30 minutes or administer 0.125 mg/kg yohimbine to speed up recovery.

### Pigs

- 0.5–3 mg/kg IM. Xylazine in pigs is best used in combination with other drugs (e.g., 2 mg/kg xylazine mixed in a syringe with 10 mg/kg of ketamine). It is unreliable used alone.

### Cattle

- 0.1–0.2 mg/kg IM.
- 0.03–0.1 mg/kg IV.

### Sheep

- 0.1–0.3 mg/kg IM.
- 0.05–0.1 mg/kg IV.

### Goats

- 0.05–0.5 mg/kg IM.
- 0.01–0.5 mg/kg IV.

## Regulatory Information

Withdrawal time for cattle: At a dosage of 0.016–0.1 mg/kg, 5 days for meat and 72 hours for milk. At a dosage of 0.05–0.3 mg/kg, 10 days for meat and 120 hours for milk. Whereas in Canada, it is listed as 3 days for meat and 48 hours for milk, in the United Kingdom, it is listed as 14 days for meat and 48 hours for milk. If yohimbine is used as a reversal agent, use a withdrawal time of 7 days for meat and 72 hours for milk.

Racing Commissioners International Classification: 3

# Yohimbine
yoe-him′been

**Trade and other names:** Yobine

**Functional classification:** Alpha$_2$-receptor antagonist

## Pharmacology and Mechanism of Action

Yohimbine is one of the older alpha$_2$-adrenergic antagonists. It is derived from several botanical sources (tree bark, roots, and other plants) and nonselectively antagonizes alpha-adrenergic receptors. It antagonizes the action of other drugs, such as anesthetic and sedative agents, that stimulate the alpha$_2$ receptor. At high doses, it may act as an agonist for other receptors such as the alpha$_1$, dopamine, and serotonin receptors. Alpha$_2$ agonists have profound effects on blood pressure, cardiac output, and intestinal motility, as well as their well-known properties of sedation and analgesia. The alpha$_2$ antagonists such as yohimbine can reverse these effects when necessary. Atipamezole is a more selective alpha$_2$ antagonist and is used preferentially in small animals to reverse the effects of alpha$_2$ agonists. (See Atipamezole for more details.)

*Pharmacokinetics:* In horses, when yohimbine is administered at 0.12 mg/kg, it has a half-life of approximately 4.4 hours and volume of distribution of 3.2 L/kg.

## Indications and Clinical Uses

Yohimbine is used primarily to reverse actions of xylazine or detomidine. Atipamezole is another alpha$_2$ antagonist that is more specific for the alpha$_2$ receptor and is preferred to use in small animals to reverse dexmedetomidine or medetomidine. Tolazoline has also been used to reverse effects of xylazine in horses.

## Precautionary Information

### Adverse Reactions and Side Effects

Yohimbine can produce a variety of responses in horses. Some horses show excitation rearing, striking, muscle tremors, and exaggerated response to stimuli. Yohimbine may cause more transient excitement than either atipamezole or tolazoline. It can produce cardiovascular events in horses such as increased heart rate.

High doses can cause tremors and seizures. If used alone (not recommended), it can produce a variety of undesirable events.

### Contraindications and Precautions

When yohimbine is administered to reverse an alpha$_2$ agonist, monitor heart rate and rhythm carefully during treatment. There is no therapeutic justification to administer an alpha$_2$ antagonist such as yohimbine as a single agent to treat horses for any diseases.

### Drug Interactions

Detomidine increases the plasma concentration and decreases clearance of yohimbine. No other interactions are reported, except the antagonism of alpha$_2$ agonists.

**Y**

## Instructions for Use

Yohimbine is used to reverse the signs of sedation and anesthesia caused by alpha$_2$ agonists. The drug concentrations of the alpha$_2$ agonist (e.g., xylazine, detomidine) may be diminished considerably by the time reversal becomes necessary in clinical practice; therefore, it may not be necessary to provide a full dose of yohimbine (or other alpha$_2$ antagonist) because a full dose may induce excitement and other undesirable events. Instead, one third of the recommended dose of yohimbine can be administered first followed by (if necessary) the same amount in 5- to 10-minute increments.

## Patient Monitoring and Laboratory Tests

Monitor heart rate and rhythm during use of yohimbine.

## Formulations

- Yohimbine is available in a 2-mg/mL injection.

## Stability and Storage

Store in a tightly sealed container, protected from light, and at room temperature.

## Small Animal Dosage

### Dogs and Cats

- 0.11 mg/kg IV.
- 0.25–0.5 mg/kg SQ or IM.

## Large Animal Dosage

### Horses

- 0.125 mg/kg IV (to reverse xylazine).
- 0.2 mg/kg IV (to reverse detomidine).
- Note about reversal: It may not be necessary to give the full dose initially. See Instructions for Use for more details.

### Cattle and Sheep

- To reverse xylazine or medetomidine: 0.125–0.2 mg/kg IV.

## Regulatory Information

Food animal withdrawal time: At least 7 days for meat and 72 hours for milk.
Racing Commissioners International Classification: 2

# Zidovudine
zye-doe′vyoo-deen

**Trade and other names:** Retrovir and azidothymidine (AZT)

**Functional classification:** Antiviral

## Pharmacology and Mechanism of Action
Zidovudine is an antiviral drug that is used infrequently in animals. Zidovudine (also known as azidothymidine or AZT) acts to inhibit the viral enzyme reverse transcriptase that prevents conversion of viral RNA into DNA. The most common use in people is for treatment of HIV/AIDS. Other drugs in this class include lamivudine, didanosine, stavudine, and zalcitabine. There are not enough clinical data on these other agents to discuss in this handbook.

## Indications and Clinical Uses
In people, AZT is used to treat HIV (AIDS). In animals, it has been experimentally used for treatment of feline leukemia virus (FeLV) and feline immunodeficiency virus (FIV) infection in cats. In cats, dosages of 25 mg/kg q12h IV or PO produced drug concentrations in the effective range to inhibit the virus. In experimentally infected cats with FeLV, it was effective to improve clinical signs. However, in naturally infected cats, it has not been effective, and the use in cats for this disease has been disappointing. In some cats, at a dosage of 5–10 mg/kg PO q12h, it may be more helpful for FIV than for FeLV and can improve quality of life, decrease virus load, and improve clinical signs in cats with FIV. AZT can reduce viral load and improve immunologic and clinical status, particularly in cats with stomatitis and neurologic signs.

## Precautionary Information
### Adverse Reactions and Side Effects
Anemia and leucopenia have been observed in treated animals. Adverse effects are more common in cats at high doses (above 10 mg/kg q12h). It has not been used often in animals; therefore a full range of potential adverse effects has not been reported.

### Contraindications and Precautions
No contraindications are reported for animals.

### Drug Interactions
No drug interactions have been reported in animals. However, the use has been infrequent, and a full range of potential drug interactions is not known.

## Instructions for Use
At this time, experience with using AZT for treating viral disease in animals is largely experimental or anecdotal. This drug may help some cats with FIV and may prevent persistent FeLV, but documentation of clinical efficacy from well-controlled clinical trials is lacking.

## Patient Monitoring and Laboratory Tests
Monitor the packed-cell volume in treated cats and perform a complete blood count. This should be done once per week initially and then once per month after the cat is stabilized.

## Formulations
- AZT is available in a 10-mg/mL syrup and a 10-mg/mL injection. The syrup has been reformulated into capsules for cats.

## Stability and Storage
Store in a tightly sealed container, protected from light, and at room temperature.

## Small Animal Dosage
### Cats
- 5–10 mg/kg PO or SQ q12h. If administered SQ, dilute in saline first to avoid injection-site irritation.

## Large Animal Dosage
- No dose has been reported for large animals.

## Regulatory Information
Do not administer to animals intended for food.

# Zilpaterol Hydrochloride
zil-pat′e-role

**Trade and other names:** Zilmax

**Functional classification:** Beta-adrenergic agonist

## Pharmacology and Mechanism of Action
Zilpaterol is a synthetic beta-receptor adrenergic agonist. Zilpaterol is administered to cattle in feed as a growth promoter and to improve feed efficiency. Zilpaterol, like other beta-adrenergic agonists, stimulates beta$_2$-adrenergic receptors in muscle and promotes muscle gain with less fat. Subsequently, if fed to cattle at approved levels, zilpaterol increases feed efficiency and improves muscle weight gain. In clinical studies, it substantially increased skeletal muscle mass and the cross-sectional area of individual muscles. It has not been used for other diseases that may benefit from beta-adrenergic stimulation.

## Indications and Clinical Uses
Zilpaterol is fed to cattle (type A medicated feed) to improve weight gain and muscle mass. It has been approved in the United States and other countries for this use. It is not approved for other uses and should not be administered to horses.

## Precautionary Information
### Adverse Reactions and Side Effects
Like other beta-adrenergic agonists, zilpaterol can produce cardiovascular problems associated with increased stimulation of receptors at high doses.

### Contraindications and Precautions
Severe adverse effects such as tachycardia, tremors, and muscle fasciculations have been observed in horses. Zilpaterol should not be administered to horses, and precautions should be taken to ensure that horses are not accidentally exposed to zilpaterol-treated cattle feed.

Because beta-adrenergic agonists such as clenbuterol are abused in humans for the purpose of promoting muscle gain and fat loss, there is a possibility that zilpaterol also could be abused in the same manner.

Labeling should include the following information: (1) Do not allow horses or other equines access to feed containing zilpaterol. (2) Not for use in animals intended for breeding. (3) Do not use in veal calves.

### Drug Interactions
Use caution when administering to animals receiving other adrenergic medications.

## Instructions for Use

Zilpaterol is used to increase rate of weight gain, improve feed efficiency, and increase carcass leanness in cattle fed in confinement for slaughter during the last 20–40 days on feed. It should be fed continuously as the sole ration during the last 20–40 days on feed.

## Patient Monitoring and Laboratory Tests

No specific monitoring is necessary.

## Formulations

• Type A medicated articles containing 21.77 g of zilpaterol hydrochloride per pound. There are several other feed additive formulations available that contain other ingredients, such as monensin, tylosin, and/or melengestrol acetate. Consult specific labeling for more details.

## Stability and Storage

Store in a tightly sealed container, protected from light, and at room temperature.

## Small Animal Dosage

• No small animal dose is established. No established uses for small animals.

## Large Animal Dosage

• Do not administer to horses.
• Cattle dose: 6.8 g/ton of feed to provide 60–90 mg of zilpaterol hydrochloride per head per day.

## Regulatory Information

Cattle withdrawal time for slaughter: 3 days.
Racing Commissioners International (RCI) Classification for horses: Class 3

# Zinc

**Trade and other names:** Zinc

**Functional classification:** Nutritional supplement

## Pharmacology and Mechanism of Action

Zinc is an essential element important in more than 200 metalloenzymes. It also is important for nucleic acid, cell membrane, and protein synthesis. In addition, it is important for growth, tissue repair, and cell division. Zinc acts as a chelating agent, and it competes with iron to inhibit fibrosis and collagen formation. It induces the production of metallothionein in intestinal mucosal cells, which binds copper from the diet and prevents uptake to the liver. The benefits have been seen in experimental animals and in humans with liver disease. One of the uses has been to manage hepatic cirrhosis. Zinc also may act as an antioxidant and prevent membrane damage.

## Indications and Clinical Uses

Zinc supplementation has been used to treat zinc-deficient diseases such as those that cause dermatologic problems. It is also used as an antifibrotic agent in liver disease. Zinc administration also may be used as a chelating agent in animals. Most commonly, zinc has been used as a cupruretic to decrease copper concentrations in animals with liver disease, often in combination with other drugs (e.g., penicillamine or trientine). When used to treat copper liver disease, it is slow acting and may take as long as 3 months for the full effect.

Z

## Precautionary Information
### Adverse Reactions and Side Effects
The most common effect is gastrointestinal (GI) problems, including nausea and vomiting. Hemolysis and anemia can be observed with high doses.

### Contraindications and Precautions
If IV forms are used (e.g., zinc sulfate), adverse effects may be more likely because it produces higher concentrations. The oral absorption is lower and more limited.

### Drug Interactions
Oral absorption is impaired from tetracyclines, iron, copper, phytates (found in bran and grains), and penicillamine.

## Instructions for Use
Administer without food to improve oral absorption, but a small meal often prevents some of the nausea associated with treatment. When considering various forms, the gluconate form may be better tolerated than the sulfate or acetate form.

## Patient Monitoring and Laboratory Tests
Monitor blood zinc concentrations at least monthly to prevent high levels, which cause hemolysis. Blood zinc concentrations should ideally be 200–500 mcg/dL. A concentration above 800 mcg/dL is considered toxic, but levels above 200 mcg/dL are needed to treat copper liver disease.

## Formulations
- Zinc is available in several forms, including zinc sulfate (23% zinc), zinc gluconate (14% zinc), and zinc acetate (35% zinc).
- Zinc gluconate is available in tablets ranging from 1.4 to 52 mg (10 mg zinc gluconate = 1.4 mg of elemental zinc).
- Zinc sulfate is available in capsules containing 25 and 50 mg of elemental zinc (110 mg of zinc sulfate = 25 mg of elemental zinc). Zinc sulfate is also available in tablets containing 15, 25, 45, and 50 mg of elemental zinc (66 mg of zinc sulfate = 15 mg of elemental zinc).
- Injectable zinc sulfate is available in a 50-mg/mL (20.2 mg of elemental zinc per milliliter) solution for IV use.

## Stability and Storage
Store in a tightly sealed container, protected from light, and at room temperature.

## Small Animal Dosage
### Dogs and Cats
Adjust dose based on measuring plasma zinc concentrations.
- Hepatic disease in dogs: 100 mg of elemental zinc per dog q12h PO, equivalent to 3 mg/kg per day of zinc gluconate, or 2 mg/kg of zinc sulfate per day PO. (Consider including vitamin E with treatment.)
- Zinc supplement: 1 mg/kg of elemental zinc gluconate or sulfate three times/day PO or 1.5–3 mg (of elemental zinc) of zinc acetate daily per animal PO.
- Dermatologic use: 10 mg/kg per day (zinc sulfate or zinc gluconate).
- IV zinc treatment: 50 mcg of elemental zinc/kg infused IV slowly per day.

## Large Animal Dosage

- No specific doses have been reported. If zinc supplementation is needed, extrapolate the dose from small animal use (approximately 1 mg/kg of elemental zinc three times per day PO) and adjust the dose by monitoring zinc concentrations.

## Regulatory Information

Because of a low risk of harmful residues in animals intended for food, no withdrawal time is suggested.

---

# Zoledronate

zoe′le-droe-nate

**Trade and other names:** Zometa, Zoledronic acid, and Reclast

**Functional classification:** Antihypercalcemic

## Pharmacology and Mechanism of Action

Zoledronate is a bisphosphonate drug. Zoledronate is also called zoledronic acid (Zometa). Other drugs in this class include pamidronate, etidronate, tiludronate, clodronate, and alendronate. These drugs belong to a group characterized by a germinal aminobisphosphonate bond. They slow the formation and dissolution of hydroxyapatite crystals. These drugs are classified as nitrogenous and nonnitrogenous bisphosphonates on the basis of whether they contain a nitrogen group. Zoledronate is a nitrogen-containing bisphosphonate, which has a hydroxyl group on carbon units opposite the nitrogen group that leads to slow metabolism and that is poorly metabolized and achieves high affinity for bone surfaces. The nitrogenous bisphosphonates such as zoledronate have much greater antiresorptive bone activity than nonnitrogenous bisphosphonates (e.g., clodronate and tiludronate). The clinical use of bisphosphonates resides in their ability to inhibit bone resorption. Inhibition of bone resorption is via inhibition of the mevalonate pathway. These drugs decrease bone turnover by inhibiting osteoclast activity, inducing osteoclast apoptosis, retarding bone resorption, and decreasing the rate of osteoporosis.

*Pharmacokinetics:* In dogs, after infusion, the half-life is approximately 2.2 hours, with a volume of distribution of 0.28 L/kg. In horses, it has a plasma half-life of 2.2 hours after IV administration. In all animals, the concentrations in bone persist for much longer than in blood or plasma.

## Indications and Clinical Uses

Zoledronate, like other bisphosphonate drugs, is used to treat refractory hypercalcemia, osteoporosis, and treatment of hypercalcemia of malignancy. In animals, bisphosphonates are helpful for managing neoplastic complications and pain associated with pathologic bone resorption. They also may provide pain relief in patients with pathologic bone disease. Other uses include osteoporosis and skeletal metastasis. It has been used in similar protocols as for pamidronate but has the advantage of a 15-minute infusion IV rather than 2–4 hours for pamidronate.

In horses, it has been administered via IV infusion for bone pain and conditions associated with bone fragility. However, other approved bisphosphonates are preferred in horses because of equine-specific labeling and experience. The agents approved for horses for treatment of navicular disease and other bone disorders include tiludronate and clodronate. See sections in this book for more information on these drugs for horses.

Z

## Precautionary Information

### Adverse Reactions and Side Effects

Zoledronate may be safer than pamidronate. Fever, joint pain, and myalgias have been observed in people, but otherwise no serious adverse effects have been identified. The use in animals has not been common enough to identify a wider range of adverse effects. In people, there is some concern that the use of bisphosphonates produces excessive mineralization and hardening of the bone, which may result in a greater risk of fractures. However, this effect has not been reported for animals.

### Contraindications and Precautions

Do not administer during pregnancy. There are also concerns about using bisphosphonates in young animals when rapid development of bone is needed. Do not administer zoledronate to young horses.

### Drug Interactions

Do not mix with calcium or other divalent cation-containing infusion solutions, such as lactated Ringer's solution. It should be administered as a single IV solution in a line separate from other drugs.

## Instructions for Use

Zoledronate is intended for IV infusion. Dilute the vial in 0.9% saline or 5% dextrose solution for IV use. If not used immediately after dilution, the solution should be refrigerated, and the refrigerated solution then should be equilibrated to room temperature prior to administration. The total time between dilution, storage in the refrigerator, and end of administration must not exceed 24 hours.

If administered to horses, which is not recommended, monitor creatinine, blood urea nitrogen (BUN), and calcium prior to administration to ensure that it is safe for the patient. However, as noted earlier, other agents are preferred for horses. Calcium supplementation in the diet is recommended.

## Patient Monitoring and Laboratory Tests

Monitor serum calcium and phosphorus. Monitor BUN, creatinine, urine-specific gravity, and food intake in treated animals.

## Formulations

- Zoledronate (zoledronic acid) is available in a 4-mg/5 mL vial for infusion and 5-mg/100 mL IV solution.

## Stability and Storage

Store in a vial at room temperature. Vials may be diluted in fluid solutions. Storage and stability information is listed in the Instructions for Use section.

## Small Animal Dosage

### Dogs

- 0.2–0.25 mg/kg IV infused over 15 minutes, diluted in 100 mL of 0.9% saline (large dogs) or 50 mL of 0.9% saline (small dogs). This dose can be administered once every 28 days.
- For osteoporosis: 5 mg (per dog) every 1–2 years IV.
- Hypercalcemia associated with cancer: 4 mg (per dog) infusion every 7 days.
- Multiple myeloma: 4 mg (per dog) infusion every 3–4 weeks.

### Cats

- 0.2 mg/kg IV over 15 minutes diluted in a volume of 25 mL every 21–28 days.
- Idiopathic hypercalcemia: 1–3 mg/kg per week.

## Large Animal Dosage
**Horses**
(Not recommended)
- 0.075 mg/kg. Dissolve each dose in 50 mL of 11.3 mg/mL citrate solution; then mix with 500 mL (400 mL of saline and 100 mL of mannitol). Administer via IV infusion to horses over 15–30 minutes. Other bisphosphonates preferred for horses include tiludronate and clodronate.

## Regulatory Information
Withdrawal times are not established for animals that produce food. For extralabel use withdrawal interval estimates, contact Food Animal Residue Avoidance Databank (FARAD) at FARAD at www.FARAD.org.

# Zolpidem
zolepi′dem
**Trade and other names:** Ambien, Edluar, Intermezzo, and Zolpimist
**Functional classification:** Sedative

## Pharmacology and Mechanism of Action
Zolpidem is a sedative and sleep aid that is used in people but infrequently used in animals. Zolpidem is a nonbenzodiazepine sedative. In people, it has effects similar to the benzodiazepines and is used as a sedative and sleep aid.

Like benzodiazepines, zolpidem potentiates the action of gamma-aminobutyric acid (GABA), an inhibitory neurotransmitter. However, it does not cause muscle relaxation or produce anticonvulsant properties. The benzodiazepines act on the $GABA_A$ and $GABA_B$ receptor. $GABA_A$ has omega-1, omega-2, and omega-3 receptors. Benzodiazepines act on all receptors, but zolpidem and other drugs known as Z-drugs only act on the omega-1 receptor to produce sedation.

## Indications and Clinical Uses
Zolpidem is used as a sedative and sleep aid in people. However, this property has not been shown in animals. It is infrequently used in animals and may produce significant adverse effects.

## Precautionary Information
**Adverse Reactions and Side Effects**
In dogs, it produced adverse effects that included vocalization, restlessness, anxiety, dysphoria, rage reaction, excitement, muscle spasticity, and hyperreflexia.

**Contraindications and Precautions**
Because of the adverse reactions observed, it is not recommended for dogs.

**Drug Interactions**
Avoid use with other sedatives, behavior-modifying drugs, or drugs that decrease drug metabolism.

## Instructions for Use
Clinical uses have not been established for veterinary patients.

## Patient Monitoring and Laboratory Tests
No monitoring has been recommended for animals.

## Formulations
• Available in 5- or 10-mg tablets.

## Stability and Storage
Store in a tightly sealed container, protected from light, and at room temperature. Stability of compounded formulations has not been evaluated.

## Small Animal Dosage
### Dogs
• 0.5 mg or 0.15 mg/kg once. (Use cautiously because of adverse effects.)

### Cats
• Dose regimens have not been defined in cats.

### Large Animal Dosage
• No dose has been reported for large animals.

## Regulatory Information
No regulatory information is available. Avoid use in food-producing animals. Do not use in racehorses.
Schedule IV controlled substance

---

# Zonisamide
zoe-nis′a-mide

**Trade and other names:** Zonegran

**Functional classification:** Anticonvulsant

---

## Pharmacology and Mechanism of Action
Zonisamide is an anticonvulsant that is used sometimes as an add-on to other drugs. The mechanism of action is uncertain. Various mechanisms have been proposed: It may suppress voltage-dependent sodium and T-type calcium channels that produce excessive excitation and stabilize membranes and suppress propagation of seizures from an epileptic foci. Zonisamide may potentiate the action of GABA, an inhibitory neurotransmitter. It may also affect dopaminergic and serotonergic systems. Its use as an anticonvulsant is usually as an add-on for refractory cases. It is rarely used as an initial sole treatment for epilepsy.

*Pharmacokinetics:* The half-life in dogs has been reported to be approximately 15 hours in one study and 16 hours (plasma) to 57 hours (red blood cells) in another study. In cats, the half-life is longer than in dogs (33 hours), with a peak at 4 hours.

## Indications and Clinical Uses
Zonisamide is used to treat refractory seizures in dogs when other drugs have not been effective. It has been effective in experimentally induced seizures in dogs and in approximately 50% of dogs with refractory epilepsy. It has been used as an add-on with other anticonvulsant drugs such as phenobarbital and potassium bromide. When used as an add-on treatment, it may reduce the dose of other anticonvulsants (e.g., phenobarbital). It has been used in cats, as an add-on, or as a single treatment. Clinical efficacy has not been reported in cats, but at the doses

listed, it suppressed electroencephalographic electrical activity in cats consistent with control of feline seizures.

## Precautionary Information

### Adverse Reactions and Side Effects

Adverse effects reported are based on limited case reports. These are usually mild and transient. In dogs, it may cause sedation, lethargy, ataxia, and vomiting. Liver injury is possible, and dogs should be monitored during treatment. Zonisamide can affect thyroid hormones in dogs, and thyroid monitoring should be performed in dogs on long-term treatment with zonisamide. Zonisamide is a sulfonamide drug, and dogs that are sensitive to sulfonamides may be at higher risk for reactions to zonisamide. In safety studies, beagles received 75 mg/kg/day for 1 year with minimal side effects. In cats, adverse effects include mild GI problems, sedation, and ataxia.

### Contraindications and Precautions

Because zonisamide resembles sulfonamides in structure, use cautiously in animals that are sensitive to these drugs. (See Sulfonamide for full details on adverse effects.)

### Drug Interactions

When administered concurrently with phenobarbital, the half-life of elimination is more rapid for zonisamide, which may necessitate higher doses. It is expected to potentiate other central nervous system depressants and anticonvulsants.

## Instructions for Use

Most experience with zonisamide in animals has been preliminary work in dogs with refractory epilepsy. Although low doses may produce plasma concentrations within the therapeutic range reported for people, when administered with phenobarbital, drug concentrations may be lower because drug metabolism is increased. Zonisamide half-life was shorter in dogs receiving phenobarbital concurrently. These observations indicate that higher doses may be needed for combination therapy with phenobarbital compared with monotherapy. (Note that higher dose is listed later when used with phenobarbital.) With chronic treatment, some tolerance that reduces efficacy after 2–3 months may develop.

Although zonisamide has been administered by the rectal route to animals, this is not recommended. The dose administered rectally was prepared by combining the contents of a capsule in water to a 100 mg/mL suspension. However, when delivered by the rectal route (20 or 30 mg/kg), it did not achieve plasma concentrations in the range that is considered therapeutic for dogs.

### Patient Monitoring and Laboratory Tests

Effective plasma concentrations in animals have been suggested to be 10–40 mcg/mL. Concentrations above 20 mcg/mL in cats have produced adverse effects. Because of the potential for zonisamide to affect thyroid hormones in dogs, monitor tetraiodothyronine ($T_4$) levels periodically during treatment.

### Formulations

• Zonisamide is available in 25-, 50-, and 100-mg capsules.

### Stability and Storage

Store in a tightly sealed container, protected from light, and at room temperature. Stability of compounded formulations has not been evaluated.

Z

## Small Animal Dosage

### Dogs

- Start with 5 mg/kg q12h PO and increase gradually as needed to maintain plasma drug concentrations and control seizures.
- 10 mg/kg q12h PO when added to phenobarbital treatment.

### Cats

- 5 mg/kg PO q12h or 10 mg/kg PO q24h and increase dose as needed by monitoring.

## Large Animal Dosage

- No dose has been reported for large animals.

## Regulatory Information

No regulatory information is available. For extralabel use withdrawal interval estimates, contact FARAD at www.FARAD.org.

RCI Classification: 3

# APPENDIX A
# Information for Pharmacists

## Excipients in Medications or Human Drugs That May Be Harmful to Pets

| Drug, Excipient, or Food | Species Affected | Toxicity |
|---|---|---|
| Acetaminophen | Dogs, cats | Hepatotoxicity (dogs) and red blood cell oxidative injury (cats) |
| Alcohols | Dogs, cats, birds | Central nervous system toxicity |
| Avocado | Birds | Pulmonary congestion; nonsuppurative inflammation of the liver, kidney, pancreas, skin, and proventriculus |
| Benzocaine | Cats | Red blood cell oxidative injury, hemolytic anemia |
| Chamomile | Cats | Emesis, diarrhea, depression, lethargy, epistaxis |
| Chocolate | Dogs, birds | Cardiovascular and central nervous system stimulation |
| Estrogen | Dogs | Bone marrow suppression |
| Ethyl glycols (diethylene glycol, ethylene glycol) | Dogs, cats | Central nervous system toxicity, nephrotoxicity |
| Fat, fatty foods | Dogs | Increased risk of pancreatitis |
| Garlic and onions | Dogs, cats | Hemolytic anemia |
| Grapes and raisins | Dogs | Renal toxicity |
| Macadamia nuts | Dogs | Neurotoxicity |
| Macrolide antibiotics, oral route | Horses, rabbits | Diarrhea, enteritis, colic |
| Methylene blue | Cats | Red blood cell oxidative injury, hemolytic anemia |
| Nonsteroidal anti-inflammatory agents for humans (naproxen, ibuprofen) | Dogs, cats | Gastrointestinal ulceration and perforation, nephrotoxicity |
| Pennyroyal | Cats | Hepatotoxicity |
| Permethrin | Cats | Neuromuscular and central nervous system toxicity |
| Phenazopyridine | Cats | Hepatotoxicity and red blood cell oxidative injury |
| Phosphate enemas | Cats | Profound hypocalcemia |
| Pseudoephedrine | Dogs, cats | Cardiovascular and central nervous system stimulation |

*Continued*

## Excipients in Medications or Human Drugs That May Be Harmful to Pets—cont'd

| Drug, Excipient, or Food | Species Affected | Toxicity |
|---|---|---|
| Raw yeast dough | Dogs | Alcohol poisoning, gastrointestinal dilatation and volvulus |
| Salt (excessive) | Dogs, cats | Hypernatremia, central nervous system toxicity |
| Tobacco products | Dogs, cats | Muscle weakness, twitching, depression, tachycardia, shallow respiration, collapse, coma, cardiac arrest |
| Xylitol | Dogs, birds | Profound hypoglycemia and hepatocellular necrosis |

This table was created with the assistance of Gigi Davidson, RPh, North Carolina State University.

# APPENDIX B
# Prescription Writing Reference

## Always Include
- Prescribing veterinarian's name
- Practice address
- Practice telephone number
- Drug Enforcement Administration (DEA) number. Include your DEA number if written for a controlled substance. But avoid sharing your DEA license number if the prescription is *not a controlled substance.*
- Current date

## Rx
- **Drug name:** Print FULL brand name or generic name; NEVER abbreviate.
- **Dosage form:** Specify tablet, capsule, suspension, or other.
- **Strength:** Specify the strength in milligrams (mg), micrograms (mcg), gram (g), or other appropriate unit of dose strength or concentration (mg/mL). Use metric units and use mcg for µg whenever possible.
- **Total quantity:** # 10 (for 10 tablets); 60 mL. Spell out the quantity if there is a risk that the prescription could be altered (for example, adding an extra zero to the quantity).
- *Sig* **(Latin for "write on label"):** Include the dose (individual), route, frequency, duration, indication, and use.
- **Number of refills:** Define the number legally permitted.
- **Substitution permitted?** Designate whether or not a generic substitution is permissible or "dispense as written" (DAW). If you indicate "no substitutions" or DAW and list the drug's brand name (proprietary name), the pharmacist cannot substitute for a generic version of the same drug. The cost of some brand name products may be 10 times higher than the generic version of the same drug, and the animal owner might have to pay much more for the prescription than anticipated.
- **Signature**

## Owner Information
### Always Include
- Patient's name (in "quotes")
- Patient's age or date of birth
- Owner's name (or that of an owner representative)
- Owner's address
- Owner's phone number

## Common Prescription Writing Errors to Avoid
- Always use metric units: for example, g (gram) for solids; ml or mL (milliliter) for liquids.
- Use per instead of a slash (/), which can be interpreted as the number 1.
- Write out "units" instead of the abbreviation u, which can be interpreted as 0, 4, or micro.
- Use "once daily" instead of SID, which has been interpreted as 5/d or 5 per day. (Note: SID is not a conventional abbreviation recognized by pharmacists.)
- Use "three times daily" instead of TID and use "four times daily" instead of QID.

- Use "every other day" instead of QOD or EOD.
- AVOID CONFUSING ABBREVIATIONS. Abbreviations such as QD, QID, and QOD are easily confused with each other.
- When prescribing grams, spell out and avoid "gr" because it can be confused with grain. (A grain is 65 mg.)

  **When writing numbers**
- Use a leading zero with decimals (e.g., use 0.5 mL rather than .5 mL).
- Avoid using a trailing zero (e.g., use 3 rather than 3.0).
- Spell out numbers in parentheses to avoid alterations.
- ALWAYS: When in doubt, spell it out.

# APPENDIX C
# Calculation of Drug Doses

### How to Calculate Milliliters (mL) Needed

$$\text{Dose (mg/kg)} \times \text{kilograms body weight} = \text{Total dose needed (mg)}$$

Strength of solution (mg/mL) = Percent (%) strength × 10 (e.g., 10% solution = 100 mg/mL)

$$\frac{\text{Total dose needed}}{\text{Strength of solution}\left(\frac{mg}{mL}\right)} = \text{mL needed}$$

### Example
- 20-kg dog needs 15 mg/kg of a 20% solution
- 20 kg × 15 mg/kg = 300 mg total dose needed
- Strength of solution = 20% × 10 = 200 mg/mL
- mL needed = 300 mg/200 mg/mL = 1.5 mL

### How to Calculate Tablets Needed

$$\text{Dose (mg/kg)} \times \text{kilograms body weight} = \text{Total dose needed (mg)}$$

$$\frac{\text{Total dose needed}}{\text{Strength of tablet}} = \text{Number of tablets needed}$$

### Example
- 20-kg dog needs 12 mg/kg
- Tablet size is 100 mg
- 15 kg × 12 mg/kg = 240 mg total dose needed
- 240 mg/100 mg tablets = 2.4 tablets

(In most instances, you would round up to 2½ tablets if the medication has sufficient safety. Refer to the end of this appendix for recommendations on splitting tablets.)

### How to Calculate Infusion Rates

$$\text{Dose (mg/kg/h)} \times \text{Body weight (kg)} = \text{Total dose (mg) needed per hour}$$

If the dose is listed in micrograms per kilogram per hour, divide by 1000 for mg/kg/h.

$$\text{Strength of solution (mg/mL)} = [\% \text{ strength}] \times 10$$

$$\text{mL needed per hour} = \frac{\text{Total dose needed per hour}}{\text{Strength of solution (mg/kg)}}$$

Administer the total milliliters of fluid administered in each hour interval. If fluid is to be administered over 24 hours: mL needed per hour × 24 = mL needed per day.

### Example
- 15-kg dog needs 2 mg/kg/h of a 10% solution
- Fluid rate (lactated Ringer's solution) is 60 mL/kg/day
- 15 kg × 2 mg/kg/h = 30 mg needed per hour
- Strength of solution = 10% × 10 = 100 mg/mL

- mL of drug needed per hour = (30 mg/h)/(100 mg/mL) = 0.3 mL/h
- 0.3 mL of medication should be added to each hour of fluids to be administered
- Fluid rate is 60 mL/kg/day = 2.5 mL/kg/h = 37.5 mL/h for a 15-kg dog

To each 37.5 mL/h of fluid volume to be infused, add 0.3 mL of medication. If the drug is stable in solution for 24 hours, the total amount can be added to a 24-hour volume of fluid:

- Total fluid needed per 24 hours = 60 mL/kg/day × 15 kg = 900 mL
- 0.3 mL per hour × 24 hours = 7.2 mL/day added to 900 mL of total fluid requirement, or 8 mL added to each liter of fluids. (Be sure to check package insert for the medication to ensure that it will remain stable for 24 hours at room temperature in a fluid administration set.)

## When Splitting Tablets, When to Round Up and When to Round Down?

- Avoid trying to split a tablet into less than one fourth of a tablet. Smaller fractions cannot be accurately measured.
- For "safe" drugs with high therapeutic indexes (e.g., antibiotics, nutritional supplements, hormones, antiparasitic agents, antacids), round up to the next highest tablet size or fraction of a tablet.
- For drugs with narrow therapeutic indexes (cardiovascular drugs, nonsteroidal anti-inflammatory drugs, drugs that act on the central nervous system, anticancer agents, anticoagulants), round down to the next lowest tablet size or fraction of a tablet. Then increase the as needed (cautiously) to obtain the desired therapeutic effect.

# APPENDIX D
## Compounded Formulations: What to Look for to Detect Incompatibility or Instability

### Liquid-Dose Forms
- Color change (amber to dark brown)
- Signs of microbial growth
- Cloudiness, haze, flocculent, or film formation
- Separation of phases (e.g., oil and water, emulsion)
- Precipitation, clumping, or crystal formation
- Droplets or fog forming on the inside of the container
- Gas or odor release
- Swelling of container

### Solid-Dose Forms
- Odor (sulfur or vinegar odor)
- Excessive powder or crumbling
- Cracks or chips in tablets
- Swelling of tablets or capsules

### "Rules of Thumb"
- Do not mix drugs that require reconstitution in a vial with other drugs. Do not add other drugs to a reconstituted vial.
- Do not mix drugs that are not in an aqueous vehicle (e.g., propylene glycol) with water-based IV fluids.
- Do not mix hydrochloride (HCl) salts or drugs with buffers (citrates, bicarbonates, phosphates).
- If a drug has HCl, acetate (acetic acid), citrate (citric acid), or sulfate (sulfuric acid) in the name, do not mix it with alkaline solutions.
- The beyond-use-dates for compounded drugs (the date after which a compounded preparation is not to be used) are 14 days for water-containing formulations (refrigerated), 6 months for nonaqueous liquids and solid formulations, and 60 days for other formulations. These times may be exceeded if there is valid scientific stability information.
- Whenever possible, compounded formulations should be prepared from a US Food and Drug Administration–approved formulation.
- Compounded formulations should retain strength of ±10% (i.e., 90%–110%) of the nominal strength of the formulation.
- Compounded formulations should be prepared in accordance with compendial standards listed in the United States Pharmacopeia (USP).

# APPENDIX E
## Controlled Substance Charts: United States and Canada

*For a complete alphabetical list, go to*
www.deadiversion.usdoj.gov/schedules/orangebook/c_cs_alpha.pdf.

| Drug Examples | United States[a] |
|---|---|
| Heroin, lysergic acid diethylamide (LSD), peyote, mescaline, methylenedioxymethamphetamine (ecstasy) | *Schedule I*<br>• High abuse potential<br>• No currently accepted medical use<br>• No veterinary uses identified |
| Morphine and morphine derivatives and synthetic opioids. Drugs used in veterinary medicine include morphine, meperidine, etorphine, hydrocodone, hydromorphone, oxymorphone, codeine (in some forms), hydrocodone, and pentobarbital. | *Schedule II*<br>• High abuse potential; potentially severe psychological or physical dependence<br>• Accepted medical use but may be severely restricted<br>• Telephone orders to a pharmacy are allowed only in emergencies if written prescription follows promptly<br>• No refills allowed<br>• There may be specific requirements for refills and orders in each state |
| Drugs used in veterinary medicine include anabolic steroids (stanozolol, oxymetholone, testosterone, methyltestosterone, boldenone, trenbolone), barbiturates (thiamylal, thiopental), opioids (buprenorphine and codeine in some forms), and ketamine and derivatives (ketamine and tiletamine zolazepam). | *Schedule III*<br>• Abuse potential less than the drugs or substances in Schedules I and II; potentially moderate or low physical dependence or high psychological dependence<br>• Accepted medical uses include anesthetics, analgesics, anabolic steroids<br>• Telephone orders to pharmacies are permitted<br>• Veterinarians may authorize limited refills |
| Drugs used in veterinary medicine include some opioids (butorphanol and pentazocine), benzodiazepines (diazepam, oxazepam, midazolam, clonazepam, clorazepate, and alprazolam), and phenobarbital. Tramadol was added in 2014. | *Schedule IV*<br>• Abuse potential relative to drugs or substances in Schedule III; potentially limited to physical or psychological dependence<br>• Accepted medical use includes sedatives, analgesics, and anticonvulsants.<br>• Telephone orders to pharmacies are permitted<br>• Veterinarians may authorize limited refills. |
| Codeine preparations used as antitussives and some opioids used as antidiarrheals (e.g., diphenoxylate), and pregabalin | *Schedule V*<br>• Lowest abuse potential; potentially very limited physical or psychological dependence<br>• Accepted medical uses include antidiarrheal, antitussive, and analgesics.<br>• Veterinarians can determine refills.<br>• Some products containing limited amounts of Schedule V substances (e.g., cough suppressants) are available over the counter |

[a]A complete list for the United States can be located at https://www.dea.gov/drug-scheduling.

| Drug Examples | Canada |
|---|---|
| Sedatives such as barbiturates and derivatives (secobarbital), thiobarbiturates (pentothal sodium), and anabolic steroids | *Part G of the Food and Drug Regulation (FDR)*<br>• Controlled drugs<br>• Misuse potential<br>• Verbal and written prescriptions under certain conditions<br>• Only prescribed if required for medical condition<br>• Specified number of refills (conditions apply)<br>• Records must be kept<br>• May be administered under emergency situations (conditions apply) |
| Amphetamines | *Part G of the FDR*<br>• Designated controlled drug<br>• May be used for designated medical conditions outlined in FDR |
| Benzodiazepine tranquilizers, such as diazepam and lorazepam | *Benzodiazepines and Other Targeted Substances Regulations*<br>• Misuse potential<br>• Verbal and written prescriptions under certain conditions<br>• Only prescribed if required for medical condition<br>• Specified number of refills (conditions apply)<br>• Records must be kept<br>• May be administered under emergency situations (conditions apply) |
| Opiates: heroin, morphine, and codeine (in some forms) and analgesics such as pentazocine and fentanyl | *Narcotic Control Regulation*<br>• High misuse potential<br>• Written prescriptions for specific medical conditions[b]<br>• Records of opiate prescription file must be kept<br>• No refills (limited amounts in a prescription)<br>• Heroin and methadone are subject to specific controls |
| Lysergic acid diethylamide (LSD), mescaline (peyote), harmaline, psilocin, and psilocybin (magic mushrooms) | *Part J of the FDR*<br>• Considered "restricted drugs"<br>• High misuse potential<br>• No recognized medical use<br>• Marijuana exemption from FDR if produced for medical reasons |

[b]Verbal prescriptions are permitted for certain opioid preparations (e.g., Tylenol No. 2 and No. 3) but not for opiate alone or opiates with one other active nonopioid ingredient.

## APPENDIX F
## Drugs for Infections Commonly Seen in Small Animals

| Infection Site | First-Choice Drugs | Alternative-Choice Drugs |
|---|---|---|
| Skin: pyoderma or other skin infection | Amoxicillin + clavulanate<br>Cephalosporin,[a] clindamycin | Trimethoprim + sulfonamides[b]<br>Fluoroquinolone,[c] lincomycin, tetracycline[d] (doxycycline or minocycline) |
| Lower urinary tract | Cephalosporin[a]<br>Amoxicillin<br>Amoxicillin + clavulanate | Trimethoprim + sulfonamides[b]<br>Fluoroquinolone[c], tetracycline (doxycycline or minocycline) |
| Respiratory tract (the choice may depend on the location of the infection [upper or lower respiratory tract]) | Amoxicillin + clavulanate<br>Fluoroquinolone[c]<br>Cephalosporin[a] (excluding cefovecin) | Macrolide (azithromycin)<br>Aminoglycosides (amikacin, gentamicin)<br>Doxycycline or minocycline<br>Clindamycin<br>Trimethoprim + sulfonamides[b]<br>Chloramphenicol<br>Ceftazidime |
| Septicemia[e] | Amoxicillin + clavulanate<br>Cephalosporin[a] (excluding cefovecin)<br>Fluoroquinolone<br>Aminoglycoside | Ceftazidime<br>Piperacillin + tazobactam<br>Carbapenem (meropenem, imipenem) |
| Bone and joint | Cephalosporin[a]<br>Amoxicillin + clavulanate | Trimethoprim + sulfonamides[b]<br>Clindamycin<br>Fluoroquinolone[c] |
| Intracellular pathogens | Doxycycline or minocycline<br>Fluoroquinolone[c] | Azithromycin<br>Clindamycin |

[a]Cephalosporin includes cephalexin, cefpodoxime proxetil, cefadroxil, or cefovecin.
[b]Trimethoprim in combination with sulfonamides includes trimethoprim in combination with sulfadiazine, trimethoprim in combination with sulfamethoxazole, and ormetoprim in combination with sulfadimethoxine.
[c]Fluoroquinolone includes enrofloxacin, marbofloxacin, orbifloxacin, or pradofloxacin (pradofloxacin is not approved for dogs in the United States). Human generic forms that are acceptable for treating dogs include levofloxacin.
[d]First confirm with a susceptibility test.
[e]Combinations of drugs are often used in acute febrile septicemia. Such combinations may include a beta-lactam plus an aminoglycoside or a fluoroquinolone plus amoxicillin + clavulanate.

# APPENDIX G
# Antibiotic Drug Selection for Equine Bacterial Pathogens

| Pathogen | Drug Choice | Alternative Choice |
|---|---|---|
| **Gram-Positive Organisms** | | |
| *Rhodococcus equi* | Rifampin, in combination with clarithromycin, azithromycin, or erythromycin | One of the macrolides used alone |
| *Streptococcus equi* | Penicillin G, ampicillin sodium, ceftiofur, trimethoprim–sulfadiazine | Erythromycin, chloramphenicol, doxycycline, or minocycline |
| *Staphylococcus aureus* | Trimethoprim + sulfonamide | Enrofloxacin, orbifloxacin, chloramphenicol, doxycycline, or minocycline |
| **Gram-Negative Organisms** | | |
| *Escherichia coli* | Gentamicin, amikacin | Ceftiofur, enrofloxacin, orbifloxacin, marbofloxacin, trimethoprim + sulfonamide |
| *Klebsiella pneumoniae* | Gentamicin, amikacin | Ceftiofur, enrofloxacin, orbifloxacin, marbofloxacin, trimethoprim + sulfonamide |
| *Enterobacter* spp. | Gentamicin, amikacin | Ceftiofur, enrofloxacin, trimethoprim + sulfonamide |
| *Pseudomonas aeruginosa* | Amikacin, piperacillin + tazobactam | Enrofloxacin, marbofloxacin, ceftazidime, meropenem |
| *Pasteurella* spp. | Ampicillin sodium, ceftiofur, trimethoprim + sulfonamide | Enrofloxacin, orbifloxacin, marbofloxacin, chloramphenicol, doxycycline or minocycline |
| *Actinobacillus* spp. | Ampicillin sodium, penicillin G, trimethoprim + sulfonamides | Enrofloxacin, amikacin, gentamicin, ceftiofur |
| **Anaerobes** | | |
| *Clostridium, Fusobacterium, Peptostreptococcus,* and *Bacteroides* spp. | Metronidazole, penicillin G | Chloramphenicol, or cefoxitin (injectable) |
| **Other** | | |
| *Lawsonia intracellularis* | Oxytetracycline, doxycycline (doxycycline, PO only), minocycline | Chloramphenicol, erythromycin, clarithromycin, azithromycin |
| *Ehrlichia* spp. | Oxytetracycline, doxycycline (doxycycline, PO only), minocycline | Chloramphenicol |
| *Neorickettsia risticii* (Potomac horse fever) | Oxytetracycline, doxycycline (doxycycline, PO only), minocycline | |

## APPENDIX H
## Drugs That May Induce Cytochrome P450 Enzymes

- Chlorinated hydrocarbons
- Diazepam (Valium)
- Diphenhydramine
- Estrogens
- Griseofulvin
- Hyperthyroidism
- Omeprazole
- Pentobarbital
- Phenobarbital
- Phenylbutazone
- Phenytoin (Dilantin)
- Progestogens
- Rifampin
- St. John's wort

# APPENDIX I
## Drugs That May Inhibit Cytochrome P450 Enzymes

- Amiodarone
- Chloramphenicol
- Cimetidine
- Cisapride
- Clarithromycin
- Clopidogrel
- Cyclophosphamide
- Diltiazem
- Erythromycin
- Esomeprazole
- Felbamate
- Fluconazole
- Fluoroquinolones (some)
- Fluoxetine
- Grapefruit juice
- Interferon (vaccines)
- Itraconazole
- Ketoconazole
- Omeprazole
- Organophosphates
- Paroxetine
- Phenylbutazone
- Posaconazole
- Quinidine
- Tetracycline
- Verapamil
- Voriconazole

# APPENDIX J
# Drugs That May Inhibit the P-Glycoprotein Membrane Transporter Coded by *ABCB1* (formerly known as *MDR1*)

- Bromocriptine
- Carvedilol
- Chlorpromazine
- Cyclosporine
- Diltiazem
- Erythromycin
- Fluoxetine
- Grapefruit juice
- Itraconazole
- Ketoconazole
- Methadone
- Paroxetine
- Pentazocine
- Quinidine
- Spinosad
- St. John's wort
- Tamoxifen
- Verapamil

### References

Mealey KL. Adverse drug reactions in veterinary patients associated with drug transporters. *Vet Clin North Am Small Anim Pract.* 2013;43:1067–1078.

Mealey KL, Fidel J. P-glycoprotein mediated drug interactions in animals and humans with cancer. *Vet Intern Med.* 2015;29:1–6.

# APPENDIX K
## Drugs That Are Substrates for the P-Glycoprotein Membrane Transporter Coded by *ABCB1* (formerly known as *MDR1*)

P-glycoprotein is a membrane transporter responsible for transporting many drugs and other chemicals across membranes. A functional p-glycoprotein at the blood–brain barrier protects the brain from harmful effects of systemically administered drugs. P-glycoprotein may also be found at other important sites, such as the liver, placenta, kidney, and intestinal mucosa. Mutation of the gene that codes for p-glycoprotein (*ABCB1*) that produces a function deletion exposes some dogs (e.g., some herding breeds) to toxic concentrations of some drugs. Alternatively, if a drug is administered that is a p-glycoprotein inhibitor (see Appendix J), it may decrease the effect of the membrane transporter and produce toxicity. Below are some of the p-glycoprotein substrates that may be affected by a mutation or drug inhibition.

- Acepromazine
- Actinomycin D
- Aldosterone
- Amitriptyline
- Butorphanol
- Cortisol
- Cyclosporine
- Dexamethasone
- Digoxin
- Diltiazem
- Docetaxel
- Doramectin
- Docetaxel
- Doxorubicin
- Doxycycline
- Eprinomectin
- Erythromycin
- Itraconazole
- Ivermectin
- Ketoconazole
- Levofloxacin
- Loperamide
- Methylprednisolone
- Milbemycin
- Morphine
- Moxidectin
- Ondansetron
- Paclitaxel
- Phenothiazines
- Quinidine
- Selamectin
- Tacrolimus
- Terfenadine
- Tetracycline
- Verapamil
- Vinblastine
- Vincristine

### References
Mealey KL. Adverse drug reactions in veterinary patients associated with drug transporters. *Vet Clin North Am Small Anim Pract.* 2013;43:1067–1078.

Mealey KL, Fidel J. P-glycoprotein mediated drug interactions in animals and humans with cancer. *J Vet Intern Med.* 2015;29:1–6.

## APPENDIX L
## Fluid Solution Composition

| Solution Type | Na+ (mEq/L) | K+ (mEq/L) | Cl— (mEq/L) | Ca²⁺ (mEq/L) | Mg²⁺ (mEq/L) | Buffer (mEq/L) | Osmolarity (mOsm/L) | pH |
|---|---|---|---|---|---|---|---|---|
| Ringer's solution | 147 | 4 | 156 | 4.4 | 0 | 0 | 310 | 5–7.5 |
| Lactated Ringer's solution | 130 | 4 | 112 | 2.7 | 0 | 29 (lactate) | 273 | 6–7.5 |
| 0.9% NaCl | 154 | 0 | 154 | 0 | 0 | 0 | 308 | 4–5 |
| 5% dextrose | 0 | 0 | 0 | 0 | 0 | 0 | 252 | 4–6.5 |
| 2.5% dextrose/0.45% NaCl | 77 | 0 | 77 | 0 | 0 | 0 | 280 | 4.5 |
| Plasma-Lyte | 140 | 5 | 98 | 0 | 3 | 27 (acetate) 23 (gluconate) | 294 | 4–6.5 |
| Dextran 6% and 0.9% NaCl | 154 | 0 | 154 | 0 | 0 | 0 | 310 | 3.0–7.0 |
| Hetastarch[a] | 154 | 0 | 154 | 0 | 0 | 0 | 309 | 5.5 |
| Pentastarch[a] | 154 | 0 | 154 | 0 | 0 | 0 | 326 | 5.0 |
| Hemoglobin glutamer (oxyglobin) | | | | | | | 300 | 7.8 |
| Normosol-R | 140 | 5 | 98 | 0 | 3 | 27 (acetate) 23 (gluconate) | 294 | 6.6 |

[a]See the Hydroxyethyl Starch section to find additional information on these solutions.

# APPENDIX M
## How to Report an Adverse Drug Reaction

1. Phone the drug sponsor to report an adverse drug experience (ADE) if it is a US Food and Drug Administration (FDA)–approved animal drug. Obtain drug sponsor phone numbers from the product label or from the company's website. When phoning the pharmaceutical company, inform them that you wish to speak with a veterinarian on their staff or technical services representative to report an ADE.
2. Contact the FDA and complete Form 1932a. This form may be completed regardless of whether the drug is an animal-approved drug or human-approved drug. The FDA can be contacted from its website at https://www.fda.gov/animal-veterinary/report-problem/how-report-animal-drug-side-effects-and-product-problems.
   Send the complete form to: CVM1932a@fda.hhs.gov. The FDA also may be contacted at this address:
   - Send email to: AskCVM@fda.hhs.gov
   - Phone: 1-888-FDA-VETS (1-888-332-8387)
   - Mail:
     Center for Veterinary Medicine
     Food and Drug Administration
     HFV-1
     7500 Standish Place
     Rockville, MD 20855

When completing Form 1932a, supply as much history and clinical data as possible, including concurrent medications administered to the animal.

### Animal Biologics: Vaccines, Bacterins

Contact the United States Department of Agriculture Animal and Plant Health Inspection Service(USDA APHIS) Center for Veterinary Biologics at 800-752-6255 or at https://www.aphis.usda.gov/aphis/ourfocus/animalhealth/veterinary-biologics/adverse-event-reporting/ct_vb_adverse_event.

### Pesticides: Topically Applied External Parasiticides

Note that some flea and tick products are regulated by the FDA, and some are regulated by the Environmental Protection Agency (EPA). To report a problem with a flea or tick product that is FDA approved, contact the FDA (see instructions above).

The label of the product will determine if the product is an FDA-approved or an EPA-registered flea and tick product or other pesticide. All FDA-approved animal drugs have a six-digit New Animal Drug Application (NADA) number, or for generic animal drugs, an Abbreviated New Animal Drug Application (ANADA) number. If it is an EPA-registered product, look for an EPA registration number on the back panel of the package, usually near the manufacturer's address: "EPA Reg. No."

If the product is regulated by the EPA, contact the National Pesticide Information Center at 800-858-7378 or http://npic.orst.edu/incidents.html#anim.

## APPENDIX N
## Drugs Prohibited from Use in Food-Producing Animals

Note: To locate the most updated list, go to www.FARAD.org.

Because they present a risk to public health, the following drugs are prohibited in food-producing animals:

- Chloramphenicol
- Clenbuterol
- Diethylstilbestrol (DES)
- Furazolidone
- Nitrofurazone (and other nitrofurans)
- Fluoroquinolones (extralabel use)
- Cephalosporins (not including cephapirin in cattle, swine, chickens, or turkeys): (1) for disease prevention purposes; (2) at unapproved doses, durations, or routes of administration; or (3) if the drug is not approved for that species and production class.
- Glycopeptide antibiotics (e.g., vancomycin)
- Ipronidazole, dimetridazole, metronidazole, and other nitroimidazoles
- Phenylbutazone in female dairy cattle younger than 20 months of age
- Sulfonamide drugs in lactating dairy cattle (with the exception of sulfadimethoxine, sulfabromomethazine, and sulfamethoxypyridazine, which are approved for use in some feeds)
- Adamantane and neuraminidase inhibitor classes of drugs approved for treating or preventing influenza A are prohibited therapy in chickens, turkeys, and ducks.

# APPENDIX O
# Performance Horse Drug Regulations and Restrictions Association of Racing Commissioners International, Inc., Uniform Classification Guidelines for Foreign Substances (Revised January 2020)

The following definitions, regulations, and restrictions are adapted from the Racing Commissioners International (RCI) website (www.arci.com) and the Fédération Equestre Internationale (FEI) Clean Sport Prohibited Substances List (www.feicleansport.org).

The RCI Drug Classification Scheme is based on (1) pharmacology, (2) drug use patterns, and (3) the appropriateness of a drug for use in the racing horse.

## Classification Definitions

### Class 1

Stimulant and depressant drugs that have the highest potential to affect performance and that have no generally accepted medical use in the racing horse. Many of these agents are Drug Enforcement Administration (DEA) Schedule II substances. These include the following drugs and their metabolites: opiates, opium derivatives, synthetic opioids and psychoactive drugs, amphetamines, and amphetamine-like drugs, as well as related drugs, including but not limited to, apomorphine, nikethamide, mazindol, pemoline, and pentylenetetrazol. Although not used as therapeutic agents, all DEA Schedule 1 agents are included in Class 1 because they are potent stimulant or depressant substances with psychotropic and often habituative actions. This class also includes all erythropoietin-stimulating substances and their analogues.

### Class 2

Drugs that have a high potential to affect performance but less of a potential than drugs in Class 1. These drugs are (1) not generally accepted as therapeutic agents in racing horses, or (2) they are therapeutic agents that have a high potential for abuse. Drugs in this class include psychotropic drugs, certain nervous system and cardiovascular system stimulants, depressants, and neuromuscular blocking agents. Injectable local anesthetics are included in this class because of their high potential for abuse as nerve blocking agents.

### Class 3

Drugs that may or may not have generally accepted medical use in the racing horse but the pharmacology of which suggests less potential to affect performance than drugs in Class 2. Drugs in this class include bronchodilators, anabolic steroids and other drugs with primary effects on the autonomic nervous system, procaine, antihistamines with sedative properties, and the high-ceiling diuretics.

### Class 4

This class includes therapeutic medications that would be expected to have less potential to affect performance than those in Class 3. Drugs in this class include less potent diuretics, corticosteroids, antihistamines and skeletal muscle relaxants without prominent central nervous system effects, expectorants and mucolytics, hemostatics, cardiac glycosides and antiarrhythmics, topical anesthetics, antidiarrheals, and mild analgesics. This class also includes the nonsteroidal anti-inflammatory drugs at concentrations greater than established limits.

## Class 5

This class includes those therapeutic medications that have very localized actions only, such as antiulcer drugs and certain antiallergic drugs. The anticoagulant drugs are also included.

### Prohibited Substances in Racing Horses

A. The possession and/or use of a drug, substance, or medication, specified here, on the premises of a facility under the jurisdiction of the regulatory body for which a recognized analytical method has not been developed to detect and confirm the administration of such substance; or the use of which may endanger the health and welfare of the horse or endanger the safety of the rider or driver; or the use of which may adversely affect the integrity of racing:
1. Erythropoietin
2. Darbepoetin
3. Oxyglobin
4. Hemopure

B. The possession and/or use of a drug, substance, or medication on the premises of a facility under the jurisdiction of the regulatory body that has not been approved by the U.S. Food and Drug Administration (FDA) for use in the United States.

C. The practice, administration, or application of a treatment, procedure, therapy, or method identified here, which is performed on the premises of a facility under jurisdiction of a regulatory body and which may endanger the health and welfare of the horse or endanger the safety of the rider or driver; or the use of which may adversely affect the integrity of racing.

### Equine Prohibited Drugs: Fédération Equestre Internationale Clean Sport Prohibited Substances Database (Revised January 2020)

The FEI has published guidelines to assist veterinarians to make a distinction between the use of routine, legitimate medication and deliberate and calculated doping to affect a horse's performance. The prohibited substance searchable database is available at http://prohibitedsubstancesdatabase.feicleansport.org.

Or access the FEI Clean Sport Prohibited Substances List (updated January 2020) at http://www.fei.org/fei/cleansport.

Page numbers followed by *t* indicate tables.